CONTENTS IN BRIEF

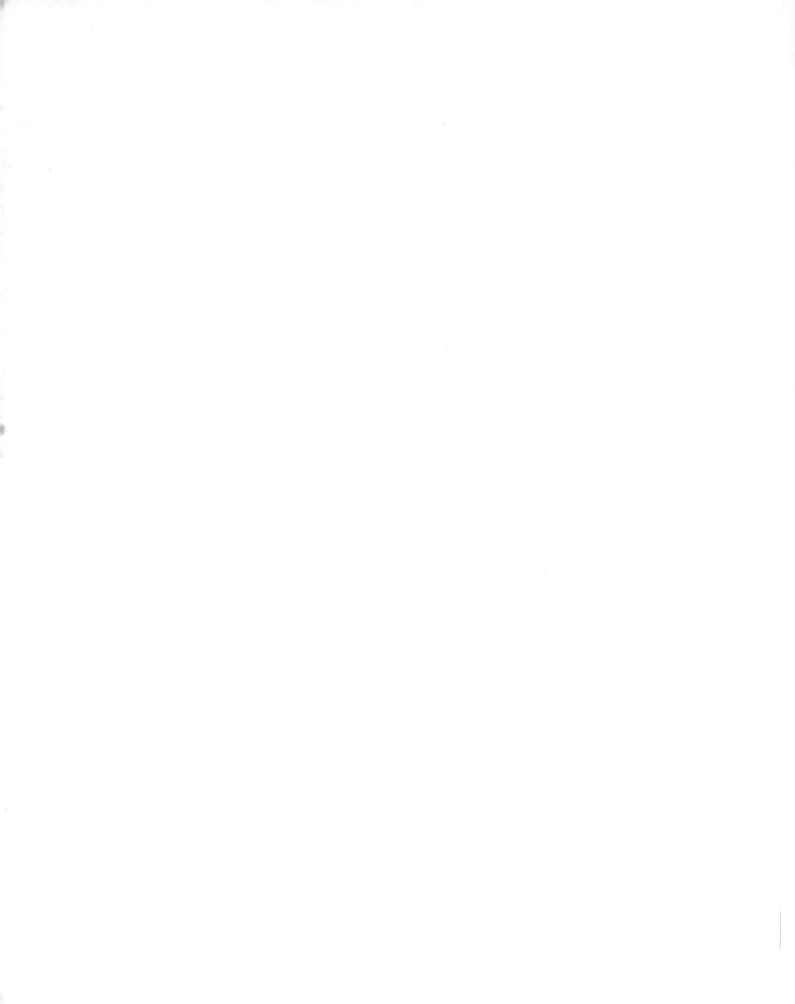

Tenth Edition

EBERSOLE & HESS'
TOWARD HEALTHY AGING
Human Needs & Nursing Response

THERIS A. TOUHY, DNP, CNS, DPNAP
Emeritus Professor
Christine E. Lynn College of Nursing
Florida Atlantic University
Boca Raton, Florida

KATHLEEN JETT, PhD, GNP-BC
Gerontological Nurse Practitioner
Clinic Coordinator
UF Health Senior Care Clinic at Oak Hammock
Department of Aging and Geriatric Research
University of Florida College of Medicine
Gainesville, Florida

ELSEVIER

EBERSOLE & HESS' TOWARD HEALTHY AGING:
HUMAN NEEDS & NURSING RESPONSE, TENTH EDITION

ISBN: 978-0-323-55422-0

Notice

Practitioners and researchers must always rely on their own experience and knowledge in evaluating and using any information, methods, compounds, or experiments described herein. Because of rapid advances in the medical sciences in particular, independent verification of diagnoses and drug dosages should be made. To the fullest extent of the law, no responsibility is assumed by Elsevier, authors, editors, or contributors for any injury and/or damage to persons or property as a matter of products liability, negligence or otherwise, or from any use or operation of any methods, products, instructions, or ideas contained in the material herein.

Previous editions copyrighted 2016, 2012, 2008, 2004, 1998, 1994, 1990, 1985, and 1981 by Elsevier.

Library of Congress Control Number: 2019946570

Content Strategist: Sandra Clark
Content Development Manager: Luke Held
Senior Content Development Specialist: Sarah Vora
Publishing Services Manager: Catherine Jackson
Senior Project Manager: Douglas Turner
Designer: Renee Duenow

Printed in Canada

Last digit is the print number: 9   8   7   6   5   4   3   2

3251 Riverport Lane
St. Louis, Missouri 63043

Working together
to grow libraries in
developing countries

www.elsevier.com • www.bookaid.org

For Danny
You touched our family and so many others in your social work practice
with your presence, caring, deep love, and your music.
Your gentle spirit lives on.

Theris A. Touhy

To my former students
who have moved gerontological nursing
in new and exciting ways—thank you.

To my patients,
who teach me every day about both the highs and lows
of the furthest reaches of age and what really matters the most in life.

To my husband, Steve,
for his patience during the years I spend
writing when I have time for little else.

To my psychiatrist, Dr. Michael Johnson,
who has taught me to look inside myself and find it good.

To my children and grandchildren,
whose smiles and laughter make life worth living.

Kathleen Jett

Theris A. Touhy, DNP, CNS, DPNAP, has been a clinical specialist in gerontological nursing, nurse practitioner, and nursing educator for more than 40 years. Her expertise is in the care of older adults in long-term care and those with dementia. Dr. Touhy received her BSN degree from St. Xavier University in Chicago, a master's degree in care of the aged from Northern Illinois University, and a Doctor of Nursing Practice from Case Western Reserve University. She is an emeritus professor in the Christine E. Lynn College of Nursing at Florida Atlantic University, where she has served as Assistant Dean of Undergraduate Programs and taught gerontological nursing and long-term, rehabilitation, and palliative care nursing in the undergraduate, graduate, and doctoral programs. Her research is focused on spirituality in aging and at the end of life, caring for persons with dementia, caring in nursing homes, and nursing leadership in long-term care. Dr. Touhy was the recipient of the Geriatric Faculty Member Award from the John A. Hartford Foundation Institute for Geriatric Nursing, is a two-time recipient of the Distinguished Teacher of the Year in the Christine E. Lynn College of Nursing at Florida Atlantic University, and received the Marie Haug Award for Excellence in Aging Research from Case Western Reserve University. Dr. Touhy was inducted into the National Academies of Practice in 2007. She is a member of the Board of Directors of the Anne Boykin Institute for the Advancement of Caring in Nursing. She is co-author with Dr. Kathleen Jett of *Gerontological Nursing and Healthy Aging* and co-author with Dr. Priscilla Ebersole of *Geriatric Nursing: Growth of a Specialty*. In addition to her professional activities, Dr. Touhy and her husband of 51 years are blessed to be involved grandparents of two grandsons and one granddaughter. This book is dedicated to all of my students who have embraced gerontological nursing as their specialty and are improving the lives of older adults through their practice, teaching, and research. Special recognition and gratitude to all the wise and wonderful older adults I have had the privilege of nursing and to their caregivers. Thank you for making the words in this book a reality for the older adults for whom you care and for teaching me how to be a gerontological nurse.

Kathleen Jett, PhD, GNP-BC, has been actively engaged in gerontological nursing for more than 40 years. Her clinical experience is broad; from her roots in public health to her clinical leadership in long-term, assisted-living and hospice care, Dr. Jett has a great deal of experience as a researcher and a teacher and has worked in advanced practice as both a clinical nurse specialist and a nurse practitioner. Dr. Jett received her bachelor's, master's, and doctoral degrees from the University of Florida, where she also holds a graduate certificate in gerontology. In 2000 she was selected as a Summer Scholar by the John A. Hartford Foundation Institute for Geriatric Nursing. In 2004 she completed a Fellowship in Ethno-Geriatrics through the Stanford Geriatric Education Center. Dr. Jett has received several awards, including recognition as an Inspirational Woman of Pacific Lutheran University in 1998 and 2000 and for her excellence in undergraduate teaching in 2005 and Distinguished Teacher of the Year Award in the Christine E. Lynn College of Nursing at Florida Atlantic University. A board-certified gerontological nurse practitioner, Dr. Jett was inducted into the National Academies of Practice in 2006. She has taught an array of courses, including public health nursing, women's studies, advanced practice gerontological nursing, and undergraduate courses in gerontology. She has coordinated two gerontological nurse practitioner graduate programs and an undergraduate interdisciplinary gerontology certificate program. The majority of her research has been in the area of reducing health disparities experienced by older adults. The thread that ties all of her work together has been a belief that nurses can make a difference in the lives of older adults. She is currently employed as a nurse practitioner and Coordinator of the UF Health Senior Care Clinic at Oak Hammock, a continuing care community in Gainesville, Florida. In addition to her professional activities, Dr. Jett is actively engaged in the lives of her children and grandchildren.

CONTRIBUTORS AND REVIEWERS

CONTRIBUTORS

Kevin W. Chamberlin, PharmD
Associate Clinical Professor
Assistant Department Head
Pharmacy Practice
University of Connecticut School of Pharmacy
Storrs, Connecticut
Residency Program Director
Pharmacy
UConn John Dempsey Hospital
Farmington, Connecticut

Lenny Chiang-Hanisko, PhD, RN
Associate Professor
Christine E. Lynn College of Nursing
Florida Atlantic University
Boca Raton, Florida

Debra Hain, PhD, APRN, AGPCNP-BC, FAANP, FNKF
Professor
Christine E. Lynn College of Nursing
Florida Atlantic University
Boca Raton, Florida
Nurse Practitioner
Nephrology
Cleveland Clinic Florida
Weston, Florida

Kathleen Jett, PhD, GNP-BC
Gerontological Nurse Practitioner
Clinic Coordinator
UF Health Senior Care Clinic at Oak Hammock
Department of Aging and Geriatric Research
University of Florida College of Medicine
Gainesville, Florida

Beth M. King, PhD, ARNP, PMHNP-BC
Assistant Professor
Christine E. Lynn College of Nursing
Florida Atlantic University
Boca Raton, Florida

María Ordóñez, DNP, ARNP/GNP-BC
Director
Louis and Anne Green Memory and Wellness Center
Assistant Professor
Christine E. Lynn College of Nursing
Florida Atlantic University
Boca Raton, Florida

Marissa Salvo, PharmD, BCACP
Associate Clinical Professor
Pharmacy Practice
University of Connecticut School of Pharmacy
Storrs, Connecticut

Theris A. Touhy, DNP, CNS, DPNAP
Emeritus Professor
Christine E. Lynn College of Nursing
Florida Atlantic University
Boca Raton, Florida

Timothy L. Wilson, DNP, APRN, PMHNP-BC
Psychiatric Nurse Practitioner
Private Practice
Dr. Timothy Wilson, LLC
Delray Beach, Florida

REVIEWERS

Susan Kay-Ransom Collins, PhD, RN, CNE
Clinical Associate Professor
Department of Adult Health Nursing
School of Nursing
University of North Carolina at Greensboro
Greensboro, North Carolina

Deborah A. Lekan, PhD, RN-BC
Assistant Professor
Department of Family and Community Health Nursing
School of Nursing
University of North Carolina at Greensboro
Greensboro, North Carolina

Angela D. Martindale PhD(c), RN
Visiting Clinical Assistant Professor
School of Nursing
The University of Tulsa
Tulsa, Oklahoma

Cheryl A. Tucker, DNP(c), RN, CNE
Clinical Associate Professor
Traditional BSN Level II Coordinator
Louise Herrington School of Nursing
Baylor University
Dallas, Texas

Tammy E. Williams, PhD, MS, RN
Assistant Professor
Department of Nursing
Longwood University
Farmville, Virginia

PREFACE

In 1981, Dr. Priscilla Ebersole and Dr. Patricia Hess published the first edition of *Toward Healthy Aging: Human Needs and Nursing Response,* which has been used in nursing schools around the globe. Their foresight in developing a textbook that focuses on health, wholeness, beauty, and potential in aging has made this book an enduring classic and the model for gerontological nursing textbooks. In 1981, few nurses chose this specialty, few schools of nursing included content related to the care of older adults, and the focus of care was on illness and problems. Today, gerontological nursing is a strong and evolving specialty with a solid theoretical base and practice grounded in evidence-based research. Dr. Ebersole and Dr. Hess set the standards for the competencies required for gerontological nursing education and the promotion of healthy aging. Many nurses, including us, have been shaped by their words, their wisdom, and their passion for care of older adults. We thank these two wonderful pioneers and mentors for the opportunity to build on such a solid foundation in the four previous editions of this book we have co-authored. We hope that we have kept the heart and spirit of their work, for that is truly what has inspired us, and so many others, to care with competence and compassion.

Toward Healthy Aging is a comprehensive gerontological nursing text. Within the covers, the reader will find information based on the latest evidence-based gerontological care available. This fosters the provision of the highest level of care to adults in settings across the continuum. The content is consistent with the Recommended Baccalaureate Competencies and Curricular Guidelines for the Nursing Care of Older Adults, the Hartford Institute for Geriatric Nursing Best Practices in Nursing Care to Older Adults, and content relevant to the gerontological nursing and adult–gerontological nurse practitioner certification exams. *Toward Healthy Aging* is an appropriate text for both undergraduate and graduate students and is an excellent reference for nurses' libraries. This edition makes an ideal supplement to health assessment, medical-surgical, community, and psychiatric and mental health textbooks in programs that do not have a freestanding gerontological nursing course.

A holistic approach—addressing body, mind, and spirit along a continuum of wellness and grounded in caring and respect for the person—provides the framework for the text. The tenth edition has been totally revised to facilitate student learning. We present aging within a cultural and global context in recognition of diversity of all kinds and health inequities that persist. We hope to encourage readers to develop a world view of aging challenges and possibilities and to fully appreciate the significant role of nursing in promoting healthy aging.

ORGANIZATION OF THE TEXT

Toward Healthy Aging is made up of 36 chapters, which are organized into five sections.

Section 1 introduces the theoretical model on which the text is based and discusses the concepts of health and wellness in aging and the roles and responsibilities of gerontological nurses to provide optimal and informed caring. It includes a discussion of the changing population dynamics around the globe as more and more persons live longer and longer.

Section 2 lays out the basic information needed to perform the day-to-day activities of gerontological nursing such as assessment, communication, provision of medication and dietary supplements, and interpretation of laboratory tests.

Section 3 explores concerns that may affect functional abilities in aging such as vision, hearing, elimination, sleep, physical activity, and safety and security. Prevention of the common geriatric syndromes and nursing interventions to enhance wellness, maintain optimal function, and prevent unnecessary disability are presented.

Section 4 goes into more depth regarding the chronic disorders that are most common in later life, with a focus on the interplay between the condition and aging. These chapters focus on common mental health disorders and neurodegenerative conditions, such as Alzheimer's and Parkinson's diseases. Emphasis is on the role of nursing in promoting the highest quality of life for older adults experiencing chronic illnesses.

Section 5 moves beyond illness and functional limitations that may occur in aging and focuses on psychosocial, legal, and ethical issues that are especially important to older adults and their families/significant others. Content ranges from the economics of health care to sexuality and palliative care. Aging is presented as a potential time of accomplishing life's tasks, developing and sharing unique gifts, and reflecting on the meaning of life. Wisdom, self-actualization, creativity, spirituality, transcendence, and legacies are discussed. The unique and important contributions of older adults to society—and to each of us—calls for nurses to foster appreciation of each older adult, no matter how frail.

KEY COMPONENTS OF THE TEXT

A Student Speaks/An Older Adult Speaks: Introduces every chapter to provide perspectives of older adults and nursing students on chapter content

Learning Objectives: Presents important chapter content and student outcomes

Promoting Healthy Aging: Implications for Gerontological Nursing: Special headings detailing pertinent assessment and interventions for practice applications of chapter content

Key Concepts: Concise review of important chapter points

Nursing Studies: Practice examples designed to assist students in assessment, planning, interventions, and outcomes to promote healthy aging

Critical Thinking Questions and Activities: Assist students in developing critical thinking and clinical judgment skills related to chapter and nursing study content and include suggestions for in-classroom activities to enhance learning

Research Questions: Suggestions to stimulate thinking about ideas for nursing research related to chapter topics

Tips for Best Practice Box

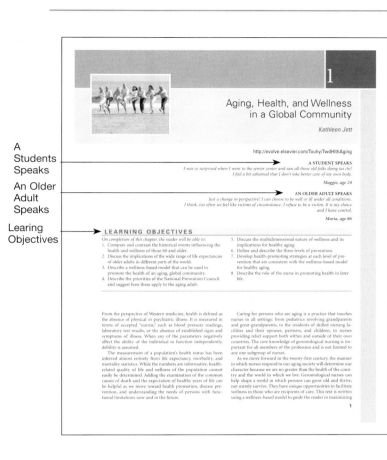

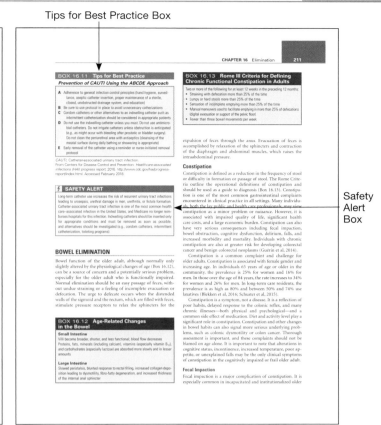

A Students Speaks

An Older Adult Speaks

Learning Objectives

Safety Alert Box

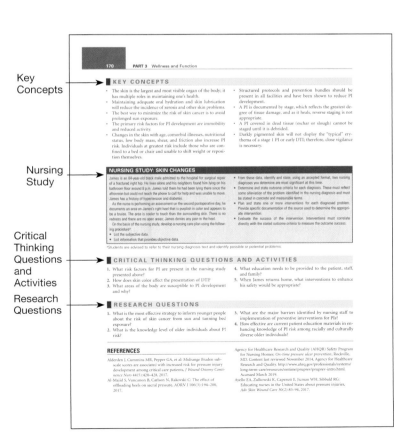

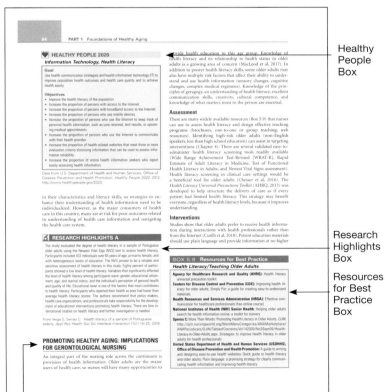

Key Concepts

Nursing Study

Critical Thinking Questions and Activities

Research Questions

Healthy People Box

Research Highlights Box

Resources for Best Practice Box

Promoting Healthy Aging: Implications for Gerontological Nursing

Boxes

Safety Alerts: Safety issues related to care of older adults

Research Highlights: Summary of pertinent current research related to chapter topics

Resources for Best Practice: Suggestions for further information for chapter topics and tools for practice

Tips for Best Practice: Summary of evidence-based nursing interventions for practice

Healthy People: Reference to the goals cited in *Healthy People 2020*

EVOLVE ANCILLARIES

Instructors

Test Bank: Hundreds of questions with rationales to use in creating exams

PowerPoint: Lecture slides for each chapter, including integrated audience response questions

Teach for Nurses Lesson Plans: Detailed listing of resources available to instructors for their lesson planning, which include unique case studies and class activities that can be shared with students

Students

Student Review Questions: Open-ended study questions covering nearly every element of each chapter

Case Studies: Accompanying select chapters, these provide short case studies with questions to help students see content put into practical use

ACKNOWLEDGMENTS

This book would not have been possible without the support and guidance of the staff at Elsevier. Special thanks also to Sandra Clark, content strategist, who has struggled with us for several editions, Sarah Vora, senior content development specialist, and Doug Turner, senior project manager, for his remarkable attention to detail, so we can give you the best product possible. We also thank our reviewers and contributors, because without their efforts this edition would not have been possible. Finally, we acknowledge past and future readers who, we hope, will provide us with enough feedback to keep us honest and relevant in any future writing.

Theris A. Touhy
Kathleen Jett

CONTENTS

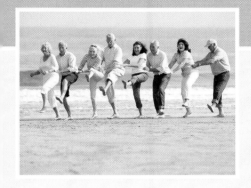

Aging, Health, and Wellness in a Global Community

Kathleen Jett

http://evolve.elsevier.com/Touhy/TwdHlthAging

A STUDENT SPEAKS

*I was so surprised when I went to the senior center and saw all those old folks doing tai chi!
I feel a bit ashamed that I don't take better care of my own body.*

Maggie, age 24

AN OLDER ADULT SPEAKS

*Just a change in perspective! I can choose to be well or ill under all conditions.
I think, too often we feel like victims of circumstance. I refuse to be a victim. It is my choice
and I have control.*

Maria, age 86

LEARNING OBJECTIVES

On completion of this chapter, the reader will be able to:

1. Compare and contrast the historical events influencing the health and wellness of those 60 and older.
2. Discuss the implications of the wide range of life expectancies of older adults in different parts of the world.
3. Describe a wellness-based model that can be used to promote the health of an aging, global community.
4. Describe the priorities of the National Prevention Council and suggest how these apply to the aging adult.
5. Discuss the multidimensional nature of wellness and its implications for healthy aging.
6. Define and describe the three levels of prevention.
7. Develop health-promoting strategies at each level of prevention that are consistent with the wellness-based model for healthy aging.
8. Describe the role of the nurse in promoting health in later life.

From the perspective of Western medicine, health is defined as the absence of physical or psychiatric illness. It is measured in terms of accepted "norms," such as blood pressure readings, laboratory test results, or the absence of established signs and symptoms of illness. When any of the parameters negatively affect the ability of the individual to function independently, debility is assumed.

The measurement of a population's health status has been inferred almost entirely from life expectancy, morbidity, and mortality statistics. While the numbers are informative, health-related quality of life and wellness of the population cannot easily be determined. Adding the examination of the common causes of death and the expectation of healthy years of life can be helpful as we move toward health promotion, disease prevention, and understanding the needs of persons with functional limitations now and in the future.

Caring for persons who are aging is a practice that touches nurses in all settings: from pediatrics involving grandparents and great-grandparents, to the residents of skilled nursing facilities and their spouses, partners, and children, to nurses providing relief support both within and outside of their own countries. The core knowledge of gerontological nursing is important for all members of the profession and is not limited to any one subgroup of nurses.

As we move forward in the twenty-first century, the manner in which nurses respond to our aging society will determine our character because we are no greater than the health of the country and the world in which we live. Gerontological nurses can help shape a world in which persons can grow old and thrive, not merely survive. They have unique opportunities to facilitate wellness in those who are recipients of care. This text is written using a wellness-based model to guide the reader in maximizing strengths, minimizing limitations, facilitating adaptation, and encouraging growth along the continuum of care. It is about helping persons move *Toward Healthy Aging*. In this tenth edition, we appreciate your willingness to join us in this challenge.

AGING

American physician Ignatz Nascher proposed the term "geriatrics" in recognition that the needs and medical care of persons in later life differed from that of other population groups, such as pregnant women or children. In 1914 he authored the first medical textbook on treatment of the "old" in the United States (Nascher, 1914). Aging was reflected in his eyes as it was in society—a problem that must be reversed, eradicated, or held at bay as long as possible.

How Old Is Old?

Each culture has its own definition of when and who is "old." Some of the terms used to name such persons are the elderly, senior citizens, elders, grannies, older adults, and tribal elders. In some cultures, elderhood is determined functionally when one is no longer able to perform one's usual activities (Jett, 2003). *Social aging* is often determined by changes in roles, such as retirement from one's usual occupation, appointment as a wise woman/man of the community, or at the birth of a grandchild. Transitions may be marked by special rituals, such as birthday and retirement parties, invitations to join groups such as the American Association of Retired Persons (AARP), eligibility for age-related pensions or income, or the qualification for "senior discounts" (Box 1.1).

Biological aging is a complex and continuous process involving every cell in the body (Chapter 3). The physical and biological traits by which we identify one as "older" (e.g., gray hair, wrinkled skin) are referred to as the aging phenotype and are the external expression of one's individual genetic makeup and internal changes.

Chronological aging may be used alone or combined with either social or biological aging. In most developed and developing areas of the world, chronological late life is recognized as beginning sometime between 50 and 65 years of age. These arbitrary numbers had been set with the expectation that persons are in the last decade or two of their lives. Yet this is no longer applicable to men and women in many developed countries where life expectancies are rising.

There is an ongoing controversy among demographers and gerontologists regarding the use and accuracy of chronological aging. In 1800 only 25% of men in Western Europe lived to the age of 60, yet in 2008, 90% of these men lived to the age of 90 (Sanderson and Scherbov, 2008, p. 3). Elderhood now has the potential to span 40 years or more, attributable in a large part to increased access to quality health services, improved sanitation, and an emphasis on improving public health. So in 1800, was one "old" at 40? Is "old age" today delayed until 70 today? How old is old and can there ever be a universal number? As life expectancy increases how will we define old age? How will these definitions, and the meaning and the perception of aging, change as the health and wellness of individuals, communities, and nations improve? How will nursing roles and responsibilities change? How can we promote wellness in those who have a much greater chance of living into their 100s?

THE YEARS AHEAD

It was projected that the number of persons at least 60 years of age worldwide will increase by almost 56% between 2015 and 2030; from 901 million to 1.4 billion and then to 2.1 billion by 2050. Fifty-four percent of those at least 60 are women (World Health Organization [WHO], 2015). With a high degree of variability by country and region (Fig. 1.1), the growth in sheer numbers of those 80 and over will grow faster than those over 65 years of age as a whole, from 69 million in 2000 to almost 379 million by 2050, an increase of 5.5 times (United Nations [UN], 2015). The

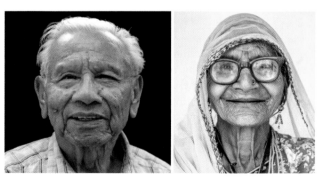

The aging phenotype. (©iStock.com/LPETTET; Mlenny.)

BOX 1.1   The Aging Phenotype

A few years ago I stopped coloring my hair, which is almost completely silver now. It was quite a surprise to me the first time the very young clerk in the booth at the movie theater assumed I was 65 and automatically gave me the "senior discount." My husband's hair is only fading to a dull brown. When he goes alone they tentatively ask, "Do you have any discounts?"

Kathleen, at age 60

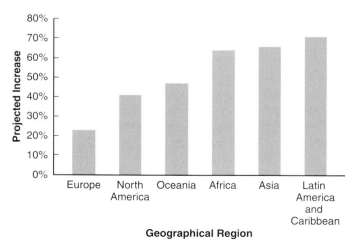

Fig. 1.1 Projected Increase in Number of Adults at Least 60 Years of Age by Geographical Region: 2015–2030. (Data from United Nations: *2030 Agenda for sustainable development,* 2015. Accessed September 15, 2017.)

world-wide number of centenarians (at least 100 years of age) is expected to be 3.7 million by 2050, up from one-half million in 2015 (Stepler, 2016).

In the United States, life expectancy at birth rose 3 years between the 2000 to 2005 and 2010 to 2015 periods. All other geographic areas of the world gained years but most notably Africa where life expectancy increased by 6 years. However, significant disparities remain from an 83.7-year life expectancy of some of those in parts of China to 49.2 years of age in Swaziland, Africa (UN, 2017).

The overall life expectancy at birth in the United States in 2015 was 78.8 years. This represents a decrease of 0.2 and 0.1 years in the life expectancy of men and women, respectively, since 2014. Life expectancy for those identifying as Hispanic of any race has been stable, at 82.0 years (Centers for Disease Control and Prevention [CDC], 2017a). The disparity between life expectancies for black and white Americans has narrowed significantly between 1999 and 2015, with the death rate for blacks (African Americans) dropping by 25% (Office of Minority Health, 2017) (Fig. 1.2).

As of 2016 there were 46 million people at least 65 years old living in the United States, and this is expected to grow to over 98 million by 2060; from 15% of the population to 24% (Mather, 2016). The population over 65 years of age will also become increasingly diverse. In 2014 those who considered themselves as "non-Hispanic white" will shrink from 78.3% to 54.6% in 2050, a drop of 24 percentage points (Mather, 2016) (Fig. 1.3).

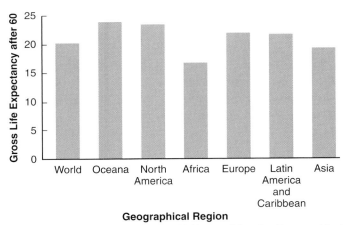

Fig. 1.2 Gross Life Expectancy at 60 Years of Age by Geographical Region, 2010–2015. (Data from United Nations: *World population prospective: the 2017 revision, key findings, and advance tables,* 2017. https://esa.un.org/unpd/wpp.)

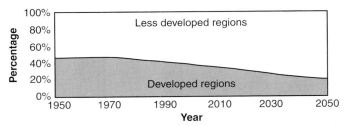

Fig. 1.3 Percentage of the Population at Least 60 Years of Age in Developed Compared With Less Developed Parts of the World, Projected to 2050.

Most of those older than 60 live in what is referred to as "less developed regions," and the percentage is expected to increase from 66% to 79% in this same time period (Fig. 1.3) (United Nations [UN], 2012a). These elders are the most likely to be very poor and in need of support to an extent that is not seen in other parts of the world. For example, many grandparents are caring for the estimated 1.3 million Zimbabwean children orphaned by acquired immunodeficiency syndrome (AIDS). They have few, if any, organizations in place to help them (UNICEF, 2010).

Population growth will change the face of aging as we know it and present many challenges today and in our future. With the increase in number of years lived comes the possibility of increased number of years living with a disability. Globally, people lost an average of 9 years of healthy life due to a disability in 2013, but the quality of life at this time is not well understood (UN, 2015).

Although healthy aging is now an achievable goal for many in developed and developing regions, it is still only a distant vision for any of those living in less developed areas of the world, where lives are shortened by persistent communicable diseases, inadequate sanitation, and lack of both nutritious food and health care. It is essential that nurses across the globe have the knowledge and skills to help people of all ages achieve the highest level of wellness possible. Some of the questions that must be asked include the following: How can global conditions change for those who are struggling? How can the years of healthy elderhood be maximized and enriched to the extent possible, regardless of the conditions in which one lives?

There is an ongoing controversy among demographers and gerontologists regarding the use and accuracy of chronological aging. In 1800 only 25% of men in Western Europe lived to the age of 60, yet today 90% of this same demographic live to the age of 90 (Sanderson and Scherbov, 2008, p. 3). In 1800, was one "old" at 40? Is "old age" delayed until 70 today? How old is old and can there ever be a universal number? As life expectancy increases, how will we define aging? How will these definitions, as well as the meaning and the perception of aging, change as the health and wellness of individuals, communities, and nations improve? How will nursing roles and responsibilities change? How can we promote wellness in those who have a much greater chance of living into their 100s?

Elderhood has the potential to span 40 years or more, attributable in a large part to increased access to quality health services and emphasis on improving the health of the public. In the countries where the average life expectancies have expanded most rapidly, the following four generational subgroups have emerged: the super-centenarians, the centenarians, the baby boomers, and those in-between. The following discussions are only overviews, and the reader must recall that there is no "typical older person."

The Super-Centenarians

The super-centenarians are those who live until at least 110 years of age. This elite group emerged in the 1960s as those first documented to have lived so long. The exact number of persons over the age of 110 is unknown as most are not known to the public. The Gerontology Research Group collects and maintains records of those documented to have lived at least 100 years to the extent possible. As of February 19, 2019, the group identified 39 supercentenarians, with an average age of 113.46 years. The oldest person at that time was Kane Tanaka of Fukuoka, Japan. She was 116 years and 50 days old (Gerontology Research Group, 2019). While some questions have arisen, the person who is still said to have lived the longest was France's almost 123-year-old Jeanne Calment (Allard, Robine, and Calment, 1999) (Box 1.2).

Many of the fathers and older siblings of the oldest of this cohort fought and died in World War I (WWI; 1914 to 1918). Too old to fight in World War II (WWII; 1939 to 1946), they saw their younger siblings and some of their children repeat this service to their countries. If living in Eastern Europe at the time, a super-centenarian of today may be a survivor of the Holocaust.

In most developed countries, especially in nontropical areas, there were no new cases of yellow fever after 1905, missing most of the supercentenarians, but cholera and typhoid still occurred during their childhoods. During the 1916 polio epidemic in New York City, many of the super-centenarians were toddlers. The sheer numbers affected by this and other communicable diseases of the 1800s and 1900s changed the view of science and the acceptance of government's role in protecting the public's health.

As teens the super-centenarians of today survived the influenza pandemic of 1918 to 1919, which killed an estimated 20 million to 40 million people, or up to one-fifth of the world's population. Referred to as the "Spanish Flu" or "Le Grippe," this outbreak began in the United States, Europe, and a small part of Asia. It spread worldwide almost overnight. The virulence was such that the period between exposure and death could be a matter of hours. In 1 year the life expectancy in the United States dropped by 10 to 12 years. It was most deadly to those 20 to 40 years old and therefore was more likely to have spared the super-centenarians of today (Gagnon et al, 2013).

A study of 32 super-centenarians in the United States found that "A surprisingly substantial portion of these individuals were still functionally independent or required minimal assistance" (Schoenhofen et al 2006, p. 1237). Most functioned

independently until after age 100, with no signs of frailty until about the age of 105. They were found to be remarkably homogeneous. None had Parkinson's disease, only 25% had ever had cancer, and stroke and cardiovascular disease were rare if they occurred at all. Few had been diagnosed with dementia. A study in Japan corroborated these findings. It is theorized that these unusual persons have survived this long for "rare and unpredictable" reasons (Willcox et al, 2008). Arai and colleagues (2017) found that those who were physically independent at 100 were the most likely to live beyond 110. While the number alive today is small, it is predicted to grow as the centenarians behind them live longer and healthier lives.

The Centenarians

Centenarians are between 100 and 109 years of age, the majority of whom are between 100 and 104 (Meyer, 2012). Only the very oldest of these fought in WWII, when approximately 55 million of their contemporaries died. In 2015 there were about 451,000 persons at least 100 years of age across the globe. It is predicted that this number will reach almost 3.7 million by 2050, or 23.6 persons per every 10,000 persons over 65. While the United States has the highest overall number of centenarians, Japan has more than double the number relative to the population as a whole (2.2 vs. 4.8 centenarians per 10,000 persons in the country) (Fig. 1.4). By 2050 it is projected that China will have the greatest overall number of centenarians, increasing 13 times the number it was in 2015 (Stepler, 2016).

Based on the U.S. Census report of 2010, centenarians in the United States were overwhelmingly white (82.5%), women (82.8%), and lived in urban areas of the Southern states (AOA, 2012). Along with the rapidly expanding numbers in this cohort, there is an exponential increase in biological and genetic research to attempt to better understand exceptional longevity in humans and the underpinnings of morbidity that is compressed toward the end of their lives (Giuliani et al, 2017;

BOX 1.2 A Well-Known Super-Centenarian

Mme Calment of Arles, France, was born in 1875 and died in 1997 at 122 years and 4.5 months old. When she was 90 years old, her lawyer recognized the value of the apartment in which she lived, and which she owned, and made her what turned out to be the deal of a lifetime. In exchange for the deed to the apartment, he would pay her a monthly "pension" for life and she could live in the apartment the rest of her life. Over the next 32 years she was paid more than double the apartment's value. She also outlived the lawyer; her husband of 55 years; her daughter; and her only grandson. An active woman, she took up fencing at 85 and was still riding a bike at 100. She smoked until she was 117 and preferred a diet rich in olive oil.

From Allard M, Robine JM, Calment J: *Jeanne Calment: from Van Gogh's time to ours, 122 extraordinary years*, Waterville, ME, 1999, Thorndike Press.

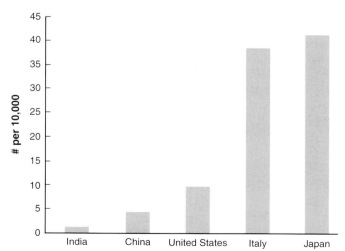

Fig. 1.4 Numbers of Persons at Least 100 years of Age per 10,000 Persons in the Population (Select Countries). (From Stepler R: *World's centenarian population projected to grow eightfold by 2050*, 2016. Pew Research Center. http://www.pewresearch.org/fact-tank/2016/04/21/worlds-centenarian-population-projected-to-grow-eightfold-by-2050/.)

Karasik and Newman, 2015). Although centenarians still carry genetic markers within their chromosomes for any number of health problems, for unknown reasons these are not "activated" until much later, if at all, when compared with other persons (Sebastiani and Perls, 2012). The relatively low number of centenarians (and super-centenarians) with dementia of some kind may be explained by the presence of some type of genetic neuroprotective factors (Takao et al, 2016). While most people have normal age-related declines in immune functioning and increases in a state of chronic inflammation, this does not appear to be the case for this group of long-lived people (Iannitti and Palmieri, 2011).

Centenarians were teenagers or young adults at the time of the Great Depression (approximately 1929 to 1940). Jobs were scarce and poverty and malnutrition were rampant. In areas where the water lacked natural fluoride, children's teeth were soft and cavity prone. "Pigeon chest," a malformation of the developing rib cage caused by lack of vitamin D, was common. Goiter and myxedema were less common but were present regionally because of unrecognized iodine deficiencies. Smallpox has been a threat to centenarians until about 35 years ago when it was essentially eradicated globally (College of Philadelphia Physicians [CPP], 2013). Many centenarians had all or most of the "childhood" diseases, such as measles, mumps, chickenpox, and whooping cough; some survivors of today also had polio as children.

Those In-Between

There is also a unique cohort born in the 30 years between the baby boomers (see later) and the centenarians; the septuagenarians (70-year-olds), octogenarians (80-year-olds), and nonagenarian (90-year-olds). The oldest were born in the last year or two of WWI and the youngest at the very end of WWII. Many of the oldest fought in WWII. Some fought in the Korean War and the youngest may have fought in the Vietnam War. This cohort includes some of the last survivors of the Holocaust. They came of age during tumultuous times. Some witnessed or had personal experience with the American Civil Rights Movement (1955–1968) or the assassination of President John F. Kennedy (1963). Most were old enough to have been drafted or volunteered to serve in Vietnam (1955–1975). The Cold War was felt by many as the tensions between the United States and the former Soviet Union reached fever pitch. Others lost friends and family to the global AIDS epidemic before the human immunodeficiency virus (HIV) was isolated in France and the United States in 1983. If born between about 1929 and 1939, they were children during the Great Depression. They have survived any number of childhood illnesses. Depending on the year they were born, they have also survived a number of communicable disease outbreaks and influenza pandemics (Table 1.1).

Polio infection was a major fear for this cohort, and for some, either they or their friends were affected. A vaccine was not available to children in the United States until 1955, providing the most benefits to the youngest of the "in-betweeners" (CPP, 2013). Penicillin, first discovered in 1928 by Alexander Fleming, became usable in humans in 1936 and likely prevented many infection-related mortalities from then to the present time (Markel, 2013).

TABLE 1.1   A Sampling of Significant Events That Occurred During the Lives of Today's Older Adults.

1906	San Francisco earthquake kills 500
1914–1918	World War I
1915	First cross-country telephone service
1916	First woman elected to the House of Representatives (Montana)
1916	New York polio epidemic
1918–1919	The Spanish Flu (La Grippe) H1N1 kills 20 million worldwide (500,000 in the United States)
1920	Women are "granted" the right to vote
1927	Charles Lindbergh makes the first solo transatlantic flight in the *Spirit of St. Louis*
1929–1940	Great Depression, creation of the Civilian Conservation Corp to provide jobs
1932	Amelia Earhart completes the first transatlantic flight by a woman
1932–1972	Tuskegee syphilis experiment is conducted
1935	Social Security is created
1939–1945	World War II
1941	Japanese bomb Pearl Harbor, Hawaii
1942	Penicillin becomes available to the public
1945	United States drops atomic bombs on Hiroshima and Nagasaki, Japan, and World War II ends
1946	Immunization against influenza becomes available
1947–1991	Cold War
1950–1953	Korean War between Communist and non-Communist forces
1952	Puerto Rico becomes a U.S. commonwealth
1952–1954	*Brown v. Board of Education:* U.S. Supreme Court rules that segregation in public schools is unconstitutional
1954	McCarthy hearings: Sen. Joseph McCarthy accuses army officials and other public figures of being communists in public forums
1955	Polio vaccine available to the public
1955–1968	Civil Rights Movement
1955–1975	Vietnam War
1957–1960	Asian Flu H2N2 epidemic
1958	Explorer I, the first American satellite, is launched
1960	Birth control pill becomes available
1961	Alan Shepard commands first spaceflight
1963	Assassination of President John F. Kennedy
1965	*Griswold v. Connecticut:* Supreme Court rules that any state laws that limit the use of contraceptives violate the right to marital privacy
1965	Medicare and Medicaid are established
1968	My Lai massacre: U.S. troops kill 300 Vietnamese villagers
1968	Assassination of Dr. Martin Luther King, Jr.
1968–1969	The Hong Kong Flu H3N2 epidemic
1969	Astronauts Neil Armstrong and Buzz Aldrin walk on the moon
1973	*Roe v. Wade:* Supreme Court rules on the legality of abortions in the first trimester
1974	Richard Nixon resigns as president due to Watergate scandal
1980	World Health Organization declares the world "smallpox free"
1981	AIDS epidemic is recognized
1983	The HIV virus, which causes AIDS, is identified
1983	Expanded pneumococcal vaccine becomes available
1991	Dr. Bernadine Healy becomes the first woman to lead the National Institutes of Health
2009–2010	Swine Flu H1N1 epidemic
2010	Catastrophic earthquake strikes Haiti

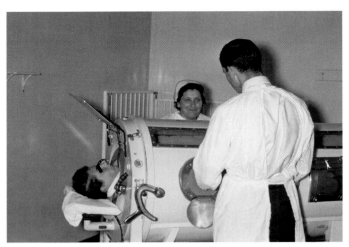

Hospital staff examining a patient in an iron lung during the Rhode Island polio epidemic, 1960. (From the Centers for Disease Control and Prevention Public Health Image Library.)

The number of persons between the ages of 70 and 99 is growing at an exponential rate as the baby boomers begin to join their ranks. At this time the population in the United States of those 85 years of age or older is expected to increase 250% between 2011 and 2040—from 5.7 million to 14.1 million. Racial and ethnic heterogeneity is slowly growing—88.5% of persons in their 90s self-identified as white alone, 87.6% in their 80s, and 84% in their 70s. Older adults who self-identify as Hispanic, as a group, are growing at the fastest rate (AOA, 2012) (Fig. 1.5).

The Baby Boomers

The youngest of the "older generation" are referred to as "baby boomers" or "boomers." They were born somewhere between approximately 1946 and 1964 depending on how they have been defined by their country. In the United States, the first to become baby boomers turned 65 in 2011; the last will do so in 2029. More babies were born in the United States in 1946, the year after the end of WWII, than any other year—3.4 million or 20% more than in 1945. These numbers increased every year until they tapered off in 1964. In just 18 years, 76.4 million babies had been born, making up 40% of the U.S. population (History, 2017).

The differences in the life experiences between those born in the late 1940s and early 1960s are quite significant. For example, the eldest had mothers and fathers who had served in WWII and as young adults they may have been drafted into the Vietnam War, obtained a "college deferment," or volunteered to serve in the military. The youngest in this cohort may have had only a childhood recollection, if any, of that period of time.

Each day another 10,000 boomers turn 65 years old (Cohn and Taylor, 2010). More than any previous cohort, baby boomers have had better access to medication and other preventive treatment regimens as they were growing up. They will nevertheless live longer with chronic disease than any of their predecessors (Chapter 21).

Of particular concern relative to chronic disease are those related to tobacco use. Obesity, diabetes, arthritis, heart disease, and dementia are all common and discussed in this text. Some of this increased rate of illness is related to a lack of importance placed on what we now consider healthful living as they were growing up. For example, in the 1950s and 1960s smoking was not only condoned, but considered a sign of status. Candy cigarettes were popular with children. Work and public places and homes were filled with smoke, affecting both the smokers themselves and those who were exposed to second-hand smoke. The use of cigarettes peaked in 1963, near the end of the baby boom. There has been a very slow but steady decline in tobacco use since then, from 21 out of 100 adults in 2005 to 15 out of 100 in 2015. This includes 8 out of 100 adults at least 65 years of age (CDC, 2017b).

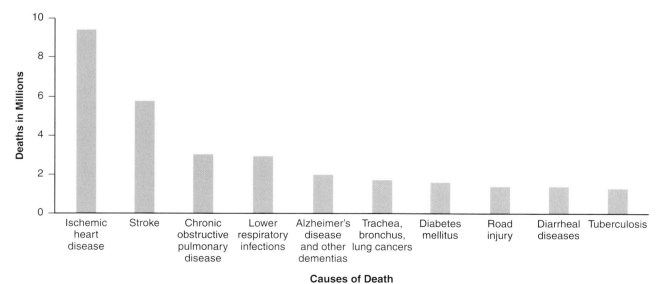

Causes of Death

Fig. 1.5 Top Ten Causes of Death Worldwide in 2016. (Data from World Health Organization: *The top 10 causes of death*, 2018. https://www.who.int/news-room/fact-sheets/detail/the-top-10-causes-of-death. Accessed April 2019.)

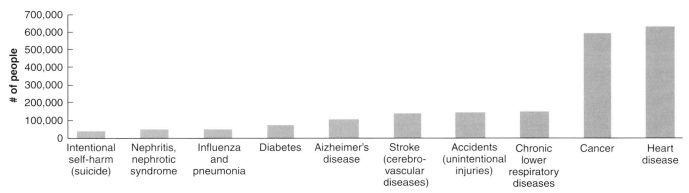

Fig. 1.6 Number of Deaths for Leading Causes of Death (U.S.). (Data from Centers for Disease Control and Prevention [CDC]: *Death and mortality,* 2016. https://www.cdc.gov/nchs/fastats/deaths.htm. Accessed 2017.)

Cigarette smoking is the number one cause of preventable deaths in the United States. Cardiovascular disease and stroke are both caused by tobacco use. These have been the top causes of non-communicable death worldwide for the past 15 years, killing almost 15 million people in 2015 (Figs. 1.5 and 1.6) (CDC, 2017c; United Nations, 2015; WHO, 2017a).

Like their older cohorts, most boomers born in 1950s contracted at least several of the childhood diseases of measles, mumps, rubella, and chickenpox. Scarlet fever was also common. The younger boomers in developed countries have had the benefit of the availability of immunizations against more and more communicable diseases, including polio. The ability to produce the potent antibiotic penicillin and those that followed has significantly influenced the survival of this cohort to the present day. The social emphasis today on healthier lifestyles will go far to help the next generation of older adults reach higher levels of wellness, but for many older adults the challenges to healthy aging are many.

Significant Events That Occurred During the Lives of Today's Older Adults

To provide the best, most sensitive care for older adults, it is necessary to have some knowledge of the historical context in which they have lived their lives. At the same time, to do so would require an entire course in history covering at least 117 years. Instead a list of events that are considered important by persons of different ages, but all at least 65 years old, is provided (Table 1.1).

A WELLNESS-BASED MODEL

The burgeoning population of persons entering the last 20 to 40 years of life presents the nurse with opportunities to make a difference in promoting wellness and stemming the tide of prolonged life accompanied by chronic disease and disability, especially for the baby boomers. While we provide the implications for nursing practice for the most common health challenges in aging, we do this from the perspective that a state of relative wellness can be an ongoing goal for both nursing practice and individuals themselves.

In this text, we use a broad view of wellness to provide nurses with a framework for addressing the needs of our aging population. A wellness-based model encompasses the idea that health is composed of multiple dimensions. Wellness is expressed in functional, environmental, intellectual, psychological, spiritual, social, and biological dimensions of the human experience within the context of culture. These dimensions are juxtaposed on myriad other factors, including normal changes of aging, income, education, sexual orientation and identity, gender, race, religion, ethnicity and country of origin, place of residence, life opportunities, and access to health care. The challenge to both living and dying in wellness is to balance each of these dimensions to the extent possible. The dimensions are like overlapping petals on a flower, anchored together at the center (Fig. 1.7). Wellness involves each of these singularly and in interaction making a fuller, richer whole.

A wellness-based model, derived from a holistic paradigm, is one in which health is viewed on a continuum. At one end there is either an absence of disease as we know it or the presence of chronic diseases that are controlled to the point where their damaging effects are minimized (e.g., a person's blood pressure reading or blood glucose level is within normal limits). At the other end of the continuum is the point when an acute episode or multiple concurrent conditions result in approaching death but one in which suffering of all kinds is minimized to the

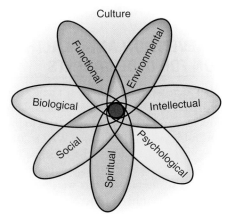

Fig. 1.7 Wellness Model.

extent possible. Age and illness influence the ease at which one moves along the continuum but do not define the individual.

The concept of healthy aging from a wellness perspective is uniquely defined by each individual and changes over time. The subcomponents within the wellness model particularly applicable to healthy aging are functional independence, self-care management of chronic illness and disability, positive outlook, personal growth, social contribution, and activities that promote one's health. The gerontological nurse has the opportunity and the responsibility when working with persons all along the continuum, including at the time of death, to promote wholeness and wellness as defined by the individual at any point in time.

Articulating Goals for Health and Wellness

In 1979 very specific goals were identified to guide the promotion of health of those living in the United States. These were described in the first document, *The Surgeon General's Report on Health and Disease Prevention* (ODPHP, 2017a). This has been updated every 10 years with the most current document *Healthy People 2020*. The over-arching goals serve as the framework from which multiple objectives are drawn and measured (Box 1.3).

Many new topical areas and objectives that are especially important to aging have been added to the 2020 edition. Among these is to increase the numbers of persons with the skills to care for vulnerable older adults and increase the percentage of persons at least 65 who receive core clinical services by 2020. Other new areas are related to dementia, health-related quality of life and well-being, and social determinants of health (ODPHP, 2017b). Throughout the text examples of objectives and the status and goals related to specific health and illness areas are presented.

DISEASE PREVENTION AND HEALTH PROMOTION FOR OLDER ADULTS

The exponential increase in the number of aging persons across the globe is a driving force behind the social and political pressure to develop, test, and implement strategies to promote wellness and healthful living (WHO, 2013; WHO, 2016). Some of these strategies have been found to be effective based on empirical evidence, others are no longer supported, and many others are believed to be helpful but we do not yet have the evidence. Because of the inherent increased vulnerability as we age, the efficacy of health-promoting strategies is especially important if we are to achieve and maintain the highest level of wellness possible along the continuum.

In an effort to increase both the length and health-related quality of life, a provision of the Affordable Care Act in the United States called for creation of the National Prevention Council. Chaired by the U.S. Surgeon General, the Council was charged with partnering community and governmental agencies in the establishment of action plans for health promotion and disease prevention (USDHHS, 2017). The document *Healthy Aging in Action* (HAIA) is a compilation of both descriptions of projects and "lessons learned" related to advancing the national strategy of health promotion for and with older adults. The projects address all levels of prevention and all address one of the three goals of healthy aging: (1) promoting health, preventing injury, and managing chronic conditions, (2) optimizing physical, cognitive, and mental health, and (3) facilitating social engagement (National Prevention Council, 2016).

Because of the paucity of research specific to health promotion and aging there are still considerable challenges to implement evidence-based practices, especially when applied to those from historically underrepresented groups. Although this may change with the next generation, the numbers of those who participate in preventive services at this time are low—only 25% of those between 50 and 64 years of age and less than 50% of those 65 years and older are up to date with potentially lifesaving preventive services (Centers for Disease Control and Prevention [CDC], 2017d).

Primary Prevention

Primary prevention refers to strategies that can and are used to prevent an illness before it occurs. For example, through a collaboration of the CDC in the United States and many worldwide partners, wellness is promoted at the primary level by reducing the incidence and prevalence of influenza infections (CDC, 2017e; WHO, 2017b). While the effectiveness of the influenza vaccination varies from person to person, one study showed that an annual immunization can reduce the risk of flu-related hospitalizations by 57% in persons over 50 (Havers et al, 2016) and reduce the risk of contracting the flu by 50% to 60% (CDC, 2017f).

Moving toward and maintaining wellness along the continuum in the context of primary prevention includes many choices that are under the control of the person. These may include never starting or stopping smoking, maintaining an ideal body weight, exercising regularly, eating a well-balanced diet, and using select age-appropriate dietary supplements such as vitamin D and calcium (Chapters 14, 18, and 26). Among other strategies at the primary level are stress management, social engagement, intellectual stimulation, and restful sleep, all of which are essential but too often not emphasized in gerontological nursing practice.

Secondary Prevention

Secondary prevention is the early detection of a disease or health problem that has already developed. The goal of early detection is to increase the likelihood that the problem can be adequately and effectively addressed and the person may return to the prior level of wellness or as close to it as possible. The majority of the strategies considered secondary prevention are in the form of health screenings of some type (e.g., eye exams,

BOX 1.4   Tertiary Prevention in Action

About 9 months ago Helen suffered a stroke that left her partially paralyzed on the right side. With extensive rehabilitation she was able to regain independent ambulation with the help of a cane and functional use of her affected hand with a brace. The left shoulder had become quite tender because of a combination of chronic arthritis and overuse, the latter occurring because she relied on it to remain mobile. She came to the clinic requesting a referral for physical therapy. There she was taught how best to use her cane, stretching exercises, and received heat and massage therapy. She has now returned to her usual activities, until she needs another "dose" of tertiary prevention.

skin screening, colonoscopy, etc.) and are particularly important in promoting healthy aging in those who are active and engaged and whose anticipated life expectancy increases with each year. Secondary prevention occurs in community and senior centers, health fairs, and in health care providers' offices. Nurses and nurse practitioners are often advocates and organizers of activities related to secondary prevention.

Tertiary Prevention

Tertiary prevention addresses the needs of persons whose wellness is already challenged. The goals of tertiary prevention are to promote wellness to the extent possible in the presence of an active health challenge. Tertiary prevention may be as "simple" as diabetic meal planning or as complex as facilitating or coordinating the skilled care needs for the person who has had a stroke. With aggressive tertiary prevention, the person may reach either a previous level of wellness or even a higher level despite the health challenges (Box 1.4).

While primary prevention is extremely important and has demonstrated efficacy, secondary and tertiary prevention take on new meaning for older adults, especially in the presence of comorbid conditions. For example, determining who should undergo health screening depends on several key factors. Will *knowing* one has a disease or condition change the course along the continuum and projected timing of death, or will aggressive treatment such as radiation or surgery is a reasonable option for someone with dementia (Box 1.5)? While one cannot entirely compensate for a lifetime of lifestyle choices that were

BOX 1.5   When Is Secondary Prevention in Question?

A breast mass was noted in a patient in a skilled nursing facility. The nurse was adamant that the patient should have a mammogram. Although the 85-year-old woman was still quite mobile and cheerful, she also had very advanced dementia. My inclination was to not pursue any further exam (secondary prevention). In conversation with her only living child, we agreed that the mammogram would most likely lead to a diagnosis of breast cancer but would be a hardship for her mother because she would not understand what was being done to her. If cancer was indeed diagnosed, questions about radiation, chemotherapy, and so on would need to be addressed. It was agreed that under the circumstances her mother would not benefit from the procedure. The patient could neither understand the diagnostic procedure nor withstand any treatment, both of which would negatively affect her current quality of life. The woman did not receive the mammogram and died of an acute myocardial event about 3 months later.

detrimental to one's health, many small health-promoting changes can ameliorate their impact in later life.

PROMOTING HEALTHY AGING: IMPLICATIONS FOR GERONTOLOGICAL NURSING

♥ HEALTHY PEOPLE 2020
Emerging Issues in the Health of Older Adults

- Person-centered care planning that includes caregivers
- Quality measures of care and monitoring of health conditions
- Fair pay and compensation standards for formal and informal caregivers
- Minimum levels of geriatric training for health professionals
- Enhanced data on subpopulations of older adults

From Office of Disease Prevention and Health Promotion (ODPHP): *Older adults*, 2017. https://www.healthypeople.gov/2020/topics-objectives/topic/older-adults. Accessed September 1, 2017.

The gerontological nurse can use the wellness-based model to promote healthy aging across the continuum of wellness and care settings. The model builds on the goals described in the strategies of the National Prevention Council and *Healthy People 2020*, expanded now to recognize emerging issues relevant to healthy aging. Gerontological nurses are active in promoting wellness at the primary level through participating in and facilitating even the simplest of activities, such as when the bedside nurse ensures that the patient is served a meal that is nutritious but also culturally appropriate. Nurses in the community promote wellness as health educators, advocates, and case managers, making sure people know the services to which they are eligible and recommended. Advanced practice nurses have become champions of the Annual Health Promotion visit for Medicare recipients (Chapter 30).

Yet both the goals and the objectives and interventions for healthy older adults will differ from those for very frail older adults or those with limited life expectancies. When select preventive approaches are questionable, the nurse can contribute to health care conversations leading to the best decision for any one person. Secondary prevention such as health screening for the most impaired or those with very short life expectancies is generally not recommended, but some primary and all tertiary prevention is appropriate. For those nearing the end of life or with advanced neurocognitive impairments the burden and benefit of lifestyle recommendations must be carefully considered. It is the responsibility of the skilled gerontological nurse to design and implement appropriate interventions for persons all along the wellness continuum; from the very active, to those with advanced cognitive impairments, to those who are nearing death.

The nurse promotes *biological wellness* by promoting regular physical activity such as playing tennis, participating in wheelchair bowling, or sitting upright for intervals throughout the day. Healthy lifestyles are encouraged: healthy eating and adequate and restful sleep, achieving control over acquired health problems such as hypertension or diabetes, and avoiding tobacco or tobacco products. Fostering maximal biological wellness also means advocating for the person to secure the highest quality of medical care when it is needed. The implementation of evidence-based care and cutting-edge research is an expectation, not an option.

The nurse promotes *social wellness* by facilitating activities in which desired interactions with others, pets, or both are possible (Box 1.6). Ongoing social interactions have been found to have a significant effect on cognition, memory, and mood (Chapters 28 and 29). Through social interaction, persons can be recognized with inherent value as men and women, regardless of sexual orientation, gender identity, age, or functional ability (Box 1.7).

Nurses promote *functional wellness* across the continuum of care and roles. The bedside nurse ensures that the physical environment is one that promotes healing and encourages the person to remain active and engaged at the highest level possible. For example, it is not appropriate to help someone out of a chair who is able to do so, albeit slower. This type of "help" negatively affects both muscle tone and self-esteem.

Addressing *environmental* wellness is individual to the person but often includes political activism. Those living in the inner city may be facing increased crime and victimization, exposure to pollution, reduced access to fresh fruits and vegetables, and greater dependence on dwindling public transportation. The nurse becomes involved in creating healthy living spaces by advocating for adequate funding for a wide range of resources such as street lighting, community gardens, or aging-related services including the American Aging Association (http://www.americanagingassociation.org), the National Society for American Indian Elderly (http://nsaie.org), or EUROFAMCARE (Family Care of Older Adults in Europe). The gerontological nurse helps create living spaces and practices that respect and support an environment where healthy aging is possible.

Addressing *psychological* wellness most often calls for identifying potential threats to this aspect of the person. Psychological health includes being aware of and accepting feelings. The nurse is often the one to observe and assess this dimension of health and challenge the view held by both persons themselves and health care providers—that declines in mental and cognitive health are "normal changes with aging." In many cases, what is thought to be dementia may be the misdiagnosis of depression (Chapter 28). The nurse can take the lead in addressing these misconceptions and helping persons who are wrestling with new or life-long psychiatric or psychological challenges as they age.

Spiritual wellness may be described as a sense that one's life has meaning. This may be a relationship with a greater source (e.g., God, Allah, The Great Spirit, Wakan Tanka, Gitche Manitou), a relationship with others, or the sense of the community or world. The nurse fosters the spiritual dimension of the person through at least openness to how others view and express their spirituality. This may be by ensuring that the person's spiritual rituals are taken into account when scheduling medical appointments or procedures or even when taking vital signs in the hospital setting. It also means that the nurse and the rest of the health care team respect and account for dying and death rituals as appropriate (Chapter 35).

The nurse promotes wellness in all dimensions within the context of the person's *culture*. When nurses address the person's needs within his or her personal perspective, they are respecting the patient's culture regardless of what it is and the form it takes. It may be ensuring the appropriate food is provided, such as a serving of pasta or rice with each meal or facilitating the inclusion of an indigenous healer in the care team.

By listening closely, nurses can hear what is most important to persons and what can be done to promote their wellness. The nurse's role across the globe is to facilitate the creation of economic, social, and physical environments that enhance the opportunity for persons to move toward wellness through the promotion of healthy lifestyles, timely health screening, and the ability to participate in tertiary prevention at every stage of life. The wellness-based approach is perhaps the most equitable in supporting the individual's potential for maximal health and functioning at all levels.

BOX 1.6   Promoting Wellness in the Face of Death

Mrs. Heinz was coming very close to the end of her life. Her symptoms were well controlled but during what turned out to be my last home visit she seemed very agitated. When asked if there was anything I could do, she was remarkably frank. "I know I have very little time left. My sister-in-law insists she wants to see me before it is 'too late.' I have never liked her and have no desire to spend one minute of my remaining time in the company of someone I do not like. Please discuss this with my husband; he doesn't seem to understand when I do." Mr. Heinz was my patient that day and after many tears he decided he had to respect his wife's wishes. She died peacefully in his arms several days later.

BOX 1.7   The Social-Sexual Dimension

There was a long-term care facility in which the staff consistently interacted with the residents, regardless of their functional or cognitive status. For many, the staff was all of the family they had left. One of the younger residents had been there a long time and would likely spend the rest of his life there because of brain damage from uncontrollable seizures. Although communication was difficult, he got much pleasure in "flirting" with the staff. One day a nurse was observed stopping by his chair and commenting on a new baseball cap he had been given. She said "you're smokin' in that cap there!" His smile could not be broader, and they each went their different directions.

KEY CONCEPTS

- Wellness is a multidimensional concept. It is human adaptation at the most individually satisfying level in response to existing internal and external conditions.
- With increasing life expectancy and numbers of persons alive, the positive outcomes of health promotion and disease prevention interventions are more important now than in any previous time in history.
- For the first time in history an individual and his or her parent and grandparent may all be of the same socially described "generation" of older adults.

- The definition of who is "old" and "elder" or a "senior citizen" is changing rapidly; this is expected to change even further as more and more of the "baby boomers" live longer.
- Health status is now recognized in unique and specific ways as noted in the U.S. document *Healthy People 2020*.
- The National Prevention Council partners with governmental and nongovernmental agencies to develop and test strategies to promote wellness.

- By using a wellness perspective as a basis of practice, the gerontological nurse can promote health regardless of where a person is on the health continuum.
- A nurse with a wellness focus designs interventions to promote optimal living, enhance healthy aging, and maximize quality of life.

NURSING STUDY: IN CELEBRATION OF LIFE

Mrs. Perraud recently celebrated her 95th birthday with a large number of family and friends attending from far and near. She shared, "That was the best day of my life! I was married three times but none of the weddings were as exciting as this. I never have thought I would live to be this old. Yes, life has been a struggle. My first husband died in the Second World War right after we were married, my second husband was abusive and I quickly got rid of him, and the last husband of 65 years was the love of my life. He developed Alzheimer's and I cared for him for six years but I never regretted a moment. My children sometimes wonder how I have managed to keep such a positive outlook. I believe my purpose in living so long is to be an example of aging well."

She is frail and thin, regularly takes acetaminophen to treat the discomfort from advanced osteoarthritis, eats sparingly but likes almost all foods and is concerned about good nutrition. Until last year she walked two brisk miles a day. She broke her hip after slipping on an acorn, has not regained her full strength, and is frustrated that she now has to use a cane. She is hoping that with enough exercise in the gym she will make it to her next birthday.

- Which of the dimensions of wellness as discussed in this chapter are reflected in the narrative provided?
- Where would you place Mrs. Perraud in the continuum of wellness? Explain your reasons for doing so.
- Identify three health promotion or disease prevention strategies to talk with Mrs. Perraud about. In doing so you will either listen as she tells you how she has addressed these over time or suggest to her how they may be incorporated into her life.

▮ CRITICAL THINKING QUESTIONS AND ACTIVITIES

1. Construct a personal definition of health that incorporates the dimensions of the wellness-based model.
2. Looking into the future, consider which decade you expect will be your last. In what state of health do you expect to be?
3. There are three levels of prevention. As science advances, so

does our knowledge of which strategies are effective in promoting health and in preventing illness and which are not. Think of a strategy you use or have heard of and believe to be effective. Then look in scientific literature (not the newspaper or Wikipedia) to see what the evidence is at this time.

▮ RESEARCH QUESTIONS

1. What factors are the most significant influences of health in aging?
2. What are the factors that indicate one is in a state of "wellness"?

3. What are the perceptions of younger people about the possibility of healthy aging?
4. How can nurses enhance wellness for older adults in various stages across the continuum?

REFERENCES

Allard M, Robine JM, Calment J: *Jeanne Calment: from Van Gogh's time to ours, 122 extraordinary years,* Waterville, ME, 1999, Thorndike Press.

Arai Y, Sasaki T, Hirose N: Demographic, phenotypic, and genetic characteristics of centenarians in Okinawa and Honshu, Japan: Part 2 Honshu, Japan, *Mech Ageing Dev* 165(Pt B):80–85, 2017.

Centers for Disease Control and Prevention (CDC): *Health, United States*, 2016, 2017a. https://www.cdc.gov/nchs/data/hus/hus16.pdf#015. Accessed September 1, 2017.

Centers for Disease Control and Prevention (CDC): *Current cigarette smoking among adults in the United States*, 2017b. https://www.cdc.gov/tobacco/data_statistics/fact_sheets/adult_data/cig_smoking/index.htm. Accessed September 1, 2017.

Centers for Disease Control and Prevention (CDC): *Smoking and tobacco use: Fast facts diseases and death*, 2017c. https://www.cdc.gov/tobacco/data_statistics/fact_sheets/fast_facts/index.htm. Accessed September 1, 2017.

Centers for Disease Control and Prevention (CDC): *Clinical preventive services,* 2017d. http://www.cdc.gov/aging/services. Accessed September 1, 2017.

Centers for Disease Control and Prevention (CDC): *International influenza,* 2017e. https://www.cdc.gov/flu/international/index.htm. Accessed September 1, 2017.

Centers for Disease Control and Prevention (CDC): *Vaccine effectiveness: How well does the flu vaccine work?* 2017f. https://www.cdc.gov/flu/about/qa/vaccineeffect.htm. Accessed September 1, 2017.

Cohn D'V, Taylor P: *Baby boomers approach 65 – glumly*, 2010, Pew Research Center. http://www.pewsocialtrends.org/2010/12/20/baby-boomers-approach-65-glumly/. Accessed September 1, 2017.

Gagnon A, Miller MS, Hallman SA, et al: Age-specific mortality during the 1918 influenza pandemic: unravelling the mystery of high young adult mortality, *PLOS One* 8(8):e69586, 2013. http://journals.plos.org/plosone/article?id=10.1371/journal.pone.0069586.

Gerontology Research Group: *GRG world supercentenarian rankings list*, 2017. http://www.grg.org/SC/WorldSCRankingsList.html. Accessed September 1, 2017.

Giuliani C, Pirazzini C, Delledonne M, et al: Centenarians as extreme phenotypes: An ecological perspective to get insight into the relationship between the genetics of longevity and age-associated diseases, *Mech Ageing Dev* 165(Pt B):195–201, 2017.

Havers F, Sokolow L, Shay DK, et al: Case-control study of vaccine effectiveness in preventing laboratory confirmed influenza hospitalizations in older adults, United States, 2010-2011, *Clin Infec Dis* 63(10):1304–1311, 2016.

History: *Baby boomers*, 2017. http://www.history.com/topics/baby-boomers. Accessed September 2017.

Iannitti T, Palmieri B: Inflammation and genetics: an insight in the centenarian model, *Hum Biol* 83(4):531–559, 2011.

Jett KF: The meaning of aging and the celebration of years, *Geriatr Nurs* 24(4):290–293, 2003.

Karasik D, Newman A: Models to explore genetics of human aging, *Adv Exp Med Biol* 847:141–161, 2015.

Mather M: *Fact sheet: aging in America*, 2016. Population Reference Bureau. http://www.prb.org/Publications/Media-Guides/2016/aging-unitedstates-fact-sheet.aspx. Accessed September 2017.

Meyer J: *Centenarians: 2010, 2010 Census Special Reports* (Report no. C2010SR-03), Washington, DC, 2012, United States Census Bureau, U.S. Government Printing Office.

Nascher I: *Geriatrics*, Philadelphia, 1914, P. Blakiston's Sons & Co.

National Prevention Council: *Healthy aging in action*, 2016. https://www.surgeongeneral.gov/priorities/prevention/about/healthy-aging-in-action-final.pdf. Accessed September 1, 2017.

Office of Disease Prevention and Health Promotion (ODPHP): *History and development of Healthy People*, 2017a. https://www.healthypeople.gov/2020/About-Healthy-People/History-Development-Healthy-People-2020. Accessed September 1, 2017.

Office of Disease Prevention and Health Promotion (ODPHP): *Older adults*, 2017b. https://www.healthypeople.gov/2020/topics-objectives/topic/older-adults. Accessed September 1, 2017.

Office of Minority Health: *African American death rate drops 25 percent*, 2017. https://minorityhealth.hhs.gov/omh/content.aspx?ID=188. Accessed September 1, 2017.

Sanderson W, Scherbov S: Rethinking age and aging. Population Bulletin, *Popul Ref Bureau* 63(4):3–16, 2008.

Schoenhofen EA, Wyszynski DF, Andersen S, et al: Characteristics of 32 supercentenarians, *J Am Geriatr Soc* 54:1237–1240, 2006.

Sebastiani P, Perls TT: The genetics of extreme longevity: lessons from the New England centenarian study, *Front Genet* 3:277, 2012.

Stepler R: *World's centenarian population projected to grow eightfold by 2050*, 2016. Pew Research Center. http://www.pewresearch.org/fact-tank/2016/04/21/worlds-centenarian-population-projected-to-grow-eightfold-by-2050/. Accessed September 1, 2017.

Takao M, Hirose N, Arai Y, Mihara B, Mimura M: Neuropathology of supercentenarians—four autopsy cases, *Acta Neuropathol Commun* 4(1):97, 2016.

United Nations (UN): *World population ageing*, 2015. http://www.un.org/en/development/desa/population/publications/pdf/ageing/WPA2015_Report.pdf. Accessed September 1, 2017.

U.S. Chamber of Commerce, Economics and Statistics Administration: *Sixty-five plus in the United States*, 2011. https://www.census.gov/population/socdemo/statbriefs/agebrief.html. Accessed September 2017.

U.S. Department of Health and Human Services(USDHHS): *National Prevention Council*, 2017. https://www.surgeongeneral.gov/priorities/prevention/about/. Accessed September 1, 2017.

Willcox DC, Willcox BJ, Wang NC, et al: Life at the extreme limit: phenotypic characteristics of supercentenarians in Okinawa, *J Gerontol A Biol Sci Med Sci* 63(11):1201–1208, 2008.

World Health Organization (WHO): *The 8th global conference on health promotion, Helsinki*, 2013. www.who.int/healthpromotion/conferences/8gchp/en/index.html. Accessed September 1, 2017.

World Health Organization (WHO): *World report on ageing and health*, 2015. http://www.who.int/ageing/events/world-report-2015-launch/en/. Accessed September 1, 2017.

World Health Organization (WHO): *9th global conference on health promotion, Shanghai*, 2016. http://www.who.int/healthpromotion/conferences/9gchp/en/. Accessed September 1, 2017.

World Health Organization (WHO): *The top 10 causes of death worldwide*, 2017a. http://www.who.int/mediacentre/factsheets/fs310/en/. Accessed September 1, 2017.

World Health Organization (WHO): *Influenza: Surveillance and monitoring*, 2017b. http://www.who.int/influenza/surveillance_monitoring/en. Accessed August 1, 2017.

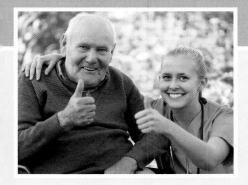

2

Gerontological Nursing: Past, Present, and Future

Theris A. Touhy

http://evolve.elsevier.com//Touhy/TwdHlthAging

A YOUTH SPEAKS

Until my grandmother became ill and needed our help, I really didn't know her well. Now I can look at her in an entirely different light. She is frail and tough, fearful and courageous, demanding and delightful, bitter and humorous, needy and needed. I'm beginning to think that old age is the culmination of all the aspects of living a long life.

Jenine, 28 years old

A PERSON AT MIDLIFE SPEAKS

Gerontological nursing brings one in touch with the most basic and profound questions of human existence: the meanings of life and death; sources of strength and survival skills; beginnings, endings, and reasons for being. It is a commitment to discovery of the self—and of the self I am becoming as I age.

Stephanie, 46 years old

AN OLDER ADULT SPEAKS

I'm 95 years old and have no family or friends that still survive. I wonder if anyone will be there for me when I leave the planet, which will be very soon I am sure. Mothers deliver, but who will deliver me into the hand of God?

Helen, 95 years old

LEARNING OBJECTIVES

On completion of this chapter, the reader will be able to:
1. Discuss strategies to prepare an adequate and competent eldercare workforce to meet the needs of the growing numbers of older adults across the globe.
2. Identify several factors that have influenced the development of gerontological nursing as a specialty practice.
3. Discuss several formal geriatric organizations and describe their significance to nurses.
4. Discuss the role of gerontological nurses in research related to aging.
5. Compare various gerontological nursing roles and requirements across the health-wellness continuum.
6. Discuss interventions to improve outcomes for older adults during transitions between health care settings.

CARE OF OLDER ADULTS: A NURSING IMPERATIVE

Healthy aging is now an achievable goal for many. It is essential that nurses have the knowledge and skills to help people of all ages, races, and cultures to achieve this goal. The developmental period of elderhood is an essential part of a healthy society and as important as childhood or adulthood (Thomas, 2004). We can expect to spend 40 or more years as older adults. Enhancing health in aging requires attention to health throughout life and expert care from nurses.

How do nurses maximize the experience of aging and enrich the years of elderhood for all individuals regardless of the physical and psychological changes that commonly occur? Nurses have a great responsibility to help shape a world in which older adults can thrive and grow, not merely survive. Most nurses care for older adults during the course of their careers. Estimates are "that by 2020, up to 75% of nurses' time

13

will be spent with older adults" (Holroyd et al, 2009, p. 374). In addition, the public will look to nurses to have the knowledge and skills to assist people to age in health. Every older adult should expect care provided by nurses with competence in gerontological nursing.

Who Will Care for an Aging Society?

By 2040, the number of older adults in the world will be at least 1.3 billion (Tolson et al, 2011) (Chapter 1). It is a critical health and societal concern that gerontological nurses, other health professionals, and direct care workers are prepared to deliver care in all settings across the globe. The aging workforce is in shortage in most of the developed world, and the increase in the number of older individuals challenges many countries to develop expanding care services. The developing countries are experiencing the most rapid growth in numbers of older adults and lack systems of care and services.

In the United States, eldercare is projected to be the fastest growing employment sector in health care. In spite of demand, the number of health care workers who are interested and prepared to care for older adults remains low (Institute of Medicine, 2008). Less than 1% of registered nurses and less than 3% of advanced practice nurses (APNs) are certified in geriatrics (Campaign for Action, 2016). "We do not have anywhere close to the number of nurses we need who are prepared in geriatrics, whether in the field of primary care, acute care, nursing home care, or in-home care" (Christine Kovner, RN, PhD, FAAN, as cited in Robert Wood Johnson Foundation, 2012).

Geriatric medicine faces similar challenges with about 7000 prepared geriatricians, 1 for every 2546 older Americans; and this number is falling with the trend predicted to be less than 5000 by 2040. Less than 3% of medical students choose to take geriatric electives (Campaign for Action, 2016). Other professions such as social work, physical therapy, and psychiatry have similar shortages. It is estimated that by 2030, 3.5 million additional health care professionals and direct care workers will be needed to meet the care needs of the older adult population. An encouraging trend is that the number of doctors and advanced practitioners in the United States who focus on nursing home care (skilled nursing facility providers–SNFs) rose by more than a third between 2012 and 2015. This suggests the rise of a significant new specialty in medical and nursing practice that will affect patient outcomes. It is very important that these providers have competency in geriatric care and the Society for Post-Acute and Long-Term Care Medicine is developing an educational program (Morley, 2017; Ryskina et al, 2017).

The geriatric workforce shortage also presents a looming crisis for the 43.5 million unpaid family caregivers providing care for someone 55 years or older. Without improvement in the eldercare workforce, even more stress will be placed on family and other informal caregivers. With smaller family sizes, the rising divorce rate, and the increase in geographical relocation, the next generation of older adults may be less able to rely on families for caregiving (Chapter 34). Will there be care workers to assist families in care of loved ones? See the *Healthy People 2020* box for an objective related to the workforce crisis.

 HEALTHY PEOPLE 2020

Objective 7.A

Increase the proportion of the health care workforce with geriatric certification (physicians, geriatric psychiatrists, registered nurses, dentists, physical therapists, registered dieticians).

Data from U.S. Department of Health and Human Services, Office of Disease Prevention and Health Promotion (2012). *Healthy People 2020.* http://www.healthypeople.gov/2020.

DEVELOPMENT OF GERONTOLOGICAL NURSING

Historically, nurses have always been in the frontline of caring for persons as they age. They have provided hands-on care, supervision, administration, program development, teaching, and research and are, to a great extent, responsible for the rapid advance of gerontology as a profession. Nurses have always been the mainstay of care of older adults. Gerontological nurses have made significant contributions to the body of knowledge guiding best practice care of older adults.

Efforts to determine the appropriate term for nurses caring for older adults have included gerontic nurses, gerontological nurses, and geriatric nurses. We prefer the term gerontological nurse because it reflects a more holistic approach encompassing both health and illness. *Gerontological* nursing has emerged as a circumscribed area of practice only within the past 6 decades. Before 1950, gerontological nursing was seen as the application of general principles of nursing to the older adult client with little recognition of this area of nursing as a specialty similar to obstetric, pediatric, or surgical nursing. Whereas most specialties in nursing developed from those identified in medicine, this was not the case with gerontological nursing because health care of the older adult was traditionally considered within the domain of general nursing (Davis, 1985). In examining the history of gerontological nursing, one must marvel at the advocacy and perseverance of nurses who have remained deeply committed to

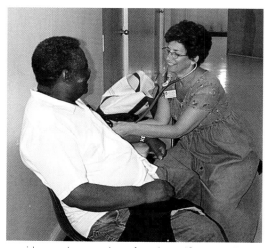
Nurses provide care in a number of settings. (Courtesy Kathleen Jett.)

the care of older adults despite struggling against insurmountable odds over the years.

The foundation of gerontological nursing as we know it today was built largely by a small cadre of nurse pioneers, many of whom are now deceased. The specialty was defined and shaped by these innovative nurses who saw, early on, that older adults had special needs and required the most subtle, holistic, and complex nursing care. These pioneers challenged the current thinking and investigated new ideas related to the care of older adults; refuted mythical tales and fantasies about aging; and found realities through investigation, clinical observation, practice, and documentation, setting in motion activities that markedly influenced the course of the aging experience. They saw new possibilities and a better future for those in the later stages of life.

The wisdom the pioneers shared is still relevant today, and we owe them a debt of gratitude for their commitment, compassion, and persistence in establishing the specialty practice. Box 2.1 presents the views of some of the geriatric nursing pioneers, and those of current leaders, on the practice of gerontological nursing and what draws them to the specialty. For a comprehensive review of the history of the specialty, including Dr. Ebersole's interviews with geriatric nursing pioneers, the reader is referred to *Geriatric Nursing: Growth of a Specialty* (Ebersole and Touhy, 2006). Nurses are proud to be the standard bearers of excellence in the care of older adults (Table 2.1).

Early History

The origins of gerontological nursing are rooted in England and began with Florence Nightingale as she accepted a position in the Institution for the Care of Sick Gentlewomen in Distressed Circumstances. Nightingale's concern for the frail and sick elderly was continued by Agnes Jones, a wealthy Nightingale-trained nurse, who in 1864 was sent to the Liverpool Infirmary, a large Poor Law institution. The care in the institution had been poor, the diet meager, and the "nurses" often drunk. Under the tutelage of Nightingale, Miss Jones was able to dramatically improve the care and reduce the costs.

In the United States, almshouses were the destination of destitute older adults and were insufferable places with "deplorable conditions, neglect, preventable suffering, contagion, and death from lack of proper medical and nursing care" (Crane, 1907, p. 873). As early as 1906, Lavinia Dock and other early leaders in nursing addressed the needs of chronically ill older adults in almshouses and published their work in the *American Journal of Nursing* (AJN). Dock and her colleagues cited the immediate need for trained nurses and pupil education in almshouses, "so that these evils, all of which lie strictly in the sphere of housekeeping and nursing—two spheres which have always been lauded as women's own—might not occur" (Dock, 1908, p. 523). In 1912, the Board of Directors of the American Nurses Association (ANA) appointed an Almshouse Committee to continue to oversee nursing in these institutions. World War I distracted them from attention to these needs. But in 1925, the ANA advanced the idea of a specialty in the nursing care of older adults.

With the passage of the Social Security Act of 1935, federal monies were provided for old-age insurance and public assistance for needy older adults not covered by insurance. To combat the public's fear of almshouse placement, Congress stipulated that the social security funds could not be used to

BOX 2.1 Reflections on Gerontological Nursing from Gerontological Nursing Pioneers and Current Leaders in the Field

Mary Opal Wolanin, Gerontological Nursing Pioneer
"I believe that one of the most valuable lessons I have learned from those who are older is that I must start with looking inside at my own thinking. I was very guilty of ageism. I believed every myth in the book, was sure that I would never live past my seventieth birthday, and made no plan for my seventies. Probably the most productive years of my career have been since that dreaded birthday and I now realize that it is very difficult, if not impossible, to think of our own aging."
—From interview data collected by Priscilla Ebersole between 1990 and 2001.

Bernita Steffl, Gerontological Nursing Pioneer
"There is always an interesting person there, sometimes locked in the cage of age. I think I have helped at least a few of my students with this approach, 'You see me as I am now, but I see myself as I've always been and all the things I've been–not just an old lady.'"
—From Ebersole P, Touhy T: *Geriatric nursing: growth of a specialty*, New York, 2006, Springer, p 52.

Terry Fulmer, Dean, College of Nursing, New York University, and Co-Director, John A. Hartford Institute for Geriatric Nursing
"I soon realized that in the arena of caring for the aged, I could have an autonomous nursing practice that would make a real difference in medical outcomes. I could practice the full scope of nursing. It gave me a sense of freedom and accomplishment. With older patients, the most important component of care, by far, is nursing care. It's very motivating."
—From Ebersole P, Touhy T: *Geriatric nursing: growth of a specialty*, New York, 2006, Springer, p 129.

Jennifer Lingler, PhD, CRNP, Assistant Professor, School of Nursing, University of Pittsburgh
"When I was in high school, a nurse I knew helped me find a nursing assistant position at the residential care facility where she worked. That experience sparked my interest in older adults that continues today. I realized that caring for frail elders could be incredibly gratifying, and I felt privileged to play a role, however small, in people's lives. At the same time, I became increasingly curious about what it means to age successfully. I questioned why some people seemed to age so gracefully, while others succumbed to physical illness, mental decline, or both. As a Building Academic Geriatric Nursing Capacity (BAGNC) alumnus, I now divide my time serving as a nurse practitioner at a memory disorders clinic, teaching an ethics course in a gerontology program, and conducting research on family caregiving. I am encouraged by the realization that as current students contemplate the array of opportunities before them, seek counsel from trusted mentors, and gain exposure to various clinical populations, the next generation of geriatric nurses will emerge. And, I am confident that in doing so, they will set their own course for affecting change in the lives of society's most vulnerable members."
—As cited in Fagin C, Franklin P: Why choose geriatric nursing? Six nursing scholars tell their stories, *Imprint* 5[4], 72-76, 2005.

TABLE 2.1 Professionalization of Gerontological Nursing.

1906	First article is published in *American Journal of Nursing* (AJN) on care of the elderly.
1925	AJN considers geriatric nursing as a possible specialty in nursing.
1950	Newton and Anderson publish first geriatric nursing textbook.
	Geriatrics becomes a specialization in nursing.
1962	American Nurses Association (ANA) forms a national geriatric nursing group.
1966	ANA creates the Division of Geriatric Nursing.
	First master's program for clinical nurse specialists in geriatric nursing developed by Virginia Stone at Duke University.
1970	ANA establishes *Standards of Practice for Geriatric Nursing*.
1974	Certification in geriatric nursing practice offered through ANA; process implemented by Laurie Gunter and Virginia Stone.
1975	*Journal of Gerontological Nursing* published by Slack; first editor, Edna Stilwell.
1976	ANA renames Geriatric Division "Gerontological" to reflect a health promotion emphasis.
	ANA publishes *Standards for Gerontological Nursing Practice*; committee chaired by Barbara Allen Davis.
	ANA begins certifying geriatric nurse practitioners.
	Nursing and the Aged edited by Burnside and published by McGraw-Hill.
1977	First gerontological nursing track funded by Division of Nursing and established by Sr. Rose Therese Bahr at University of Kansas School of Nursing.
1979	*Education for Gerontic Nursing* written by Gunter and Estes; suggested curricula for all levels of nursing education.
1980	*Geriatric Nursing* first published by AJN; Cynthia Kelly, editor.
1983	Florence Cellar Endowed Gerontological Nursing Chair established at Case Western Reserve University, first in the nation; Doreen Norton, first scholar to occupy chair.
	National Conference of Gerontological Nurse Practitioners is established.
1984	National Gerontological Nurses Association is established.
	Division of Gerontological Nursing Practice becomes Council on Gerontological Nursing (councils established for all practice specialties).
1989	ANA certifies gerontological clinical nurse specialists.
1992	Terry Fulmer of the John A. Hartford Foundation founds a major initiative to improve care of hospitalized older patients: Nurses Improving Care for Healthsystem Elders (NICHE). NICHE is an international nursing education and consultation program designed to improve geriatric care in healthcare organizations. Later NICHE introduced an online Leadership Training Program (LTP) to increase the flexibility and affordability of starting a NICHE program in a health care facility.
1996	John A. Hartford Foundation establishes the Institute for Geriatric Nursing at New York University under the direction of Mathy Mezey.
2000	Recommended baccalaureate competencies and curricular guidelines for geriatric nursing care published by the American Association of Colleges of Nursing and the John A. Hartford Foundation Institute for Geriatric Nursing.
	The American Academy of Nursing established Building Academic Geriatric Nursing Capacity (BAGNC) in 2000 with support from the John A. Hartford Foundation.
2001	Hartford Coalition of Geriatric Nursing Associations formed.
2002	Nurse Competence in Aging (funded by the Atlantic Philanthropies Inc.) initiative to improve the quality of health care to older adults by enhancing the geriatric competence of nurses who are members of specialty nursing.
2004	Nurse Practitioner and Clinical Nurse Specialist Competencies for Older Adult Care published by the American Association of Colleges of Nursing and the Hartford Institute for Geriatric Nursing.
	Atlantic Philanthropies committed its resources to postdoctoral fellowships in gerontology nursing.
2007	Atlantic Philanthropies provides a grant to the American Academy of Nursing of $500,000 to improve care of older adults in nursing homes by improving the clinical skills of professional nurses (Nursing Home Collaborative).
	American Association for Long-Term Care Nurses formed.
2008	Four new Centers of Geriatric Nursing Excellence (CGNE) are funded by the John A. Hartford Foundation, bringing the total number of Centers to nine. Existing Centers are at the University of Iowa, University of California San Francisco, Oregon Health Sciences University, University of Arkansas, University of Pennsylvania, Arizona State University, Pennsylvania State University, University of Minnesota, and University of Utah.
	Research in Gerontological Nursing launched by Slack Inc; Dr. Kitty Buckwalter, Editor.
	Geriatric Nursing Leadership Academy established by Sigma Theta Tau International with funding from the John A. Hartford Foundation.
	John A. Hartford Foundation funds the Geropsychiatric Nursing Collaborative (Universities of Iowa, Arkansas, Pennsylvania, American Academy of Nursing).
	Institute of Medicine publishes *Retooling for an aging America: building the health care workforce* report and addresses the need for enhanced geriatric competencies for the health care workforce.
	Consensus Model for Advanced Practice Registered Nurses (APRN) Regulation: Licensure, Accreditation, Certification & Education designates adult-gerontology as one of six population foci for APRNs
2009	*Sigma Theta Tau's Center for Nursing Excellence in Long-Term Care* launched.
	John A. Hartford Foundation funds Phase 2 of the Fostering Geriatrics in Pre-Licensure Nursing Education, a partnership between the Community College of Philadelphia and the National League for Nursing.

	TABLE 2.1 Professionalization of Gerontological Nursing.—cont'd
2010	Adult-gerontology primary care nurse practitioner competencies published by the John A. Hartford Foundation Institute for Geriatric Nursing, the American Association of Colleges of Nursing (AACN), and National Organization of Nurse Practitioner Faculties (NONPF). Sigma Theta Tau's Center for Nursing Excellence established. ANCC Pathways to Excellence–Long-Term Care Program established. *ANA Gerontological Nursing Scope and Standards of Practice* published.
2012	The Gerontological Society of America is now home to the Coordinating Center for the National Hartford Centers of Gerontological Nursing Excellence (HCGNE), also known as the Building Academic Geriatric Nursing Capacity Initiative. U.S. Department of Health and Human Services provides funding to five designated medical center hospitals for clinical training to newly enrolled APRNs to deliver primary care, preventive care, transitional care, chronic case management, and other services appropriate for Medicare recipients.
2013	Adult-Gerontology Acute Care Nurse Practitioner and Adult-Gerontology Primary Care Nurse Practitioner certifications through ANCC begin. Hartford Institute of Geriatric Nursing (HIGI) receives a $1.5 million Nurse Education, Practice, Quality, and Retention (NEPQR) Grant from HRSA to enhance interprofessional education, leadership, and team-building skills for practitioners and students to help address the complexity of medication management for frail older adults in the community. The grant is a practice/education partnership between HIGI, New York University (NYU) College of Nursing, NYU Silver School of Social Work, Touro College of Pharmacy, and Visiting Nurse Service of New York. Primary Care for Older Adults Initiative e-learning clinical training modules released; supported by funds from the U.S. Department of Health and Human Services (DHHS), Health Resources and Service Administration (HRSA), Bureau of Health Professions (BHPr), and Division of Public Health and Interdisciplinary Education (DPHIE). Modules available on GenerationNP.com.
2016	$3.7 million grant awarded to Harvard Medical School (with nurse researcher involvement) to establish the Network for Investigation of Delirium Across the U.S. (NIDUS): Advancing the field of delirium with a new interdisciplinary research network.
2017	*Journal of Gerontological Nursing, Geriatric Nursing, Research in Gerontological Nursing, Annals of Long-term Care,* and *Journal of the American Geriatrics Society* adopt new manuscript submission guidelines to reframe the current image of aging and make meaningful change in communication about aging. Examples include adopting older adult as the preferred term for men and women who benefit from geriatrics expertise and providing a specific age range (e.g., older adults between the ages of 65 and 75 when describing research or making recommendations about patient care or the health of the population). See the Leaders of Aging Organizations Frameworks Institute for a toolkit to assist in reframing concepts and skills to better advance the conversation about older adults in the United States (http://www.frameworkinstitute.org/toolkits/aging). Fifty-five Schools of Nursing and Related Organizations have joined as members of the Centers for Geriatric Nursing Excellence (CHNE) and join the nine founding CGNE to total 64 National Hartford Centers of Gerontological Excellence around the world

pay for care in almshouses or other public institutions. This move is thought to have been the genesis of commercial nursing homes. During the next 10 years, many almshouses closed and the number of private boarding homes providing care to older individuals increased. Because retired and widowed nurses often converted their homes into such living quarters and gave care when their boarders became ill, they can be considered the first geriatric (gerontological) nurses in the community and their homes the first nursing homes.

In the 1940s, two nursing journals described centers of excellence for geriatric care: the Cuyahoga County Nursing Home in Ohio and the Hebrew Home for the Aged in New York. An article in the *American Journal of Nursing (AJN)* by Sarah Gelbach (1943) recommended that nurses should have not only an aptitude for working with the elderly but also specific geriatric education. The first textbook on nursing care of older adults, *Geriatric Nursing*, was published by Newton and Anderson in 1950, and the first published nursing research on chronic disease and older adults (Mack, 1952) appeared in the premier issue of *Nursing Research* in 1952.

In 1962 a focus group was formed to discuss geriatric nursing, and in 1966 a geriatric practice group was convened. Also in 1966, the ANA formed a Division of Geriatric Nursing. The first geriatric standards were published by the ANA in 1968, and soon after, geriatric nursing certification was offered. Geriatric nursing was the first specialty to establish standards of practice

within the ANA and the first to provide a certification mechanism to ensure specific professional expertise through credentialing (Ebersole and Touhy, 2006). In 1976 the Division of Geriatric Nursing changed its name to the Gerontological Nursing Division to reflect the broad role nurses play in the care of older adults. In 1984 the Council on Gerontological Nursing was formed and certification for geriatric nurse practitioners (GNPs) and gerontological clinical nurse specialists (GCNSs) became available. The most recent edition of *Gerontological Nursing: Scope and Standards of Practice* was published in 2010 and identifies levels of gerontological nursing practice (basic and advanced) and standards of clinical gerontological nursing care and gerontological nursing performance.

Current Initiatives

The most significant influence in enhancing the specialty of gerontological nursing has been the work of the Hartford Institute for Geriatric Nursing, established in 1996 and funded by the John A. Hartford Foundation. It is the only nurse-led organization in the country seeking to shape the quality of the nation's health care for older Americans by promoting geriatric nursing excellence to both the nursing profession and the larger health care community. Initiatives in nursing education, nursing practice, nursing research, and nursing policy include enhancement of geriatrics in nursing education programs through curricular reform and faculty development, the development of the National Hartford Centers of Gerontological Nursing Excellence, predoctoral and postdoctoral scholarships for study and research in geriatric nursing, and clinical practice improvement projects to enhance care for older adults (www.hartfordign.org).

Another significant influence on improving care for older adults was the Nurse Competence in Aging (NCA) project. This initiative addressed the need to ensure competence in geriatrics among nursing specialty organizations. The initiative provided grant and technical assistance to more than 50 specialty nursing organizations, developed a free web-based comprehensive gerontological nursing resource center where nurses can access evidence-based information on topics related to the care of older adults, and conducted a national gerontological nursing certification outreach (Stierle et al, 2006).

There are two iPad/iPhone apps that give access to information and tools to treat common problems encountered in the care of older adults, including one specific to dementia (https://itunes.apple.com/us/app/consultgeri-dementia/id962437779; https://itunes.apple.com/us/app/consultgerirn/id578360141). The Resourcefully Enhancing Aging in Specialty Nursing (REASN) project extended this work and focused on building intensive collaborations with 13 hospital-based specialty associations to create geriatric educational products and resources to ensure the geriatric competencies of their members.

Sigma Theta Tau's Center for Nursing Excellence in Long-Term Care was launched in 2009. The center sponsors the Geriatric Nursing Leadership Academy (GNLA) and offers a range of products and services to support the professional development and leadership growth of nurses who provide care to older adults in long-term care. In 2013, The Hartford Institute for Geriatric Nursing, in collaboration with several other organizations, began several initiatives focusing on interprofessional education, leadership, and team building skills, and improving the knowledge and skill sets of primary care providers caring for older adults (Table 2.1).

GERONTOLOGICAL NURSING EDUCATION

According to the ANA's *Gerontological Nursing: Scope and Standards of Practice* (2010), "Nurses require the knowledge and skills to assist older adults in a broad range of nursing care issues, from maintaining health and preventing illnesses, to managing complex, overlapping chronic conditions and progressive/protracted frailty in physical and mental functions, to palliative care" (pp. 12–13).

Essential educational competencies and academic standards for care of older adults have been developed by national organizations such as the American Association of Colleges of Nursing (AACN) for both basic and advanced nursing education (ANA, 2010). *The Essentials of Baccalaureate Education for Professional Nursing Practice* (AACN, 2008) specifically address the importance of geriatric content and structured clinical experiences with older adults across the continuum in the education of students. In 2010, AACN and the Hartford Institute for Geriatric Nursing, New York University, published the *Recommended Baccalaureate Competencies and Curricular Guidelines for the Nursing Care of Older Adults,* a supplement to the *Essentials* document (Appendix 2.A). In addition, gerontological nursing competencies for advanced practice graduate programs have also been developed. All of these documents can be accessed from the AACN website. "Despite these lists of competencies, however, there remains a lack of consistency among nursing schools in helping students gain needed gerontological nursing information and skills" (ANA, 2010, p. 12).

There has been some improvement in the amount of gerontology-related content in nursing school curricula, but it is still uneven across schools and hampered by lack of faculty expertise in the subject (Institute of Medicine [IOM], 2011; Robert Wood Johnson Foundation, 2012). The vast majority of schools of nursing have no faculty members certified by the American Nurse Credentialing Center in gerontological nursing. Faculty with expertise in gerontological nursing are scarce and there is a critical need for nurses with master's and doctoral preparation and expertise in care of older adults to assume faculty roles. Most schools still do not have freestanding courses in the specialty similar to courses in maternal/child or psychiatric nursing. This means that a substantial number of graduating nurses have not had the education needed to competently meet the needs of the growing number of older adults for whom they will care.

A 2007 AACN report stated: "In the past, nursing education has been dogged about assuring that every student has the opportunity to attend a birth, but has never insisted that every student have the opportunity to manage a death, even though the vast majority of nurses are more likely to practice with clients who are at the end of life" (p. 7). Best practice recommendations for nursing education include provision of a stand-alone course, and integration of content throughout the curriculum to ensure that gerontology is valued and viewed as an integral part of nursing care (Garbrah et al, 2017; Kydd et al, 2014). Curriculum and clinical experiences have to be inspirational, and so do faculty and clinical mentors teaching students. Care of older adults now covers a 50-year age span of ages 60 to 110 and older so there needs to be practice experiences in a wide range of settings including community and long-term care settings (Kydd et al, 2014).

Experiences with well older adults in the community and opportunities to focus on health promotion should be the first experience for students. This will assist them to develop more positive attitudes, understand the full scope of nursing practice with older adults, and learn nursing responses to enhance health and wellness. Practice in rehabilitation centers, subacute and skilled nursing facilities, and hospice settings are suited for more advanced students and provide opportunities for leadership experience, nursing management of complex problems, interprofessional teamwork, and research application (Sherman and Touhy, 2017).

ORGANIZATIONS DEVOTED TO GERONTOLOGY RESEARCH AND PRACTICE

The Gerontological Society of America (GSA) demonstrates the need for interdisciplinary collaboration in research and practice. The divisions of Biological Sciences, Health Sciences,

Behavioral and Social Sciences, Social Research, Policy and Practice, and Emerging Scholar and Professional Organization include individuals from myriad backgrounds and disciplines who affiliate with a section based on their particular function rather than their educational or professional credentials. Nurses can be found in all sections and occupy important positions as officers and committee chairs in the GSA.

This mingling of the disciplines based on practice interests is also characteristic of the American Society on Aging (ASA). Other interdisciplinary organizations have joined forces to strengthen the field. The Association for Gerontology in Higher Education (AGHE) has partnered with the GSA, and the National Council on Aging (NCOA) is affiliated with the ASA. These organizations and others have encouraged the blending of ideas and functions, furthering the understanding of aging and the interprofessional collaboration necessary for optimal care. International gerontology associations, such as the International Federation on Aging and the International Association of Gerontology and Geriatrics, also have interdisciplinary membership and offer the opportunity to study aging internationally.

Organizations specific to gerontological nursing include the National Gerontological Nursing Association (NGNA), the Gerontological Advanced Practice Nurses Association (GAPNA), the National Association Directors of Nursing Administration in Long Term Care (NADONA/LTC) (also includes assisted-living registered nurses [RNs], licensed practical nurses [LPNs], and licensed vocational nurses [LVNs] as associate members), the American Association of Directors of Nursing Services (AADNS), American Assisted Living Nurses Association (AALNA), the International Consortium on Professional Nursing Practice in Long-Term Care Homes, and the Canadian Gerontological Nursing Association (CGNA).

RESEARCH ON AGING

Inquiry into and curiosity about aging is as old as curiosity about life and death itself. Gerontology began as an inquiry into the characteristics of long-lived people, and we are still intrigued by them. Anecdotal evidence was used in the past to illustrate issues assumed to be universal. Only in the past 60 years have serious and carefully controlled research studies flourished.

The impact of disease morbidity and impending death on quality of life and the experience of aging have provided the impetus for much of the study by gerontologists. Many ideas about aging have been found to be erroneous, and early research was conducted with older adults who were ill. As a result, aging has been inevitably seen through the distorted lens of disease. However, we are finally recognizing that aging and disease are separate entities, though frequent companions.

Aging has been seen as a biomedical problem that must be reversed, eradicated, or controlled for as long as possible. The trend toward the medicalization of aging has also influenced the general public. The biomedical view of the "problem" of aging is reinforced on all sides. A shift in the view of aging to one that centers on the potential for health, wholeness, and quality of life, and the significant contributions of older adults to society, is increasingly the focus in the research, popular literature, and the public portrayal of older adults, and is the theme of this text.

The National Institute on Aging (NIA), the National Institute of Nursing Research (NINR), the National Institute of Mental Health (NIMH), and the Agency for Healthcare Research and Quality (AHRQ) continue to make significant research contributions to our understanding of older adults. Research and knowledge about aging are strongly influenced by federal bulletins that are distributed nationwide to indicate the type of research most likely to receive federal funding. These are published in requests for proposals (RFPs). Ongoing and projected budget cuts are of concern in the adequate funding of aging research and services in the United States.

Nursing Research

Gerontological nursing research and practice have evolved to such a point that the best practice standards are being published and distributed widely. Nurses have generated significant research on the care of older adults and have established a solid foundation for the practice of gerontological nursing. Many nursing research studies and evidence-based protocols are featured in this text. Some of the most important nursing studies have investigated methods of caring for individuals with dementia, reducing falls and the use of restraints, incontinence prevention and management, delirium, pain management, care transitions, and end-of-life care. Research with older adults receives considerable funding from the NINR and their website (www.nih.gov/ninr) provides information about results of studies and funding opportunities. Improving quality of life for individuals with chronic illness, caregiving, and end-of-life and palliative care are current areas of scientific focus in the NINR strategic plan that are important in care of older adults (NINR, 2016).

Gerontological nurse researchers publish in many nursing journals and journals devoted to gerontology such as *The Gerontologist* and *Journal of Gerontology* (GSA), and there are several gerontological nursing journals including *Journal of Gerontological Nursing*, *Research in Gerontological Nursing*, *Geriatric Nursing*, and the *International Journal of Older Adult Nursing*.

Knowledge about aging and the lived experience of aging has changed considerably and will continue to change in the future. Past ideas and current practices will not be acceptable to a generation of healthier and better-educated individuals who expect a much higher quality of life than older individuals from other generations. Nursing research will continue to examine the best practices for care of older adults who are ill and living in institutions but increasing emphasis will be placed on strategies to maintain and improve health while aging, especially in light of the increasing numbers of older adults across the globe. Translational research and continued attention to interprofessional studies are increasingly important. Some suggestions for nursing research directions are presented in Box 2.2.

BOX 2.2   Suggestions for Gerontological Nursing Research

- Staffing patterns and the most appropriate mix to improve care outcomes in long-term care settings; role of the registered nurse in residential long-term care settings
- Strategies to increase preparation in gerontological nursing and increased recruitment into the specialty
- Gay, lesbian, bisexual, transgender couples/families/relationships
- Retirement decisions of current and future older adults, how they are made and how they are changing
- Dementia as a chronic illness and staying well with the disease
- Developing the science behind other pain management devices such as transcutaneous electrical nerve stimulation (TENS), acupuncture, distraction, and various skin stimulation techniques
- Caregiving, particularly intergenerational and cross-cultural
- Interventions for drug and alcohol abuse and mental health problems of current and future generations of older adults
- Integration of current best practice protocols into settings across the continuum in cost-effective and care-efficient models
- Health promotion and illness management interventions in the assisted living setting; role of professional nurses and advanced practice nurses in this setting
- Development of models for end-of-life care in the home and nursing home
- Aging in war-torn societies
- Aging in developing countries
- Older adults in the context of natural disaster management

From Resnick B, Kovach C, McCormack B: Personal email communication, December 18, 2003.

GERONTOLOGICAL NURSING ROLES

Gerontological nursing roles encompass every imaginable venue and circumstance. The opportunities are limitless because we are a rapidly aging society. "Nurses have the potential to improve elder care across settings through effective screening and comprehensive assessment, facilitating access to programs and services, educating and empowering older adults and their families to improve their health and manage chronic conditions, leading and coordinating the efforts of members of the health care team, conducting and applying research, and influencing policy" (Young, 2003, p. 9).

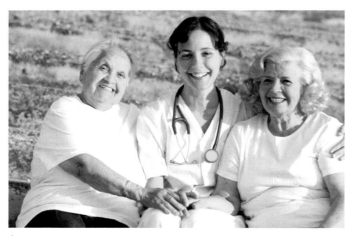

Gerontological nursing is important in this rapidly aging society. (©iStock.com/DianaHirsch.)

A gerontological nurse may be a generalist or a specialist. The generalist functions in a variety of settings (primary care, acute care, home care, subacute and long-term care, and the community), providing nursing care to individuals and their families. National certification as a gerontological nurse is a way to demonstrate one's special knowledge in care for older adults and should be encouraged (http://www.nursecredentialing.org/GerontologicalNursing). The gerontological nursing specialist has advanced preparation at the master's level and performs all of the functions of a generalist but has developed advanced clinical expertise, an understanding of health and social policy, and proficiency in planning, implementing, and evaluating health programs.

Specialist Roles

Under the Consensus Model for APRN Regulation: *Licensure, Accreditation, Certification and Education* (2008), advanced practice registered nurses (APRNs) must be educated, certified, and licensed to practice in a role and a population. APRNs may specialize but may not be licensed solely within a specialty area. APRNs are educated in one of four roles, one of which is adult-gerontology. This population focus encompasses the young adult to the older adult, including the frail older adult. Certification is available as an Adult-Gerontology Acute Care Nurse Practitioner (NP); Adult-Gerontology Primary Care NP; and Adult-Gerontology Clinical Nurse Specialist (CNS). Nurses educated at the master's level for NP roles in gerontological nursing and nationally certified prior to this change retain titles of gerontological nurse practitioners (GNPs) or gerontological clinical nurse specialists (GCNSs).

Advanced practice nurses with certification in adult-gerontology will find a full range of opportunities for collaborative and independent practice both now and in the future. Direct care sites include geriatric and family practice clinics, long-term care, acute and subacute care facilities, home health care agencies, hospice agencies, continuing care retirement communities, assisted living facilities, managed care organizations, and specialty care clinics (e.g., Alzheimer disease, heart failure, diabetes). Specialty gerontological nurses are also involved with community agencies such as local Area Agencies on Aging, public health departments, and national and worldwide organizations such as the Centers for Disease Control and Prevention and the World Health Organization. They function as care managers, eldercare consultants, educators, and clinicians.

One of the most important advanced practice nursing roles that emerged over the past 40 years is that of the GNP and the GCNS in skilled nursing facilities. The education and training programs arose from evident need, particularly in the long-term care (LTC) setting (Ploeg et al, 2013). Nurse practitioners have been providing care in nursing homes in the United States since the 1970s, in Canada since 2000, and only recently in the United Kingdom. Numbers remain small and there is a need for continued attention at the policy and funding levels for increased use of nurse practitioners in LTC. Family nurse practitioner programs must ensure that students receive adequate content and practice experiences in LTC since many enter this setting for practice. Recommendations from expert groups in the United States and Canada have called for a nurse practitioner in every nursing home (Harrington et al, 2000; Ploeg et al, 2013). This role is well established and there is strong research to support the impact of advanced practice nurses working in LTC settings (Bakerjian, 2008; Dwyer et al, 2017; Melillo et al, 2015; Oliver et al, 2014; Ploeg et al, 2013).

🔱 RESEARCH HIGHLIGHTS A

Outcomes of Advanced Practice Nurses Working in Long-Term Care Settings

Improvement in or reduced rate of decline in incontinence, pressure ulcers, aggressive behavior, and loss of affect in cognitively impaired residents
Lower use of restraints with no increase in staffing
Reduced psychoactive drug use and serious fall-related injuries
Improved or slower decline in some health status indicators including depression
Improvements in meeting personal goals
Lower hospitalization rates and costs
Fewer emergency department visits and lower costs
Improved satisfaction with care

Data from Ploeg J, Kaaslainen S, McAiney C, et al: Resident and family perceptions of the nurse practitioner role in long term care settings, *BMC Nurs* 12(24), 2013.

The Evercare Care Model, a federally funded Medicare demonstration project, originally designed by two nurse practitioners, is a very successful innovative model with a long history of positive outcomes. This model utilizes APRNs, either certified in gerontology or specially trained by Evercare, for care of long-term nursing home residents and individuals with severe or disabling conditions (www.innovativecaremodels.com). Research Highlights B presents findings from a study examining resident and family perceptions of the nurse practitioner role in long-term care settings.

🔱 RESEARCH HIGHLIGHTS B

In-depth and focus group interviews were conducted with residents and family members in four Canadian nursing homes to explore their perceptions of the nurse practitioner (NP) role. The major themes that emerged were as follows:
NPs were seen as providing resident and family-centered care and providing enhanced quality of care. Residents and families perceived the NP as improving availability and timeliness of care and helping to prevent unnecessary hospitalization. Participants spoke eloquently about the NP role as a "catalyst," "light switch," and "bridge" in shaping the culture and working relationships in long-term care (LTC). "She [NP] helps me and my sister a lot just by listening and providing suggestions . . . not just communicating but she is also listening. It's almost like having a midwife or doula or something like that, from an emotional point of view" (p. 7).
Residents and families valued the caring relationship with the NP and this was a central means through which enhanced quality of care occurs. Increased use of NPs in LTC settings can enhance outcomes and satisfaction. Including the concepts of caring relationships and person-centered care in NP education is important.

Data from Ploeg J, Kaaslainen S, McAiney C, et al: Resident and family perceptions of the nurse practitioner role in long term care settings, *BMC Nurs* 12(24), 2013.

Generalist Roles
Acute Care
Older adults often enter the health care system with admissions to acute care settings. Older adults comprise 60% of the medical-surgical patients and 46% of the critical care patients. Acutely ill older adults frequently have multiple chronic conditions and comorbidities and present many challenges. Even though most nurses working in acute care are caring for older adults, many have not had gerontological nursing content in their basic nursing education programs and few are certified in the specialty. "Only a small number of the country's 6000 hospitals have institutional practice guidelines, educational resources, and administrative practices that support best practice care of older adults" (Boltz et al, 2008, p. 176).

Kagan (2008) reminds us that "older adults are the work of hospitals but most nurses practicing in hospitals do not say they specialize in geriatrics . . . We, as a profession and a force in an aging society, must make the transformation to understanding care of older adults **is** acute care nursing . . . Care of older adults would be the rule instead of the exception" (2008, p. 103). Kagan goes on to suggest that such a transformation would mean that acute care nurses would proudly describe themselves as geriatric nurses with subspecialties (geriatric vascular nurses, geriatric emergency nurses) and, along with geriatric nurse generalists, would populate hospital nursing services across the country.

Nurses caring for older adults in hospitals may function in the direct care provider role; as care managers, discharge planners, care coordinators, or transitional care nurses; or in leadership and management positions. Many acute care hospitals are adopting new models of geriatric and chronic care to meet the needs of older adults. These include geriatric emergency rooms and specialized units such as acute care for the elderly (ACE), geriatric evaluation and management units (GEM), and transitional care programs. This will increase the need for well-prepared geriatric professionals working in interprofessional teams to deliver needed services. Box 2.3 presents guiding principles for the elder-friendly hospital.

NICHE. The Nurses Improving Care for Health System Elders (NICHE), a program developed by Dr. Terry Fulmer of the Hartford Geriatric Nursing Institute in 1992, was designed to improve outcomes for hospitalized older adults and offers many opportunities for new roles for acute care nurses such as the geriatric resource nurse (GRN). The GRN role emphasizes the pivotal role of the bedside nurse in influencing outcomes of care and coordination of interprofessional activities. "All geriatric models of care include a high level of nursing input but only NICHE stresses nurse involvement in hospital decision-making regarding care of older adults. This professional nursing practice perspective supports nurse competencies related to the complex interdisciplinary care management of older adults and the resources they need to improve the safety and outcomes of hospitalized older adults" (Capezuti et al, 2012, p. 3117).

NICHE especially targets the prevention of iatrogenic complications, which occur in as many as 29% to 38% of hospitalized older adults, a rate three to five times higher than that seen in younger patients (Inouye et al, 2000). Common iatrogenic complications include functional decline, pneumonia, delirium, new-onset incontinence, malnutrition, pressure ulcers, medication reactions, and falls. Recognizing the impact of iatrogenesis, both on patient outcomes and on the cost of care, the Centers for Medicare and Medicaid Services (CMS) has instituted changes that will reduce payment to hospitals relative to

BOX 2.3 Guiding Principles for the Elder-Friendly Hospital/Facility

For the Patient
- Each patient is a unique individual and should be evaluated as such.
- Measures are taken to accommodate the patient's and family's special needs.

For the Staff
- Nurses demonstrate clinical competence in geriatric nursing.
- Nurses provide therapeutic response, patience, and presence when caring for geriatric patients.
- Nurses and staff who provide direct care identify and address the patient's individual needs and preferences; staff creates a positive experience for the patient and family.
- Nurses coordinate care across the continuum and "manage the journey" of the patient and family.
- Excellent communication, tailored to meet the needs of the geriatric patient, results in a "climate of confidence" for the patient and the nurse.
- The organization provides appropriate resources and systems that support best practice in geriatric nursing care.

For the Environment
- The physical environment supports the needs of the geriatric patient and family and the staff who care for them.
- An elder-friendly environment, as defined by the patient and family, also enhances the practice environment for the staff.
- The elder-friendly environment is embraced hospital wide.

From American Association of Nurse Executives: *The guiding principles for creating elder-friendly hospitals.* Copyright 2010 by the American Organization Nurse Executives (AONE). All Rights Reserved.

these often preventable outcomes. The changes target conditions that are high cost or high volume, result in a higher payment when present as a secondary diagnosis, are not present on admission, and could have reasonably been prevented through the use of evidence-based guidelines. Targeted conditions include catheter-associated urinary tract infection, pressure ulcers, and falls (Chapters 13, 16, and 19). Expertise in gerontological nursing is essential in prevention of these conditions.

NICHE has been the most successful acute care geriatric model in recruiting hospital membership and contributing to the depth of geriatric hospital programming. NICHE programs have been implemented in 566 hospitals in more than 40 states, as well as parts of Canada, and are involved in NICHE projects (www.nicheprogram.org). NICHE also provides an online Leadership Training Program (LTP) to increase flexibility and affordability of starting a NICHE program in a health care facility.

Community-Based and Home-Based Care

Nurses will care for older adults in hospitals and long-term care facilities, but the majority of older adults live in the community. Community-based care occurs through home and hospice care, provided in persons' homes, independent senior housing complexes, retirement communities, residential care facilities such as assisted living facilities, and adult day health centers. It also takes place in primary care clinics and public health departments. Care will continue to move out of hospitals and long-term care institutions into the community because of rapidly

escalating health care costs and the person's preference to "age in place." Gerontological nurses will find opportunities to create practices in community-based settings with a focus not only on care for those who are ill but also health promotion and community wellness.

Nurses in the home setting provide comprehensive assessments including physical, functional, psychosocial, family, home, environmental, and community. Care management and working with interprofessional teams are integral components of the home health nursing role. Nurses may provide and supervise care for older individuals with a variety of care needs (including chronic wounds, intravenous therapy, tube feedings, unstable medical conditions, and complex medication regimens), and for those receiving rehabilitation and palliative and hospice services. Schools of nursing must increase education and practice experiences for nursing students in home-based and community-based care. Nurse practitioners are now Medicare-accepted providers of the annual wellness visits for beneficiaries. Advances in technology for remote monitoring of health status and safety and the development of point-of-care testing devices show promise in improving outcomes for older individuals who want to age in place (Chapter 20). These technologies present exciting opportunities for nurses in the management and evaluation of care.

Case and care management roles. Nurses are especially well suited for roles as case managers and care managers. There are increasing opportunities for these roles both in care of individuals with chronic illnesses and in transitional care (discussed later in the chapter). Although the terms case manager and care manager have slightly different connotations, in practice the roles are seldom that clear and there is much overlap. Both of these roles include that of advocate, broker, leader, manager, counselor, negotiator, administrator, and communicator. Ideally the care manager follows the person through the entire continuum of care. Care managers must be experts regarding community resources and understand how these can best be used to meet the person's needs. They are expected to make appropriate referrals within the person's expectations and abilities and to monitor the quality of arranged services. The care or case manager is a resource person whom the older adult or caregiver can seek for advice and counsel and for brokering (negotiating, arranging) the flow of services. As a gatekeeper, the care or case manager controls the entrances and exits to services to make sure that the individual gets what is needed without wasting resources.

Care managers are usually paid privately. Those who cannot afford the out-of-pocket expenses of purchased care management services must rely on services available through Medicaid-managed care plans or nonprofit community agencies, such as Catholic Senior Services, if available. Access to publicly funded programs varies by state and areas within the state and is dependent on state, county, and agency budget and priorities. Hospitals, skilled nursing facilities, and insurance agencies also utilize care/case managers. Care that is well managed is believed to be a solution to both the spiraling costs and the fragmentation of care often experienced by older individuals with multiple needs. The care manager works to optimize the resources

BOX 2.4 Resources for Best Practice: Care Management

American Association of Managed Care Nurses: Certification, educational resources

Case Management Society of America: Standards of Practice, certification, educational resources

RNCaseManager.com: Resources, education, job assistance for job seekers and employers

BOX 2.5 Caring Nurse and Resident Relationships in Long-Term Care

"The residents become our friends and surrogate family. . . . Nowhere else in healthcare are relationships formed the way they are in LTC. I would say that we have more value for our residents as people and patients than they are given elsewhere in healthcare."

From Sherman R, Touhy T: Unpublished data from a study of nurse leader challenges and opportunities in nursing home settings 2017.

and outcome for the client and the agency or community in which the person resides. There are Standards of Practice and certifications available for care/case manager roles (Box 2.4).

Certified Nursing Facilities (Nursing Homes)

Certified nursing facilities, commonly called nursing homes, have evolved into significant locations where health care is provided across the continuum, part of a range of long-term post-acute care (LTPAC) services. Over a quarter of Medicare patients admitted to the hospital are discharged to postacute care (PAC) facilities, many with acute health conditions (Horney et al, 2017). The old images of nursing homes caring for older adults in a custodial manner is no longer valid. Today, most facilities have subacute care units that more closely resemble the general medical-surgical hospital units of the past. Most people enter nursing facilities for short stays that last no more than 1 week to 3 months (Toles et al, 2013). "Nursing homes are no longer just a destination but rather a stage in the recovery process" (Thaler, 2014). Postacute care in nursing facilities will continue to grow with health care reform, and there are many new roles and opportunities for professional nursing in the setting.

Roles for professional nursing include nursing administrator, manager, supervisor, charge nurse, educator, infection control nurse, Minimum Data Set (MDS) coordinator, case manager, transitional care nurse, quality improvement coordinator, and direct care provider. Professional nurses in nursing facilities must be highly skilled in the complex care concerns of older adults, ranging from subacute care to end-of-life care. Excellent assessment skills; ability to work with interprofessional teams in partnership with residents and families; skills in acute, rehabilitative, and palliative care; and leadership, management, supervision, and delegation skills are essential.

Practice in this setting calls for independent decision-making and is guided by a nursing model of care because there are fewer physicians and other professionals on site at all times. In addition, stringent federal regulations governing care practices and greater use of licensed practical nurses and nursing assistants influence the role of professional nursing in this setting. The opportunity to form long-term relationships with individuals and families is valued by nurses and cited as one of the most rewarding aspects of practice in LTC facilities (Box 2.5). Many new graduates will be entering this setting upon graduation so it is essential to provide education and practice experiences to prepare them to function competently in this setting, particularly leadership and management skills. Research Highlights C presents findings of a study of RN perceptions of their professional work in nursing homes and

RESEARCH HIGHLIGHTS C

Registered Nurses' Perceptions of Their Professional Work in Nursing Homes and Home-Based Care: A Focus Group Study

The qualitative focus group study examined how nurses in nursing homes and home-based care perceived their professional role. Thirty nurses working with older individuals in rural areas and in a larger city in southern Sweden participated in the focus groups. Data from the focus groups were analyzed in line with the tradition of naturalistic inquiry. Findings included the following:
- Nursing practice in these settings is a complex advanced professional role.
- Nurses are attracted to this specialty because of the autonomous and person-centered nature of the nursing.
- The nurses were highly committed to their jobs.
- The decision to practice in the specialty was a conscious career choice and they described a great deal of professional pride.
- Long-lasting relationships with patients and families added to job satisfaction
- Nursing in long-term care (LTC) was seen as multifaceted and holistic in nature, addressing the physical, emotional, mental and spiritual well-being of the individual. The nurses considered their work to be more complex than in an acute-care setting.

Implications include the importance of providing clinical practice opportunities in LTC in nursing education programs. The authors state that "these placements can provide a learning environment where the essence of caring and nursing can be explicit in helping student nurses shape and develop professional identity" (p. 766). Additional implications include exposure to positive role models in gerontological nursing and discussion of the skills and attitudes required for practice in LTC. LTC is an essential component of the health care system and students need to be prepared to care for individuals in this setting with competence.

Data from Carlson E, Ramgard M, Bolmsjo I, et al: Registered nurses' perceptions of their professional work in nursing homes and home-based care: a focus group study, *Int J Nurs Studies*. 51:761–767, 2014.

home-based care. Chapter 32 provides comprehensive information about long-term care.

TRANSITIONS ACROSS THE CONTINUUM: ROLE OF NURSING

Care transition refers to the movement of patients from one health care practitioner or setting to another as their condition and care needs change. Older adults may have complex health care needs and often require care in multiple settings across the health-wellness continuum. This makes them and their family and/or caregivers vulnerable to poor outcomes during transitions (Naylor, 2012). An older adult may be treated by a family practitioner or internist in the community and by a hospitalist and specialists in the hospital; discharged to a nursing home and followed by another practitioner; and then discharged home or to a less care-intensive setting (e.g., assisted living facilities/residential care settings) where their original providers may or may not resume care. The lack of coordinated care often contributes to serious consequences and frequent readmissions. Approximately one in four patients experiences an adverse event from medical mismanagement within 3 weeks of discharge from the hospital; 66% of those events are drug-related (Jusela et al, 2017). Most health care providers practice in only one setting and are not familiar with the specific requirements of other settings. Each setting is seen as a distinct provider of services and little collaboration exists (Jones et al, 2017). This is changing with health care reform initiatives such as accountable care organizations, health homes, value-based purchasing, and bundled care payments (Chapters 30 and 32).

Readmissions: The Revolving Door

Avoidable readmissions are one of the leading problems facing the U.S. health care system. Hospital readmission is a critical event for both the patients and the health care system with extraordinary associated costs. One in four Medicare patients is readmitted to the hospital within 30 days of discharge. Ninety percent of these readmissions for Medicare patients are unplanned, resulting in annual costs of more than $17 billion, paying for return trips that need not happen if patients had received the right care. Readmissions have been a critical quality indicator for more than 2 decades because they cost the health care system money and because they indicate incomplete discharge planning (Carnahan et al, 2016; Horney et al, 2017; Jones et al, 2017; Robert Wood Johnson Foundation, 2013).

Medicare patients admitted to a PAC facility following hospital discharge have an increased risk of readmission, with more than a quarter readmitted to the hospital in the first week and one-fifth readmitted within 30 days. Up to two-thirds of these hospital transfers are rated as potentially avoidable by expert long-term care health professionals (http://interact2.net/). However, the rate of potentially avoidable hospitalizations among SNF residents has fallen by nearly a third in recent years as a result of many quality improvement initiatives (Chapter 32) (Brennan, 2017; Morgan, 2017).

The federal government has several initiatives designed to address avoidable readmission and care transitions. The Hospital Readmission Reduction Program (HRRP) was established as a provision in the Affordable Care Act (ACA) requiring Medicare to reduce payments to hospitals with relatively high readmission rates for selected conditions for patients in traditional Medicare (Box 2.6). The HRRP was established in 2013 as a permanent component of Medicare's inpatient hospital payment system. Under the HRRP, hospitals with readmission rates that exceed the national average are penalized by a reduction in payments from the CMS across all of their Medicare admissions, not just those which resulted in readmissions.

Since the HRRP, readmission rates for the selected conditions have dropped nationwide but estimates are that in 2018, about 80% of hospitals evaluated by CMS will face penalties totaling $564 million (Advisory Board, 2017). Additionally, the

---

BOX 2.6 Conditions Included in the Hospital Readmission Reduction Program

- Acute myocardial infarction
- Heart failure
- Pneumonia
- Total hip and knee replacement
- Chronic obstructive pulmonary disease
- Coronary artery bypass surgery

HRRP has been the impetus for many hospitals to institute system-wide interventions to prevent readmissions that have also contributed to the decline in readmission rates. Hospital readmission rates are posted on the CMS Hospital Compare website (Boccuti and Casillas, 2017; Zuckerman et al, 2016).

Skilled nursing facilities will also face penalties for high readmission rates. The Protecting Access to Medicare Act (PAMA) is legislation intended to address several concerns with SNF care and ensure that SNFs will share the responsibility with hospitals for 30-day readmissions. SNFs will receive value-based incentive payments beginning October 2019 based on their ranking with regard to readmission rates. Readmission concerns have encouraged the development of closer alliances (e.g., accountable care organizations) and communication between hospitals and posthospital care providers, including SNFs, home health, and primary care.

Multiple factors contribute to poor outcomes during transitions: patient, provider, and system. Many are the result of a fragmented system of care that too often leaves discharged patients to their own devices, unable to follow instructions they did not understand, and not taking medications or getting the necessary follow-up care (Box 2.7 and 2.8). Other factors identified in the literature are presented in Box 2.9.

BOX 2.7 Patient Story

John is a 68-year-old retired farm laborer who was readmitted for heart failure 10 days after hospital discharge. He lives alone in a rural community and has no friends or family to assist in his care and was not given a referral for home health care follow-up. His medical records document teaching about medication usage and his ability to repeat back the instructions correctly. He brought all of his pill bottles in a bag; all of the bottles were full, not one was opened. When questioned why he had not taken his medication, he looked away and began to cry, explaining he had never learned to read and could not read the instructions on the bottles.

Adapted from The Joint Commission: *Hot topics in health care: transitions of care: the need for a more effective approach in continuing patient care,* 2012. http://www.jointcommission.org/assets/1/18/Hot_Topics_Transitions_of_Care.pdf. Accessed February 10, 2014.

BOX 2.8 Tips for Best Practice

Some hospitals began giving low-income patients free medications prescribed for their recovery. Combined with nurse follow-up in the home, these practices resulted in a drop in readmission rates.

From Miller A: Once again, Medicare penalizing most hospitals for patient readmission rates. http://www.georgiahealthnews.com/2017/08/again-medicare-penalizing-hospitals-patient-readmission-rate/. Accessed October 17, 2017.

BOX 2.9   Factors Associated With Readmission Risk

- The presence of complex comorbidities
- Sensory impairment
- Functional decline
- Cognitive dysfunction
- Poor communication between disciplines and across sites of care
- Inadequate discharge planning and involvement of caregivers
- Shorter hospital stays
- Increasing acuity of patients in skilled nursing facilities (SNFs)
- Scarcity of geriatric trained health care professionals

- Inadequate knowledge and use of evidence-based protocols for geriatric care
- Certain disease states such as cancer and respiratory diseases
- Social concerns (isolation, living situation, lack of caregiver support)
- Language and literacy
- Culture
- Socioeconomic factors
- Place of residence and the health care available
- Inadequate funding for postacute care (PAC) and staff shortages.

⚡ SAFETY ALERT

Medication discrepancies are the most prevalent adverse events following hospital discharge and the most challenging component of a successful hospital-to-home transition (Hain et al, 2012; Tong et al, 2017). Nurses' attention to an accurate prehospital medication list; medication reconciliation during hospitalization, at discharge and after discharge; and patient and family education about medications are required to enhance safety.

Improving Transitional Care

Transitional care "refers to a broad range of time-limited services to ensure health care continuity, avoid preventable poor outcomes among at-risk populations, and promote the safe and timely transfer of these patient groups from one level of care (e.g., acute to subacute) or setting (e.g., hospital to home) to another" (Naylor, 2012, p. 116). National attention to improving patient safety during transfers and preventing avoidable readmissions is increasing, and a growing body of evidence-based research provides data for design of care to improve transition outcomes.

Nurse researchers Dorothy Brooten and Mary Naylor, along with their colleagues, have significantly contributed to knowledge in the area of transitional care and the critical role of nurses in transitional care improvement. The Transitional Care

Model (TCM) is a nurse-led intervention targeting older adults at risk for poor outcomes as they move across health care settings and between clinicians. Over the past 20 years, TCM has been one of the most rigorously studied transitional care approaches and has demonstrated reductions in preventable hospital readmissions, improvements in health outcomes, enhancement in patient satisfaction, and reductions in total health care costs (Garcia, 2017; Hirschman et al, 2015). Key components of the model are presented in Box 2.10.

Nurses in acute and long-term care are uniquely positioned to play a lead role in transitional care to improve outcomes and form a "bridge across settings" (Jones et al, 2017, p. 18). This will require closer collaboration and knowledge of the settings and valuing of the different nursing practice roles. In addition to roles as care managers and transition coaches, nurses play a key role in many of the elements of successful transitional care models, such as medication management, patient and family caregiver education, comprehensive discharge planning, and adequate and timely communication between providers and sites of service.

BOX 2.10   Components of the Transitional Care Model

- **Screening:** Identify older adults at high risk for poor outcomes
- **Staffing:** Uses advanced practice registered nurses who are responsible for care management throughout the acute care stay
- **Maintaining relationships:** Establishes a trusting relationship with patient and caregivers
- **Engaging patients and caregivers:** Engages older adults/caregivers in the design and implementation of the plan of care consistent with their value, preferences, goals
- **Assessing/managing risks and symptoms:** Identifies and addresses priority risk factors and symptoms using core geriatric principles
- **Educating/promoting self-management:** Prepares patient and family to identify and respond quickly to worsening symptoms
- **Collaborating:** Promotes consensus on plan of care between patient and members of the care team; utilizes an interprofessional team approach
- **Promoting continuity:** Prevents gaps in care by having the same clinician involved in care from hospital to home/skilled nursing facility (SNF)
- **Fostering confidence:** Promotes communication and connections between health care and community-based practitioners

From Hirschman K, Shaid E, McCauley K, Pauly M, Naylor M. Continuity of care: the Transitional Care Model. *Online J Issues Nurs* 20(3):1, 2015.

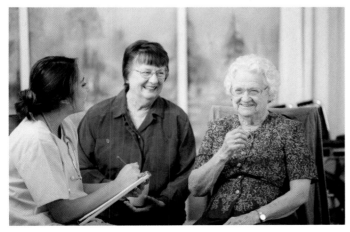

Working with the patient and the caregiver to provide education to enhance self-care abilities and to facilitate linkages to resources is important to promote safe discharges and transitions to home and other care settings. (©iStock.com/Pamela Moore.)

The nursing role in discharge planning and patient and family education is critical. Engaging patients and families in learning about care required after discharge contributes to improved outcomes. Teaching must be based on a complete assessment of the unique needs of the individual and adapted to ensure understanding (Chapter 5). Patients who lack the knowledge, skills, and confidence to manage their own care after discharge have nearly twice the rate of readmissions as patients with the highest level of engagement (Kangovi et al, 2014; Schneidermann and Critchfield, 2012–2013). Nursing education must prepare graduates to effectively work across the care continuum and be well prepared in gerontological nursing competencies.

Box 2.11 presents Resources for Best Practice and Box 2.12 gives Tips for Best Practice for transitional care nursing.

BOX 2.11   Resources for Best Practice: Transitional Care

- **Hospital Admission Risk Profile (HARP):** Hartford Institute for Geriatric Nursing (Try This, General Assessment Series). https://consultgeri.org/try-this/general-assessment/issue-24
- **Transitional Care Model:** http://evidencebasedprograms.org/1366-2/transitional-care-model-top-tier; https://www.nursing.upenn.edu/ncth/transitional-care-model/
- **The Joint Commission:** Speak Up: Planning Your Follow-Up Care
- **NICHE:** Need to Know for Patients and Families Series: Discharge, Dementia Transitions, Managing Medications
- **Agency for Healthcare Research and Quality:** Taking Care of Myself: A Guide for When I Leave the Hospital. https://www.ahrq.gov/patients-consumers/diagnosis-treatment/hospitals-clinics/goinghome/index.html

---

BOX 2.12   Tips for Best Practice: Transitional Care

- Identify patients at high risk for poor outcomes (e.g., low literacy, living alone, frequent hospitalizations, complex chronic illness, cognitive impairment, socioeconomic deprivation).
- Coach patient in self-care skills and encourage active involvement in care.
- Educate and support family caregivers and informal and formal caregivers.
- Adapt patient teaching for health literacy, language, culture, cognitive function, and sensory deficits.
- Prepare patient and family for what to expect at next site of care.
- Provide a complete and updated medication record; explain purpose of all medications, side effects, correct dosing, and how to obtain more medication.
- Perform a medication reconciliation.
- Assist in establishing regimen for proper administration of medication.
- Discuss symptoms that should be reported after discharge and how to contact provider; provide follow-up plan for how outstanding tests and follow-up appointments will be completed.
- Be aware of community resources in your area to assist with needs following discharge and how to link patient to resources.

Further research is needed to evaluate which transitional care models are most effective in various settings and for which group of patients, particularly those who are most frail or cognitively impaired and for medically underserved populations. Chapter 32 discusses transitional care in the nursing home setting.

PROMOTING HEALTHY AGING: IMPLICATIONS FOR GERONTOLOGICAL NURSING

The rapid growth of the older population brings forth opportunities and challenges for the world now and in the future. With the promise of a healthier old age, health care professionals, particularly nurses, will play a significant role in creating systems of care and services that enhance the possibility of healthy aging for an increasingly diverse population. Nurses have the skills needed to create a more person-centered, coordinated health care system and improve outcomes in health and illness. Continued attention must be paid to the recruitment and education of health professionals and direct care staff prepared to care for older adults to meet critical shortages that threaten health and safety.

Exciting roles for nurses with preparation in gerontological nursing are increasing in settings across the continuum of care, with increasing emphasis on community-based and long-term care settings. Nursing education is called upon to prepare graduates for practice in these settings. Of particular importance is improving outcomes during transitions of care for older adults. Dare we say that gerontological nursing will be the most needed specialty in nursing as the number of older adults continues to increase and the need for our specialized knowledge becomes even more critical in every specialty and every health care setting?

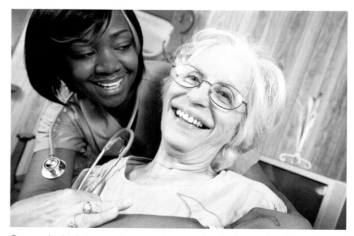

Gerontological nurses have a significant role in the healthy aging of older adults. (©iStock.com/Pamela Moore.)

KEY CONCEPTS

- The eldercare workforce is dangerously understaffed and unprepared to care for the growing numbers of older adults.
- Nursing has led the field in gerontology, and nurses were the first professionals in the nation to be certified as geriatric specialists.
- Certification assures the public of nurses' commitment to specialized education and qualification for the care of older adults.
- Research in gerontological nursing has provided the foundation for improved care of older adults.

- Health care reform initiatives and a growing older adult population offer many exciting opportunities for nurses with competence in care of older adults.
- Advanced practice role opportunities for nurses are numerous and are seen as potentially cost-effective in health care delivery while facilitating more holistic health care.
- Professional nursing involvement is an essential component in models to improve transitions of care across the continuum.

CRITICAL THINKING QUESTIONS AND ACTIVITIES

1. What content and clinical experiences on care of older adults is included in your nursing program?
2. Reflect on the Recommended Baccalaureate Competencies for Care of Older Adults (Appendix 2.A). Which have you had the opportunity to meet in your nursing program?
3. Review one of the gerontological nursing journals (*Geriatric Nursing, Journal of Gerontological Nursing, Research in Gerontological Nursing*) and choose a research study of interest to you. How could you use the findings of the study in your clinical practice with older adults?
4. You are asked to write a small proposal for a research project related to care of older adults. What would be the focus of your research and why?
5. What programs to improve transitional care are being implemented in the acute care setting where you are studying?
6. What settings for care of older adults are of interest to you as you consider a nursing practice area after graduation?

RESEARCH QUESTIONS

1. What aspects of gerontological nursing roles do practicing nurses find most rewarding and which do they find most challenging?
2. Why do so few students choose gerontological nursing as an area of practice? What factors might encourage more interest in the specialty?
3. What is the actual amount of time in the curriculum of baccalaureate nursing schools spent on content and practice experiences related to the care of older adults?
4. What is the phenomenon of interest in nursing research? How does it differ from other disciplines?
5. What roles in gerontological nursing and which settings of practice are of most interest to new graduates?

REFERENCES

Advisory Board: *2,573 hospitals will face readmission penalties this year. Is yours one of them?* 2017. https://www.advisory.com/daily-briefing/2017/08/07/hospital-penalties. Accessed October 17, 2017.

American Association of Colleges of Nursing: *White paper on the education and role of the clinical nurse leader,* 2007. https://www.aacnnursing.org/News-Information/Position-Statements-White-Papers/CNL. Accessed November 2018.

American Association of Colleges of Nursing: *The essentials of baccalaureate education for professional nursing practice,* 2008. https://www.aacnnursing.org/Faculty/Teaching-Resources/Curriculum-Guidelines. Accessed November 2018.

American Association of Colleges of Nursing: *Adult-gerontology primary care nurse practitioner competencies,* 2010. https://www.aacnnursing.org/Faculty/Teaching-Resources/Curriculum-Guidelines. Accessed November 2018.

American Association of Colleges of Nursing: *Recommended baccalaureate competencies and curricular guidelines for the nursing care of older adults, a supplement to The Essentials of Baccalaureate Education for Professional Nursing Practice,* 2010. https://www.aacnnursing.org/Faculty/Teaching-Resources/Curriculum-Guidelines. Accessed November 2018.

American Nurses Association: *Gerontological nursing: scope and standards of practice,* ed 3. Silver Spring, MD, 2010, American Nurses Association.

APRN Consensus Work Group & National Council of State Boards of Nursing APRN Advisory Committee: *Consensus model for APRN regulation: licensure, accreditation, certification & education,* 2008. https://www.ncsbn.org/aprn-consensus.htm. Accessed November 2018.

Bakerjian D: Care of nursing home residents by advanced practice nurses. A review of the literature, *Res Gerontol Nurs* 1:177–185, 2008.

Boccuti C, Casillas G: Aiming for fewer hospital U-turns: The Medicare hospital readmission reduction program, *Issue Brief,* 2017. https://www.kff.org/medicare/issue-brief/aiming-for-fewer-hospital-u-turns-the-medicare-hospital-readmission-reduction-program/. Accessed October 12, 2017.

Boltz M, Capezuti E, Bower-Ferris S, et al: Changes in the geriatric care environment associated with NICHE, *Geriatr Nurs* 29(3): 176–185, 2008.

Brennan N: Data brief: sharp reduction in avoidable hospitalizations among long-term care facility residents, *The CMS Blog,* 2017. https://blog.cms.gov/2017/01/17/data-brief-sharp-reduction-in-avoidable-hospitalizations-among-long-term-care-facility-residents/. Accessed October 19, 2017.

Campaign for Action: *Not enough nurses prepared to care for those older than 65,* 2016. https://campaignforaction.org/not-enough-nurses-prepared-to-care-for-americas-65/. Accessed February 2019.

Capezuti E, Boltz M, Cline D, et al: Nurses improving care for health system elders—a model for optimizing the geriatric nurse practice environment, *J Clin Nurs* 21(21–22):3117–3125, 2012.

Carnahan JL, Unroe KT, Torke AM: Hospital readmission penalties: coming soon to a nursing home near you, *J Am Geriatr Soc* 64:614–618, 2016.

Crane C: Almshouse nursing: the human need, *Am J Nurs* 7:872, 1907.

Davis B: Nursing care of the aged: historical evolution, *Bull Am Assoc Hist Nurs* 47, 1985.

Dock L: The crusade for almshouse nursing, *Am J Nurs* 8:520, 1908.

Dwyer T, Craswell A, Rossi D, Holzberger D: Evaluation of an aged care nurse practitioner service: quality of care within a residential aged care facility hospital avoidance service, *BMC Health Serv Res,* 2017. doi:10.1186/s12913-017-1977-x.

Ebersole P, Touhy T: *Geriatric nursing: Growth of a specialty,* New York, 2006, Springer.

Garbrah W, Välimäki T, Palovaara M, Kankkunen P: Nursing curriculums may hinder a career in gerontological nursing: an integrative review, *Int J Older People Nurs* 12:e12152, 2017.

Garcia C: A literature review of heart failure: Transitional care interventions, *Am J Accountable Care,* 2017. http://www.ajmc.com/journals/ajac/2017/2017-vol5-n3/a-literature-review-of-heart-failure-transitional-care-interventions. Accessed October 20, 2017.

Gelbach S: Nursing care of the aged, *Am J Nurs* 43;1112–1114, 1943.

Golden R, Shier G: What does "care transitions" really mean? *Generations* 36(4):6–12, 2012–2013.

Hain DJ, Tappen R, Diaz S, Ouslander JG: Characteristics of older adults rehospitalized within 7 and 30 days of discharge: implications for nursing practice, *J Gerontol Nurs* 38(8):32–44, 2012.

Harrington C, Kovner C, Mezey M, et al: Experts recommend minimum nurse staffing standards for nursing facilities in the United States, *Gerontologist* 40(1):5–16, 2000.

Hirschman KB, Shaid E, McCauley K, Pauly MV, Naylor MD: Continuity of care: The transitional care model, *Online J Issues Nurs* 20(3):1, 2015.

Holroyd A, Dahlke S, Fehr C, Jung P, Hunter A: Attitudes toward aging: implications for a caring profession, *J Nurs Educ* 48(7): 374–380, 2009.

Horney C, Capp R, Boxer R, Burke RE: Factors associated with early readmission among patients discharged to post-acute care facilities, *J Am Geriatr Soc* 65(6):1199–1205, 2017.

Inouye SK, Bogardus ST, Baker DI, Leo-Summers L, Cooney LM Jr: The Hospital Elder Life Program: a model of care to prevent cognitive and functional decline in older hospitalized patients. Hospital Elder Life Program, *J Am Geriatr Soc* 48(12):1697–1706, 2000.

Institute of Medicine, National Academies: *Retooling for an aging America: building the health care workforce,* 2008. http://www.nationalacademies.org/hmd/reports/2008/retooling-for-an-aging-america-building-the-health-care-workforce.aspx/. Accessed March 2018.

Jones J, Lawrence E, Ladebue A, Leonard C, Ayele R, Burke RE: Nurses' role in managing "the fit" of older adults in skilled nursing facilities, *J Gerontol Nurs* 43(12):11–19, 2017.

Jusela C, Struble L, Gallagher N, Redman RW, Ziemba RA: Communication between acute care hospitals and skilled nursing facilities during care transitions: A retrospective chart review, *J Gerontol Nurs* 43(3):19–28, 2017.

Kagan SH: Moving from achievement to transformation, *Geriatr Nurs* 29:102–104, 2008.

Kangovi S, Barg FK, Carter T, et al: Challenges faced by patients with low socioeconomic status during the post-hospital transition, *J Gen Intern Med* 29(2):283–289, 2014.

Kydd A, Engstrom G, Touhy T, et al: Attitudes of nurses, and student nurses towards working with older people and to gerontological nursing as a career in Germany, Scotland, Slovenia, Sweden, Japan and the United States, *Int J Nurs Educ* 6(2):33–40, 2014.

Mack M: The Personal adjustment of chronically ill old people under home care, *Nurs Res* 1:9–30, 1952.

Melillo KD, Remington R, Abdallah L, et al: Comparison of nurse practitioner and physician practice models in nursing facilities, *Ann Longterm Care.* 23(12):19–24, 2015.

Morgan E: CMS reports sharp drop in avoidable hospitalizations among long-term care residents, *McKnights Long-term Care News,* 2017. http://www.mcknights.com/news/cms-reports-sharp-drop-in-avoidable-hospitalizations-among-long-term-care-residents/article/632414/. Accessed October 19, 2017.

Morley J: The future of long-term care, *J Am Med Dir Assoc* 18:1–7, 2017.

National Institute of Nursing Research: *The NINR strategic plan: advancing science: improving lives,* 2016. NIH publication #16-NR-7783. https://www.ninr.nih.gov/sites/www.ninr.nih.gov/files/NINR_StratPlan2016_reduced.pdf. Accessed October 2018.

Naylor M: Advancing high value transitional care: the central role of nursing and its leadership, *Nurs Adm Q* 36(2):115–126, 2012.

Oliver G, Pennington L, Revelle S, Rantz M: Impact of nurse practitioners on health outcomes of Medicare and Medicaid patients, *Nurs Outlook* 62(6):440–447, 2014.

Ploeg J, Kaasalainen S, McAiney C, et al: Resident and family perceptions of the nurse practitioner role in long term care settings: a qualitative descriptive study, *BMC Nurs* 12(1):24, 2013. http://www.biomedcentral.com/content/pdf/1472-6955-12-24.pdf. Accessed September 16, 2014.

Robert Wood Johnson Foundation: *United States in search of nurses with geriatrics training,* 2012. http://www.rwjf.org/en/about-rwjf/newsroom/newsroom-content/2012/02/united-states-in-search-of-nurses-with-geriatrics-training.html. Accessed March 2018.

Robert Wood Johnson Foundation: *The revolving door: a report on U.S. hospital readmission,* 2013. http://www.rwjf.org/content/dam/farm/reports/reports/2013/rwjf404178. Accessed March 2018.

Ryskina K, Polsky D, Werner R: Physicians and advanced practitioners specializing in nursing home care, 2012-2015, *JAMA* 318(20):2040–2042, 2017.

Schneidermann M, Critchfield J: Customizing the "teachable moment": ways to address hospital transitions in a culturally conscious manner, *Generations* 36(4):94–97, 2012–2013.

Sherman R, Touhy T: An exploratory descriptive study to evaluate Florida nurse leader challenges and opportunities in nursing homes settings, *SAGE Open Nurs* 3:1–7, 2017.

Stierle LJ, Mezey M, Schumann MJ, et al: The Nurse Competence in Aging initiative: encouraging expertise in the care of older adults, *Am J Nurs* 106:93–96, 2006.

Thaler M: The need for SNFs for baby boomers, *McKnight's long-term care news and assisted living,* 2014. http://www.mcknights.com/the-need-for-snfs-for-baby-boomers/article/327724/. Accessed February 5, 2014.

Thomas W: *What are old people for? How elders will save the world,* Acton, MA, 2004, VanderWyk & Burnham.

Toles M, Young H, Ouslander J: Improving care transitions in nursing homes, *Generations* 36(4):78–85, 2013.

Tolson D, Rolland Y, Andrieu S, et al: International Association of Gerontology and Geriatrics: a global agenda for clinical research and quality of care in nursing homes, *J Am Med Dir Assoc* 12: 184–189, 2011.

Tong M, Thomas J, Patel S, Hardesty JL, Brandt NJ: Nursing home medication reconciliation: A quality improvement initiative, *J Gerontol Nurs* 43(4):9–14, 2017.

Young H: Challenges and solutions for care of frail older adults, *Online J Issues Nurs* 8(2):5, 2003.

Zuckerman R, Sheingold S, Orav J, Ruhter J, Epstein AM: Readmissions, observation, and the hospital readmissions reduction program, *N Engl J Med* 374:1543–1551, 2016.

Recommended Baccalaureate Competencies and Curricular Guidelines for the Nursing Care of Older Adults
Gerontological Nursing Competency Statements

1. Incorporate professional attitudes, values, and expectations about physical and mental aging in the provision of patient-centered care for older adults and their families.

Corresponding to Essential VIII

2. Assess barriers for older adults in receiving, understanding, and giving of information.

Corresponding to Essentials IV and IX

3. Use valid and reliable assessment tools to guide nursing practice for older adults.

Corresponding to Essential IX

4. Assess the living environment as it relates to functional, physical, cognitive, psychological, and social needs of older adults.

Corresponding to Essential IX

5. Intervene to assist older adults and their support network to achieve personal goals, based on the analysis of the living environment and availability of community resources.

Corresponding to Essential VII

6. Identify actual or potential mistreatment (physical, mental, or financial abuse, and/or self-neglect) in older adults and refer appropriately.

Corresponding to Essential V

7. Implement strategies and use online guidelines to prevent and/or identify and manage geriatric syndromes.

Corresponding to Essentials IV and IX

8. Recognize and respect the variations of care, the increased complexity, and the increased use of health care resources inherent in caring for older adults.

Corresponding to Essentials IV and IX

9. Recognize the complex interaction of acute and chronic comorbid physical and mental conditions and associated treatments common to older adults.

Corresponding to Essential IX

10. Compare models of care that promote safe, quality physical and mental health care for older adults such as PACE, NICHE, Guided Care, Culture Change, and Transitional Care Models.

Corresponding to Essential II

11. Facilitate ethical, noncoercive decision-making by older adults and/or families/caregivers for maintaining everyday living, receiving treatment, initiating advance directives, and implementing end-of-life care.

Corresponding to Essential VIII

12. Promote adherence to the evidence-based practice of providing restraint-free care (both physical and chemical restraints).

Corresponding to Essential II

13. Integrate leadership and communication techniques that foster discussion and reflection on the extent to which diversity (among nurses, nurse assistive personnel, therapists, physicians, and patients) has the potential to impact the care of older adults.

Corresponding to Essential VI

14. Facilitate safe and effective transitions across levels of care, including acute, community-based, and long-term care (e.g., home, assisted living, hospice, nursing homes), for older adults and their families.

Corresponding to Essentials IV and IX

15. Plan patient-centered care with consideration for mental and physical health and well-being of informal and formal caregivers of older adults.

Corresponding to Essential IX

16. Advocate for timely and appropriate palliative and hospice care for older adults with physical and cognitive impairments.

Corresponding to Essential IX

17. Implement and monitor strategies to prevent risk and promote quality and safety (e.g., falls, medication mismanagement, pressure ulcers) in the nursing care of older adults with physical and cognitive needs.

Corresponding to Essentials II and IV

18. Use resources/programs to promote functional, physical, and mental wellness in older adults.

Corresponding to Essential VII

19. Integrate relevant theories and concepts included in a liberal education into the delivery of patient-centered care for older adults.

Corresponding to Essential I

From American Association of Colleges of Nursing, Hartford Institute for Geriatric Nursing, New York University College of Nursing: *Recommended baccalaureate competencies and curricular guidelines for the nursing care of older adults* [supplement to *The essentials of baccalaureate education for professional nursing practice*], September 2010. Retrieved from https://www.pogoe. org/NursingCompetencies. Accessed February 2019.

3

Theories and Processes of Aging

Kathleen Jett

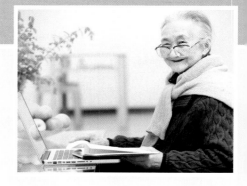

http://evolve.elsevier.com/Touhy/TwdHlthAging

A STUDENT SPEAKS

Until I started learning about the science of the aging process I had no idea how complicated it could be. We seem to have learned so much but still have so much more to learn.

Helena, age 23

AN OLDER ADULT SPEAKS

When I was a young girl Einstein was proposing the molecular theory of matter, and we had never heard of DNA or RNA. We only knew of genes in the most rudimentary theoretical sense. Now I hear that scientists believe there is a gene that is controlling my life span. I really hope they find it before I die.

Beatrice, age 72

LEARNING OBJECTIVES

On completion of this chapter, the reader will be able to:

1. Describe the evolving knowledge regarding the processes and theories of aging.
2. Compare and contrast the major psychosocial theories of aging.
3. Describe the cultural and economic limitations of the current psychosocial theories associated with aging.
4. Use at least one psychosocial theory of aging to support or refute commonly provided social services for older adults living in the community.
5. Create theory-based strategies to foster the highest level of wellness while aging.

Theories are attempts to explain phenomena, to give a sense of order, and to provide a framework from which one can interpret and simplify the world (Einstein, 1920). While some theories of biological aging were developed in the early 1950s, more recently the focus has been on attempts to understand the cellular changes within organisms as they age. In some cases, the associations between biological processes and an organism's aging have become clearer. However, what triggers these processes remains largely theoretical—at least for now.

Psychosocial theories of aging focus on the psychological and social experiences of aging. Although they are more subjective and ethnocentric, they can still provide potential context for aging and social behavior.

This chapter provides the reader with an overview of several prominent biological and psychosocial theories and frameworks of aging. The nurse can use the biological theories to help understand the physical changes of aging and the genetic underpinnings of some of the most common disorders. The nurse can use the psychosocial theories to plan activities which promote healthy and successful aging. Taken together, the nuances of the bio-psychosocial being can be better understood.

BIOLOGICAL AGING

Biological aging, referred to as *senescence*, is an exceedingly complex interactive process of change, resulting in decreased physiological reserves, increased rate of cellular deterioration, and increased vulnerability to disease (Fougère et al, 2019). Aging changes are made visible in what is referred to as the aging phenotype.

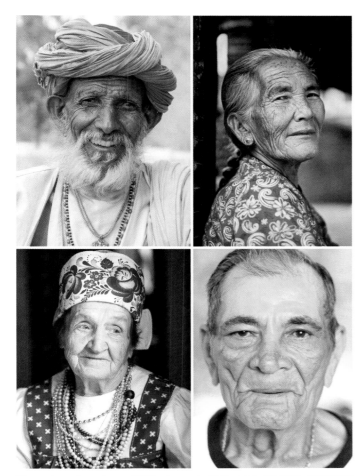

The aging phenotype. (©iStock.com/kailash soni; Bartosz Hadyniak; De Visu; ProArtWork.)

The genome or genetic components of each cell (DNA and RNA) lie within the nucleus of the cell and the mitochondria. They serve as templates for cellular reproduction and direct cellular metabolism. Maintaining the integrity of the genome is the most important function of the cell. This includes regulation of reproduction, repair of damaged DNA, and senescence (MacRae et al, 2015). Survival of an organism depends on successful cellular reproduction (mitosis). If reproduction were always perfect, the organism would never age. Instead, the ability of some cells to reproduce decreases, errors occur in the process, and, ultimately, the ability to reproduce ceases altogether.

While there is a growing body of knowledge about the genomics of aging, complex questions remain. What triggers the changes at the cellular or organ level? Are the changes orderly and predictable or random and chaotic? What are the roles of cellular mutation and epigenetics, that is, the effect of the environment on the RNA? What are the effects of lifestyle choices and how do they influence the aging phenotype?

Evolution and Aging

Evolution theories are recognized as important tools in the understanding of the genetic influence on cellular aging and the understanding of longevity. These theories draw heavily on

conversations about the concept of "natural selection," that is, those who live long enough to reproduce are the fittest of a population. Since we become less fit as we age, we now must address the questions, why some persons live to very late life, and what are the genetic and cellular factors influencing who survives and who does not?

The most developed of these theories is that of the "Disposable Soma [cell]." According to this theory, growth is viewed in terms of the utilization of metabolic resources. These are either spent in the preparation for and the production of offspring or in "keeping … going from one day to the next" (Kirkwood, 2017, p. 23). Theoretically, those whose metabolic resources are spent almost entirely on procreation die earlier than those with fewer offspring. During procreation fewer metabolic resources are available to repair naturally occurring cellular damage. Additionally, there are several metabolic needs (Box 3.1). If any of these needs are unmet the organism will die. Studies have shown that longevity is proportionate to an organism's ability to balance its somatic systems and metabolic needs (Kirkwood, 2017).

Free Radicals

Free radicals are molecules within the cell which are physiologically unstable (missing an electron). Reactive oxygen species (ROS) are also found in the cell, some of which are already free radicals or cause their formation. Both are formed spontaneously during cell metabolism. While both free radicals and ROS are necessary for some cellular activities, they are capable of damaging lipids, proteins, and other macromolecules (Speakman and Selman, 2017). They have been found to cause mutations within the mitochondrial DNA (mtDNA) (Lai et al, 2017).

The number of ROS is increased by several external factors, such as pollution and cigarette smoke, and by internal factors, such as inflammation (Dato et al, 2013). A dramatic rise in the level of ROS, referred to as oxidative stress, has been well documented to lead to cell damage and an accumulation of senescent (aging) cells. These cells have been found to be associated with a number of diseases (Kirkland, 2017; Lobo et al, 2010; Speakman and Selman, 2011) (Box 3.2). The damage from oxidative stress appears to be random and unpredictable, varying from one cell to another, from one person to another (Speakman and Selman, 2011).

BOX 3.1   Examples of Somatic Maintenance Needs

Ability to repair damaged DNA
Ability to remove antioxidants
Ability to control stress proteins
Ability to accurately replicate DNA and proteins
Ability to suppress tumor growth
Ability to maintain a healthy immune system

Adapted from Kirkwood TB: Evolution theory and the mechanisms of aging. In Fillit H, Rockwood K, Young JB, editors: *Brocklehurst's textbook of geriatric medicine and gerontology*, ed 8. Philadelphia, 2017, Elsevier, pp 22–26.

The free radical theory of aging has its origins in the 1950s when scientists were studying the effect of radiation following the use of atomic weapons by the United States in Japan. It was discovered that the extensive damage done by the radiation was primarily caused by free radical's damage to the body's macromolecules (e.g., DNA, proteins, and lipids). Subsequently the paradigm emerged that the molecular damage seen in aging was from the same source, free radicals. It was postulated that any actions that increase the protection against free radicals or decrease oxidative damage would slow aging and hence prolong life (Speakman and Selman, 2011).

For many years it has been promoted in the popular press that the consumption of some supplements can delay or minimize the effects of aging by counteracting the oxidative stress caused by free radicals. However, some antioxidant supplements such as beta-carotene and vitamins C and E have been found to be harmful (Box 3.3). High doses of beta-carotene supplements may increase the risk of lung cancer in smokers and high doses of vitamin E may increase the risk for hemorrhagic stroke and prostate cancer. At the same time evidence has been consistent that *diets* high in antioxidants (high in fruits and vegetables) or a Mediterranean diet rich with red wine and olive oil may prevent or delay some cell damage and several diseases. It is not yet known if this is the effect of the antioxidants themselves or something else, such as lifestyle. (National Center for Complementary and Alternative Medicine [NCCAM], 2013).

As research has become more sophisticated, this theory has been called into question. Using animal models, decreasing cellular protection through a reduction in antioxidants or increasing oxidative damage has not been shown to affect longevity. While the free radical theory may not answer our questions about how long we live, there are considerable data associating oxidative stress with various degenerative disease processes (Speakman and Selman, 2011).

"Inflamm-aging"

The human immune system is a complex network of cells, tissues, and organs that function separately. The body maintains homeostasis through the actions of this protective, self-regulatory system, controlled by B lymphocytes (humoral immunity) and T lymphocytes (a type of white blood cell). Together they protect the body from the invasion of exogenous substances, such as exposure to bacteria, and endogenous conditions, such as emotional stress. The function of the immune system decreases with age, leading to increased risk for infection, cancers, autoimmune disorders, and associated mortality (Kirkland, 2017).

Acute inflammation is the immune system's response to a sudden insult such as trauma. When inflammation is present, several *cellular* mediators (e.g., macrophages) are activated. In turn these cells release *molecular* mediators which are responsible for the inflammatory cascade designed to destroy pathogens, begin tissue repair, and promote physiological homeostasis. The molecular mediators include cytokines, tumor necrosis factor (TNF-α), and interleukin-6 (IL-6) in particular. The nurse observes an inflammation response in the assessment of erythema, edema, and pain.

It has been well documented that aging is accompanied by chronic, low-level, subclinical inflammation (and an increase in mediators such as cytokines). This is referred to as "inflamm-aging" and is theorized to accelerate biological aging and increase the risk for a number of "age-related" diseases and cellular senescence (Fougère et al, 2019; Ventura et al, 2017) (Box 3.4). The inflammatory response is exacerbated by oxidative stress and impaired antioxidant defense. While some of the effects of chronic inflammation are well known, others remain theoretical.

Mitochondrial Dysfunction

Mitochondrial DNA, or mtDNA, is key to the production of adenosine triphosphate (ATP), the precursor to the energy needed

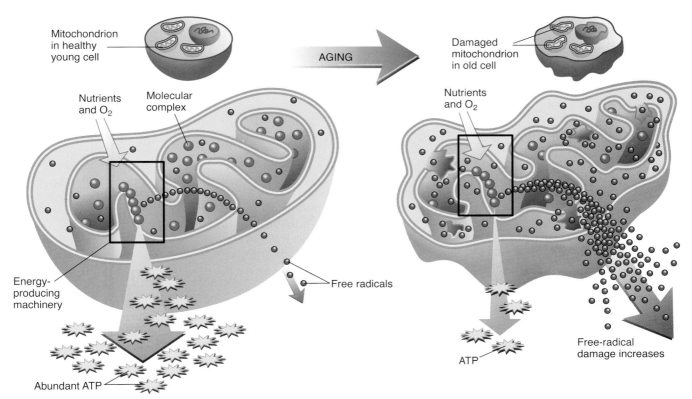

Fig. 3.1 Mitochondria in Young and Old Cells. *ATP,* Adenosine triphosphate. (From McCance KL, Huether SE: *Pathophysiology: the biologic basis for disease in adults and children,* ed 6. St Louis, 2010, Mosby.)

for physiological processes (Fig. 3.1). mtDNA are also necessary for the reproduction of the mitochondria themselves. When damage occurs it is in the form of mutation and resultant replicative errors (Kirkland, 2017B; Lagouge and Larsson, 2013; Wang et al, 2013). mtDNA mutations have been found in both normal aging cells and those associated with neurodegenerative disorders such as Alzheimer's disease (Chapter 23) (Fougère et al, 2019).

Telomeres and Aging

Telomers are sequences of DNA wrapped in proteins found at the end of each chromosome (Fig. 3.2). With each reproduction the telomers shorten. When a critical length is reached the cell ages and ultimately dies (apoptosis). Initial telomere length has been found to be determined by genetic factors; however, the rate of shortening is influenced by other factors, including psychosocial, environmental, and behavioral (Starkweather et al, 2014) (Box 3.5). Shortened telomers have been associated with decreased longevity and several chronic diseases, including cardiovascular disease, hypertension, diabetes, and dementia (Fougère et al, 2019; Lai et al, 2017) (Box 3.6). There is evidence associating this shortening with oxidative stress and inflammation. The enzyme telomerase prevents telomere shortening but is only present in human stem cells, reproductive cells, and cancer cells (Kirkland, 2017; Lai et al, 2017). Length has been proposed as a potentially reliable measure of age.

Although the current biological theories provide a growing understanding of aging, there is still not a definitive answer to what triggers the process. However there has been considerable

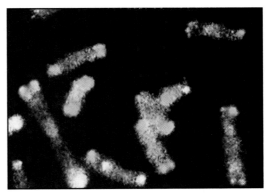

Fig. 3.2 Chromosomes With Telomere Caps. (Modified from Jerry Shay and the University of Texas Southwestern Medical Center at Dallas, Office of News and Publications, 5323 Harry Hines Blvd, Dallas, TX 75235.)

progress in illuminating the association between what appears to be cellular aging and "age-related diseases." Perhaps what will become more important than understanding the triggers of aging will be understanding the triggers of the diseases and thereby the ability to improve health while aging.

PROMOTING HEALTHY AGING: IMPLICATIONS FOR GERONTOLOGICAL NURSING

In the application of our growing knowledge of biological aging, it appears reasonable to expect that slowing or reducing

BOX 3.5   Examples of Factors That Have Been Suggested to Accelerate Telomere Shortening

Chronic stress (perceived)
Pessimism
Interpartner violence
Long-term caregiving (e.g., in Alzheimer's disease)
≤6 hours of sleep a night
Self-reported poor quality of sleep
Higher body mass index and lack of exercise
History of childhood neglect or adverse events
Smoking
Major depressive disorder

From Astuti, Y., Wardhana, A., Watkins, J., et al. (2017). Cigarette smoking and telomere length: A systematic review of 84 studies and meta-analysis. *Environ Res, 158*, 480–489.
Starkweather, A. R., Alhaeeri, A., A., & Montpetit, A. (2014). An integrative review of factors associated with telomere length and implications for biobehavioral research. *Nur Re 63*(1), 36–50.

BOX 3.6   Telomeres, Aging, and Longevity

Telomere length decreases at a rate of 24.8 to 27.7 base pairs per year. A number of lifestyle factors can increase the rate of shortening. Smoking one pack of cigarettes a day for 40 years is associated with the loss of five additional base pairs a year or 7.4 years of life. Obesity also causes accelerated telomere shortening, resulting in 8.8 years of life lost. Excessive emotional stress results in the release of glucocorticoids by the adrenal glands. They have been shown to reduce antioxidants and thereby increase oxidative and premature shortening of telomeres. Shorter telomeres are suggested as greatly increasing one's vulnerability to early onset of age-related health problems such as heart disease.

From Shammas MA: Telomeres, lifestyle, cancer and aging. *Curr Opin Clin Nutr Metab Care* 14(1):28–34, 2011.

cellular damage may have the potential to promote healthy aging. Although we do not know if this will lead to increased longevity, it may be a way to ultimately delay those diseases commonly acquired by many as they age. Helping persons reduce external factors (e.g., pollutants in the environment such as second-hand smoke) that are known to increase the development of ROS is one important approach. One approach to this is through facilitating improved nutrition for all persons, as this has been found to reduce the speed of telomere shortening (Box 3.7). Levels of *naturally* occurring antioxidants can be increased through regular exercise and diet (NCCAM, 2013). Because we have realized the deleterious effects of supplemental antioxidants such as vitamin E, the gerontological nurse can use this knowledge to encourage persons to abandon long-held habits and beliefs and replace these with the healthiest diets and

BOX 3.7   Tips for Best Practice

Finding ways for all persons to have access to nutritious food is an important nursing intervention.

judicious use of herbs and dietary supplements (Chapters 10 and 14).

Of significant importance in the clinical setting is inflamm-aging and implications for its increased susceptibility to infections, autoimmune disorders, and cancers with aging. Observing for early signs and symptoms of infections in older adults is a particularly important contribution nurses can make to facilitate a return to wellness (Chapter 1).

With an understanding of the changes in immunity, the conscientious nurse can take an active role in promoting specific preventive strategies such as the use of immunizations (especially influenza and pneumococcal) and the avoidance of exposure to others with infections. It is nurses' responsibility to not only promote healthy lifestyles but also to serve as role models.

PSYCHOSOCIAL THEORIES OF AGING

A person is not just a biological being but a multidimensional whole (Chapter 1, Fig. 1.7). Only when life is considered in its totality can we begin to truly understand aging. Here we discuss a selection of psychosocial theories of aging. We acknowledge that most are more accurately conceptual models relating to aging or more simply, approaches to understanding. Because they are most often referred to as "theories" in the gerontological literature, we will do so here for the ease of discussion. Each proposes the meaning of successful aging.

Early psychosocial theories of aging were an attempt to explain and predict the changes in middle and late life. The theories began appearing in the gerontological literature in the 1940s and 1950s. They were based on little research and primarily on "face validity," that is, emerging from the personal and professional experience of both scientists and clinicians and appearing to be reasonable explanations of their perceptions of successful aging.

Role Theory

Role theory, an approach drawn from sociology and social psychology, was one of the earliest propositions of what it means to age successfully (Cottrell, 1942). According to this theory, self-identity is defined by one's role in society (e.g., nurse, teacher, banker). As individuals evolve through the various stages in life, so do their roles. Successful aging means that as one role is completed it is replaced by another one of comparative value to the individual and society. For example, the wage-earning work role is replaced by that of a volunteer or a parent becomes a grandparent. The ability of an individual to adapt to changing roles is a predictor of successful aging. Resistance to change is seen as a harbinger of difficulty at the end of life.

Role theory is operationalized in the phenomenon of age norms otherwise referred to as *social stereotypes*. These are culturally constructed expectations of what is deemed acceptable behavior and are internalized by the individual. Age norms are based on the assumption that chronological age and gender, in and of themselves, imply roles; for example, one may hear, "If only they would act their age," or "You are too old to do/say/behave like that." Although beliefs in age- and gender-segregated roles are still present, challenges began with the socially controversial but popular television show of the 1970s *Maude* (1972–1978) and later in *The Golden Girls* (1985–1993). In both of these, the characters behaved in ways that challenged long-established age norms for white middle- and late-aged women. While older men have long served as role models (albeit unrealistic ones) in movies and television, they are now becoming available to women, such as those performed by Dame Judi Dench (born in 1934), Dame Helen Mirren (born in 1945), and Meryl Streep (1949).With the aging of the baby boomers (Chapter 1), popular culture is challenging age norms; for example, older persons are now depicted as still sexually active; from advertisements for genital lubricants and medications to treat erectile dysfunction featuring actors with graying hair. These images replace the historical view that persons become asexual as they age, or so their grandchildren hope!

Activity Theory

Based on data from the Kansas City Studies of Adult Life, Havinghurst and Albrecht (1953) proposed that continued activity and the ability to "stay young" were indicators of successful aging. It is expected that the productivity and activities of middle life are replaced with equally engaging pursuits in later life (Maddox, 1963). The theory assumed that it is better to be active (and young) than inactive (Havinghurst, 1972). Further increased activity leads to a greater sense of well-being due to a higher level of satisfaction (Heinz et al, 2017). *Activity theory* is consistent with Western society's emphasis on work, wealth, and productivity and therefore continues to influence the perception of both successful and unsuccessful aging (Wadensten, 2006).

Disengagement Theory

Disengagement theory contrasts with both role and activity theories. In 1961, Cumming and Henry proposed that in the natural course of aging the individual does, and should, slowly withdraw from society to allow the transfer of power to younger generations. The transfer is viewed as necessary for the maintenance of social equilibrium and a benefit to the older adult (Hooyman and Kiyak, 2011; Wadensten, 2006). A belief in the appropriateness of disengagement provides the basis of age discrimination when an older employee is replaced by a younger one. While this practice has been overtly outlawed in the workplace (in the United States), it is still present covertly and must be challenged socially and legally. An older adult's withdrawal is no longer considered an indicator of successful aging. It is not *necessarily* a good thing for society, and does not consider the needs of the individual or culture in which one lives. Disengagement theory is no longer widely accepted in gerontology.

Continuity Theory

Continuity theory has similarities to both activity and role theory. Atchley (1989) proposed that individuals develop and maintain a consistent pattern of behavior over a lifetime. Aging, as an extension of earlier life, reflects a *continuation of the patterns* of roles, responsibilities, and activities. Personality influences the roles and activities chosen and the level of satisfaction drawn from these. Successful aging is associated with

one's ability to maintain and continue previous behaviors and roles or to find suitable replacements (Wadensten, 2006) (Box 3.8).

Social Exchange Theory

Social exchange theory conceptualizes aging from an economic perspective. The presumption is that as one ages, one has fewer and fewer economic resources to contribute to society. This paucity results in loss of social status, self-esteem, and political power (Hooyman and Kiyak, 2011). Only those who can maintain control of their financial resources have the potential to remain fully participating members of society and anticipate successful aging. Although this may have some applicability in the communities in the world that have been able to develop a stable economy for its citizens, this theory marginalizes those in communities and countries who struggle for the barest necessities now and into the foreseeable future (World Health Organization [WHO], 2017).

Modernization Theory

Although not usually associated with social exchange theory, *modernization theory* can be used to consider nonmaterial aspects of exchange. This theory is an attempt to explain the social changes that have resulted in devaluing the contributions of older adults (Cowgill and Holmes, 1972). In the United States before about 1900, material and political resources were controlled by the older members of a society (Achenbaum, 1978). The resources included their knowledge, skills, experience, and wisdom (Fung, 2013). In agricultural cultures and communities, the oldest members held power through property ownership and the right to make decisions related to food distribution. Older men and women often held valuable religious and cultural roles of instructing youth and controlling ceremony (Sokolovsky, 1997).

According to modernization theory successful aging would mean that older adults maintain status, their skills are valued, and kinship groups remain intact. In contemporary society, the status and value of older adults are lost, labors are no longer valued, and kinship networks are dispersed (Hendricks and Hendricks, 1986). Modernization has had a notable effect on cultures such as those in China and Japan where filial duty predominated as an underlying construct of eldercare (Fung, 2013). As more and more adult children enter the marketplace or emigrate for social or economic reasons, conflicts between traditional values mount (see *The Bonesetter's Daughter* [2001] by Amy Tan). It is proposed that these changes are the result of advancing technology, urbanization, and mass education (Cowgill, 1974).

Gerotranscendence Theory

Gerotranscendence theory is similar to that of disengagement yet the reason for the withdrawal is not for societal needs but to give the person time for self-reflection, exploration of the inner self, contemplation of the meaning of life, and movement away from the material world (Chapter 36) (Maslow, 1954; Moody, 2004; Tornstam, 1989, 2000, 2005; Wadensten, 2007). Aging is viewed as movement from birth to death and maturation toward wisdom, an ever-evolving process that alters one's view of reality, sense of spirituality, and meaning beyond the self. Inasmuch, gerotranscendence implies achieving wisdom through personal transformation. Tornstam (2005), Erikson (1993), and Peck (1968) describe the necessity of transcending individual identity (Table 3.1). With aging, time becomes less important, as do superficial relationships.

Transcendence is viewed as a universal goal, the highest goal any person can achieve, and a marker of successful aging. This theory is based on a highly ethnocentric approach to aging. It is less likely to be applicable in cultures based on the quality of interpersonal relationships (Chapters 4 and 34). It also does not account for differences in economic resources, which may or may not provide the individual the "luxury" of time for introspection.

Socioemotional Selectivity Theory

Carstensen's *Theory of Socioemotional Selectivity* proposes that as people age they become increasingly selective with their emotions, goals, and activities. Aging is associated with a preference for positive over negative information (Carstensen, 1992). Called the "positivity effect," there is the potential for successful aging and improved emotional well-being by selectively choosing positive rather than negative memories (Mather and Carstensen, 2005; Reed and Carstensen, 2012).

Valuing emotional satisfaction highly, time is spent with those persons who share a history of rewarding relationships. When one's life expectancy is viewed as limited, as it is in late life, the focus is present-oriented; life's goals become focused on making the most of the "time left" rather than the distant future (Carstensen, Isaacowitz, et al, 1999).

Selective Optimization With Compensation

The *selective optimization with compensation theory* proposes that successful aging lies in the ability to adapt and cope with the common losses in late life by focusing on strengths; compensatory strategies are used when challenges occur (Baltes and Baltes, 1993). It has been suggested that it can be useful for understanding aging from a number of perspectives (Heinz et al, 2017).

PROMOTING HEALTHY AGING: IMPLICATIONS FOR GERONTOLOGICAL NURSING

Some of the theories of aging have been criticized because of their limited applicability, problems with intersubjectivity of meaning, and inability to be tested. In some cases they fail to consider social class, education, health, and economic and cultural diversity as influencing factors (Hooyman and Kiyak, 2011; Marshall, 1994). But this may be simply consistent with the historical period of their development. Nonetheless, except for disengagement theory, the expressions of how successful aging is defined may prove useful (Table 3.2).

TABLE 3.1   Comparison of Conceptual Perspectives Related to the Developmental Tasks Associated With Aging: Erikson and Peck.

ERIKSON		PECK	
Concept	**Description**	**Concept**	**Description**
Generativity	Establishing oneself as one who contributes to society in meaningful ways	Ego differentiation	Begins to define self as separate from work role
vs. Stagnation	Identifying oneself as restricted to that of one's major role (e.g., nurse)	vs. Work role preoccupation	Difficulty identifying oneself outside of a work role
Ego integrity	Attaining a sense of completeness and cohesion of the self	Body transcendence and ego transcendence	Body changes accepted as part of life. Sees oneself as part of a greater whole
vs. Despair	A sense that one's self no longer has purpose in life, physically or mentally	vs. Body preoccupation and ego preoccupation	Body changes as a source of focus. Sees oneself as an individual needing special attention

TABLE 3.2   The Meaning of Successful Aging, by Psychosocial Theory.

Role theory	As one role is completed it is replaced by another one of comparative value to the individual and society
Activity theory	Ability to maintain an active lifestyle
Disengagement	Natural course of aging; the individual does, and should, slowly withdraw from society to allow the transfer of power to the younger generations
Continuity	The ability to maintain and continue previous behaviors and roles or to find suitable replacements. Productivity and activities of middle life are replaced with equally engaging pursuits in later life
Social exchange theory	Ability to maintain control of their financial resources in order to remain fully participating members of society
Modernization theory	Status is maintained, skills remain valuable, and kinship groups remain intact
Gerotranscendence	To achieve wisdom through personal transformation
Socioemotional selectivity theory	Selectively choosing positive rather than negative memories, companions, and activities
Selective optimization with compensation	The ability to adapt and cope with the common losses in late life by focusing on strengths; compensatory strategies are used when challenges occur

Psychosocial theories and perspectives of aging provide the gerontological nurse with useful information to serve as a backdrop for the development of one's philosophy of care. Although they have been neither proved nor disproved, some have stood the test of time but may have applicability limited to privileged persons wherever they live. They have been used as the rationale for many things, from the creation of senior activity centers to laws regulating employment. They do not, per se, address "crucial issues regarding the attitudes and structure of good nursing" (Wadensten, 2006, p. 347). However, nurses have a unique opportunity to work with multiple approaches to understanding aging. In doing so, they can have an important voice in testing, modifying, and discussing psychosocial theories and frameworks and how they apply to worldwide diversity.

Many questions about late life development remain unanswered. Do biological differences exist between persons of different races and ethnicities, and how does this influence the aging of the human body and the psyche? How do people change in the later years? What is the reason for and purpose of aging? What is the meaning of aging and can this ever be generalized? What is meant by successful aging? These are not new questions, but they still beg answers. The answers may be the essence of maturity in later life.

KEY CONCEPTS

- The timing of when one begins to have features that are identified as "old" is significantly affected by one's genetic makeup and environmental stressors experienced over a lifetime.
- There is no longer one exclusive explanation for aging or for adaptation to aging.
- Regardless of the theory, biological aging results in damage within the cell itself, resulting in a decrease in or loss of its ability to function or reproduce.

- The increased incidence of many chronic diseases in later life can be explained by biological theories of aging.
- While the psychosocial theories in use today apply to some populations, this applicability is limited by socioeconomic, educational, and cultural factors.

CRITICAL THINKING QUESTIONS AND ACTIVITIES

1. What is meant by the phrase "later life is culturally and socially determined"?
2. Consider the psychosocial theories of aging and discuss how each would or would not apply to the oldest person with whom you most commonly interact.
3. Identify at least two "older persons" among your family or friends and ask them their own theories of why the body ages. In a classroom discussion, compare their responses to the current state of the science of biological aging.

4. Discuss the meanings and the thoughts triggered by the student's and older adult's viewpoints as expressed at the beginning of the chapter. How do these vary from your own experience?
5. Imagine yourself at 90 years old and describe the lifestyle you will have and the factors that you believe will account for your long life.
6. Organize a debate in which each individual attempts to convince others of the logic of one particular generation of the psychosocial theories of aging.

RESEARCH QUESTIONS

1. What environmental factors have the potential to affect longevity?
2. What factors in relationships have the potential to contribute to survival?

3. What factors have been associated with extreme longevity?

REFERENCES

Achenbaum WA: *Old age in a new land*, Baltimore, 1978, Johns Hopkins University Press.

Atchley RC: A continuity theory of normal aging, *Gerontologist* 29;183–190, 1989.

Baltes PB, Baltes MM: *Successful aging: perspectives from the behavioural sciences*, Cambridge, UK, 1993, Cambridge University Press.

Carstensen LL: Motivation for social contact across the life span: a theory of socioemotional selectivity, *Nebr Symp Motiv* 40: 209–254, 1992.

Carstensen LL, Isaacowitz DM, Charles ST: Taking time seriously. A theory of socioemotional selectivity, *Am Psychol* 54(3):165–181, 1999.

Cottrell L: The adjustment of the individual to his age and sex roles, *Am Sociol Rev* 7:617–620, 1942.

Cowgill D: Aging and modernization: a revision of the theory. In Gubrium JF, editor: *Late life communities and environmental policy*, Springfield, IL, 1974, Charles C Thomas.

Cumming E, Henry W: *Growing old, the process of disengagement*, New York, 1961, Basic Books.

Dato S, Crocco P, D'Aquila P, et al: Exploring the role of genetic variability and lifestyle in oxidative stress response for healthy aging and longevity, *Int J Mol Sci* 14:16443–16472, 2013.

Einstein A: *Relativity: the special and the general theory*, New York, 1920, Henry Holt.

Erikson E: *Childhood and society*, 1950, Reprint. New York, 1993, Norton.

Fougère B, Boulanger E, Nourhashèmi F, Guyonnet S, Cesari M: Retraction to chronic inflammation: accelerator of biological aging, *J Gerontol A Biol Sci Med Sci* 72(9):1218–1225, 2019.

Fung HH: Aging in culture, *Gerontologist* 53(3):369–377, 2013.

Grune T, Shringarpure R, Sitte N, Davies K: Age-related changes in protein oxidation and proteolysis in mammalian cells, *J Gerontol A Biol Sci Med Sci* 56:B459–B467, 2001.

Havinghurst RJ: *Developmental tasks and education*, New York, 1972, David McKay.

Havinghurst RJ, Albrecht R: *Older people*, New York, 1953, Longmans, Green and Co.

Heinz M, Cone N, da Rosa G, et al: Examining supportive evidence for psychosocial theories of aging with the oral history narratives of centenarians, *Societies* 7(8):1–21, 2017.

Hendricks J, Hendricks CD: *Aging in mass society: myths and realities*, Boston, 1986, Little, Brown.

Hooyman NR, Kiyak HA: *Social gerontology: a multidisciplinary approach*, New York, 2011, Allyn & Bacon.

Kirkland JL: Cellular mechanisms of aging. In Fillit HM, Rockwood K, Young J, editors: *Brocklehurst's Textbook of Geriatric Medicine and Gerontology*, ed 8, Philadelphia, 2017, Elsevier, pp 47–52.

Kirkwood TB: Evolution theory and the mechanisms of aging. In Fillit HM, Rockwood K, Young J, editors: *Brocklehurst's textbook of geriatric medicine and gerontology*, ed 8, Philadelphia, 2017, Elsevier, pp 22–26.

Lagouge M, Larsson NG: The role of mitochondrial DNA mutations and free radicals in disease and ageing, *J Int Med* 273:529–543, 2013.

Lai CQ, Parnell LD, Ordovás JM: Genetic mechanisms of aging. In Fillit HM, Rockwood K, Young J, editors: *Brocklehurst's textbook of geriatric medicine and gerontology*, ed 8, Philadelphia, 2017, Elsevier, pp 43–46.

Lobo V, Patil A, Phatak A, Chandra N: Free radicals, antioxidants and functional foods: impact on human health, *Pharmacogn Rev* 4(8):118–126, 2010.

MacRae SL, Croken MM, Calder RB, et al: DNA repair in species with extreme lifespan differences, *Aging* 7(12):1171–1182, 2015.

Maddox G: Activity and morale: a longitudinal study of selected elderly subjects, *Soc Forces* 42:195–204, 1963.

Marshall VW: Sociology, psychology, and the theoretical legacy of the Kansas City studies, *Gerontologist* 34(4):768–774, 1994.

Maslow A: *Motivation and personality*, New York, 1954, Harper & Row.

Mather M, Cartensen LL: Aging and motivated cognition: the positivity effect in attention and memory, *Trends Cogn Sci* 9(10):496–502, 2005.

Moody HR: From successful aging to conscious aging. In Wykle M, Whitehouse P, Morris D, editors: *Successful aging through the life span*, New York, 2004, Springer, pp 55–68.

National Center for Complementary and Alternative Medicine (NCCAM): *Antioxidants and health: an introduction*, 2013. http://nccam.nih.gov/health/antioxidants/introduction.htm. Accessed February 20, 2019.

Peck R: Psychological developments in the second half of life. In Neugarten B, editor: *Middle age and aging*, Chicago, 1968, University of Chicago Press.

Reed AE, Carstensen LL: The theory behind the age-related positivity effect, *Front Psychol* 3:339, 2012.

Sokolovsky F, editor: *The cultural context of aging: worldwide perspectives*, ed 2, Westpoint, CT, 1997, Plenum Press.

Speakman JR, Selman C: The free-radical damage theory: Accumulating evidence against a simple link of oxidative stress to ageing and lifespan, *Bioessays* 33(4):255–259, 2011.

Starkweather AR, Alhaeeri AA, Montpetit A, et al: An integrative review of factors associated with telomere length and implications for biobehavioral research, *Nurs Res* 63(1):36–50, 2014.

Tan A: *The Bonesetter's daughter*, New York, 2001, Random House.

Tornstam L: Gerotranscendence: a meta-theoretical reformulation of the disengagement theory. *Aging Clin Exp Res* 1:55–64, 1989.

Tornstam L: Transcendence in later life, *Generations* 23:1014, 2000.

Tornstam L: *Gerotranscendence: a developmental theory of positive aging*, New York, 2005, Springer.

Ventura MT, Casciaro M, Gagemi S, Buquicchio R: Immunosenescence in aging: between immune cells depletion and cytokines up-regulation, *Clin Mol Allergy* 15(21), 2017. https://www.ncbi.nlm.nih.gov/pmc/articles/PMC5731094/pdf/12948_2017_Article_77.pdf. Accessed February 24, 2019.

Wadensten B: An analysis of psychosocial theories of ageing and their relevance to practical gerontological nursing in Sweden, *Scand J Caring Sci* 20:347–354, 2006.

Wadensten B: The theory of gerotranscendence as applied to gerontological nursing—part 1, *Int J Older People Nurs* 2:289–294, 2007.

Wang CH, Wu SB, Wu YT, Wei YH: Oxidative stress response elicited by mitochondrial dysfunction: implication in the pathophysiology of aging, *Exp Biol Med* 238:450–460, 2013.

World Health Organization: *Global financial crisis and the health of older people*, 2017. http://www.who.int/ageing/economic_issues/en.

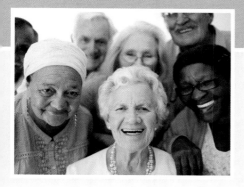

4

Cross-Cultural Caring and Aging

Kathleen Jett

http://evolve.elsevier.com/Touhy/TwdHlthAging

A STUDENT SPEAKS

We are trying to do our work with the patient, but her daughter keeps getting in the way and keeps saying that it "is not the way we do things." I don't understand, we are just trying to do what we were taught to do.

Sandy, age 20

AN OLDER ADULT SPEAKS

It seems like I don't fit in anywhere anymore. My children do their best, but they have to work, and my grandchildren don't have the same respect for me that I had for my grandparents. I know they love me, but it is just not the same.

Yi Liu, age 87

LEARNING OBJECTIVES

On completion of this chapter, the reader will be able to:

1. Compare the major paradigms of health and illness.
2. Identify strategies one might take to move toward cultural proficiency in the delivery of cross-cultural care.
3. Accurately identify situations in which expert interpretation is essential.
4. Be prepared to work with interpreters effectively.
5. Formulate a care plan incorporating culturally sensitive interventions.
6. Develop gerontological nursing interventions geared toward reducing health disparities.

CULTURE, AGING, AND HEALTH CARE

Culture is most often referred to in terms of the shared and learned values, beliefs, expectations, behaviors, and often religion of a group of people. Culture guides thinking, decision-making, and beliefs about aging, health and health-seeking, illness, treatment, and prevention (Jett, 2003; Spector, 2017). Cultural values extend into health care delivery any time the "seeker" and "giver" meet. The "seekers" determine the perceived seriousness of the problem. The "giver" determines the problems that are present (if any), the treatments that are appropriate, and the way they expect seekers to respond. In turn, seekers decide if they agree with the problems the givers have identified, the value of the treatment, if they will accept the "prescription," and if they will act on it (e.g., get the "prescription" filled).

Culture provides directions for individuals as they interact with family and friends within the same group and outside of their group, such as during health care encounters. Culture allows members of the group to predict each other's behavior and respond in ways that are considered appropriate. Cultural beliefs are passed down from one generation to another through *enculturation* and involve the family, the community, and even the political and structural aspects of an environment, such as where they live.

In contrast, *acculturation* is the process by which persons from one culture adjust to another culture. There has been much concern about immigrants who moved to their adopted country in later life. Adjustments needed to find late life satisfaction in their adopted countries are significant. Some aspects of acculturation were more critical to functional adaptation than others. For example, outward adaptations that incorporate language and dress are expressions of cultural identity, but many have less importance than attitudes toward aging, health, illness and treatment, use of time, and interactions with others (Fung, 2013; Spector, 2017).

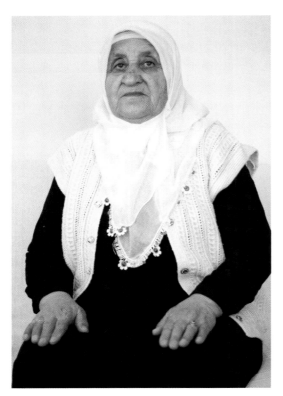

Common attire of Muslim women as expressions of culturally expected modesty. (©iStock.com/Reddiplomat.)

This chapter provides an overview of cross-cultural health care, diversity, inequity, and the aging adult. It is important to note that an encyclopedic approach is not used. In other words, the reader will not find lists of "what term is used to refer to a German elder," etc. Many texts devoted solely to culture can serve as resources for this if desired. Instead, larger concepts are discussed that may refer to more than any one "group" of people, such as health beliefs systems.

Strategies are provided to help the gerontological nurse respond to the changing face of older adults, regardless of their backgrounds, but particularly those with beliefs and values that differ from those of the nurse. The goal of cross-cultural caring is to move toward cultural proficiency and thereby optimize health outcomes and promote healthy aging.

DIVERSITY

Extending the idea of culture is that of *cultural diversity* or simply the existence of more than one group with differing values and perspectives. Morin (2013) describes the extent of diversity in the world, comparing those countries with the least amount of cultural diversity to those with the most. In Argentina, 97% of the citizens are white (of European descent), Roman Catholic, and Spanish is their primary language.

At the other end of the spectrum are many of the countries on the African continent. The 37 different tribal groups in Togo speak 39 different languages and share little in common other than geography. Canada is the only "Western" country in the top 20 in terms of diversity. The United States ranks near the middle, but with considerable changes anticipated in the years to come (Morin, 2013) (Fig. 4.1).

Diversity in the United States usually refers to the six major ethno-racial groups: Black/African American, Asian American, Native Hawaiian/Pacific Islander, American Indian/Alaskan Native, White (of northern European descent), the ethnic group who self-identify as "Hispanic" (regardless of race), and more recently "mixed race." Of note: Most of the persons referred to as Black/African American were brought to the United States against their will to service as slaves in the 17th century (Spector, 2017). The elders of today are descendants of "slavery time."

Except for those classified as "White," the relative percentage of persons who identify with one of these groups is growing rapidly. While the immigration policies of the administration of President Trump have the potential to significantly affect who and when persons immigrate to the United States, it is still expected that diversity will increase. Older adults of today either arrived as children or young adults or late in life joining their children who have become naturalized citizens.

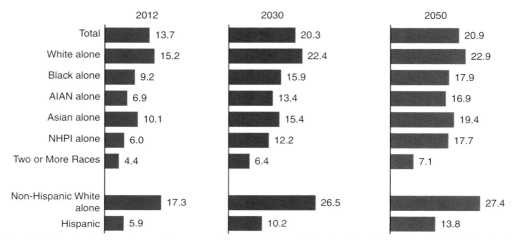

Fig. 4.1 Projected Percentage of Persons at least 65 Years of Age by Race/Ethnicity, 2012, 2030, 2050. (From https://www.census.gov/prod/2014pubs/p25-1140.pdf. Ortman JM, Velkoff VA, Hogan H: *An aging nation: the older population in the United States, current population reports,* Washington, DC, 2014, U.S. Census Bureau, pp 25–1140.)

In 2010 the U.S. Census began working toward means of providing individuals an opportunity to better self-identify their heritage in the 2020 Census (Krogstad, 2014). In 2016 a notice was posted (National Registry) seeking feedback specifically for persons of North African and Middle Eastern roots. It is anticipated that further discussions will be related to persons in sub-ethno-racial groups such as Hispanic (e.g., Mexican, Cuban, etc.) and mixed race (U.S. Census Bureau, 2016). This may prove to be very empowering to older adults who are recent immigrants or who still strongly identify with their country of origin.

It is important to note that within any one group, culturally similar or disparate, there is diversity of gender, power, social status, sexual orientation, gender identity, and an untold number of factors. These factors, in particular, greatly influence the delivery and receipt of health care in all places in the world.

HEALTH INEQUITIES AND DISPARITIES

The terms *health inequities* and *health disparities* are often used interchangeably. Although they are somewhat different, both have implications for health care outcomes. "Health disparities" is the term used in discussions of the results of inequities (Braveman, 2014). One of the most dramatic examples is the discrepancy in life expectancies between low- and high-income nations. A child born in Sierra Leone can expect to live 50 years and one in Japan can expect to live 84 years (WHO, 2017a). However, there is a significant gender disparity in Japan; women have a life expectancy of 86.8 years and men only 80.5 years. Life expectancy varies greatly by neighborhood within countries, as well. In Glasgow, Scotland, the life expectancy of men varies from 60 to 74 years (GCPH, 2017). It is always important to note that health disparities are not limited to those between geographic area, gender, and ethnicity/race. African Americans make up 13% of the population of the United States but almost half of those with HIV.

The term *health inequalities* refer to differences in avoidable, unnecessary, and unjust differences in health outcomes between groups; specifically, poor health outcomes of disadvantaged groups, such as many older adults. Health inequities are often the result of unequal distribution of wealth. Most often one group holds most of the power and influence in a culture, including control of a resource such as health care.

In 2002 the Institute of Medicine published the landmark report of the state of the science of health disparities in the United States, aptly titled *Unequal Treatment: Confronting Racial and Ethnic Disparities in Health Care* (Smedley et al, 2002). Previous research had demonstrated an irrefutable differential in access to health care between white Americans and all others (Box 4.1). Hence, researchers were charged with determining the state of care with this disparity already known.

Among the results of the study were that health care treatment in and of itself was unequal (Smedley et al, 2002). The barriers were found regardless of insurance status, intensity of symptoms, geographical location, age, gender, and sexual orientation. Disparities occurred in all clinical settings, including public hospitals, private hospitals, and teaching hospitals. Most

---

BOX 4.1 The Tuskegee Experiment

Among some older African Americans today there remains mistrust of white health care providers, especially those conducting research. This distrust will continue at some level until the memory of the infamous "Tuskegee Experiment" fades. In 1932 a study to understand the "natural history of syphilis" was conducted. Nearly 600 black men from Macon County, Mississippi, were recruited to participate in a study conducted jointly by the U.S. Public Health Service and the Tuskegee Institute. About half of the men had documented syphilis and were told they were being treated for "bad blood," a phrase with several meanings in the U.S. Southern dialect. The men were never treated, even when penicillin became the evidenced-based practice in 1947. While concerns were raised in 1968, the study was not discontinued until 1972 when it was deemed to be unethical for being misleading and for failing to inform the subjects of the risks of participation. In 1973 a class action suit was filed, and in 1974 $10 million was provided to the survivors and surviving families. In 1997 President Clinton apologized on behalf of the nation, and not long afterward strict rules on the conduct of research were created. The last participant died on January 16, 2004. The last widow died on January 27, 2009.

From Centers for Disease Control and Prevention: *The Tuskegee timeline*, 2017. http://www.cdc.gov/tuskegee/timeline.htm. Accessed November 2017.

---

notable was that the disparities in care resulted in higher mortality among persons of color compared with their white counterparts and were exacerbated with age.

In any country where older adults are marginalized simply because of their age, they are especially vulnerable to health disparities. If the person has other characteristics (e.g., skin color, religion, sexual orientation) that differentiate him or her further from those with power and status, the disparities are amplified. While health disparities have lessened between non-Hispanic whites and Hispanics, American Indians/Alaskan Natives, and blacks in recent years (in the United States), this is not always the case (AHRQ, 2016). For example, older adults are at higher risk for influenza than most other age groups. African American older adults have higher rates of influenza-related hospitalizations than any other ethnic or racial group. African Americans also have the largest proportion of inequality in life expectancy due to cardiovascular disease (USHHS, 2016).

In the years since *Unequal Treatment* was published, the U.S. Agency for Healthcare Research and Quality has produced an annual report, the *National Healthcare Quality and National Healthcare Disparities* (2017), to track the prevailing trends in health care quality and access for vulnerable populations especially those who are statistical minorities, *including the older adults*. The World Health Organization contributes to this knowledge base by monitoring special needs groups such as migrants, migrant workers, and asylum seekers (WHO, 2017b).

OBSTACLES TO CROSS-CULTURAL CARING

Providing cross-cultural care does not always mean addressing disparities or inequities, but it does mean overcoming common obstacles to reach at least culturally competent care (WHO, 2017c). Both overt and covert barriers to care include ethnocentrism and stereotyping, both of which lead to significant

BOX 4.2   Intercultural Conflicts in Nursing Care

A newly immigrated Korean nurse is instructed to ambulate an 80-year-old male patient. He says that he is tired and wants to remain in bed. The nurse does not insist. The nurse manager reprimands the nurse for not getting the patient out of bed. The Korean nurse says to another Korean nurse: "Those Americans do not respect their elders; they treat them as if they were children." The nurse manager complains to another nurse, "Those Asian nurses allow patients to walk all over them." In the traditional Korean culture, elders are revered.

From McHale JP, Dinh KT, Rao N: Understanding co-parenting and family systems among East and Southeast Asian–heritage families. In Selin H, editor: *Parenting across cultures: childrearing, motherhood and fatherhood in non-Western cultures,* Dordrecht, 2014, Springer, pp 163–173.

conflict and decreased quality of care. Conflict can occur in the nursing situation any time one person interacts with another whose beliefs, values, customs, languages, behavior patterns, or expectations differ from their own (Box 4.2). Gerontological nurses will have to find ways to overcome these obstacles in their workplaces and communities to promote healthy aging.

Ethnocentrism

Both nurses in Box 4.2 denigrated the other's nationality as a proxy for culture. These are examples of what is known as *ethnocentrism*, or the belief that one ethnic/cultural group is superior to that of another. This belief may be acquired through enculturation learned at an early age or acculturation later in life. In health care in developed countries, it is expected that seekers adapt to the rules of the givers: to be on time for appointments; to listen and follow the directions that are relayed by their caregivers. In an institutional setting, acculturated older adults will accept the type, frequency, and timing of such things as bathing and personal grooming and sleep and rest schedules. The more acculturated an older adult is to the culture of the institution and individual nurse and aides, the less the potential for conflict. The older adult will eat the meals provided, even if the food does not look or taste like what he or she is accustomed to eating. A "compliant" non–English-speaking resident will accommodate the staff, with or without the help of an interpreter.

Stereotyping

Stereotyping is the application of limited knowledge of a race, ethnicity, age, or culture to an individual. The nurse may hear or say something about what "old people are like" without getting to know the person as a unique individual and member of a tribe, clan, or family, for example. When stereotypes are used, the identification of the heterogeneity *within* the group is not recognized. However, the use of some stereotypes can be a helpful starting point in the provision of the fast-paced health care expected today. For example, a common stereotype about Hispanic elders is that they live with a child and grandchildren and that a male in the family is the decision-maker. If the nurse simply assumes this to be true, it could have a negative outcome, such as fewer referrals for support (e.g., home-delivered

meals). On the other hand, this stereotype can be used to shortcut the assessment. In discussing discharge plans, the non-Hispanic nurse may say, "I have always understood that many Hispanic elders [or Latino/Latina] live with family members. Do I understand this correctly? Is this the case for you and is anyone at home to help you if you need help?" This same approach would be appropriate for most racial/ethnic groups. This must be done with utmost tact to avoid the patient from embarrassment if the stereotype does not apply. This applies regardless of the racial or ethnic group.

PROVIDING CROSS-CULTURAL HEALTH CARE

Providing cultural and linguistically appropriate services (CLAS) and care in a way that challenges ethnocentrism and negative stereotyping is no longer an option; it is an expectation and a necessity as we move to a world community (The Joint Commission, 2017). It is also a means to an end—of reducing health disparities and inequities experienced by vulnerable populations, among them, many older adults (Kirmayer, 2012). Gerontological nurses can learn to do this more expertly as they move along a continuum from cultural destructiveness to cultural proficiency (Fig. 4.2). This requires a willingness to become more self-aware, to learn to know others from their perspectives (i.e., "where they are coming from"), and finally by applying new skills to more effectively work with individuals to support and strengthen, rather than hinder, their cultural strengths (Georgetown University, n.d.) (Box 4.3).

Cultural Destructiveness

Cultural destructiveness is the systematic elimination of the recognized culture of another. There are many well-known examples of this: the genocide of the Jews in Eastern Europe, of

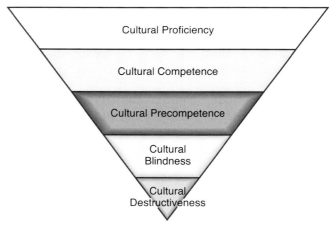

Fig. 4.2 A Model for Cross-Cultural Caring. (Adapted from Cross T, Bazron B, Dennis K, et al: *Toward a culturally competent system of care,* vol 1. Washington, DC, 1989, CASSP Technical Assistance Center, Center for Child Health and Mental Health Policy, Georgetown University Child Development Center; Goode TD: *Cultural competence continuum,* revised ed, Washington, DC, 2004, National Center for Cultural Competence, Georgetown University Center for Child and Human Development, University Center for Excellence in Developmental Disabilities; and Lindsey R, Robins K, Terrell R: *Cultural proficiency: a manual for school leaders,* Thousand Oaks, 2003, Corwin Press.)

BOX 4.3 Moving Toward Cultural Proficiency and Healthy Aging

- Become familiar with your own cultural perspectives, including beliefs about disease etiology, treatments, and factors leading to outcomes.
- Examine your personal and professional behavior for signs of bias and the use of negative stereotypes.
- Remain open to viewpoints and behaviors that are different from your expectations.
- Appreciate the inherent worth of all persons from all groups.
- Develop the skill of attending to both nonverbal and verbal communication.
- Develop sensitivity to the clues given by others, indicating the paradigm from which they face health, illness, and aging.
- Learn to negotiate, rather than impose, strategies to promote healthy aging consistent with the beliefs of the persons to whom we provide care.

BOX 4.4 Unrecognized Privilege and Ethnocentrism

A gerontological nurse responded to a call from an older patient's room. While she was with him, he repeatedly, and without comment, dropped his watch on the floor. She calmly picked it up, handed it back to him, and continued talking. One time an aide walked in the room when the patient dropped the watch. The aide picked it up and handed it back to him just as the nurse had done. The patient immediately started yelling and cursing at the aide for attempting to steal his watch. When telling this story, the nurse thought the whole situation odd, but not too remarkable.

The patient and nurse were white and the aide was black. The nurse did not realize that the behavior of the patient was both ethnocentric and culturally destructive until the nurse learned of the concepts while taking a formal class on cross-cultural health care.

the Hutu in Rwanda, and of many American Indians in the United States. In both Australia (Australian Human Rights Commission, n.d.) and the United States cultural destructiveness occurred by the removal of indigenous children from their homes to boarding schools where the language, dress, and food expressive of their heritages were forbidden (Bear, 2008; Little, 2017). American Indian healing ceremonies, performed by tribal elders, were forbidden. Practices referred to as "traditional" or "folk" healing were and continue to be discounted. Suspiciousness of Western medicine is still present among many African American and American Indians, especially those in their 80s and 90s who may have first- or second-hand knowledge of the cultural destruction (Grandbois et al, 2012).

Cultural Blindness

It is hoped by this point the reader has begun to understand that there are multiple cultures coexisting in countries and continents and that such things as skin color, socioeconomic, political, and educational power affect the health care experience. Yet some people, including health care providers, voice that they see a person's difference from themselves (such as age) but depend on stereotypes such as "all old people are the same" or "all old people are grumpy." They are blind to the fact that life experiences such as prejudice and historical trauma, including ageism, influence both the pursuit and the receipt of health care. It is not possible to provide cross-cultural care or reduce health disparities in the context of cultural destructiveness or cultural blindness unless individual and community health belief paradigms, factors such as ageism, poverty, and racism, are considered (Feagin and Bennefield, 2014; Williams and Mohammed, 2009). Cultural blindness prevents the nurse from providing sensitive and, more importantly, effective care. It prevents even the possibility of reducing health disparities and inequities.

Cultural Pre-Competence

The development of pre-competence begins in the cross-cultural setting with self-awareness of one's personal biases, prejudices, attitudes, and behaviors toward persons different from oneself. For persons whose culture or status places them in a position of power, such as health care providers, cultural awareness is realizing that this alone often means special privilege and freedoms (Box 4.4). Achieving cultural pre-competence requires a willingness to learn how health is viewed by others. It means playing an active role to combat ageism in society.

Cultural Competence

The nurse who moves beyond pre-competence is able to step outside of one's biases and accept that others bring a different set of values and priorities to the health care setting. The nurse who is able to provide competent cross-cultural care accepts that all persons are deserving of respect. The nurse has some knowledge of other cultures, particularly those she or he is most likely to encounter in the health care setting. This is especially important when the nurse and the older adults are of different ages or have different religions, values, backgrounds, and cultures. The acquisition of cross-cultural knowledge takes place in the classroom, at the bedside, and in the community. Cultural knowledge is both what the nurse brings to the caring situation and what the nurse learns from others (Fung, 2013).

Cultural Knowledge

Cross-cultural knowledge has the potential to optimize health care and minimize frustration and conflict between older patients and other health care providers (Kirmayer, 2012). It is expected that knowledge will allow the nurse to more appropriately and effectively improve health outcomes (Campinha-Bacote, 2011; Kirmayer, 2012). Some nurses prefer to use what can be called an "encyclopedic" approach in learning the details of an *individual* culture group, such as proper name usage, greeting, eye contact, gender roles, foods, and attitudes toward aging.

Although this information is important, it should be combined with conceptual knowledge of others as whole persons. In the nursing setting, such as in acute and long-term care facilities, basic knowledge of what is important to someone from a specific culture, such as dietary preference or patterns of interaction, starts the conversation. For example, older adults of Italian descent are often accustomed to having pasta with their major meal, usually midday. Many older adults in the Filipino culture eat rice with all three meals. Providing for choices and then ensuring these are met are factors that allow the delivery of competent cross-cultural nursing care (Fung, 2013).

Definitions of terms. Cultural knowledge includes the appropriate use of terms, especially race and ethnicity. Often used interchangeably, each has a separate meaning. *Race* is a phenotype as expressed in observable traits, such as eye color, facial structure, hair texture, and especially skin tones. However, at this time it is best used as a proxy for geographical origins and lineage such as Africa, Central Europe, or the Pacific Rim (Specter, 2017).

Ethnicity refers to the culture group with which one self-identifies. Persons may share a common nationality, migratory status, language or dialect, religion, or even geographical location (e.g., rural versus urban). Traditions, symbols, literature, folklore, food preferences, and dress are often expressions of ethnicity. Persons from a specific ethnic group may not share a common race. For example, persons who identify themselves as "Hispanic" may be from any race and from a number of countries. However, most Hispanic persons share the Catholic religion and the Spanish language. Instead of Hispanic, the terms "Latino" and "Latina" are increasing heard but are not necessarily interchangeable. The latter specifically refers to a person residing in or from counties in Latin America. It is more accurate to ask an older adult to self-identify ethnicity rather than make assumptions (Box 4.5).

Orientation to family and self. A useful concept in providing cross-cultural health care to older adults is orientation to self and family. Many of those of northern European descent place

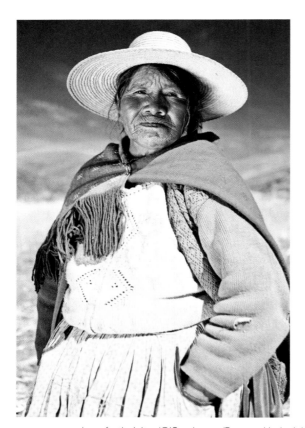

Dress as an expression of ethnicity. (©iStock.com/Bartosz Hadyniak.)

great value on independence, that is, personal autonomy and individuality (Fung, 2013). Identity is closely bound to oneself. In a classic study, Rathbone-McCune (1982) found that a large group of Americans living in a segregated ("white") senior apartment building went to great lengths and lived with significant discomforts rather than ask for help. To seek or receive help was considered a sign of weakness and dependence, something to be avoided at all costs.

In the United States the cultural expression of autonomy was institutionalized in the passing of the Patient Self-Determination Act of 1990 wherein individuals were recognized as the sole decision-makers regarding their health. Health care providers are now legally bound to restrict access to health care information only to the patient, without the person's explicit permission.

This approach conflicts with many other cultures such as that of a collectivist or interdependent culture, a norm in most parts of the world. In the Latino/Latina culture this is referred to as "familismo" (Savage et al, 2016). Self-identity is drawn from family ties (broadly defined) rather than the individual. The "family" (e.g., extended, tribe, clan) is of primary importance; decisions are made by the group or designee based on the needs and beliefs of the group rather than those of the individual (Box 4.6). Within families, the exchange of help and resources is both expected and commonplace. In African American families, fictive kin (persons considered family but are not related by blood or marriage) are especially important. The cultural beliefs and behaviors around families is particularly significant for healthy aging because it relates to eldercare and health-related decision-making. *When a nurse from a culture in which independent decision-making is expected cares for*

BOX 4.6   Opportunities for Cultural Conflicts: Independent Versus Interdependent Health Care Decision-Making

An older Chinese woman is seen in her home by a Euro-American public health nurse and found to have a blood pressure reading of 210/100 mm Hg and a blood glucose level of 380 mg/dL. The nurse insists on calling the patient's nurse practitioner and arranging immediate transportation to an acute care hospital. The woman insists that she must wait until her son-in-law and daughter return home from work so she can discuss it with them before any decisions are made. They will decide if, where, and when she will go for treatment. She is concerned about the welfare of the family and wants to ensure that income is not lost and the family can afford a provider's visit and a possible hospitalization. They would need to make alternate arrangements for childcare and meal preparation. The nurse's main concern is the health of the individual elder, and the elder's concern is her family. The nurse is operating from the value that says an individual is independent and responsible for personal health care decisions, inconsistent with that of the older adult.

BOX 4.7   Cultural Orientations to Time as Applied to Health Care

A past orientation to health and health problems views both as dependent on the actions in the past (such as a past life or earlier in this life) or on events or circumstances of one's ancestors. For example, dishonoring ancestors by failure to perform certain rituals or having poor interactions with others earlier in one's life may result in illness today. Illness today may be considered punishment for past deeds, and it may be prevented by living an honorable life.

A present orientation means that when a health care problem occurs, immediate treatment is needed. Future treatment is considered potentially too late for a positive outcome. The success of freestanding "immediate care centers" or those associated with pharmacy chains in the United States may be a reflection of a present orientation. In general, preventive actions for future health are not consistent with a present orientation toward illness and need for treatment.

Future time orientation is consistent with a belief that when one is ill today, a health care appointment can be made for the future (e.g., the "next available" appointment). In other words, the health problem and its treatment can "wait." The problem will still be there and the delay will not necessarily affect the outcome. Prevention is important because of its effect on future health days, years, and even decades later, for example weight control.

an elder whose dominant value is interdependence or vice versa, the potential for cultural conflict and poor outcomes is great.

Orientation to time.   Orientation to time is often overlooked as a culturally constructed factor influencing the use of health care and the attitudes toward preventive practices (Belgrave and Allison, 2014). Time orientations are culturally described as future, past, or present (Box 4.7).

Conflicts between the future-oriented Westernized medical care and those with past or present orientations are many. This is especially true when working with older adults who have a life time of "habits." Patients are likely to be labeled as *noncompliant* for failing to keep an appointment set tomorrow for a health problem of today, or for failing to participate in preventive measures, such as a "turning schedule" for a bed-bound patient to prevent a (future) pressure ulcer or immunizations to prevent future infections. Members of present-oriented cultures are often accused of overusing hospital emergency departments in the United States, when in fact it may be considered the only reasonable option available for today's treatment of today's problems (Belgrave and Allison, 2014).

Regardless of the health and illness orientation of an individual or members of a culture, community or geographic area and a country's infrastructure have significantly confounding effects. In many developing countries, health care may only be available when provided by outside organizations such as Doctors without Borders *(Medecins Sans Frontieres)* (www.doctorswithoutborders.com).

Obtaining health care may mean a walk of many days, and once at the clinic the waiting time may be hours to days. Such a walk may be impossible for frail or ill older adults. Those living in remote areas, such as those in the state of Montana or the Inuit living near the Arctic, have to wait until the public health nurses make their next rounds by helicopter. For older adults living with chronic diseases, this infrequency of contact may result is persistent health disparities. In such circumstances, older adults are much more dependent on their own resources to deal with illness. Increasing use of technology, such as telemedicine, may ultimately decrease some of the disparities between those near health care services and those at a distance.

In providing cross-cultural care, the nurse can listen closely, determine which orientation has the *most* value to the individual, and find ways to work with it rather than expecting conformity to the cultural model in which the health care is provided. In this way we are reaching out beyond our own perspectives and ethnocentrism to improve the quality of gerontological nursing care.

Beliefs about health, illness, and treatment.   The diversity of the population has brought the strong potential for a clash of health belief systems, languages, and attitudes about health and illness in the delivery of care. Aging itself further increases the diversity of beliefs because of the life-long experiences with illness of self, family, and others. The major health belief paradigms are the biomedical, magico-religious, and naturalistic/holistic. The biomedical paradigm is consistent with what is referred to as "Western" medicine (allopathic). The magico-religious paradigm is often referred to as "folk" medicine. Many naturalistic/holistic practices are referred to as "Eastern medicine" when contrasted to the biomedical (Western) model.

Biomedical.   The biomedical health paradigm espouses that disease is the result of abnormalities in structure and function of body organs or illness/disease caused by the intrusion of pathogens (e.g., bacteria or a virus) into the body. Clinicians use what is referred to as the *scientific method*, such as quantitative laboratory tests and other procedures, to make a diagnosis. Treatment involves repairing the abnormality, destroying the pathogen, or at least ameliorating the damage caused by its presence. Surgery, medications, and rehabilitation programs are typical treatments. Health is viewed as the absence of illness or abnormalities. Biomedical care is considered highly impersonal because the focus is on the abnormality and disease rather than on the person. Preventive strategies are those in which pathogens, chemicals, activities, and dietary agents known to cause malfunction are avoided. Health screenings, as described in Chapter 1, are those activities that identify the disease in an early stage and are consistent with this paradigm.

Magico-religious.   In the magico-religious health belief paradigm, illness is believed to be caused by the actions of a higher power, a supernatural force such as God(s), ghosts, ancestors, or evil spirits (Kail, 2008). This belief system can be traced back thousands of years to ancient Egypt and persists in whole or in part in many groups. Health is viewed as a blessing or reward and illness as punishment for breaking a rule or taboo or displeasing or failing to honor the source of power. Beliefs that illness and disease are attributed to the wrath of the higher power are prevalent among members of many groups, including the Holiness, Pentecostal, and Fundamentalist Baptist churches in the United States. Examples of magical causes of illness are voodoo, especially among persons from the Caribbean; root work among southern African Americans; hexing among Mexican Americans and African Americans; Gaba among Filipinos, cuarnderismo in Mexico and much of Latin America, Santeria in Brazil and Cuba, and espiritismo in Puerto Rico (Junckett, 2013).

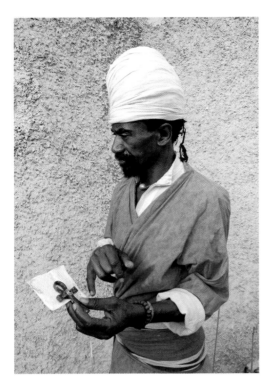

The "ankh" is sometimes used in healing practices. (©iStock.com/tapuzina.)

Magico-religious healing is often in the form of rituals lead by culturally trained and appointed persons such as Faith Healers, brujos(as), yerberas, Shaman, Curanderos, and others. The healers are most often a designated elder or elders in a community.

Treatments may consist of, or include, religious practices such as meditating, fasting, wearing amulets, burning candles, "laying of hands" and prayer circles, or establishing family altars. Such practices may be used both curatively and preventively. Another preventive strategy is to ensure that one maintains good relationships with others, especially elders in the family and community. The "others" may also include Western health care providers (Samovar et al, 2017).

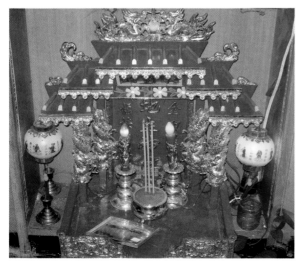

Buddhist shrine. (Courtesy Rachel E. Spector, 2006.)

Some patients refuse biomedical treatments because of the belief that to participate in the treatment is disrespectful to ancestors or challenging "God's will." As a result, significant conflict with Western-trained nurses can occur.

Most of us adhere to magico-religious practices to some extent. How many nurses and their patients have prayed to a higher power that health be restored or maintained? It is not uncommon to hear an older adult pray for a cure or to lament "What did I do to cause/deserve this?" or "God please help me."

Naturalistic or holistic. The naturalistic or holistic health belief system is based on the concept of balance. The balance is between the Yin and the Yang, dark and light, male and female. The ancient health practice based on the concept of Yin-Yang stems from the ancient civilizations of China, India, and Greece (Young and Koopsen, 2005).

Many people throughout the world view health as a sign of balance—of the right amount of exercise, food, sleep, evacuation, interpersonal relationships, or geophysical and metaphysical forces in the universe, such as Qi in the Chinese culture.

Disturbances in this balance result in disharmony and subsequent illness. Diagnosis requires the determination of the type of imbalance and treatment requires a specific strategy to restore balance. Treatments include the use of herbs, acupuncture, acupressure, controlled deep-breathing exercises, and lifestyle changes as appropriate. When one is in balance there is the serenity of inner and outer peace.

Another naturalistic approach is based on a balance between hot and cold. It is a common paradigm throughout the world, especially in the Latino culture, and combines with the magico-religious beliefs already discussed. Illness is classified as either hot or cold and believed to be the result of an imbalance between the two. Many common age-related illnesses are classified as such (Table 4.1). Diagnosis is the determination of the cause of the imbalance (e.g., too much cold) and treatment is usually through countering this with a substance with the opposite properties (e.g., something hot).

Ayurveda is the oldest known medical paradigm in the naturalistic system, practiced in India and many other countries. Like others in this category, health is in terms of balance of key elements. In this case the major foci are earth, wind, water, and air. Illness is again the result of imbalance. However, both diagnosis and selection of appropriate treatments are very complex. Health promotion and disease prevention are key aspects in the

TABLE 4.1 **Hot and Cold Conditions That Are Particularly Relevant to Older Adults.**	
Cold Conditions	**Hot Conditions**
Cancer	Diabetes
Pneumonia	Gastric reflux
Upper respiratory infections	Hypertension
Indigestion	Sore throat or infection

Data from Juckett G: Caring for Latino patients, *Am Fam Phys* 87(1), 48–54, 2013.

lives of those who practice Ayurveda; strategies to maintain health and live a long life include good hygiene, yoga, and meditation (National Center for Complementary and Alternative Medicine [NCCAM], 2016).

Cultural Skills: Communication

Communication and language are foundational skills and intimately tied to the concept of the self. The self is continuously constructed and inextricably intertwined with the linguistic categories available in any given culture. We can conceive of ourselves only within the language we know. Promoting healthy aging and providing the highest quality of cross-cultural care for older adults require not only awareness and knowledge but also the ability to communicate in new and expert ways. In doing so, the person's self-esteem is enhanced, and health-related quality of life is increased to the extent possible.

Communication means listening carefully to the person, especially for his or her perception of the situation, and attending not just to the words but also to nonverbal expressions and the meaning behind both. If the person communicates verbally, it includes attention to idiom, style, jargon, voice tone, and inflection. When the person is nonverbal due to a condition such as dementia and communicating with speech or sign, attention to body language is necessary to make each contact meaningful. Communication begins long before a word is spoken. In many cultures the unspoken message may be as, or more important than, what is said.

The application of cross-cultural communication skills plays an essential part in assessment, in relationship and trust building, and in the development of the plan of care. Expert communication skills are especially important in cross-cultural gerontological nursing. For example, there may be very strict rules of communication between genders or persons who differ in age. Without these skills only less than optimal outcomes can be achieved.

The handshake/bow. A handshake is the customary and expected greeting in most of North America. A firm handshake is thought to be a sign of good character and strength. Yet this is not always the case and the types of acceptable physical contact vary widely. Traditional American Indian elders may interpret firm or vigorous handshakes as signs of aggression. Their handshake may instead be more of a passing of the hand with a light touch as a sign of respect rather than of weakness. In the Muslim culture, cross-gender physical contact (including handshakes) may be considered highly inappropriate or even forbidden. Before the nurse makes physical contact with an older adult of any culture, he or she should ask the person's permission or follow his or her lead, such as an outstretched hand. In a number of East Asian cultures, the handshake is used in the business setting, but it is expected to be slight and accompanied by a bow (eDiplomat, 2017). In non-business settings a bow is expected and accompanied by a nod in some Asian cultures, especially China and Japan. The depth of the bow is an expression of the status afforded each other. A deep bow at the waist is usually expected when greeting an elder.

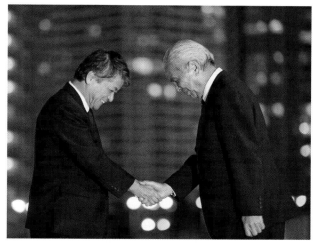
The bow is a gesture of respect in many East Asian cultures and religions. (©iStock.com/stockstudioX.)

Eye contact. Eye contact is another highly culturally constructed behavior. In some cultures, direct eye contact is believed to be a sign of honesty and trustworthiness. Nursing students in the United States are taught to establish and maintain eye contact when interacting with patients, but this behavior may also be misinterpreted. Some persons avoid eye contact, not as a sign of deceit, but as a sign of respect. A more traditional American Indian elder may not allow the nurse to make eye contact, moving his or her eyes slowly from the floor to the ceiling and around the room. During a health care encounter, in most Asian cultures, direct eye contact is considered disrespectful (eDiplomat, 2017). Looking one directly in the eye implies equality. Older adults may avoid eye contact with physicians and nurses if health professionals are viewed as authority figures. In other cultures, direct eye contact between men and women is considered a sexual advance. The gerontological nurse can follow the lead of the older adults by being open to eye contact but neither forcing it nor assigning it any inherent value to it.

The use of silence. The value, use, and interpretation of silence also vary markedly from one culture to another and between ages. In many Eastern cultures, especially those in which the Confucian philosophy is embraced, silence is highly valued. It is expected of young family members and family members with less authority. Silence may be considered a sign of respect for the wisdom of an elder. In traditional Japanese and Chinese families, silence during a conversation may indicate the speaker is giving the listener time to ponder what has been said before moving on to another idea. In traditional American Indian cultures, it is believed that one learns self-control, courage, patience, and dignity from remaining silent. In contrast, Western cultures place much importance on verbal communication. French, Spanish, and older adult immigrants from the former Soviet Union may interpret silence as a sign of agreement (Purnell and Paulanka, 2003; Tripp-Reimer and Lauer, 1987).

Spoken communication. If the nurse and the older adults share the same spoken language, communication is facilitated,

---

BOX 4.8 When a Professional Interpreter Is Needed

An interpreter is needed any time the nurse and the patient speak different languages, when the elder has limited proficiency in the language used in the health care setting, or when cultural tradition prevents the elder from speaking directly to the nurse. The more complex the decision-making, the more important are the interpreter and his or her skills. In gerontological nursing these circumstances are many, such as when discussions are needed about the treatment plan for a new condition, the options for treatment, advanced care planning, or even preparation for care after discharge from a health care institution. The use of a specially trained interpreter is even more important if the elder has lowered levels of health literacy.

BOX 4.10 Guidelines for Working With Interpreters

- Before an interview or session with a client, meet with the interpreter to:
  - Explain the purpose of the session.
  - Instruct the interpreter to use the person's own words and avoid paraphrasing.
  - Instruct the interpreter to avoid inserting his or her own ideas or omitting any information.
- Look and speak directly to the person, not the interpreter.
- Be patient. Interpreted interviews take more time because of the need for three-way communication.
- Use short units of speech. Long, involved sentences or complex discussions create confusion.
- Use simple language. Avoid technical terms, professional jargon, slang, abbreviations, abstractions, metaphors, and idiomatic expressions.
- Listen to the person and watch nonverbal communication (facial expression, voice intonation, body movement) to learn about emotions regarding a specific topic.
- Clarify the person's understanding and the accuracy of the interpretation by asking the person to tell you in his or her own words what he or she understands, facilitated by the interpreter.

Modified from Lipson JG, Dibble SL, Minarik PA, editors: *Culture and nursing care: a pocket guide*, San Francisco, 1996, UCSF School of Nursing Press.

---

although attention to cross-cultural factors is not precluded, such as the appropriate use of specific words and phrases. In health care, recognition of this is especially important such as in the appropriateness of directions (e.g., related to assessment techniques), requests, and instructions (Box 4.8).

Interpretation and translation are needed when different languages are spoken. *Interpretation* is the processing of one *spoken* language into another in a manner that preserves the meaning and tone of the original language without adding or deleting anything. The job of the interpreter is to work with two different linguistic codes in a way that will produce equivalent messages, that is, without adding meaning or opinion.

It is ideal to engage those who are trained in medical interpretation who are adults and of the same culture and gender (Box 4.9). Unfortunately, too often children or even grandchildren are called on to fulfill this role. When they are not available, secretaries or housekeepers may be asked to interpret. When depending on these interpreters, the nurse must realize that either the interpreter or the elder may "edit" his or her comments because of cultural restrictions about the content, that is, what is or is not appropriate to speak about to, or in front of, a parent, child, or stranger. When there are no other reasonable options, "interpreter lines" via the phone or computer are used. Due to the frequency of hearing loss in aging, the use of high-quality head phones or visual imaging of the speaker will maximize the accuracy of the communication. Regardless of who is available to assist, there are guidelines available to maximize the quality and acceptability of the communication (Box 4.10). *Translation* is the exchange of one *written* language for another, such as in the translation of patient education materials. It is recommended that a "back translation" is done for accuracy. This is to first translate the

material into the language needed and then translate it back to the original language in which it was written to ensure accuracy. There are many patient education materials in multiple languages available on the websites www.cdc.gov and www.ahrq.gov. However, it is essential that the nurse remember that many older adults across the globe have low or no literacy. Many of the oldest African Americans in the southern United States have only a third grade education for financial and political reasons.

Cultural Proficiency

To provide the best care to all persons regardless of race, ethnicity, or culture, it is now expected that the nurse demonstrate at least cultural competence but can go further and move toward cultural proficiency (Fig. 4.2). The culturally proficient nurse can move smoothly between two worlds for the promotion of health and the promotion of healthy aging. Culturally proficient care to older adults is that which is respectful, compassionate, and relevant. Cultural proficiency includes putting cultural knowledge to use in assessment, communication, negotiation, and intervention.

It includes the recognition of factors beyond culture, such as the effect of past and current trauma, social status, and poverty leading to health disparities and inequities. The nurse providing proficient cross-cultural health care can work with, and build relationships with, members from a variety of cultural groups as a natural part of daily practice. The relationship building results in the ability to communicate effectively, sensitively assess the individual's state of health, formulate mutually acceptable goals, and support interventions that are culturally acceptable and empowering.

BOX 4.9 Cross-Cultural Health Care

A Haitian woman about 70 years old came to the clinic where I was working, complaining of vaginal itching. I explained that I needed to examine her before I would be able to treat her correctly. When I started to step out of the room after the examination so that she could re-dress, she smiled and said (through an interpreter), "No need for that, you just saw where only my mother and God ever saw, you might as well stay."

Kathleen

PROMOTING HEALTHY AGING: IMPLICATIONS FOR GERONTOLOGICAL NURSING

To provide proficient cross-cultural care, one must enter into an unknown conceptual world in which time, space, religion, tradition, and wellness are expressed through a unique language that conveys the perceived nature of the health, illness, and humanity. It requires sensitive and effective assessment, mutual goal setting, and acceptable interventions that are possible within the limitations of available resources.

Assessment

Many "cultural assessment" tools have been created to detail an individual's beliefs and practices in very specific and comprehensive ways, especially that of Leininger's Sunshine Model and Spector's Heritage Assessment Tool (Murphy, 2006; Spector, 2017). However, adding one of the larger tools, such as that of Leininger, to the already inherently complex and lengthy assessments required in working with aging adults may be too burdensome for all involved, especially older adults who are frail or ill. The Explanatory Model can serve as a guide to assessment questions that have helped nurses and other health care professionals more quickly obtain relevant assessment information in a culturally sensitive manner (Kleinman, Eisenberg, and Good, 1978) (Box 4.11).

The assessment should include a discussion of which of the overall health belief paradigms are most meaningful to the individual. Some ascribe to only one, but many find parts of them or some of the practices of one or the other to have meaning to them.

BOX 4.11   Kleinman's Explanatory Model for Culturally Sensitive Assessment

1. How would you describe the problem that has brought you here? (What do you call your problem; does it have a name?)
   a. Who is involved in your decision-making processes about health concerns?
2. How long have you had this problem?
   a. When do you think it started?
   b. What do you think started it?
   c. Do you know anyone else with it?
   d. Tell me what happened to that person when dealing with this problem.
3. What do you think is wrong with you?
   a. How severe is it?
   b. How long do you think it will last?
4. Why do you think this happened to you?
   a. Why has it happened to the involved part?
   b. What do you fear most about your sickness?
5. What are the chief problems your sickness has caused you?
6. What do you think will help this problem? (What treatment should you receive and what are the most important results you hope to receive?)
   a. If specific tests, medications are listed, ask what they are and do.
7. Apart from me, who else do you think can make you feel better?
   a. Are there therapies that make you feel better that I do not know? (Maybe in another discipline?)

Modified from Kleinman A: *Patient and healers in the context of culture: an exploration of the borderland between anthropology, medicine, and psychiatry,* Berkeley, 1980, University of California Press.

Interventions

The On Lok Program

The most well-known model for the provision of gerontological cross-cultural care in the United States is the On Lok Lifeways PACE Program (All-inclusive Care for the Elderly) in San Francisco and surrounding areas. It has long been recognized for its cultural relativism. Services are provided in the language of the older adult and in a manner that optimizes each person's cultural heritage. Nurses can learn from the work of On Lok Lifeways and other programs to promote wellness and healthy aging and to help reduce health disparities and inequities. It is suggested that modifications of existing long-term care services that enhance the well-being of aging persons regardless of their language, race, ethnicity, culture, or heritage, should include the following:

1. A professional interpreter if needed.
2. A program that reflects the diversity of the participants or residents.
3. Staff reflective of the diversity of residents/clients/patients.

The LEARN Model

Regardless of the assessment model chosen, this information must be operationalized into a plan of care that addresses the special needs of the person and is realistic and consistent with the person's cultural patterns and beliefs. The LEARN model (Box 4.12) (Berlin and Fowkes, 1983) is simple and highly effective and can be used not only in the cross-cultural encounter but also any time the nurse wants to increase the probability that the highest level of wellness is achieved.

The LEARN model is used to negotiate a plan of care and includes the identification of the availability of culturally appropriate and sensitive resources, including those in the person's community. When working with older adults, resources may also include the identification of others who will be part of the care team, such as indigenous healers, priests, monks, rabbis, or ministers, if their presence is desired or believed to be helpful.

Through the skilled use of this simple model, gerontological nurses can provide culturally sensitive care regardless of setting. When caring for persons from marginalized groups, including many older adults, using the model has the potential to reduce health disparities and increase health equity.

BOX 4.12   LEARN Model

L Listen carefully to what the person is saying. Attend not just to the words but to the nonverbal communication and the meaning behind them. Listen to the perception of the person's situation, desired goals, and ideas for treatment.

E Explain your perception of the situation and the problems.

A Acknowledge and discuss both the similarities and the differences between your perceptions and goals and those of the elder and their significant other/decision-makers as appropriate.

R Recommend a plan of action that takes both perspectives into account.

N Negotiate a plan that is mutually acceptable and possible.

Adapted from Berlin E, Fowkes W: A teaching framework for cross-cultural health care: application in family practice, *West J Med* 139:934–938, 1983.

INTEGRATING CONCEPTS

Promoting cross-cultural healthy aging provides the gerontological nurse with new challenges and opportunities to learn from new perspectives (Butler et al, 2016). Unfortunately, poverty is very common in many households of persons who are not of the dominant culture in a country and can be exacerbated when the person is in later life. Meeting basic needs, especially food and health care, may be difficult. Some older adults immigrated to the United States or other adopted countries much earlier in their lives and their moves were not traumatic. Others have experienced horrific events in their home country or during their immigration process and hold a unique and perhaps life-long concern for safety and security. The nurse must be sensitive to this possibility without stereotyping or making assumptions. The nurse can assess the components of biological integrity and, if necessary, facilitate the older adults or family obtaining support services (e.g., food stamps, home-delivered meals) that are possible and appropriate.

The increasing diversity of the health care work force provides further challenges. When the nurse or aide speaks with an accent or uses tones and phrases reflective of their background, communication may be difficult with older adults who speak a different language (Georgetown University, n.d. b). Most people with presbycusis (normal age-related hearing loss) depend on lip-reading to some extend to augment what they are hearing. The words may be the same but the physical (oral) way they are spoken differs making understanding difficult.

Cultural identity is one of the major elements of self-concept and a key to self-esteem, increasingly so as a person ages or becomes more mentally or physically frail (Fung, 2013). Older adults may be closely tied to family and community and, often, religious beliefs. Estrangement from their country of origin may be ameliorated if they live in homogeneous communities and may be exacerbated if they live in social isolation or away from persons with similar backgrounds. The monoethnic community (e.g., barrio, Nihonmachi, Chinatown) serves as a buffer and a means of strengthening cohesiveness for older adults from similar cultural groups. Within the community, elders are protected from discrimination and the language and customs of the society outside.

Family support is highly variable among groups, social classes, and subcultures, yet the nuclear or extended family is the chief avenue of transmitting cultural values, beliefs, customs, and practices. The family may provide stability and sanctuary to the aging individual. Making the broadest of generalizations, we may say that persons from Asian cultures value familial piety rooted in Confucianism. This means that a fundamental value is respect for older adults (McHale et al, 2014). It has long been a Korean custom to celebrate one's 60th and 70th birthdays. The 60th (hwan-gap) is the celebration into old age. The 70th birthday (kohCui) is a celebratory recognition of the "old and rare." It has been the traditional expectation that younger members of the family care for older members of family although this is challenged more and more with changes in employment (Healthy Living, 2015). Hispanic families, and

those from the Mediterranean rim, often function within large, extended networks and church affiliations. For example, in the Greek (and Greek-American) culture old-age is honored and celebrated, respect for older members of the community is expected. Decision-making, including that related to health, is the responsibility of the oldest male in many families. African Americans embrace extended families and fictive kin with the oldest woman usually holding the most power in day-to-day life. During times of celebration (e.g., family reunions) all of the older adults share their wisdom through stories of survival during the civil rights conflicts of the 1950s and 1960s and the ongoing discrimination in their lives (McCoy, 2011). While attitudes vary among the more than 500 American Indian tribes (First People), there is a consistent expectation that older adults will pass down their wisdom to younger members of the family (Healthy Living, 2015). A group of elders hold political and decision-making power within the tribe. In striking contrast, adults in the typical culture of many of those of northern Europe remain highly independent when younger and become more and more dependent with age, more so with frailty. Physical signs of aging are often avoided resulting in a very lucrative business of "antiaging" products (Applewhite, 2016).

Spirituality or religiosity plays a major role in defining many cultures. Religion may function as a consistent experience that affords psychic support in the individual's life. Early Japanese immigrants (Issei) sought religious tradition in the face of aging and death (Kitano, 1969). Hispanic/Latino/Latina older adults may seek Spanish-speaking clergy rather than mental health professionals when they have emotional problems (Junckett, 2013).

Changes are threatening the historical role of aging in families across the globe. Different degrees of assimilation between generations create a communication gap between the young and older immigrants, as they join their families in new countries where the language and customs may be unknown to them. This may cause isolation and estrangement between the oldest and youngest generations. Enculturated and acculturated expectations may clash (see any of the books by author Amy Tan). In marginalized groups of older adults, illness, poverty, and migration are destroying the insulation previously afforded by the family and community (Jett, 2006) (Box 4.13). Members of minorities in any community are extremely vulnerable as they age. They may experience triple jeopardy when devalued because of age, race, and ethnicity.

The study of aging is one of the most complex and intriguing opportunities of our day. Realistically, it will be almost

---

BOX 4.13 Where Did the Community Go?

A middle-aged African American woman talked about her community and care of persons with dementia. She said that when she grew up "it was expected that the neighbor would watch out for you. Like if someone saw you out and about and knew you would get lost they would just take you home again. . . . That just doesn't seem to be happening anymore . . . we don't even know each other!"

From Jett KF: Mind-loss in the African American community: dementia as a normal part of aging, *J Aging Studies* 20(1):1–10, 2006.

BOX 4.14 A Cross-Cultural Caring Encounter

Determine the following about the older adult:
- Preferred cultural, ethnic, and racial identity
- Expectations concerning formality of the encounter
- Expectations concerning use of names, titles, addressing the patient and the nurse
- Preferred language
- Level of health and reading literacy and availability of assistance if needed
- Past personal experience with the Western health care model
- Level of acculturation, adherence to traditional approaches, openness to new approaches
- Factors influencing decision-making: who, how, when, what

impossible to become familiar with the whole range of clinically relevant cultural differences of older adults one may encounter. Attempting to provide care holistically and sensitively is the most challenging opportunity leading to personal growth for both the nurse and the person receiving care.

Today's nurse is expected to provide culturally proficient care to persons regardless of their age, health beliefs, experiences, values, and styles of communication (Box 4.14). Cross-cultural communication is especially important because of the inherent complexity of health while aging and the combination of generational and cultural differences between the person and the nurse. The nurse will need to communicate effectively with persons regardless of the languages spoken. In doing so, the nurse may depend on limited verbal exchanges and attend more to facial and body expressions, postures, and gestures and know how to work with the many aspects of communication. Effective gerontological nurses provide cross-cultural care through the application of cultural knowledge and skills needed to optimize intercultural communication.

To skillfully assess and intervene, nurses must develop cultural proficiency through awareness of their own ethnocentricities. They must be acutely sensitive to the cues suggested (e.g., eye contact) to know how best to respond. Promoting healthy aging in cross-cultural settings includes the ability to develop a plan of action that considers the perspective of both the older adult/family and the nurse/health care system to negotiate an outcome that is mutually acceptable. Skillful cross-cultural nursing means developing a sense of mutual respect between the nurse and the person. A sense of caring is conveyed in gestures of personal recognition. It is working "with" the person rather than "on" the person; and in doing so, health disparities and inequities, if they exist, can begin to be reduced and movement toward healthy aging can be facilitated. Unbiased caring can surmount cultural differences.

KEY CONCEPTS

- Global population diversity is rapidly increasing and will continue to do so. This suggests that nurses will be caring for a greater number of older adults from a broader number of cultural backgrounds and older adults will encounter caregivers from a greater number of places of origin.
- Recent research has shown that significant disparities and inequities in the outcomes of health care persist. Those who bear the greatest burden of morbidity and mortality are those who are the most marginalized from those in control of health care resources, this includes older adults, especially those who are frail.
- Nurses can contribute to the reduction of health disparities and the promotion of social justice by increasing their own cultural awareness, knowledge, and skills.
- Cultural proficiency and sensitivity require awareness of issues related to culture, race, social class, and economic situations.
- Ethnicity is a complex phenomenon of self-identity expressed as language, dress, traditions, symbols, and folklore.

- Stereotyping can negate the fact that significant heterogeneity exists within cultural groups.
- Health beliefs of various groups emerge from three general belief systems: biomedical (allopathic), magico-religious, and naturalistic. Older adults may adhere to one or more of these systems.
- Effective cross-cultural care to older adults includes skills related to both verbal and nonverbal communication.
- The more complex the decision-making, the more important the quality of communication. For those with limited English proficiency, expert interpretation is needed whenever serious decisions are needed (e.g., end-of-life care or treatment changes).
- The use of family, children, or support staff as interpreters is not recommended and may result in censored interpretation because of rules of cultural etiquette that may be unknown to the nurse.
- The LEARN model provides a useful framework for working to reach mutually agreeable and possible health care goals.

NURSING STUDY: Where Do I Belong? Who Am I?

Georgia thought she was a misfit. She had always thought this. She was born in China in 1920 where her parents had built and managed a school for orphaned children in Shanghai. When she was 15 the family returned to the United States and moved to an Appalachian mining village to manage a small school and clinic. Having grown to adolescence in China, she felt more Chinese than American.

She had a difficult adjustment in the poverty-stricken rural mining village in Appalachia, so different from Shanghai. In a few years, her parents sent her to a private religious college, attended mainly by the children of the affluent older adults of her church. She married a young army officer, and they were immediately sent to France. Her life from then on seemed to consist of nothing but

Continued

NURSING STUDY: Where Do I Belong? Who Am I?—cont'd

moves as she followed her husband. She was widowed at 70 when her only son was 45. She thought she would continue to live in her home but her son insisted that she move to an assisted living facility immediately. He worked all day and his wife was busy. At her new "home" she found that most of the staff were Filipino and talked among themselves in Tagalog. Again, she felt disconnected with the prevailing culture in which she found herself. She became very difficult to get along with, and the staff members were at their wits' end trying to please her. You recently went to work as director of nursing in the facility. How will you help her and the staff maximize life satisfaction?

On the basis of this nursing study, propose:
- How best to reach out to Georgia and attempt to understand the story behind her current behavior.
- A method to work with Georgia to develop a plan of care that meets both her physical and her psychological needs.
- A means of working with the staff to facilitate optimizing Georgia's life satisfaction while minimizing the demands on their already heavy workload.

CRITICAL THINKING QUESTIONS AND ACTIVITIES

1. Define the terms *culture*, *ethnicity*, *ethnocentricity*, and *cultural proficiency*.
2. Identify several personal values or beliefs that are derived from your ethnic roots.
3. Privately list your stereotypes and "ethnocentrisms" for various ethno-racial cultural groups, and explore the basis of these beliefs (e.g., taught, fear, experience, lack of knowledge). Then consider what you can do to address these stereotypes.
4. Describe the advocacy role of nurses to reduce health disparities.
5. What are the primary difficulties in providing nursing care for individuals from a different background from one's own?

RESEARCH QUESTIONS

1. What are the factors that identify a group as an ethnic minority?
2. What are the enduring cohort differences that are unlikely to change throughout life?
3. What are the outcomes of an integrated cultural approach versus a separate-culture approach in a curriculum?

REFERENCES

Agency for Healthcare Research Quality: 2016 *National healthcare quality and disparities report*, 2017. https://www.ahrq.gov/research/findings/nhqrdr/nhqdr17/index.html. Accessed February 24, 2019.

Applewhite A: *This chair rocks: a manifesto against ageism*, New York, NY, 2016, Networked Books.

Australian Human Rights Commission: *Track the timeline: the stolen generation. History of separation of Aboriginal and Torres Strait Islander children from their parents*. https://www.humanrights.gov.au/timeline-history-separation-aboriginal-and-torres-strait-islander-children-their-families-text. Accessed February 1, 2018.

Bear C: *American Indian boarding schools haunt many*, 2008. http://www.npr.org/templates/story/story.php?storyId=16516865.

Belgrave FZ, Allison K: *African American Psychology: from Africa to America*, Thousand Oaks, CA, 2014, Sage.

Berlin EA, Fowkes WC: A teaching framework for cross-cultural health care: application in family practice, *West J Med* 139:934–938, 1983.

Braveman P: What are health disparities and health equity? We need to be clear, *Public Health Rep* 129(Suppl 2):5–8, 2014.

Butler M, McCreedy E, Schwer N, et al: Improving cultural competence to reduce health disparities, *Comparative Effectiveness Reviews* 170, 2016. Rockville MD, Agency for healthcare research and quality, report no. 16-EHC0066-EF. Accessed February 1, 2018.

Campinha-Bacote J: Delivering patient-centered care in the midst of a cultural conflict: the role of cultural competence, *Online J Issues Nurs* 16(2):5, 2011.

eDiplomat: *Japan*, 2017. http://www.ediplomat.com/np/cultural_etiquette/ce_jp.htm#topnav. Accessed November 2017.

Feagin J, Bennefield Z: Systematic racism in U.S. healthcare, *Soc Sci Med* 103:7–14, 2014.

Fung HH: Aging in culture, *Gerontologist* 53(3):369–377, 2013.

Georgetown University National Center for Cultural Competence (a): *Self-Assessments*. https://nccc.georgetown.edu/assessments/. Accessed November 2017.

Georgetown University National Center for Cultural Competence (b): *Cultural and linguistic competence health practitioner assessment (CLCHPA)*. https://www.clchpa.org/. Accessed November 2017.

Glasgow Centre for Population Health: *Building understanding, evidence and new thinking for a healthier future*, 2017. https://www.gcph.co.uk/population_health_trends/life_expectancy_in_glasgow. Accessed November 2017.

Grandbois DM, Warne D, Eschiti V: The impact of history and culture on nursing care of Native American elders, *J Gerontol Nurs* 38(10):3–5, 2012.

Healthy Living: *Seven cultures that celebrate aging and respect their elders*, 2015. https://www.huffingtonpost.com/2014/02/25/what-other-cultures-can-teach_n_4834228.html. Accessed November 2017.

Jett KF: The meaning of aging and the celebration of years among rural African American women, *Geriatr Nurs* 24:290–293, 2003.

Jett KF: Mind-Loss in the African American community: a normal part of aging, *J Aging Stud* 20(1):1–10, 2006.

Juckett G: Caring for Latino patients, *Am Fam Physician* 87(1):48–54, 2013.

Kail TM: *Magico-religious groups and ritualistic activities: a guide for first responders*, Boca Raton, FL, 2008, Taylor & Francis.

Kirmayer LJ: Rethinking cultural competence, *Transcult Psychiatry* 49(2):149–164, 2012.

Kitano H: *Japanese Americans*, Englewood Cliffs, NJ, 1969, Prentice-Hall.

Kleinman A, Eisenberg L, Good B: Culture, illness, and care: clinical lessons from anthropologic and cross-cultural research, *Ann Intern Med* 88:251–258, 1978.

Krogstad JM, Cohn DV: U.S. Census looking at big changes in how it asks about race and ethnicity. *Pew Research Center*, 2014. http://www.pewresearch.org/fact-tank/2014/03/14/u-s-census-looking-at-big-changes-in-how-it-asks-about-race-and-ethnicity. Accessed November 2017.

Little B: *How boarding schools tried to "kill the Indian" through assimilation*, 2017. http://www.history.com/news/how-boarding-schools-tried-to-kill-the-indian-through-assimilation. Accessed November 2017.

McCoy R: African American elders, cultural traditions and the family reunion, *Journal of the American Society on Aging*, 2011. http://www.asaging.org/blog/african-american-elders-cultural-traditions-and-family-reunion. Accessed November 2017.

McHale JP, Dinh KT, Rao N: Understanding co-parenting and family systems among East and Southeast Asian–heritage families. In Selin H, editor: *Parenting across cultures: childrearing, motherhood and fatherhood in non-western cultures*, Dordrecht, Netherlands, 2014, Springer, pp 163–173.

Morin R: The most (and least) culturally diverse countries in the world, *Pew Research Center*, 2013. www.pewresearch.org/fact-tank/2013/07/18/the-most-and-least-culturally-diverse-countries-in-the-world. Accessed October 2017.

Murphy SC: Mapping the literature of transcultural nursing, *J Med Libr Assoc* 94(Suppl 2):E143–E151, 2006.

National Center for Complementary and Alternative Medicine: *Ayurvedic medicine: in depth*, 2016. http://nccam.nih.gov/health/ayurveda/introduction.htm. Accessed November 2017.

Rathbone-McCune E: *Isolated elders: health and social intervention*, Rockville, MD, 1982, Aspen.

Samovar LA, Porter RE, McDaniel ER, Roy CS: *Communicating between cultures*, Boston, 2017, Cengage.

Savage B, Foli KJ, Edwards NE, Abrahamson K: Familism and health care provision to Hispanic older adults, *J Gerontol Nurs* 42(1):21–29, 2016.

Population Reference Bureau: *Elderly immigrants in the United States*, 2019. https://www.prb.org/us-elderly-immigrants/. Accessed February 2019.

Smedley B, Stith AY, Nelson AR, editors: *Unequal treatment: confronting racial and ethnic disparities in health care*, Washington, DC, 2002, National Academy Press.

Spector RE: *Cultural diversity in health and illness*, ed 9, New York, NY, 2017, Pearson.

The Joint Commission: *Health equity*, 2017. https://www.jointcommission.org/topics/health_equity.aspx. Accessed November 2017.

U.S. Census Bureau: *Research to improve data on race and ethnicity*, 2016. https://www.census.gov/about/our-research/race-ethnicity.html. Accessed October 2017.

U.S. Health and Human Services: *HHS action plan to reduce racial and ethnic health disparities: a nation free of disparities in health and health care*, 2016. https://minorityhealth.hhs.gov/assets/pdf/hhs/HHS_Plan_complete.pdf. Accessed November 2017.

Williams DR, Mohammed SA: Discrimination and racial disparities in health: evidence and needed research, *J Behav Med* 32(1):20–47, 2009.

World Health Organization: *World health statistics 2017: monitoring health for the SDGs* [Sustainable development goals], 2017a. http://www.who.int/gho/publications/world_health_statistics/2017/en/. Accessed November 2017.

World Health Organization: *Frequently asked questions on migration and health*, 2017b. http://www.who.int/features/qa/88/en/. Accessed November 2017.

World Health Organization: *10 facts on health inequities and their causes*, 2017c. http://www.who.int/features/factfiles/health_inequities/en/. Accessed November 2017.

Young C, Koopsen C: *Spirituality, health and healing*, Sudbury, MA, 2005, Jones & Bartlett.

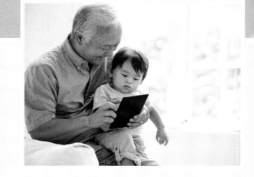

5

Cognition and Learning

Theris A. Touhy

http://evolve.elsevier.com/Touhy/TwdHlthAging

A STUDENT SPEAKS

I was shocked the other day when I got a message on my Facebook page from my grandmother. I had no idea that older adults even knew about Facebook but my Gram says she has 30 friends and has reconnected with some of her classmates from high school. She's been pretty lonely since Grandpa died and I wouldn't be surprised if she finds her old boyfriend next. Older adults can be pretty cool.

Kate, age 19

AN OLDER ADULT SPEAKS

Imagine, they tell us now that our brain continues to develop even though we are older. I thought it was all downhill to dementia when I turned 70. My nurse practitioner advised me to get involved in some activities for stimulating my brain and improving my memory. I found a free class at the high school where I could learn French, something I have always wanted to do. I am having such fun and am already looking at brochures for river cruises through France.

Marie, age 74

LEARNING OBJECTIVES

On completion of this chapter, the reader will be able to:

1. Explain cognitive changes with age and strategies to enhance cognitive health.
2. Identify nursing responses to assist older adults to maintain or improve cognitive abilities.
3. Discuss factors influencing learning in late life, including health literacy, and appropriate teaching and learning strategies.

The processes of normal cognition and learning in late life and strategies to enhance cognitive health and effective teaching-learning are discussed in this chapter. Assessment of cognition is discussed in Chapters 7 and 23, and care of older adults with mild and major neurocognitive disorders is discussed in Chapter 29.

ADULT COGNITION

Cognition is the process of acquiring, storing, sharing, and using information. Components of cognitive function include language, thought, memory, executive function, judgment, attention, and perception. The determination of intellectual capacity and performance has been the focus of a major portion of gerontological research. Developing knowledge today suggests that cognitive function and intellectual capacity are a complex interplay of age-related changes in the brain and nervous system and many other factors such as education, environment, nutrition, life experiences, physical function, emotions, biomedical and physiological factors, and genetics (Agency for Healthcare Research and Quality, 2017; National Institute on Aging, 2017a).

Before the development of sophisticated neuroimaging techniques, conclusions about brain function with aging were based on autopsy results (often on diseased brains) or results of cross-sectional studies conducted with older adults who were institutionalized or had coexisting illnesses. Changes seen were considered unavoidable and the result of the biological aging process rather than disease. As a result, the bulk of research has focused on the inevitable cognitive declines rather than on

56

BOX 5.1 Myths About Aging and the Brain

MYTH: People lose brain cells every day and eventually just run out.

FACT: Most areas of the brain do not lose brain cells. Although you may lose some nerve connections, it can be part of the reshaping of the brain that comes with experience.

MYTH: You cannot change your brain.

FACT: The brain is constantly changing in response to experiences and learning, and it retains this "plasticity" well into aging. Changing our way of thinking causes corresponding changes in the brain systems involved; that is, your brain believes what you tell it.

MYTH: The brain does not make new brain cells.

FACT: Certain areas of the brain, including the hippocampus (where new memories are created) and the olfactory bulb (scent-processing center), regularly generate new brain cells.

MYTH: Memory decline is inevitable as we age.

FACT: Many people reach old age and have no memory problems. Participation in physical exercise, stimulating mental activity, socialization, healthy diet, and stress management helps maintain brain health. The incidence of dementia does increase with age, but when there are changes in memory, older adults need to be evaluated for possible causes and receive treatment.

MYTH: There is no point in trying to teach older adults anything because "you can't teach an old dog new tricks."

FACT: Basic intelligence remains unchanged with age, and older adults should be provided with opportunities for continued learning. Minimizing barriers to learning such as hearing and vision loss and applying principles of geragogy enhance learning ability.

Modified from American Association of Retired Persons: *Myths about aging and the brain*, April 10, 2006. https://www.aarp.org/health/brain-health/info-2017/common-myths-aging-brains-fd.html. Accessed February 2019.

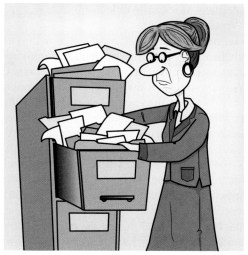

Alex Comfort, an early gerontologist, described the slowed response time of an older adult: By the time you are 80, you have a lot of files in the file cabinet. Your secretary is 80 so it also takes her a lot longer to locate the files, go through them, find the one you want, and bring it to you.

cognitive capacities. Many old myths about aging and the brain are still believed by both older adults and health professionals. It is important to understand cognition and memory in late life and dispel the myths that can have a negative effect on wellness (Box 5.1). Ramscar et al. suggest that "ideas about cognitive decline are likely to have been exerting a strong, negative influence on the lives of many millions of older adults" (2014, p. 35).

Changes in the aging nervous system (Box 5.2) cause a general slowing of many neural processes, but they are not consistent with deteriorating mental function, nor do they interfere with daily routines. Age-related changes in brain structure, function, and cognition are also not uniform across the whole brain or across individuals. Cognitive functions may remain stable or decline with increasing age. Recent research suggests that the reason older brains slow down is because they take longer to process constantly increasing amounts of information (Ramscar et al, 2014). Overall cognitive abilities remain intact, and it is important to remember that if brain function becomes impaired in old age, it is the result of disease, not aging (Crowley, 1996).

Neuroplasticity

It is very important to know that the aging brain maintains resiliency or the ability to compensate for age-related changes. Past thinking was that we are born with a fixed number of neurons that die as we age. We now know that the brain has the capacity for neuronal replacement (Fick, 2016). Developing

knowledge also refutes the myth that the adult brain is less plastic than the child's brain and less able to strengthen and increase neuronal connections (Petrus et al, 2014). The old adage "use it or lose it" applies to cognitive and physical health. Stimulating the brain increases brain tissue formation, enhances synaptic regulation of messages, and enhances the development of cognitive reserve (CR).

CR is based on the concept of neuroplasticity and refers to the strength and complexity of neuronal/dendrite connections from which information is transmitted and cognition/mentation emerges. The greater the strength and complexity of these connections, the more the brain can absorb damage before cognitive functioning is compromised. "CR can be increased or decreased due to two complex, overarching processes—positive or negative neuroplasticity. Positive neuroplasticity is the brain's ability to make more and stronger connections between neurons in response to novel situations. Negative neuroplasticity refers to the atrophy of

BOX 5.2 Changes in the Central Nervous System

Neurons
- Shrinkage in neuron size and gradual decrease in neuron numbers
- Structural changes in dendrites
- Deposit of lipofuscin granules, neuritic plaque, and neurofibrillary bodies within the cytoplasm and neurons
- Loss of myelin and decreased conduction in some nerves, especially peripheral nerves

Neurotransmitters
- Changes in the precursors necessary for neurotransmitter synthesis
- Changes in receptor sites
- Alteration in the enzymes that synthesize and degrade neurotransmitters
- Significant decreases in neurotransmitters, including acetylcholine, glutamate, serotonin, dopamine, and γ-aminobutyric acid

such connections in response to low stimulation or physiological insults" (Vance, 2012, p. 28).

To maximize brain plasticity and CR, it is important to engage in challenging cognitive, sensory, and motor activities and meaningful social interactions on a regular basis throughout life. People vary in the CR they have, and this variability may be because of differences in genetics, overall health, education, occupation, lifestyle, leisure activities, or other life experiences. Brain diseases and injuries may be less apparent in those with greater CR because they are able to tolerate lost neurons and synapses. For example, people who have attained more years of education may have high levels of Alzheimer pathology, but few, if any, clinical symptoms (Pinto and Tandel, 2016).

Dementia incidence rates have decreased significantly among individuals born after 1929 during the past 10 to 20 years in the United States and Western Europe. Better nutrition, improved health care, especially vascular risk and control of diabetes, healthier environment, enhanced intellectual stimulation, and better general living conditions may have contributed to the decline. Additional studies are needed to determine whether the decreasing rate will continue with the aging of the world population (Derby et al, 2017).

Changes in the brain with aging, once seen only as compensation for declining skills, are now thought to indicate the development of new capacities. These changes include using both hemispheres more equally than younger adults, thus enhancing bilateral communication potential, greater density of synapses, and more use of the frontal lobes, which are thought to be important in abstract reasoning, problem solving, and concept formation (Davis et al, 2017; Grossman et al, 2010). The scaffolding theory of aging and cognition suggests that the increased frontal lobe activation with age is a marker of an adaptive brain that engages in compensatory scaffolding in response to the challenges of declining neural structures and function. The scaffolding can be considered a form of positive plasticity that accompanies aging (Reuter-Lorenz and Park, 2014).

Later adulthood is no longer seen as a period when growth has ceased and cognitive development has halted; rather, it is seen as a life stage programmed for plasticity and the development of unique capacities. The renewed emphasis on the development of cognitive capabilities that can develop with age provides a view of aging that reflects the history of many cultures and provides a much more hopeful view of both aging and human development. While "some areas experience decline (e.g., memory and processing speed), improvements are noted in areas such as wisdom, knowledge, and resilience" (Fick, 2016, p. 6) (Chapter 36).

Fluid and Crystallized Intelligence

Fluid intelligence and crystallized intelligence are factors of general intelligence that can be measured in standardized IQ tests. Fluid intelligence (often called *native intelligence*) consists of skills that are biologically determined, independent of experience or learning. It involves the capacity to think logically and solve problems in novel situations, independent of acquired knowledge. Fluid intelligence can be likened to "street smarts." Crystallized intelligence is composed of knowledge and abilities that the person acquires through education and life ("book smarts") and is demonstrated largely through one's vocabulary and general knowledge. Crystallized intelligence is long-lasting and improves with experience.

Older adults perform more poorly on performance scales (fluid intelligence), but scores on verbal scales (crystallized intelligence) remain stable. This has been known as the classic aging pattern. The tendency to do poorly on performance tasks was attributed to changes in sensory and perceptual abilities and psychomotor skills. However, research by Rascar et al. (2014) questions this and postulates that older adults need more time to process the knowledge they have gained from their experiences. "In other words, you get slower when you're older because you're smarter" (Hill, 2017). Testing methods may also contribute to differences.

Memory

Memory is defined as the ability to retain or store information and retrieve it when needed. Memory is a complex set of processes and storage systems. Three components characterize memory: immediate recall; short-term memory (which may range from minutes to days); and remote or long-term memory. Biological, functional, environmental, and psychosocial influences affect memory development throughout adulthood. Recall of newly encountered information seems to decrease with age, and memory declines are noted in connection with complex tasks and strategies. Even though some older adults show decrements in the ability to process information, reaction time, perception, and capacity for attentional tasks, the majority of functioning remains intact and sufficient. Tips for improving your memory are presented in Table 5.1.

Familiarity, previous learning, and life experience compensate for the minor loss of efficiency in the basic neurological processes. In unfamiliar, stressful, or demanding situations, however, these changes may be more marked (e.g., hospitalization). Healthy older adults may complain of memory problems, but their symptoms do not meet the criteria for mild or major neurocognitive impairment (Chapter 23). The term *age-related cognitive decline (ARCD)* has been used to describe memory loss that is considered normal in light of a person's age and educational level. This may include a general slowness in processing, storing, and recalling new information and difficulty remembering names and words. However, these concerns can cause great anxiety in older adults who may fear dementia (Box 5.3). Many medical or psychiatric difficulties (delirium, depression) also influence memory abilities, and it is important for older adults with memory complaints to have a comprehensive evaluation (Chapters 7, 23, and 29).

Cognitive Health

Cognitive health is defined as "the development and preservation of the multidimensional cognitive structure that allows the older adult to maintain social connectedness, an ongoing sense of purpose, and the abilities to function independently, to permit functional recovery from illness or injury, and to cope with residual functional deficits" (Hendrie et al, 2006, p. 12).

TABLE 5.1 Tips for Improving Your Memory.

Technique	Example
Pay attention to the task at hand; minimize distractions, avoid multitasking.	When listening to someone giving you directions while you are driving, do not keep the radio on.
Involve your senses.	To help remember the names of people you are meeting, look them in the eye, shake their hand, and repeat their name. Use auditory cues such as timers, alarm clocks, cell phone reminders.
Use repetition.	Say what you are trying to remember several times. Say things aloud ("I am putting my car keys on the hall table"). Review new learning at the end of the day.
Chunk it and organize it.	When trying to remember a telephone number, chunk it into 3 pieces of information (area code, 3-digit prefix, and a 4-digit number). Write things down, organize routine tasks, try to prepare things in advance when you have time to concentrate.
Use mnemonic devices (clues to help you remember) (visual images, acronyms, rhymes, and alliterations).	Use the word HOMES to remember the names of the Great Lakes: Huron, Ontario, Michigan, Erie, and Superior. Remember the months of the year with 30 days using the rhyme "Thirty days has September…" Search the alphabet when trying to remember something. Do an Internet search for what you are trying to remember.
Relate information to what you already know.	Remember a new address by thinking of someone you know who lives on the same street.
Get adequate sleep; use stress-relieving techniques; and engage in physical activity.	Sleep is necessary for memory consolidation, and the key memory-enhancing activity occurs during the deepest stages of sleep. Cognitive training and memory training exercises may improve sleep. Mindfulness meditation encourages more connections between brain cells and increases mental acuity and memory ability. Exercise increases oxygen to the brain, reduces the risk of illness, enhances helpful brain chemicals, and protects brain cells.

Adapted from Grobol J: 8 tips for improving your memory. *Psych Central,* 2010. http://psychcentral.com/blog/archives/2010/09/03/8-tips-for-improving-your-memory. Accessed February 17, 2014; Smith M, Robinson L: *How to improve your memory.* http://www.helpguide.org/articles/memory/how-to-improve-your-memory.htm. Accessed February 17, 2014.

BOX 5.3 Memory and Thinking: What's Normal and What's Not?

Normal Aging/ARCD
Making a bad decision once in a while
Missing a monthly payment
Forgetting which day it is and remembering it later
Sometimes forgetting names or what word to use
Losing things from time to time

Dementia
Making poor judgments and decisions a lot of the time
Problems taking care of monthly bills/managing finances
Losing track of the date, year, or time of year
Trouble having a conversation
Misplacing things often and being unable to find them

ARCD, Age-related cognitive decline.
From National Institute on Aging: *Memory and thinking: what's normal and what's not?* https://www.nia.nih.gov/health/memory-and-thinking-whats-normal-and-whats-not. Accessed February 2019.

A healthy brain is "one that can perform all mental processes that are collectively known as cognition, including the ability to learn new things, intuition, judgment, language, and remembering" (CDC, 2017b).

Cognitive health is influenced by many of the factors that comprise the multiple dimensions of wellness discussed in Chapter 1. Attention to cognitive health, beginning at conception and continuing throughout life, is just as important as attention to physical and emotional health. Many of the behaviors influencing physical and emotional health also promote cognitive health (Fig. 5.1). This view of healthy cognitive aging is comprehensive and proactive; it implies that cognitive health is much more than simply a lack of decline with aging (Desai et al, 2010). The National Center for Creative Aging campaign, *Beautiful Minds: Finding Your Lifelong Potential,* describes four steps to a beautiful mind (Box 5.4).

PROMOTING HEALTHY AGING: IMPLICATIONS FOR GERONTOLOGICAL NURSING

Several national studies have examined the existing evidence related to interventions to promote cognitive health and prevent dementia. At present, there is not sufficient strength to establish benefit or encourage people to adopt specific interventions to prevent cognitive decline or dementia. There is no magic bullet to prevent late-life dementia (Larson, 2018). Encouraging evidence suggests that blood pressure management, particularly in midlife, physical activity (twice-weekly exercise training) (Chapter 18), adherence to a Mediterranean diet (MetDiet) and a combined MetDiet and Dietary Approaches to Stop Hypertension (DASH) diet plan (Mediterranean-DASH Intervention for Neurodegenerative Delay [MIND]), and cognitive stimulation may reduce the risk of ARCD but further research is needed (McEvoy et al, 2017) (Chapter 14). Other areas of research that may hold promise include the

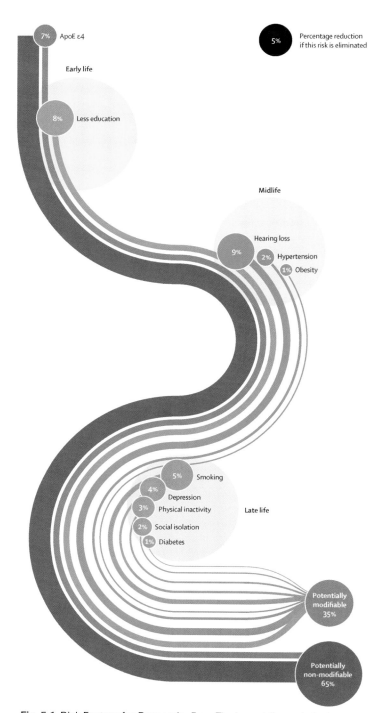

Fig. 5.1 Risk Factors for Dementia. From The Lancet Commission's new life-course model, showing potentially modifiable—and nonmodifiable—risk factors for dementia. *ApoE*, Apolipoprotein E. (Reprinted from Livingston G, Sommerlad A, Orgeta V, Costafreda SG, Huntley J, Ames D, et al: Dementia prevention, intervention, and care, *Lancet* 390(10113):2673–2674, 2017. Copyright 2017, with permission from Elsevier.)

and Quality, 2017; National Academies of Sciences, Engineering, Medicine, 2017; Petersen et al, 2018). The effect of uncorrected hearing loss on cognitive decline and dementia also requires further investigation (Liu et al, 2013; National Institute on Aging, 2017b) (Chapter 12).

Nurses can educate people of all ages about effective strategies to enhance cognitive health and vitality and to promote CR and brain plasticity. Fig. 5.2 presents a checklist to promote healthy brain aging that can be used by clinicians. Box 5.5 presents resources for the public and professionals about brain health. While the evidence is inconclusive about the benefits of cognitive stimulation on brain health, remaining intellectually engaged throughout life is important. Game playing (Scrabble, Trivial Pursuit, cards), puzzles, learning a new language, developing a new hobby, taking a class, volunteering, reading, and engaging in interesting conversations are all ways to stimulate the brain. Among the various types of cognitive stimulating activities, games such as cards or puzzles seem to be particularly useful (Jeffrey, 2014; Rebok et al, 2014).

The brain exercising activity chosen should meet the following criteria: (1) it is new, unfamiliar, and out of your comfort zone; (2) it is challenging and takes some mental effort; and (3) it is fun and stimulates your interest and enjoyment. At present, there is no evidence that long-term cognitive effects are obtained with commercial computer-based "brain training" applications and no evidence that cognitive training can delay dementia (AHRQ, 2017). Tips for Best Practice are presented in Box 5.6.

Education provided about cognitive health should be tailored to specific communities and cultural subgroups because there are differences in perceptions about cognitive health among these groups. Results of a study examining perceptions about aging well in the context of cognitive health among a large and diverse group of older adults suggest that there are common themes about aging well among groups but also differences (Centers for Disease Control and Prevention, 2017c; Laditka et al, 2009). More research is needed to understand adaptations of interventions for specific communities and cultural subgroups (Chapter 4).

following: new dementia treatments that can delay or slow disease progression; diabetes treatment; depression treatment; dietary interventions; lipid-lowering treatments; sleep quality interventions; social engagement interventions; vitamin B$_{12}$ plus folic acid supplementation (Agency for Healthcare Research

1	Counseled regarding smoking cessation	☐
	Comments:	
2	Advised to follow guidelines proposed jointly by the American Heart Association and the American College of Sports Medicine regarding daily physical activity	☐
	Comments:	
3	Counseled regarding healthy nutrition (e.g., Mediterranean diet, DASH [Dietary Approaches to Stop Hypertension] diet)	☐
	Comments:	
4	Counseled regarding the importance of intellectually challenging and creative leisure activities	☐
	Comments:	
5	Counseled regarding strategies to promote emotional resilience and reduce psychological distress and depression (e.g., relaxation exercises, mindfulness-meditation practices)	☐
	Comments:	
6	Advised to maintain an active, socially integrated lifestyle	☐
	Comments:	
7	Discussed strategies to achieve and maintain optimal daily sleep	☐
	Comments:	
8	Provided education about strategies to reduce risk of serious head injury (e.g., wearing seat belts, wearing helmets during contact sports, bicycling, skiing, skateboarding)	☐
	Comments:	
9	Provided education about strategies to reduce exposure to hazardous substances (e.g., wearing protective clothing during the administration of pesticides, fumigants, fertilizers, and defoliants)	☐
	Comments:	
10	Provided education and counseling regarding negative health effects of alcohol consumption more than recommended as safe by the National Institute of Alcoholism and Alcohol Abuse	☐
	Comments:	
11	Provided education about importance of achieving and maintaining healthy weight to promote overall health	☐
	Comments:	
12	Discussed and implemented strategies to achieve optimal blood pressure control	☐
	Comments:	
13	Discussed and implemented strategies to achieve optimal control of dyslipidemia (e.g., high cholesterol)	☐
	Comments:	
14	Discussed and implemented strategies to achieve optimal control of blood sugar/diabetes	☐
	Comments:	
15	Discussed risks and benefits of medications, supplements, herbal remedies, and vitamins to promote brain health	☐
	Comments:	
16	Discussed and implemented secondary prevention of stroke strategies (e.g., daily baby aspirin)	☐
	Comments:	

Fig. 5.2 Promoting Healthy Aging: Cognitive Health. (Courtesy Center for Healthy Brain Aging, St Louis University School of Medicine, St Louis, MO. From Desai A, Grossberg G, Chibnall J: Healthy brain aging: a road map, *Clin Geriatr Med* 26:1–16, 2010.)

BOX 5.5 Resources for Best Practice

Cognitive Health
- **National Institutes of Health:** Cognitive and Emotional Health Project: The Healthy Brain
- **Centers for Disease Control and Prevention:** The Healthy Brain Initiative: A National Public Health Road Map to Maintaining Cognitive Health
- **National Institute on Aging:** Alzheimer's Disease Education and Referral Center: Understanding Memory Loss: What to Do When You Have Trouble Remembering
- **National Center for Creative Aging:** Beautiful Minds: Finding Your Lifelong Potential; 2014, America's Brain Health Index

BOX 5.6 Tips for Best Practice

Cognitive Health
- Dispel myths about brain aging and teach about cognition and aging.
- Educate people of all ages about factors that influence cognitive health.
- Be aware of cultural differences in perceptions of cognitive health and adapt education accordingly.
- Advise older adults to have comprehensive assessment if they are experiencing cognitive decline.
- Encourage socialization and participation in intellectual stimulating activities, exercise, healthy diets (e.g., Mediterranean, Dietary Approaches to Stop Hypertension [DASH] diet).
- Teach chronic illness prevention strategies and ensure good management of chronic illnesses.
- Share resources for cognitive training (memory enhancing techniques, computer games, puzzles, card games).

LEARNING IN LATER LIFE

Basic intelligence remains unchanged with increasing years, and older adults should be provided with opportunities for continued learning. Adapting communication and teaching to enhance understanding requires knowledge of learning in late life and effective teaching-learning strategies with older adults. *Geragogy* is the application of the principles of adult learning theory to teaching interventions for older adults.

The older adult demands that teaching situations be relevant; new learning must relate to what the person already knows and should emphasize concrete and practical information. Aging may present barriers to learning, such as hearing and vision losses and cognitive impairment. Pain and discomfort can also interfere with learning. Moreover, the process of aging may accentuate other challenges that had already been factors in a person's life, such as cultural and cohort variations and education. Many older adults may have special learning needs based on educational deprivation in their early years and consequent anxiety about formalized learning.

Attention to literacy level and cultural variations is important to enhance learning and the usefulness of what is learned. Mood is extremely important in terms of what individuals (both young and old) will recall. In other words, when we attempt to measure recall of events that may have occurred in a crisis situation or an anxiety state, recall will be impaired. This is significant for health care professionals who give information to older adults who are ill or upset, particularly at times of crisis such as hospital discharge.

Learning Opportunities

Opportunities for older adults to learn are available in many formal and informal modes: self-teaching, college attendance, participation in seminars and conferences, public television programs, audio classes, Internet courses, and countless others. In most colleges and universities, older adults are taking classes of all types. Fees are usually lower for individuals older than 60 years of age, and individuals may choose to work toward a degree or audit classes for enrichment and enjoyment. Senior centers and local school districts often also provide a wide array of adult education courses. The Road Scholar (formerly Elderhostel) program is an example of a program designed for older adults that combines continued learning with travel. The program offers trips to all 50 states and 150 countries. Road Scholar offers intergenerational programs for grandparents and grandchildren ages 4 and older (https://www.roadscholar.org/).

Information Technology and Older Adults

Older adults comprise the fastest growing population using computers and the Internet. According to Hill (2017), the digital divide is shrinking. In 2000, only 14% of older adults were using the Internet; in 2016, 64% use the Internet and 80% own a cell phone, 34% use social media. More than half (56%) of Internet users ages 65 and older use Facebook (Pew Research Center, 2018). More than any other age group, older adults perceive the Internet as a valuable resource to help them more easily obtain information and connect to loved ones. This could

range from using a cell phone to set medication reminders to using Skype and FaceTime to interact with long-distance grandchildren. Many individuals are also using email to communicate with their health care providers (Box 5.7). Organizations such as Cyber Seniors and the American Association of Retired Persons (AARP) provide basic computer and Internet training for older adults.

With the aging of the baby boomers and the young tech-savvy adults, the future of technology in care and services for older adults can only be imagined. Technology has the

---

BOX 5.7   This Is What 90 Looks Like

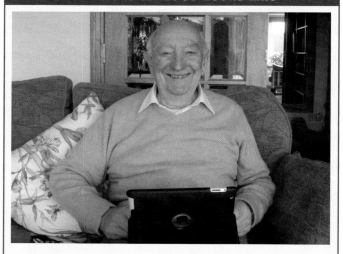

"When Britain entered the war in Europe, I decided that further attendance at formal schooling was out, and as soon as I was old enough I volunteered for aircrew duties in the Royal Air Force and was accepted and trained as a pilot. Following an injury, I left the RAF in 1951 and soon found that entering the industrial market was not easy. Soon after my return to civilian status I married a nurse whom I had met while I was at the RAF rehabilitation unit, and over the 50 years of our marriage we raised 6 children.

"I eventually found employment in the new plastics industry and was surprised to find how short of background knowledge the new factories and their management were; therefore, having gained some knowledge in processing I joined an engineering group that intended to manufacture processing machinery. Fortunately I had received good background training in hydraulics and electrics in the services. I was able to take an active part in improving their equipment.

"During my employment the Rubber and Plastics Institute elected me a fellow for my service to the industry. When I retired I was the director of development and technical training. After retirement I worked for a further 17 years as a consultant specializing in processing and training.

"Losing my wife while we were both in our mid-80s was a double blow. Living alone after more than 50 years of shared companionship was difficult but the restriction of advancing years in my new solitary state made the years ahead look very bleak. My children all helped me at this difficult period and I learned to live with what I had and modify my life to suit. Now that I am 90 years of age I no longer fly my own plane but I still feel confident driving, so I do have a degree of mobility that I feel is helping me deal with life's problems. I find learning to recognize what is possible and what is hazardous and to realize that these factors do change is an important lesson when growing old."

Skype communication with Victor T. Gardner

potential to improve the quality of life across settings by enhancing access to health information and resources, making communication with family and friends easier, providing cognitive stimulation and enjoyable activities, and alleviating isolation among community-dwelling older adults and those in nursing homes (Culley et al, 2013; Tak et al, 2007). Hill (2017) suggests that nurses need to utilize a person-centered approach in using technology. This includes involving older adults in development, testing, and evaluation of technology, considering individual needs, preferences, and characteristics, and customizing the approach for each individual's identified goals. Chapter 20 further discusses the use of technology in practice.

PROMOTING HEALTHY AGING: IMPLICATIONS FOR GERONTOLOGICAL NURSING

Traditional ways of providing health information and services are changing, and both public and private institutions are increasingly using the Internet and other technologies. This presents challenges for people with limited experience using computers and for those with limited literacy. Nurses can share resources available for older adults who want to learn computer skills and adaptations that can be made to make computers as user-friendly as possible (e.g., touch screens, voice systems) for those who may have limitations. Nurses and other health professionals need to develop skills in the understanding and use of consumer health information and teach clients how to evaluate the reliability and validity of health information on the Internet (Box 5.8). Using social media as a platform for health promotion and health education presents exciting possibilities. Continued attention to access to technology, especially among disadvantaged groups, and also efforts to enhance culturally and language-appropriate materials are important (Culley et al, 2013).

HEALTH LITERACY

Health literacy is defined as the degree to which individuals have the capacity to obtain, process, and understand basic health information and services needed to make appropriate health decisions (CDC, 2017a). Limited health literacy has been linked to increased health disparities, poor health outcomes, inadequate preventive care, increased use of health care services, higher health care costs, higher risk of mortality for older adults, and several health care safety issues, including medical and medication errors (Cutilli et al, 2018).

Health literacy plays a major role in improving health and health care quality for all Americans. In the past, health literacy has been viewed in terms of individual patient deficits (lack of knowledge regarding health issues) but is now recognized as a complex issue that involves the patient, the health care professional, and the health care system. *Healthy People 2020* includes goals and objectives to improve health literacy and use of information technology.

Nearly 9 of 10 adults do not have the level of proficiency in health literacy skills necessary to successfully navigate the health

> ### BOX 5.8 Evaluating Internet Health Information
>
> - SPONSORSHIP: Consider the source: use only recognized authorities. Government agencies have .gov in the address; educational institutions or medical schools have .edu in the address; professional organizations will be identified as .org. These are usually the best websites to use to obtain health information. MedlinePlus, NIH Senior Health, Centers for Disease Control and Prevention, and Healthfinder provide credible information and can get you started by pointing to other credible sites.
> - The site should clearly identify the sponsor of the site, including the identities of commercial and noncommercial organizations that have contributed to funding, service, or material on the site. Some commercial websites (.com) have valuable or credible information (e.g., www.mayoclinic.com), but others may represent a specific company using the web for commercial reasons—to sell products. Advertisements should be labeled.
> - PURPOSE: Is the purpose of the site to inform? Is it to sell a product? Is it to raise money? Be cautious about sites trying to sell a product or service. If it sounds too good to be true, it probably is.
> - CURRENCY: The site should be updated frequently and be consistently available, with the date of the latest revision clearly posted (usually at the bottom of the page).
> - FACTUAL INFORMATION: Information should be presented in a clear manner capable of being verified. Information presented as opinion should be clearly stated and the source should be identified as a qualified professional or organization.
> - AUDIENCE: The website should state if information is intended for the consumer or health professional.
> - OTHER: Reliable websites have a policy about how they establish links to other sites. Look for the site's linking policy, often found in a section titled "About This Web Site."
> - Check the Privacy Policy and be cautious about providing personal information until you determine what is done with your information.
> - Check with your health care provider before using information found on web searches.

Adapted from Medline Plus: *Medline Plus guide to healthy Web surfing*, 2012. http://www.nlm.nih.gov/medlineplus/healthywebsurfing.htm; Medical Library Association: *Find and evaluate health information on the Web*, 2014. https://www.mlanet.org/resources/userguide.html. Accessed March 23, 2014.

care system. Income and education are the strongest predictors of health literacy. However, anyone can have low health literacy, including people with good literacy skills. Most people will have trouble understanding health information at some point in their lives. In today's complex health care system health literacy also includes the ability to obtain and apply relevant information, understand visual information, operate a computer, search the Internet and evaluate websites, calculate or reason numerically, and interact with health professionals.

Health Literacy and Older Adults

Some older adults may be disproportionately affected by inadequate health literacy. Chronic illness and sensory impairments further contribute to challenges related to communication and understanding. Older adults have lower health literacy scores than all other age groups. Today, more than half of individuals older than 65 years of age are at the below-basic level (MacLeod et al, 2017). Older adults are a heterogeneous group

HEALTHY PEOPLE 2020

Information Technology, Health Literacy

Goal

Use health communication strategies and health information technology (IT) to improve population health outcomes and health care quality and to achieve health equity.

Objectives

- Improve the health literacy of the population.
- Increase the proportion of persons with access to the Internet.
- Increase the proportion of persons with broadband access to the Internet.
- Increase the proportion of persons who use mobile devices.
- Increase the proportion of persons who use the Internet to keep track of personal health information, such as care received, test results, or upcoming medical appointments.
- Increase the proportion of persons who use the Internet to communicate with their health provider.
- Increase the proportion of health-related websites that meet three or more evaluation criteria disclosing information that can be used to assess information reliability.
- Increase the proportion of online health information seekers who report easily accessing health information.

Data from U.S. Department of Health and Human Services, Office of Disease Prevention and Health Promotion: *Healthy People 2020*, 2012. http://www.healthypeople.gov/2020.

in their characteristics and literacy skills, so strategies to enhance their understanding of health information need to be individualized. However, as the major consumers of health care in this country, many are at risk for poor outcomes related to understanding of health care information and navigating the health care system.

RESEARCH HIGHLIGHTS A

The study evaluated the degree of health literacy in a sample of Portuguese older adults using the Newest Vital Sign (NVS) test to assess health literacy. Participants included 433 individuals over 65 years of age, primarily female, and with heterogeneous levels of education. The NVS proved to be a reliable and sensitive assessment of health literacy in this study. Eighty percent of participants showed a low level of health literacy. Variables that significantly affected the level of health literacy among participants were: gender, educational attainment, age, and marital status, and the individual's perception of general health and quality of life. Educational level is one of the factors that most contributes to health literacy. Participants who reported their health as poor had lower than average health literacy scores. The authors recommend that policy makers, health care organizations, and professionals take responsibility for the development of educational interventions promoting health literacy. There are few international studies on health literacy and further investigation is needed.

From Veiga S, Serrao C: Health literacy of a sample of Portuguese elderly, *Appl Res Health Soc Sci Interface Interaction* 13(1):14–25, 2016.

PROMOTING HEALTHY AGING: IMPLICATIONS FOR GERONTOLOGICAL NURSING

An integral part of the nursing role across the continuum is provision of health information. Older adults are the major users of health care, so nurses will have many opportunities to provide health education to this age group. Knowledge of health literacy and its relationship to health status in older adults is a growing area of concern (MacLeod et al, 2017). In addition to poorer health literacy skills, some older adults may also have multiple risk factors that affect their ability to understand and use health information (sensory changes, cognitive changes, complex medical regimens). Knowledge of the principles of geragogy, an understanding of health literacy, excellent communication skills, creativity, cultural competence, and knowledge of what matters most to the person are essential.

Assessment

There are many widely available resources (Box 5.9) that nurses can use to assess health literacy and design effective teaching programs (brochures, one-to-one or group teaching, web resources). Identifying high-risk older adults (non-English speakers, less than high school education) can assist in targeting interventions (Chapter 4). There are several validated easy-to-administer health literacy screening tools readily available (Wide Range Achievement Test-Revised [WRAT-R], Rapid Estimate of Adult Literacy in Medicine, Test of Functional Health Literacy in Adults, and Newest Vital Signs assessment). Health literacy screening in clinical care settings would be a beneficial tool for older adults (Chesser et al, 2016). The *Health Literacy Universal Precautions Toolkit* (AHRQ, 2013) was developed to help structure the delivery of care as if every patient had limited health literacy. This strategy may benefit everyone, regardless of health literacy levels, because it improves understanding.

Interventions

Studies show that older adults prefer to receive health information during interactions with health professionals rather than from the Internet (Cutilli et al, 2018). Patient education materials should use plain language and provide information at no higher

BOX 5.9 Resources for Best Practice

Health Literacy/Teaching Older Adults

Agency for Healthcare Research and Quality (AHRQ): Health literacy universal precaution toolkit

Centers for Disease Control and Prevention (CDC): Improving health literacy for older adults; Simply Put: a guide for creating easy-to-understand materials

Health Resources and Services Administration (HRSA): Effective communication for healthcare professionals (free online course)

National Institutes of Health (NIH) Senior Health: Helping older adults search for health information online: a toolkit for trainers

Speros C: More Than Words: Promoting Health Literacy in Older Adults, *OJIN*: http://ojin.nursingworld.org/MainMenuCategories/ANAMarketplace/ANAPeriodicals/OJIN/TableofContents/Vol142009/No3Sept09/Health-Literacy-in-Older-Adults.aspx. Strategies to improve health literacy in older adults for health professionals

United States Department of Health and Human Services (USDHHS), Office of Disease Prevention and Health Promotion: A guide to writing and designing easy-to-use health websites; Quick guide to health literacy and older adults; Plain language: a promising strategy for clearly communicating health information and improving health literacy

than a sixth-grade level in the person's language (may vary depending on person's abilities), be culturally appropriate, and use varying methods to communicate information (pictures, videos). The Centers for Medicare and Medicaid Services (CMS) describes written material as clear and effective when it meets the following criteria: (1) attracts the intended reader's attention; (2) holds the reader's attention; (3) makes the reader feel respected and understood; (4) helps the reader understand the messages in the material; and (5) moves the reader to take action. Translation of materials should be done by certified medical interpreters or a native speaker of the target language rather than by the literal translation of English to another language because many concepts cannot be translated (Pearce and Clark, 2013).

RESEARCH HIGHLIGHTS B

Discharge instructions for low-literate diverse older adults following hip replacement surgery were designed using pictographs (simple line drawings with stick figures showing explicit care actions). The pictographs were evaluated for acceptability and comprehension. All were well received by all participants of various races/ethnicities and they felt the pictograph instructions helped them understand the health care messages, particularly for step-by-step procedures and postdischarge care. Pictographs are culturally and language neutral, making them appropriate for different ethnicities, ages, languages, and genders. The pictograph approach is an effective strategy for discharge instructions for patients with low literacy levels and also for immigrants with significant communication challenges. Using pictographs may also be appropriate as a supplement to written instructions.

Further research is needed to evaluate this approach and compare it with text-based instructions on adherence to instructions and health outcomes.

From Choi J: Older adults' perceptions of pictograph-based discharge instructions after hip replacement surgery, *J Gerontol Nurs* 39(7), 48–54, 2013.

BOX 5.10 Tips for Best Practice

Strategies to Improve Health Literacy in Older Adult Learners

Manage the Teaching Environment
- Schedule appointment when individual is rested
- Ensure comfort (appropriate seating, room temperature, pain medication if needed).
- Limit session to 10 to 15 minutes
- Observe for signs of fatigue, discomfort during session

Improve Oral Communication
- Pay attention to vision and hearing deficits (face individual, speak slowly, keep pitch of voice low, eliminate background noise)
- Adapt materials for culture, language, health literacy
- Limit content to three to five points and repeat key points frequently
- Be specific and concrete; use plain language
- Connect new learning to past experiences
- Conclude with brief summary of essential points

Modify Written Communication
- Use 16–18 point Arial font for written material with both uppercase and lowercase letters
- Use high contrast on printed materials (dark colors for text and lighter for background, black print on white)
- Use gestures, demonstrations, and pictures in addition to printed material
- Bold key points
- Avoid charts with rows and columns
- Use lots of white space

Evaluate Comprehension
- Use "teach-back" methods to ensure understanding
- Have individual paraphrase instructions
- Have individual demonstrate and provide feedback
- Encourage individual to teach family/caregivers in your presence

Individuals should be able to both understand and use the information presented. Using the "teach-back" (also known as "show-me" or "closing the loop") method involves having people explain back to you or demonstrate what you have told them. For example, you might say "I want to be sure you understand your medication correctly. Can you tell me how you are going to take this medicine?" (Box 5.10). Because medication management is a high-risk activity for older adults, attention to improving older adults' ability to understand their medications and take them correctly is essential. In addition to effective teaching, simplified drug regimens, and use of assistive medication management devices, pharmaceutical companies should be encouraged to develop educational materials at lower literacy levels to ensure comprehension.

There are relatively few studies specifically examining health literacy in older adults and strategies to improve the health literacy of older adults (Chesser et al, 2016). Nurses should be advocates for continued development and research on the most effective age-specific, culturally appropriate health literacy materials and interventions. Interventions for diverse populations are particularly important (Lee et al, 2017).

KEY CONCEPTS

- Although there are changes in the aging brain, cognitive function, in the absence of disease, remains adequate. Any changes in cognitive function require adequate assessment.
- The aging brain maintains resiliency or the ability to compensate for age-related changes. Developing knowledge refutes the myth that the adult brain is less plastic than the child's brain and can strengthen and increase neuronal connections.
- Late adulthood is no longer seen as a period when growth has ceased and cognitive development halted; rather, it is seen as a life stage programmed for plasticity and the development of unique capacities.
- Attention to brain health throughout life is just as important as attention to physical health.
- Learning in late life can be enhanced by utilizing principles of geragogy and adapting teaching strategies to minimize barriers such as hearing and vision impairment and low literacy.
- Older adults are disproportionally affected by inadequate health literacy, and nurses must ensure that health information is provided in an appropriate manner to ensure understanding.

CRITICAL THINKING QUESTIONS AND ACTIVITIES

1. Review the myths about aging and the brain (Box 5.1). Were any of the facts surprising to you?
2. Partner with another student and use the checklist of promoting cognitive health (Fig. 5.2). Discuss what areas may need improvement to enhance cognitive health in aging.
3. What types of health teaching would you provide to a young adult to enhance cognitive health in aging?
4. Work with another student and design a brochure to teach older adults about interventions to enhance cognitive health. What adaptations would you incorporate to ensure understanding for individuals with low health literacy?

RESEARCH QUESTIONS

1. What do older adults of different cultures believe about aging and brain function?
2. What types of cognitive stimulating activities do older adults report engaging in on a daily basis?
3. What strategies to improve the understanding of health information are most effective for older adults?
4. What are the learning needs of older adults related to the use of computers?
5. What do older adults perceive as the benefits of participation in social networking sites such as Facebook?

REFERENCES

Agency for Healthcare Research and Quality: *Health literacy universal precautions toolkit,* 2013. www.ahrq.gov/professionals/quality-patient-safety/quality-resources/tools/literacy-toolkit/index.html. Accessed October 30, 2017.

Agency for Healthcare Research and Quality: Interventions to prevent age-related cognitive decline, mild cognitive impairment and clinical Alzheimer's-type dementia, *Comp Eff Rev* 188, 2017. https://effectivehealthcare.ahrq.gov/topics/cognitive-decline/research-2017/. Accessed October 22, 2017.

Centers for Disease Control and Prevention (CDC): *Health literacy,* 2017a. https://www.cdc.gov/healthliteracy/index.html. Accessed October 30, 2017.

Centers for Disease Control and Prevention (CDC): *Healthy Brain Initiative,* 2017b. https://www.cdc.gov/aging/healthybrain/index.htm. Accessed January 2019.

Centers for Disease Control and Prevention (CDC): *What is a healthy brain? New research explores perceptions of cognitive health among diverse older adults,* 2017c. https://www.cdc.gov/aging/pdf/Perceptions_of_Cog_Hlth_factsheet.pdf. Accessed October 2017.

Chesser AK, Keene Woods N, Smothers K, Rogers N: Health literacy and older adults, *Gerontol Geriatr Med* 2:2333721416630492, 2016.

Crowley SL: Aging brain's staying power, *AARP Bulletin* 37:1, 1996.

Culley JM, Herman JA, Smith D, Tavakoli A: Effects of technology and connectedness on community-dwelling older adults, *Online J Nurs Inform* 17(3), 2013.

Cutilli CC, Simko LC, Colbert AM, Bennett IM: Health literacy, health disparities, and sources of health information in U.S. older adults, *Orthop Nurs* 37(1):54–65, 2018.

Davis SW, Luber B, Murphy DLK, Lisanby SH, Cabeza R: Frequency-specific neuromodulation of local and distant connectivity in aging and episodic memory function, *Hum Brain Mapp* 38(12):5987–6004, 2017.

Derby CA, Katz MJ, Lipton RB, Hall CB: Trends in dementia incidence in a birth cohort analysis of the Einstein Aging Study, *JAMA Neurol* 74(11):1345–1351, 2017.

Desai AK, Grossberg GT, Chibnall JT: Healthy brain aging: a road map, *Clin Geriatr Med* 26(1):1–16, 2010.

Fick DM: Promoting cognitive health, *J Gerontol Nurs* 42(7):4–6, 2016.

Grossman I, Na J, Varnum ME, Park DC, Kitayama S, Nisbett RE: Reasoning about social conflicts improves into old age, *Proc Natl Acad Sci USA* 107(16):7246–7250, 2010.

Hendrie HC, Albert MS, Butters MA, et al: The NIH Cognitive and Emotional Health Project: report of the Critical Evaluation Study Committee, *Alzheimers Dement* 2:12–32, 2006.

Hill NL: Person-centered technology for older adults, *J Gerontol Nurs* 43(4):3–4, 2017.

Jeffrey S: More evidence brain games boost cognitive health, *Medscape Medical News from the Alzheimer's Association International Conference,* 2014. http://www.medscape.com/viewarticle/828285#3. Accessed July 2014.

Laditka SB, Corwin SJ, Laditka JN, et al: Attitudes about aging well among a diverse group of older Americans: implications for promoting cognitive health, *Gerontologist* 49(Suppl 1):S30–S39, 2009.

Larson EB: Prevention of late-life dementia: no magic bullet, *Ann Intern Med* 168(1):77–79, 2018.

Lee SJ, Song M, Im EO: Effect of a health-literacy-considered diabetes self-management program for older adults in South Korea, *Res Gerontol Nurs* 10(5):215–225, 2017.

Lin FR, Yaffe K, Xia J, et al: Hearing loss and cognitive decline in older adults, *JAMA Intern Med* 173(4):293–299, 2013.

MacLeod S, Musich S, Gulyas S, et al: The impact of inadequate health literacy on patient satisfaction, healthcare utilization, and expenditures among older adults, *Geriatr Nurs* 38(4):334–341, 2017.

McEvoy CT, Guyer H, Langa KM, Yaffe K: Neuroprotective diets are associated with better cognitive function: the Health and Retirement Study, *J Am Geriatr Soc* 65:1857–1862, 2017.

National Academies of Science, Engineering, Medicine: *Preventing cognitive decline and dementia: A way forward,* 2017, National Academies of Science. http://www.nationalacademies.org/hmd/Reports/2017/preventing-cognitive-decline-and-dementia-a-way-forward.aspx. Accessed October 27, 2017.

National Institute on Aging: *Cognitive health and older adults,* 2017a. https://www.nia.nih.gov/health/cognitive-health-and-older-adults. Accessed October 22, 2017.

National Institute on Aging: *What's the connection between hearing and cognitive health?* 2017b. https://www.nia.nih.gov/news/whats-connection-between-hearing-and-cognitive-health. Accessed October 27, 2017.

Pearce T, Clark D: Strategies to address low health literacy in the older adult, *Top Geriatr Rehabil* 29(2):98–106, 2013.

Petersen RC, Lopez O, Armstrong MJ, et al: Practice guideline update summary: mild cognitive impairment, *Neurology* 90(3):126–135, 2018.

Petrus E, Isaiah A, Jones A, et al: Crossmodal induction of thalamocortical potentiation leads to enhanced information processing in the auditory cortex, *Neuron* 81(3):664–673, 2014.

Pew Research Center: *Social media fact sheet,* 2018. http://www.pewinternet.org/fact-sheet/social-media/. Accessed October 27, 2017.

Pinto C, Tander K: Review article: Cognitive reserve: concept, determinants and promotion, *J Geriatr Ment Health* 3(1):44–51, 2016.

Ramscar M, Hendrix P, Shaoul C, Milin P, Baayen H: The myth of cognitive decline: non-linear dynamics of lifelong learning, *Top Cogn Sci* 6(1):5–42, 2014.

Rebok GW, Ball K, Guey LT, et al: Ten-year effects of the advanced cognitive training for independent and vital elderly cognitive training trial on cognition and everyday functioning in older adults, *J Am Geriatr Soc* 62:16–24, 2014.

Reuter-Lorenz PA, Park DC: How does it STAC Up? Revisiting the scaffolding theory of aging and cognition, *Neuropsychol Rev* 24(3):366–370, 2014.

Tak SH, Beck C, McMahon E: Computer and Internet access for long-term care residents, *J Gerontol Nurs* 33:32–40, 2007.

The National Academies of Sciences, Engineering, Medicine: *Preventing cognitive decline and dementia: A way forward,* 2017. http://nationalacademies.org/hmd/reports/2017/preventing-cognitive-decline-and-dementia-a-way-forward.aspx. Accessed October 22, 2017.

Vance DE: Potential factors that may promote successful cognitive aging, *Nursing (Auckl)* 2:27–32, 2012.

6

Communicating With Older Adults

Theris A. Touhy

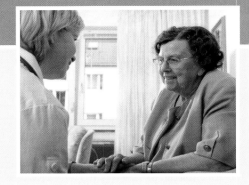

http://evolve.elsevier.com/Touhy/TwdHlthAging

A STUDENT SPEAKS

When they told us we were going to a senior center to interview an older person about their life, I was really nervous. My grandparents are no longer living and I really wasn't close to them when they were alive. I have little contact with older people and to tell you the truth, I find them a little boring. Seems to me they are always complaining and criticizing and talking about the good old days. I am just not sure what I am going to learn from this assignment. I plan to go into pediatrics, so it isn't very relevant to me.

James, age 22

AN OLDER ADULT SPEAKS

I love living in my retirement community but I tell you I miss being around younger people. My grandchildren live far away and I don't see them often. I would enjoy being around the young folks more. They really bring a new perspective on things and have a lot of enthusiasm and energy. It's good to keep up on the new things they are involved in. I think older people and younger people could learn a lot from each other.

Frances, age 82

LEARNING OBJECTIVES

On completion of this chapter, the reader will be able to:

1. Describe the importance of communication to the lives of older adults.
2. Discuss how ageist attitudes affect communication with older adults.
3. Understand the significance of the life story in coming to know older adults.
4. Discuss the modalities of reminiscence and life review.
5. Identify effective methods to facilitate communication with older adults individually and in groups.

Communication is the single most important capacity of human beings. Few things are more dehumanizing than the inability to communicate effectively and engage in social interaction with others. The need to communicate, to be listened to, and to be heard does not change with age or impairment. Meaningful communication and active engagement with society contributes to healthy aging and improves an older adult's chances of living longer, responding better to health care interventions, and maintaining optimal function (Herman and Williams, 2009; Rowe and Kahn, 1998; Van Leuven, 2010; Williams et al, 2008).

For some individuals, opportunities for social interaction may be more limited as a result of loss of family and friends, illnesses, and sensory and cognitive losses. The ageist attitudes of the public, and of health professionals, also present barriers to communicating effectively with older adults (Fick and Lundebjerg, 2017; Saliba, 2017). Good communication skills are the basis for accurate assessment, care planning, and the development of caring relationships between the nurse and the older adult.

This chapter discusses the effect of health professionals' attitudes toward aging on their communication with older adults and communication skills essential to therapeutic interaction. The significance of the life story, reminiscence, life review, and communication with groups of older adults are also included in this chapter. Communication with individuals with hearing and vision loss is discussed in Chapters 11 and 12, and communicating with individuals with cognitive impairment is discussed in Chapter 29.

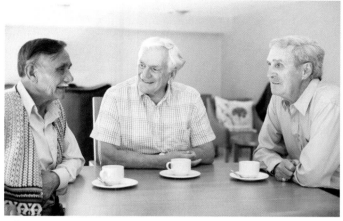

Group of older men talking over coffee. (©iStock.com/Squaredpixels.)

AGEISM AND COMMUNICATION

Beliefs in myths and stereotypes about aging and ageist attitudes on the part of health professionals, society, and older adults themselves can interfere with the ability to communicate effectively. For example, if the nurse believes that all older adults have memory problems or are unable to learn or process information, he or she will be less likely to engage in conversation, provide appropriate health information, or treat the individual with respect and dignity. If an older individual believes that illness is inevitable with increased age, he or she may fail to report changes in health or adopt health promotion strategies.

Robert Butler (1969), the first director of the National Institute on Aging (Bethesda, MD), defined ageism as the systematic stereotyping of and discrimination against people because they are old, in the way that racism and sexism discriminate against color and gender. The FrameWorks Institute (https://frameworksinstitute.org/toolkits/aging/) proposes a current definition that includes both interpersonal and societal effects of ageism. "Ageism is discrimination based on prejudices about age. When ageism is directed at older adults, it often involves the assumptions that older adults are less competent, less attractive, and less vigorous than younger people. Ageism has a huge negative impact on older adults throughout all areas of life" (Sweetland et al, 2017, p. 22) (Box 6.1).

While ageism is found cross-culturally, it is more prevalent in the United States, where aging is viewed with sadness, fear, and anxiety (International Longevity Center, 2006). Some research indicates that individuals in many non-Western cultures are more tolerant toward their elders, perceive older adults as significantly more important to their society, and engage in less avoiding behaviors toward older adults (Bergman et al, 2013).

Ageism also affects health professionals and, with few exceptions, studies of attitudes of students in the health professions toward aging reflect negative views. Examples of the effect of ageism include the small number of students who choose to work in the field of aging and the lack of education of health professionals in the care of older adults, even though the majority of their patients are older (Kydd et al, 2014). Other effects include spending less time with older patients, taking a more authoritarian role, having less patience, providing less information, and neglecting to address important psychosocial and preventive factors (Gerontological Society of America, 2017).

It is important for nurses who care for older adults to be aware of their own attitudes and beliefs about aging and the effect of these attitudes on communication and care provision. Enhancing one's interpersonal communication skills and examining personal and societal attitudes toward aging are the foundation for therapeutic interactions with older adults. Educators play an important part in shaping attitudes of students in the health professions towards older adults (Kydd et al, 2014) (Chapter 2).

Elderspeak

Elderspeak is a form of patronizing speech, similar to "baby talk," which is often used to talk to very young children (Box 6.2). Elderspeak is most likely a cognitive component of ageism (Williams et al, 2017). It is especially common in communication between health care professionals and older adults in hospitals and nursing homes but also occurs in non-health care settings (Corwin, 2017; Williams et al, 2003, 2004, 2016, 2017). Recent research reported that at least one example of elderspeak was identified in 84% of video recording transcripts of interactions between residents and staff during daily care activities. Collective pronoun substitution (e.g., "We are going to take a bath"), and inappropriate terms of endearment such as honey/hon, sweetheart/sweetie were most commonly used (Williams et al, 2017).

Elderspeak is most often used without maliciousness or conscious awareness and nurses may view it as an effective way to communicate with older adults, especially those with cognitive impairment. However, research has shown that use of this form of speech conveys messages of dependence, incompetence, and control. A majority of older adults interpret elderspeak as disrespectful or patronizing. Elderspeak is associated with lower rates of communication ability, social isolation, increased dependence, and cognitive decline.

Use of elderspeak doubles the rates of challenging behaviors of individuals with dementia (Corwin, 2017; Lombardi et al, 2014; Williams et al, 2017) (Chapter 29). Some features of elderspeak (speaking more slowly, repeating, or paraphrasing) may be beneficial in communication with older adults with dementia, and further research is needed. Other examples of communication that conveys ageist attitudes are ignoring the older adult and talking to family and friends as if the person were not present, and limiting interaction to task-focused communication only (Touhy and Williams, 2008).

Communication training offered to nurses in nursing homes reduced their use of some features of elderspeak such as simple vocabulary, reduced grammatical complexity, slow speech rate, and repetition (Williams et al, 2003; Williams et al, 2016; Williams et al, 2017). In addition to avoiding elderspeak, engaging in linguistically complex interaction is a key component in the maintenance of language ability and cognitive and emotional well-being among older adults (Corwin, 2017).

THERAPEUTIC COMMUNICATION WITH OLDER ADULTS

Basic communication strategies that apply to all situations in nursing, such as attentive listening, authentic presence, nonjudgmental attitude, clarifying, giving information, seeking validation of understanding, keeping focus, and using open-ended questions, are all applicable in communicating with older adults. Basically, older adults may need more time to give information or answer questions simply because they have a larger life experience from which to draw information. Sorting thoughts requires intervals of silence, and therefore listening carefully without rushing the older adult is important. Word retrieval may be slower, particularly for nouns and names (Chapter 5).

Open-ended questions are useful but can also be difficult. Those who wish to please, especially when feeling vulnerable or somewhat dependent, may wonder what it is you want to hear rather than what it is they would like to say. The most productive communication will initially focus on the issue of major concern to the individual, regardless of the priority of the nursing assessment. When using closed questioning to obtain specific information, be aware that the individual may feel on the spot, and thus the appropriate information may not be immediately forthcoming. This is especially true when asking questions to determine mental status. The older adult may develop a mental block because of anxiety or feel threatened if questions are asked in a quizzing or demeaning manner.

Older adults may also be reluctant to disclose information for fear of the consequences. For example, if they are having problems remembering things or are experiencing frequent falls, sharing this information may mean that they might have to relinquish desired activities or even leave their home and move to a more protective setting. When communicating with individuals in a bed or wheelchair, position yourself at their level rather than talking over a side rail or standing above them. Pay attention to their gaze, gestures, body language, and the pitch, volume, and tone of their voice, to help you understand what they are trying to communicate. Thoughts unstated are often as important as those that are verbalized. You may ask, "What are you thinking about right now?" Clarification is essential to ensure that you and the individual have the same framework of understanding. Many generational, cultural, and regional differences in speech patterns and idioms exist. Frequently seek validation of what you hear. If you tend to speak quickly, particularly if your accent is different from that of the patient, try to speak more slowly and give the person time to process what you are saying.

THE LIFE STORY

As we age, we accumulate complex stories from the long years lived. Storytelling is a complementary and alternative therapy that nurses can use to enhance communication with older adults (Moss, 2014; Westerhof and Bohlmeijer, 2014). The life story can tell us a great deal about the person and is an important part of the assessment process. Stories provide important information about etiology, diagnosis, treatment, prognosis, and experience of living with an illness from the patient's point of view. Listening to stories is also a way of demonstrating cultural competence (Chapter 4). The nurse can learn much about an older adult's history, communication style, relationships, coping mechanisms, strengths, fears, affect, and adaptive capacity by listening thoughtfully as the life story is constructed.

Listening to memories and life stories requires time and patience and a belief that the story and the person are valuable and meaningful. A memory is an incredible gift given to the nurse, a sharing of a part of oneself when one may have little else to give. The more personal memories are saved for persons who will patiently wait for their unveiling and who will treasure them. Stories are important. "The people who come to see us bring us their stories. They hope they tell them well enough so that we understand the truth in their lives. They hope we know how to interpret their stories correctly" (Coles, 1989, p. 7).

The life story as constructed through reminiscing, journaling, life review, or guided autobiography has held great fascination for gerontologists in the past 30 years. The universal appeal of the life story as a vehicle of culture, a demonstration of caring and generational continuity, and an easily stimulated activity has held allure for many professionals. The most exciting aspect of working with older adults is being a part of the emergence of the life story: the shifting and blending patterns.

Reminiscing

Reminiscing is an umbrella term that can include any recall of the past. Reminiscing occurs from childhood onward, particularly at life's junctures and transitions. Robert Butler (2002) emphasized that in the past, reminiscing was thought to be a sign of senility or what we now call Alzheimer disease. Older adults who talked about the past and told the same stories again and again were said to be boring and living in the past. However, reminiscing is now considered a key developmental skill across the entire life span but an especially important psychological task of older adults. The focus of reminiscing changes as we age and older adults reminisce more frequently for death preparation and to teach/inform others (Westerhof and Bohlmeijer, 2014). The emerging model of reminiscence and well-being has been evaluated with Eastern and Western cultures, but further research is needed about ways of reminiscing among other cultures (Bergman et al, 2013; Cappeliez, 2013; O'Rourke et al, 2012).

For the nurse, reminiscing is a therapeutic intervention important in assessment and understanding. The work of several gerontological nursing leaders, including Irene Burnside, Priscilla Ebersole, and Barbara Haight, has contributed to the body of knowledge about reminiscence and its importance in nursing. There is an official interest group of the Gerontological Society of America, a biannual international conference, and an International Institute for Reminiscence and Life Review. These are valuable resources for nurses and members of other disciplines involved in research and practice. This group also publishes a journal, the *International Journal of Reminiscence and Life Review*.

Reminiscence can have many goals. It not only provides a pleasurable experience that improves quality of life but also improves well-being, alleviates depression symptoms, increases socialization and connectedness with others, provides cognitive stimulation, improves communication, and helps individuals find meaning (Kris et al, 2017; Westerhof and Bohlmeijer, 2014). The process of reminiscence can occur in individual conversations with older adults, be structured as in a nursing history, or can occur in a group where each person shares his or her memories and listens to others sharing their memories. Recent research examined the effect of a story-sharing intervention to improve depression and well-being in older adults transitioning to long-term care (Sullivan et al, 2019). Some suggestions for encouraging reminiscence are presented in Box 6.3.

Intergenerational reminiscence activities could have benefits for both older and younger individuals. In several studies, benefits include increased engagement, enthusiasm, appreciation, respect, and empathy for the older adult (Gammonley et al, 2015; Yamashita et al, 2017). "Nurses in long-term care facilities who engaged in reminiscence activities reported knowing older adults better, thereby enhancing their personhood" (Kris et al, 2017, p. 36 (Research Highlights box). Reminiscence can also be used by family caregivers to enhance communication and strengthen relationships with family members experiencing cognitive impairment (Karlsson et al, 2017; Latha et al, 2014).

Digital storytelling is another medium that can be used with older adults to record their stories and memories across a variety of platforms including tablets and smartphones in a format that can be shared with others. The digital story is a first-person narrative created by combining personal narration, video, animation, artifacts, and music or other sounds. Several studies have examined the use of digital stories to assist nurses and other health care workers to enhance their relationship with residents and contribute to building a sense of community. Digital storytelling is an excellent tool for intergenerational

---

BOX 6.3   Suggestions for Encouraging Reminiscence

- Listen actively without correction or criticism. Older adults are presenting their version of their reality; our version belongs to another generation.
- Encourage older adults to discuss various ages and stages of their lives. Use questions such as, "What was it like growing up on that farm?", "What did teenagers do for fun when you were young?", or "What was World War II like for you?"
- Be patient with repetition and do not interrupt. Sometimes people need to tell the same story often to come to terms with the experience, especially if it was meaningful to them. If they have a memory loss, it may be the only story they can remember, and it is important for them to be able to share it with others.
- Be attuned to signs of depression in conversation (dwelling on sad topics) or changes in physical status or behavior, and provide appropriate assessment and intervention.
- If a topic arises that the person does not want to discuss, change to another topic.
- If individuals are reluctant to share because they do not feel their life was interesting, reassure them that everyone's life is valuable and interesting and tell them how important their memories are to you and others.
- Keep in mind that reminiscing is not an orderly process. One memory triggers another in a way that may not seem related; it is not important to keep things in order or verify accuracy.
- Keep the conversation focused on the person reminiscing, but do not hesitate to share some of your own memories that relate to the situation being discussed. Participate as equals, and enjoy each other's contributions.

- Respond positively and give feedback by making caring, appropriate comments that encourage the person to continue.
- Use props and triggers such as photographs, memorabilia (e.g., a childhood toy or antique, short stories or poems about the past, favorite foods, YouTube videos, old songs).
- Use open-ended questions to encourage reminiscing. If working with a group, you can prepare questions ahead of time, or you can ask the group members to pick a topic that interests them. One question or topic may be enough for an entire group session.
- Consider using questions such as the following:
  - How did your parents meet?
  - What do you remember most about your mother? Father? Grandmother? Grandfather?
  - What are some of your favorite memories from childhood?
  - What was the first house you remember?
  - What were your favorite foods as a child?
  - Did you have a pet as a child?
  - What do you remember about your first job?
  - How did you celebrate birthdays or other holidays?
  - If you were married, what are your memories of your wedding day?
  - What was the greatest accomplishment or joy in your life?

▗▖ RESEARCH HIGHLIGHTS

The purpose of this study was to understand the extent to which reminiscence is used by nursing home staff with cognitively impaired individuals, the reasons why nursing home staff engage in reminiscence activities, and the value they attribute to these activities. The degree to which engagement in reminiscence activities by nursing staff contributed to knowledge about residents was also explored. Participants included 23 licensed nursing staff and 20 certified nursing assistants (CNAs) in three suburban nursing homes in Connecticut. Homes ranged in size from 107–353 beds. Instruments used included a survey that utilized key elements and ideas from previously validated reminiscence surveys and a modified version of the Reminiscence Functions Scale Brief Version. Most of the participants found reminiscence to be enjoyable and valuable in their personal and professional lives (86%). However, fewer than half reported engaging in these activities frequently or very frequently. The authors stated that there may be many reasons for this (lack of time, belief that it is not valuable, or the view that engaging in reminiscence activities or sharing personal experiences with residents is unprofessional). The most frequently used functions of reminiscence were to calm anxiety, help residents to see meaning in life, and reorient confused residents. Those who engaged in reminiscence activities more often reported knowing residents better—a hallmark of high-quality care. Exploring the impediments to reminiscing in this setting and strategies to increase this practice requires further study. A key finding from previous research indicates that residents would prefer to reminisce with staff more frequently and the intervention of reminiscence enhances nurse-patient relationships.

Adapted from Kris A, Henkel L, Krauss K, Birney S: Functions and value of reminiscence for nursing home staff, *J Gerontol Nurs* 43(6):35–44, 2017.

connection that can help nursing students begin to know and value older adults and their life journeys. Technological advances can ease the incorporation of digital stories into regular care delivery and the electronic medical record (Flottemesch, 2013; Gammonley et al, 2015; Karlsson et al, 2017). There are many resources available for those interested in digital storytelling, and community centers and educational institutions, as well as the Internet, provide instruction on this medium (Box 6.4).

BOX 6.4 Resources for Best Practice

Center for Digital Storytelling, Berkeley, CA
Gerontological Society of America: Communicating with older adults: an evidence-based review of what really works, https://www.geron.org/programs-services/alliances-and-multi-stakeholder-collaborations/communicating-with-older-adults.
International Institute for Reminiscence and Life Review, University of Wisconsin, Superior, WI.
Laurenhue K: *Getting to know the life stories of older adults: activities for building relationships,* Baltimore, 2007, Health Professions Press.
Link A: *Group work with older adults: 85 therapeutic exercises for reminiscence, validation, and remotivation,* Sarasota, 2013, Professional Resource Press.
Roberts B: *I remember when: activity ideas to help people reminisce,* Herefordshire, 2000, Elder Books.
TimeSlips: Examples of storytelling with individuals with dementia, training and certification. http://www.timeslips.org/

Reminiscing and Storytelling With Individuals Experiencing Cognitive Impairment

Cognitive impairment does not necessarily preclude older adults from participating in reminiscence or storytelling groups. Opportunities for telling the life story, enjoying memories, and achieving ego integrity should not be denied to individuals on the basis of their cognitive status. Modifications must be made according to the cognitive abilities of the person, and although individual life review from a psychotherapeutic approach is not an appropriate modality, individuals with mild to moderate memory impairment can enjoy and benefit from group work focused on reminiscence and storytelling.

Emerging evidence suggests that reminiscence is an important nonpharmacological intervention for individuals with dementia. Reminiscence and storytelling provide a structure and mechanism for communication and engaging in interaction and can enhance quality of life and improve mood (Cooney et al, 2014; O'Shea et al, 2014; Testad et al, 2014). Results of a study examining the use of reminiscence with people with dementia living in long-term care (Cooney et al, 2014) reported positive outcomes for the residents, staff, and family members. Outcomes for the resident included increased opportunities to socialize and interact, increased enjoyment, and potential changes in behavior (e.g., being more talkative and engaging with residents and staff more). For the staff, increased knowledge about the resident and engaging in relationships were associated with job satisfaction. Family members felt their relative was better known and cared about (as opposed to cared for). For family caregivers, communication skills training that involves reminiscence and life review activities between the caregiver and family member with dementia can increase the quantity and quality of communication between care recipients and caregivers; lower caregiver stress and burden; and reduce behavioral problems.

When the nurse is working with a group of persons who are cognitively impaired, the emphasis in reminiscence groups is on sharing memories, however they may be expressed, rather than specific recall of events. There should be no pressure to answer questions such as "Where were you born?" or "What was your first job?" Rather, discussions may center on jobs people had and places they have lived. Displaying additional props, such as music, pictures, familiar objects (e.g., an American flag, an old coffee grinder) and doing familiar activities that trigger past memories (e.g., having a tea party, folding linens) can prompt many recollections and sharing. The leader of a group with participants who have memory problems must assume a more active approach.

The TimeSlips program (Basting, 2003, 2006, 2013, 2014) is an evidence-based innovation, cited by the Agency for Healthcare Research and Quality (AHRQ, 2014), that uses storytelling to enhance the lives of people with cognitive impairment. Positive outcomes associated with the program include enhanced verbal skills and provider reports of positive behavioral changes, increased communication, increased sociability, and less confusion (Basting, 2013; Phillips et al, 2010). TimeSlips is a beneficial and cost-effective therapeutic intervention that can be used in many settings. See http://www.timeslips.org/ for more information and examples and online training and certification (Box 6.4).

Using the TimeSlips format, group members looking at a picture are encouraged to create a story about the picture. The pictures can be fantastical and funny, such as from greeting cards, or more nostalgic, such as Norman Rockwell paintings. All contributions are encouraged and welcomed, there are no right or wrong answers, and everything that the individuals say is included in the story and written down by the scribe. Stories are read back to the participants during the session, using their names to identify their contributions. At the beginning of each session, the story from the last session is read to the participants. Care is taken to compliment each member for his or her contribution to the wonderful story. The stories that emerge are full of humor and creativity and often include discussions of memories and reminiscing.

One of the authors of this text (T. Touhy) has used the storytelling modality extensively with mild to moderately impaired older adults with great success as part of a research study on the effect of therapeutic activities for persons with memory loss. Qualitative responses from group participants and families indicated their enjoyment with the process. At the end of the 16-week group, the stories were bound into a book and given to the participants with a picture of the group and each member's name listed. Many of the participants and their families have commented on the pride they feel at their "book" and have even shared them with grandchildren and great-grandchildren.

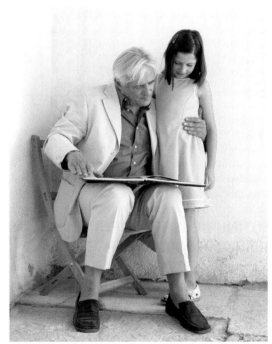

Grandfather sharing stories with his granddaughter. (©iStock.com/ IS_ImageSource.)

Life Review

Robert Butler (1963) first noted and brought to public attention the review process that normally occurs in the older person as the realization of his or her approaching death creates a resurgence of unresolved conflicts. Butler called this process *life review*. Life review occurs quite naturally for many persons

during periods of crisis and transition. However, Butler (2003) noted that in old age, the process of putting one's life in order increases in intensity and emphasis. Life review occurs most frequently as an internal review of memories, an intensely private, soul-searching activity.

Life review is a more formal therapy technique than reminiscence and takes a person through his or her life in a structured and chronological order. Life review therapy (Butler and Lewis, 1983), guided autobiography (Birren and Deutchman, 1991), and structured life review (Haight and Webster, 2002) are psychotherapeutic techniques based on the concept of life review. Gerontological nurses participate with older adults in both reminiscence and life review, and it is important to acquire the skills to be effective in achieving the purposes of both of these techniques. Life review may be especially important for older adults experiencing depressive symptoms and those facing death (Chan et al, 2014; Kris et al, 2017; Pot et al, 2010).

Life review should occur not only when we are old or facing death but also frequently throughout our lives. This process can assist us to examine where we are in life and change our course or set new goals. Butler (2003) commented that ongoing life review by an individual may help avoid the overwhelming feelings of despair that may surface for some individuals at the end of life when there may not be time to make changes.

COMMUNICATING WITH GROUPS OF OLDER ADULTS

Group work with older adults has been used extensively in institutional settings to meet their myriad needs in an economical manner. Nurses have led groups of older adults for a variety of therapeutic reasons. Expert gerontological nurses, such as Irene Burnside and Priscilla Ebersole, have extensively discussed advantages of group work both for older adults and for group leaders and have provided in-depth guidelines for conducting groups. Box 6.5 presents some of the benefits of group work.

BOX 6.5 Benefits of Group Work With Older Adults

- Group experiences provide older adults with an opportunity to try new roles—those of teacher, expert, storyteller, or even clown.
- Groups may improve communication skills for lonely, shy, or withdrawn older people and those with communication disorders or memory impairment.
- Groups provide peer support and opportunities to share common experiences, and they may foster the development of warm friendships that endure long after the group has ended.
- The group may be of interest to other residents, staff, and relatives and may improve satisfaction and morale. Staff, in particular, may come to see their patients in a different light—not just as persons needing care but as persons.
- Active listening and interest in what older people have to say may improve self-esteem and help them feel like worthwhile persons whose wisdom is valued.
- Group work offers the opportunity for leaders to be creative and use many modalities, such as music, art, dance, poetry, exercise, and current events.
- Groups provide an opportunity for the leader to assess the person's mood, cognitive abilities, and functional level on a weekly basis.

Adapted from Burnside IM: Group work with older persons, *J Gerontol Nurs* 20:43, 1994.

BOX 6.6 Special Considerations in Group Work With Older Adults

- The leader must pay special attention to sensory losses and compensate for vision and hearing loss.
- Pacing is different, and group leaders must slow down in both physical and psychological actions depending on the group's abilities.
- Group members often need assistance or transportation to the group, and adequate time must be allowed for assembling the members and assisting them to return to their homes or rooms.
- Time of day a group is scheduled is important. Meeting time should not conflict with bathing and eating schedules, and evening groups may not be good for older people, who may be tired by then. For community-based older people, transportation logistics may become complicated in the evening.
- Groups generally should include people with similar levels of cognitive ability. Mixing cognitively intact older adults with those who have memory and communication impairments calls for special skills. In groups of people with varying abilities, alert persons tend to ask, "Will I become like them?" whereas the people with memory and communication impairments may become anxious when they are aware that they cannot perform as well as the other members.
- Many older people likely to be in need of groups may be depressed or have experienced a number of losses (health, friends, spouse). Discussion of losses and sad feelings can be difficult for group leaders. A leader prone to depression would not be appropriate.
- Remind members of the termination date for the group so that they can prepare and not experience another loss.
- Leaders must be prepared for some members to become ill, deteriorate, and die. Plans regarding recognition of missing members will need to be clear.
- Leaders are continually confronted with their own aging and attitudes toward it. Coleaders are ideal and can support each other. If leading the group alone, locate someone with expertise in group work with elders who can discuss the group experiences with you and provide support and direction. Students generally should work in pairs and will need supervision.
- Evaluate each group session and the total group experience. Involve the group members in the evaluation.

From Burnside IM: Group work with older persons, *J Gerontol Nurs* 20:43, 1994; Stinson C: Structured group reminiscence: an intervention for older adults, *J Contin Educ Nurs* 40(11):521–528, 2009.

Many groups can be managed effectively by staff with clear goals and guidance and training. Volunteers, nursing assistants, students, and recreational staff can be taught to conduct many types of groups, but groups with a psychotherapy focus require a trained and skilled leader. Some basic considerations for group work are presented in this chapter, but nurses interested in working with groups of older adults should consult a text on group work for more in-depth information.

Groups can be implemented in many settings, including adult day health programs, retirement communities, assisted living facilities, nutrition sites, and nursing homes. Examples of groups include reminiscence groups, psychoeducational groups, caregiver support groups, and groups for people with memory impairment or other conditions such as Parkinson disease or stroke. Groups can be organized to meet any level of human need; some meet multiple needs.

Group Structure and Special Considerations

Implementing a group intervention follows a thorough assessment of environment, needs, and the potential for various group strategies. Major decisions regarding goals will influence the strategy selected. For instance, individuals with diabetes in an acute care setting may need health care teaching regarding diabetes. The nurse sees the major goal as education and restoring order (or control) in each individual's lifestyle. The strategy best suited for that would be motivational or educational. A group of people experiencing mild neurocognitive impairment may benefit from a support group to express feelings or a group that teaches memory-enhancing strategies. Successful group work depends on organization, attention to details, agency support, assessment and consideration of the older person's needs and status, and caring, sensitive, and skillful leadership.

Group work with older adults is different from that with younger age groups; and there are some unique aspects that require special skills and training and an extraordinary commitment on the part of the leader. Irene Burnside's (1994)

BOX 6.7 Group Work: The Wisdom of Older Adults

While the chapter author was conducting a weekly reminiscence group with cognitively impaired older adults, we were told by the supervisor that one of our members had died. One of the group members had been a priest so we asked him to say a prayer for our deceased group member. He did so beautifully, and the group was grateful. The next week, to our surprise, the supposedly deceased member showed up for the group (she had been in the hospital). We didn't know how to handle the situation, but the other members came to our rescue by saying, "Father's prayers really worked this time." Older people's wisdom and humor can teach us a lot.

pioneering work in this area remains a model for group work with older adults. Although these unique aspects may not apply to all types of groups of older adults, some strategies are presented in Box 6.6. Box 6.7 shares a story about the wisdom and humor of older adults.

PROMOTING HEALTHY AGING: IMPLICATIONS FOR GERONTOLOGICAL NURSING

Throughout this chapter we have tried to convey the potential for honest and hopeful communication with individuals as they age. Communicating with older adults requires special skills, patience, and respect. We must break through the barriers and continue to reach toward the humanity of the individual with the belief that communication is the most vital service we offer. This is the heart of nursing. Skilled, sensitive, and caring individual and group communication strategies with older adults are essential to meeting needs and are the basis for therapeutic nursing relationships. Just as all people have the need to communicate and have their basic needs met, they also have the right to experiences that are meaningful and fulfilling. Age, language impairment, or mental status does not change these needs. Communication with individuals with cognitive impairment is discussed in Chapter 29.

KEY CONCEPTS

- Communication is a basic need regardless of age or impairment.
- It is important for nurses who care for older adults to be aware of their own attitudes and beliefs about aging and the effect of these attitudes on communication, care provision, and health and well-being.
- The life history of an individual is a story to be developed and treasured. This is particularly important toward the end of life.

- Storytelling is a complementary and alternative therapy that nurses can use to come to know older adults and enhance communication.
- In a rapidly changing society, the shared life histories of older adults provide a sense of continuity among the generations.
- Group work can meet many needs and is satisfying and rewarding for both the older adult and the group leader.

CRITICAL THINKING QUESTIONS AND ACTIVITIES

1. Observe communication styles of people talking to older adults (e.g., in restaurants, stores, and in the health care setting). Do you see examples of elderspeak?
2. Watch some commercials on television that feature older adults. What image do they portray?
3. Ask an older adult whom you know to tell you his or her life story. Reflect on whether or not you learned anything surprising.

4. If you were going to create a digital life story of your own life, what kinds of music, pictures, and artifacts would you include to help people know about your life?
5. Sit with another student and share your life stories. Reflect on what this exercise meant to you and to the other person.

RESEARCH QUESTIONS

1. Are there particular care settings and activities in which elderspeak is more prevalent?
2. What benefits do older adults experience in sharing their life stories?

3. Can digital storytelling be used to promote more positive attitudes toward older adults among nursing students?
4. Does the use of reminiscence and storytelling lead to more holistic assessment of older adults?

REFERENCES

Agency for Healthcare Research and Quality: Weekly group storytelling enhances verbal skills, encourages positive behavior change, and reduces confusion in patients with Alzheimer's and related dementias, 2014, AHRQ Innovations Exchange. https://innovations.ahrq.gov/profiles/weekly-group-storytelling-enhances-verbal-skills-encourages-positive-behavior-change-and/. Accessed November 2017.

Basting AD: Reading the story behind the story: context and content in stories by people with dementia, *Generations* 27:25–29, 2003.

Basting AD: Arts in dementia care: "This is not the end . . . it's the end of this chapter," *Generations* 30:16–20, 2006.

Basting AD: Time Slips: creativity for people with dementia, *Age Action* 28(4):1–5, 2013.

Bergman YS, Bodner E, Cohen-Fridel S: Cross-cultural ageism: ageism and attitudes toward aging among Jews and Arabs in Israel, *Int Psychogeriatr* 25(1):6–15, 2013.

Birren JE, Deutchman DE: *Guiding autobiography groups for older adults: exploring the fabric of life,* Baltimore, 1991, Johns Hopkins University Press.

Burnside IM: Group work with older persons, *J Gerontol Nurs* 20:43, 1994.

Butler R: The life review: an interpretation of reminiscence in the aged, *Psychiatry* 26:65–76, 1963.

Butler R: Age-ism: another form of bigotry, *Gerontologist* 9:243–246, 1969.

Butler R: Age, death and life review. In Doka K, editor: *Living with grief: loss in later life,* Washington, DC, 2003, Hospice Foundation.

Butler R, Lewis M: *Aging and mental health: positive psychosocial approaches,* ed 3, St Louis, MO, 1983, Mosby.

Cappeliez P: Neglected issue and new orientations for research and practice in reminiscence and life review, *Int J Reminiscence Life Rev* 1(1):19–25, 2013.

Chan MF, Leong KS, Heng BL, et al: Reducing depression among community-dwelling older adults using life-story review: a pilot study, *Geriatr Nurs* 35:105–110, 2014.

Coles R: *The call of stories,* Boston, 1989, Houghton Mifflin.

Cooney A, Hunter A, Murphy K, et al: 'Seeing me through my memories': a grounded theory study on using reminiscence with people with dementia living in long-term care, *J Clin Nurs* 23:3564–3574, 2014.

Corwin AI: Overcoming elderspeak: a qualitative study of three alternatives, *Gerontologist* 58:724–729, 2017.

Fick DM, Lundebjerg NE: When it comes to older adults, language matters, *J Gerontol Nurs* 43(9):2–4, 2017.

Flottemesch K: Learning through narratives: the impact of digital storytelling on intergenerational relationships, *Acad Educ Leadersh J* 17(3):53–60, 2013.

FrameWorks Institute: *Framing strategies to advance aging and address ageism as policy issues,* 2017. https://frameworksinstitute.org/toolkits/aging/elements/items/aging_frame_brief.pdf. Accessed November 5, 2017.

Gammonley D, Lester C, Fleishman D, Duran L, Cravero G: Using life history narratives to educate staff members about personhood in assisted living, *Gerontol Geriatr Educ* 36:109–123, 2015.

Gerontological Society of America: *Communicating with older adults: an evidence based review of what really works,* 2012. https://www.geron.org/programs-services/alliances-and-multi-stakeholder-collaborations/communicating-with-older-adults. Accessed November 2017.

Haight B, Webster J: *Critical advances in reminiscence work: from theory to application,* New York, 2002, Springer.

Heliker D: Enhancing relationships in long-term care through story-sharing, *J Gerontol Nurs* 35(6):43–49, 2009.

International Longevity Center, Anti-ageism Task Force: *Ageism in America,* New York, 2006, International Longevity Center.

Karlsson E, Zingmark K, Axelsson K, Sävenstedt S: Aspects of self and identify in narrations about recent events: communication with individuals with Alzheimer's disease enabled by a digital photograph diary, *J Gerontol Nurs* 43(6):25–31, 2017.

Kris AE, Henkel LA, Krauss KM, Birney SC: Functions and value of reminiscence for nursing home staff, *J Gerontol Nurs* 43(6):35–44, 2017.

Kydd A, Touhy T, Newman D, Fagerberg I, Engstrom G: Attitudes toward caring for older adults in Scotland, Sweden and the United States, *Nurs Older People* 26(2):33–40, 2014.

Levy BR, Zonderman AB, Slade MD, Ferrucci L: Age stereotypes held earlier in life predict cardiovascular events in later life, *Psychol Sci* 20:296–298, 2009.

Lombardi NJ, Buchanan JA, Afierbach S, Campana K Sattler A, Lai D: Is elderspeak appropriate? A survey of certified nursing assistants, *J Gerontol Nurs* 40:44–52, 2014.

Moss M: Storytelling. In Lindquist R, Snyder M, Tracy M, editors: *Complementary and alternative therapies in nursing,* ed 7, New York, 2014, Springer, pp 215–228.

O'Rourke N, Carmel S, Chaudhury H, Polchenko N, Bachner YG: A cross-national comparison of reminiscence functions between Canadian and Israeli older adults, *J Gerontol B Psychol Sci Soc Sci* 68(2):184–192, 2012.

O'Shea E, Devane D, Cooney A, et al: The impact of reminiscence on the quality of life of residents with dementia in long-stay care, *Int J Geriatr Psychiatry* 29:1062–1070, 2014.

Perese EF, Simon MR, Ryan E: Promoting positive student clinical experiences with older adults through the use of group reminiscence therapy, *J Gerontol Nurs* 34(12):46–51, 2008.

Phillips LJ, Reid-Arndt SA, Pak Y: Effects of a creative expression intervention on emotions, communication, and quality of life in persons with dementia, *Nurs Res* 59(6):417–425, 2010.

Pot AM, Bahlmeijer ET, Onrust S, Melenhorst AS, Veerbeek M, De Vries W: The impact of life review on depression in older adults: a randomized controlled trial, *Int Psychogeriatr* 22:572–585, 2010.

Rowe JW, Kahn RL: *Successful aging,* New York, 1998, Pantheon Books.

Saliba D: Looking at our words as if seeing them for the first time, *J Gerontol Nurs* 43(9):47–48, 2017.

Stinson CK: Structured group reminiscence: an intervention for older adults, *J Contin Educ Nurs* 40(11):521–528, 2009.

Sullivan GJ, Hain DJ, Williams C, Newman D: Story-sharing intervention to improve depression and well-being in older adults transitioning to long-term care. *Res Gerontol Nurs* 29(1):1-10, 2019.

Sweetland J, Volmert A, O'Neill M: *Finding the frame: an empirical approach to reframing aging and ageism,* 2017, FrameWorks Institute. http://frameworksinstitute.org/assets/files/aging_elder_abuse/aging_research_report_final_2017.pdf. Accessed November 10, 2017.

Testad I, Corbett A, Aarsland D, et al: The value of personalized psychosocial interventions to address behavioral and psychological symptoms in people with dementia living in care home settings: a systematic review, *Int Psychogeriatr* 26:1083–1098, 2014.

Touhy T, Williams C: Communicating with older adults. In Williams C, editor: *Therapeutic interaction in nursing,* ed 2, Boston, 2008, Jones & Bartlett.

Van Leuven KA: Health practices of older adults in good health: engagement is the key, *J Gerontol Nurs* 36:38–46, 2010.

Westerhof GJ, Bohlmeijer ET: Celebrating fifty years of research and applications in reminiscence and life review: state of the art and new directions, *J Aging Stud* 29:107–114, 2014.

Williams KN: Improving outcomes of nursing home interactions, *Res Nurs Health* 29:121–133, 2006.

Williams KN, Herman R, Gajewski B, Wilson K: Elderspeak communication: impact on dementia care, *Am J Alzheimers Dis Other Demen* 24(1):11–20, 2009.

Williams K, Kemper S, Hummert L: Enhancing communication with older adults: overcoming elderspeak, *J Gerontol Nurs* 30:17–25, 2004.

Williams K, Kemper S, Hummert L: Improving nursing home communication: an intervention to reduce elderspeak, *Gerontologist* 43:242–247, 2003.

Williams KN, Perkounkova Y, Herman R, Bossen A: A communication intervention to reduce resistiveness to dementia care: a cluster randomized controlled trial, *Gerontologist* 57:707–718, 2017.

Williams K, Shaw C, Lee A, et al: Voicing ageism in nursing home dementia care, *J Gerontol Nurs* 43(9):16–20, 2017.

Yamashita T, Hahn S, Kinney J, Poon L: Impact of life stories on college students' positive and negative attitudes toward older adults, *Gerontol Geriatr Educ* 39(3):326–340, 2018.

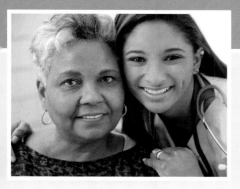

7

Health Assessment

Kathleen Jett

http://evolve.elsevier.com/Touhy/TwdHlthAging

A STUDENT SPEAKS

It takes so long to get a health history from older adults—they have so many stories. I have learned to listen carefully, and I will find out what I need to know to give good nursing care. After all, most of them have had their health problems longer than I have been alive!

Michelle, age 20

AN OLDER ADULT SPEAKS

Whenever I go to one of my doctors I feel like they are rushing through and never really give me a good examination. Then I had an appointment with a nurse practitioner who specializes in us older folks. I couldn't believe the difference. I not only felt listened to, but I also felt like I got the best exam I have had in a long time. I am sure she will help me get better!

Henry, age 76

LEARNING OBJECTIVES

On completion of this chapter, the reader will be able to:

1. Identify the findings of the physical assessment of older adults that differ in meaning from those for younger adults.
2. List the essential components of a comprehensive health assessment of an older adult.
3. Discuss the advantages and disadvantages of the use of standardized assessment instruments.
4. Describe the purpose of the functional assessment when caring for an older adult.

In the promotion of healthy aging, gerontological nurses conduct skilled and detailed assessments of, and with, the persons who entrust themselves to their care. The process is strikingly different from that of younger adults in that it is more complex, even when it is limited to a single problem. Assessment takes more time than it does with younger adults because of their increased medical, functional, and social complexities, and of simply having lived longer. When it is necessary to use a medical interpreter, approximately double the amount of time will be needed (Chapter 4).

Assessment of the older adult requires that the gerontological nurse must be able to listen patiently, allow for pauses, ask questions that are not often asked, observe details, obtain data from all available sources, and recognize the normal changes associated with late life that might be considered abnormal in one who is younger. The quality and speed of the assessment are arts born of experience. Novice nurses should neither be expected to nor expect themselves to do this quickly but should expect to see their skills and efficiency increase over time.

According to Benner (1984), assessment is a task for the expert. However, an expert is not always available. Nurses at all skill levels can learn to conduct health assessments that promote healthy aging by using a high degree of compassion, being aware of the normal changes with aging, and knowing how and when to use reliable instruments.

The assessment provides information critical to goal setting and leads to the development of a plan of care that enhances healthy aging, decreases the potential for complications related to chronic conditions, and increases older adults' self-efficacy and self-care empowerment. The nurse uses the results of the initial assessment as a baseline, in other words, a snapshot of the person's health status at that point in time. Subsequent assessments are used for comparison and modification of goals as the person moves along the wellness trajectory. Health assessment is a complex process that requires entire textbooks to address in detail; often the books have short sections relative to the older adult. In this chapter we provide an overview of key aspects of the geriatric assessment and a discussion of instruments that are unique to, or helpful in, caring for the older adult. Specialized aspects of the geriatric assessment can be found in chapters in this text specific to the issue, such as falls, continence, caregiver burden, and safety.

THE HEALTH HISTORY

The health history marks the beginning of the nurse-patient relationship in the assessment process. The health history in an older adult will take longer because of both the high number of concurrent illnesses and the unknown etiologies of some of these. It is collected through the completion of a form by the patient in advance of the health care contact, through a face-to-face interview, or, most often, through a combination of the two (Box 7.1). The data needed for the health history include demographic information, a past medical history, current medications and dietary supplements (prescribed, over-the-counter, "home remedies," and herbals), functional status, and social histories. Too often an incomplete aspect of the health history is the presence or absence of advance directives (Chapter 35). Copies of these and other related documents should be obtained. All other medical information is transferred into an electronic medical record (EMR).

A discussion of functional status may be one of the more difficult parts of the health history because it deals with the degree of a person's ability to manage independently. It includes histories, such as falls, ability to manage every day activities, such as cooking, and driving record. These must be discussed with the utmost tact to avoid embarrassing the person who has developed limitations, such as the inability to hold a spoon without spilling its contents because of tremors. In many Asian cultures such an admission runs counter to the concept of "saving face," where it is necessary to preserve dignity, or at least its appearance, at all costs (Kim et al, 2004). Most often, the history of functional status is in the form of a screening tool, several of which are discussed later in this chapter.

The social component of the health history is often a part of the functional assessment. Several of the instruments discussed later in this chapter address the collection of these data. It includes a discussion of social networks and specifically who would be available, if support, physical care, or transportation were needed. It is very important that the social history includes information about those who are involved in health care decision-making, such as health care proxies or surrogates (Chapter 31). The gerontological nurse must be cognizant of the fact that persons in their 90s and 100s may have outlived children and perhaps all other relatives.

BOX 7.1   Factors Affecting the Collection of Information for the Health History

Visual and auditory acuity
Manual dexterity
Language and health fluency
Adequacy of translation of materials
Availability of a trained interpreter
Cognitive ability and reading level

Review of Systems

The final part of the health history is the review of systems (ROS), or the person's report of symptoms (or lack of them) in each body system. In a younger adult it is likely to be quick with most systems asymptomatic. However, as one ages and collects health problems, this review becomes more complex and time consuming because one system affects another. Very often the systems reviewed are limited to those associated with the symptom(s) and other relevant systems. When no symptoms are mentioned by the patient, the ROS begins with the systems associated with the person's chronic conditions or the problems are most likely to be problematic in the country, race, ethnicity, socioeconomic class, or age of the patient (Box 7.2).

It is ideal to obtain the history from the person himself or herself. This allows the gerontological nurse to better understand the person's priorities. If this is not possible, it is necessary to obtain the information from a proxy, that is, someone who knows the person well and has permission to speak on the person's behalf. In some cases, the person with a cognitive impairment can still be part of the process when simple language is used, such as "Are you having any pain today?" or "Where are you hurting?"

Kleinman's explanatory model provides questions to supplement the usual data collected in the health history. It will enable the nurse to better understand the older adult and plan individually designed and effective interventions (Box 4.11) (Kleinman, 1980).

PHYSICAL ASSESSMENT

The ROS is followed by or accompanies the physical assessment, depending on the stamina of the patient or other time constraints. When a comprehensive examination is needed, this is often done over the course of two appointments depending on the level of complexity of the current health problems and functional status.

Many of the manual techniques of the physical examination, such as the use of the otoscope, do not differ from those used with younger adults; however, it is always necessary to consider the normal changes with aging and their effect on both the exam and the findings (Box 7.3). When either physical or cognitive limitations are present it is not always possible to perform these tests as precisely as is ideal in all settings (Box 7.4). For example, in the outpatient setting, a thorough abdominal exam may not be possible if the person cannot assume a lying position because of arthritis, kyphosis, or other skeletal deformity. Instead, the best that can be done is for the person to lean as far back in the chair as possible and then for the examiner to auscultate, percuss, and palpate as usual. (This is documented as a "limited abdominal exam.") It is highly unlikely that a complete "head-to-toe" exam is done, except under special circumstances, such as the "Welcome to Medicare" visit (Box 7.5) (Zambas, 2010). It is always best that the exam begins with the presenting problem(s), the associated systems, and the problems/symptoms that place the person at most risk, such as evidence of any of the geriatric syndromes (Box 7.6). In many cases, the aspects of the exam that require special attention are determined by the setting and purpose of the assessment. It is always necessary to be aware of cultural rules of etiquette and taboos that influence the physical examination (Box 7.7).

BOX 7.2 Tips for Best Practice

Review of Systems With Older Adults

Areas of Emphasis

Constitutional

- Changes in the level of energy? Change in appetite?

Senses

- Changes in vision? Sudden or slowly and what type?
- Changes in hearing acuity? In certain situations or noted by others? Recent check for cerumen impaction? Recent hearing aid "checkup"?
- Increase in dental caries; changes in taste, bleeding gums, or level of current dental care?
- Changes in smell?
- Changes in sensation? Less or more? Pain[a]?

Respiratory

- Shortness of breath and, if so, under what circumstances?
- Need to sleep in chair or elevated on pillows?
- If taking "inhalers/puffers" are more doses required to achieve the same result?

Cardiac

- Chest, shoulder, or jaw pain and under what circumstances?
- Sense of heart palpitations?
- If using anticoagulants, including aspirin, any evidence of bruising or bleeding?

Vascular

- Cramping or pain in extremities?
- Edema, what time of the day and how much (can still wear usual shoes)?
- Change of color of the skin, if so, what color?

Urinary

- Changes in urine stream or difficulty starting stream?
- Incontinence, if this is new, under what circumstances and amount?

Sexual

- Change in usual desire or ability to participate in physical sexual activity?
- Changes with aging that may affect sexual activity (e.g., vaginal dryness, erectile dysfunction)?

Musculoskeletal

- Pain in joints, back, or muscles?[a]
- Changes in gait and sense of safety in ambulation?
- If stiffness is present, when is it the worst and is it relieved by activity?
- If limited mobility or movement, effect on day-to-day life? Independence?

Neurological

- Changes in sensation, especially in extremities?
- Changes in memory other than very minimal?
- Ability to continue usual cognitive activities? Change in memory?
- Changes in sense of balance or episodes of dizziness?
- History of falls, trips, slips?

Gastrointestinal

- Incontinence, constipation, bloating, anorexia?
- Dyspepsia or reflux?

Integument

- Dryness, frequency of injury, and speed of healing?
- Itching, dryness, history of skin cancer?

[a]If reports having pain then thorough pain assessment must be completed, see Chapter 27.
Adapted from Elsawy B, Higgins KE: The geriatric assessment. *Am Fam Physician* 83(1):48-56, 2011.

BOX 7.3 Tips for Best Practice

Special Considerations When Conducting a Physical Assessment With an Older Adult

Height and Weight

- Monitor for changes in weight.
- Weight gain: especially important if the person has any heart disease; be alert for early signs of heart failure.
- Weight loss: be alert for indications of malnutrition from dental problems, depression, or cancer. Check for mouth lesions from ill-fitting dentures. There is an increased rate of mortality for rapid weight loss in persons with dementia.

Temperature

- Even a low-grade fever could be an indication of a serious illness. Temperatures as low as 100° F may indicate pending sepsis.

Blood Pressure

- Positional blood pressure readings should be obtained because of the high occurrence of orthostatic hypotension (drop of 20/10 mm Hg or more when changing from sitting to standing). Isolated systolic hypertension is common. Common auscultatory gap heard due to high rate of hypertension.

Skin

- Check for skin cancer especially in those with solar damage. Due to thinning, "tenting" is not a good indicator of hydration status.

Ears

- Increased hair in the canals may make visualization of the tympanic membrane difficult.

- It may not be possible to straighten out the canal completely. Begin by pulling back gently with otoscope in canal until tympanic membrane is visible.

Hearing

- Cerumen dries and impactions are common. These must be removed before hearing and tympanic membrane can be adequately assessed.
- High-frequency hearing loss (presbycusis) is common.
- Evaluate functional hearing by determining the volume needed by nurse for consistent understanding.

Eyes

- Small pupils common (miosis). Normal if equal bilaterally. Gray ring around the iris (arcus senilis) normal. Sagging of upper lids.

Vision

- If Snellen chart is not available, a newspaper can be used for test of visual acuity, recording heading level that is easy to read (with reading glasses if worn).
- Increased glare sensitivity, decreased contrast sensitivity, and need for more light to see and read can be expected.
- Decreased color discrimination may affect ability to self-administer medications safely.

Mouth

- Excessive dryness common and exacerbated by many medications. Periodontal disease common. Decreased sense of taste and thirst. Tooth surface abraded.

Continued

BOX 7.3 Tips for Best Practice—cont'd

Special Considerations When Conducting a Physical Assessment With an Older Adult

Neck
- Because of loss of subcutaneous adipose tissue it may appear that carotid arteries are enlarged when they are not.

Chest/pulmonary
- Any kyphosis or barrel chest will alter the location of the lobes, making careful assessment more important. Crackles in lower lobes may clear with cough.
- Risk for aspiration pneumonia increased and therefore the importance of the lateral exam and measurement of oxygen saturation.

Heart
- Listen carefully for murmurs and third and fourth heart sounds. Fourth heart sounds are somewhat common. A third heart sound is suggestive of heart failure.
- Presence of edema, especially lower extremities.

Extremities
- Dorsalis pedis and posterior tibial pulses very difficult to palpate. Must look for other indications of vascular integrity. Edema common.

Abdomen/Gastrointestinal
- Because of deposition of fat in the abdomen, auscultation of bowel tones may be difficult.
- If concerned about incontinence or constipation, gentle rectal exam may be needed, hemorrhoids common. Occult blood test can be done at same time.

Musculoskeletal
- Osteoarthritis very common and pain often undertreated. Ask about pain and function in joints. Conduct very gentle passive range-of-motion (ROM) exercises if active ROM exercises not possible. Do not push past comfort level. Observe for gait disorders. Observe the person get in and out of chair to assess independent function and fall risk.
- Although there is a gradual decrease in muscle strength, it still should remain equal bilaterally.
- Observe for Heberden's nodes.
- Observe gait.

Neurological
- Greatly diminished or absent ankle jerk (Achilles) tendon reflex is common and normal. Decreased or absent vibratory sense of the lower extremities are common. Slowed reflexes are normal but should be equal. Verbal fluency should be intact; assess quality of conversation. Slight memory loss common.

Genitourinary: Male
- Pendulous scrotum with less rugae; smaller penis; thin and graying pubic hair.

Genitourinary: Female
- Small to nonpalpable ovaries; short, dryer vagina; decreased size of labia and clitoris; sparse pubic hair. Use utmost care with exam to avoid trauma to the tissues.

BOX 7.4 An Abbreviated Exam

Alice has severe dementia. She spends most of her time walking around the unit where she lives. When she gets tired she lays down in whatever bed she is near, occupied or not. When an exam in the outpatient clinic was needed, the only way we could examine her was to very quietly and gently "follow her around" as she wandered. An aide was with her and knew exactly how to redirect her back to the clinic hallway.

BOX 7.5 Select Components of the Welcome to Medicare Exam[a]

Comprehensive review of medical and social history
Assessment of risk for depression
Assessment of functional ability and safety
Brief education related to the identified risk factors and the development of a plan to address these factors

[a]These are often conducted by advanced practice gerontological nurse practitioners. There is no charge to the patient. See Chapter 30 for more detail.
For more information see www.cms.gov/Outreach-and-Education/Medicare-Learning-Network-MLN/MLNProducts/downloads/AWV_Chart_ICN905706.pdf.

BOX 7.6 Geriatric Syndromes[a]

Falls and gait abnormalities
Frailty
Delirium
Urinary incontinence
Sleep disorders
Pressure ulcers

[a]Note that there is considerable discussion about the exact "conditions" that are considered "geriatric syndrome." There is agreement that a syndrome is something that does not neatly fit into another disease category.
From Brown-O'Hara T: Geriatric syndromes and their implications for nursing. *Nursing* 43(1):1–3, 2013.

BOX 7.7 Key Points to Consider in Observing Cultural Rules and Etiquette

- Be aware of past experiences in the health care setting.
- Ask if there are persons (e.g., males in the family) who need to be present or involved in some way with the exam.
- Respect the communication style used in the health care setting.
- Do not intrude into personal space without permission.
- Determine general health orientation related to time (past, present, future).
- Inquire as to appropriate wording reference to the person; presume use of last name unless otherwise welcomed (e.g., Mrs. Jones).
- Inquiry as to acceptability of touch during appropriate parts of the exam.
- Inquire as to the acceptability of the gender of provider.

Instruments for Use When Conducting a Physical Assessment

To address the complex interrelationship between parts of the physical assessment, standardized, evidence-based instruments have proven helpful. The website of the Hartford Institute for Geriatric Nursing (https://hign.org/what-we-do/resources/consultgeri) provides a compilation of many tools for individual use. In many cases videos demonstrating their use are included.

Two mnemonics to assist gerontological nurses to remember the parts of the exam are *SPICES* and *FANCAPES*. The resultant findings will indicate the domain where more detailed assessments are needed, many of which are discussed in subsequent chapters.

FANCAPES

The mnemonic *FANCAPES* stands for Fluids, Aeration, Nutrition, Communication, Activity, Pain, Elimination, and Socialization. The guide was developed by Barbara Bent (2005) in her work as a geriatric resource nurse at Missouri Hospital in Ashville, North Carolina. It has broad applicability in any setting.

F: Fluids. An assessment of a person's state of hydration (fluids) includes those physiological, situational, functional, and mental factors that contribute to the maintenance of its adequacy. Attention is directed to the ability of the person to obtain adequate fluids, to express thirst, and to swallow effectively. Medications are reviewed to identify those with the potential to affect intake. This is especially important when working with older adults who are not able to independently access fluids because of functional limitations or for anyone with the reduced sense of thirst, a common change with aging (Chapters 14 and 15).

A: Aeration. Because of the close relationship between pulmonary function (aeration) and cardiovascular function, these are assessed simultaneously. Careful pulmonary auscultation in the older adult should include the lateral aspects of the lower lobes. The measurement of the oxygen saturation rate is a part of this exam and easily done in any setting with a small, inexpensive fingertip device. Many people with heart disease already have these at home and can provide the nurse with very useful information. Those with any amount of chronic peripheral cyanosis will have artificially low readings. It may be necessary to use the toes to check saturation if the person has latex fingernail polish. Assessment of the respiratory rate and depth at rest and with activity should be done any time respiratory or cardiac compromise is suspected (Chapter 25). Assessment of the cardiovascular system is addressed in more detail in Chapter 22.

N: Nutrition. Protein-calorie malnutrition is common among the frail and those who live alone or are socially isolated. Nutritional assessment is a complex process but especially important in frail older adults or those with dementia. For the frail older adult who is losing weight, even with an adequate intake, the risk for mortality escalates considerably.

Assessment of nutritional status and gerontological nurses' responses to alterations in nutrition are addressed in Chapter 14.

C: Communication. While the assessment of communication in the healthy older adult may be the same as that of a younger adult, many of those who are aging today will have or already have some level of communication impairment. Assessment includes the physical capacity to negotiate the environment, meet self-care needs, and communicate effectively, orally, visually, and aurally. With the high rate of hearing loss (presbycusis) and visual compromise (e.g., glaucoma, macular degeneration, presbyopia) this is an important area of assessment that is often overlooked.

A: Activity. The ability to continue to ambulate safely and the capacity to participate in enjoyable physical activities are important parts of healthy living. This does not change with aging. However, an activity assessment is exceedingly complex because of the range of abilities among those referred to as "older adults." As more baby boomers join this group, the complexity of assessment increases. It ranges from the risk for falling; to the need for, and correct use of, assistive devices; to the degree to which one can participate in aerobic exercises. Assessment of activity abilities are often accomplished by the combined efforts of nurses, physical therapists, and personal trainers (Chapters 18 and 19).

P: Pain. The assessment of pain includes that which is physical, psychological, and spiritual. One rarely occurs in isolation. Many nurses hear their patients implore, "What did I do to deserve this [pain]?" Because of the increasing amount of pain common with each decade of life (e.g., progression of arthritis or number of losses), this deserves particular attention by gerontological nurses (Chapter 27).

E: Elimination. Although difficulties with bowel and bladder functioning are not normal parts of aging, they are more common than they are in younger adults and can be triggered by such things as immobility attributable to physical limitations (e.g., post-stroke) or medications (e.g., diuretics). Incontinence can result from cognitive changes that may cause a reduced, or even nonexistent, sensation indicating a need to void or defecate. There are many elimination problems for older adults living in institutional settings where they are dependent on others for assistance to maintain continence (e.g., getting to the toilet in time). If the person is having a problem with bowel or bladder functioning, including incontinence and constipation, and it has not been discussed, the assessment begins by "opening the door" to communication about problems that may be embarrassing to admit, much less discuss. The observant nurse may notice the upper edge of an incontinence brief when examining the chest or the advanced practice nurse may notice peri-genital irritation when conducting a gynecological exam. Providing a safe and nonjudgmental avenue of communication and finding mutually acceptable and understandable language are ways to approach this difficult topic (Chapter 6). Sensitivity is required to determine if such conversations are even culturally acceptable at all.

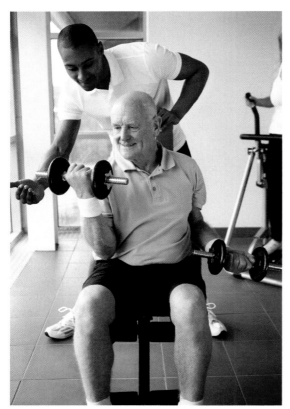

©iStock.com/Dean Mitchell.

S: Social skills. Socialization and social skills include the individual's ability to navigate in society, to give and receive love and friendship, and to feel self-worth. Who is included in one's social network is highly culturally influenced (Box 7.8). Assessment of social skills can be quite complex. It is addressed in more detail in Chapters 33 and 34.

SPICES

As with FANCAPES, the mnemonic *SPICES* helps the nurse remember key aspects of the assessment (Fulmer and Wallace, 2012; Montgomery et al, 2008). *SPICES* refers to six common and very serious geriatric syndromes that require nursing interventions: *S*leep disorders, *P*roblems with eating, *I*ncontinence, *C*onfusion, *E*vidence of falls, and *S*kin breakdown. As with FANCAPES, anything that indicates a problem in one of the categories alerts the nurse to problems that are interfering with the person's health and well-being, particularly those who have

one or more unstable medical conditions or are at risk for further physical and functional decline.

FUNCTIONAL ASSESSMENT

Whereas FANCAPES and SPICES address primarily physical parameters, a functional assessment is the evaluation of a person's ability to carry out the tasks needed for self-care and those needed to support independent living. Other aspects of the functional assessment include the individual's ability to negotiate physical and social environments. The functional assessment helps the gerontological nurse work with the individual to move toward healthy aging by accomplishing the following:

- Identifying the specific areas in which help is needed or not needed
- Identifying changes in abilities from one time to another
- Providing information that may be useful in assessing the safety of a living situation

Evidence-based instruments are available to screen, describe, monitor, and predict an individual's ability to perform the activities or tasks needed for daily living. The activities are considered mutually exclusive and the scoring is arbitrary on most tools. For example, drinking is not broken down into its component parts, such as picking up a cup or swallowing water. It is measured as a total task, when a person may be able to perform one part and not the other. Several of the tools rate and score as (1) can do the task alone, (2) needs assistance, or (3) is not able to perform the task at all. The ratings are done by self-report, proxy, or observation. This type of scoring is not sensitive to small changes and can only be used as part of a holistic assessment. It should be noted that some research has found that self-reports overestimate functional ability and differ from that of proxy report (Sakurai et al, 2013; Stratford et al, 2010). While all the activities of daily living (ADL) tasks are universal human needs, the way they are met are socially and culturally determined. However, the tools are beneficial in that they provide caregivers with a common nomenclature and therefore have the potential to increase the quality of care. When deficits are found in any aspect of functional status, a more detailed assessment is expected of the gerontological nurse or care team.

Activities of Daily Living

The day-to-day functions related to personal needs are referred to as the *ADLs* (Box 7.9). Two of these tasks (dressing [including grooming] and bathing) require higher cognitive function than the others. The ability to feed oneself, in at least some rudimentary manner, remains intact until late in dementia, assuming other health problems do not interfere, such as a dominant-side stroke.

BOX 7.8   **Culturally Constructed Support**

"I grew up in a large extended Catholic family. As a growing child, all of our activities, and even lives, revolved around the Church and the family. Now my cousins have grown and have families of their own. While we have been able to hold on to our affection, we live scattered across the country. Over the years I have also grown apart from the Church. Now that I need support, I don't really have any experience reaching out for it—it was 'just always there.' I stay connected with my family through Facebook, but it is not the same."

Helen, age 52

BOX 7.9   **Activities of Daily Living**

- Bathing
- Dressing
- Toileting
- Transferring
- Continence
- Feeding/eating

Katz Index

ADLs were first classified as such by Sidney Katz and colleagues in 1963 (Katz et al, 1963). The *Katz Index* has served as a basic framework for most of the subsequent measures. The ADLs are considered only in dichotomous terms: the ability to complete the task independently (one point) or the complete inability to do so (zero points) (Skelkey and Wallace, 2012). With equal weight on all activities, this index cannot be used to identify specific areas of need and cannot show change in any one task. Over the years this instrument has been refined to afford more sensitivity to the nuances of, and changes in, functional status (Nikula et al, 2003).

Barthel Index (BI)

The *Barthel index* (BI) (Mahoney and Barthel, 1965) is a quick and reliable instrument for the assessment of both mobility and the ability to perform ADLs. It can be completed in 2 to 3 minutes using self-report or in about 20 minutes when direct observation is necessary. The items are rated in various ways, depending on the item. The BI has been found to be sensitive enough to identify when a person first needs help and to measure progress or decline, especially following a stroke (Quinn et al, 2011).

Functional Independence Measure

The Functional Independence Measure (FIM) was designed to assess a person's need for assistance with ADLs during inpatient stays and for discharge planning, especially following a stroke (Cournan, 2011; Rayegani et al, 2016). In some studies, the BI and FIM were found to be comparable (Sangha et al, 2005). In others the FIM was deemed preferable. The FIM is a highly sensitive instrument and includes measures of ADLs, mobility, cognition, and social functioning. The tasks are rated using a seven-point scale from totally independent to totally dependent. It is a required tool in the rehabilitation setting in Veterans' Administration hospitals in the United States (Shulkin, 2017). Information about this tool is easily found on the Internet.

Functional Assessment Staging Tool

The Functional Assessment Staging Tool (FAST) is unique in that it is descriptive in nature and specific to the functional changes seen and anticipated in persons with a progressive dementia such as Alzheimer's disease (Table 7.1). It was designed by geriatrician Barry Reisberg (1988) to assist clinicians to identify the level (stage) of ability and, in doing so, help the family know what to expect and how to prepare for the changes ahead. It uses an ordinal scale from stage 1 (no functional impairment, associated with any cognitive impairment) to 7 (unable to perform any ADLs, associated with very severe [late stage] cognitive impairment). It has been found to be a reliable and valid instrument for the evaluation and staging of functional decline in persons with Alzheimer's disease (Sclan and Reisberg, 1992).

Instrumental Activities of Daily Living

Those activities considered necessary for independent living in many cultures are referred to as *instrumental activities of daily living or IADLs* (Box 7.10). This does not mean that the person

TABLE 7.1 **Functional Assessment Staging Tool (FAST).**	
Stage 1—Normal adult	Shows no functional decline.
Stage 2—Normal older adult	Shows personal awareness of some functional decline.
Stage 3—Early Alzheimer's disease	Demonstrates noticeable deficits in demanding job situations.
Stage 4—Mild Alzheimer's disease	Requires assistance in complicated tasks such as handling finances or planning parties.
Stage 5—Moderate Alzheimer's disease	Requires assistance in choosing proper attire.
Stage 6—Moderately severe Alzheimer's disease	Requires assistance dressing, bathing, and toileting. Experiences urinary and fecal incontinence.
Stage 7—Severe Alzheimer's disease	Speech ability declines to about a half-dozen intelligible words. Demonstrates progressive loss of abilities to walk, sit up, smile, and hold up head.

From Reisberg B: Functional Assessment Staging (FAST), *Psychopharmacol Bull* 24:653–659, 1998. Copyright ©1984 by Barry Reisberg, MD. Reproduced with permission.

BOX 7.10   Instrumental Activities of Daily Living

- Ability to use telephone
- Abilities related to travel
- Shopping
- Self-medication administration
- Food preparation
- Handling finances
- Housekeeping
- Laundry

BOX 7.11   Evelyn: Moving From Dependence to Independence

When I first met Evelyn, she was 65 and recently widowed. She had married young, moving from her parents' home into that of her husband's. During their entire marriage she had never driven, pumped gas, shopped alone, or taken care of anything but personal and child care, cooking, and house cleaning. She knew nothing about their finances. She had significant instrumental activities of daily living (IADL) deficits but had no choice but to learn how to take care of herself independently after her husband died. She never did learn how to drive very well!

---

performs the tasks, just that he or she could perform them if called upon to do so (Box 7.11). It is generally agreed that the ability to perform IADLs requires higher cognitive and physical functioning than do the ADLs.

The Lawton IADL Scale

The original *Lawton IADL scale* rated the IADLs from zero (lowest functioning) to eight (highest functioning) (Lawton and Brody, 1969). The level of functioning is determined by a summary score. It may be useful as a screening tool to establish an overall baseline of general functioning but, like the Katz Index, it is not sensitive to changes in any one area. The original tool and the subsequent iterations take about 15 minutes to administer using self-report, proxy, or observation. Persons with dementia will progressively lose the ability to perform IADLs beginning with those associated with the highest neuropsychological functioning, such as handling finances and shopping. Unfortunately, it may be biased by age and culture (Cress, 2017; LaPlante, 2010).

FUNCTION AND COGNITION

When conducting health screenings of both function and cognition simultaneously, a slightly different tool is necessary.

Cognition

In a comprehensive assessment, baseline measures of cognition are obtained. For those with potential problems, any screening or testing is often particularly stressful to the person and significant others. An environment and relationship of trust leads to the most accurate assessment possible with the least amount of embarrassment. A cognitive assessment may be honestly described as similar to auscultation of the heart, to "see how the brain is doing." Like most other assessments, these are best administered when the person is comfortable, rested, and free of pain. Gerontological nursing requires the sensitivity to note subtle changes that may indicate a reversible health problem or the need for a more in-depth assessment (Chapter 29).

Mini-Mental State Examination

For many years the Mini-Mental State Examination (MMSE) has been the mainstay for the gross screening of cognitive status (Folstein et al, 1975; Mitchell, 2009). It has been translated into 10 languages (Folstein and Folstein, n.d.). The original 30-item instrument has been revised into a briefer 16-item instrument (MMSE-2) that is used to screen for and monitor a wide range of cognitive skills (orientation, short-term memory and attention, calculation ability, language, and construction). It requires functional vision and manual dexterity. The score can be adjusted for those with low education levels. It has been tested and found comparable to similar cognitive tests. To ensure reliability,

the nurse must be able to administer them correctly each time they are used. The instruments, permission for use, and instructions can be purchased from the Psychological Assessments Resources Company (www.parinc.com).

Clock Drawing Test

The *Clock Drawing Test*, in use since 1992, also tests a range of cognitive skills. It is quick and easy to administer and score. The results have been highly correlated with the MMSE across the world (Aprahamian et al, 2010; Ehreke et al, 2010). It is not appropriate for use with those who are blind or who have limiting conditions such as tremors, or a stroke that affects their dominant hand. While reading fluency is not necessary, completion of the clock test requires number fluency, the ability to hear and see, manual dexterity adequate to hold a pencil, and experience with analog clocks (Fig. 7.1). Scoring is based on the position of both the numbers and the hands. This tool cannot be used as the sole measure for dementia, but it does test for constructional apraxia, an early indicator (Nair et al, 2010). It has been found by some to be useful for ruling-out dementia (Janssen et al, 2017). The clock test is an evidence-based instrument that has been found to be useful across cultures and languages (Borson et al, 1999).

Mini-Cog

In some settings the *Mini-Cog* is being used as a screening tool for cognitive impairment (Borson et al, 2000). It has been found to be as accurate and reliable as the MMSE but less biased, easier to administer, and possibly more sensitive to dementia (Mitchell and Malladi, 2010). The Mini-Cog combines the test of short-term memory with the executive function of the clock test (Boxes 7.12 and 7.13). It has been found to be equally reliable with English-speaking and non–English-speaking individuals (Doerflinger, 2013). It takes 3 to 5 minutes to administer and like the other screening tools discussed in this chapter, only serves as an indicator of the need for more detailed assessments leading to diagnosis. It requires number fluency and the ability

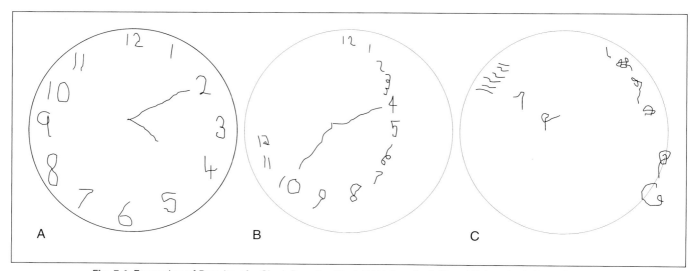

Fig. 7.1 Examples of Results of a Clock Drawing Test. (A) Unimpaired. (B and C) Impaired. (From Stern TA, Rosenbaum JF, Fava M, et al: *Massachusetts General Hospital comprehensive clinical psychiatry*, St Louis, 2008, Mosby.)

BOX 7.12 Instructions for the Administration of the Mini-Cog and Clock Drawing Tests

1. State three unrelated words, such as "chair," "coin," "tree"; state each word clearly and slowly, about 1 second for each.
2. Ask the person to repeat these words; if the person is unable to do so, you may repeat the words up to 3 times to give the person three attempts to say them back to you correctly.
3. The person is asked to draw a clock as in the Clock Drawing Test.
   a. Provide the person with a piece of plain white paper with a circle drawn on it.
   b. Ask the person to draw numbers in the circle so that it looks like a clock, and then to put the hands in the circle to read "10 after 4."
4. The person is asked to recall the three words from step 1.

BOX 7.13 Scoring of the Mini-Cog and Clock Drawing Tests

Scoring

Points are awarded for recalled words first. The following scoring system is used: none remembered, dementia likely; all three words remembered, dementia unlikely; recall of either one or two words then results of the clock drawing must be taken into consideration: normal (all numbers and hands correct) or abnormal (any errors).

There are several suggestions by psychologists about how the clocks are scored. All consider (1) the symmetry of the numbers (able to plan ahead): if all the numbers are included, repeated, or missed; whether they are inside or outside of the circle; if they appear as numbers; and (2) the hands of the clock: whether the numbers appear at all and if they are in the correct place relative to the numbers (abstract thinking).

to hear and see, hold a pencil, and have experience with analog clocks. For a copy of the tool and instructions in its use, see https://www.alz.org/documents_custom/minicog.pdf.

Montreal Cognitive Assessment

The Montreal Cognitive Assessment (MoCA) was designed to be a brief screening instrument to identify mild cognitive impairment. Like the MMSE it is intended to evaluate the person's ability to perform activities in a number of categories: attention and concentration, executive function, memory, language, visuo-constructional skills, conceptual thinking, calculations, and orientation (Nasreddine, 2010). However, the MoCA has proven to be more sensitive than the MMSE (Ciesielska et al, 2016; Nasreddine et al, 2005). It has been found to be applicable in several countries (Fujiwara et al, 2010; Memoria et al, 2013). Due to the complexity of the tests within each category, understandable speech, past math abilities, vision, functional hearing, and ability to use a pencil or pen are necessary.

ASSESSMENT OF MOOD

Assessment of mood is especially important because of the number of illnesses that are common in late life and are associated with depression, such as stroke (33%) and Parkinson's disease (up to 75%). Another group with high rates of depression are those living in long-term care facilities. Rates have been

found from 5% to 82%. Being female and socially isolated increase the person's risk (Fox et al, 2017). Older adults with untreated or undertreated depression are more functionally impaired and will have prolonged hospitalizations and nursing home stays, lowered quality of life, and overall increased morbidity and mortality. Persons with depression may appear to have dementia and many persons with dementia are also depressed (Bowker et al, 2012). The interconnection between the two calls for skill and sensitivity on the part of the nurse to ensure that older adults receive the most appropriate, effective, and timely care possible. Although several tools have been used, the most common one is the Geriatric Depression Scale. The Cornell Scale is an observational tool specifically for persons with dementia (Chapter 28).

Geriatric Depression Scale

The Geriatric Depression Scale (GDS) was developed as a 30-item tool specifically for screening older adults (Brink, 1982; Yesavage et al, 1983). A shortened 15-item version is now used (Table 7.2). It has also been suggested that the short version can be used by some who are aphasic but are able to use a point-board. A score of 5 or greater indicates the potential of a major depressive disorder and indicates the need for a more detailed clinical assessment by a psychiatrist or a mental health advanced practice nurse. The GDS has been extremely successful in identifying depression because it deemphasizes physical complaints, libido, and appetite (Lach et al, 2010). It has been tested extensively with translations in multiple languages (Ortiz and Romero, 2008). With the free resources provided by Drs. Yesavage and Brink, the instrument can be completed on an iPhone or Android with an automatic

TABLE 7.2 Geriatric Depression Scale (Short Form).

Are you basically satisfied with your life?	Yes	No*
Have you dropped many of your activities and interests?	Yes*	No
Do you feel that your life is empty?	Yes*	No
Do you often get bored?	Yes*	No
Are you in good spirits most of the time?	Yes	No*
Are you afraid that something bad is going to happen to you?	Yes*	No
Do you feel happy most of the time?	Yes	No*
Do you often feel helpless?	Yes*	No
Do you prefer to stay at home, rather than going out and doing new things?	Yes*	No
Do you feel you have more problems with memory than most?	Yes*	No
Do you think it is wonderful to be alive?	Yes	No*
Do you feel pretty worthless about the way you are now?	Yes*	No
Do you feel full of energy?	Yes	No*
Do you feel that your situation is hopeless?	Yes*	No
Do you think that most people are better off than you?	Yes*	No

*Each answer indicated by an asterisk counts as 1 point. Scores greater than 5 indicate need for further evaluation. Contact Dr. Yesavage directly at Stanford University in Palo Alto, Calif, or see http://www.stanford.edu/~yesavage/GDS.html.
From Yesavage J, Brink TL, Rose TL, et al: Development and validation of a Geriatric Depression Screening Scale: a preliminary report, *J Psychiatric Res* 17:37, 1982–1983.

calculation of the results that can be downloaded to a computer. Dr. Yesavage may be contacted directly at Stanford University in the United States for more information and the products he has available. See http://www.stanford.edu/~yesavage/GDS.html.

Cornell Scale for Depression in Dementia

The Cornell Scale for Depression in Dementia (CSD-D) was designed to identify major depressive disorders (Alexopoulos et al, 1988; Lim et al, 2012). It can be used with persons with or without dementia. The first person to be interviewed is a proxy followed by an attempted interview with the patient. If he or she is unable to respond to the questions, many of these can be completed through observation. The questions refer to the presence or absence of symptoms of depression in the *week* before the interview. It is considered the gold standard of assessing mood in persons with dementia (Sheehan, 2012). For a downloadable instructions and document, see http://geropsychiatriceducation.vch.ca/docs/edu-downloads/depression/cornell_scale_depression.pdf.

COMPREHENSIVE GERIATRIC ASSESSMENT

In some cases, an integrated approach is used rather than an individual or collection of separate instruments, that is, one that combines physical, functional, and psychosocial components. The most well-known comprehensive tools have been the OARS Multidimensional Functional Assessment Questionnaire (OMFAQ), the Resident Assessment Instrument (RAI), and the Outcomes and Assessment Information Set (OASIS). All are quite comprehensive and therefore lengthy but once completed can serve as a basis for a detailed plan of care. They are all very labor intensive and therefore expensive to administer. The RAI is required for persons in skilled nursing facilities and the OASIS is required for persons receiving skilled care from a home health agency.

The OARS Multidimensional Functional Assessment Questionnaire

The classic *Older Americans Resources and Services* (OARS) was developed at the Center for the Study of Aging and Human Development at Duke University. It was later updated as the OMFAQ (Duke University Center for the Study of Aging and Human Development, 2014). The updated instrument includes (1) an evaluation of the ability, disability, and capacity level at which the person can function and (2) the determination of the extent and intensity of the utilization of resources. In the first section, the assessment is divided into five subscales that may be used separately or alone. The person's functional capacity in each area is rated on a scale of one (excellent functioning) to six (totally impaired functioning). A cumulative impairment score (CIS) is calculated ranging from the most capable (6) to total disability (30). It takes approximately 45 minutes to administer and requires some training. The subscales are described in the following sections. It has been considered one of best tools for the assessment of function (Haywood, 2006).

Social Resources

Social skills and the ability to negotiate and make friends are measures of social resources. Is the person able to ask for things from friends, family, and strangers? Who are the caregivers and how long are they available? Does the person belong to any social network or group, such as a church, synagogue, ashram, or temple that serves as a source of support?

Economic Resources

Information about monthly income and sources to determine the adequacy of income compared with needs. This will provide insight into the older adult's relative standard of living and highlight areas of need that might be alleviated using additional resources (e.g., food stamps).

Mental Health

Consideration is given to intellectual function in the presence or absence of psychiatric symptoms and the amount of enjoyment the person gets from life (Chapter 28).

Physical Health

The current diagnoses, prescribed and over-the-counter medications used, and the person's perception of his or her health status are all parts of assessment of physical health. Excellent physical health includes participation in vigorous activities, such as walking, dancing, or biking at least twice each week. The presence of one or more illnesses or disabilities that are very painful or life-threatening, or that require extensive care indicate seriously impaired physical health.

ADLs and IADLs

The ADLs included in this instrument are the ability to walk, get into and out of bed, bathe and groom oneself (e.g., combing hair, shaving), dress, eat, and get to the bathroom on time. The IADLs include tasks such as dialing the telephone, driving a car, hanging up clothes, obtaining groceries, taking medications, and having the correct knowledge of medication dosages.

The OMFAQ and training materials can be purchased for a nominal fee from the Center for the Study of Aging and Human Development at Duke University (www.sites.duke.edu/centerforaging/?s=OMFAQ&submit=).

Resident Assessment Instrument

In 1986 the Institute of Medicine (IOM) completed a study indicating that although there was considerable variation, residents in skilled nursing facilities in the United States were receiving unacceptably poor care. As a result, nursing home reform was legislated as part of the Omnibus Budget Reconciliation Act (OBRA) of 1987. The creators of OBRA recognized the challenging work of caring for progressively sicker persons discharged from acute care settings to nursing homes and, along with this, the need for comprehensive assessments, complex decision-making, and documentation regarding the care that was needed, planned, implemented, and evaluated.

In 1990 a resident assessment instrument (RAI) was created and mandated for use in all skilled nursing facilities that receive compensation from either Medicare or Medicaid (Chapter 30).

BOX 7.14   Quality Indicators: Factors Considered in the Measurement of Quality of Care Provided in a Skilled Nursing Facility[a]

Short-Term Stay Residents	Long-Term Stay Residents
• Self-report severe pain • Pressure ulcers: new or worsened • Assessed for/given seasonal influenza vaccination • Assessed for/given pneumococcal vaccine • Newly received antipsychotic medication	All of the indicators for short stays **plus**: • One or more falls with major injury • Developed urinary tract infection(s) • Developed incontinence • Had catheter inserted into and left in bladder • Was physically restrained • Increased need for assistance with activities of daily living • Showed excessive weight loss • Showed depressive symptoms • Received an antipsychotic medication

[a]Note that indicators are measured in percentage of residents.
From Centers for Medicare and Medicaid Services: *Quality measures,* 2017. https://www.cms.gov/Medicare/Quality-Initiatives-Patient-Assessment-Instruments/NursingHomeQualityInits/NHQIQualityMeasures.html. Accessed January 2018.

In 2017 both the RAI and the Quality Measures, a portion of the RAI, were updated (CMS, 2017). The Quality Measures provide information to the public regarding specific factors indicative of the care provided and give nursing homes information about specific areas in need of improvement. The Quality Measures are divided into "short stay" (<100 days) and "long stay" (Box 7.14).

Now in its third version, the 450-item *Minimum Data Set* (MDS 3.0), part of the RAI, is the basis for the assessment. As the MDS is analyzed, specific areas of need are identified and guide the development of and revisions to the plan of care (CMS, 2014). Evidence-based assessment tools are included whenever possible (Saliba and Buchanan, 2008). In a significant change from the MDS 2.0, care recipient interviews are now included.

The RAI provides a comprehensive health, social, and functional profile of persons as they enter skilled nursing facilities and at designated times thereafter. The initial assessment serves as the framework for the initial goals and outcomes for the individual. As assessments are repeated at set periods of time and as needed, the nurse and other members of the care team can track the progress toward the resolution of identified problems and make changes to the plan of care as appropriate. As goals are met and resources are available, the assessment leads to discharge to a lower level of care, such as returning home or to an assisted living facility. For a person whose condition is one of progressive decline, the RAI leads to a plan of care focused on comfort. The RAI process is dynamic and care oriented. It is used to gather definitive information and promote healthy aging in a specific care setting and in a holistic manner. The RAI is coordinated by a nurse and requires his or her signature attesting to its accuracy.

OASIS D

The plan for the skilled nursing care provided in the home is based on, and documented in, the OASIS. The most recent version became effective on January 1, 2019 (CMS, 2019). OASIS includes at least the measurement of functional, behavioral and physical status, and service utilization. The assessment is very

BOX 7.15   Risk for Hospitalization From the Outcomes and Assessment Information Set Assessment

1: History of falls (two or more falls—or any fall with an injury—in the past 12 months)
2: Unintentional weight loss of a total of 10 pounds or more in the past 12 months
3: Multiple hospitalizations (two or more) in the past 6 months
4: Multiple emergency department visits (two or more) in the past 6 months
5: Decline in mental, emotional, or behavioral status in the past 3 months
6: Reported or observed history of difficulty complying with any medical instructions (e.g., medications, diet, exercise) in the past 3 months
7: Currently taking five or more medications
8: Currently reports exhaustion
9: Other risk(s) not listed in 1–8
10: None of the above

comprehensive and focuses on the development of nursing interventions to improve post-acute care, prevent rehospitalization, and ensure safety in the home setting. Among the items on the instrument are those that identify the person's risk for hospitalization (Box 7.15). Most of the documentation takes place in the patient's home and is entered into a laptop or tablet for transmission to the agency database and ultimately the Centers for Medicare and Medicaid Services. As with other instruments, the assessment is completed at the time the care is begun and at intervals thereafter. Nurses supplement the OASIS data with information necessary to personalize the care provided. It is exceedingly complex, and training is required.

PROMOTING HEALTHY AGING: IMPLICATIONS FOR GERONTOLOGICAL NURSING

Whether the nurse is working with a standardized instrument or creating a new one, the goal is always to assist the person to move along the wellness trajectory toward healthy aging, regardless of the care setting or health status. The nurse is expected to collect data that are accurate and to do so in the most efficient yet caring manner possible. The use of assessment instruments serves to organize the data and enable them to be compared at various points in time. Each tool has strengths and weaknesses, as does each completed assessment. Many factors complicate assessment of the older adult: differentiating the effects of aging from those originating from disease, determining the presence of comorbidities, underreporting of symptoms by older adults, manifesting atypical presentations or nonspecific presentations of illnesses, and increasing numbers of iatrogenic illnesses.

Over-diagnosis and under-diagnosis occur when the normal age changes are not considered and assessments are inadequate. Assessing the person in later life with multiple chronic conditions is a complex task at the least. Many symptoms or complaints are ascribed to normal aging rather than to a disease entity that may be developing, necessitating careful and often problem-oriented assessments. Symptoms of one condition can exacerbate or mask symptoms of another. The gerontological nurse is challenged to provide the highest level of excellence in the assessment of the older adult without burdening the person in the process.

KEY CONCEPTS

- Assessment of the physical, cognitive, psychosocial, functional, and environmental status is essential to identifying specific needs, leading to implementation of appropriate interventions designed to enhance quality of life while aging.
- The quality and quantity of assessment data are affected by the source of collection, whether by self-report, report by proxy, or through nurse observation.

- Evidence-based instruments are available for most aspects of the assessment of the older adult.
- Knowledge of, and sometimes training in, the use of an assessment instrument is needed to accurately administer it.
- Multiple factors complicate obtaining and interpreting assessment data and providing the highest quality of care to older adults.

NURSING STUDY: Is a Comprehensive Assessment Needed?

Eighty-year-old Señora Hernandez is newly admitted to your acute care hospital unit. She is there for evaluation after a witnessed syncopal episode. She lives with her 90-year-old husband, who has mild dementia, and her 60-year-old daughter. Her daughter admits to you that neither of her parents have been doing well and that the doctors "just haven't been able to figure it out." You know that Señora Hernandez will be receiving both neurological and cardiac testing. However, as a gerontological resource nurse you also know that she and her family may benefit from a comprehensive evaluation. The decision of which aspects of the assessment to complete is within your scope of practice at your facility.

- Of the assessment instruments available to you, which do you think is most important in determining the immediate needs of Señora Hernandez?
- To prepare Señora Hernandez for discharge, which one or which selection of instruments will you use to collect the data needed to promote her well-being and safety?
- What information will you collect to supplement the information that you obtain using standardized instruments?

CRITICAL THINKING QUESTIONS AND ACTIVITIES

1. Of the assessment tools that are available to you, which are the most reasonable to perform within the limitations of an acute care setting? Give your rationale for the choices.
2. How would any of your answers to the preceding question change in a skilled nursing facility? In an assisted living facility? In the home setting? What is your rationale?
3. If you cannot do a complete head-to-toe examination and detailed history, list the parts that are essential when assessing an older adult, in order of priority.

4. Review the literature and present to your class two instruments that are applicable for use in cultures or languages other than the ones for which they were created.
5. Select the instrument or the portion of an instrument you are the least comfortable with and role-play with a classmate in conducting the assessment until you become comfortable.

RESEARCH QUESTIONS

1. What is the importance of measuring ADLs and IADLs in older adults?

2. What makes an assessment tool effective?

REFERENCES

Alexopoulos GS, Abrams RC, Young RC, Shamoian CA: Cornell Scale for Depression in Dementia, *Biol Psychiatry* 23:271–284, 1988.

Aprahamian I, Martinelli JE, Neri AL, Yassuda MS: The accuracy of the Clock Drawing Test compared to that of standard screening tests for Alzheimer's disease: results from a study of Brazilian elderly with heterogeneous educational backgrounds, *Int Psychogeriatr* 22:64–71, 2010.

Benner P: *From novice to expert*, Menlo Park, CA, 1984, Addison-Wesley.

Bent B: FANCAPES Assessment: increases in longevity lead to need for expertise in geriatric care, *Adv Healthcare Netw Nurs* 7(14):10, 2005.

Borson S, Brush M, Gil E, et al: The Clock Drawing Test: utility for dementia detection in multiethnic elders, *J Gerontol A Biol Sci Med Sci* 54(11):M534–M540, 1999.

Borson S, Scanlan J, Brush M, Vitaliano P, Dokmak A: The Mini-Cog: a cognitive "vital signs" measure for dementia screening in multilingual elderly, *Int J Geriatr Psychiatry* 15(11):1021–1207, 2000.

Bowker LK, Price JD, Smith SC, editors: *Oxford handbook of geriatric medicine*, ed 2, Oxford, 2012, Oxford University Press.

Brink TL, Yesavage JA, Lum O, Heersema PH, Adey M, Rose TL: Screening tests for geriatric depression, *Clin Gerontol* 1:37–43, 1982.

Centers for Medicare & Medicaid Services: *OASIS Data Sets,* 2019. https://www.cms.gov/Medicare/Quality-Initiatives-Patient-Assessment-Instruments/HomeHealthQualityInits/OASIS-Data-Sets.html. Accessed February, 2019.

Centers for Medicare & Medicaid Services: *MDS 3.0 RAI Manuel,* 2017. https://www.cms.gov/Medicare/Quality-Initiatives-Patient-Assessment-Instruments/NursingHomeQualityInits/MDS30RAIManual.html. Accessed December 2017.

Ciesielska N, Sokołowski R, Mazur E, Podhorecka M, Polak-Szabela A, Kedziora-Kornatowska K: Is the Montreal Cognitive Assessment (MoCA) test better suited than the Mini-Mental State Examination (MMSE) in mild cognitive impairment (MCI) detection among people aged over 60? Meta-analysis, *Psychiatr Pol* 50(5):1039–1052, 2016.

Cournan M: Use of the Functional Independence Measure for outcomes measurement in acute inpatient rehabilitation, *Rehabil Nurs* 36(3):111–117, 2011.

Cress CJ: *Handbook of geriatric care management*, ed 4, Burlington MA, 2017, Jones and Bartlett.

Doerflinger DM: *Mental status assessment of older adults: The Mini-Cog™*. Issue 3, 2013. https://consultgeri.org/try-this/general-assessment/issue-3.1.pdf. Accessed December 2017.

Duke University Center for the Study of Aging and Human Development: *Older Americans resources and services*, 2015. https://sites.duke.edu/centerforaging/services/older-americans-resources-and-services/. Accessed December 2017.

Folstein MF, Folstein SE: *Mini-Mental State Examination*, ed 2. http://www4.parinc.com/WebUploads/samplerpts/Fact%20Sheet%20MMSE-2.pdf. Accessed December 2017.

Folstein MF, Folstein SE, McHugh PR: Mini-Mental State: a practical method for grading the cognitive state of patients for the clinician, *J Psychiatr Res* 12:189–198, 1975.

Fujiwara Y, Suzuki H, Yasunaga M, et al: Brief screen tool for mild cognitive impairment in older Japanese: validation of the Japanese version of the Montreal Cognitive Assessment, *Geriatr Gerontol Int* 10(3):225–232, 2010.

Fulmer T, Wallace M: *Fulmer SPICES: an overall assessment tool for older adults*, New York, NY, 2012, Hartford Institute for Geriatric Nursing. https://consultgeri.org/try-this/general-assessment/issue-1.

Janssen J, Koekkoek PS, Moll van Charante EP., Jaap Kappelle L, Biessels GJ, Rutten GEHM: How to choose the most appropriate cognitive test to evaluate cognitive complaints in primary care, *BMC Fam Pract* 18:101, 2017. https://bmcfampract.biomedcentral.com/articles/10.1186/s12875-017-0675-4.

Katz S, Ford AB, Moskowitz RW, Jackson BA, Jaffe MW: Studies of illness in the aged: the index of ADL: a standardized measure of biological and psychosocial function, *JAMA* 185:914–919, 1963.

Kim EY, Bean RA, Harper JM: Do general treatment guidelines for Asian American families have applications to specific ethnic groups? The case of culturally-competent therapy with Korean American, *J Marital Fam Ther* 30(3):359–372, 2004.

Kleinman A: *Patient and healers in the context of culture: an exploration of the borderland between anthropology, medicine, and psychiatry*, Berkeley, CA, 1980, University of California Press.

Lach HW, Chang YP, Edwards D: Can older adults accurately report depression using brief forms? *J Gerontol Nurs* 36:30–37, 2010.

LaPlante MP: The classic measure of disability of activities of daily living is biased by age but an expanded IADL/ADL measure is not, *J Gerontol B Psychol Sci Soc Sci* 65(6):720–732, 2010.

Lawton MP, Brody EM: Assessment of older people: self-maintaining and instrumental activities of daily living, *Gerontologist* 9:179–186, 1969.

Mahoney FI, Barthel DW: Functional evaluation: the Barthel Index, *Md State Med J* 14:61–65, 1965.

Memória CM, Yassuda MS, Nakano EY, Forlenza OV: Brief screen for mild cognitive impairment: validation of the Brazilian version of the Montreal cognitive assessment, *Int J Geriatr Psychiatry* 28(1):34–40, 2013.

Mitchell AJ: A meta-analysis of the accuracy of the Mini-Mental Status Examination in the detection of dementia and mild cognitive impairment, *J Psychiatr Res* 43:411–431, 2009.

Mitchell AJ, Malladi S: Screening and case finding tools for the detection of dementia. Part 1. Evidence-based meta-analysis of multidomain tests, *Am J Geriatr Psychiatry* 18:759–782, 2010.

Montgomery J, Mitty E, Flores S: Resident condition change: should I call 911? *Geriatr Nurs* 29:15–26, 2008.

Nair AK, Gavett BE, Damman M, et al: Clock Drawing Test ratings by dementia specialists: interrater reliability and diagnostic accuracy, *J Neuropsychiatry Clin Neurosci* 22(1):85–92, 2010.

Nasreddine Z: *Montreal cognitive assessment: administration and score instructions,* 2010. www.mocatest.org. Accessed December 2017.

Nasreddine ZS, Phillips NA, Bédirian V, et al: The Montreal Cognitive Assessment, MoCA: a brief screen tool for mild cognitive impairment, *J Am Geriatr Soc* 53(4):695–699, 2005.

Nikula S, Jylhä M, Bardage C, et al: Are ADLs comparable across countries? Sociodemographic associates of harmonized IADL measures, *Aging Clin Exp Res* 15(6):451–459, 2003.

Ortiz I, Romero L: Cultural implications for assessment and treatment of depression in Hispanic elderly individuals, *Ann Longterm Care* 16:45, 2008.

Quinn TJ, Langhorne P, Stott DJ: Barthel Index for stroke trials: development, properties and application, *Stroke* 42:1146–1151, 2011.

Rayegani SM, Raeissadat SA, Alikhani E, Bayat M, Bahrami MH, Karimzadeh A: Evaluation of complete functional status of patients with stroke by Functional Independence Scale on admission, discharge, and six months post-stroke, *Iran J Neurol* 15(4):202–208, 2016.

Reisberg B: Functional Assessment Staging (FAST), *Psychopharmacol Bull* 24:653, 1988.

Sakurai R, Fujiwara Y, Ishihara M, Higuchi T, Uchida H, Imanaka K: Age-related self-overestimation of step-over ability in the healthy older adults and its relationship to fall risk, *BMC Geriatr* 13:44, 2013.

Saliba D, Buchanan J: *Development and validation of a revised nursing home assessment tool: MDS 3.0*. Santa Monica, CA, 2008, RAND Corporation.

Sangha H, Lipson D, Foley N, et al: A comparison of the Barthel Index and the functional independence measure as outcome measures in stroke rehabilitation: patterns of disability scale usage in clinical trials, *Int J Rehabil Res* 28:135–139, 2005.

Sclan SG, Reisberg B: Functional Assessment Staging (FAST) in Alzheimer's disease: reliability, validity, and ordinality, *Int Psychogeriatr* 4:55–69, 1992.

Sheehan B: Assessment scales in dementia, *Ther Adv Neurol Disord* 5(6):349–358, 2012.

Shelkey M, Wallace M: *Katz Index of Independence in Activities of Daily Living (ADL). No. 2 try this: Best practices in nursing care of older adults,* 2012. https://consultgeri.org/try-this/general-assessment/issue-2.pdf. Accessed December 2017.

Shulkin DJ: Physical medicine and rehabilitation outcomes for inpatient rehabilitation units. *VHA Directive 1225,* 2017. https://www.va.gov/search/?query=VHA+directive+1225. Accessed February 2019.

Stratford PW, Kennedy DM, Maly MR, Macintyre NJ: Quantifying self-report measures' overestimation of mobility scores post-arthroplasty, *Phys Ther* 90(9):1288–1296, 2010.

Yesavage JA, Brink TL, Rose TL, et al: Development and validation of a geriatric depression screening scale: a preliminary report, *J Psychiatr Res* 17:37–49, 1983.

Zambas SI: Purpose of the systematic physical assessment in everyday practice: critique of a "sacred cow," *J Nurs Educ* 49(6):305–311, 2010.

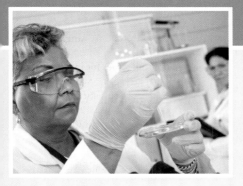

8

Laboratory Diagnostics and Geriatrics

Kathleen Jett

http://evolve.elsevier.com/Touhy/TwdHlthAging

A STUDENT SPEAKS

I always thought that as people got older, their blood sugars went up a little and that was okay. Now I realize that an elevation in fasting glucose means a problem regardless of one's age.

Susan, age 20

AN OLDER ADULT SPEAKS

Every time I turn around somebody wants my blood. They say that they need to "watch me closely" but I am not sure what that has to do with my blood. What if they take too much and it causes me to get sick?

Sung Ye, age 92

LEARNING OBJECTIVES

On completion of this chapter, the reader will be able to:

1. Discuss the key laboratory tests used to monitor common health problems in later life.
2. Understand the implications of deviations in key abnormal diagnostic laboratory values that can occur in the older adult.
3. Define precautions the nurse should take when interpreting laboratory values for the older adult.

Since ancient times the diagnosis of medical problems was based, in part, on the results of laboratory tests. The results were thought to be quantitative measures of health or illness. "Standards" or "reference ranges" were statistically determined based on the results drawn from normal healthy adults.

However, a comparable "reference range" for older adults has not been established (Lapin and Mueller, 2017). First, the older one is, the more likely he or she is to have acquired at least one or more chronic disease (multimorbidity), any of which could influence laboratory findings. Second, it has been well established (Chapter 3) that aging is a continuous and progressive decline in physiological function, some of which can be seen in alterations of the findings from laboratory testing. Finally, age-related reference ranges cannot account for the high degree of individual variability that occurs during senescence. Factors to consider include physical endurance, nutritional status, mobility, cognitive status, and predominant diseases (Lapin and Mueller, 2017).

Unfortunately, structural factors influence laboratory results that are particularly relevant to frail older adults. For example, Laboratory A performs phlebotomy services for Nursing Home

A. One day the phlebotomist is late, arriving after breakfast, but "fasting" tests are drawn nonetheless, and the discrepancy may or may not make it to the attention of the provider. On most days Nursing Home A is the first of several stops for Laboratory A and specimens are chronically late getting to the analytical laboratory. If any abnormalities are found are they reflections of structure or health or disease or aging? With the increasing number of "point-of-care tests" (POCTs) available some of these problems will be resolved.

The nurse's knowledge related to laboratory values assumes special meaning when working with older adults. The older the person is, the more common the abnormalities. In this chapter the more common laboratory tests are reviewed with a discussion of why they may be done and how normal changes with aging may affect the results.

HEMATOLOGICAL TESTING

Hematological testing refers to that associated with the blood and lymph and their component parts: red blood cells (RBCs), white blood cells (WBCs), and cell fragments called *platelets*.

Together the cells float in a fluid matrix called *plasma*. A basic complete blood count (CBC) provides the number of RBCs, WBCs, platelets, and the hematocrit and hemoglobin indices. A CBC with a "differential" refers to the inclusion of the subtypes of the WBCs: granulocytes (neutrophils, basophils, and eosinophils) and agranulocytes (lymphocytes and monocytes).

Hematological laboratory tests are often used to diagnose anemia or check for the presence of potential side effects of treatment such as chemotherapeutic agents. They are also used to evaluate symptoms such as fatigue, weakness, shortness of breath, increased heart rate, headache, low blood pressure, or pallor. Several conditions more common in the older adult affect the results, especially dehydration, malnutrition, infection, and inflammation.

Red Blood Cell Count

The primary function of the RBCs (erythrocytes) is to transport molecules of hemoglobin. With an average life span of 120 days, the RBCs are constantly being replenished. They are produced primarily by the bone marrow of the long bones. If the person is dehydrated the RBC will be artificially high. Once the person is hydrated, anemia may be found. As it is normal for the sense of thirst to decrease with age, this is always something to attend to before making any conclusions.

Hemoglobin and Hematocrit

Hemoglobin (Hgb), a conjugated protein, is the main component of the RBC. It contains iron and the red pigment porphyrin. The iron is part of protein synthesis in the mitochondria, essential for generating cellular energy, and transports oxygen from the lungs to the tissues and carbon dioxide from the tissues to the lungs. A hemoglobin level equal to or less than 5 g/dL, or more than 20 g/dL, is considered a "critical value" regardless of age and requires urgent intervention (Box 8.1). If the drop in the hemoglobin occurs suddenly it is most likely the result of trauma, such as a subdural hematoma following a fall. If it drops slowly (a "slow bleed") an older adult may complain of fatigue. A common cause is gastrointestinal (GI) in nature. Older adults may begin to show signs of physiological distress well before these values are reached.

The term *hematocrit* means "to separate blood." It is the *relative percentage* of packed RBCs to the plasma in blood, after the two have been separated (often referred to as "spun down"). Although they measure different aspects of the RBCs, the hematocrit and hemoglobin values are comparative numbers, with the hemoglobin level approximately one-third of the hematocrit value. For example, a person with a hemoglobin level of 12 g/dL will have a hematocrit of approximately 36% (Chernecky and Berger, 2013).

There is no indication that there is a change in RBCs in healthy aging; however, the speed at which new blood cells can be produced in late life is reduced *(decreased marrow reserve)*. This becomes a potential problem with a loss of blood such as after repeated phlebotomy or with frank bleeding. Recovery from the loss takes much longer, increasing the risk of falling, delirium, and other geriatric syndromes (Chapter 21).

Iron. The primary source of iron is through the consumption of iron-containing foods such as dark-green leafy vegetables and red meats. Iron is transported into bone marrow by the plasma protein *transferrin* for storage and later use. The serum concentration of iron is determined by a combination of its absorption and storage and the breakdown and synthesis of hemoglobin. Iron studies include measurements of serum iron, total iron binding capacity (TIBC), ferritin, and transferrin levels.

The TIBC is a measure of the combination of the amount of iron already in the blood and the amount of transferrin available in the blood serum. Ferritin is a complex molecule made up of ferric hydroxide and a protein; its measurement reflects body iron stores. If the person has adequate iron, the body can respond quickly to the demand for increased oxygen and energy and to replenish iron lost through bleeding.

Anemia. Anemia is defined as a hematocrit below 41% in males and below 36% in women (Damon and Andreadis, 2017). Although not a normal part of aging, anemia has been found in between 10% and 24% of those living in the community who are at least 65 years of age. For those residing in nursing homes the numbers are much higher at 48% to 54%. The prevalence is highest among African Americans compared with whites and Hispanics (Ershler, 2017). The most common types of anemia in late life are iron deficiency, vitamin B_{12}/folate deficiency, as a result of renal insufficiency, in the presence of chronic inflammation, and those that remain unexplained.

Screening for anemia is rarely done in the younger, healthy population. In geriatrics it is more common but rarely done unless one of several signs or symptoms is present (Box 8.2). Diagnostic testing for anemia includes a CBC with differential, iron studies, and the measurement of several vitamins, especially the levels of folic acid and vitamin B_{12}.

BOX 8.1   Caution With the Interpretation of Hematocrit and Hemoglobin Levels

Elevations in hematocrit and hemoglobin levels may be the result of a pathological process but are more often an early sign of hypovolemia from malnutrition, dehydration, or severe diarrhea. The volume depletion must be corrected before an accurate interpretation can be done.

BOX 8.2   Potential Effects of Reduced Hemoglobin in Older Adults

Reduced quality of life
Clinical depression
Falls
Functional impairment
Reduced walking speed
Loss of mobility
Reduced grip strength
Loss of mobility

From Lapin A, Mueller E: Laboratory diagnosis and geriatrics: more than just reference intervals for older adults. In Fillit HM, Rockwood K, Young R, editors: *Brocklehurst's textbook of geriatric medicine and gerontology*, Philadelphia, 2017, Elsevier, pp 220-225.

Anemia that is progressive and untreated or not responsive to treatment will result in the person's death. The advanced practice gerontological nurse must be able to recognize the need to consider anemia as a causative factor in several vague complaints, such as fatigue. The nurse should be able to recognize the potential for anemia and to monitor its treatment.

White Blood Cells

WBCs (leukocytes) are the cells of the immune system that primarily function to protect the body from infection and other foreign invaders. They are produced by the bone marrow and thymus and are stored in the lymph nodes, spleen, and tonsils, then travel to the site of invasion or infection. The average adult has 5000 to 10,000 WBCs/mm^3. The number of WBCs and the type of WBC are regulated largely by the endocrine system and by the body's need for a particular type of cell at a point in time. Each cell has a life span of 13 to 20 days, after which it is destroyed in the lymphatic system and excreted in feces. An excess is referred to as leukocytosis and a deficiency as leukopenia. Both conditions are more common in the older adult because of adverse side effects of medications. Leukopenia can be caused by common medical conditions and commonly prescribed medications, such as some antibiotics, anticonvulsants, antihistamines, analgesics, sulfonamides, or diuretics. On the other hand, leukocytosis may be a side effect of other drugs including allopurinol, aspirin, heparin, or steroids (Dugdale, 2013).

⚡ SAFETY ALERT

Due to the decreased immune function in the older adult, laboratory indicators of infection may be delayed. Waiting for the "usual signs" of infection in an older adult may result in his or her death. Instead, the nurse must be alert for more subtle signs of illness such as new-onset or increased confusion, falling, or incontinence, and respond to these changes earlier rather than later.

Granulocytes

Neutrophils. Neutrophils are produced in the bone marrow every 7 to 14 days and are in circulation for about 6 hours. They fight illness by phagocytizing bacteria and other products perceived to be foreign. *Neutrophilia*, or increased numbers of neutrophils, is a nonspecific finding. It may be an indicator of several conditions more common in late life, including infections and connective tissue diseases, such as rheumatoid arthritis; a side effect of medications, such as corticosteroids; or a result of trauma such as a fall (Chernecky and Berger, 2013).

Eosinophils and basophils. Eosinophils ingest antigen-antibody complexes induced by immunoglobulin-E–mediated reactions to attack allergens and parasites. High eosinophil counts are found in people with type I allergies such as hay fever and asthma. Eosinophils are known to diminish in late life due to age-related reductions in immune function (Liesveld and Reagan, 2014). Basophils transport histamine, a factor in immune and antiinflammatory responses. Like eosinophils, they play a role in allergic reactions but are not involved in bacterial or viral infections (Chernecky and Berger, 2013).

Agranulocytes

Lymphocytes. Lymphocytes play key roles in the immune system (Lin et al, 2016). Among the types are T and B cells. T cells are produced by the thymus and are active in cell-mediated immunity; B cells are produced in the bone marrow and are involved in the production of antibodies (humoral immunity). While T-cell activity is especially important in late life, due in part to the naturally occurring immunosenescence, T-cell responses and T-cell–macrophage activity are slowed (Chapter 3). Measurement of the number of T cells is included in the monitoring of the health status and treatment response of persons who are immunocompromised such as those who are receiving chemotherapeutic agents or are infected with the human immunodeficiency virus (HIV).

Monocytes. Monocytes are the largest of the leukocytes. When matured they become macrophages and help defend the body against foreign substances or, more importantly, what the body believes are foreign substances. The macrophages migrate to a site in the body where they can remove microorganisms, dead RBCs, and foreign debris through the physiological process of phagocytosis. If the number of monocytes is low, the person has reduced physiological capacity to fight infection. This value must be watched carefully, especially in ill or frail older adults.

Infection

Due to age-related decreases or delayed responses in the immune system, an infection in an older adult is particularly dangerous. A simply bothersome viral infection (e.g., cold) can quickly become bacterial bronchitis or even life-threatening pneumonia.

One way to theoretically determine the intensity of an infection is through the measurement of the WBCs. A WBC count greater than 10,000/mm^3 alone is indicative of a potential infection, especially in an older adult. However up to 50% of those with pneumonia will initially have WBCs that are within normal limits. Up to 95% will have a *left shift*—that is, an abnormally high number of immature neutrophils (Reuben et al, 2017). Unfortunately, with aging it becomes more and more difficult to detect early signs of infection. The WBC elevation as the traditional signs of an infection is not immediately apparent and a fever is often absent. These changes have significant implications for the gerontological nurse.

Platelets

Platelets are small, irregular particles known as thrombocytes, an essential ingredient in clotting. They are formed in the bone marrow, lungs, and spleen and are released when a blood vessel is injured. As they arrive at the site of injury, they become "sticky," forming a plug at the site to stop the bleeding and to help trigger what is known as the *clotting cascade* (Leavitt and Minichiello, 2017). Although the platelet count does not change with aging, there is an increase in the concentrations of coagulation enzymes (factors VII and VIII and fibrinogen). This and other developments indicate a greater possibility of hypercoagulability. At the same time, older adults are more likely to have blood diatheses, resulting in unexplained bruising, nosebleeds, or excessive bleeding with surgery. If any of these signs are present, a platelet count and coagulation studies may be done. Counts of 150,000 to 400,000/mm^3 are considered normal. Counts less than 100,000/mm^3 are considered thrombocytopenia and spontaneous hemorrhage may occur when the count falls below 20,000/mm^3. There is a significantly exacerbated risk of excessive bleeding when anticoagulants (e.g., warfarin, apixaban [Eliquis]) are used in the presence of thrombocytopenia. *Thrombocythemia* indicates a platelet count greater than 1 million/mm^3; bleeding still may occur because of abnormal functioning.

The gerontological nurse caring for older adults, especially those who are frail or who have vague symptoms, is expected to monitor patients at risk for bleeding. A basic understanding of the meaning of the patient's hematological laboratory findings is expected. For frail older adults, such as those in long-term care facilities, thrombocytopenia can quickly lead to death should bleeding occur, such as from nonsteroidal antiinflammatory drug (NSAID)–related gastric bleeding or from an unrecognized subdural hematoma following a fall.

MEASURES OF INFLAMMATION

Erythrocyte Sedimentation Rate

The *erythrocyte sedimentation rate* (ESR), also referred to as the "sed rate," is a proxy measure for the degree of inflammation, infection, necrosis, infarction, or advanced neoplasm that is present. It is slightly elevated in many older adults, most likely attributable to the prevalence of long-standing chronic disease and consequential inflammation (Ferri, 2015). An ESR greater than 100 mm/h is strongly associated with a serious illness, however when there is no obvious reason for the elevation, the test should be repeated before further testing is done. The ESR may be useful for monitoring several inflammatory diseases and their treatments, such as polymyalgia rheumatica, temporal arteritis, or rheumatoid arthritis (Chapter 26). An ESR which becomes elevated due to a sudden event such as heart failure will stay elevated for weeks (Litao and Kamat, 2014). However, the ESR is a nonspecific test and this must always be taken into consideration when evaluating the results.

VITAMINS

Vitamin deficiencies are common in later life and should be considered any time the person complains of vague symptoms (especially fatigue), cognitive impairment develops, wound healing is delayed, or anemia is suspected. Those at highest risk are persons with protein-calorie malnutrition. Vitamin B deficiencies are more likely in persons undernourished for long periods of time such as many of those living in low-income countries (Mathew and Jacobs, 2014). Vitamin D deficiencies are now being found in both apparently healthy and ill adults.

B Vitamins

The two B vitamins that are especially important in aging are folic acid (folate) and B$_{12}$.

Folate (B$_9$)

Folate is formed by bacteria in the intestines; it is necessary for the normal functioning of both RBCs and WBCs, and for DNA synthesis (Rote and McCance, 2012). It is stored in the liver and can be found in eggs, milk, green leafy vegetables, yeast, liver, and fruit. Decreases in folate may indicate protein-energy malnutrition, several types of anemia, and liver and renal disease. It is common among persons with chronic alcohol abuse and persons who take any one of several medications. Prolonged deficiencies can result in cognitive impairment and depression.

Due to the number of foods that are enriched with folic acid, the deficiencies and associated anemias are much less common than they were in the past. Nonetheless, the nurse must be alert for potential folate deficiencies when the person has significant nutritional deficits, such as those who are very frail or abuse alcohol.

Vitamin B$_{12}$

Vitamin B$_{12}$ (cyanocobalamin) is a water-soluble vitamin required for the normal development of RBCs, for several neurological functions, and for the synthesis of DNA. It cannot be synthesized in the human body and thus must be provided by the diet or supplementation. B$_{12}$ deficiency is common in older adults and is estimated to affect about 3.2% of those older than age 51. Conditions that lead to folate and B$_{12}$ deficiency can result in megaloblastic anemia (large RBCs that do not functional properly). Tests of B$_{12}$ and folate levels are now part of the standard workup for dementia, or unexplained neurological or functional decline (Damon and Andreadis, 2017).

Vitamin B$_{12}$ is found in the proteins of foods such as eggs, fish, shellfish, and meat; typically, only half of the B$_{12}$ ingested by healthy adults with normal gastric function is absorbed. It is primarily extracted from proteins in the stomach in the presence of gastric acid and other compounds including intrinsic factor (IF). Pernicious anemia is a type of anemia characterized by lowered IF production by gastric cells. The age-related decrease in the production of gastric acid and IF significantly increases the risk for vitamin B$_{12}$ deficiency. There is not a clear numerical cut-off for the determination of serum B$_{12}$ (Wong, 2015).

Vitamin D

Vitamin D is produced in the skin when exposed to ultraviolet light (UV) through the conversion of 7-dehydrocholesterol to vitamin D$_3$ (cholecalciferol) (NHLBI, 2011). Levels are measured in the blood considering vitamin D$_2$, D$_3$, and total levels. A total of more than 30 ng/mL indicates a minimally acceptable level. Vitamin D deficiencies have been found to be common among all ages. Vitamin D is a key component in maintaining bone strength.

Those with decreased exposure to UV light, such as many who live in institutional settings or at the extremes of the hemispheres (e.g., the Inuit living near the Arctic circle), are at higher than usual risk for vitamin D deficiencies. The changes in the aging skin (i.e., decreased ability to synthesize vitamin D in the skin) exacerbate the risk considerably. Ensuring adequate intake of calcium and vitamin D is essential for healthy aging through food, sun exposure, and dietary supplements. There is a universal recommendation of 1200 mg a day of calcium for women over 50 years old and 1000 mg a day for men over 70 years old (divided doses). This should be taken with vitamin D_3 800 to 1000 units daily (Reuben, 2017).

BLOOD CHEMISTRY STUDIES

Blood chemistry studies include an assortment of laboratory tests used to identify and measure circulating elements and particles in the plasma and blood including thyroxin-stimulating hormone, glucose, proteins, amino acids, nutritive materials, excretion products, hormones, enzymes, vitamins, and minerals. Due to the number of medications taken and common chronic diseases in older adults, typical tests include lipids (cholesterol and triglycerides), vitamins D and B_{12} (see earlier), and thyroid-stimulating hormone. Some of these tests are used for screening and others for monitoring specific health problems or treatments. All tests are individually selected and must be justified by a current diagnosis for reimbursement (Table 8.1). The nurse must become familiar with the names and test components used by the laboratory that provides services to her or his patients. The advanced practice nurse is expected to know when urgent and disease-monitoring blood chemistry studies are needed and what to do with the results.

Basic and Comprehensive Panels

A basic metabolic panel may be referred to as a BMP (8 tests) or a Chem-7. It measures the health of the kidneys (creatinine and blood urea nitrogen [BUN]), overall metabolism, blood glucose, electrolytes, and acid-base balance. The comprehensive metabolic panel (CMP) includes all of the measures found in the BMP plus measures of nutritional status (albumin) and several measures of liver function.

Electrolytes are inorganic substances that help maintain cellular homeostasis. They regulate hydration and blood pH and are critical for nerve and muscle function. For example, if there is an imbalance of calcium, sodium, or potassium levels, muscle weakness or contractions may occur. Because older adults are more sensitive to electrolyte imbalances, these should be checked any time there is a sudden change in mental status, an adjustment or addition of a medication (e.g., potassium), a change in fluid intake, or a transfer of the patient from one setting to another (e.g., home to hospital, nursing home to hospital, general unit to intensive care unit). Excessive diuresis, medication interactions (such as the use of both potassium and a potassium-sparing medication), and dehydration are probably the most common causes of electrolyte imbalances in older adults.

All the electrolytes are excreted by the kidneys. If kidney function is compromised imbalances can quickly occur. Those who are frail, residing in long-term care facilities, or taking multiple medications are at the highest risk. The most common electrolyte disturbances seen in gerontological nursing are sodium and potassium.

⚡ SAFETY ALERT

A minor electrolyte imbalance may have little effect in a younger adult but may have significantly deleterious effects in older adults, especially those who are medically or cognitively fragile. The signs and symptoms of an imbalance in the older adult include weakness, fatigue, immobility, falling, or delirium (altered mental status).

Sodium

Serum sodium (Na^+) is necessary for the maintenance of blood pressure, the transmission of nerve impulses, and the regulation of body fluids into and out of the cells (Filippatos et al, 2017) (Table 8.2). Sodium is always accompanied by chloride (Cl^-) and are found in combination as sodium chloride. Both are included in the BMP and CMP.

Hyponatremia. The causes of hyponatremia, or serum sodium 130 mmol/L or less, can be divided into three types: increased extracellular fluid (ECF) volume, impaired water

---

TABLE 8.1 Examples of Laboratory Testing and Associated Diagnoses.

Diagnosis	Examples of Justified Laboratory Test
Hypertension	Basic metabolic panel (monitoring renal function and electrolytes related to treatment)
Altered mental status	Comprehensive metabolic panel, vitamin D, vitamin B_{12}, thyroid-stimulating panel, urine analysis (culture and sensitivity if positive)
Dyslipidemia	Lipid panel, liver function (usually part of the comprehensive metabolic panel)

TABLE 8.2 Signs and Symptoms of Disturbances in Sodium Levels.

	Hyponatremia	Hypernatremia
Signs	Plasma Na^+ ≤130 mmol/L (approximately)	Plasma Na^+ ≥150 mmol/L (approximately)
	Drop in BP (in hypovolemia)	Poor skin turgor
	Tachycardia (in hypovolemia)	Dry mucous membranes
Symptoms	Mental status changes	Mental status changes

BP, Blood pressure.

Data from Doig AK, Huether SE: The cellular environment fluids and electrolytes, acids and bases. In McCance KL, Huether SE, Brashers VL, et al, editors: *Pathophysiology: the biological basis for disease in adults and children*, St Louis, 2014, Elsevier, pp 103–134.

excretion (e.g., renal insufficiency), and least often in late life, the syndrome of inappropriate antidiuretic hormone (SIADH) secretion. In most cases the cause of hyponatremia is multifactorial in older adults. Several medications, including thiazide diuretics and several antidepressants, including mirtazapine, place a person at higher risk. Those with poor diets (i.e., low salt and protein accompanied by *increased* intake of water) are also at risk (Filippatos et al, 2017).

Hyponatremia is usually asymptomatic until the plasma sodium concentration drops slightly below 130 mEq/L. Mental status and central nervous changes can be seen with levels 125 to 130 mEq/L or less. With further loss of sodium, other CNS symptoms may quickly develop including seizures and coma secondary to cerebral edema. Hypovolemic hyponatremia is always accompanied by a significant drop in postural blood pressure and tachycardia as the body attempts to compensate. In the most severe cases, hyponatremia can result in a high rate of morbidity and mortality. Hyponatremia is one of the more common causes of delirium in older adults. *Slow replacement is necessary.*

Hypernatremia. Hypernatremia is an elevation of plasma sodium concentration (>145 mEq/L) and indicates a deficit in total body water relative to total body sodium (i.e., less water intake than output). It is usually caused by either reduced or impaired thirst (normal part of aging) or limited access to water. It is common among older adults especially those who are frail, hospitalized, or living in long-term care facilities. Contributing factors include dependence on others for fluids, impaired thirst mechanism, reduced body water, and use of fluid wasting medications such as furosemide, all of which are common in later life. Signs and symptoms of hypernatremia include confusion, thirst, weakness, nausea, and muscle twitching (Lewis, 2016a).

The prevalence of hypernatremia among those living in the community is as high as 3.7%, approximately 2% for those admitted to the hospital but up to 30% of those admitted with a febrile illness. In the older adult the mortality rate is considerable unless detected and treated promptly (Shah et al, 2014).

Potassium

Potassium (K^+) is an electrolyte found primarily within the cells. It is essential in maintaining cell osmolality, ensuring muscle functioning, and transmitting nerve impulses. It is a key component in the maintenance of the acid-base balance. Serum potassium levels decrease as lean body mass decreases, a normal part of aging. When the person is taking any K^+-sparing or wasting medications, as is common in later life, potassium level must be closely monitored.

Hypokalemia. Excess renal or gastrointestinal tract loss (diarrhea) are the most common causes of hypokalemia (K^+ <3.5 mEq/L). Renal loss is usually a side effect of "potassium-wasting" medications such as furosemide (Lewis, 2016). Mild hypokalemia is asymptomatic but as the loss increases muscle weakness and polyuria develop. Potassium levels less than 3.0 mEq/L are critical and produce cramping, confusion, fatigue, paralytic ileus, electrocardiogram (ECG) changes and tachycardia, fibrillation, and sudden death (Chernecky and

BOX 8.3	Signs and Symptoms of Disturbances in Potassium Levels
Hypokalemia	**Hyperkalemia**
Generalized muscle weakness	Impaired muscle activity
Fatigue	Weakness
Muscle cramps	Muscle pain/cramps
Constipation	Increased GI motility
Ileus	Bradycardia
Flaccid paralysis	Cardiac arrest
Hyporeflexia	ECG changes:
Hypercapnia	P wave flattened
Tetany	T wave large, peaked
ECG changes:	QRS broad
Q-T interval prolonged	Biphasic QRS-T complex
T wave flattened or depressed	
ST segment depressed	

ECG, Electrocardiogram; *GI*, gastrointestinal.
For additional information, see Cho KC: Electrolyte and acid-base disorders. In Papadakis MA, McPhee SJ, editors: *Current medical diagnosis and treatment*, New York, 2017, McGraw-Hill, pp 884–912.

Berger, 2013). Chronic low levels of potassium may lead to significant renal tubular dysfunction.

Hyperkalemia. Hyperkalemia (K^+ >5.5 mEq/L) most often results when potassium is not adequately excreted via the kidneys. However, it is also found in those with acidosis, inadequate monitoring of potassium-sparing medications such as angiotensin-converting enzyme (ACE) inhibitors, or excessive potassium supplementation, all highly relevant to older adults. The signs and symptoms of a disturbance in potassium levels may not be evident until cardiac toxicity occurs (Box 8.3) (Cho, 2017).

Glucose

Glucose is a complex sugar produced by the pancreas. Glucose and fat circulate in the blood as sources of physiological energy. Most of the glucose is used by the brain. When not in use, it is stored in skeletal muscle and the liver as glycogen. The level of fasting glucose in the body is between about 70 and 126 mg/dL. Although the required levels do not change with aging, the signs and symptoms of persons with elevations or reductions may change. The fasting blood glucose levels are in the high normal range and it takes longer to return to normal levels after eating. These changes appear to be most likely related to a decrease in the insulin sensitivity of the tissues. For many older adults, even slight hypoglycemia can result in confused and depressed central nervous system activity. Elevations may not be evident until the person is in a hyperosmolar hyperglycemic state (HHS), or coma. Interpretation of findings and related nursing interventions must always be done within the context of time since the person has eaten. Due to a blunted reaction to hyperglycemia, older adults are particularly at risk for coma.

Glycosylated hemoglobin A_{1C}. Laboratory testing of blood glucose or plasma glucose levels provides "snapshot" information at any one time. For more accurate measurement and monitoring of glucose concentration, as is done in persons with diabetes, the glycosylated hemoglobin A_{1C} (Hb A_{1C}) is used. About 6.5% of the hemoglobin in the RBCs can combine with glucose through the process of glycosylation. The glucose attachment is not easily reversible and therefore stays for the life of the RBC, approximately 120 days, and provides a good estimate of the overall average blood glucose. In nondiabetics less than 6.5% is the normal range regardless of one's age; less than 7% indicates good diabetic control, 8% to 9% fair control, and more than 9% poor control. Nine percent or more correlates with a mean glucose of 200 mg/dL (Ferri, 2015). The A_{1C} can be skewed in persons with conditions that alter the life span of the RBC. This includes those taking erythropoietin (to stimulate RBC growth) as many very frail older adults do. Ethnicity is an additional factor that can affect the results (ADA, 2018).

URIC ACID

Uric acid is a naturally occurring end-product of purine metabolism. It is usually measured in specific serum chemistry studies but is also found in the urine. Two-thirds of the amount normally produced is excreted by the kidneys and the rest via the stool. Elevations in uric acid levels (>7 mg/dL) are found when there is either *overproduction* or *underexcretion*. It is used in, but not a requirement for, diagnosing gout. Warfarin, frequently taken by older adults, represses the uric acid level (Ferri, 2015). While all persons with gout have an elevated uric acid level (>13 mg/dL), others with elevated uric acid levels do not have gout (Nakasato and Christensen, 2014). A number of conditions and situations can result in increased uric acid levels such as hypothyroidism; binge alcohol drinking; medications, especially thiazide diuretics; surgery; or acute medical illness. The use of thiazide diuretics in the person with preexisting elevations in uric acid levels may trigger an episode or recurrence of gout. The levels also increase slightly with age (Chernecky and Berger, 2013).

PROSTATE-SPECIFIC ANTIGEN

The primary screening tool for prostate cancer has been a blood test to measure the prostate-specific antigen (PSA). After detailed analysis of the science it had been concluded that while there was a slight benefit to this testing there were also significant potential harms. The harms all relate to the large number of false positives. The false positives led to additional aggressive testing or treatment when cancer was not actually present. Common harms of treating the "cancer" included impotence, incontinence (bowel and bladder), or death from unnecessary surgery. In 2018 the U.S. Preventive Services Task Force (USPSTF) recommended that it no longer be used for screening except in certain circumstances.

The guidelines recommend against screening for men over 70 years of age. Screening for others is to be considered. African American men more often develop more aggressive forms of prostate cancer and at a younger age than their white counterparts. While there is still inadequate research relating to African American men, screening may be somewhat helpful. There also may be some benefit for screening men with a strong family history of prostate cancer. Those with two to three close relatives may be at risk for a genetic type of the cancer. The evidence is not yet conclusive. The PSA does continue to be used as a gross measure of men's responsiveness to *treatment* of prostate cancer. For those who select to be screened for prostate cancer using the PSA this usually begins at the age of 55.

LABORATORY TESTING FOR CARDIAC HEALTH

Heart disease remains the primary cause of death for all persons. As a result, the gerontological nurse must be knowledgeable about the most common laboratory testing related to cardiac function. These include measures performed after acute cardiac events and those used in the determination of cardiac health and health risk.

Acute Cardiac Events

Older adults who appear to have acute and unexpected changes may be having an ischemic event and need immediate transportation to an emergency department for evaluation. At the emergency department, initial testing for an acute myocardial infarction (AMI) will include at least an ECG and measurement of cardiac enzymes or tissue markers (creatinine kinase and troponin). Measurement of inflammation with the high-sensitivity C-reactive protein (hs-CRP) and ESR are often used in combination.

Creatinine Kinase

The cardiac enzyme creatinine kinase (CK) is present in various parts of the body and in several forms (called isoenzymes). An elevation in isoenzyme CK-MB is associated with cardiac tissue, and laboratory values for CK-MB are used in the diagnosis of an AMI and several conditions. Among these are rhabdomyolysis and cerebrovascular accidents, both of which are common among older adults (Ferri, 2015). The CK-MB level rises in the first 6 hours after the onset of AMI symptoms. It peaks at 12 to 24 hours (unless the infarction extends) and returns to normal in 12 to 48 hours; therefore, it is not a useful measure after that period. A number of medications used to manage chronic diseases can cause false CK-MB testing results (Box 8.4). For the best

BOX 8.4 **Medications That Can Cause False CK-MB Results**	
Anticoagulants	Alcohol
Aspirin	Lovastatin
Dexamethasone	Lidocaine
Furosemide	Propranolol
Captopril	Morphine
Colchicine	

CK, Creatinine kinase.

diagnosis, CK-MB is used as a comparative measure with troponin (Reuben, 2017).

Troponin

A troponin is a cardiac and skeletal protein. Either transient or persistent troponin I and troponin T elevations can be caused by both acute cardiac and noncardiac events or conditions. These include hypertension, acute congestive heart failure, sepsis, rhabdomyolysis, and acute central nervous events (Reuben et al, 2017). Of the multiple causes, these are the most relative to the older adult and therefore most important to the gerontological nurse. A troponin T of 0.50 ng/mL or less indicated a strong probability of an AMI. This sensitive marker is seen within the first 48 hours after the AMI and remains elevated for 5 to 7 days. The cardiac troponin I can be seen in the first 8 hours, peaking at 24 hours and persisting for up to 7 days. The higher the troponin I the higher the risk of mortality (Ferri, 2015).

Due to the asymptomatic ("silent") nature of the AMI in many older adults, the troponins may be measured incidentally to another acute health problem (Chapter 22). An elevated troponin with a normal CK-MB can be used to identify reinfarction both in the first week after an AMI and in the ensuing 5 years (Reuben et al, 2017).

Monitoring Cardiovascular Risk and Health

Increasing attention has been given to three biochemical markers that are believed to have value in the detection of heart disease, in the assessment for risk of cardiovascular disease, or for decreasing the risk of future cardiac events. These are hs-CRP, homocysteine, and brain natriuretic peptide (BNP). Detection and monitoring of dyslipidemia and elevated triglyceride levels are important for determining both health and health risk (Takata et al, 2014).

hs-CRP

C-reactive protein (CRP) is produced by the liver, increasing whenever there is inflammation somewhere in the body. It is recommended that persons with at least one risk factor for coronary artery disease have at least one measurement of serum CRP (Reuben et al, 2017).

Although originally used to determine cardiac events, it has been found to be a useful indicator for other forms of inflammation, such as after an injury, following surgery, or in the presence of infection. The CRP can also be used as a marker for cardiac risk, such as identifying those with "silent" atherosclerosis prior to a cardiac event (Ferri, 2015). Tests of both CRP and ESR are used at the time of an acute event for the determination of tissue damage associated with an AMI. It normalizes in 3 to 7 days (Litao and Kamat, 2014). The high-sensitivity assay hs-CRP has increased the accuracy of the measurement even at low levels.

Homocysteine

Serum homocysteine is a naturally occurring amino acid produced during the metabolism of proteins such as meat. The range considered normal increases with age (>59 years old: 5.8–11.9 μmol/L). Elevations are associated with and increase the risk for dementia, atherosclerosis, strokes, AMI,

and peripheral vascular disease. Elevations are present in B_6, B_{12}, and folic acid deficiencies (Ferri, 2015). The gerontological nurse can work with the older adult to avoid these deficiencies and therefore promote cognitive and cardiac health (Beckett et al, 2017).

B-type Natriuretic Peptide

B-type natriuretic peptide (BNP) and the N-terminal pro b-type natriuretic peptide (NT-proBNP) are produced by the heart and released when it is stretched. The values increase with age and are higher in women (Ferri, 2015). Elevations are found in several cardiac conditions but most often in acute heart failure. BNP and NT-proBNP levels are also used to monitor the effectiveness of treatment. An elevated BNP is a predictor of mortality from sudden death (Mayo Clinic, n.d.).

Lipid Panels

Elevated cholesterol and triglycerides have been found to be health risks regardless of age. When uncontrolled, they are major predictors of coronary heart disease. Laboratory testing is usually done as a lipid panel. A lipid panel provides a total cholesterol, a low-density lipoprotein (LDL), a high-density lipoprotein (HDL), and a triglyceride level. It is done both as a routine health screen and as a means of monitoring the response to treatment. Fasting 12 to 15 hours before the test is required for accuracy.

Cholesterol. Cholesterol is a sterol compound used by the body to stabilize cell membranes. It is metabolized in the liver, where it is combined with LDL, HDL, and very-low-density lipoprotein (VLDL). According to considerable evidence, cholesterol levels have not been found to be associated with heart disease in persons over the age of 75 (Baron, 2017).

Although lipid panels are usually conducted for the management of statin therapy, according to the most recent guidelines of the American Heart Association there is no longer a "one size fits all" in the consideration of the component parts of lipids. For many years there has been widespread belief in the relationship between high cholesterol and the development of heart disease at any age. Instead, the American Heart Association now recommends that multiple factors be considered when the "numbers" are reviewed. These include family history, other risk factors for heart disease, and long-term risk/benefit ratios (Grundy et al, 2018). Nonetheless, total cholesterol level less than 160 mg/dL in a frail older adult is a risk factor for increased mortality. A total cholesterol level 200 mg/dL or more has also been suggested to increase neuropsychiatric symptoms in Alzheimer's disease, especially in men (Hall et al, 2014).

Triglycerides are produced in the liver and circulated in the blood. Most of the serum triglycerides combine with the VLDL. Excess blood levels are deposited into fatty tissue. Reasons for elevated levels include chronic renal failure and poorly controlled diabetes. Severely elevated triglyceride levels (>2000 mg/dL) are a strong risk factor for pancreatitis (Mathew and Jacobs, 2014).

Albumin

Serum albumin has been used as a biomarker for visceral protein, therefore it was always part of a nutritional assessment.

More recent research indicates that a low level reflects chronic inflammation (measured by the hs-CRP) rather than protein stores or weight (Alves et al, 2018). The concentration of serum albumin depends on many factors such as body losses, hepatic synthesis, and rate and extent of protein breakdown. The concentration declines with low intake but this is not particularly dangerous unless accompanied by inflammation.

Although serum protein measurements are commonly ordered, they are neither sensitive nor specific for nutritional health and are often in the low range of normal in older adults. Dehydration will show a deceptive increase in albumin levels at the same time albumin levels appear to decrease with overhydration, liver and renal disease, malabsorption, and changes from an upright position to a supine position during the blood draw (Ferri, 2016). The half-life of albumin is about 3 weeks, so changes are not quickly apparent except in sudden and acutely severe conditions. However, albumin levels are most useful as an indicator of the severity of illness and the risk of mortality. Prealbumin (transthyretin) has a half-life of only 2 to 3 days and is therefore a more sensitive marker for change. A low prealbumin level can confirm poor nutritional status and serve as a monitor for active treatment.

LABORATORY TESTS OF RENAL HEALTH

Renal function decreases substantially with age, but in most cases the body can adequately compensate and laboratory findings stay "within normal limits." However, laboratory findings may be *unreliable* in those with reduced lean body mass (a normal change with aging), excessive dietary intake of protein, alterations in metabolism, and strenuous physical activity before measurement. Because of the frequency of health problems and medications that affect renal health, measuring and monitoring renal functioning are particularly important to the older adult and the gerontological nurse. Laboratory indices particularly diagnostic of renal disease are elevated BUN and creatinine levels. These are included in a basic metabolic panel.

Blood Urea Nitrogen

Urea nitrogen is the end-product of protein metabolism. The BUN is used as a gross measurement for renal functioning and level of hydration. Blood levels are often in the high-normal range because of the age-related changes to the liver and kidney. Changes over time in the BUN level may be more important than any one laboratory result, especially in the assessment of dehydration, renal insufficiency, or renal failure. *Azotemia* is an elevation of BUN level. Prerenal azotemia refers to elevations before blood reaches the kidneys; causes include shock, severe dehydration, congestive heart failure, and excessive protein catabolism such as in starvation. Normal BUN findings for adults are approximately 8 to 18 mg/dL (Ferri, 2015).

Creatinine

Creatinine is a waste product resulting from the breakdown of muscle that is normally produced in energy metabolism; its level is highly dependent on muscle mass. If muscle mass remains the same, the serum creatinine level should be constant. The reduced lean muscle mass of normal aging will result in a decreased creatinine level. The BUN and creatinine are usually considered together in the evaluation of renal function.

The glomerular filtration rate (GFR) is a measure of the flow of filtered fluid through the kidneys. As the GFR normally decreases with aging, the nurse must take this into consideration any time a nephrotoxic medication is administered or prescribed. The GFR is an estimated number and is usually calculated by the laboratory.

An alternate way to estimate renal function is to use creatinine clearance (CrCl). It is calculated number that includes age, sex, weight, and serum creatinine. There are multiple calculators that are available online, for example http://nephron.com/cgi-bin/CGSI.cgi (Chapter 9).

MONITORING FOR THERAPEUTIC BLOOD LEVELS

The monitoring of physiological levels of certain medications is especially important at any time but more so in later life not only because more are prescribed but also because inappropriate dosing can more easily have a life-threatening effect. At levels too low, the effects of medications may be negligible and at levels too high they may easily result in adverse events (Chapter 9).

Anticoagulants

Anticoagulation therapy has become the mainstay of stroke prevention for persons with atrial fibrillation and artificial heart valves (Chapter 22) and in the treatment or prevention of deep vein thrombosis. When the blood is excessively anticoagulated, the person is at risk for life-threatening bleeding. When the levels of anticoagulants in the blood are too low, the protective qualities are lost.

At the time of writing, there were nine oral and one subcutaneous anticoagulants available in the United States, but only the blood levels of warfarin and heparin can be monitored. Anyone who is taking warfarin or heparin must have their coagulability measured regularly because of these drugs' narrow therapeutic windows. The results are important for prompt adjustment of an individual's dosage for the anticoagulants as needed.

The partial thromboplastin time (PTT) and occasionally the test for anti-Xa activity are used to monitor coagulation status of heparin. The results of the PTT test vary somewhat. The laboratory's normal range is used to determine if the dose used is correct. Heparin is used primarily in the acute care setting.

In the past, precise monitoring of the anticoagulation effects of warfarin (Coumadin, Jantoven) was difficult because of the amount of variation in test results between laboratories. An international normalized ratio (INR) is now used to overcome these difficulties. The INR can be measured by a laboratory or at the point of care (POC), such as in a clinic or a care facility, using a device similar to a blood glucose monitor. Most of the time standard ranges are used: 2.0 to 3.0 for those treated for atrial fibrillation or flutter and 2.5 to 3.5 for persons with a mechanical heart valve, deep vein thrombosis, or pulmonary embolism. Some persons self-monitor, with their cardiologists receiving the results and adjusting the dose of the warfarin as needed. Specially trained pharmacists and registered nurses often perform the POC INR test.

Antiarrhythmics: Digoxin

Digoxin (Lanoxin) is a drug that is used to control ventricular response to chronic atrial fibrillation. It is initiated slowly and carefully to prevent too rapid a reduction in heart rate. Once the patient's dose is stabilized, the nurse monitors the effect of the medication by measuring the heart rate before drug administration and by observing for signs of adverse effects. Monitoring may include periodic determination of blood levels. The normal therapeutic range is 0.9 to 2.0 ng/mL with toxicity occurring at levels greater than 3.0 ng/mL. However, because of the normal changes with aging that affect pharmacokinetics, toxicity may be evident at levels well below 3.0 ng/mL. Observing for signs of toxicity, regardless of laboratory results, is probably more meaningful; this is especially important for an older adult who is receiving a dose higher than 0.125 mg/day (not recommended). The nurse can use the blood level only as a general guide, and it must be combined with the clinical presentation (including heart rate) of the person being treated.

Thyroid Panels

Thyroid panels are used to both diagnose and monitor thyroid disorders and their treatment. The panel includes measurement of the level of thyroid-stimulating hormone (TSH), free triiodothyronine (T_3), and free thyroxin (T_4). The levels of each of these, considered relative to each other, are used to make a diagnosis (Chapter 24). In most cases, treatment (especially thyroid replacement) can be monitored easily based on TSH levels alone. Testing is repeated initially at 6- to 8-week intervals until a euthyroid state is reached and confirmed. After that, only annual reevaluations are necessary unless there is a change in the person's condition. The nurse is in a key position to monitor the thyroid function of the patient by ensuring timely and appropriate laboratory testing of TSH level.

URINE STUDIES

Urine is the end-product of metabolism and should only contain products that have exceeded the body's threshold of usefulness. If the kidneys are working well and the urine level of a compound is elevated, there should be a corresponding elevation in the blood. However, if the kidney is diseased, urine levels may be deceptively low. The most common urine test in the everyday care of older adults is a urinalysis.

A macroscopic urinalysis may be performed in the outpatient primary care setting, but more often is done by a diagnostic laboratory. In healthy aging, the findings do not differ by age, but abnormalities are frequently found because of the high rate of diabetes, renal insufficiency, subclinical bacteriuria, and proteinuria.

⚡ SAFETY ALERT

A finding of hematuria, even in outpatient macroscopy, always requires further evaluation.

A urine specimen is collected either by using the clean-catch method or via catheterization. In the outpatient setting, it is best that the specimen be collected at the laboratory or sent to the lab immediately. If absolutely necessary, it may be collected and refrigerated for up to 2 hours. Any specimen that has not been properly stored or tested promptly must be disposed of and a new one obtained. The cleaner and fresher the specimen, the more accurate the analysis will be. There is a long history of conflicting evidence of the accuracy and reliability of urine testing using a "dip stick" method in the outpatient setting. Both laboratory and outpatient office analyses will yield results for urine specific gravity, pH, and the presence of urine protein, glucose, ketones, blood, bilirubin, nitrates, and leukocytes.

The specific gravity is a measure of the adequacy of the renal concentrative mechanism; it measures hydration and therefore is a useful measure when caring for frail older adults. Specific gravity in the adult is normally between 1.005 and 1.030. These values decrease with aging because of the 33% to 50% decline in the number of nephrons, which impairs the ability of the kidney to concentrate urine. The urine pH indicates its acid-base balance. An alkaline pH is usually caused by bacteria (which may indicate a urinary tract infection), a diet high in citrus fruits and vegetables, or the intake of sodium bicarbonates. Acidic urine occurs with starvation, dehydration, and diets high in meats and cranberries. A urine albumin level of almost 30 mg/dL translates into a considerably high rate of proteinuria and always indicates a need for further evaluation of renal function. Ascorbic acid and aspirin can cause false-negative results for glucose. Ketones may be positive in high-protein diets, "crash" diets, or starvation.

Nitrates and/or leukocytes are often found in the presence of infection. A urinalysis suggestive of the presence of bacteria usually results in further testing, most often a culture of the urine and a subsequent testing of sensitivity of the bacteria to select antibiotics. This is often ordered as a "U/A (urine analysis) C & S (culture and sensitivity) as indicated." However, because of the potential lethality of any infection in ill older adults, empirical clinical evidence of a potential infection may require treatment before the 3 or 4 days needed to obtain culture results.

PROMOTING HEALTHY AGING: IMPLICATIONS FOR GERONTOLOGICAL NURSING

The bedside or home health nurse is expected to have skills in basic laboratory interpretation, knowledge of the appropriate timing of the testing, and awareness of factors that could affect the results. For nurses working in long-term care settings, knowledge of interpretation is especially important to ensure that when abnormalities are identified, the person is treated promptly and appropriately. Advanced practice nurses are responsible for knowing when and what testing to order and to use the results for prescriptive responses to promote healthy aging.

Laboratory findings are often reported in relationship to a range of normalized values or reference ranges referred to as "within normal limits" (WNL). Special diligence is needed to interpret the results within the context of the person's overall health and normal changes with aging.

Laboratory tests and regular screening tests are commonly employed when caring for a resident of a nursing home. Protocols for establishing routine laboratory testing procedures for long-term care vary widely from one institution to the next and from one laboratory to the next. Gerontological nurses advocate good resident care by requesting laboratory tests and developing protocols to comply with recommended evidence-based standards for screening and monitoring for both long-term and short-term residents in residential settings.

Knowledge about the use, frequency, and basic interpretations of laboratory findings is important to the quality of care provided. These skills are especially important in

gerontological nursing practice—not because of the expected normal changes in laboratory results but because of the potential influence of commonly prescribed medications in the presence of chronic diseases often prevalent in the older adult.

Laboratory values are helpful tools in understanding clinical signs and symptoms, although clinical decisions based on laboratory values alone are not enough for treatment of the whole person. Abnormal laboratory results trigger comprehensive patient assessments, obtaining information about clinical signs and symptoms, patient history, and psychosocial and physical examination. The nurse combines this information with the interpretation of laboratory values to establish the most appropriate care in collaboration with the person's nurse practitioner or physician. The nurse practitioner quickly and accurately interprets the findings and translates these into the plan of care.

KEY CONCEPTS

- The normal range of diagnostic laboratory results does not differ by age.
- Because of more limited reserves, the older adult is often more sensitive to slight variations in biological parameters.

- The nurse is often responsible for the initial interpretation of laboratory results. The nurse cannot depend entirely on laboratory values when considering the possibility of medication toxicity.
- The interactions between medications and chronic disorders complicate the interpretation of laboratory values in older adults.

NURSING STUDY: Evaluating Laboratory Results

An 84-year-old white male, Mr. Jones, is being admitted to the nursing home where you work. He has a history of heart disease, hypertension, diabetes, constipation, and anemia of chronic inflammation. You find that he denies any fever, chest pain, numbness or tingling, leg swelling, or palpitations. His diabetes has been under fairly good control while at home, but he has difficulty telling you how much insulin he has been taking. His skin is slightly warm to the touch. He is lethargic, but you notice that he also has some muscle twitching. He has an order to have blood tests done today, including a CBC and a complete metabolic panel. You request it and get the following results later in the evening. Medications include lisinopril, 20 mg/day; Lasix, 40 mg/day; potassium, 5 mEq/day; Lantus insulin, 12 units every morning; laxative as needed; multivitamin daily. Blood sugar before supper is 243.

	Result	Normal Range
Sodium	135 mEq/L	136–48 mEq/L
Potassium	5.8 mEq/L	3.5–5.3 mEq/L
Chloride	110 mEq/L	97–108 mEq/L
Glucose	60 mg/dL	70–110 mg/dL

	Result	Normal Range
BUN	25 mg/dL	10–20 mg/dL
Creatinine	1.8 mg/dL	0.6–1.2 mg/dL
Albumin	2.4 g/dL	3.5–5.8 g/dL
WBCs	7000/mm^3	5000–10,000/mm^3
RBCs	$4.0 \times 10^6/\mu L$	$4.4–5.8 \times 10^6/\mu L$
Hgb	10.2 g/dL	14–18 g/dL
Hct	30.6%	39–48%

- Considering Mr. Jones and his current health status, which of the preceding lab results concerns you most?
- Are there any deviations in the results that are consistent with normal aging?
- Which of these deviations from normal are potentially the most dangerous for Mr. Jones at this time? If so, why?
- Could any of the abnormal blood tests be related to his medications?
- Are there any results that need prompt referral to the primary care provider for Mr. Jones? If so, which one(s)?

BUN, Blood urea nitrogen; *CBC*, complete blood count; *Hgb*, hemoglobin; *Hct*, hematocrit; *RBCs*, red blood cells; *WBCs*, white blood cells.

CRITICAL THINKING QUESTIONS AND ACTIVITIES

1. The next time you are working with an older adult either as his or her nurse/nurse practitioner or as a student nurse, review the most recent laboratory report and determine which variations are more likely a reflection of the person's disease state rather than age.
2. In a classroom discussion, consider a 90-year-old with increasing dyspnea (shortness of breath) and fatigue. If you

were ordering laboratory tests for this person, which ones would you choose in order of priority?
3. Summarize laboratory values that are considered the most "critical" in older adults and require some type of immediate response.

RESEARCH QUESTIONS

1. In what way does food and alcohol intake affect the accuracy of laboratory test results?

2. If someone has had several chronic diseases for an extended period of time and yet the person is active and "healthy," what laboratory finding(s) may still be outside of the normal limits?

REFERENCES

Alves FC, Sun J, Qureshi AR, et al: The higher mortality associated with low serum albumin is dependent on systemic inflammation in end-stage kidney disease, *PLoS One* 13(1):e0190410, 2018. Accessed January 2018.

American Diabetes Association: Classification and diagnosis of diabetes: standards of medical care in diabetes—2018, *Diabetes Care* 41(Suppl 1):S13–S27, 2018.

Beckett EL, Martin C, Boyd L, et al: Reduced plasma homocysteine levels in elderly Australians following mandatory folic acid fortification—a comparison of two cross-sectional cohorts, *J Nutr Intermed Metab* 8:14–20, 2019.

Chernecky CC, Berger BJ: *Laboratory tests and diagnostic procedures,* ed 6, St Louis, MO, 2013, Elsevier.

Cho KC: Electrolyte and acid-base disorders. In Papadakis MA, McPhee SJ, editors: *Current medical diagnosis and treatment 2017,* New York, NY, 2017, McGraw-Hill, pp 884–912.

Damon LE, Andreadis CB: Blood disorders. In Papadakis MA, McPhee SJ, editors: *Current medical diagnosis and treatment 2017,* New York, NY, 2017, McGraw-Hill, pp 499–545.

Dugdale DC: *Blood differential,* 2017, MedlinePlus. https://medlineplus.gov/lab-tests/blood-differential/. Accessed February 2019.

Ershler WB: Blood disorders in older adults. In Fillit HM, Rockwood K, Young JB, editors: *Brocklehurst's Textbook of geriatric medicine and gerontology,* Philadelphia, PA, 2017, Elsevier, pp 757–771.

Ferri FF: *Ferri's best test: a practical guide to clinical laboratory medicine and diagnostic imaging,* Philadelphia, PA, 2015, Saunders.

Filippatos TD, Makri A, Elisaf MS, Liamis G: Hyponatremia in the elderly: challenges and solutions, *Clin Interv Aging* 12:1957–1965, 2017.

Grundy SM, Stone NJ, Bailey AL, et al: *Guideline on the management of blood cholesterol,* 2018. Retrieved from https://www.acc.org/~/media/Non-Clinical/Files-PDFs-Excel-MS-Word-etc/Guidelines/2018/Guidelines-Made-Simple-Tool-2018-Cholesterol.pdf Accessed April 2019.

Hall JR, Wiechmann AR, Johnson LA, et al: Total cholesterol and neuropsychiatric symptoms in Alzheimer's disease: the impact of total cholesterol level and gender, *Dement Geriatr Cogn Disord* 38(5–6):300–309, 2014.

Lapin A, Mueller E: Laboratory diagnosis and geriatrics: more than just reference intervals for older adults. In Fillit HM, Rockwood K, Young JB, editors: *Brocklehurst's textbook of geriatric medicine and gerontology,* Philadelphia, PA, 2017, Elsevier, pp 220–225.

Leavitt AD, Minichiello T: Disorders of hemostasis, thrombosis, & antithrombotic therapy. In Papadakis MA, McPhee SJ, editors: *Current medical diagnosis and treatment 2017,* New York, NY, 2017, McGraw-Hill, pp 884–912.

Lewis JL: *Hypernatremia. Merck manual: Professional version,* 2016a. http://www.merckmanuals.com/professional/endocrine-and-metabolic-disorders/electrolyte-disorders/hypernatremia. Accessed January 2018.

Lewis JL: *Hypokalemia. Merck manual: Professional version,* 2016b. http://www.merckmanuals.com/professional/endocrine-and-metabolic-disorders/electrolyte-disorders/hypokalemia. Accessed January 2018.

Lin Y, Kim J, Metter EJ, et al: Changes in blood lymphocyte numbers with age in vivo and their association with the levels of cytokines/cytokine receptors, *Immun Ageing* 13:24, 2016.

Litao MK, Kamat D: Erythrocyte sedimentation rate and C-reactive protein: how best to use them in clinical practice, *Pediatr Ann* 43(10):417–420, 2014.

Mathew MK, Jacobs MS: Malnutrition and feeding problems. In Ham RJ, Sloane PD, Warshaw GA, Potter J, Flaherty E, editors: *Ham's primary care geriatrics: a case-based approach,* ed 6, Philadelphia, PA, 2014, Elsevier, pp 315–322.

Mayo Clinic: *Test ID: PBNP: NT-Pro B-type natriuretic peptide (BNP), serum.* https://www.mayomedicallaboratories.com/test-catalog/Clinical+and+Interpretive/84291. Accessed January 2018.

Nakasato Y, Christensen M: Arthritis and related disorders. In Ham RJ, Sloane PD, Warshaw GA, Potter J, Flaherty E, editors: *Ham's primary care geriatrics: a case-based approach,* ed 6, Philadelphia, PA, 2014, Elsevier, pp 456–465.

Reuben DB, Herr KA, Pacala JT, Pollock BG, Potter JF, Semla TP: *Geriatrics at your fingertips,* ed 19, New York, NY, 2017, American Geriatric Society.

Rote NS, McCance KL: Structure and function of the hematologic system. In McCance KL, Huether SE, Brashers VL, Rote NS, editors: *Pathophysiology: the biologic basis for disease in adults and children,* ed 7t, St Louis, MO, 2014, Elsevier, pp 945–981.

Shah MK, Workeneh B, Taffet GE: Hypernatremia in the geriatric population, *Clin Interv Aging* 9:1987–1992, 2014.

Takata Y, Ansai T, Soh I, et al: Serum total cholesterol concentration and 10-year mortality in an 85-year-old population, *Clin Interv Aging* 9:293–300, 2014.

U.S. Preventive Services Task Force: *Final recommendation statement: prostate cancer: Screening,* 2018. https://www.uspreventiveservicestaskforce.org/Page/Document/RecommendationStatementFinal/prostate-cancer-screening1. Accessed February 2019.

Wong CW: Vitamin B12 deficiency in the elderly: is it worth screening? *Hong Kong Med J* 21(2):155–164, 2015.

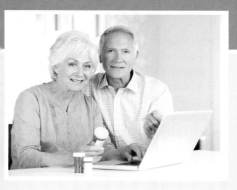

9

Geropharmacology

Kathleen Jett

http://evolve.elsevier.com/Touhy/TwdHlthAging

A STUDENT SPEAKS

Whenever I see patients in the clinic I try to think very carefully before adding any medications, but since most of them have so many illnesses at the same time, I sometimes wonder where I can start!

Helen, age 32, gerontological nurse practitioner student

AN OLDER ADULT SPEAKS

Every time I go to the clinic I get another prescription. It just doesn't seem like I need to take so many medications, so sometimes I don't.

Annie, age 72

LEARNING OBJECTIVES

On completion of this chapter, the reader will be able to:
1. Describe the pharmacokinetic and pharmacodynamic changes that are normal changes with aging.
2. Describe potential problems associated with medication therapy in late life.
3. Identify medications that are more commonly used in late life.
4. Identify inappropriate use of medication and explain how it interferes with healthy aging.
5. Identify the early signs of adverse medication reactions and events and develop strategies to prevent these.
6. Discuss barriers to medication adherence in older adults.
7. Develop a nursing plan to promote safe medication practices and prevent medication toxicity.

In the United States, persons 65 years of age and older are prescribed more medications than any other age group. Although the exact statistics vary from study to study, all findings indicate that as one ages, the number of prescribed medications, dietary supplements, and herbal products taken increases. In one survey of persons at least 55 years of age, 53% reported taking at least four medications; the use of supplements has increased from 14% in 1998 to 49% in 2006 (Slattum et al, 2017).

When used appropriately, pharmacological interventions can enhance the quality of life and promote healthy aging. When used inappropriately, they can contribute to both morbidity and mortality at any age. Unfortunately, even when medications are prescribed, administered, and taken appropriately, adverse medication reactions and events can and do occur, especially in older adults. The reasons for this are many and include reduced organ function and physiological reserve and varying levels of skills of health care providers.

This chapter reviews the effect of aging on pharmacokinetics and pharmacodynamics. Issues in medications are discussed including polypharmacy, medication interactions, adverse medication reactions and events, and the uses of psychoactive agents relative to the aging adult.

PHARMACOKINETICS

Pharmacokinetics is the study of the movement and action of a medication in the body from the time it is administered to the time it is excreted. Pharmacokinetic processes determine the concentration of medications in the body, which in turn determines the effect. The concentration of the medication at different times depends on how the medication is taken into the body (absorption), where the medication is dispersed (distribution), how the medication is broken down (metabolism), and how the body gets rid of the medication (excretion) (Box 9.1).

Absorption

There are several normal age-related changes that have the potential to affect absorption and therefore the amount of the

BOX 9.1 Physiological Changes With Aging and Effect on Pharmacokinetics and Pharmacodynamics

Absorption
Reduced saliva
Presbyphagia
Decreased gastric acid
Delayed stomach emptying
Slowed intestinal motility

Distribution
Reduced cardiac output and reduced circulation
Reduced body water
Reduced extracellular volume
Increased adipose tissue
Reduced serum albumin and other body protein levels
Metabolism
Reduced liver mass
Reduced liver circulation
Reduced enzyme activity

Excretion
Reduced glomerular filtration and creatinine clearance

medication available for both therapeutic and adverse effects. Most medications are administered orally. This is potentially problematic due to an age-related reduction in saliva. When combined with medication with strong anticholinergic properties, swallowing is sometimes very difficult. Age-related decreases in esophageal motility (presbyphagia) further contribute to swallowing difficulties and, in extreme cases, tissue erosions (Shim et al, 2017). With sublingual administration, medication is absorbed directly into the systemic circulation through the mucous membrane, but a dry mouth will reduce or delay buccal absorption. Transdermal and rectal administration may be useful when the patient cannot tolerate oral or sublingual medications, such as for those nearing the end of life.

Age-related changes in the stomach have several potential effects. Decreases in the amount of gastric acid may retard the action of acid-dependent medications. Delayed stomach emptying may diminish or negate the effectiveness of short-lived medications that could become inactivated before reaching the small intestine. Some enteric-coated formulations of medications, such as aspirin, which are specifically meant to bypass stomach acidity, may be delayed so long that their action begins in the stomach and may cause gastric irritation or nausea.

Once a medication has been administered orally (or enterally), it may be absorbed directly into the bloodstream from the stomach (e.g., alcohol), but usually absorption begins in the duodenum of the small intestine and continues in the large intestine. Slowed intestinal motility, while not a normal change of aging, is frequently encountered in late life. This additional time the medication has contact with the intestinal walls increases the risk for adverse reactions and unpredictable effects.

Nurses working with older adults are usually familiar with the transdermal drug delivery system (TDDS). Designed for the slow absorption of fat-soluble medications, it has been found to

be extremely useful for those who require very small doses of a medication over a longer period (usually more than 72 hours). This route overcomes any first-pass problems and is more convenient, more acceptable, and potentially more reliable than other routes, especially for persons with cognitive disorders. Ideally, the TDDS provides for a more constant rate of medication administration and eliminates concern about gastrointestinal absorption variation, gastrointestinal intolerance, and medication interaction. However, the use of these patches requires manual dexterity that is not always possible, especially for persons with orthopedic deformities such as osteoarthritis. Additionally, for the person who is underweight or overweight, absorption may be unreliable. The characteristic thin, dry older skin also may affect absorption of the intended dose at the intended time. Finally, due to reduced natural immunity there is an increased risk for an allergic reaction to the patch (Castelo-Branco and Soveral, 2014).

Distribution

The systemic circulation transports a medication throughout the body to receptors on the cells of the target organ where a therapeutic effect is initiated. The organs of high blood flow (e.g., brain, kidneys, lungs, and liver) rapidly receive the highest concentrations. Distribution to organs of lower blood flow (e.g., skin, muscles, fat) occurs more slowly and results in lower concentrations of the medication in these tissues. The circulatory diseases common in late life, such as peripheral vascular disease, can negatively affect medication distribution.

Normal changes with aging include lower total body water and higher body fat (as fat replaces lean tissue). By the age of 70 adipose tissue increases to 36% in healthy older men and 45% in older women. Lipophilic (fat-soluble) medications concentrate in adipose tissue more than in other tissues. If the medication accumulates to an excess in the adipose tissue, it may increase medication effect and can even result in a potentially fatal overdose. Extracellular volume decreases by 40% between the ages of 20 and 65 and body water decreases by 17% (Slattum et al, 2017).

Distribution also depends on the availability of plasma protein in the form of lipoproteins, globulins, and especially albumin (Box 9.2). Several medications are bound to plasma protein for distribution (Cambridge, 2017). In healthy adults of any age, a predictable percentage of an absorbed medication is inactivated as it is bound to the protein. The remaining free medication is available in the bloodstream for therapeutic effect when an effective concentration is reached in the plasma.

Serum albumin levels decrease with age (Lapin and Mueller, 2017) (Fig. 9.1). They are further reduced in those

BOX 9.2 Medications That Bind Strongly to the Plasma Protein Albumin

Ceftriaxone	Valproic acid
Ibuprofen	Warfarin
Naproxen	

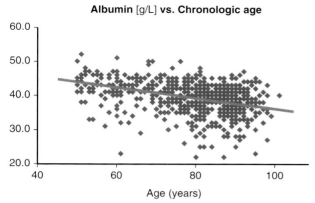

Albumin [g/L] vs. Chronologic age

Fig. 9.1 Correlation of Albumin Levels With Age. (From Lapin A, Mueller E: Laboratory diagnosis and geriatrics: more than just reference intervals for older adults. In Fillit HM, Rockwood K, Young JB, editors: *Brocklehurst's textbook of geriatric medicine and gerontology*, ed 8, Philadelphia, PA, 2017, Elsevier, pp 220–225.)

with acute illness or a long-standing chronic condition. This reduction is especially common among those who are frail and in need of skilled care at home or in long-term care settings (Chapter 32). This decrease in serum albumin reduces binding capacity and therefore increases the amount of free medication, with the subsequent amount available for therapeutic action being unpredictable. Signs of medication toxicity can occur quickly; this is especially dangerous in medications that bind with albumin and have a narrow therapeutic window, such as warfarin.

Metabolism

Drug metabolism, or biotransformation, is the process wherein a pharmaceutical substance can be eliminated from the body more easily. In the transformation the medication becomes a metabolite. This usually occurs in the liver and is facilitated by enzymes. Several factors (e.g., smoking, frailty, sex) are key factors affecting drug metabolism. Aging results in reduced liver mass. As a result liver perfusion is reduced by 30% to 40%, further limiting the amount and speed of biotransformation (Lavan et al, 2016). The medications make a "first pass" through the liver but are not metabolized and remain available for therapeutic action (Slattum et al, 2017).

Excretion

Medications are excreted either unchanged or as metabolites. A few are eliminated through the lungs, in bile and feces, or in breast milk. A small amount is eliminated through hair, sweat, saliva, tears, and semen. The renal system is the primary site of excretion as a medication or metabolite passes through the kidneys and into the bladder. Excretion depends on both the rate and extent of protein binding of the medication; only unbound medications are filtered. The effectiveness of excretion depends on health of all parts; the efficiency of excretion can be measured by the glomerular filtration rate (GFR).

Age-related changes in renal function have a significant effect on medication/metabolite excretion. Most people lose 1% of their GFR a year starting at about 20 years of age (Slattum

et al, 2017). This change reduces the body's ability to eliminate medications in a timely manner by prolonging their half-life, that is, the amount of time it takes for a medication's therapeutic effect to be reduced by one-half. This results in more opportunities for accumulation and can lead to potential toxicity or other adverse events.

Renal filtration can be approximated by calculating a creatinine clearance rate (CrCl) (Chapter 8). Many free automatic calculators are available online (http://nephron.com/cgi-bin/CGSI.cgi). The CrCl allows the nurse to determine which person needs medication dosage adjustment due to renal impairment.

PHARMACODYNAMICS

Pharmacodynamics refers to the physiological interactions between a medication and the body, specifically the chemical compounds introduced into the body and the receptors on cell membranes. These receptors are cellular proteins with unique shapes and ionic charges that bind to a very specific medication, like a glove to a hand. When this binding occurs, a structural change in the receptor protein is initiated, which in turn leads to a biochemical cascade and resultant therapeutic effect.

The older a person becomes, the more likely he or she will have unreliable pharmacodynamics. Although it is not always possible to explain or predict all of the alterations, several are well known. Those of special note in aging are the side effects associated with sedating or anticholinergic medications. These side effects can significantly increase the rate of functional decline and the risk for accidental injury (Box 9.3) (Reuben et al, 2017). Baroreceptor reflex responses decrease with age, causing increased susceptibility to orthostatic hypotension and the need to pay special attention to antihypertensive medications. Age-related decreases in thirst sensation may lead to dehydration and subsequent alterations in drug metabolism. A decreased responsiveness of the α-adrenergic system results in decreased sensitivity to β-agonist and β-antagonist medications (e.g., beta-blockers).

BOX 9.3 Medications With Strong Anticholinergic and Sedating Properties and Select Side Effects

Examples of Medications	Select Potential Effects
Antihistamines	Constipation
Antimuscarinics (for urinary incontinence)	Dry mouth
	Blurred vision
Antispasmodics	Dizziness
Benzodiazepines	Confusion
Antipsychotics	Urinary retention
Antidepressants	Functional impairment
Opioids	Increased heart rate

Data from Kouladjian L, Gnjidic D, Chen TF, et al: Drug burden index in older adults: theoretical and practical issues, *Clin Interv Aging* 9, 1503–1515, 2014.

ISSUES IN MEDICATION USE

Polypharmacy

Polypharmacy has been defined in many ways but the most commonly used definition is the use of approximately five or more medications, more medications than are medically necessary, or the use of multiple medications for the same problem (Levy, 2017; Maher et al, 2014). The rate of polypharmacy varies by country. In the United States, 53% of persons over 55 years of age and living in the community took at least four medications daily (Slattum et al, 2017). In a study of persons at least 65 years of age, 41.4% were taking five to eight at the time of hospital discharge and 58.6% were taking one or more medications that could be considered unnecessary. U.S. nursing homes have been under pressure to reduce the number of medications to below nine per person (Maher et al, 2014).

If the patient has multiple chronic conditions, simple polypharmacy may be necessary, even if the prescribing provider is following evidence-based guidelines. It may occur unintentionally, if an existing medication regimen is not considered when new prescriptions are given. When any number of the hundreds of over-the-counter (OTC) supplements such as vitamins and herbs are added to those prescribed, the polypharmacy is exacerbated.

Polypharmacy is exacerbated by the combination of a high use of health care specialists and a reluctance of prescribers to discontinue potentially unnecessary medications that have been prescribed by someone else. This can lead to the continued use of medications that may no longer be necessary. When communication among patients, nurses, other health care providers, and caregivers becomes fragmented, the risk for duplicative medications, inappropriate medications, potentially unsafe dosages, and potentially preventable interactions is heightened. Polypharmacy is extremely common among older adults and a source of multiple potential morbidities and mortality (Box 9.4). The issues of polypharmacy are the increased risk for medication interactions and the increased risk for adverse events. The more the medications, the more risk.

Medication Interactions

The more prescribed medications and any other substances a person takes (e.g., herbs, vitamins, dietary supplements, foods),

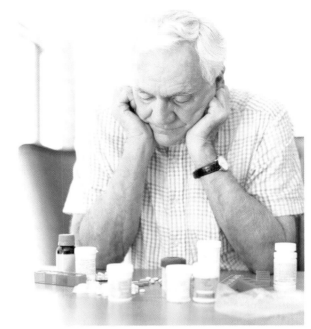

Polypharmacy. (From ©iStock.com/Squaredpixels.)

the greater the possibility one or more will interact with another. At the same time, the more chronic conditions one has, the more likely it is that a medication for one condition will affect the body in such a way as to influence another condition. For example, a person takes ibuprofen for arthritis pain and subsequently has an increase in his or her already high blood pressure. When two or more medications (or products of any kind, including food) are taken at the same time or closely together, one substance may potentiate another (i.e., cause it to have stronger effects than when given alone) or antagonize (lower the potency) the other, even to the point that the medication is inactivated.

Medication-Herb/Supplement Interactions

As the popularity of medicinal herbs and other dietary supplements rises, so does the risk for interactions with prescribed medications. Although much remains unknown, new knowledge is added almost daily upon which the gerontological nurse may base her or his practice. For example, a number of herbs have a direct effect on coagulability. When these herbs are taken with warfarin, the risk of bleeding may significantly increase. If the herb influences the results of the international normalized ratio (INR) or other measure of coagulation, adjustments to the warfarin dose will lead to inappropriate and potentially dangerous consequences. The interactions presented in Table 9.1 represent only a small fraction of the many real and potential problems when prescribed medications are combined with an herb or a dietary supplement. See Chapter 10 for in-depth coverage of this important topic.

Medication-Food Interactions

Many foods interact with medications, producing increased, decreased, or variable effects. For example, calcium in dairy

BOX 9.4   **Consequences of Polypharmacy**
Increased health care cost
Adverse drug reactions and events
Drug interactions (drug, supplement, disease)
Difficulty with compliance
Reduced functional status
Cognitive impairment
Falls
Urinary incontinence
Poor nutrition

Adapted from Maher RL, Hanlon JT, Hajjar ER: Clinical consequences of polypharmacy in elderly, *Expert Opin Drug Saf* 13(1):57–65, 2014.

TABLE 9.1 Select Herb-Medication Interactions.[a]

Herb	Medication	Complication	Nursing Action
Echinacea	**Any anticoagulant drug** such as warfarin sodium; digoxin	Risk of bleeding may increase; therapeutic digoxin level may be altered	Advise person not to take without provider approval
Garlic	**Any anticoagulant or antiplatelet drug** such as warfarin sodium, streptokinase, aspirin, other NSAIDs	Risk of bleeding may increase	Advise person not to take without provider approval
	Antihypertensives	Increased hypotensive effect	Advise provider approval with use
	Antivirals, such as ritonavir	Altered drug effect	Advise against use
	Antimetabolites such as cyclosporine	Risk of less effective response	Advise against use
	Insulin or oral hypoglycemic agent such as pioglitazone or tolbutamide	Serum glucose control may improve; less antidiabetic drug needed	Monitor blood glucose levels
Ginkgo	Aspirin, other NSAIDs, heparin sodium, warfarin sodium, **any anticoagulant**	Risk of bleeding may occur	Teach person not to take without approval of provider
	Antiplatelet drugs such as ticlopidine		
	Antidiabetic drugs: insulin, oral DMT2 drugs such as metformin	May alter blood glucose levels	Monitor blood glucose level closely
	Antidepressants, MAOIs, SSRIs	May cause abnormal response or decrease effectiveness	Advise not to take with these drugs
	Antihypertensives	May cause increased effect	Monitor blood pressure
	Antiseizure drugs	Risk for seizure if history of seizure	Advise against use
Ginseng	Insulin and oral antidiabetic drugs	Blood glucose levels may be altered	Monitor blood glucose levels closely
	Anticoagulant and antiplatelet drugs Aspirin and other NSAIDs	May increase bleeding	Advise use with caution and provider oversight
	MAOIs such as isocarboxazid	Headaches, tremors, mania	Advise against use
	Antihypertensives, cardiac drugs such as calcium channel blockers	May alter effects of drug	Advise against use unless provider monitors closely
	Immunosuppressants	May interfere with action	Advise against use
	Stimulants	May cause additive effect	Advise against use
	Fenugreek	Decreased blood glucose	Monitor closely
Green tea	**Warfarin sodium**	May alter anticoagulant effects	Advise against use
	Stimulants	May cause additive effect	Advise to use with care
Hawthorn	Digoxin	May cause a loss of potassium, leading to drug toxicity	Monitor blood levels
	Beta-blockers and other drugs lowering blood pressure and improving blood flow	May be additive in effects	Monitor blood pressure meticulously; advise that this concern holds true for erectile dysfunction drugs also
Red yeast rice	Fibrate drugs; other cholesterol drugs	May cause additive effects	Avoid concomitant use
	Drugs for diabetes management	May alter blood sugar levels	Monitor blood sugar carefully
	Anticoagulants, antiplatelet drugs, NSAIDs	May increase risk of bleeding	Warn patient and monitor carefully
St. John's wort	Triptans such as sumatriptan, zolmitriptan	May increase risks of serotonergic adverse effects, serotonin syndrome, cerebral vasoconstriction	Advise against use
	HMG-CoA reductase inhibitors	May decrease plasma concentrations of these drugs	Monitor levels of lipids
	MAOIs	May cause similar effects as with use with any SSRI	Advise against use
	Digoxin	Decreases the effects of the drug	Advise against use
	Alprazolam	May decrease effect of drug	Advise against use
	Ketoprofen	Photosensitivity	Advise sun block use
	Tramadol and some SSRIs	May increase risk for serotonin syndrome	Advise against use
	Olanzapine	May cause serotonin syndrome	Advise against use
	Paroxetine	Sedative-hypnotic intoxication	Advise against use
	Theophylline	Increases metabolism; decreases drug blood level	Monitor drug effects
	Albuterol		
	Warfarin	May decrease anticoagulant effect	Advise against use
	Amlodipine	Lowers efficacy of calcium channel	Advise against use
	Estrogen or progesterone	May decrease effect of hormones	Advise that this effect may occur

[a]The interactions listed represent only a few of the possible herb-drug interactions. Use of herbs that interfere with metabolism of drugs by the liver's cytochrome P450 enzyme system should be avoided or monitored closely by the provider.

DMT2, Diabetes mellitus type 2; *FDA,* U.S. Food and Drug Administration; *HMG-CoA,* 3-hydroxy-3-methylglutaryl coenzyme-A; *MAOIs,* monoamine oxidase inhibitors; *NSAIDs,* nonsteroidal antiinflammatory drugs; *SSRIs,* selective serotonin reuptake inhibitors.

Data from Shiel WC: *Herbs: toxicities and drug interactions,* 2016. https://www.medicinenet.com/herbs__toxicities_and_drug_interactions/views. htm. Accessed February 2017; Anderson L: *18 herbal supplements with risky drug interactions,* 2017. https://www.drugs.com/slideshow/herb-drug-interactions-1069. Accessed February 2018.

products will bind to levothyroxine, tetracycline, and ciprofloxacin, greatly decreasing their absorption; lovastatin absorption is increased by a high-fat, low-fiber meal. Grapefruit juice contains substances that inhibit CYP3A4 isoenzyme 3A4-mediated metabolism in the gut wall and liver and either increase or decrease the bioavailability of a medication (Table 9.2).

Spironolactone, prescribed for end-stage heart failure, increases potassium (K^+) reabsorption by the renal tubule. If a patient ingests a diet high in potassium (e.g., KCl salt substitute, molasses, oranges, bananas) or other potassium-sparing agents (e.g., lisinopril) at the same time, K^+ levels can rise significantly and quickly reach toxic levels. The vitamin K^+ in leafy green vegetables antagonizes (decreases) the anticoagulant effects of warfarin and may have a significant effect on the coagulability of the blood (Reuben, 2017). It is recommended that patients who choose to eat greens while taking warfarin ingest a consistent amount of greens to avoid variations in their warfarin levels (Box 9.5) (www.cc.nih.gov/ccc/patient_education/drug_nutrient/coumadin1.pdf).

Medication-Medication Interactions

The polypharmacy that may be a necessary part of health care in later life significantly increases both the risk for and the frequency of medication-medication interactions. These may occur at any time from preparation to excretion. For example, persons who cannot swallow after a stroke may receive all feedings and medications enterally. Medications intended for oral administration must be converted to a soluble form for passage through the tube without clogging and yet also remain in their original form. When several medications are crushed, mixed

TABLE 9.2 Common Drug-Food Interactions.

Food	Drug	Potential Effect
Fiber	Digoxin	Absorption of drug into fiber, reducing drug action
Foods with vitamin K	Warfarin	Decreased effect of drug
Food	Many antibiotics	Reduced absorption rate of drug
Vitamin B₆ supplements	Levodopa-carbidopa	Reverses antiparkinsonian effect
Grapefruit juice	Multiple medications	Altered metabolism and elimination can increase concentration of drug
Citrus juice	Calcium channel blockers	Gastric reflux exacerbated

BOX 9.5 Top 10 Foods to Avoid When Taking Warfarin

Kale	Turnip greens
Spinach	Parsley
Collards	Broccoli
Swiss chard	Brussels sprouts
Mustard greens	Brussels sprouts, cooked

See for expanded list and for patient information: www.cc.nih.gov/ccc/patient_education/drug_nutrient/coumadin1.pdf

together, and then dissolved in water for administration, a new product is created, and medication-medication interactions may have already begun.

⚡ SAFETY ALERT

Safe Administration of Medications Through Enteral Feeding Tubes

Persons who receive their medications via the enteral route are at high risk for medication errors. Safe administration of such drugs is a time-consuming process that requires detailed knowledge of the medications (and their formulation) and the skill to prepare them appropriately. Most often this preparation occurs at the bedside, further increasing the risk for errors. The possible outcomes of such errors may include the following: occluded tube, reduced medication effect, medication toxicity, patient harm, and patient death. The three most common errors are incompatible route, improper preparation, and improper administration.

Altered absorption can occur when one medication binds another medication in the small intestine to form a nonabsorbable compound. For example, ciprofloxacin and iron compounds are both taken frequently by older adults. They bind together, and both lose their therapeutic effect. Other medications may compete for the same receptor site, creating varied bioavailability of one or both drugs. Interference with enzyme activity may alter metabolism and cause deficiencies or toxicities. Antispasmodic medications slow gastric and intestinal motility even further than that present in normal aging. In some instances, this may be useful if a prolonged effect is beneficial but may prove harmful when it leads to an accumulation and potential medication intoxication.

Altered distribution may be caused by displacement of one medication from its receptor site by another medication. Altered distribution is a common cause of adverse medication reactions in older adults and is an especially important issue in patients with lowered albumin levels. Thus, it is common among chronically ill, frail older adults, such as many of those residing in long-term care facilities (Slattum et al, 2017).

Altered excretion coupled with age-related decreases in renal function can occur when one medication changes the urinary pH such that another medication is either reabsorbed or excreted to a greater extent than is desired. Another mechanism may involve one medication increasing or decreasing active transport in the renal tubules (e.g., probenecid decreases the active transport of penicillin, thereby prolonging its half-life).

Pharmacodynamic medication interactions can be especially dangerous for older adults, including the additive pharmacological effects of two or more similar medications; that is, together they are more potent than they are separately (e.g., central nervous system [CNS] effects of sedative-hypnotic medications and anticholinergic medications) (Slattum et al, 2017). Due to the frequency of polypharmacy, medication-medication interactions can have a significant effect on everyday prescribing, administration, and monitoring of effects of medications taken by older adults (Box 9.6).

BOX 9.6 Tips for Best Practice

Examples of Medication Combinations With a High Potential for Adverse Interactions

- ACE inhibitors and potassium-sparing diuretics
- ACE inhibitors or ARBs and Septra (Bactrim)
- Macrolide antibiotics (e.g., Cipro) and either calcium channel blockers or digoxin
- Warfarin and any of the antibiotics or NSAIDs

ACE, Angiotensin-converting enzyme; *ARB,* α-receptor blocker; *NSAID,* nonsteroidal antiinflammatory drug.

Adverse Drug Reactions and Events

Adverse drug reactions (ADRs) and *adverse drug events* (ADEs) occur when there is a noxious response to a medication. The effects of such reactions may range from a minor annoyance to death and are a common cause of hospitalization. In an analysis of 178,000 emergency room visits, 3.6 % were related to potentially inappropriate medications. Three medications (warfarin, digoxin, and insulin) accounted for one-third of these. When considering emergency hospitalizations, four types of medications (warfarin, insulin, oral antiplatelet drugs, oral hypoglycemics) accounted for 67% of the cases (Rochon, 2018). At the same time, rates of overall in-hospital ADE declined 19% between 2010 and 2013 attributed to the implementation of "meaningful use" requirements and consequences (Furukawa et al, 2017).

Sometimes an ADR can be predicted from the pharmacological action of the medication, such as bone marrow suppression from chemotherapeutic agents or bleeding from anticoagulants. At other times they are unpredictable, such as in an allergic reaction to antibiotics. Allergic reactions become more common in older adults as the immune system decreases in function (Chapter 24). It is reasonable to assume that many ADRs in older adults go unrecognized because of their nonspecific nature, their similarity to some of the subtle changes with aging, and to the vague signs and symptoms of many of the chronic conditions common in later life.

When a response reaches the level of harm, it is referred to as an *adverse drug event* (ADE). Many of these must be reported to the U.S. Food and Drug Administration or other regulatory body. ADEs can result either from the administration of a single medication or from the interaction of multiple medications as previously discussed. Although the reporting of ADEs had previously been limited to prescribed substances, this reporting has now been expanded to include any other products (such as dietary supplements) for which health-related claims are made (FDA, 2017). Most reporting is voluntary. However, it is strongly encouraged because reporting ADEs and product quality problems contributes to the protection of the public from harm.

Although ADRs and ADEs still occur, there has been considerable progress in the development of strategies to reduce their likelihood, especially in the recognition of age-related pharmacokinetic and pharmacodynamic changes in later life. We now know that in many cases an older adult should be prescribed lower dosages of several of the medications commonly needed, especially when beginning a new medication regimen. To minimize the likelihood of an ADR, the dose can be slowly increased until it safely reaches a therapeutic level. A common adage related to medication dosing in older adults is, "Start low, go slow, but go." There has also been a recognition that the risk of ADEs is so high with some medications that they are simply not recommended for use in persons with any known risk factors.

Beers' Criteria

The appropriate use of medications in the older adult means that such products are used only as needed, at the minimum dose necessary to achieve the desired effects, and in a way the risks relative to benefits have been considered within the greater context of the person's life expectancy, health, lifestyle, and values. Beers published a list of "potentially inappropriate medications (PIMs)" for the nursing home setting in 1997 (Beers, 1997). It was expanded several times to cover all care settings, and most recently by the American Geriatrics Society (AGS, 2019).

The Beers' Criteria is the result of an exhaustive analysis of medications considered to be frequently prescribed to older adults. The 2019 list includes those medications that are "potentially inappropriate" for use with older adults, potentially inappropriate for older adults with certain conditions, those that should only be used with caution, medications to be avoided or have their dose changed for people with impaired renal function, and a list of drug-drug interactions documented to be harmful to older adults. The American Geriatric Society has created a list of alternatives that is intended to be used along the use of the Beers Criteria (AGS, 2019).

While the Beers' Criteria have been incorporated into regulatory policy, the authors of the 2019 document emphasize the need to have it serve as a guide rather absolute direction. The Criteria are a part of the quality measures for the National Committee for Quality Assurance (NCQA) and the Healthcare Effectiveness Data and Information Set (HEDIS) (NCQA, 2018). When a potentially inappropriate medication is prescribed in the long-term care setting without documentation of an overwhelming benefit of its use, it can be considered a form of medication misuse by the prescribing practitioner (Box 9.7). The use of PIMs has been found to be associated with confusion, falls, other syndromes (Chapter 21), and death.

PSYCHOACTIVE MEDICATIONS

Psychoactive medications are those that affect mental function, which in turn affects behavior and how the world is experienced. The gerontological nurse, especially one working in a long-term care setting, is likely to be responsible for older adults who are receiving psychoactive medications, especially those for the treatment of depression, anxiety, and bipolar disorder (Chapter 28). Medications with psychoactive properties have a higher than usual risk for adverse events and must be prescribed and administered with an acute awareness of how age-related changes affect their absorption, distribution, excretion, and hepatic function.

To control the burgeoning use of psychotropic medications in nursing homes, the Centers for Medicare and Medicaid

---

BOX 9.7 Examples of Medications From the Beers' Criteria for Potentially Inappropriate Medications for Use in Older Adults (>65 Years of Age)

Potentially Inappropriate in Most Circumstances

Meclizine
Dipyridamole (short acting)
Nitrofurantoin
Digoxin (especially as first line)
Tricyclic antidepressants
Antipsychotics except under limited circumstances
Benzodiazepines except under limited circumstances
Sulfonylureas
Meperidine
NSAIDS (except for brief use)
Amiodarone
Zaleplon
Zolpidem
Sliding scale insulin
Proton pump inhibitors longer than 8 weeks
Desmopressin
Opioids (especially in persons with history of falls)

Should Be Avoided or Dose Adjusted Based on Renal Function

Anticoagulants
Spironolactone

Triamterene
Apixaban
Edoxaban
Rivaroxaban
Gabapentin
Tramadol
Ranitidine
Colchicine

Drug Disease or Drug-Syndrome Interactions That May Exacerbate the Condition in Older Adults

Anticholinergics
First-generation antihistamines
Alpha$_1$-blockers
H2 receptor antagonists
Corticosteroids
Nifedipine, immediate release
Tricyclic antidepressants
Barbiturates
Benzodiazepines
Sliding scale insulin
Demerol
Non–COX-selective NSAIDs

For full list and details see American Geriatrics Society (AGS) Expert Panel: American Geriatrics Society 2019 updated Beers Criteria for potentially inappropriate medication use in older adults, *J Am Geriatr Soc* 67(4):674–694, 2019.

Services issued a clarification of instructions to guide those who were responsible for monitoring the quality of patient care (usually state surveyors) (CMS, 2013). This classification of medications may never be used as a "quick fix" and should only be used when a thorough assessment had been completed, nonpharmacological approaches had been proven ineffective, and the patient would clearly benefit from their use.

One specific class of psychoactive medications, antipsychotics, is sometimes prescribed to persons with neurodegenerative disorders and behavior disturbances that place those around the person in danger, due to hallucinations and delusions. These should never be used unless all nonpharmacological means have been tried. Persons taking these medications must be monitored with special care.

Antipsychotics

Antipsychotic medications are tranquilizing and used to treat major depressive disorders, bipolar disorders, and psychoses, including those associated with the dementias. Their mechanism of action centers on blocking dopamine receptor pathways in the brain and they also affect the hypothalamic and thermoregulatory pathways. They are often ranked in relation to their side effects, especially sedation, hypotension, and extrapyramidal (and anticholinergic) side effects (EPSEs). Other side effects of these medications include neuroleptic malignant syndrome (NMS) and movement disorders.

The first such medications to be produced (in the 1950s) are now referred to as "typical antipsychotics" (e.g., haloperidol, chlorpromazine), and the newer, second-generation medications (developed since the 1990s) are classified as the "atypicals" (e.g., quetiapine [Seroquel]). The dangers associated with the use of any of these requires that their use be significantly justified and that a careful cost/benefit analysis be done. *Typical antipsychotics can never be used for someone with the diagnosis of dementia with Lewy bodies.*

When used appropriately and cautiously, antipsychotics can provide a person with relief from what may be frightening and incapacitating symptoms. Inappropriate use of antipsychotic medications may mask a reversible cause for the psychosis (such as delirium, infection, dehydration, fever, or electrolyte imbalance), an adverse medication effect, or a sudden change in the environment. Because of the seriousness, frequency, and number of the side effects and associated complications, these medications are prescribed at the lowest dose possible and for the shortest time possible. When antipsychotic medications are prescribed, more caution than usual must be used and the patient must be monitored closely.

⚡ **SAFETY ALERT**

Examples of side effects of antipsychotic medications include drowsiness, dizziness, weight gain, constipation, low blood pressure, tremors, restlessness, rigidity, and muscle spasms (National Institute of Mental Health, 2016).

Malignant Syndrome

Because antipsychotics affect the thermoregulatory pathway, patients taking them cannot tolerate excess environmental heat. Even mild elevations of core temperature can result in liver damage, called *neuroleptic malignant syndrome* (NMS). Acute

NMS is characterized by high fever, rigidity, altered mental status, and other symptoms of autonomic instability such as tachycardia and pallor. The nurse or caregiver must therefore protect the person from NMS by making sure the environment is cool at all times and the person is adequately hydrated. Direct sunlight should be avoided. Because the patient may not share or be able to share his or her discomfort about the heat, regular assessment of body temperature is essential. Any circumstance resulting in dehydration greatly increases the risk of heat stroke, which in late life is associated with high death rates.

Movement Disorders

NMS is not commonly seen in older adults taking antipsychotics. The more common side effects are movement disorders, also referred to as *extrapyramidal syndrome* (EPS). These include acute dystonia, akathisia, parkinsonian symptoms, and tardive dyskinesia (TD). Although more common with the typical antipsychotics, they can occur with any of the antipsychotics. The prescribing provider should be notified immediately any time such symptoms or signs are seen. Many of them are potentially life-threatening. In most cases the offending medication must be stopped immediately, with a potential need for hospitalization.

Acute Dystonia

An acute dystonic reaction is an abnormal involuntary movement consisting of a slow and continuous muscular contraction or spasm of the mouth, jaw, face, and neck. The jaw may lock (trismus), the tongue may roll back and block the airway, the neck may arch backward (opisthotonos), or the eyes may close. In an oculogyric crisis, the eyes are fixed in one position. Often this creates a feeling of needing to look up constantly without the ability to gaze downward. These reactions may occur hours or days after the initiation of a medication or after a dose increase and may continue from a few minutes to many hours.

Akathisia

Akathisia is a compulsion to be in motion, a sense of restlessness, being unable to be still, having an unrelenting desire to move, and feeling "like crawling out of my skin." The patient is seen pacing, fidgeting, and markedly restless. Often this symptom is mistaken for worsening psychosis instead of the adverse medication reaction that it is. It may occur at any time during therapy.

Parkinsonian Symptoms

The use of antipsychotics may cause a collection of symptoms that are like those of Parkinson's disease: a bilateral tremor (as opposed to a unilateral tremor in true Parkinson's disease), bradykinesia, and rigidity that may progress to the inability to move. The patient may have an inflexible facial expression and appear bored and apathetic and thus be mistakenly diagnosed as depressed. These are more common with the higher potency antipsychotics: these side effects may begin within weeks to months of initiation of antipsychotic therapy.

Tardive Dyskinesia

When antipsychotics have been used continuously for at least 3 to 6 months, patients are at risk for the development of the irreversible movement disorder called tardive dyskinesia (TD). Several psychotropic medications aside from the antipsychotics can either result in TD or increase the risk. TD symptoms usually appear first as wormlike movements of the tongue and other facial movements include grimacing, blinking, and frowning. Slow, maintained, involuntary twisting movements of the limbs, trunk, neck, face, and eyes (involuntary eye closure) have been reported (Williams and DeBattista, 2017). Risk factors for the development of TD are increased age, female, dementia, African, or African American. No treatment completely reverses the effect of TD. Therefore, it is essential that the nurse be attentive for early detection so that the health care provider can make prompt changes to the psychotropic regimen. The scheduled and repeated use of a standardized monitoring instrument is recommended (Cornett et al, 2017).

PROMOTING HEALTHY AGING: IMPLICATIONS FOR GERONTOLOGICAL NURSING

The gerontological nurse is a key person in ensuring that the medications used are appropriate, effective, and as safe as possible. The knowledgeable nurse is alert for potential medication interactions and for signs or symptoms of adverse medication effects. Nurses in the long-term care setting are responsible for monitoring the overall health of the residents, including fluid and dietary intake, and for being alert to the need for laboratory tests and other measures to ensure correct medication dosage. They are responsible for prompt attention to changes in the patient's or resident's condition (such as potassium level) that either are the result of the medication regimen or are affected by the regimen. The nurse is often the person to initiate assessment of medication use, evaluate outcomes, and provide the teaching necessary for safe medication use and self-administration.

In all settings, a vital nursing function is to educate patients and to ensure that they understand the purpose and side effects of the medications and assist the patient and family in adapting the medication regimen to functional ability and lifestyle.

Assessment

The initial step in ensuring that medication use is safe and effective is to conduct a comprehensive medication assessment. Although in some settings clinical pharmacists interview patients about their medication history, more often such reviews are completed through the combined efforts of the licensed nurse and the health care provider (e.g., a physician or a nurse practitioner).

The gold standard of assessment, especially important to use with the older adult, is the "brown bag" approach in which the person is asked to show the nurse the bottles of all of the medications that he or she is taking, including OTCs, herbals, and other dietary supplements. As each product container is removed from the bag, the necessary information can be obtained and compiled. To prevent possible misunderstandings or to determine misuse, it is best to ask the person how he or she takes the medicine rather than depend on how it is the labeled. By completing the assessment in this manner, the nurse can discover discrepancies between the prescribed dosage and the dosage taken, spot potential interactions, and identify potential or actual ADRs. The basics of the comprehensive medication assessment are the same as those for younger adults (Box 9.8). For details of the information needed in such an assessment that are particularly important for older adults, see Box 9.9.

The analysis by the nurse or the advanced practice nurse (APN) should be centered on identifying unnecessary or inappropriate medications, establishing safe usage, determining the patient's self-medication management ability, monitoring the effect and interactions of current medications and other products (e.g., herbals), and evaluating effectiveness of any education provided. Ideally, the nurse should know what resources are available for teaching about medications, such as the clinical pharmacist. The nurse is well situated to coordinate care, identify the patient's goals, determine what the patient needs to learn in order to understand his or her medications, and arrange for follow-up care to determine the outcome of medication teaching (Chapter 7).

Education

Patient education is used to promote safe medication use. Because of the complex needs of the older patient, education can

---

BOX 9.8 Basic Analysis of Assessment Findings Related to Medication Use

1. Is the medication working to improve the patient's symptoms?
   a. What are the desired therapeutic effects of the medication?
   b. What is the time frame for the therapeutic effects?
   c. Have the appropriate medication and dose been prescribed?
   d. Has the length of time been appropriate to determine efficacy?
2. Is the medication harming the patient?
   a. What physiological changes are occurring?
   b. What laboratory values are changing?
   c. What mental status changes are occurring?
   d. What functional changes are occurring?
   e. Is the patient experiencing side effects?
   f. Is the medication interacting with any other medication?
3. Does the patient understand the following?
   a. Why is the medication being taken?
   b. How is the medication is supposed to be taken?
   c. What are the side effects and who to report these to should any occur?
   d. How do you reduce or manage side effects?
   e. What limitations are imposed by taking the medication (e.g., sedative effects)?

BOX 9.9 Tips for Best Practice

Components of a Medication Assessment With Special Emphasis for Older Adults

- Ability to pay for medications
- Ability to obtain medications and refills
- Persons involved in decision making regarding medication use
- Medications obtained from others
- Recently discontinued medications or "leftover" prescriptions
- Strategies used to remember when to take medications
- Recent medication blood levels as appropriate
- Recent measurement of liver and kidney functioning
- Ability to remove packaging, manipulate medication, and store supply

---

BOX 9.10 Knowing Whom You Are Talking To

M. François came to the clinic as a new patient with uncontrolled hypertension. The nurse practitioner, through an interpreter, spent a lot of time with him explaining how to take his medications, what they were for, and so on. He and his presumed caregiver sat quietly and appeared to understand. When he returned a month later his blood pressure was still out of control. There was a different person with him who asked all of the questions that were addressed at the first appointment. On further inquiry it was determined that the person who brought M. François the first time was just a neighbor helping and not involved in his day-to-day life at all! His niece who "takes care of things" had been unavailable during the previous appointment and was now present.

---

be particularly challenging. The following tips may be helpful in the promotion of healthy aging related to medication use:

Key persons: Find out who, if anyone, manages the person's medications, helps the person, or assists with decision making; and with the person's permission, make sure that the helper is present when any teaching is done (Box 9.10).

Environment: Minimize distraction, and avoid competition with television, grandchildren, or others demanding the patient's attention; make sure the person is comfortable and is not hungry, thirsty, tired, too warm or too cold, in pain, or in need of the toilet.

Timing: Provide the teaching during the best time of the day for the person, when he or she is most engaged and energetic. Keep the education sessions short and succinct.

Communication: Ensure that you are understood. Make sure the learners have their glasses or hearing aids on, if they are used. Use simple and direct language, and avoid medical or nursing jargon (e.g., "intake"). Speak clearly, facing the person and with light on your face, at head level. Use formal language (e.g., Mr. Jones) unless you have permission to do otherwise. Do not touch the patient unless he or she indicates to you that it is acceptable to do so (e.g., patient lays his or her hand on yours (Chapter 4). If the person is blind, braille instructions may be available from the pharmacy. If the person has limited language proficiency in the country in which care is delivered, a trained medical interpreter is needed.

Reinforce teaching: Although there are a wide array of teaching tools and medication reminders available on the market today, many older adults continue to use the strategies they have developed over the years to remember to take their medications. These may be as simple as a using an egg carton as a storage box or turning a bottle upside down once it has been taken for the day, or as intense as having a family member or friend call the person at designated times. Encourage the person to use techniques that have worked in the past or to develop new strategies to ensure correct and timely medication use when needed. All education is supported by written or graphic material in the language that the person (if literate) can read or in the language of the person who helps.

Safe Medication Use

A safe, optimal, and feasible medication plan is one which the patient can adhere to. Appropriate nursing interventions include those that minimize polypharmacy, avoid adverse medication reactions, and promote adherence to medication regimens that promote healthy aging (or comfort while dying) (Box 9.11). The nurse caring for frail elders is especially challenged because of the physical and social vulnerability and medical complexity common in late life; medication interactions are more likely and adverse reactions more lethal. The use of a screening tool such as STOPP/START may be helpful for a quick assessment of potentially inappropriate medications (Hill-Taylor et al, 2016; O'Mahony et al, 2015).

The promotion of safe medication use requires attention to the potential for ADRs/ADEs, misuse, including overuse, underuse, erratic use, and contraindicated use. Computer-based drug-interaction programs and electronic medical records are important tools used to minimize the risk for ADEs. Misuse by patients may be unintentional, such as misunderstanding, or purposeful, such as when trying to make a prescription last longer because of cost or believing that it is not appropriate for the believed cause of illness (Box 9.12) (Lavan et al, 2016). A person may have considerable difficulty adhering to a medication regimen that is inconsistent with his or her established life patterns or beliefs. For example, the individual cannot follow the instruction to take medication three times per day with meals if he or she eats only two meals each day. In late life adherence is made significantly more complicated when the complexity of a medication regimen is combined with difficulties with self-administration due to normal changes with aging (Table 9.3).

TABLE 9.3 Examples of Changes With Aging That May Interfere With Medication Self-Administration.

Change in Aging	Consequence
Sensory	
Decreased visual acuity	Greater difficulty in reading instructions
Decreased sensation	Greater difficulty in manipulating medications
Decreased salivation	Greater difficulty in swallowing
Mechanical	
Decreased fine motor coordination	Greater difficulty in manipulating medications and packaging
Stiffening of large joints	Greater difficulty in self-administering medications

All medications have indications, side effects, interactions, and individual patient reactions. The nurse must determine whether side effects are minimal and tolerable or serious (Table 9.4). Asking subjective questions and observing the patient's interactions, behavior, mood, emotional responses, and daily habits can provide essential objective data. By compiling the information obtained in this manner, patient problems can be delineated, nursing diagnoses developed, outcome criteria planned, and interventions initiated.

Lastly, it is necessary for the gerontological nurse to monitor and evaluate prescribed treatments for both side effects and efficacy (Table 9.5). Monitoring and evaluating involve making

BOX 9.11 Tips for Best Practice
Reducing Adverse Medication Events

By paying attention to the following principles for prescribing and monitoring medications for older adults, the advanced practice nurse can reduce the risk for adverse medication events:
- Give the lowest dose possible.
- Discontinue unnecessary therapy.
- Attempt nonpharmacological interventions first.
- Give the safest medication possible.
- Assess renal function.
- Always consider the risk-to-benefit ratio when adding medications.
- Assess for new interactions with any new prescription or supplement.
- Avoid the prescribing cascade (i.e., new medications without consideration of those to be discontinued).
- Avoid inappropriate medications.

BOX 9.12 A Potentially Lethal Misunderstanding

I was making a visit to Mrs. Helena to enroll her in a research study. As we were reviewing her health and current medications she shared that she had not been feeling well and thought it was her heart, and that she had been told to "take the little white pills" until she felt better. When I looked at her pill bottle she had already taken five or more digoxin in the space of about 2 hours. I called an ambulance.

TABLE 9.4 Indications of Toxicity of Medications Commonly Prescribed to Older Adults.

Medication(s)	Signs and Symptoms
Benzodiazepines (e.g., Ativan)	Ataxia, restlessness, confusion, depression, anticholinergic effect
Cimetidine (Tagamet)	Confusion, depression
Digitalis (digoxin)	Confusion, headache, anorexia, vomiting, arrhythmias, blurred vision or visual changes (halos, frost on objects, color blindness), paresthesia
Furosemide (Lasix)	Electrolyte imbalance, hepatic changes, pancreatitis, leukopenia, thrombocytopenia
Levodopa (L-Dopa)	Muscle and eye twitching, disorientation, asterixis, hallucinations, dyskinetic movements, grimacing, depression, delirium, ataxia
Nonsteroidal antiinflammatory medications (NSAIDs) such as Advil and Naprosyn	Photosensitivity, fluid retention, anemia, nephrotoxicity, visual changes, bleeding, blood pressure elevations
Ranitidine (Zantac)	Liver dysfunction, blood dyscrasias
Sulfonylureas—first generation (e.g., Diabinese)	Hypoglycemia, hepatic changes, heart failure, bone marrow depression, jaundice

TABLE 9.5   Monitoring Parameters and Evaluation of Effectiveness for Medications Commonly Prescribed to Older Adults.

Class of Medication	Monitoring Activity
Antibiotics and antivirals	Improvement of infection: symptom reduction
Antihyperlipidemics	Lipid profile: lipids and triglycerides within normal limits for this person Liver function testing: no changes in function Blood glucose: no elevation
Cardiac medications	Measurement of heart rate and rhythm: within optimal parameters for that person
Anticoagulants	Clotting times (international normalized ratio [INR], prothrombin time): no bleeding; if using INR, kept between 2.0 and 3.0 in most cases
Antihypertensives	Measurement of blood pressure: maintained within set limits and without the development of orthostatic hypotension Weight: no unexplained weight gain
Antihyperglycemics	Hemoglobin A_{1C}: maintained between 6.0 and 7.0 for all but frail patients (controversy regarding a combination of goal and health status)
Antiarthritics	Relief from arthritis symptoms such as pain and inflammation
Antiparkinsonians	Improved functional status Less visible immobility
Analgesics	Improved symptoms of pain and inflammation

astute observations and documenting those observations, noting changes in physical and functional status (e.g., vital signs, performance of activities of daily living, sleeping, eating, hydrating, eliminating) and mental status (e.g., attention and level of alertness, memory, orientation, behavior, mood, emotional display and affect, and content and characteristics of interactions). Monitoring also means ensuring that blood levels are measured when they are needed—for example, regular thyroid-stimulating hormone (TSH) levels for all persons taking thyroid replacement therapy, INRs for all persons taking warfarin, or periodic hemoglobin A_{1C} levels for all persons with diabetes (Chapter 24). Proper patient care requires nurses to promptly communicate

their findings of potential problems to the patient's nurse practitioner or physician. Accurate monitoring is dependent on the nurse possessing and understanding the relevant information about the treatments and medications that are administered.

Medications occupy a central place in the lives of many older persons: cost, acceptability, interactions, adverse reactions and events, and the need to schedule medications appropriately all combine to create many difficulties. The nurse can promote healthy aging through knowledge of the effect of normal age-related changes on pharmacodynamics and pharmacokinetics, and by awareness of the key issues in medication use in older adults in all care settings.

KEY CONCEPTS

- The therapeutic goal of pharmacological intervention is to reduce the targeted symptoms and control disease conditions without undesirable side effects.
- One must always be alert for medication-medication, medication-herb, and medication-food interactions; whereas some are known and anticipated, others can be unexpected.
- Polypharmacy significantly increases the risk of medication interactions and adverse events. Polypharmacy increases with each prescriber seen.
- Any time there is a change in the patient's status, it is reasonable to first consider the possibility of a medication effect; this is of paramount importance when caring for older adults and those who are frail.
- Medication misuse may be triggered by prescriber practices, individual self-medication, physiological idiosyncrasies, altered biodegradability, nutritional and fluid states, and inadequate assessment before prescribing.
- Nurses must investigate medications immediately if a change in mental status is observed. Patients cannot comply with a prescription or treatment when it interferes with the practicalities of life or is distressful to the individual's well-being

or when actual misinformation or disability prevents compliance.
- The side effects of psychotropic medications vary significantly; thus, these medications must be selected with care when prescribed for the older adult.
- The response of the older adult to treatment with psychotropic medications should show reduced distress, clearer thinking, and enhanced safety for the person and those around him or her.
- It is always expected that psychotropic pharmacological approaches augment rather than replace nonpharmacological approaches.
- Older adults are particularly vulnerable to develop movement disorders (extrapyramidal symptoms, parkinsonian symptoms, akathisia, dystonia) with the use of antipsychotics.
- The Health Care Financing Administration (HCFA) and the congressional Omnibus Budget Reconciliation Act (OBRA) have severely restricted the use of psychotropic medications for the elderly unless they are truly needed for specific disorders and to maintain or improve function. Careful monitoring and continued justification are required.

NURSING STUDY: At Risk for an Adverse Event

Rosa was a 78-year-old woman who lived alone in a large city. She had been widowed for 10 years. Her children were grown, and all were successful. She was very proud of them because she and her husband had immigrated to the United States when the children were small and had worked very hard to establish and maintain a home. She had only a few years of primary education and still clung to many of her "old country" ways. She spoke a mixture of English and her native language, and her children were somewhat embarrassed by her. They thought she was somewhat of a hypochondriac because she constantly complained to them about various aches and pains, her knees that "gave out," her "sugar" and "water" problems, and her heart palpitations. She had been diagnosed with mild diabetes and heart failure. She was a devout Catholic and attended mass each morning. Her treks to church events, to the senior center at church, and to her various physicians (internist; orthopedic, cardiac, and ophthalmic specialists) constituted her social life. One day the recreation director at the senior center noticed her pulling a paper bag of medication bottles from her purse. She sat down to talk with Rosa about them and soon realized that Rosa had only a vague idea of what most of them were for and tended to take them whenever she felt she needed them.

- What factors about Rosa's probable medication misuse would be most alarming to you?
- List two of Rosa's strengths that you have identified from the information presented in the study.
- Develop three nursing diagnoses appropriate to this nursing study. These must be stated in concrete and measurable terms.
- Plan and state one or more interventions for each diagnosed problem. Provide specific documentation of the source used to determine the appropriate intervention and how the effectiveness can be evaluated.

CRITICAL THINKING QUESTIONS AND ACTIVITIES

1. As a student visiting the center for a 6-week assignment, how would you begin to help someone like Rosa?
2. Who should be responsible for teaching and monitoring medication use in persons such as Rosa? In any case?
3. Mrs. J., a patient of yours in a long-term care setting, is calling out repeatedly for a nurse; other patients are complaining, and you simply cannot be available for long periods to quiet her. Considering the setting and the OBRA guidelines, what would you do to manage the situation?
4. When you are given a prescription for medication, what do you ask about it?
5. Do you think most older adults seek adequate information about their medications before taking them?

RESEARCH QUESTIONS

1. Where would you obtain sufficient medication information for persons with limited English proficiency (LEP)?
2. What symptoms do elders most often self-treat with OTC and herbal medicines?
3. What are nursing roles in preventing adverse medication events in elders?
4. Among the following three teaching strategies, which works the best: computer-assisted medication teaching, telephone teaching, or in-person medication teaching? Why?
5. What aspects of Rosa's situation related to medications do you think are common among isolated elders?

REFERENCES

American Geriatrics Society 2019 Beers Criteria Update Expert Panel: American Geriatrics Society 2019 updated Beers Criteria for potentially inappropriate medication use in older adults, *J Am Geriatr Soc* 67(4):674–694, 2019.

Beers MH: Explicit criteria for determining potentially inappropriate medication use by the elderly. An update, *Arch Intern Med* 157:1531–1536, 1997.

Cambridge MedChem Consulting: *Distribution and plasma protein binding*, 2017. https://www.cambridgemedchemconsulting.com/resources/ADME/distribution.html. Accessed January 2018.

Castelo-Branco C, Soveral I: The immune system and aging: a review, *Gynecol Endocrinol* 30(1):16–22, 2014.

Centers for Medicare & Medicaid Services: *Atypical antipsychotic medications: use in adults*, 2013. https://www.cms.gov/medicare-medicaid-coordination/fraud-prevention/medicaid-integrity-education/pharmacy-education-materials/downloads/atyp-antipsych-adult-factsheet.pdf. Accessed February 2018.

Cornett EM, Novitch M, Kaye AD, Kata V, Kaye AM: Medication-induced tardive dyskinesia: a review and update, *Ochsner J* 17(2):162–174, 2017.

Furukawa MF, Spector WD, Rhona Limcangco M, Encinosa WE: Meaningful use of health information technology and declines in in-hospital adverse drug events, *J Am Med Inform Assoc* 24(4):729–736, 2017.

Hill-Taylor B, Walsh KA, Stewart S, Hayden J, Byrne S, Sketris IS: Effectiveness of the STOPP/START (Screening Tool of Older Persons' potentially inappropriate Prescriptions/Screening Tool to Alert doctors to the Right Treatment) criteria: systematic review and meta-analysis of randomized controlled studies, *J Clin Pharm Ther* 41(2):158–169, 2016.

Kouladjian L, Gnjidic D, Chen TF, Mangoni AA, Hilmer SN: Drug burden index in older adults: theoretical and practical issues, *Clin Interv Aging* 9:1503–1515, 2014.

Lavan AH, Gallagher PE, O'Mahony D: Methods to reduce prescribing errors in elderly patients with multimorbidity, *Clin Interv Aging* 11:857–866, 2016.

Levy HB: Polypharmacy reduction strategies: tips on incorporating American Geriatrics Society Beers and Screening Tool of Older People's Prescriptions Criteria, *Clin Geriatr Med* 33(2):177–187, 2017.

Maher RL, Hanlon J, Hajjar ER: Clinical consequences of polypharmacy in elderly, *Expert Opin Drug Saf* 13(1):57–65, 2014.

National Institute of Mental Health: *Mental health medications,* 2016. https://www.nimh.nih.gov/health/topics/mental-health-medications/index.shtml. Accessed February 2018.

Reuben DB, Herr KA, Pacala JT, Pollock BG, Potter JF, Semla TP: *Geriatrics at your fingertips,* ed 19, New York, NY, 2017, American Geriatrics Society.

Rochon PA: *Drug prescribing for older adults, UpToDate,* 2018. https://www.uptodate.com/contents/drug-prescribing-for-older-adults. Accessed February 2018.

Shim YK, Kim N, Park YH, et al: Effects of age on esophageal motility: use of high-resolution esophageal impedance manometry, *J Neurogastroenterol Motil* 23(2):229–236, 2017.

Slattum PW, Ogbonna KC, Peron EP: The pharmacology of aging. In Fillit HM, Rockwood K, Young JB, editors: *Brocklehurst's textbook of geriatric medicine and gerontology,* ed 8, Philadelphia, PA, 2017, Elsevier, pp 160–165.

U.S. Food and Drug Administration: *FDA 101: Dietary supplements,* 2017. https://www.fda.gov/ForConsumers/ConsumerUpdates/ucm050803.htm. Accessed February 2018.

Williams N, DeBattista C: Psychiatric disorders. In Papadakis MA, McPhee SJ, editors: *CURRENT Medical diagnosis and treatment,* ed 56, New York, NY, 2017, McGraw-Hill Education, pp 1050–1107.

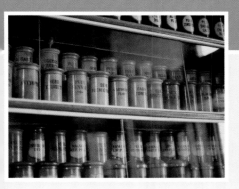

10

The Use of Dietary Supplements: Focus on Herbal Products

Kevin W. Chamberlin and Marissa C. Salvo

http://evolve.elsevier.com/Touhy/TwdHlthAging

A STUDENT SPEAKS

I had no idea how many different things people take. Older adults have so many remedies! All sorts of herbal teas and vitamins . . . I wonder if they work.

Kelly, age 18

AN OLDER ADULT SPEAKS

I try to take the medicines that the nurse practitioner gives me, but I can't always afford them, so I ask my friend what I should do because she knows a lot about herbs and teas. I take them instead of my medicines. Sometimes they really help.

Jean, age 65

LEARNING OBJECTIVES

On completion of this chapter, the reader will be able to:
1. Identify the legal standards that affect dietary supplement use.
2. Discuss the information that older adults should know about the use of select dietary supplements.
3. Discuss the role of the gerontological nurse when assisting the older adult who uses dietary supplements.
4. Describe the effects of selected commonly used dietary supplements on the older adult and their chronic disease.
5. Develop a nursing care plan to prevent adverse reactions related to dietary supplement use.

Various terms are used to describe dietary supplements (DS), including nutraceuticals, natural products, supplements, herbs, botanicals, and phytochemicals. The U.S. Food and Drug Administration (FDA) classifies DS as vitamins, minerals, herbs, and other botanical and amino acids that are used to supplement the diet (NCCIH, 2015; NIH, 1994). DS have been used for thousands of years to promote health and treat illness. According to a 2016 report, $38.8 billion was spent by Americans on DS; of which, 18% was spent on herbs and botanicals (Nutrition Business Journal, 2016). Estimates indicate the highest use is in those ages 50 to 59 years (Barnes et al, 2008; Nahin et al, 2009).

While DS use occurs across races and ethnicities, a National Health and Nutrition Examination Survey indicated the highest rate of use was in non-Hispanic white, older, educated (college education or higher) females with a current self-rated health of "very good to excellent" (Barnes et al, 2008). The most commonly used nonvitamin, nonmineral DS in the 30 days prior to the survey were fish oil/omega 3 fatty acids/docosahexaenoic acid (DHA) (37%), glucosamine (20%), echinacea (20%), flaxseed (16%), and ginseng (14%) (Barnes et al, 2008).

In the United States, the increasing use of DS by older adults may be related to their hopes of preventing illness, promoting and maintaining health, treating a health problem, or replacing some currently missing dietary component (Bruno and Ellis, 2005; Cheung et al, 2007; Yoon and Horne, 2001; Yoon et al, 2004). Older adults with chronic conditions are more likely to use DS with their prescription medication therapy (Nieva et al, 2012; Ryder et al, 2008; Yoon and Schaffer 2006). Combining DS with prescription and over-the-counter (OTC) medications increases the likelihood of adverse reactions in older adults (Lam and Bradley, 2006; Loya et al, 2009). While historically patients have not been likely to disclose the use of DS to their health care providers (Bruno and Ellis, 2005; Cheung et al, 2007), persons older than 50 years of age may be more likely than younger persons to share information about their use (Durante et al, 2001; Israel and Youngkin, 2005; Ryder et al, 2008). Regardless, gerontological nurses should always inquire about DS use and can anticipate that older adults may use a variety of complementary and alternative therapies, including DS, in addition to prescribed and OTC medications. The nurse

117

has a significant obligation to ask the right questions and obtain specific information related to their use—reason, formulation, frequency, duration, dose, any side/adverse effects, and plans for continuing. The nurse is then expected to be aware of any interactions that may occur.

STANDARDS IN MANUFACTURING

In 1994 the Dietary Supplement Health and Education Act was signed into law and required that DS only meet the standards applied to food preparation, implying safety, rather than the purity and potency standards, which applied to prescription and nonprescription drugs (National Registry, 1994). With the lack of strict good manufacturing practices, consumers were left at risk. To improve the quality of DS, the FDA put Good Manufacturing Practices (GMPs) into place in 2007. This set of guidelines for the preparation and storage of DS stipulates that manufacturers are now required to guarantee the identity, purity, strength, and composition of DS. Some manufacturers are also ensuring standardization by having their products tested by external quality assurance programs, such as the U.S. Pharmacopeia, to verify compliance with GMP. A symbol can be found on the product's label to indicate such compliance (USP). As this is not a requirement, commercially marketed DS products are difficult to study systematically, because of differences in plant products used (parts of plant, such as whole plant or extract), different combination products and proprietary blends, and/or differences in manufacturing processes.

By regulation, all DS marketed in the United States must include the following on its label: name of the product and the word "supplement"; the net quantity of contents; the manufacturer's, packer's, or distributor's name and place of business; and directions for use in addition to a supplement facts panel (http://www.herbalnutritionhealth.com/CRNlabel0302.pdf) (CRN, 2008; National Registry, 1994). Labels *cannot* claim that the product will cure, mitigate, treat, or prevent disease; unless the claim has been substantiated by research and recognized by the FDA—and in this case the product would need to meet the regulations of a drug (USFDA, 2017a). Products may make a structure-function claim on the label by notifying the FDA of such some claim 30 days after the product is marketed and describing how the product is intended to affect or maintain normal structure or function of the body. For example, if a claim such as "helps maintain joint function" is made, the following must also appear on the product label: "This statement has not been evaluated by the FDA. This product is not intended to diagnose, treat, cure, or prevent disease" (USFDA, 2017b). To further protect consumers, the Dietary Supplement and Nonprescription Drug Consumer Protection Act of 2006 required manufacturers/packers/distributors of DS to submit reports of serious adverse events to the FDA. Consumer and health care professionals may also report adverse events through the FDA MedWatch program (https://www.fda.gov/Safety/MedWatch/default.htm) (National Registry, 1994).

Nurses can alert and educate individuals to potential risks and adverse effects of DS, and to interactions. Nurses must maintain current knowledge about DS so that when they conduct a complete medication review (Chapter 9), potential and actual harmful effects may be recognized. Consideration of each product's intended use, dose, possible adverse effects, and possible interactions with other substances based on the person's health or illness conditions is required. Nurses should urge their patients to be aware of these issues, purchase products from reputable distributors, and discuss DS use with all their health care providers and pharmacists.

PRODUCT FORMULATIONS

DS come in a variety of formulations, depending on the raw material used. For example, plant-based DS (i.e., garlic) have more available formulations, due to the chemical composition and plant factors (i.e., time of harvest, plant species, part of plant used) compared to nonbotanical DS (i.e., glucosamine) (Gurib-Fakim, 2006). Common formulations include extracts, tinctures, capsules, tablets, teas, salves, and essential oils (Khalsa, 2007). Efficacy varies with each, depending on the part of the herb used and its preparation; this should be considered when evaluating the published literature on its efficacy (Khalsa, 2007).

An *extract* is a concentrated fluid or solid form of the fresh or dried herb that is made by soaking the crude plant in alcohol, water, alcohol/water mixtures, or oil which is then distilled or evaporated (Khalsa, 2007). *Tinctures* are fluid extracts that use alcohol as the extract medium (Khalsa, 2007). Tinctures should be used with caution in the elderly and/or those taking sedative medications or medications with a disulfiram reaction warning. Evaporating the extract fluid and drying the remaining product allows tablets or capsules to be made. A *salve* is a type of ointment that is used topically (Khalsa, 2007). *Teas* are commonly prepared as an infusion, pouring boiling water over a fresh or dried portion of the plant (i.e., leaf, root, bark) and letting it steep. The steeping time and amount of plant used will contribute to the tea's potency. *Essential oils* are aromatic, volatile compounds derived from various parts of the fresh plant, and are commonly used in aroma or massage therapy (Tillett and Ames, 2010).

SELECTING COMMONLY USED DIETARY SUPPLEMENTS

Although potential benefits of various products may have been reported, it must be noted that in many cases the scientific evidence supporting DS benefits is limited or inconclusive (Basch and Ulbricht, 2005). It is recommended that formulation selection and dosing follow available literature. For reliable and up-to-date information about DS research and use, consider referring to one of the resources listed in Table 10.1. This section provides an overview of some commonly used DS.

Echinacea

Echinacea (Echinacea angustifolia, Echinacea purpurea, Echinacea pallida) is a very popular product, especially for treatment and prevention of respiratory infections such as common colds (Shah et al, 2007). It is available commercially in single- and multiple-ingredient formulations, including capsules, tablets,

TABLE 10.1 Reliable Resources for Information About Dietary Supplements.

Resource	Website
AltMedDEx, Micromedex[a]	www.micromedexsolutions.com/home/dispatch
Cochrane Library	www.cochranelibrary.com/cochrane-database-of-systematic-reviews
Dietary Supplement Label Database	www.dsld.nlm.nih.gov/dsld/index.jsp
MedlinePlus	www.medlineplus.gov
National Center for Complementary and Integrative Health	www.nccih.nih.gov
Natural Medicines Comprehensive Database/Natural Standard[a]	http://naturaldatabase.therapeuticresearch.com/home.aspx?cs=&s=ND
Office of Dietary Supplements, National Institutes of Health	https://ods.od.nih.gov and https://ods.od.nih.gov/Research/CARDS_Database.aspx
PubMed Subset for Dietary Supplements	https://ods.od.nih.gov/Research/PubMed_Dietary_Supplement_Subset.aspx

[a]Paid subscription needed for access.

tea, juice, extract, and throat sprays. Products may contain different chemical plants and plant parts, making comparison difficult, and often available products are less concentrated than those used in trials.

A 2013 Cochrane review of 24 double-blinded studies compared single-ingredient *Echinacea* products to placebo for the prevention and treatment of the common cold. While some studies found a shortened cold duration (1 to 2 days when started at symptom onset) with *Echinacea* use, the overall clinically relevant treatment effect was weak. However, nearly all prevention trials with *E. purpurea* found a small preventative effect; although, clinical relevance is questionable (Karsch-Völk et al, 2014; Therapeutic Research Center, 2018a). Adverse reactions include fever, sore throat, diarrhea, nausea and vomiting, abdominal pain, and dry eyes (Askeroglu et al, 2013). *Echinacea* exhibits some cytochrome P450 (CYP) and P-glycoprotein effects; however, these are likely not significant unless used with narrow therapeutic range medications (Hermann, 2012).

> **SAFETY ALERT**
> *Echinacea* should not be used in those with a history of asthma or atopy, severe allergy to ragweed or chrysanthemums, severe systemic illness (HIV/AIDS, tuberculosis, multiple sclerosis, autoimmune disorders), or when taking immunosuppressants (Lee, 2004).

Elderberry

Elderberry, juice or extract of the *Sambucus nigra* berry, has been used for the treatment or prevention of influenza and other upper respiratory illnesses. Formulations include a spray, dried juice, standardized syrup, and encapsulated extract (Murkovic et al, 2004). Elderberry extract (Sambucol) was studied in both influenza A and B outbreaks and found to

decrease the duration of fever and improve symptom resolution in a shorter amount of time compared to placebo (Zakay-Rones et al, 1995, 2004).

> **SAFETY ALERT**
> Commercially available elderberry products are well tolerated. Use of insufficiently cooked or unripe berries, stems, or leaves can result in nausea, vomiting, dizziness, and weakness (Vlachojannis et al, 2010).

Coenzyme Q10

Coenzyme Q10, also known CoQ10 or ubiquinone, is converted to ubiquinol in the body and found within the mitochondria of cells. CoQ10 is involved in energy production and generation of antioxidants. It is thought that CoQ10 impacts vasodilatory and inotropic effects, with the highest concentration of CoQ10 in the heart. Statins, although to varying extents, lower CoQ10 concentrations (Laaksonen et al, 1995; Rundek et al, 2004; Toyama et al, 2001; Turunen et al, 2004). Mild GI effects and elevated liver function tests (LFTs) are possible adverse events.

CoQ10 has been studied for an array of cardiovascular (CV) conditions, including heart failure, high blood pressure, and primary prevention of CV disease (CVD). Due to varying outcomes, a review of seven small randomized controlled trials was unable to evaluate the impact of CoQ10 on clinically relevant endpoints in heart failure (Madmani et al, 2014). There is moderate-quality evidence that CoQ10 does not have a clinically significant effect on blood pressure lowering (Ho et al, 2016). Further, in several trials evidence the role of CoQ10 in primary prevention of CVD is not clear (Flowers et al, 2014). While statins lower CoQ10 concentrations, the clinical significance is not well understood and use of CoQ10 may or may not reverse some statin-related adverse events (Langsjoen et al, 2005).

Fish Oil

The American Heart Association recommends eating two servings (3.5 ounces cooked fish) of oily fish, such as mackerel, sardines, albacore tuna, and salmon, per week (AHA, 2019). Fish oil is a major source of omega-3 polyunsaturated fatty acids (PUFA), which include eicosapentaenoic acid (EPA) and DHA. Available products contain varying amounts of EPA and DHA. Studies often include products with an EPA:DHA ratio of 1.2:1 to 1.5:1, respectively, in each capsule. Individuals who decide to use omega-3 PUFA products should be advised that products vary in ratios; a prescription product may be more reliable for consistency in ratios. Side effects include gastrointestinal (GI) upset, belching, and fishy taste (de Leiris et al, 2009). Patients taking anticoagulants or antiplatelets should not consume more than 3 g/day of fish oil due to the increased risk of bleeding with higher doses. Box 10.1 details some selected DS interactions with anticoagulants and antiplatelet medications.

Omega-3 PUFA have been studied for cardiac health and improvement of inflammatory conditions, given their action on increasing noninflammatory and decreasing proinflammatory cytokines, and lowering cholesterol, based on their ability

BOX 10.1 Select Dietary Supplement Interactions With Anticoagulant and Antiplatelet Medications and Perioperative Management

Several dietary supplements should be used with caution and/or avoided when used in combination or with concomitant anticoagulant or antiplatelet use, due to the increased risk for bleeding or prolonged bleeding time. These include:

- Ginseng
- Garlic
- Ginkgo biloba
- Saw palmetto
- Coenzyme Q10

The American Society of Anesthesiologists suggests all herbal products be stopped 2 to 3 weeks before an elective surgical procedure and with provider monitoring if discontinuation may cause harm.

Data from Kuhn MA: Herbal remedies: drug-herb interactions, *Crit Care Nurse* 22 (2):22–28, 2002; Basch E, Ulbricht C: *Natural standard herb & supplement handbook: the clinical bottom line*, St Louis, MO, 2005, Mosby; Stanger MJ, Thompson LA, Young AJ, Lieberman HR: Anticoagulant activity of select dietary supplements, *Nutr Rev* 70: 107–117, 2012; Engelsen J: Effect of coenzyme Q10 and ginkgo biloba on warfarin dosage in stable, long-term warfarin treated outpatients. A randomised, double blind, placebo-crossover trial, *Thromb Haemost* 87(6):1075–1076, 2002; Kaye AD, Kucera I, Sabar R: Perioperative anesthesia clinical considerations of alternative medicines, *Anesthesiol Clin North America* 22:125–139, 2004.

to decrease intestinal cholesterol absorption (Adkins and Kelley, 2010). Prescription omega-3 PUFA products are approved for hypertriglyceridemia and studies support up to a 30% reduction in triglycerides (TGs) (Hartweg et al, 2007).

The American Heart Association's advisory group on the use of omega-3 PUFA for patients' supplementation is reasonable. Additionally, they recommend omega-3 PUFA supplementation in patients with heart failure without preserved left ventricular ejection fraction to decrease mortality and hospitalizations (Siscovick et al, 2017). It should be noted that supplementation is *not* recommended in patients with diabetes or prediabetes, to prevent coronary heart disease, patients with high CV risk, and patients with recurrent atrial fibrillation to prevent incident stroke (Siscovick, et al, 2017).

Garlic

Garlic (*Allium sativum*), derived from dried or fresh bulbs, contains a sulfur compound called *allicin*, which is released when the garlic clove is crushed, chewed, or chopped. Allicin is used as a quality marker in standardization. Research often involves powdered garlic, in a tablet or capsule form, standardized to 1% to 1.6% allicin content. Studies have focused on garlic for the treatment of hyperlipidemia and hypertension (Stabler, 2012). Reductions in low-density lipoprotein (LDL) (up to 16%), TG (up to 22%), and total cholesterol (TC) (up to 12%) have been reported (Alder and Reinhart 2009; Sobenin et al, 2010). Two metaanalyses have shown that garlic helps reduce blood pressure in persons with hypertension (Reinhart et al, 2008; Ried et al, 2008, 2013). However there is not yet sufficient evidence to broadly recommend its use in the treatment (Simons et al, 2009; Stabler et al, 2012). The use of garlic

for reduction of CV morbidity and mortality is unclear (Stabler et al, 2012).

As one may anticipate, garlic's smell, resulting in bad breath and body odor, is a limitation of its use. Increased flatulence, nausea, and heartburn are side effects at higher doses (Tachjian et al, 2010).

⚡ SAFETY ALERT

Garlic may interact with medications metabolized through CYP 3A4 and 2D6.

Red Yeast Rice

Red yeast rice has been a traditional Chinese culinary and medicinal product for centuries and has been shown in multiple studies to decrease lipid (LDL, TG, and TC) concentrations (Liu et al, 2006). Its effect comes from monacolin K, which is naturally occurring lovastatin analogue. The dose is 1.2 grams to 2.4 grams, divided twice daily. However, if the product includes more than a trace amount of monacolin K, it is considered an unapproved *medication* and cannot be sold legally in the United States (NCCIH, 2017a), making reliable product selection a limitation of use. It is not known if other red yeast products that do not contain monacolin K have any effect on cholesterol levels (Gordon et al, 2010). Red yeast rice may cause headache, heartburn, increased LFT results, and myalgias. Regular LFT monitoring is suggested.

⚡ SAFETY ALERT

Red yeast rice can generate citrinin during fermentation, which can cause kidney failure. It is important to purchase it from a reliable and reputable source; one that has been tested to be free of citrinin. Patients with kidney disease should not use red yeast rice.

Ginkgo Biloba

Ginkgo (*Ginkgo biloba*) is a standardized concentrated leaf extract from the oldest living tree species (Sierpina et al, 2003). It is prepared in capsule, tablet, and extract forms. The dose varies depending on its purpose and is administered in two or three divided doses (Therapeutic Research Center, 2017a). The flavonoids, glycosides, and terpenoids, such as gingkolide B and bilobalide, are the primary active ingredients (Jiang et al, 2011). It is often marketed as EGb 761, a standardized extract containing 22% to 27% flavone glycosides and 5% to 7% terpenoids.

Many studies, often very small, have investigated ginkgo for conditions ranging from vertigo, tinnitus, macular degeneration, depression, to altitude sickness and acute hemorrhoids. Adequate scientific evidence to support its use for those noted above is unclear and inconsistent (Therapeutic Research Center, 2017a). Some of the reported side effects of ginkgo include increased blood pressure, intestinal upset, headache, palpitations, dizziness, muscle weakness, and constipation (Jalili et al, 2013).

It is widely believed that ginkgo benefits cognition in dementia or with cognitive decline. However, there is no scientific evidence that ginkgo impacts cognitive impairment, memory, attention, language, visual-spatial ability, executive functions or reduces the development of dementia and Alzheimer's disease in older adults with normal cognition (Amieva et al, 2013; Birks et al, 2009; Canter and Ernst, 2007). A study of community dwelling older adults with either no cognitive impairment or mild disease treated with ginkgo twice daily or placebo were followed for 6 years showed no differences on the Mini-Mental State Examination, which includes tests of memory, attention, and executive function (Chapter 7) (Snitz et al, 2009).

St. John's Wort

St. John's wort (SJW) *(Hypericum perforatum)* is a yellow-flowered plant, whose flowers and leaves contain the highest level of useful compounds used to prepare teas, tablets and capsules, extracts, and salves. The proposed active ingredients in SJW include hypericin and hyperforin. One available standardized product, known as WS 5570, contains 0.1% to 0.3% hypericin and 3% to 6% hyperforin; however, like other DS the content of these active ingredients varies in commercially prepared products. SJW appears to play a role in serotonin, dopamine, and norepinephrine activity, activation of gamma-aminobutyric acid (GABA) and glutamate receptors and inhibition of monoamine oxidase (MAO) (Butterweck and Schmidt, 2007).

SJW is most often used as a self-treatment for depression, although it is used by some without clear evidential support for a large variety of illnesses such as seasonal affective disorder, anxiety, pain relief, and premenstrual syndrome (Ernst, 2002; Lawvere and Mahoney, 2005; NCCIH, 2017b; Ravindran et al, 2009; van der Watt et al, 2008). The concern of many experts is that its use could endanger the individual with depression by increasing the risk of suicide when other treatment is delayed.

A Cochrane review evaluated SJW in 18 placebo-controlled and 17 active-controlled studies, SJW was found to have a significant benefit over placebo and similar efficacy compared to commonly used antidepressants (e.g., citalopram, sertraline, etc.) for mild or moderate depression with better tolerability; its therapeutic effect takes several weeks (Linde et al, 2008; Therapeutic Research Center, 2018b). SJW has been found to be ineffective in treating major depression (NCCIH, 2018; Shelton, 2009).

Unless otherwise contraindicated, SJW is considered relatively well tolerated in recommended doses when taken for a maximum of 1 to 3 months (Brattström, 2009; Therapeutic Research Center, 2018b). As with prescribed antidepressants, side effects are common but not often severe, occurring in about one in three patients. Side effects include dermatitis, GI upset, restlessness, anxiety, headache, dry mouth, and possible sexual dysfunction (Therapeutic Research Center, 2018b). Patients taking SJW should be aware of photosensitivity and be advised to wear sunscreen and seek shade in prolonged outdoor exposure. Hypomania with bipolar disorder and suicidal and homicidal thoughts have been reported. Hypertension has also been reported (Jalili et al, 2013).

> ⚡ **SAFETY ALERT**
>
> St. John's wort is a known inducer of the CYP 3A4 enzyme and cannot be taken with medications metabolized by this route, including warfarin and digoxin, because it may decrease the effectiveness of these medications (NCCIH, 2015).

Melatonin

Melatonin is endogenously produced by the pineal gland and is an important signal in regulating the sleep-wake cycle. Melatonin levels are low during the day, increase during the evening, remain high throughout the night, and decrease again by morning; thus, it is commonly used to promote sleep. Numerous studies, including metaanalyses and systematic reviews, have shown supportive evidence for its use in prevention of jet lag; insomnia in children, adults, and the elderly; and delayed sleep phase syndrome (Ferracioli-Oda et al, 2013; Krystal et al, 2013; Ramar and Olson, 2013; Wilhelmsen-Langeland et al, 2013). Often melatonin is dosed at 3 to 5 mg 30 minutes prior to bed for insomnia and 2 mg to 5 mg for jet lag. Adverse effects include headache, nausea, and irritability (Therapeutic Research Center, 2017b).

Melatonin can decrease sleep onset latency, increase sleep duration, and improve sleep quality; although its effects are generally not as strong as those for benzodiazepines and benzodiazepine receptor agonists, the latter are contraindicated for use in older adults (AGS, 2019; Ferracioli-Oda et al, 2013). Melatonin is available in both immediate and extended release forms, and both have been found to be effective. A metaanalysis specifically looking at an extended-release melatonin preparation in patients older than 55 found that a dose of 2 mg orally 2 hours before bed was effective at decreasing sleep onset latency, improving quality of sleep, and improving morning wakefulness (Lemoine and Zisapel, 2012).

> ⚡ **SAFETY ALERT**
>
> Care should be taken if a patient is taking other medications that may increase endogenous melatonin concentrations, such as tricyclic antidepressants, selective serotonin reuptake inhibitors, or monoamine oxidase inhibitors. Other medications such as calcium channel blockers, benzodiazepines, and valproate have variable effects on melatonin concentrations (Therapeutic Research Center, 2017b).

Cinnamon

Cinnamon (*Cinnamomum cassia* or *Cinnamomum aromaticum*), available as a ground spice, capsule, and aqueous extract, contains flavonoids responsible for lowering blood glucose. A teaspoonful has about 2 grams. Studies vary in quantities and range from 1 to 6 grams daily in divided doses.

There are varying results of the lowering effect of cinnamon on blood glucose, along with the formulation used. One trial found that when 2 grams/day of ground cinnamon was added to standard diabetes medications, the mean hemoglobin A1C was significantly reduced from 8.22% to 7.86% in 12 weeks when compared to placebo (Akilen et al, 2010). However, a Cochrane review of 10 prospective randomized controlled trials of cinnamon (mean dose of 2 grams) in a tablet or capsule form for 4 to 16 weeks, found no statistically significant difference in hemoglobin A1C compared to control groups (placebo or active medication) (Leach and Kumar, 2012). If no benefit is seen after 3 to 4 months of use, consider stopping cinnamon. Other than the potential for hypoglycemia when used with other blood glucose lowering agents, few adverse events are reported with cinnamon at usual doses. However, high doses may result in hepatotoxicity due to varying concentration of coumarin (Abraham et al, 2010).

Ginseng

Two of the main categories of ginseng are American and Asian. *Asian ginseng* is also referred to as Chinese, Korean, and Asiatic; the Latin name is *Panax ginseng*. Another herb called Siberian ginseng or *eleuthero* is not true ginseng. The ginseng root is dried and used to make tablets, capsules, extracts, teas, and tinctures. The most active constituents are ginsenosides or panaxosides, but ginseng also contains other compounds that may play a role in its efficacy (Therapeutic Research Center 2017c). Dosages vary with the type of ginseng, the preparation, the frequency of consumption, the strength of dose, and the indication for use.

Ginseng has had numerous applications over thousands of years' use and has long been believed to improve well-being, help with stress adaptation, enhance immune function, and decrease oxidative cell damage. It has also been thought to improve mental and physical performance, lower blood glucose level and blood pressure, regulate symptoms related to menopause (NCCIH, 2017d), and treat erectile dysfunction (Hong et al, 2002).

A systematic review of seven randomized controlled trials found significant benefit with Asian ginseng on erectile dysfunction (Jang et al, 2008). Whereas, a systematic review of four trials assessing Asian ginseng's effect on fasting and 2-hour postprandial glucose found a lack of overall benefit (Kim et al, 2014). There is not enough evidence to support its use for improving memory and enhancing feelings of well-being (Therapeutic Research Center, 2017c).

Short-term use for most people at recommended doses appears to be safe; however, benefits are limited. Long-term use of ginseng is not recommended. Adverse effects include blood pressure changes, insomnia, and headache (Amico et al, 2013; Jalili et al, 2013; Lee and Ahn et al, 2008; Therapeutic Research Center 2017c; Tachjian et al, 2010). Avoid using ginseng with phenelzine, MAO-inhibitors, corticosteroids, imatinib, or large amounts stimulants, including caffeine (Izzo, 2012; Ulbricht et al 2008).

> ⚡ **SAFETY ALERT**
>
> Allergic reaction to ginseng can occur in people allergic to plants in the Araliaceous family.

Green Tea

Green tea comes in an array of formulations, including as a tea, chewable candy, extract, and topical. Tea leaves from the shrub, *Camellia sinensis*, are heated immediately after harvesting, rolled, and crushed before drying to produce green tea. As a tea, it contains caffeine, flavanols, flavonoids, and phenolic acids, which is reported to contribute to its antioxidant and antitumor effects, weight loss, and performance enhancement (Henning et al, 2004; Jurgens et al, 2012). A Cochrane review found green tea to have a small, statistically nonsignificant decrease in weight in overweight and obese adults. No effect on maintenance of weight loss was noted (Jurgens et al, 2012).

In a systematic review of the effects of green tea on CVD, potential mechanisms include antiinflammatory, antioxidant, and antiproliferative effects, but findings are confounded by lifestyle and dietary factors (Deka and Vita, 2011). A Cochrane review evaluated the effectiveness of green tea in healthy individuals and those with high CVD risk. Results indicate a beneficial effect in lowering blood pressure and LDL cholesterol; however, long-term studies are warranted to fully evaluate green tea's benefit in primary prevention of CVD (Hartley et al, 2013).

Limited, moderate to strong evidence has supported its consumption for the prevention of lung, pancreatic, and colorectal cancer (Boehm et al, 2009). It should be noted that most studies were conducted in Asia, where tea drinking is high, and consumption neared three to five cups per day (Boehm et al, 2009).

While the consumption of green tea can be considered safe at moderate and regular use, excessive consumption can lead to adverse GI effects and central nervous system and cardiac stimulation due to the caffeine content. As with any caffeinated beverage, users should be aware of caffeine content. One 8-ounce cup of green tea has less caffeine (25 to 29 mg) compared to that of coffee (95 to 165 mg) (Mayo Clinic, 1998–2018). However, all teas vary in caffeine content; therefore, it is recommended that patients check the label to assess the caffeine content of each product.

> ⚡ **SAFETY ALERT**
>
> Limit green tea intake when using other stimulating drugs due to green tea's caffeine content.
> Green tea products have been associated with liver toxicity (Sarma et al, 2008).

Glucosamine and Chondroitin Sulfate

Glucosamine works endogenously to increase components for cartilage synthesis; whereas, chondroitin sulfate is found in cartilage and inhibits its degradation while serving as a building material for cartilage production (Martel-Pelletier et al, 2010; Nagaoka et al, 2012; Volpi, 2011). While they can be purchased separately, they are often combined in tablet or capsule formulations and typically used for osteoarthritis (OA) and joint health (Therapeutic Research Center, 2018c). Major studies have been conducted regarding the safety and efficacy of these products both individually and together. It is important to note that glucosamine is available in two salt formations: sulfate and hydrochloride. Each has different efficacy and outcomes in trials.

The Glucosamine/Chondroitin Arthritis Intervention Trial (GAIT) found that while well tolerated and without significant adverse effects, neither glucosamine hydrochloride or chondroitin sulfate, alone or in combination, was more effective than placebo or celecoxib (a nonsteroidal antiinflammatory drug) (Sawitzke et al, 2010). However, it was found that patients in the glucosamine hydrochloride and celecoxib groups had better odds of achieving a 20% reduction in the Western Ontario McMaster Universities Osteoarthritis (WOMAC) scale (standardized questionnaire that measures five items for pain) (Bruyere and Reginster, 2007; Clegg et al, 2006). Despite this, glucosamine hydrochloride is not recommended for use as monotherapy.

Significant reduction in pain and improved movement has been shown in trials using glucosamine sulfate with or without chondroitin sulfate for knee OA (Reginster et al, 2012). A Cochrane review found that specifically the Rotta Laboratories crystalline glucosamine sulfate-containing products were superior to placebo in the treatment of pain and functional impairment with OA (Towheed et al, 2005). Another Cochrane review found that chondroitin sulfate alone or in combination with glucosamine was better than placebo in improving pain in the short term (6 months). Furthermore, scores on pain and functional scales was more favorable when taking chondroitin sulfate alone (Singh et al, 2015).

If supplement therapy is selected for use, consider recommending glucosamine sulfate as initial therapy, at a total daily dose of 1500 mg. It may take 6 to 8 weeks to see an initial effect with full effect not being seen for 4 to 6 months. The addition of chondroitin sulfate at a total daily dose of 1200 mg may be considered around 4 months if benefit is noted but symptoms persistent. Glucosamine and chondroitin both may cause nausea and GI upset; thus, patients should be instructed to take with food.

> ⚡ **SAFETY ALERT**
>
> Persons with a severe shellfish allergy should not use glucosamine. Those with a less severe allergy should use caution, as glucosamine is manufactured from shellfish chitin or produced synthetically. Those who eat a vegetarian or vegan diet should be informed that chondroitin is often derived from animal cartilage, in case they do not wish to consume these products.

Methylsulfonylmethane

Methylsulfonylmethane (MSM) is a natural compound found in humans that when broken down by intestinal bacteria releases sulfur; sulfur is key for bonding cartilage. Research is emerging investigating the use of MSM in conjunction with glucosamine and chondroitin sulfate. In a pilot study of 32 participants, this combination was found to significantly reduce pain and oxidative stress (Nakasone et al, 2011). Other clinical trials support the safety and use of MSM alone in reducing pain and functional impairment (Debbi et al, 2011; Kim et al, 2006). However, a meta-analysis of three studies indicated there was no significant benefit of MSM in OA of the knee, indicating additional research is needed before recommending it in clinical practice (Brien et al, 2011).

MSM can be purchased alone or in combination with glucosamine sulfate and chondroitin and should not exceed a total daily dose of 3000 mg. A few mild side effects have been reported including GI upset, insomnia, headache, and skin reactions. Caution should be used in combination with antiglycemics or anticoagulants (Burks, 2005).

Cranberry

Cranberry, an evergreen bush known as *Vaccinium macrocarpon*, is native to the United States and contains proanthocyanins, specifically epicatechin. Cranberry juice and its concentrate in tablet form are available; however, efficacy is related to the proanthocyanins content, which varies. It is thought that cranberry may prevent urinary tract infections (UTIs) by blocking *Escherichia coli* bacteria from adhering to the bladder, kidneys, and urethra (Howell, 2007).

Early evidence suggested some benefit of cranberry for UTI prevention in women with recurrent infections. However, this changed following the inclusion of 14 additional studies in a Cochrane review. In the review of 24 studies, no statically significant difference in decreasing the number of symptomatic UTIs over a 12-month period in women with recurrent UTIs was found with the use of cranberry juice for UTI prevention. The main limitation in all studies and in available products is the inconsistency in proanthocyanins content (Jepson et al, 2012).

Safety considerations include diarrhea with high doses, potential increase in kidney stone formation with regular use of cranberry concentrate tablets, and the potential increased bleeding risk in patients taking warfarin (Haber et al, 2012; Izzo, 2012; Terris et al, 2001).

Saw Palmetto

Saw palmetto, a fruit-bearing palm tree known as *Serenoa repens*, grows wild in the southern United States. The ripe fruit or berries are dried and ground into tablets or capsules or made into extracts or teas. Saw palmetto has been used for a variety of symptoms, most notably for those related to benign prostatic hyperplasia (BPH) (Tacklind et al, 2009). It inhibits 5α-reductase and androgen receptors and has local antiestrogenic effects and antiinflammatory effects on the prostate. Mild GI side effects are most commonly reported (Therapeutic Research Center, 2018d).

Despite its common use for BPH, evidence does not support its use. A Cochrane review of 32 randomized controlled trials found that its use did not improve urinary flow or prostate size (Tacklind et al, 2012). Several additional studies, including those funded by the NIH, have found no more of an effect than placebo (Barry et al, 2011; Kim et al, 2012; MacDonald et al, 2012).

> ⚡ **SAFETY ALERT**
>
> Saw palmetto must not be taken with other drugs used for the treatment of benign prostatic hyperplasia or prostate cancer or with any drug or supplement that can affect testosterone (Therapeutic Research Center, 2018d). Patients should seek medical evaluation to rule out prostate cancer prior to considering use of saw palmetto.

USE OF DIETARY SUPPLEMENTS FOR SELECT CONDITIONS

Hypertension

Many DS have the potential to lower blood pressure but need more research to support their use in treatment. Some of those already listed and with evidence include coenzyme Q10, fish oil, garlic, green tea, and melatonin (Therapeutic Research Center, 2017d, 2017e).

Some research suggests that taking coenzyme Q10 50–100 mg by mouth twice daily, with or without other antihypertensives, may significantly lower blood pressure after 12 weeks (Therapeutic Research Center, 2017b). However, a Cochrane Database review of blood pressure and coenzyme Q10 disputed whether it reduces blood pressure in the long-term management of primary hypertension, since only three clinical trials with 96 participants met quality inclusion criteria (Ho and Li, 2016). Patients and providers should be mindful that coenzyme Q10 should not be taken with warfarin (Heck et al, 2000).

Reviews of clinical research suggest that fish oil reduces systolic blood pressure by 2.5 to 5 mm Hg and diastolic blood pressure by 1.5 to 3.5 mm Hg in individuals with hypertension, though evidence is conflicting as to whether the hypotensive effect of fish oil is dose dependent (Therapeutic Research Center, 2017c).

Green tea has contradictory evidence relating to hypertension, with some evidence suggesting that green tea may help prevent the development of hypertension and lower blood pressure in patients with or without diagnosed hypertension. Metaanalyses show that green tea reduces systolic blood pressure by 1.94 to 3.2 mm Hg and diastolic by 1.7 to 3.4 mm Hg in patients with or without diagnosed hypertension, whereas smaller studies on both normotensive and hypertensive patients showed green tea had no effect on blood pressure (Therapeutic Research Center, 2017e).

Immediate-release melatonin did not demonstrate effects on blood pressure; however, controlled-release melatonin 2 to 3 mg by mouth at bedtime for up to 4 weeks demonstrated a systolic blood pressure lowering of 3.8 to 6 mm Hg and a diastolic lowering of 3.6 to 4 mm Hg in patients with essential or nocturnal hypertension (Therapeutic Research Center, 2017b).

HIV-Related Symptoms

The number of persons entering late life who are living with a HIV infection is increasing, many of whom use complementary and alternative therapies, including herbs, to manage their symptoms. In one study herbal therapies were used by 92% (Eller et al, 2005). Another study showed that *Aloe vera* (n = 54, 49.1%), ginger (*n* = 33, 30.0%), and garlic (*n* = 23, 20.9%) were the medicinal herbs most used by HIV patients (Bahall, 2017). Of concern is the potential that some herbal products may alter the metabolic action of antiretroviral drugs used in treatment (Ladenheim et al, 2008; Walubo, 2007). For example, SJW is commonly used for depression, but research indicates it may lower the blood level of antiretroviral medications such as indinavir, protease inhibitors, nonnucleoside reverse transcriptase inhibitors (NNRTIs), and maraviroc when taken together (Therapeutic Research Center, 2018b).

Gastrointestinal Disorders

Older adults with GI disorders such as irritable bowel syndrome (IBS) are likely to use alternative therapies, including herbs (Tillisch, 2006). The Chinese have used herbal therapies

for thousands of years to treat IBS. Liu and colleagues (2006) found 75 randomized clinical trials for IBS that indicated it was improved by some of the herbal therapies. Psyllium (*Plantago ovata* and *Plantago ispaghula*) is used as a bulk laxative (Natural Standard, 2018b) that is generally well tolerated and may decrease IBS symptoms, although results are conflicting (Basch and Ulbricht, 2005). Calcium is approved by the FDA and scientifically well supported for use in reducing gastric acidity; probiotic products help control harmful organisms in the gut, such as *Helicobacter pylori* (Natural Standard, 2018b). Milk thistle has been shown to possibly improve dyspepsia (Melzer et al, 2004), but has insufficient reliable evidence in alcohol-related liver disease (Rambaldi, Jacobs, and Gluud, 2007).

Cancer

Cancer is common in late life. When treatments such as chemotherapy and radiation are not effective, many people turn to complementary and alternative approaches. Many of the herbs need more scientific study for helping patients with cancer and their possible roles in decreasing risk for cancer. Supplements with limited efficacy support include but are not limited to calcium (colorectal), fish oil (endometrial), garlic (colorectal, prostate), and ginseng (breast, stomach, lung, liver, ovarian, skin) (Therapeutic Research Center, 2017f).

Drinking black or green tea is thought to help reduce the risk for ovarian cancer by as much as 46% (Larsson and Wolk, 2005) and for endometrial cancer by 21% (Tang et al, 2009) over non-users, but evidence is conflicting and insufficient (Boehm et al, 2009). Claims are often made that a substance or an herb will help the patient with cancer, even though no data support such claims. Gerontological nurses must be sensitive to this situation and work with all concerned to provide the best evidence-based care possible.

Alzheimer's Disease

According to a 2016 report, $38.8 billion was spent by Americans on OTC supplements in 2015, including $91 million on ginkgo biloba marketed as a memory booster (Nutrition Business Journal, 2016). A systematic review of the literature summarizes evidence on efficacy and harms of OTC supplements used to prevent cognitive decline, mild cognitive impairment (MCI), or Alzheimer's dementia (Butler et al, 2018). The authors concluded that a lack of evidence prevented any OTC supplement for cognitive protection in adults with normal cognition or MCI but cited high attrition rates and variable cognitive outcome measurements across included studies (Butler et al, 2018).

Among 82 elderly veterans with dementia and depression, nearly one-fifth of the veterans and their caretakers used herbs and supplements (Kales et al, 2004). Ginkgo is often used by older persons with dementia because it is thought it may increase cerebral blood supply (Mashayekh et al, 2011). Three randomized studies (*n* = 5559) have looked at ginkgo biloba's effects in older adults with presumed normal cognition for up to 6 years. While two of the trials suggested low-strength of evidence on Alzheimer-type dementia incidence (DeKosky et al, 2008; Snitz et al, 2009; Vellas et al, 2012), neither demonstrated protective benefits of gingko biloba versus placebo. Similarly, evidence was lacking to support benefits for executive function (Snitz et al, 2009), attention, or memory (Dodge et al, 2008). Ginkgo is also not without risk, with all three studies reporting adverse events that included stroke and cardiac events, the smaller study by Dodge et al showed a larger number of strokes or transient ischemic attacks (TIA) in the ginkgo group versus placebo over 3.5 years (7 vs. 0; $p = 0.001$) (Dodge et al, 2008).

Further study is advised in the use of sage with dementia and Alzheimer's disease. According to William Thies, chief medical and scientific officer of the Alzheimer's Association, engaging in moderate to heavy physical activity levels, drinking tea one to four times per day, and maintaining normal serum levels of vitamin D have all been associated with decreased risk for cognitive decline. Currently, additional studies are needed to substantiate these associations, and the use of melatonin for sleep benefits and lemon balm for agitation with patients with Alzheimer's disease or dementia (Natural Standard, 2013a).

The omega-3 fatty acid DHA is the chief omega-3 found in the fatty membranes that surround nerve cells in the brain. Theories about why omega-3s might influence dementia risk include their benefit for the heart and blood vessels, antiinflammatory effects, and support and protection of nerve cell membranes (Alzheimer's Association, 2019). A study of 295 individuals comparing DHA 2 grams per day ($n = 171$) vs. placebo for 18 months did not slow the rate of cognitive or functional decline in patients with mild to moderate Alzheimer's disease (Quinn et al, 2010).

Caprylic acid is a medium-chain triglyceride (fat) produced by processing coconut oil or palm kernel oil. The theory behind caprylic acid is that the ketone bodies produced through metabolism may provide an alternate energy source for brain cells that have lost their ability to use glucose because of Alzheimer's (Henderson et al, 2009).

Huperzine A is a moss extract used in traditional Chinese medicine with properties like cholinesterase inhibitors (e.g., Aricept). However, large-scale trial of huperzine A in mild to moderate Alzheimer's disease demonstrated no greater benefit than placebo (Alzheimer's Disease Cooperative Study, 2017).

Diabetes

Herbal approaches to diabetes management were in place before the discovery of insulin in 1921. As many as 400 herbs and supplements have been reported as beneficial in treating diabetes (Kasuli, 2011), and the Natural Medicines database lists more than 20 with possible efficacy for use in persons with the disease (Therapeutic Research Center, 2017g). Much of the supportive data exist in cellular and animal models with mechanisms of actions that include increased insulin secretion and sensitivity, improved glucose uptake in adipose and muscle tissue, and decreased intestinal glucose absorption and hepatocyte glucose production and antiinflammatory actions (Li et al, 2012). However, human studies are often not well designed and have yielded either negative or mixed results.

Fenugreek *(Trigonella foenum-graecum),* a seed powder, when consumed as a cup of tea three times daily or taken orally in a capsule can induce a hypoglycemic response and must be used carefully (Basch and Ulbricht, 2005). It can cause diarrhea and flatulence and may increase anticoagulant activity of other drugs the person is taking. Research suggests a dose-dependent benefit of caffeinated coffee in reducing the risk of type 2 diabetes (Iso et al, 2006; Salazar-Martinez et al, 2004; Tuomilehto et al, 2004). Consuming more than 6 to 10 cups/day of coffee is associated with a 54% lower risk of diabetes development in North American men and 29% lower risk in North American women (Salazar-Martinez et al, 2004). Europeans and Japanese adults see comparable, if not even better, numbers in risk reduction of diabetes (Iso et al, 2006; Tuomilehto et al, 2004;). However, several possible adverse effects may occur with increased caffeine intake, including headache, insomnia, anxiety and nervousness, hypertension, and heart rhythm disturbance.

Cinnamon is another herb that has been linked with lowering blood glucose level, but scientific evidence is mixed and overall the results do not support its effectiveness in diabetes (Baker et al, 2008; Kirkham et al, 2009; Leach and Kumar, 2012; Pham et al, 2007). Other herbs or supplements linked with some scientific evidence of lowering blood glucose level are alpha-lipoic acid, American ginseng, berberine, chromium, flaxseed, ginseng, gymnema, magnesium, milk thistle, and resveratrol (Kasuli, 2011; Lee and Dugoua, 2011).

Numerous other substances are said to have unclear or conflicting scientific evidence for lowering blood sugar, such as astragalus, bilberry, red yeast rice, honey, and even the parasitic vine kudzu, but the evidence is not sufficient to support that these are effective in treating or reducing the development of type 2 diabetes mellitus (Therapeutic Research Center: Natural Medicines, 2017f). To date, there are insufficient data to support the use of herbal supplements in the primary treatment of diabetes. If any herb or supplement is used by the patient for diabetes management, health care professionals need to urge careful blood glucose monitoring and direct appropriate dose adjustments for prescribed medications.

INTERACTIONS WITH STANDARDIZED DRUGS

A major issue in the use of DS is the risk for interactions, especially considering the number of medications already taken by older adults (Tsai et al, 2012). A 22-month study of more than 3000 U.S. adults, ages 75 years or older, found that almost 2250 of the study participants combined at least one prescription drug with one dietary supplement daily, and approximately 10% to 33% combined up to five prescription drugs and five supplements daily (Nahin et al, 2009). The more prescription, OTC, and DS that the person is taking, the more likely it is that an interaction will occur (Chapter 9) (Kuhn, 2002). In a study of 58 women 65 years and older, nearly 75% of them were taking herbs, prescription drugs, and/or OTC drugs that could interact at a moderate- or high-risk level (Yoon and Schaffer, 2006). And remember that the contents of DS vary considerably based on their manufacturer and formulation; therefore, the therapeutic outcome and potential for interaction also vary.

PROMOTING HEALTHY AGING: IMPLICATIONS FOR GERONTOLOGICAL NURSING

The gerontological nurse can promote healthy aging in several ways among persons who use or are considering the use of DS. It begins with creating a safe and nonjudgmental relationship wherein the person feels comfortable describing his or her use and understanding of DS. Any verbal or nonverbal action from the provider that may block this openness may lead to a potentially dangerous lack of assessment data. Once the conversation has begun, both the nurse and the older adult can begin to evaluate the existing knowledge regarding safe use of DS. This includes the name and manufacturer of the DS, its intended use, outcome, potential side effects, and interactions. The conversation is a useful venue for teaching about the safe use of DS. The LEARN Model discussed in Chapter 4 may be particularly helpful.

Additionally, the gerontological nurse may aid in determining if a DS is being used in an appropriate manner. Encourage the older adult to bring the specific DS product to an upcoming visit and discuss its use; the goal is to ensure safety. Sometimes, DS use may provide a placebo effect. That is, the taking of the product, and not the action of the DS itself, may produce a positive effect on the person. In this instance, if the DS causes no harm, it may be decided to continue use; however, the safety of a DS is often difficult to determine, and a placebo effect is impossible to measure. Ultimately, it is the health care professional's responsibility to assess appropriateness and safety of DS use. Table 10.1 provides reliable resources for gathering DS information to help in the decision-making process. Pharmacists are additional, readily accessible resources.

Important interventions of the gerontological nurse in the promotion of healthy aging include assessing DS use; checking for side effects, adverse reactions, and interactions between DS and medications, foods, and disease states; and providing education, especially if DS use is not safe. In instances where an adverse reaction or harmful interaction is suspected, the person must be urged to stop taking the DS and to see his or her prescribing health care provider or seek emergency care, if indicated. Educating patients about available DS evidence is a powerful intervention that must be provided in the context of the person's age and learning needs.

Several additional issues need to be addressed with persons who are taking DS:

- Stress the importance of reporting the use of all DS to *all* health care providers before beginning a DS.
- Regarding product safety: (1) There is no universal standardization among manufacturers, so the amount of active ingredient per dose among brands may be inconsistent; (2) DS should be purchased from reputable sources; (3) DS are available in different formulations, making accurate dosing difficult; (4) research on both the potential adverse and the beneficial effects of most DS is inadequate, making recommendations about specific products difficult; and (5) persons who have allergies to certain plants may have allergies to products in the same plant family.
- Older adults may react differently to DS than a younger adult. If side effects occur within 1 or 2 hours of taking the DS, it should be discontinued immediately. If the side effects continue or worsen, the person should report them to a health care provider or go to the nearest emergency department.
- Many adults take DS along with prescribed and OTC medications. Thus, the communication approach must be open and encouraging for effective assessment, evaluation of risks, appropriate teaching-learning applications, intervention, and monitoring. The gerontological nurse must be knowledgeable and continue to determine the latest information about DS use.

■ KEY CONCEPTS

- Many older adults continue to use prescription and nonprescription medications along with complementary and alternative medicines, including DS.
- No manufacturing or quality assurance standards for DS are in place or enforced by the U.S. government.
- Nurses and other health care providers should always ask about the use of DS when conducting a patient interview.
- Nurses and other health care providers should provide an open, nonjudgmental environment to foster education on dietary supplement use with prescription and nonprescription medications.

NURSE STUDY: COMMON USE OF DIETARY SUPPLEMENTS

Anna is an 80-year-old woman of French descent who lives in a suburb of a large city. She is a widow. She has two grown children and six grandchildren. Anna is very proud of all of them. She taught high school English for 20 years but was raised with many of the "old country" traditions, speaking French for most of her formative years. As part of her background, she would rather use supplements and "home treatments" than prescribed "pills." She has been diagnosed with hypertension, diabetes mellitus, and arthritis. She often complains of symptoms that are related to these chronic conditions, but she refuses to consistently follow her diet or take any prescribed medications. Anna attends mass daily and takes part in community activities. On a visit to her health care provider, she mentions the use of supplements. After some discussion, the nurse realizes that Anna has little information about supplements and has some incorrect assumptions about them.

- What questions would you ask Anna about her dietary supplement use?
- What are some educational opportunities regarding dietary supplement use?
- How would you address Anna's expectations of the benefits of dietary supplements?

CRITICAL THINKING QUESTIONS AND ACTIVITIES

1. Interview a member of your health care community who recommends the use of DS along with prescription medications.
2. Read the labels of the more commonly used DS. Do the labels list the information you expected? How would you make sure that your patients have the necessary information to select an appropriate product?
3. Visit a senior citizen center. Talk with members about their use of DS. Keep track of the more commonly used products and the reasons for their use.

RESEARCH QUESTIONS

1. How do older adults decide which DS to use?
2. Are older adults aware of possible negative effects of dietary supplement use?
3. What do older adults see as the rewards (positive factors) and costs (negative factors) of using DS?
4. What strategies can health care providers use to bridge the gap in knowledge between dietary supplement use and prescribed medications?

REFERENCES

Abraham K, Wöhrlin F, Lindtner O, Heinemeyer G, Lampen A: Toxicology and risk assessment of coumarin: focus on human data, *Mol Nutr Food Res* 54(2):228–239, 2010.

Adkins Y, Kelley DS: Mechanisms underlying the cardioprotective effects of omega-3 polyunsaturated fatty acids, *J Nutr Biochem* 21(9):781–792, 2010.

Akilen R, Tsiami A, Devendra D, Robinson N: Glycated haemoglobin and blood pressure-lowering effect of cinnamon in multi-ethnic type 2 diabetic patients in the UK: a randomized, placebo-controlled, double-blind clinical trial, *Diabet Med* 27(10):1159–1167, 2010.

Alzheimer's Association: *Alternative treatments,* 2019. https://www.alz.org/alzheimers_disease_alternative_treatments.asp. Accessed April 2019.

Alzheimer's Disease Cooperative Study: *Huperzine A,* 2017. https://www.adcs.org/huperzine-a-study. Accessed December 2017.

American Geriatrics Society Beers Criteria Update Expert Panel: American Geriatrics Society 2019 updated Beers Criteria for potentially inappropriate medication use in older adults, *J Am Geriatr Soc* 67(4):674–694, 2019.

American Heart Association: *Fish and omega-3 fatty acids,* 2019. https://www.heart.org/en/healthy-living/healthy-eating/eat-smart/fats/fish-and-omega-3-fatty-acids?s=q%253Dfish%252520and%252520omega%2525203%252520fatty%252520acids%2526sort%253Drelevancy. Accessed April 2019.

Amico AP, Terlizzi A, Damiani S, Ranieri M, Megna M, Fiore P: Immunopharmacology of the main herbal supplements: a review, *Endocr Metab Immune Disord Drug Targets* 13:283–288, 2013.

Amieva H, Meillon C, Helmer C, Barberger-Gateau P, Dartigues JF: Ginkgo biloba extract and long-term cognitive decline: a 20-year follow-up population-based study, *PLoS One* 8(1):e52755, 2013.

Askeroglu U, Alleyne B, Guyuron B: Pharmaceutical and herbal products that may contribute to dry eyes, *Plast Reconstr Surg* 131:159–167, 2013.

Bahall M: Prevalence, patterns, and perceived value of complementary and alternative medicine among HIV patients: a descriptive study, *BMC Complement Altern Med* 17:422, 2017.

Barnes PM, Bloom B, Nahin RL: Complementary and alternative medicine use among adults and children: United States, 2007, *Natl Health Stat Report* (12):1–23, 2008.

Barry MJ, Meleth S, Lee JY, et al: Effect of increasing doses of saw palmetto extract on lower urinary tract symptoms: a randomized trial, *JAMA* 306:1344–1351, 2011.

Basch E, Ulbricht C: *Natural standard herb & supplement handbook: the clinical bottom line,* St Louis, MO, 2005, Mosby.

Birks J, Grimley Evans J: Ginkgo biloba for cognitive impairment and dementia, *Cochrane Database Syst Rev* (1):CD003120, 2009.

Boehm K, Borrelli F, Ernst E, et al: Green tea (*Camellia sinensis*) for the prevention of cancer, *Cochrane Database Syst Rev* (3):CD005004, 2009.

Brattström A: Long-term effects of St. John's wort (*Hypericum perforatum*) treatment: a 1-year safety study in mild to moderate depression, *Phytomedicine* 16:277–283, 2009.

Brien S, Prescott P, Lewith G: Meta-analysis of the related nutritional supplements dimethyl sulfoxide and methylsulfonylmethane in the treatment of osteoarthritis of the knee, *Evid Based Complement Alternat Med* 2011:528403, 2011.

Bruno JJ, Ellis JJ: Herbal use among US elderly: 2002 National Health Interview Survey, *Ann Pharmacother* 39:643–648, 2005.

Bruyere O, Reginster JY: Glucosamine and chondroitin sulfate as therapeutic agents for knee and hip osteoarthritis, *Drugs Aging* 24:573–580, 2007.

Burks K: Osteoarthritis in older adults: current treatments, *J Gerontol Nurs* 31:11–19, 2005.

Butler M, Nelson VA, Davila H, et al: Over-the-counter supplement interventions to prevent cognitive decline, mild cognitive impairment, and clinical Alzheimer-type dementia: a systematic review, *Ann Intern Med* 168(1):52–62, 2018. doi:10.7326/M17-1530.

Butterweck V, Schmidt M: St. John's wort: role of active compounds for its mechanism of action and efficacy, *Wien Med Wochenschr* 157(13-14):356–361, 2007.

Canter PH, Ernst E: Ginkgo biloba is not a smart drug: an updated systematic review of randomised clinical trials testing the nootropic effects of G. biloba extracts in healthy people, *Hum Psychopharmacol* 22:265–278, 2007.

Cheung CK, Wyman JF, Halcon LL: Use of complementary and alternative therapies in community-dwelling older adults, *J Altern Complement Med* 13:997–1006, 2007.

Clegg DO, Reda DJ, Harris CL, et al: Glucosamine, chondroitin sulfate, and the two in combination for painful knee osteoarthritis, *N Engl J Med* 354:795–808, 2006.

Council for Responsible Nutrition: *How do you read a supplement label?* 2008. www.herbalnutritionhealth.com/CRNlabel0302.pdf. Accessed January 2018.

de Leiris J, de Lorgeril M, Boucher F: Fish oil and heart health, *J Cardiovasc Pharmacol* 54:378–384, 2009.

Debbi EM, Agar G, Fichman G, et al: Efficacy of methylsulfonylmethane supplementation on osteoarthritis of the knee: a randomized controlled study, *BMC Complement Altern Med* 11:50, 2011.

Deka A, Vita JA: Tea and cardiovascular disease, *Pharmacol Res* 64:136–145, 2011.

DeKosky ST, Williamson JD, Fitzpatrick AL, et al: Ginkgo biloba for prevention of dementia: a randomized controlled trial, *JAMA* 300:2253–2262, 2008.

Dodge HH, Zitzelberger T, Oken BS, Howieson D, Kaye J: A randomized placebo-controlled trial of Ginkgo biloba for the prevention of cognitive decline, *Neurology* 70:1809–1817, 2008.

Durante KM, Whitmore B, Jones CA, Campbell NR: Use of vitamins, minerals and herbs: a survey of patients attending family practice clinics, *Clin Invest Med* 24:242–249, 2001.

Engelsen J, Nielsen JD, Winther K: Effect of coenzyme Q10 and Ginkgo biloba on warfarin dosage in stable, long-term warfarin treated outpatients. A randomised, double blind, placebo-crossover trial, *Thromb Haemost* 87(6):1075–1076, 2002.

Ernst E: The risk-benefit profile of commonly used herbal therapies: ginkgo, St. John's wort, ginseng, echinacea, saw palmetto, and kava, *Ann Intern Med* 136:42–53, 2002.

Federal Registry. Current good manufacturing practice in manufacturing, packaging, labeling, or holding operations for dietary supplements. Final rule, *Federal Register* 72:34752–34958, 2007. https://www.federalregister.gov/documents/2007/06/25/07-3039/current-good-manufacturing-practice-in-manufacturing-packaging-labeling-or-holding-operations-for. Accessed April 2019.

Ferracioli-Oda E, Qawasmi A, Bloch MH: Meta-analysis: melatonin for the treatment of primary sleep disorders, *PLoS One* 8:e63773, 2013.

Flowers N, Hartley L, Todkill D, Stranges S, Rees K: Co-enzyme Q10 supplementation for the primary prevention of cardiovascular disease, *Cochrane Database Syst Rev* (12):CD010405, 2014.

Gordon RY, Cooperman T, Obermeyer W, Becker DJ: Marked variability of monacolin levels in commercial red yeast rice products: buyer beware! *Arch Intern Med* 170(19):1722–1727, 2010.

Gurib-Fakim A: Medicinal plants: traditions of yesterday and drugs of tomorrow, *Mol Aspects Med* 27(1):1–93, 2006.

Haber SL, Cauthon KA, Raney EC: Cranberry and warfarin interaction: a case report and review of the literature, *Consult Pharm* 27(1):58–65, 2012.

Hartley L, Flowers N, Holmes J, et al: Green and black tea for the primary prevention of cardiovascular disease, *Cochrane Database Syst Rev* (6):CD009934, 2013.

Hartweg J, Farmer AJ, Perera R, Holman RR, Neil HA: Meta-analysis of the effects of n-3 polyunsaturated fatty acids on lipoproteins and other emerging lipid cardiovascular risk markers in patients with type 2 diabetes, *Diabetologia* 50(8):1593–1602, 2007.

Heck AM, DeWitt BA, Lukes AL: Potential interactions between alternative therapies and warfarin, *Am J Health Syst Pharm* 57:1221–1227, 2000.

Henderson ST, Vogel JL, Barr LJ, Garvin F, Jones JJ, Costantini LC: Study of the ketogenic agent AC-1202 in mild to moderate Alzheimer's disease: a randomized, double-blind, placebo-controlled, multicenter trial, *Nutr Metab (Lond)* 6:31, 2009.

Henning SM, Niu Y, Lee NH, et al: Bioavailability and antioxidant activity of tea flavanols after consumption of green tea, black tea, or a green tea extract supplement, *Am J Clin Nutr* 80(6):1558–1564, 2004.

Hermann R, von Richter O: Clinical evidence of herbal drugs as perpetrators of pharmacokinetic drug interactions, *Planta Med* 78(13):1458–1477, 2012.

Ho MJ, Li EC, Wright JM: Blood pressure lowering efficacy of coenzyme Q10 for primary hypertension, *Cochrane Database Syst Rev* 3:CD007435, 2016.

Hong B, Ji YH, Hong JH, Nam KY, Ahn TY: A double-blind crossover study evaluating the efficacy of Korean red ginseng in patients with erectile dysfunction: a preliminary report, *J Urol* 168:2070–2073, 2002.

Howell AB: Bioactive compounds in cranberries and their role in prevention of urinary tract infections, *Mol Nutr Food Res* 51(6):732–737, 2007.

Iso H, Date C, Wakai K, Fukui M, Tamakoshi A, JACC Study Group: The relationship between green tea and total caffeine intake and risk for self-reported type 2 diabetes among Japanese adults, *Ann Intern Med* 144:554–562, 2006.

Israel D, Youngkin E: Herbal therapies for common health problems. In Youngkin EQ, Sawin KB, Kissinger JF, Israel DS, editors: *Pharmacotherapeutics: a primary care clinical guide*, ed 2, Upper Saddle River, NJ, 2005, Pearson Prentice Hall.

Izzo AA: Interactions between herbs and conventional drugs: overview of the clinical data, *Med Princ Pract* 21(5):404–428, 2012.

Jalili J, Askeroglu U, Alleyne B, Guyuron B: Herbal products that may contribute to hypertension, *Plast Reconstr Surg* 131:168–173, 2013.

Jang DJ, Lee MS, Shin BC, Lee YC, Ernst E: Red ginseng for treating erectile dysfunction: a systematic review, *Br J Clin Pharmacol* 66(4):444–450, 2008.

Jepson RG, Williams G, Craig JC: Cranberries for preventing urinary tract infections, *Cochrane Database Syst Rev* (10):CD001321, 2012.

Jiang W, Qiu W, Wang Y, et al: Ginkgo may prevent genetic-associated ovarian cancer risk: multiple biomarkers and anticancer pathways induced by ginkgolide B in BRCA1-mutant ovarian epithelial cells, *Eur J Cancer Prev* 20:508–517, 2011.

Jurgens TM, Whelan AM, Killian L, Doucette S, Kirk S, Foy E: Green tea for weight loss and weight maintenance in overweight or obese adults, *Cochrane Database Syst Rev* (12):CD008650, 2012.

Karsch-Völk M, Barrett B, Kiefer D, Bauer R, Ardjomand-Woelkart K, Linde K: Echinacea for preventing and treating the common cold, *Cochrane Database Syst Rev* (2):CD000530, 2014.

Khalsa KP: Preparing botanical medicines, *J Herb Pharmacother* 7:267–277, 2007.

Kim LS, Axelrod LJ, Howard P, Buratovich N, Waters RF: Efficacy of methylsulfonylmethane (MSM) in osteoarthritis pain of the knee: a pilot clinical trial, *Osteoarthritis Cartilage* 14:286–294, 2006.

Kim TH, Lim HJ, Kim MS, Lee MS: Dietary supplements for benign prostatic hyperplasia: an overview of systematic reviews, *Maturitas* 73:180–185, 2012.

Krystal AD, Benca RM, Kilduff TS: Understanding the sleep-wake cycle: sleep, insomnia, and the orexin system, *J Clin Psychiatry* 74(Suppl 1):3–20, 2013.

Kuhn MA: Herbal remedies: drug-herb interactions, *Crit Care Nurse* 22:22–28, 2002.

Laaksonen R, Jokelainen K, Sahi T, Tikkanen MJ, Himberg JJ: Decreases in serum ubiquinone concentrations do not result in reduced levels in muscle tissue during short-term simvastatin treatment in humans, *Clin Pharmacol Ther* 57:62–66, 1995.

Lam A, Bradley G: Use of self-prescribed nonprescription medications and dietary supplements among assisted living facility residents, *J Am Pharm Assoc* 46:574–581, 2006.

Langsjoen PH, Langsjoen JO, Langsjoen AM, Lucas LA: Treatment of statin adverse effects with supplemental coenzyme Q10 and statin drug discontinuation, *Biofactors* 25:147–152, 2005.

Larsson SC, Wolk A: Tea consumption and ovarian cancer risk in a population-based cohort, *Arch Intern Med* 165:2683–2686, 2005.

Lawvere S, Mahoney MC: St. John's wort, *Am Fam Physician* 72: 2249–2254, 2005.

Leach MJ, Kumar S: Cinnamon for diabetes mellitus, *Cochrane Database Syst Rev* (9):CD007170, 2012.

Lee AN, Werth VP: Activation of autoimmunity following use of immunostimulatory herbal supplements, *Arch Dermatol* 140(6): 723–727, 2004.

Lee SH, Ahn YM, Ahn SY, Doo HK, Lee BC: Interaction between warfarin and *Panax ginseng* in ischemic stroke patients, *J Altern Complement Med* 14:715–721, 2008.

Lemoine P, Zisapel N: Prolonged-release formulation of melatonin (Circadin) for the treatment of insomnia, *Expert Opin Pharmacother* 13:895–905, 2012.

Linde K, Berner MM, Kriston L: St. John's wort for major depression, *Cochrane Database Syst Rev* (4):CD000448, 2008.

Liu J, Zhang J, Shi Y, Grimsgaard S, Alraek T, Fønnebø V: Chinese red yeast rice (*Monascus purpureus*) for primary hyperlipidemia: a meta-analysis of randomized controlled trials, *Chin Med* 1:4, 2006.

Loya AM, González-Stuart A, Rivera JO: Prevalence of polypharmacy, polyherbacy, nutritional supplement use and potential product interactions among older adults living on the United States–Mexico border: a descriptive, questionnaire-based study, *Drugs Aging* 26:423–436, 2009.

MacDonald R, Tacklind JW, Rutks I, Wilt TJ: Serenoa repens monotherapy for benign prostatic hyperplasia (BPH): an updated Cochrane systematic review, *BJU Int* 109:1756–1761, 2012.

Madmani ME, Yusuf Solaiman A, Tamr Agha K, et al: Coenzyme Q10 for heart failure, *Cochrane Database Syst Rev* (6):CD008684, 2014.

Martel-Pelletier J, Kwan Tat S, Pelletier JP: Effects of chondroitin sulfate in the pathophysiology of the osteoarthritic joint: a narrative review, *Osteoarthritis Cartilage* 18:S7–S11, 2010.

Mashayekh A, Pham DL, Yousem DM, Dizon M, Barker PB, Lin DD: Effects of Ginkgo biloba on cerebral blood flow assessed by quantitative MR perfusion imaging: a pilot study, *Neuroradiology* 53(3):185–191, 2011.

Mayo Clinic: *Caffeine content for coffee, tea, soda and more*, 1998-2018. https://www.mayoclinic.org/healthy-lifestyle/nutrition-and-healthy-eating/in-depth/caffeine/art-20049372.

Melzer J, Rösch W, Reichling J, Brignoli R, Saller R: Meta-analysis: phytotherapy of functional dyspepsia with the herbal drug preparation STW 5 (Iberogast), *Aliment Pharmacol Ther* 20:1279–1287, 2004.

Murkovic M, Abuja PM, Bergmann AR, et al: Effects of elderberry juice on fasting and postprandial serum lipids and low-density lipoprotein oxidation in healthy volunteers: a randomized, double-blind, placebo-controlled study, *Eur J Clin Nutr* 2004;58: 244–249.

Nagaoka I, Igarashi M, Sakamoto K: Biological activities of glucosamine and its related substances, *Adv Food Nutr Res* 65:337–352, 2012.

Nahin RL, Barnes PM, Stussman BJ, Bloom B: Costs of complementary and alternative medicine (CAM) and frequency of visits to CAM practitioners: United States, 2007, *Natl Health Stat Report* 18:1–14, 2009.

Nakasone Y, Watabe K, Watanabe K, et al: Effect of a glucosamine-based combination supplement containing chondroitin sulfate and antioxidant micronutrients in subjects with symptomatic knee osteoarthritis: a pilot study, *Exp Ther Med* 2:893–899, 2011.

National Center for Complementary and Integrative Health: *6 tips: how herbs can interact with medicines*, 2015. https://nccih.nih.gov/health/tips/herb-drug. Accessed February 2018.

National Center for Complementary and Integrative Health: *Red yeast rice*, 2017a. https://nccih.nih.gov/health/redyeastrice. Accessed February 2018.

National Center for Complementary and Integrative Health: *St. John's wort and depression: in depth*, 2017b. https://nccih.nih.gov/health/stjohnswort/sjw-and-depression.htm. Accessed March 2018.

National Center for Complementary and Integrative Health: *St. John's wort*, 2017c. https://nccih.nih.gov/health/stjohnswort. Assessed February 2018.

National Center for Complementary and Integrative Health: *Ginseng*, 2017d. https://nccih.nih.gov/health/asianginseng. Accessed February 2018.

National Center for Complementary and Integrative Health: *St. John's wort and depression: in depth*, 2018. https://nccih.nih.gov/health/stjohnswort/sjw-and-depression.htm. Accessed February 2018.

National Institute of Health: *Dietary Supplement Health and Education Act of 1994. Public Law 103-417. 103rd Congress*, 1994. https://ods.od.nih.gov/About/DSHEA_Wording.aspx. Accessed April 2019.

Nieva R, Safavynia SA, Lee Bishop K, Laurence S: Herbal, vitamin, and mineral supplement use in patients enrolled in a cardiac rehabilitation program, *J Cardiopulm Rehabil Prev* 32:270–277, 2012.

Nutrition Business Journal: *2016 Supplement Business Report*, New York, NY, 2016, Penton Media.

Quinn JF, Raman R, Thomas RG, et al: Docosahexaenoic acid supplementation and cognitive decline in Alzheimer disease: a randomized trial, *JAAM* 304(17):1903–1911, 2010.

Ramar K, Olson EJ: Management of common sleep disorders, *Am Fam Physician* 88:231–238, 2013.

Rambaldi A, Jacobs BP, Gluud C: Milk thistle for alcoholic and/or hepatitis B or C virus liver diseases, *Cochrane Database Syst Rev* (4):CD003620, 2007.

Ravindran AV, Lam RW, Filteau MJ, et al: Canadian Network for Mood and Anxiety Treatments (CANMAT) clinical guidelines for the management of major depressive disorder in adults. V. Complementary and alternative medicine treatments, *J Affect Disord* 117(Suppl 1):S54–S64, 2009.

Reginster JY, Neuprez A, Lecart MP, Sarlet N, Bruyere O: Role of glucosamine in the treatment for osteoarthritis, *Rheumatol Int* 32:2959–2967, 2012.

Reinhart KM, Coleman CI, Teevan C, Vachhani P, White CM: Effects of garlic on blood pressure in patients with and without systolic hypertension: a meta-analysis, *Ann Pharmacother* 42:1766–1771, 2008.

Reinhart KM, Talati R, White CM, Coleman CI: The impact of garlic on lipid parameters: a systematic review and meta-analysis, *Nutr Res Rev* 22:39–48, 2009.

Ried K, Frank OR, Stocks NP: Aged garlic extract reduces blood pressure in hypertensives: a dose-response trial, *Eur J Clin Nutr* 67:64–70, 2013.

Ried K, Frank OR, Stocks NP, Fakler P, Sullivan T: Effect of garlic on blood pressure: a systematic review and meta-analysis, *BMC Cardiovasc Disord* 8:13, 2008.

Rundek T, Naini A, Sacco R, Coates K, DiMauro S: Atorvastatin decreases the coenzyme Q10 level in the blood of patients at risk for cardiovascular disease and stroke, *Arch Neurol* 61:889–892, 2004.

Ryder PT, Wolpert B, Orwig D, Carter-Pokras O, Black SA: Complementary and alternative medicine use among older urban African Americans: individual and neighborhood associations, *J Natl Med Assoc* 100:1186–1192, 2008.

Salazar-Martinez E, Willett WC, Ascherio A, et al: Coffee consumption and risk for type 2 diabetes mellitus, *Ann Intern Med* 140:1–8, 2004.

Sarma DN, Barrett ML, Chavez ML, et al: Safety of green tea extracts: a systematic review by the US Pharmacopeia, *Drug Saf* 31(6): 469–484, 2008.

Sawitzke AD, Shi H, Finco MF, et al: Clinical efficacy and safety of glucosamine, chondroitin sulphate, their combination, celecoxib or placebo taken to treat osteoarthritis of the knee: 2-year results from GAIT, *Ann Rheum Dis* 69:1459–1464, 2010.

Shah SA, Sander S, White CM, Rinaldi M, Coleman CI: Evaluation of echinacea for the prevention and treatment of the common cold: a meta-analysis, *Lancet Infect Dis* 7:473–480, 2007.

Shelton RC: St. John's wort (Hypericum perforatum) in major depression, *J Clin Psychiatry* 70(Suppl 5):23–27, 2009.

Sierpina VS, Wollschlaeger B, Blumenthal M: Ginkgo biloba, *Am Fam Physician* 68:923–926, 2003.

Simons S, Wollersheim H, Thien T: A systematic review on the influence of trial quality on the effect of garlic on blood pressure, *Neth J Med* 67:212–219, 2009.

Singh JA, Noorbaloochi S, MacDonald R, Maxwell LJ: Chondroitin for osteoarthritis, *Cochrane Database Syst Rev* (1):CD005614, 2015.

Siscovick DS, Barringer TA, Fretts AM, et al: Omega-3 polyunsaturated fatty acid (fish oil) supplementation and the prevention of clinical cardiovascular disease: a science advisory from the American Heart Association, *Circulation* 135(15), e867–e884, 2017.

Snitz BE, O'Meara ES, Carlson MC, et al. Ginkgo Evaluation of Memory (GEM) Study Investigators. Ginkgo biloba for preventing cognitive decline in older adults: a randomized trial, *JAMA* 302:2663–2670, 2009.

Sobenin IA, Pryanishnikov VV, Kunnova LM, Rabinovich YA, Martirosyan DM, Orekhov AN: The effects of time-released garlic powder tablets on multifunctional cardiovascular risk in patients with coronary artery disease, *Lipids Health Dis* 9:119, 2010.

Stabler SN, Tejani AM, Huynh F, Fowkes C: Garlic for the prevention of cardiovascular morbidity and mortality in hypertensive patients, *Cochrane Database Syst Rev* (8):CD007653, 2012.

Tachjian A, Maria V, Jahangir A: Use of herbal products and potential interactions in patients with cardiovascular diseases, *J Am Coll Cardiol* 55:515–525, 2010.

Tacklind J, MacDonald R, Rutks I, Stanke JU, Wilt TJ: Serenoa repens for benign prostatic hyperplasia, *Cochrane Database Syst Rev* 12:CD001423, 2012.

Tacklind J, MacDonald R, Rutks I, Wilt TJ: Serenoa repens for benign prostatic hyperplasia, *Cochrane Database Syst Rev* (2):CD001423, 2009.

Tang NP, Hua L, Zhou YL, Zhou GM, Ma J: Tea consumption and risk of endometrial cancer: a metaanalysis, *Am J Obstet Gynecol* 201(6):e1-8, 2009.

Terris MK, Issa MM, Tacker JR: Dietary supplementation with cranberry concentrate tablets may increase the risk of nephrolithiasis, *Urology* 57:26–29, 2001.

Therapeutic Research Center: *Natural medicines: ginkgo*, 2017a. https://naturalmedicines.therapeuticresearch.com/databases/food,-herbs-supplements/professional.aspx?productid=333. Accessed March 22, 2018.

Therapeutic Research Center: *Natural medicines: melatonin*, 2017b. https://naturalmedicines.therapeuticresearch.com/databases/food,-herbs-supplements/professional.aspx?productid=940. Accessed March 22, 2018.

Therapeutic Research Center: *Natural medicines: Ginseng Panax*, 2017c. https://naturalmedicines.therapeuticresearch.com/databases/food,-herbs-supplements/professional.aspx?productid=1000. Accessed March 22, 2018.

Therapeutic Research Center: *Natural medicines: coenzyme Q10*, 2017d. https://naturalmedicines.therapeuticresearch.com/. Accessed December 28, 2017

Therapeutic Research Center: *Natural medicines: green tea*, 2017e. https://naturalmedicines.therapeuticresearch.com/search.aspx?q=green+tea. Accessed December 28, 2017.

Therapeutic Research Center: *Natural medicines: diabetes*, 2017f. https://naturalmedicines.therapeuticresearch.com/search.aspx?q=diabetes. Accessed December 29, 2017.

Therapeutic Research Center: *Natural Medicines—Effectiveness Checker, 2017—"garlic"*, 2017g. https://naturalmedicines.therapeuticresearch.com/databases/food,-herbs-supplements/professional.aspx?productid=300. Accessed December 28, 2017.

Therapeutic Research Center: *Natural medicines: echinacea*, 2018a. https://naturalmedicines.therapeuticresearch.com/databases/food,-herbs-supplements/professional.aspx?productid=981. Accessed March 22, 2018.

Therapeutic Research Center: *Natural medicines: St. John's wort*, 2018b. https://naturalmedicines.therapeuticresearch.com/databases/food,-herbs-supplements/professional.aspx?productid=329. Accessed March 22, 2018.

Therapeutic Research Center: *Natural medicines: chondroitin sulfate*, 2018c. https://naturalmedicines.therapeuticresearch.com/databases/food,-herbs-supplements/professional.aspx?productid=744. Accessed March 22, 2018.

Therapeutic Research Center: *Natural medicines: saw palmetto*, 2018d. https://naturalmedicines.therapeuticresearch.com/databases/food,-herbs-supplements/professional.aspx?productid=971. Accessed March 22, 2018.

Tillett J, Ames D: The uses of aromatherapy in women's health, *J Perinat Neonatal Nurs* 24:238–245, 2010.

Towheed TE, Maxwell L, Anastassiades TP, et al: Glucosamine therapy for treating osteoarthritis, *Cochrane Database Syst Rev* (2):CD002946, 2005.

Toyama K, Sugiyama S, Oka H, et al: Rosuvastatin combined with regular exercise preserves coenzyme Q10 levels associated with a significant increase in high-density lipoprotein cholesterol in patients with coronary artery disease, *Atherosclerosis* 217: 158–164, 2001.

Tuomilehto J, Hu G, Bidel S, Lindström J, Jousilahti P: Coffee consumption and risk of type 2 diabetes mellitus among middle-aged Finnish men and women, *JAMA* 291:1213–1219, 2004.

Turunen M, Olsson J, Dallner G: Metabolism and function of coenzyme Q, *Biochim Biophys Acta* 1660(1-2):171–199, 2004.

U.S. Food and Drug Administration: *Dietary supplements*, 2017a. http://www.fda.gov/Food/Dietarysupplements/default.htm. Accessed January 2018.

U.S. Food and Drug Administration: *Structure/function claims*, 2017b. https://www.fda.gov/Food/LabelingNutrition/ucm2006881.htm. Accessed January 2018.

Ulbricht C, Chao W, Costa D, Rusie-Seamon E, Weissner W, Woods J: Clinical evidence of herb-drug interactions: a systematic review by the Natural Standard Research Collaboration, *Curr Drug Metab* 9(10):1063–1120, 2008.

van der Watt G, Laugharne J, Janca A: Complementary and alternative medicine in the treatment of anxiety and depression, *Curr Opin Psychiatry* 21:37–42, 2008.

Vellas B, Coley N, Ousset PJ, et al: Long-term use of standardised Ginkgo biloba extract for the prevention of Alzheimer's disease (GuidAge): a randomised placebo-controlled trial, *Lancet Neurol* 11:851–859, 2012.

Vlachojannis JE, Cameron M, Chrubasik S: A systematic review on the Sambuci fructus effect and efficacy profiles, *Phytother Res* 24(1):1–8, 2010.

Volpi N: Anti-inflammatory activity of chondroitin sulphate: new functions from an old natural macromolecule, *Inflammopharmacology* 19(6):299–306, 2011.

Wilhelmsen-Langeland A, Saxvig IW, Pallesen S, et al: A randomized controlled trial with bright light and melatonin for the treatment of delayed sleep phase disorder: effects on subjective and objective sleepiness and cognitive function, *J Biol Rhythms* 28:306–321, 2013.

Yoon SL, Horne CH, Adams C: Herbal product use by African American older women, *Clin Nurs Res* 13:271–288, 2004.

Yoon SJ, Horne CH: Herbal products and conventional medicines used by community-residing older women, *J Adv Nurs* 33:51–59, 2001.

Yoon SL, Schaffer SD: Herbal, prescribed, and over-the-counter drug use in older women: prevalence of drug interactions, *Geriatr Nurs* 27:118–129, 2006.

Zakay-Rones Z, Thom E, Wollan T, Wadstein J: Randomized study of the efficacy and safety of oral elderberry extract in the treatment of influenza A and B virus infections, *J Int Med Res* 32(2): 132–140, 2004.

Zakay-Rones Z, Varsano N, Zlotnik M, et al: Inhibition of several strains of influenza virus in vitro and reduction of symptoms by an elderberry extract (Sambucus nigra L.) during an outbreak of influenza B Panama, *J Altern Complement Med* 1(4):361–369, 1995.

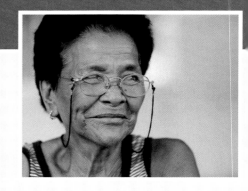

11

Vision

Theris A. Touhy

http://evolve.elsevier.com/Touhy/TwdHlthAging

A STUDENT SPEAKS

I kind of understand the problems vision impairment can cause as one ages. I am pretty blind without my glasses. I can't even see the alarm clock numbers. I worry about what my vision will be when I am older. I took care of a woman in the assisted living facility with macular degeneration. I asked her how the disease affects her vision. The woman put her hand in front of my face and said, "I can see your hair, the color, and some of the space around you, but I cannot see your face or the color of your skin." She seems to cope pretty well and uses low-vision devices to help her manage her life. It frightened me a little but also gave me hope that even with this kind of vision loss, she is able to function and stay in pretty good spirits. I am going to get some information about how to keep my eyes healthy. I hadn't thought about the things I could do now that might help as I age.

Debbie, age 27

AN OLDER ADULT SPEAKS

One of the great frustrations is the matter of eyesight. One can get used to large print and hope for black letters on white paper, but why do modern publishers seem to prefer the shiny, slick off-white paper and pale ink in minuscule print? Thank goodness for restaurants with lighted menus and my new iPhone with a bright light.

Lyn, age 85

LEARNING OBJECTIVES

On completion of this chapter, the reader will be able to:

1. Identify age-related changes in the eye that affect vision and discuss recommendations to promote eye health throughout life.
2. Discuss diseases of the eye that may occur in older adults.
3. Describe the importance of screening, health education, and treatment of eye diseases to prevent unnecessary vision loss.
4. Identify effective communication strategies for older adults with vision impairments.
5. Gain awareness of assistive devices to enhance vision.

CHANGES IN VISION WITH AGE

Changes in eye structure begin early, are progressive in nature, and are both functional and structural. The structures most affected are the cornea, anterior chamber, lens, ciliary muscles, and retina. All of the age-related changes affect visual acuity and accommodation. Although presbyopia (decreased near vision as a result of aging) is first seen between 45 and 55 years of age, 80% of those older than 65 years have fair to adequate far vision past 90 years of age. Nearly 95% of adults older than 65 years wear glasses for close vision.

Extraocular Changes

Like the skin elsewhere, the eyelids lose elasticity and drooping (senile ptosis) may result. In most cases, this is only a cosmetic concern. In some cases, it can interfere with vision if the lids sag far enough over the lower lid margin. Spasms of the orbicular muscle may cause the lower lid to turn inward. If it stays this way, it is called *entropion*. With the curling of the lid, the lower lashes also turn inward, causing irritation and scratching of the cornea. Surgery may be needed to prevent permanent injury. Decreases in orbicular muscle strength may result in *ectropion*,

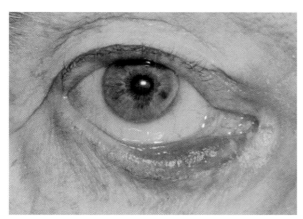

Fig. 11.1 Ectropion. (From Swartz MH: *Textbook of physical diagnosis: history and examination,* ed 6, Philadelphia, 2009, Saunders.)

or an out-turning of the lower lid (Fig. 11.1). Without the integrity of the trough of the lower lid, tears run down the cheek instead of bathing the cornea. This, along with an inability to close the lid completely, leads to excessively dry eyes (xerophthalmia) and the need for use of artificial tears. The individual also may need to tape the eyes shut during sleep. A reduction of goblet cells in the conjunctiva is another cause for drying of the eyes in the older adult. Goblet cells produce mucin, which slows the evaporation of tear film and is essential for eye lubrication and movement.

Ocular Changes

The cornea is the avascular transparent outer surface of the eye globe that refracts (bends) light rays entering the eye through the pupil. With aging, the cornea becomes flatter, less smooth, and thicker, with the changes noticeable by its lackluster appearance or loss of sparkling transparency. The result is the increased incidence of astigmatism. The anterior chamber is the space between the cornea and the lens. The edges of the chamber include the canals that control the volume and movement of aqueous fluid within the space. With aging, the chamber decreases slightly in size and volume capacity because of thickening of the lens. Resorption of the intraocular fluid becomes less efficient and may lead to eventual breakdown in the absorption process. If the change is greater, it can lead to increased intraocular pressure (IOP) and the development of glaucoma.

The iris is a ring of muscles inside the anterior chamber. The iris surrounds the opening into the eye (the pupil), gives the eye color, and regulates the amount of light that reaches the retina. With age the iris becomes paler in color as a result of pigment loss and increases in the density of collagen fibers. A normal age-related change in the iris is related to other neurological changes—that is, slowed response to sensory stimuli, in this case, to light and dark. Slowness to dilate in dark environments creates moments when older adults cannot see where they are going (e.g., moving from a well-lit area to a dark area such as in a movie theater).

Because of the slow ability of the pupils to accommodate to changes in light, glare can be a major problem. Glare is caused by not only sunlight but also reflection of light on any shiny object, such as headlights or polished floors. The use of sunglasses outdoors (and indoors if considerable glare exists) can be helpful. The effect of glare from headlights of oncoming vehicles increases safety risks with driving (night blindness). Persistent pupillary constriction is known as *senile miosis*. It is often noted during the physical exam but often a normal finding if it is bilateral. At the edges of the cornea and the iris is a small ring known as the **limbus**. In some older adults, a gray-white ring or partial ring, known as **arcus senilis**, forms 1 to 2 mm inside the limbus. It does not affect vision and is composed of deposits of calcium and cholesterol salts.

The lens, a small, flexible, biconvex, crystal-like structure just behind the iris, is responsible for visual acuity as it adjusts the light entering the pupil and focuses it on the retina. Age-related changes in the lens are probably universal, but many of the changes are thought to result from exposure to ultraviolet light. The constant compression of lens fibers with age, the yellowing effect, and the inefficiency of the aqueous humor, which provides the lens with nutrition, all have a role in altered lens transparency. Lens cells continue to grow but at a slower rate than previously. The lens can no longer focus (refract) close objects effectively, described as decreased accommodation.

Changes to the suspensory ligaments, ciliary muscles, and parasympathetic nerves also contribute to the decreased accommodation. Finally, light scattering increases and color perception decreases. For the person who was myopic (near-sighted) earlier in life, this change may actually improve vision. Lens opacity (cataracts) begins to develop around the fifth decade of life. The origins are not fully understood, although ultraviolet light contributes, with cross-linkage of collagen creating a more rigid and thickened lens structure.

Intraocular Changes

The vitreous humor, which gives the eye globe its shape and support, loses some of its water and fibrous skeletal support with age. Opacities other than cataracts can be seen by the person as lines, webs, spots, or clusters of dots moving rapidly across the visual field with each movement of the eye. These opacities are called "floaters" and are bits of coalesced vitreous humor that have broken off from the peripheral or central part of the retina. Most are harmless but annoying until they dissipate or one gets used to them. However, if the person sees a shower of these and a flash of light, immediate medical attention is required and this is always considered an ocular emergency (retinal detachment).

The retina, which lines the inside of the eye, has less distinct margins and is duller in appearance than in younger adults. Fidelity of color is less accurate with blues, violets, and greens of the spectrum; warm colors such as reds, oranges, and yellows are more easily seen. Color clarity diminishes by 25% in the sixth decade and by 59% in the eighth decade. Some of this difficulty is linked to the yellowing of the lens and the impaired transmission of light to the retina, and the fovea may not be as bright. The average 80-year-old needs more than twice as much light as a 20-year-old to see equally well (Huether et al, 2014).

Drusen (yellow-white) spots may appear in the area of the macula. As long as these changes are not accompanied by

TABLE 11.1   Changes in the Eye Caused by Aging.

Structure	Change	Consequence
Cornea	Thicker and less curved	Increase in astigmatism
	Formation of a gray ring at the edge of cornea (arcus senilis)	Not detrimental to vision
Anterior chamber	Decrease in size and volume caused by thickening of lens	Occasionally exerts pressure on Schlemm canal and may lead to increased intraocular pressure and glaucoma
Lens	Increase in opacity	Decrease in refraction with increased light scattering and decreased color vision (green and blue); decreased dark adaptation; cataracts
	Loss of elasticity	Loss of accommodation (presbyopia: loss of focus for near objects)
Ciliary muscles	Reduction in pupil diameter, atrophy of radial dilation muscles	Persistent constriction (senile miosis); decrease in critical flicker frequency[a]
Retina	Reduction in number of rods at periphery, loss of rods and associated nerve cells	Increase in the minimum amount of light necessary to see an object
Macula	Atrophy (age-related macular degeneration)	Loss of vision
Vitreous	Liquefaction of vitreous and decrease in gel volume	Posterior vitreous detachment causing "floaters"; risk for retinal detachment

[a]The rate at which consecutive visual stimuli can be presented and still be perceived as separate.

From McCance KL, Huether SE: *Pathophysiology*, ed 7, St Louis, 2014, Mosby.

distortion of objects or a decrease in vision, they are not clinically significant. Finally, the number of rods and associated nerves at the periphery of the retina is reduced, resulting in peripheral vision that is not as discrete or is absent. Arteries in the back of the eye may show atherosclerosis and slight narrowing. Veins may show indentations (nicking) at the arteriovenous crossings if the person has a long history of hypertension. Table 11.1 summarizes changes in the eye with age.

VISUAL IMPAIRMENT

Incidence and Prevalence

Vision loss is not an inevitable part of the aging process, but age-related changes contribute to decreased vision. Even older adults with good visual acuity (20/40 or better) and no significant eye disease show deficits in visual function and need accommodations to enhance vision and safety. As we age there is a higher risk of developing age-related eye diseases and other conditions (hypertension, diabetes) that can result in vision losses if left untreated.

Vision loss is a leading cause of age-related disability. More than two-thirds of those with visual impairment are more than 65 years of age, and adults older than 80 years account for 70% of the cases of severe visual impairment. The World Health Organization (WHO, 2019) defines visual impairment as visual acuity worse than 20/70 but better than 20/400 (legal blindness) in the better eye, even with corrective lenses.

Visual impairment worldwide has decreased since the 1990s as a result of increased availability of eye care services (particularly cataract surgery), promotion of eye care education, and improved treatment of infectious diseases. However, vision impairment is a major public health problem across the globe that is expected to increase substantially with the aging of the population. Rates of blindness and visual impairment in disadvantaged, minority populations, particularly African American and Latino subpopulations who have an increased prevalence of diabetes and hypertension, are expected to increase even

further. In the United States, the leading causes of visual impairment are cataracts, glaucoma, diabetic neuropathy, and age-related macular degeneration (AMD). Globally, uncorrected refractive errors (myopia, hyperopia, or astigmatism) and unoperated cataract and glaucoma are the leading causes of visual impairment.

Vision loss from eye disease is particularly a concern in the developing countries, where 90% of the world's blind individuals live. Cataracts are the leading cause of blindness in economically challenged countries, largely as a result of limited service and treatment (World Health Organization, 2019). The World Health Organization's Universal Eye Health: A Global Action Plan 2014–2019 (http://www.who.int/blindness/actionplan/en/) proposes to achieve a measurable reduction of 25% of avoidable visual impairments by 2019. Other goals include securing access to vision rehabilitation services by improving access to comprehensive eye care services that are integrated into health systems (World Health Organization, 2017). Estimates are that 80% of all visual impairment can be avoided or cured. See the *Healthy People 2020* box for objectives for vision in older adults.

♥ HEALTHY PEOPLE 2020

Objectives Vision—Older Adults

- Increase the proportion of adults who have had a comprehensive eye examination, including dilation, within the past 2 years.
- Reduce visual impairment due to diabetic retinopathy.
- Reduce visual impairment due to glaucoma.
- Reduce visual impairment due to cataracts.
- Reduce visual impairment due to age-related macular degeneration.
- Increase the use of vision rehabilitation services by persons with visual impairment.
- Increase the use of assistive and adaptive devices by persons with visual impairment.

Data from U.S. Department of Health and Human Services, Office of Disease Prevention and Health Promotion: *Healthy People 2020*, 2012. http://www.healthypeople.gov/2020.

Consequences of Visual Impairment

Visual problems have a negative impact on quality of life, equivalent to that of life-threatening conditions such as heart disease and cancer. Loss of vision impacts an individual's quality of life and ability to function in most daily activities such as driving, reading, maneuvering safely, dressing, cooking, taking medications, and participating in social activities. Decreased vision has also been found to be a significant risk factor for falls and other accidents and is associated with cognitive decline and depression, increased risk of institutionalization, and death. "Vision loss not only severely impairs one's ability to be independent and self-sufficient, but it also has a 'snowball effect' on the health and well-being of older adults, families, caregivers, and society at large. This cumulative effect is severely underestimated" (International Federation on Ageing, 2012, p. 4).

Prevention of Visual Impairment

Many age-related eye diseases have no symptoms in the early stages but can be detected early through a comprehensive dilated eye exam. However, knowledge about eye disease and treatments remains inadequate among both laypersons and medical professionals. Socioeconomic position and educational position are important social determinants that may influence access to and use of effective and appropriate eye care, thus influencing disease identification and treatment (MacLennan et al, 2014; Zhang et al, 2013).

At all ages, attention to eye health and protection of your vision are important (Box 11.1). Prevention and treatment of eye disease are important priorities for nurses and other health professionals. The National Eye Health Education Program (NEHEP) of the National Eye Institute (NEI) provides a program for health professionals with evidence-based tools and resources that can be used in community settings to educate older adults about eye health and maintaining healthy vision. Educational materials and outreach activities targeted to populations at high risk for eye diseases, including African Americans, American Indians, Alaska natives, Hispanics/Latinos, and individuals with diabetes and a family history of glaucoma are available (NEI, NEHEP, 2017) (http://www.nei.nih.gov/SeeWellToolkit) (Box 11.2).

BOX 11.1 Promoting Healthy Eyes

- Have a comprehensive eye dilated eye exam
- Know your family's eye health history
- Eat right to protect your sight (diet rich in green leafy vegetables, fruit, and fish)
- Maintain a healthy weight
- Wear protective eyewear
- Quit smoking or never start
- Be cool and wear your shades
- Give your eyes a rest when doing computer work or focusing on any one thing. Every 20 minutes look away 20 feet in front of you for 20 seconds. This will help reduce eyestrain
- Clean your hands and your contact lenses properly
- Practice workplace eye safety (protective eye wear if required)

From National Eye Institute: *Information for healthy vision.* https://nei.nih.gov/healthyeyes/eyehealthtips. Accessed November 2017.

BOX 11.2 Resources for Best Practice

Vision

Centers for Disease Control and Prevention: Education, videos illustrating vision with age-related macular degeneration (AMD), glaucoma, diabetic retinopathy
Eye Care America: On-line referral center for eye care resources
Lighthouse International: Educational resources, professional development, public policy center
National Eye Health Education Program (NEHEP) and National Eye Institute (NEI): Educational and professional resources, vision and aging program; See Well for a Lifetime Toolkit, vodcasts on common visual problems, videos on eye health and eye diseases (https://nei.nih.gov/videos)
National Federation for the Blind: Educational information, resources
United States Department of Health and Human Services /Agency for Healthcare Research and Quality (USDHHS/AHRQ): Evidence-based practice guideline: care of the patient with open angle glaucoma.
Vision Aware (American Foundation for the Blind): Resources for independent living with vision loss; Getting started kit for people new to vision loss; How to walk with a guide
World Health Organization plan

DISEASES AND DISORDERS OF THE EYE

Cataracts

A cataract is an opacification (cloudiness) in the eye's normally clear crystalline lens, causing the lens to lose transparency or scatter light. Cataracts can occur at any age (babies can be born with them), but they are most common later in life. In the United States, about 70% of people older than age 75 have cataracts. Cataracts are categorized according to their location within the lens: nuclear, cortical, and posterior subcapsular (in the rear of the lens capsule). Nuclear cataracts are the most common type and their incidence increases with age and cigarette smoking. Cortical cataracts also are more common with age, and their development is related to a lifetime of exposure to ultraviolet light. Older adults with diabetes are 60% more likely to develop cataracts than individuals without diabetes. Cataracts are also more likely to occur after glaucoma surgery or other types of eye surgery.

Cataracts form painlessly over time. The most common symptom is cloudy or blurred vision. Everything becomes dimmer, as if seen through glasses that need cleaning. Other symptoms include glare, halos around lights, poor night vision, a perception that colors are faded or that objects are yellowish, and the need for brighter light when reading. The red reflex may be absent or may appear as a black area. Fig. 11.2A illustrates normal vision; Fig 11.2B illustrates the effects of a cataract on vision. The NEI (https://nei.nih.gov/videos) provides videos on eye disorders and eye health (see Box 11.2).

Treatment of Cataracts

The treatment of cataracts is surgical, and cataract surgery is the most common surgical procedure performed in the United States. The surgery involves removal of the lens and placement of a plastic intraocular lens (IOL). Most often, cataract surgery involves only local anesthesia and is done on an outpatient

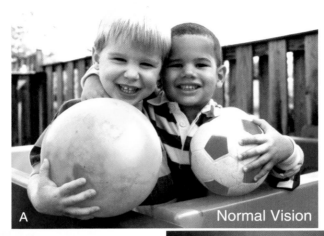

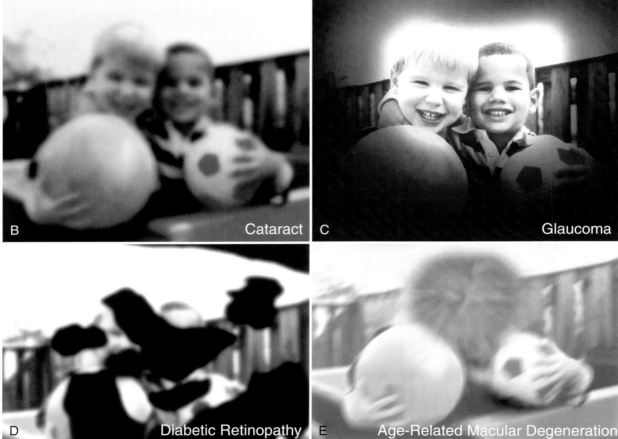

Fig. 11.2 (A) Normal vision. (B) Simulated vision with cataracts. (C) Simulated vision with glaucoma. (D) Simulated vision with diabetic retinopathy. (E) Simulated loss of vision with age-related macular degeneration. (From National Eye Institute, National Institutes of Health, 2010.)

basis. If the eye is normal except for the cataract, surgery will improve vision in 95% of cases. Significant postsurgical complications such as inflammation, infection, bleeding, retinal detachment, swelling, and glaucoma are rare. Individuals with medical problems such as diabetes and other eye diseases are most at risk for complications.

Presurgical and Postsurgical Interventions

Nursing interventions when caring for the person experiencing cataract surgery include preparing the individual for significant changes in vision and adaptation to light and ensuring that the individual has received adequate counseling regarding realistic postsurgical expectations. Most people experience a small amount of discomfort after surgery. Some redness, scratchiness, or discharge from the eye may occur during the first day after surgery. There may also be a few black spots or shapes (floaters) drifting through the field of vision. Vision remains blurred for several days or weeks and then gradually improves as the eye heals.

If the person has bilateral cataracts, surgery is performed first on one eye with the second surgery on the other eye a month or so later to ensure healing. Following surgery, the individual needs to avoid heavy lifting, straining, and bending at the waist. Eye drops may be prescribed to aid healing and prevent infection. Teaching fall prevention techniques and ensuring home safety modifications are also important because some research suggests that the risk of falls increases after surgery, particularly between first and second cataract surgeries. The vision imbalance that can occur if the person has one "good" eye and one "bad" eye contributes to the risk of falls.

Glaucoma

Glaucoma is a group of diseases that can damage the optic nerve. Glaucoma is the second leading cause of blindness in the United States. Glaucoma affects as many as 2.3 million Americans age 40 years and older and 6% of those older than age 65. Because the most common form of the condition, primary open-angle glaucoma (POAG), affects side vision first, it may remain unnoticed for years. At least half of all persons with glaucoma are unaware they have the disease.

Individuals at higher risk for glaucoma include African Americans over age 40 years; people with a family history of glaucoma; and everyone over 60 years, especially Mexican Americans. The condition is four times more common in Hispanics and five times more common in blacks than whites. African Americans are at risk of developing glaucoma at an earlier age than other racial and ethnic groups and blindness from glaucoma is four to five times more common than among whites. Type 2 diabetes is associated with an 82% higher risk of POAG. Other risk factors include trauma to the eye, severe myopia, or previous eye surgeries. Other high-risk groups are individuals with a history of corticosteroid use, trauma to the eye, myopia, or previous eye surgeries (NEI, 2017a). Some genetic variants may be associated with elevated IOP; thus family history is an important risk factor (Sussman, 2016). Research into genes that could explain how glaucoma damages the eye is underway (NEI, 2016).

The damage to the optic nerve in glaucoma is irreversible and regenerative attempts have been unsuccessful, so early diagnosis is essential. If detected early, glaucoma can usually be controlled and serious vision loss prevented. Signs of glaucoma can include headaches, poor vision in dim lighting, increased sensitivity to glare, "tired eyes," impaired peripheral vision, a fixed and dilated pupil, and frequent changes in prescriptions for corrective lenses. Fig. 11.2C illustrates the effects of glaucoma on vision.

Angle-closure glaucoma is not as common as POAG and occurs when the angle of the iris causes obstruction of the aqueous humor through the trabecular network. Individuals with smaller eyes, Asians, and women are most susceptible. It may occur as a result of infection or trauma. IOP rises rapidly accompanied by redness and pain in and around the eye, severe headaches, nausea and vomiting, and blurring of vision. It is a medical emergency and blindness can occur in 2 days. Treatment is an iridectomy to ease pressure. Many drugs with anticholinergic properties, including antihistamines, stimulants, vasodilators, and sympathomimetics, are particularly dangerous for individuals predisposed to acute-closure glaucoma.

⚡ SAFETY ALERT

Redness and pain in and around the eye, severe headaches, nausea and vomiting, and blurring of vision occur with angle-closure glaucoma. It is a medical emergency and blindness can occur in 2 days.

Screening and Treatment of Glaucoma

A dilated eye examination and tonometry are necessary to diagnose glaucoma. Adults older than age 65 should have annual eye examinations with dilation, and those with medication-controlled glaucoma should be examined at least every 6 months. Annual screening is also recommended for African Americans and other individuals with a family history of glaucoma who are older than 40 years. Although standard Medicare does not cover routine eye care, it does cover 80% of the cost for dilated eye exams for individuals at higher risk for glaucoma and those with diabetes.

Management of glaucoma involves medications (oral or topical eye drops) to decrease IOP and/or laser trabeculoplasty and filtration surgery. Medications lower eye pressure either by decreasing the amount of aqueous fluid produced within the eye or by improving the flow through the drainage angle. Beta-blockers are the first-line therapy for glaucoma followed by prostaglandin analogues. Second-line agents include topical carbonic anhydrase inhibitors and α_2-agonists. The patient may need combinations of several types of eye drops. There is ongoing research on the development of a contact lens to deliver glaucoma medication in a continuous-release dose. Further research is needed before use on humans but this may become an option for the treatment of glaucoma and improve outcomes for individuals who struggle with imprecise, difficult to administer eye drops (Ciolino et al, 2016).

In the hospital or long-term care setting, it is important to obtain a medical history to determine if the person has glaucoma and to ensure that eye drops are given according to the person's treatment regimen. Without the eye drops, eye pressure can rise and cause an acute exacerbation of glaucoma. Usually medications can control glaucoma, but laser surgery (trabeculoplasty) and filtration surgery may be recommended for some types of glaucoma. Surgery is usually recommended only if necessary to prevent further damage to the optic nerve.

Diabetic Eye Disease

Diabetic eye disease includes diabetic retinopathy (DR) and diabetic macular edema (DME). Cataracts and glaucoma are also more prevalent in individuals with diabetes. All forms of diabetic eye disease have the potential to cause severe vision loss and blindness (NEI, 2017c).

Diabetic Retinopathy

Diabetes has become an epidemic in the United States, and DR occurs in both type 1 and type 2 diabetes mellitus (Chapter 24). Risk increases the longer an individual has diabetes. Almost all people with type 1 diabetes will eventually develop retinopathy. People with type 2 diabetes are less likely to develop more advanced retinopathy than those with type 1. Chronically high blood sugar from diabetes is associated with damage to the tiny blood vessels in the retina, leading to DR. Blood and lipid leakage leads to macular edema and hard exudates (composed of lipids). In advanced disease, new fragile blood vessels form and hemorrhage easily. Because of the vascular and cellular changes accompanying diabetes, there is often also rapid worsening of other pathologic vision conditions (Fig. 11.2D). DR progresses through four stages (Box 11.3).

Screening and Treatment of Diabetic Retinopathy

Early detection and treatment of diabetic DR is essential. There are no symptoms in the early stages of DR. The disease often progresses unnoticed until it affects vision. Bleeding from abnormal retinal blood vessels can cause the appearance of "floating" spots that sometimes clear on their own. Without prompt treatment, bleeding often recurs, increasing the risk of permanent vision loss. Early signs are seen in the fundoscopic examination and include microaneurysms, flame-shaped hemorrhages, cotton wool spots, hard exudates, and dilated capillaries. Constant, strict control of blood glucose levels, cholesterol levels, and blood pressure measurements and laser photocoagulation (LPC) treatments can halt progression of the disease.

BOX 11.3 Stages of Diabetic Retinopathy

1. **Mild nonproliferative retinopathy.** At this earliest stage, microaneurysms occur. They are small areas of balloon-like swelling in the retina's tiny blood vessels.
2. **Moderate nonproliferative retinopathy.** As the disease progresses, some blood vessels that nourish the retina are blocked.
3. **Severe nonproliferative retinopathy.** Many more blood vessels are blocked, depriving several areas of the retina with their blood supply. These areas of the retina send signals to the body to grow new blood vessels for nourishment.
4. **Proliferative retinopathy.** At this advanced stage, the signals sent by the retina for nourishment trigger the growth of new blood vessels. This condition is called proliferative retinopathy. These new blood vessels are abnormal and fragile. They grow along the retina and along the surface of the clear, vitreous gel that fills the inside of the eye. By themselves, these blood vessels do not cause symptoms or vision loss. However, they have thin, fragile walls. If they leak blood, severe vision loss and even blindness can result (NEI, 2017c).

Annual dilated fundoscopic examination of the eye is recommended beginning 5 years after diagnosis of diabetes type 1 and at the time of diagnosis of diabetes type 2. Nurses need to provide education to diabetic patients about the risk of DR, the importance of early identification, and good control of diabetes. An increased likelihood of falls has been reported in individuals with mild to moderate nonproliferative DR. Fall prevention education should be provided to individuals with early-stage disease (Gupta et al, 2017). Some experts are encouraging mass screening efforts. There is good treatment that can reverse vision loss and improve vision, but individuals must have access to screenings and eye examinations.

Diabetic Macular Edema

DME is the buildup of fluid (edema) in a region of the retina called the macula. DME is the most common cause of visual loss attributable to diabetes and the leading cause of legal blindness. The disease affects 1 in 25 adults aged 40 years and older with diabetes and the incidence is higher in African Americans and Hispanics. About half of people with DR will develop DME. People with a history of high blood pressure and atherosclerosis are at a high risk of developing DME. Although it is more likely to occur as DR becomes worse, it can happen at any stage of the disease. Symptoms include blurred vision, loss of contrast, and patches of vision loss which may appear a black dots or lines "floating" across the front of the eye (Genentech, 2017).

Treatment includes medications (often cortisone-type drugs), anti-VEGF (vascular endothelial growth factor) injection therapy, and laser therapy to cauterize leaky blood vessels and reduce accumulated fluid within the macula. Anti-VEGF therapy (Lucentis) is used alone or in conjunction with laser treatment to treat DR in individuals with DME. The treatment appears to be well tolerated but requires about 12 to 15 injections into the eye over 36 months (NEI, 2017c).

Strict control of blood glucose, cholesterol, and blood pressure values; completion of annual dilated retinal examinations; and education about eye disease and diabetes are essential. However, in a recent study, only 44.7% of adults 40 years and older with DME reported that they were told by a physician that diabetes had affected their eyes and 59.7% had received a dilated eye examination in the past year. Approximately 55% of individuals with DME are unaware they have the condition (Genentech, 2017). Advances in stem cell technology and tissue engineering in the past several years have opened the possibility of replacing lost retinal neurons that occur as a result of glaucoma, DR, and AMD (Levin et al, 2017).

Detached Retina

A retinal detachment can occur at any age but is more common after the age of 40 years. Emergency medical treatment is required or permanent visual loss can result. There may be small areas of the retina that are torn (retinal tears or breaks) and will lead to retinal detachment. This condition can develop in persons with cataracts or recent cataract surgery or trauma, or it can occur spontaneously. Symptoms include a gradual increase in the number of floaters and/or light flashes in the eye. It also manifests as a curtain coming down over the person's field of vision. Small holes or tears are treated with laser surgery or a freeze treatment called *cryopexy*. Retinal detachments are treated with surgery. More than 90% of individuals with a retinal detachment can be successfully treated, although sometimes a second treatment is needed. However, the visual outcome is not always predictable and may not be known for several months following surgery. Visual results are best if the detachment is repaired before the macula detaches, so immediate treatment of symptoms is essential (NEI, 2017d).

Age-Related Macular Degeneration

AMD is the most common cause of new visual impairment among people age 50 years and older, although it is most likely to occur after age 60 (NEI, 2017e). The prevalence of AMD increases drastically with age, with more than 15% of white women older than age 80 years having the disease. Whites and Asian Americans are more likely to lose vision from AMD than African Americans or Hispanics/Latinos. With the number of affected older adults projected to increase over the next 20 years, AMD has been called a growing global epidemic.

AMD is a degenerative eye disease that affects the macula, the central part of the eye responsible for clear central vision. The disease causes the progressive loss of central vision, leaving only peripheral vision intact. The early and intermediate stages usually start without symptoms and only a comprehensive dilated eye exam can detect AMD. Objects may not appear to be as bright as they used to be and individuals may attribute their vision problems to normal aging or cataracts.

As AMD progresses, a blurred area near the center of vision is a common symptom. Over time, the blurred areas may grow larger and blank spots can develop in the central vision. AMD does not lead to complete blindness, but the loss of central vision interferes with everyday activities such as the ability to see faces, read, drive, or do close work, and can lead to impaired mobility, increased risk of falls, depression, and decreased quality of life (NEI, 2017e). Fig. 11.2E illustrates the effects of AMD on vision.

AMD results from systemic changes in circulation, accumulation of cellular waste products, atrophy of tissue, and growth of abnormal blood vessels in the choroid layer beneath the retina. Fibrous scarring disrupts nourishment of photoreceptor cells, causing their death and loss of central vision. Risk factors for AMD are similar to those for coronary artery disease (hypertension, atherosclerosis), inflammation, and diet. High glycemic diets are associated with AMD onset and progression (Rowan et al, 2017). Smoking doubles the risk of AMD. Individuals with a family history of AMD are at higher risk. At least 20 genes have been identified that affect the risk of developing AMD and many more genetic risk factors are suspected (NEI, 2017e).

There are three stages of AMD, defined in part by the size and number of drusen under the retina (Box 11.4). An individual can have AMD in one eye only or have one eye with a later stage than the other. Not everyone with early AMD will develop the later stage of the disease. In individuals with early AMD in one eye and no signs of AMD in the other eye, about 5% will develop advanced AMD after 10 years. For people who

RESEARCH HIGHLIGHTS

The intent of this interpretive phenomenological study was to understand the individual's experience of neovascular age-related macular degeneration (AMD), including ongoing treatment with anti-vascular endothelial growth factor (anti-VEGF). The study took place in an Australian public hospital clinic. Thirteen female and 12 male participants between 67 and 90 years of age with a diagnosis of neovascular AMD in at least one eye who were receiving anti-VEGF therapy on a routine basis were interviewed. Thematic analysis identified two major themes: *Life negotiated by neovascular AMD* and *Uncertainty*.

For most participants a diagnosis of AMD that required ongoing anti-VEGF injection was a life-changing event that evoked a range of feelings and fears from high anxiety to pragmatic acceptance. Participants expressed relief that the condition could be treated but they experienced apprehension at the thought of "having a needle into the eye." Positive experiences of the injection process helped with coping but anxiety increased if a new clinician was to give the injection or there were unexpected symptoms/complications (e.g., pain, intraocular bleeding). It was difficult for the participants to have to structure their lives around appointments and they described sadness at the loss of enjoyment of life that occurred as a result of the treatment and vision limitations. A fear of blindness was pervasive. Many experienced a significant halt in disease progression and for some, improvement in vision. However, they struggled with the uncertainty about prognosis.

The relationship between the health care facility staff and participants was critical in helping overcome anxieties. Reassurance, caring, communication, and feeling supported and known helped participants endure the rigors of the treatment and they were grateful for the treatment being available. Continuity of providers and treatment techniques and coming to know the patient and their unique experience are important.

From McCloud C, Lake S: Understanding the patient's lived experience of neovascular age-related macular degeneration: a qualitative study, *Eye (Lond)* 29(12), 1561–1569, 2015.

BOX 11.4 Three Stages of Age-Related Macular Degeneration

There are three stages of age-related macular degeneration (AMD) defined in part by the size and number of drusen under the retina. It is possible to have AMD in one eye only, or to have one eye with a later stage of AMD than the other.

- **Early AMD.** Early AMD is diagnosed by the presence of medium-sized drusen, which are about the width of an average human hair. People with early AMD typically do not have vision loss.
- **Intermediate AMD.** People with intermediate AMD typically have large drusen, pigment changes in the retina, or both. Again, these changes can only be detected during a dilated eye exam. Intermediate AMD may cause some vision loss, but most people will not experience any symptoms.
- **Late AMD.** In addition to drusen, people with late AMD have vision loss from damage to the macula. There are two types of late AMD:
  - In geographic atrophy (also called dry AMD), there is a gradual breakdown of the light-sensitive cells in the macula that convey visual information to the brain, and of the supporting tissue beneath the macula. These changes cause vision loss.
  - In neovascular AMD (also called wet AMD), abnormal blood vessels grow underneath the retina. ("Neovascular" literally means "new vessels.") These vessels can leak fluid and blood, which may lead to swelling and damage of the macula. The damage may be rapid and severe, unlike the more gradual course of geographic atrophy. It is possible to have both geographic atrophy and neovascular AMD in the same eye, and either condition can appear first.

From National Eye Institute: *Facts about age-related macular degeneration.* https://nei.nih.gov/health/maculardegen/armd_facts. Accessed November 2017.

have early AMD in both eyes, about 14% will develop late AMD in at least one eye after 10 years. Having late AMD in one eye puts an individual at increased risk for late AMD in the other eye.

In late AMD, there is vision loss attributable to damage to the macula. There are two types of late AMD: geographic atrophy (dry AMD) and neovascular AMD (wet AMD). Neovascular AMD occurs when abnormal blood vessels behind the retina start to grow under the macula. These new blood vessels are fragile and often leak blood and fluid, which raise the macula from its normal place at the back of the eye. With wet AMD, the severe loss of central vision can be rapid and many people will be legally blind within 2 years of diagnosis.

Screening and Treatment of AMD

Early diagnosis is the key. An Amsler grid (Fig. 11.3) is used to determine clarity of vision. A perception of wavy lines is diagnostic of beginning macular degeneration. In the advanced forms, the person may see dark or empty spaces that block the center of vision. People with AMD are usually taught to test their eyes daily using an Amsler grid so that they will be aware of any changes. AMD occurs less in individuals who exercise, avoid smoking, and consume a diet high in green, leafy vegetables and fruits. In early AMD, adopting some of these habits may help keep vision longer (NEI, 2017e).

The NEI Age-Related Eye Disease Studies (AREDS/AREDS2) found that daily intake of certain high-dose vitamins and minerals can slow progression of the disease in individuals with intermediate AMD and those with late AMD in one eye. Supplementation with these formulations will not help people with early AMD and will not restore vision already lost. Individuals should discuss the supplementation with AREDS formulations with their eye care professional.

Treatment of wet AMD includes photodynamic therapy (PDT), LPC, and anti-VEGF therapy. In 2010 the FDA approved an implantable telescope (IMT) to help individuals 65 years of age and older with vision loss attributable to AMD. The IMT helps individuals with advanced AMD by enlarging objects in the center of the visual field (Duffy, 2017).

Lucentis and Avastin (anti-VEGF therapy) are biological drugs that are the most common form of treatment in neovascular AMD. Abnormally high levels of a specific growth factor occur in eyes with wet AMD, which promote the growth of abnormal blood vessels. Anti-VEGF therapy blocks the effect of the growth factor. These drugs are injected into the eye as often as once a month and can help slow vision loss from AMD and, in some cases, improve sight. PDT with laser treatment is also used to manage AMD (NEI, 2017e).

Charles Bonnet Syndrome

Charles Bonnet syndrome (visual hallucinations) is a common side effect of vision loss in individuals with AMD. Individuals may see simple patterns of colors or shapes, or detailed pictures of people, animals, buildings, or landscapes. Sometimes these images fit logically into a visual scene but often they do not. Nurses are cautioned to understand the syndrome and not attribute symptoms to cognitive impairment or mental illness.

The condition is similar to phantom limb syndrome, a condition in which individuals with a missing limb still feel their fingers or toes or experience itching. Similarly, when the brain loses input from the eye, it may fill the void by generating visual images on its own. The syndrome often goes away a year to 18 months after it begins. Interventions to lessen the symptoms include adequate lighting and encouraging the individual to blink, close the eyes, or focus on a real object for a few moments (NEI, 2017e).

Dry Eye

Dry eye is not a disease of the eye but is a frequent complaint among older adults. Tear production normally diminishes as we age. The condition is termed *keratoconjunctivitis sicca*. It occurs most commonly in women after menopause. There may be age-related changes in the mucin-secreting cells necessary for surface wetting, in the lacrimal glands, or in the meibomian glands that secrete surface oil, and all of these may occur at the same time. The individual will describe a dry, scratchy feeling in mild cases (xerophthalmia). There may be marked discomfort and decreased mucus production in severe situations.

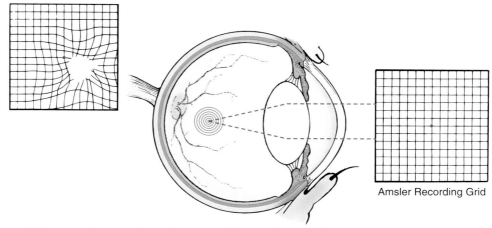

Amsler Recording Grid

Fig. 11.3 Macular Degeneration: Distortion of Center Vision (*left*), Normal Peripheral Vision (*right*).
(Illustration by Harriet R. Greenfield, Newton, MA.)

Medications can cause dry eye, especially anticholinergics, antihistamines, diuretics, beta-blockers, and some hypnotics. Sjögren syndrome is a cell-mediated autoimmune disease whose manifestations include decreased lacrimal gland activity. The problem is diagnosed by an ophthalmologist using a Schirmer tear test, in which filter paper strips are placed under the lower eyelid to measure the rate of tear production. A common treatment is artificial tears or a saline gel, but dry eyes may be sensitive to them because of preservatives, which can be irritating. The ophthalmologist may close the tear duct channel either temporarily or permanently. Other management methods include keeping the house air moist with humidifiers, avoiding wind and hair dryers, and using artificial tear ointments at bedtime. Vitamin A deficiency can be a cause of dry eye, and vitamin A ointments are available for treatment.

PROMOTING HEALTHY AGING: IMPLICATIONS FOR GERONTOLOGICAL NURSES

Assessment

Vision impairment is common among older adults in connection with aging changes and eye diseases and can significantly affect communication, functional ability, safety, and quality of life. To promote healthy aging and quality of life, nurses who care for older adults in all settings can improve outcomes for visually impaired elders by assessing for vision changes, adapting the environment to enhance vision and safety, communicating appropriately, and providing appropriate health teaching and referrals for prevention, treatment, and assistive devices.

Interventions

General principles in caring for persons with visual impairment include the following: use warm incandescent lighting; increase intensity of lighting; control glare by using shades and blinds; suggest yellow or amber lenses to decrease glare; suggest sunglasses that block all ultraviolet light; recommend reading materials that have large, dark, evenly spaced printing; and select colors with good contrast and intensity. Color contrasts are used to facilitate location of items. Sharply contrasting colors

assist the partially sighted. For instance, a bright towel is much easier to locate than a white towel hanging on a beige wall. When choosing color, it is best to use primary colors at the top end of the spectrum rather than those at the bottom. If you think of the colors of the rainbow, it is more likely that people will see reds and oranges better than blues and greens. Fig. 11.4 beautifully illustrates the use of color in a nursing home in Copenhagen, Denmark. Box 11.5 presents Tips for Best Practice in care for elders with visual impairment.

Special Considerations in Long-Term Care Settings

Visual impairment among nursing home residents ranges from 3% to 15% higher than for adults of the same age living in the community (Johnson and Record, 2014). Cognitive and hearing impairments often accompany visual impairment and can severely affect communication, safety, functional status, and quality of life. A 2017 study (Jensen and Tubaek, 2017) reported that cataracts and AMD were the most frequent causes of impaired vision. Information on eye diagnoses was often lacking in medical records and staff were often unaware of vision impairment. Recommendations are that individuals should have an eye examination prior to entering the nursing home and information on needed visual aids that the individual uses (glasses, need for lighting, optical aids) needs to be in the plan of care. Ongoing assessment is important and if function declines, a referral made to an ophthalmologist is indicated. Treatments to improve visual acuity such as cataract removal, if needed, should be accessible. Even in individuals with dementia who have clinically significant cataracts, surgery was found to improve visual acuity, slow the rate of cognitive decline, decrease neuropsychiatric symptoms, and reduce caregiver stress (Cassels, 2014).

Although it may sound like common sense, it is especially important that individuals who wear glasses are wearing them and that the glasses are cleaned regularly. Also important is asking the person or the person's family/significant other if the person routinely wears glasses and if the person is able to see well enough to function. There is limited research on visual impairment in nursing homes and assisted living facilities in

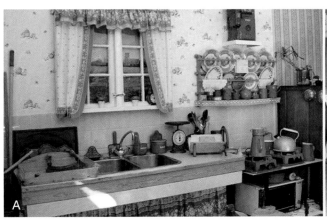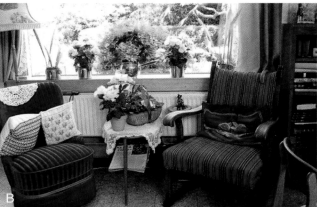

Fig. 11.4 (A) Reminiscence kitchen (Højdevang Sogns Plejejem, Copenhagen, Denmark). (B) Sitting room (Højdevang Sogns Plejejem, Copenhagen, Denmark). (Photos courtesy Christine Williams, PhD, RN.)

BOX 11.5   Tips for Best Practice

Communicating With Older Adults Who Have Visual Impairment

- Assess for vision loss.
- Make sure you have the person's attention before speaking.
- Clearly identify yourself and others with you. State when you are leaving to make sure the person is aware of your departure.
- Position yourself at the person's level when speaking.
- Ensure adequate lighting and eliminate glare.
- When others are present, address the visually impaired person by prefacing remarks with his or her name or a light touch on the arm.
- Select colors for paint, furniture, pictures with rich intensity (e.g., red, orange).
- Use large, dark, evenly spaced printing.
- Use contrast in printed material (e.g., black marker on white paper).
- Use a night light in bathroom and hallways and use illuminated switches.
- Do not change room arrangement or the arrangement of personal items without explanations.

- If in a hospital or nursing home, use some means to identify individuals who are visually impaired and include visual impairment in the plan of care.
- Use the analogy of a clock face to help locate objects (e.g., describe positions of food on a plate in relation to clock positions, such as meat at 3 o'clock, dessert at 6 o'clock).
- Label eyeglasses and have a spare pair if possible; make sure glasses are worn and are clean.
- Be aware of low-vision assistive devices such as talking watches, talking books, and magnifiers, and facilitate access to these resources.
- If the person is blind, ask the person how you can help. If walking, do not try to push or pull. Let the person take your arm just above the elbow, and give directions with details (e.g., the bench is on your immediate right); when seating the person, place his or her hand on the back of the chair.
- Recommend screening for vision loss and annual dilated eye exams for older adults.

spite of the scope of the concern and the need for improved interventions.

Low-Vision Optical Devices

Technology advances in the past decade have produced some low-vision devices that may be used successfully in the care of the visually impaired individual. These devices are grouped into devices for "near" activities (such as reading, sewing, and writing) and devices for "distance" activities (such as attending movies, reading street signs, and identifying numbers on buses and trains). Nurses can refer individuals with low vision or blindness to vision rehabilitation services, which may include assistance with communication skills, counseling, independent living and personal management skills; independent movement and travel skills; training with low-vision devices; and vocational rehabilitation. It is important to be familiar with agencies in your community that offer these services. Persons with severe visual impairment may qualify for disability and financial and social services assistance through government and private programs including vision rehabilitation programs.

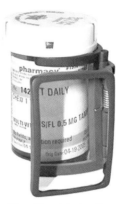

Prescription bottle magnifier. (Reprinted with permission from Carson Optical.)

An array of low-vision assistive devices is now available, including insulin delivery systems, talking clocks and watches, large-print books, magnifiers, telescopes (handheld or mounted on eyeglasses), electronic magnification through closed circuit television or computer software, and software that converts text into artificial voice output. iPods have a setting for audio menus; Microsoft and Apple computer programs allow a person to change color schemes, select a high-contrast display, and magnify and enlarge print. Many websites also have an option for audio text. The e-Reader product from Kindle allows the user to increase font sizes up to 40 points in e-books and offers a Text-to-Speech feature. The iPad from Apple can enlarge text up to 56 points and includes VoiceOver, a feature that reads everything displayed on the screen for you, making it fully usable for people with low to no vision. More and more mobile phones have speech-enabled features, and the Jitterbug phone comes with a live operator whose actions can be directed. As individual needs are unique, it is recommended that before investing in vision aids, the individual consult with a low-vision center or low-vision specialist. Other vision resources are presented in Box 11.2.

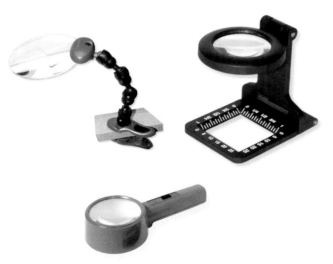

Magnifiers. (Reprinted with permission from Carson Optical.)

KEY CONCEPTS

- Vision loss is a leading cause of age-related disability.
- The leading causes of visual impairment in the United States are diseases that are common in older adults: AMD, cataract, glaucoma, and DR.
- Many causes of visual impairment are preventable, so attention to keeping eyes healthy throughout life and early detection and treatment of eye disease are essential.
- Visual impairment significantly affects quality of life and a person's ability to perform activities of daily living and function independently.

- Nurses who care for visually impaired older adults in all settings can improve outcomes by assessing for vision changes, adapting the environment to enhance vision and safety, communicating appropriately, and providing appropriate health teaching and referrals for prevention, treatment, and assistive devices.

CRITICAL THINKING QUESTIONS AND ACTIVITIES

1. How can nurses enhance awareness and education about vision disorders?
2. Have students attempt to ambulate, read, or take simulated medications while wearing sunglasses with lenses covered in Vaseline or with one lens covered.
3. What is the role of the nurse in the acute care setting/long-term setting in screening and assessment of vision?
4. Develop a teaching plan for an individual with a new diagnosis of glaucoma.
5. What community resources are available in your area for individuals with vision impairment?

RESEARCH QUESTIONS

1. What do people think is helpful in enhancing communication with the visually impaired?
2. What content on visual impairment and nursing interventions is included in curricula of BSN nursing programs?
3. What are the factors influencing the decisions of older adults to seek help for visual problems?
4. Which types of educational programs and outreach activities are most effective in educating older adults about prevention and treatment of eye diseases?
5. Are there differences in the views about visual health in aging among diverse groups of older adults?
6. What is the effect of visual rehabilitation services on performance of activities of daily living (ADLs) and instrumental activities of daily living (IADLs) and quality of life for visually impaired older adults?
7. Formulate a research question related to caring for visually impaired older adults in long-term care settings.

REFERENCES

Cassels C: Cataract surgery may cut cognitive decline in dementia, *Medscape Medical News,* 2014. http://www.medscape.com/viewarticle/828188. Accessed July 2014.

Ciolino JB, Ross AE, Tulsan R, et al: Latanoprost-eluting contact lenses in glaucomatous monkeys, *Opthalmology* 123(10):2085–2092, 2016. http://www.aaojournal.org/article/S0161-6420(16)30506-1/fulltext. Accessed November 2017.

Duffy M: *The implantable miniature telescope (IMT) for end-stage age-related macular degeneration,* 2017. http://www.visionaware.org/info/your-eye-condition/age-related-macular-degeneration-amd/new-fda-approved-implantable-telescope-for-end-stage-amd/125. Accessed November 2017.

Genentech: *Retinal diseases fact sheet,* 2017. https://www.gene.com/stories/retinal-diseases-fact-sheet. Accessed November 2017.

Gupta P, Aravindhan A, Gand ATL, et al: Association between the severity of DR and falls in an Asian population with diabetes: the Singapore epidemiology of eye diseases study, *JAMA Ophthalmol* 135(12):1410–1416, 2017.

Huether S, Rodway G, DeFriez C: Pain, temperature regulation, sleep, and sensory function. In McCance K, Huether S, editors: *Pathophysiology,* ed 7, St Louis, 2014, Elsevier, p 516.

International Federation on Ageing: *The high cost of low vision: the evidence on ageing and the loss of sight,* 2012. https://www.ifa-fiv.org/publication/vision/the-high-cost-of-low-vision-the-evidence-on-ageing-and-the-loss-of-sight/. Accessed December 2017.

Jensen H, Tubæk G: Elderly people need an eye examination before entering nursing homes, *Dan Med J* 64(2), 2017. https://www.ncbi.nlm.nih.gov/pubmed/28157061. Accessed November 2017.

Johnson K, Record S: Visual impairment and eye problems. In Ham R, Sloane R, Warshaw G, et al, editors: *Primary care geriatrics,* ed 6, Philadelphia, 2014, Elsevier Saunders, pp 301–305.

Levin LA, Miller JW, Zack DJ, Friedlander M, Smith LEH: Special commentary: early clinical development of cell replacement therapy: considerations for the National Eye Institute Audacious Goals Initiative, *Ophthalmology* 124(7):926–934, 2017.

MacLennan PA, McGivin G Jr, Heckemeyer C, et al: Eye care use among a high-risk diabetic population seen in a public hospital's clinics, *JAMA Ophthalmol* 132(2):162–167, 2014.

National Eye Institute, National Eye Health Education Program: *Facts about glaucoma,* 2015. https://nei.nih.gov/health/glaucoma/glaucoma_facts. Accessed November 2017a.

National Eye Institute: *Researchers discover three glaucoma-related genes*, 2016. https://nei.nih.gov/news/pressrelease/three_glaucoma_related_genes. Accessed November 2017b.

National Eye Institute: *Facts about diabetic eye disease*. https://nei.nih.gov/health/diabetic/retinopathy. Accessed November 2017c.

National Eye Institute, National Eye Health Education Program: *Facts about retinal detachment*. https://nei.nih.gov/health/retinaldetach. Accessed November 2017d. http://www.nei.nih.gov/health/retinaldetach. Accessed July 2014.

National Eye Institute: *Facts about age-related macular degeneration*. https://nei.nih.gov/health/maculardegen/armd_facts. Accessed December 2017e.

National Eye Institute, National Eye Health Education Program: *Vision and aging: See Well for a Lifetime Toolkit*. https://nei.nih.gov/nehep/programs/visionandaging/toolkit. Accessed November 2017.

Rowan S, Jiang S, Korem T, et al: Involvement of a gut-retina axis in protection against dietary glycemia-induced age-related macular degeneration, *Proc Natl Acad Sci USA* 114(22):E4472–E4481, 2017.

Sussman R: *Understanding glaucoma: epidemiology and pathophysiology*, 2016. https://www.medpagetoday.com/resource-center/Ocular-Health/Understanding-Glaucoma/a/60891. Accessed November 2017.

World Health Organization: *Visual impairment and blindness*, 2017. https://www.who.int/news-room/fact-sheets/detail/blindness-and-visual-impairment. Accessed February 2019.

World Health Organization: Prevention of blindness and visual impairment: *Universal eye health: a global action plan 2014–2019*, 2013. https://www.who.int/blindness/actionplan/en/. Accessed February 2019.

Zhang X, Beckles GL, Chou CF, et al: Socioeconomic disparity in use of eye care services among US adults with age-related eye diseases: National Health Interview Survey, 2002 and 2008, *JAMA Ophthalmol* 131(9):1198–1206, 2013.

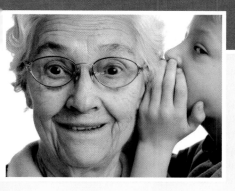

12

Hearing

Theris A. Touhy

http://evolve.elsevier.com/Touhy/TwdHlthAging

A STUDENT SPEAKS

My dad has had a hearing problem for a couple of years and it has driven us all crazy. He won't admit he can't hear. It's always us mumbling or some other excuse. When you go in the house the TV is so loud no one can talk and visit. When I call him on his cell phone, he gets half of what I am saying. His responses are off the wall a lot of the time. I am sure there is something that would help him if he would accept it—it would sure help us!

Sophia, age 21

AN OLDER ADULT SPEAKS

A great annoyance of hearing loss is in the subtle aspects of living with a partner, who most probably has a hearing loss as well. You must often repeat what you say, and in lovemaking, whispering sweet words becomes a gesture for yourself alone.

Bob, age 80

LEARNING OBJECTIVES

On completion of this chapter, the reader will be able to:

1. Discuss changes in hearing with age and describe their impact on quality of life and function.
2. Describe the types of hearing loss and contributing factors.
3. Describe the importance of health education and screening for hearing problems.
4. Identify the components of a focused assessment to evaluate hearing and hearing loss.
5. Identify effective communication strategies for individuals with hearing impairment.
6. Increase awareness of the resources available to assist individuals with hearing loss.
7. Discuss the role of the nurse in assisting individuals to utilize hearing aids and assistive technology to improve hearing.

Although both vision and hearing impairment significantly affect all aspects of life, Oliver Sacks (1989), in his book *Seeing Voices*, presents a view that blindness may in fact be less serious than loss of hearing. Hearing loss interferes with communication with others and the interactional input that is so necessary to stimulate and validate. Helen Keller was most profound in her expression: "Never to see the face of a loved one nor to witness a summer sunset is indeed a handicap. But I can touch a face and feel the warmth of the sun. But to be deprived of hearing the song of the first spring robin and the laughter of children provides me with a long and dreadful sadness" (Keller, 1902).

HEARING IMPAIRMENT

Hearing loss is the third most prevalent chronic condition and the foremost communicative disorder of older adults in the United States. Hearing loss is an underrecognized public health issue. Nearly two-thirds of adults aged 70 years and older have a hearing loss significant enough to impair daily communication. In all age groups, men are more likely than women to be hearing impaired and black Americans have a lower prevalence of hearing impairment than either white or Hispanic Americans (Lin and Whitson, 2017). The *Healthy People 2020* box presents objectives related to hearing impairment and older adults.

Age-related hearing loss (ARHL) is a complex disease caused by interactions between age-related changes (Table 12.1), genetics, lifestyle, and environmental factors. Factors associated with hearing loss include noise exposure, ear infections, smoking, and chronic disease (e.g., diabetes, chronic kidney disease, heart disease) (Bainbridge and Wallhagen, 2014). Hearing loss may not be an inevitable part of aging and increased attention

TABLE 12.1	Changes in Hearing Related to Aging.	
Changes in Structure	**Changes in Function**
Cochlear hair cell degeneration; loss of auditory neurons in spiral ganglia of organ of Corti	Inability to hear high-frequency sounds (presbycusis, sensorineural loss); interferes with understanding speech; hearing may be lost in both ears at different times
Degeneration of basilar (cochlear) conductive membrane of cochlea	Inability to hear at all frequencies, but more pronounced at higher frequencies (cochlear conductive loss)
Decreased vascularity of cochlea; loss of cortical auditory neurons	Equal loss of hearing at all frequencies (strial loss); inability to disseminate localization of sound

From McCance KL, Huether SE: *Pathophysiology*, ed 7, St Louis, 2014, Mosby.

 HEALTHY PEOPLE 2020

Objectives: Hearing—Older Adults

- Increase the proportion of persons with hearing impairment who have ever used a hearing aid or assistive listening device or who have cochlear implants.
- Increase the proportion of adults 70 years of age who have had a hearing examination in the past 5 years.
- Increase the number of persons who are referred by their primary care physician or other health care provider for hearing evaluation and treatment.
- Increase the proportion of adults bothered by tinnitus who have seen a doctor or other health care professional.
- Increase the proportion of persons with hearing loss and other sensory communication disorders who have used Internet resources for health care information, guidance, or advice in the past 12 months.

Data from U.S. Department of Health and Human Services, Office of Disease Prevention and Health Promotion: *Healthy People 2020*, 2012. http://www.healthypeople.gov/2020.

is being given to the links between lifestyle factors (e.g., smoking, poor nutrition, hypertension) and hearing impairment (Box 12.1).

Consequences of Hearing Impairment

The broad consequences of hearing loss have functional and clinical significance and should not be viewed as something a person accepts as part of aging. Hearing loss diminishes quality of life and is associated with multiple negative outcomes, in-

BOX 12.1	Promoting Healthy Hearing
Avoid exposure to excessively loud noises.
Avoid cigarette smoking.
Maintain blood pressure/cholesterol levels within normal limits.
Eat a healthy diet.
Have hearing evaluated if any changes.
Avoid injury with cotton-tipped applicators and other cleaning materials.

cluding decreased function, miscommunication, depression, falls, loss of self-esteem, safety risks, poor cognitive function, and possible increased health service utilization secondary to unmet health care needs (Strawbridge and Wallhagen, 2017; Wallhagen and Strawbridge, 2017). Failures in clinical communication are considered to be the leading cause of medical errors and ARHL has a negative effect on clinical communication across both hospital and primary care clinical settings (Cohen et al, 2017; Cudmore et al, 2017). ARHL has also been linked with late-life cognitive disorders and correcting hearing loss may have a long-term protective effect against cognitive decline (Logroscino and Panza, 2016).

Hearing loss increases feelings of isolation and may cause older adults to become suspicious or distrustful or to display feelings of paranoia. Because older adults with a hearing loss may not understand or respond appropriately to conversation, they may be inappropriately diagnosed with dementia. Older adults who are hospitalized are at risk for adverse outcomes such as being labeled confused, experiencing a loss of control, heightened fear and anxiety, and misunderstanding the plan of care (Funk et al, 2018). All of these consequences of hearing impairment further increase social isolation and decrease opportunities for meaningful interaction and stimulation.

Types of Hearing Loss

The two major forms of hearing loss are *conductive* and *sensorineural*. Sensorineural hearing loss results from damage to any part of the inner ear or the neural pathways to the brain. Presbycusis (also called age-related hearing loss or ARHL) is a form of sensorineural hearing loss that is related to aging and is the most common form of hearing loss. Presbycusis progressively worsens with age and is usually permanent. The cochlea appears to be the site of pathogenesis, but the precise cause of presbycusis is uncertain.

Noise-induced hearing loss (NIHL) is the second most common cause of sensorineural hearing loss among older adults. Direct mechanical injury to the sensory hair cells of the cochlea causes NIHL, and continuous noise exposure contributes to damage more than intermittent exposure (Lewis, 2014). NIHL is permanent but considered largely preventable. The rate of hearing impairment is expected to rise because of the growing number of older adults and also because of the increased number of military personnel who have been exposed to blast exposure in combat situations. NIHL may be reduced through the development of better ear-protection devices, education about exposure to loud noise, and emerging research into interventions that may protect or repair hair cells in the ear, which are key to the body's ability to hear (National Institute on Deafness and Other Communication Disorders [NIDCD], 2017).

Presbycusis is a slow, progressive hearing loss that affects both ears equally. Because of its slow progression, many individuals ignore their hearing loss for years, considering it "just part of aging." Only about 10% to 25% of Americans with hearing loss wear hearing aids, depending on the extent of the loss (Strawbridge and Wallhagen, 2017). It is common to hear older adults deny hearing impairment and accuse others of mumbling. Their spouse or significant other, however, often voices frustration over the hearing loss long before the individual acknowledges it.

One of the first signs of presbycusis is difficulty hearing and understanding speech in noisy environments. A hallmark of presbycusis is difficulty separating the incoming speech signal from background noise (Cohen et al, 2017). Presbycusis begins in the high frequencies and later affects the lower frequencies. High-frequency consonants are important to speech understanding. Changes related to presbycusis make it difficult to distinguish among some of the sibilant consonants such as z, s, sh, f, p, k, t, and g. People often raise their voices when speaking to a hearing-impaired person. When this happens, more consonants drop out of speech, making hearing even more difficult. Without consonants, the high-frequency–pitched language becomes disjointed and misunderstood. Older adults with presbycusis have difficulty filtering out background noise and often complain of difficulty understanding women's and children's speech (higher pitched) and conversations in large groups. Sensorineural hearing loss is treated with hearing aids and, in some cases, cochlear implants.

Conductive Hearing Loss

Conductive hearing loss usually involves abnormalities of the external and middle ear that reduce the ability of sound to be transmitted to the middle ear. Otosclerosis, infection, perforated eardrum, fluid in the middle ear, tumors, or cerumen accumulations cause conductive hearing loss. Cerumen impaction is the most common and easily corrected of all interferences in the hearing of older adults (Fig. 12.1).

Cerumen interferes with the conduction of sound through air in the eardrum. The reduction in the number and activity of cerumen-producing glands results in a tendency toward cerumen impaction. Long-standing impactions become hard, dry, and dark brown. Individuals at particular risk of impaction are African Americans, individuals who wear hearing aids, and older men with large amounts of ear canal tragi (hairs in the ear) that tend to become entangled with the cerumen. One-third to two-thirds of nursing home residents and patients older than 65 years have cerumen impaction. Among individuals with cognitive impairment, the impaction rate is estimated at 28% to 36% (Sun, 2017). It is very important to assess the ears for cerumen impaction in primary care evaluation and among long-term care residents (Schwartz et al, 2017).

When hearing loss is suspected, or a person with existing hearing loss experiences increasing difficulty, it is important first to check for cerumen impaction as a possible cause. After accurate assessment, if cerumen removal is indicated, it may be removed through irrigation, cerumenolytic products, or manual extraction (Schwartz et al, 2017) (Safety Alert box). Box 12.2 presents evidence-based recommendations for managing cerumen impaction.

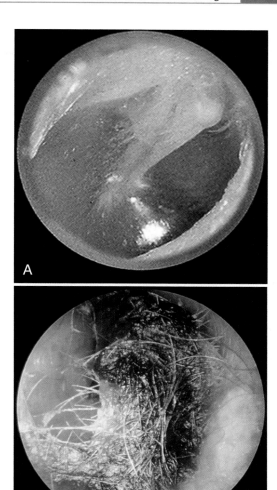

Fig. 12.1 (A) Normal eardrum. (B) Eardrum impacted with cerumen. (A, From Ball JW, Dains JE, Flynn FA, et al: (2015). *Seidel's guide to physical examination*, ed 8, St Louis, 2015, Mosby. B, From Swartz MH: *Textbook of physical diagnosis*, ed 7, Philadelphia, 2014, Saunders.

⚡ SAFETY ALERT

Do not attempt ear lavage or cerumen removal if the person has a history of ear surgery, ruptured tympanic membrane, otitis externa (swimmer's ear), or ear trauma. Use sterilized equipment to avoid infection and spreading bacteria and use caution in patients with diabetes because of an increased risk of infection.

BOX 12.2   Guidelines for Cerumen Impaction Management

- Explain proper ear hygiene to prevent cerumen impaction
- Diagnose cerumen impaction when an accumulation of cerumen that prevents assessment of the ear is seen with an otoscope
- Perform otoscopy to detect the presence of cerumen in patients with hearing aids
- Assess factors that modify management (e.g., anticoagulant therapy, immunocompromised state, diabetes, prior radiation therapy to head/neck, ear canal stenosis, nonintact tympanic membrane)
- Treat or refer to a clinician who can treat the patient with cerumen impaction with an appropriate intervention which may include one or more of the following: cerumenolytic agents, irrigation, or manual removal requiring instrumentation.

From Schwartz S, Magit A, Rosenfeld R: Clinical practice guideline (update): earwax (cerumen impaction), *Otolaryngol Head Neck Surg* 156(1S):S1–S29, 2016.

INTERVENTIONS TO ENHANCE HEARING

Hearing Aids

A hearing aid is a personal amplifying system that includes a microphone, an amplifier, and a loudspeaker. There are numerous types of hearing aids with either analog or digital circuitry. The size, appearance, and effectiveness of hearing aids have greatly improved (decreasing stigma), and many can be programmed to meet specific needs. Digital hearing aids are smaller and have better sound quality and noise reduction, and less acoustic feedback; however, they are expensive. Completely-in-the-canal (CIC) hearing aids fit entirely in the ear canal. These types of devices are among the most expensive and require good dexterity. Some models are invisible and placed deep in the ear canal and replaced every 4 months. New hearing aids can be adjusted precisely for noisy environments and telephone usage through software built into smartphones.

Most individuals can obtain some hearing enhancement with a hearing aid but among adults aged 70 years and older, fewer than one in three have ever used a hearing aid (Kimball et al, 2017). The kind of device chosen depends on the type of hearing impairment and the cost, but most users will experience hearing improvement with a basic to midlevel hearing aid. The investment in a good hearing aid is considerable, and a good fit is critical. Accessibility and affordability of hearing care are massive barriers for those with hearing impairment. The average cost of bilateral hearing aids in the United States is $4700 and requires several visits to a hearing professional's office. The cost of hearing aids is usually not covered by health insurance or Medicare, another barrier to purchase.

The way hearing aids are regulated and sold is also a deterrent to use. The National Academies of Sciences, Engineering, and Medicine (2016) made the following recommendations for hearing health care: (1) include options for more coverage for hearing care under Medicare; (2) eliminate the regulation for medical evaluation prior to hearing aid purchase; (3) create a new regulatory classification for hearing aids that could be sold over the counter for adults with mild to moderate hearing loss (Lin and Whitson, 2017; Warren and Grassley, 2017).

Adjustment to Hearing Aids

Nearly 50% of people who purchased hearing aids either never began wearing them or stopped wearing them after a short period. Factors contributing to low hearing aid use after purchase include difficulty manipulating the device, annoying loud noises, being exposed to sensory overload, developing headaches, and perceiving stigma. Hearing aids amplify all sounds, making things sound different. ARHL is like any other physical impairment and requires counseling, rehabilitative training, patient education, environmental accommodations, and patience. The Internet may be a valuable tool for aural rehabilitation and for improving adjustment to hearing aids and communication (Lewis, 2014). More research about factors that influence the decision to seek help for hearing loss is needed (Wallhagen and Strawbridge, 2017).

It is important for nurses who work with individuals wearing hearing aids to be knowledgeable about their care and maintenance. They can teach the individual, family, or formal caregiver proper use and care of hearing aids. Many older adults experience unnecessary communication problems when in the hospital or nursing home because their hearing aids are not inserted and working properly, need batteries, or because they are lost. Additionally, individuals who wear hearing aids often come to the hospital in emergent situations without their hearing aids or don't bring them because they fear they will be lost or broken (Kimball et al, 2018).

Cochlear Implants

Cochlear implants are increasingly being used for older adults with sensorineural loss who are not able to gain effective speech recognition with hearing aids. Cochlear implants are safe and well tolerated and improve communication. A cochlear implant is a small, complex electronic device that consists of an external portion that sits behind the ear and a second portion that is surgically placed under the skin (Fig. 12.2). Unlike hearing aids that magnify sounds, the cochlear implant bypasses damaged portions of the ear and directly stimulates the auditory nerve. Hearing through a cochlear implant is different from normal hearing and takes time to learn or relearn. Most insurance plans cover the cochlear implant procedure. The transplant carries some risk because the surgery destroys any residual hearing. Therefore, cochlear implant users can never revert to using a hearing aid. Individuals with cochlear implants need to be advised to never have an MRI (magnetic resonance imaging) because it may dislodge the implant or demagnetize its internal magnet.

Assistive Listening and Adaptive Devices

Assistive listening devices (also called personal listening systems) should be considered as an adjunct to hearing aids or used in place of hearing aids for people with hearing impairment. These devices are available commercially and can be used to enhance face-to-face communication and to better understand speech in large rooms such as theaters, to use the telephone, and to listen to television. Many movie theaters have both sound amplifiers and personal subtitle devices available. Hearing loop conduction systems are newer technology and consist of a copper wire that is installed around the periphery of a room or other venue to transmit the microphone or TV sound signal to hearing aids and cochlear implants that have "telecoil" receivers (built into most hearing aids and cochlear implants). Sound from the microphone or TV is received but not background noises. This transforms the hearing aid into loudspeakers delivering sound for one's own hearing loss. These devices are widely used in Europe and becoming more available in the United States in places such as theaters, churches, subway information booths, taxi back seats, and home TV rooms.

Other examples of assistive listening and adaptive devices include text messaging devices for telephones and closed-caption television, now required on all televisions with screens 13 inches and larger. Alerting devices, such as vibrating alarm clocks that shake the bed or activate a flashing light, and sound lamps that respond with lights to sounds, such as doorbells and telephones, are also available. Special service dogs ("hearing dogs") are trained to alert people with a hearing impairment about sounds and intruders. Dogs are trained to respond to different sounds, such as the telephone, smoke alarms, alarm clock, doorbell/door knock, and name call, and lead the individual to the sound.

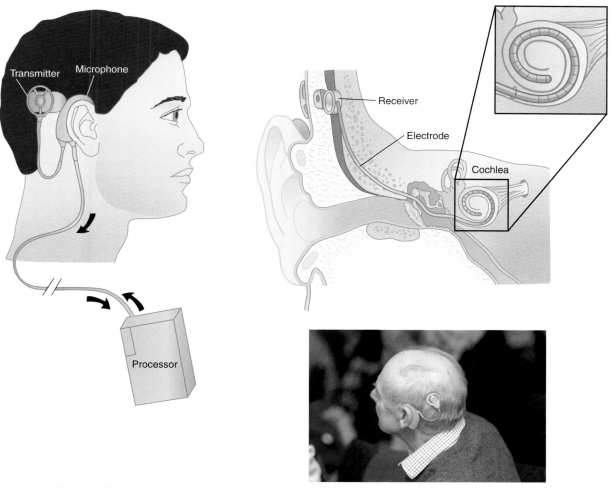

Fig. 12.2 Cochlear Implant. (Photo courtesy of the patient. Available at http://ais.southampton.ac.uk/
new-programme-launched-help-cochlear-implant-users-enjoy-music/.)

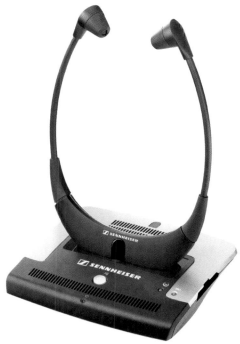

Voice-clarifying headset system for TV listening. (With permission from
TV Ears, Inc.)

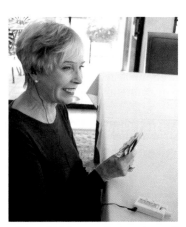

Pocket-sized amplifier. (With permission from Sonic Technology
Products, Inc.)

The use of computers and email also assists individuals with
hearing impairment to communicate more easily. Programs
such as Skype and FaceTime are also beneficial because they
may allow the person to lip read and to adjust volume. Pocket-
sized amplifiers (available at retail stores) are especially helpful
in improving communication in health care settings, and nurses

in a clinical setting should be able to obtain appropriate devices for use with hearing-impaired individuals. A recent study reported that these devices are safe and easy to use in inpatient settings and both patients and nurses were very satisfied with their use (Kimball et al, 2018).

PROMOTING HEALTHY AGING: IMPLICATIONS FOR GERONTOLOGICAL NURSING

Assessment

Hearing impairment is underdiagnosed and undertreated in older adults. There is a low rate of hearing screening in primary care in spite of the high prevalence of hearing loss among older adults. Older adults may be initially unaware of hearing loss because of the gradual manner in which it develops and, therefore, may not report any problems. Screening for hearing impairment and appropriate treatment are essential parts of primary care for older adults (Wallhagen and Strawbridge, 2017). In hospitals and long-term care facilities, bedside screening for hearing impairment is important.

Nurses should note any nonverbal signs of a hearing deficit (e.g., cupping the ear, turning the head to one side when asked questions, or misunderstanding questions). Ask the individual directly if he or she has a hearing impairment. Since many individuals are unaware of or deny hearing impairment, the screening should include a short discussion rather than yes-or-no questions. A suggested question is: "Can you tell me about any problems you have with hearing or misunderstanding questions?" It is important to identify barriers to hearing such as background noise, unfamiliar accents, and call system speakers. The individual should also be asked his or her preferred method for enhancing hearing such as writing or using personal sound amplifiers. All of this information needs to be incorporated into the plan of care (Funk et al, 2018).

Assessment of hearing includes a focused history and physical examination and screening assessment for hearing impairment. Ask the individual if he or she has any difficulty understanding speech in noisy situations, during telephone use, or in daily conversation. Obtaining information from the significant other about hearing problems can also be useful. Self-assessment instruments (Box 12.3) and the Hearing

BOX 12.4 Resources for Best Practice
Hearing Impairment

- **American Tinnitus Association:** Listen to the sounds of tinnitus; patient and professional information
- **Experience hearing loss:** Unfair hearing test: https://www.youtube.com/watch?v=9vqY7cJpwRs
- **Hartford Institute for Geriatric Nursing:** Hearing Handicap Inventory for the Elderly: Screening Version (HHIE-S). https://consultgeri.org/try-this/general-assessment/issue-12.
- **National Institute on Deafness and Other Communication Disorders (NIDCD):** https://www.nidcd.nih.gov/health/hearing-ear-infections-deafness: Hearing loss and older adults patient information; Interactive hearing test; "It's a noisy planet: protect their hearing"; resources for health professionals.
- **National Institute Health (NIH):** Senior Health: Hearing Loss (patient information)

Handicap Inventory for the Elderly Screening Version (HHIT-S) can also be included (Box 12.4). Question the person about prolonged noise exposure, past ear injuries, and use of potentially ototoxic medications.

Physical examination includes assessing the external ear to determine any evidence of infection and using an otoscope to visualize the inner ear, looking for any possible causes of conductive hearing loss, such as cerumen impaction or foreign objects. Inspect the tympanic membrane (TM) for integrity. Depending on findings, the patient may need to be referred for follow up by a specialist. Results of a recent study reported that the finger rub test showed high sensitivity and requires little time and no special equipment, making it an effective screening tool in primary care (Srawbridge and Wallhagen, 2017).

Interventions

Nursing actions are based on assessment findings and may include referral to an audiologist, education on hearing loss (including prevention and consequences), hearing aids, assistive listening devices, and communication techniques. If cerumen impaction is found, cerumen removal may be indicated (Box 12.2). Providing education to individuals and family members about hearing loss, how it affects one's communication, why it is important to address hearing loss early in the process,

BOX 12.3 Do I Have a Hearing Problem?

- Do I have a problem hearing on the telephone?
- Do I have trouble hearing when there is noise in the background?
- Is it hard for me to follow a conversation when two or more people talk at once?
- Do I have to strain to understand a conversation?
- Do many people I talk to seem to mumble (or not speak clearly)?
- Do I misunderstand what others are saying and respond inappropriately?
- Do I have trouble understanding the speech of women and children?
- Do people complain that I turn the TV volume up too high?
- Do I hear a ringing, roaring, or hissing sound a lot?
- Do some sounds seem too loud?

From National Institute on Deafness and Other Communication Disorders: *Hearing loss and older adults,* 2014. http://www.nidcd.nih.gov/health/hearing/pages/older.aspx#2. Accessed October 31, 2014.

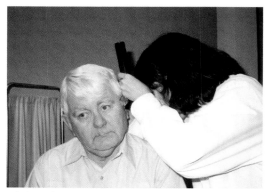

Proper technique for an otoscopic examination. (From Ignatavicius DD, Workman ML: *Medical-surgical nursing: patient-centered collaborative care,* ed 6, St Louis, 2014, Saunders.)

BOX 12.5   Tips for Best Practice

Communication With Individuals With Hearing Impairment

- Never assume hearing loss is from age until other causes are ruled out (infection, cerumen buildup).
- Inappropriate responses, inattentiveness, and apathy may be symptoms of a hearing loss.
- Face the individual, and stand or sit on the same level; do not turn away while speaking (e.g., face a computer).
- Gain the individual's attention before beginning to speak. Look directly at the person at eye level before starting to speak.
- Determine if hearing is better in one ear than another, and position yourself appropriately.
- If hearing aid is used, make sure it is in place and batteries are functioning.
- Ask patient or family what helps the person to hear best.
- Keep hands away from your mouth and project voice by controlled diaphragmatic breathing.
- Avoid conversations in which the speaker's face is in glare or darkness; orient the light on the speaker's face.
- Lower your tone of voice, articulate clearly, and use a moderate rate of speech.
- If the person is in a hospital or nursing facility, label the chart, note on the intercom button, and inform all caregivers that the patient has a hearing impairment.
- Use nonverbal approaches: gestures, demonstrations, visual aids, and written materials.
- Pause between sentences or phrases to confirm understanding.
- When changing topics, preface the change by stating the topic.
- Reduce background noise (e.g., turn off television, close door).
- Utilize assistive listening devices such as pocket talker.
- Verify that the information being given has been clearly understood. Be aware that the person may agree to everything and appear to understand what you have said even when he or she did not hear you (listener bluffing).
- Share resources for the hearing-impaired and refer as appropriate.

From Adams-Wendling L, Pimple C: Evidence-based guideline: nursing management of hearing impairment in nursing facility residents, *J Gerontol Nurs* 34(11):9–16, 2008.

what hearing aids can and cannot do, and alternatives to the use of hearing aids is important and may enhance the effective use of hearing health care services (Wallhagen and Srawbridge, 2017). Recommendations offered by participants in a qualitative study on the hospital experience of older adults with hearing impairment included the following: staff being more patient, using paper and pencil to convey information, repeating things more than once, and sharing information about patients' hearing deficits at shift handoffs so patients don't have to keep reminding staff (Funk et al, 2018). There are many evidence-based resources available that can be used to educate the patient and family and assist the nurse in designing educational materials (Box 12.4). Using the information presented in this chapter, nurses can play an important role in providing older adults the information they need to improve their hearing and avoid the negative consequences of untreated hearing loss. Effective communication strategies when working with individuals who are hearing-impaired are presented in Box 12.5.

TINNITUS

Tinnitus is defined as the perception of sound in one or both ears or in the head when no external sound is present. It is often referred to as "ringing in the ears" but may also manifest as buzzing, hissing, whistling, cricket chirping, bells, roaring, clicking, pulsating, humming, or swishing sounds. The sounds may be constant or intermittent and are more acute at night or in quiet surroundings. The most common type is high-pitched tinnitus with sensorineural loss; less common is low-pitched tinnitus with conduction loss such as is seen in Ménière disease. Tinnitus affects about one in five people. Tinnitus is the number one service-related disability for U.S. veterans military personnel and is the leading cause of service-connected disability of veterans returning from Iraq or Afghanistan (American Tinnitus Association, 2017).

The exact physiological cause or causes of tinnitus are not known, but there are several likely factors that are known to trigger or worsen tinnitus. Exposure to loud noises is the leading cause of tinnitus, and the exposure can damage and destroy cilia in the inner ear. Once damaged, the cilia cannot be renewed or replaced. Other possible causes of tinnitus include head and neck trauma, certain types of tumors, cerumen accumulation, jaw misalignment, cardiovascular disease, and ototoxicity from medications. More than 200 prescription and nonprescription medications list tinnitus as a potential side effect, aspirin being the most common. There is some evidence that caffeine, alcohol, cigarettes, stress, and fatigue may exacerbate the problem.

Interventions

Some persons with tinnitus will never find the cause; for others the problem may arbitrarily disappear. Hearing aids can be prescribed to amplify environmental sounds to obscure tinnitus, and there is a device that combines the features of a masker and a hearing aid, which emits a competitive but pleasant sound that distracts from head noise. Therapeutic modes of treating tinnitus include transtympanal electrostimulation, iontophoresis, biofeedback, tinnitus masking with alternative sound production (white noise), cochlear implants, and hearing aids. Some have found hypnosis, cognitive behavioral therapy, acupuncture, and chiropractic, naturopathic, allergy, or drug treatment to be effective.

Nursing actions include discussions with the client regarding times when the noises are most irritating and having the person keep a diary to identify patterns. Assess medications for possibly contributing to the problem. Discuss lifestyle changes and alternative methods that some have found effective. Also, refer clients to the American Tinnitus Association for research updates, education, and support groups (Box 12.4).

KEY CONCEPTS

- Hearing impairment is the third most prevalent chronic condition among older Americans and the foremost communicative disorder.
- Age-related hearing loss (AHRL) is a complex disease caused by interactions among age-related changes, genetics, lifestyle, and environment.
- The two major forms of hearing loss are conductive and sensorineural.
- Presbycusis (also called age-related hearing loss or ARHL) is a form of sensorineural hearing loss that is related to aging and is the most common form of hearing loss.
- Hearing aids and cochlear implants are used to improve hearing, and both require a period of adjustment and education.

- Hearing loss diminishes quality of life and is associated with multiple negative outcomes including decreased function, increased likelihood of hospitalizations, miscommunication, medical errors, depression, falls, loss of self-esteem, safety risks, and cognitive decline.
- Screening for hearing loss is an essential component of assessment in older adults.
- Nurses need to provide education about hearing health, care of hearing aids, and assistive listening devices to enhance communication.

NURSING STUDY: HEARING IMPAIRMENT

Sonya is a 66-year-old high school nurse/consultant. She retired from the Army Nurse Corps with an officer's rank after serving 20 years, much of it in the Korean conflict with heavy exposure to shelling in the early part of her career. She became aware of hearing loss at about age 45, and by age 55 it had become severe. While in the service she had considerable assistance from noncommissioned personnel and functioned well. When she entered civilian life, it became more difficult for her to manage but she was unwilling to admit to others her major hearing deficit. During those years she simply attempted to cover it as much as possible, and some of her coworkers thought she was rather obtuse; others suspected her deafness. When she took the position with the school district, she was involved with three high schools, numerous faculty members, and students, and interpersonal communication was a major aspect of her position. When she was evaluated at the end of the first year, it was pointed out that feedback indicated she was inattentive. She did then admit her hearing problem and was advised to get a hearing aid. She said, "I've known several people over the years who have hearing aids, and none of them were really satisfied with them. I guess that is why I have not gotten them before now." She complied but, after a few weeks, rarely wore her hearing aids. The personnel officer of the school board, after hearing several more complaints of inappropriate communication, told her she must wear the hearing aids if she wished to continue in her position. Sonya knew that hearing aids were essential, not only for communication but also for safety—she had almost been hit by a car while walking because she simply did not hear it coming. Yet she did not want to go back to

the audiology clinic, because they did not seem to know what they were doing, and each time she saw someone, the person gave her different information. She tried three different types of aids that seemed of little help. She lost confidence in her ear, nose, and throat specialist because he had been unable to help her resolve the ringing in her ears. Now her school district had contracted with a health maintenance organization, and she was not even sure which health care provider she should see.

On the basis of the nursing study, develop a nursing care plan using the following procedure[a]:

- List Sonya's comments that provide subjective data.
- List information that provides objective data.
- From these data identify and state, using accepted format, two nursing diagnoses you determine are most significant to Sonya at this time. List two of Sonya's strengths that you have identified from data.
- Determine and state outcome criteria for each diagnosis. These must reflect some alleviation of the problem identified in the nursing diagnosis and must be stated in concrete and measurable terms.
- Plan and state one or more interventions for each diagnosed problem. Provide specific documentation of the source used to determine the appropriate intervention. Plan at least one intervention that incorporates Sonya's existing strengths.
- Evaluate the success of the intervention. Interventions must correlate directly with the stated outcome criteria to measure the outcome success.

[a]Students are advised to refer to their nursing diagnosis text and identify possible or potential problems.

CRITICAL THINKING QUESTIONS AND ACTIVITIES

1. What are some of the possible reasons Sonya suffered severe hearing loss at so young an age?
2. Discuss the stigma of hearing loss and hearing aids.
3. Obtain a "hearing aid loaner." Instruct students to wear it for several hours and report their reactions in writing. List difficulties experienced.
4. How would you advise Sonya if you were her nurse/friend?
5. Discuss the various kinds of hearing aids and explain how they differ.
6. Discuss reasons Sonya may have discontinued wearing her hearing aids.
7. What might you suggest that would be helpful in adapting to wearing a hearing aid?
8. Which of the various sensory/perceptual changes of aging would you find most difficult to handle?
9. Discuss the meanings and the thoughts triggered by the student's and older adult's viewpoints expressed at the beginning of the chapter. How do these vary from your own experience?

RESEARCH QUESTIONS

1. What do older adults think is helpful in enhancing communication with individuals experiencing hearing impairment?
2. What strategies are most effective in facilitating adaptation to hearing aids?
3. What are the challenges for older adults and their families/significant others in living with hearing loss?

4. What is the knowledge level of professional nurses related to hearing impairment and communication strategies to enhance communication?
5. What is the relationship between stigma and denial of hearing loss and wearing hearing aids?

REFERENCES

American Tinnitus Association: *Understanding the facts:* Tinnitus. https://www.ata.org/understanding-facts. Accessed December 2017.

Bainbridge KE, Wallhagen MI: Hearing loss in an aging American population: extent, impact, and management, *Annu Rev Public Health* 35:139–152, 2014.

Cohen JM, Blustein J, Weinstein BE, et al: Studies of physician-patient communication with older patients: how often is hearing loss considered? A systematic literature review, *J Am Geriatr Soc* 65:1642–1648, 2017.

Cudmore V, Henn P, O'Tuathaigh CMP, Smith S: Age-related hearing loss and communication breakdown in the clinical setting, *JAMA Otolaryngol Head Neck Surg* 143(10):105–1055, 2017.

Funk A, Garcia C, Mullen T: Original research: understanding the hospital experience of older adults with hearing impairment, *Am J Nurs* 118(6):28–34, 2018.

Keller H: *The story of my life,* Garden City, NY, 1902, Doubleday.

Kimball AR, Roscigno CI, Jenerette CM, Hughart KM, Jenkins WW, Hsu W: Amplified hearing device use in acute care settings for patients with hearing loss: a feasibility study, *Geriatr Nurs* 39: 279–284, 2018.

Lewis T: Hearing impairment. In Ham R, Sloane P, Warshaw G, et al, editors: *Primary Care Geriatrics,* ed 6, Philadelphia, 2014, Elsevier Saunders, pp 291–300.

Lin FR, Whitson HE: The common sense of considering the senses in patient communication, *J Am Geriatr Soc* 65:1659–1660, 2017.

Logroscino G, Panza F: The role of hearing impairment in cognitive decline: need for the special sense assessment in evaluating cognition in older age, *Neuroepidemiology* 6(46):290–291, 2016.

National Academies of Sciences, Engineering, and Medicine: *Hearing health care for adults: priorities for improving access and affordability,* Washington, DC, 2016, The National Academies Press.

National Institute on Deafness and Other Communication Disorders (NIDCD): *Hearing, ear infections, and deafness.* https://www.nidcd.nih.gov/health/hearing-ear-infections-deafness. Accessed December 2017.

Sacks O: *Seeing voices: a journey into the world of the deaf,* Berkeley, 1989, University of California Press.

Schwartz S, Magit A, Rosenfeld R, et al: Clinical practice guideline (update): earwax (cerumen impaction), *Otolaryngol Head Neck Surg* 156(1S):S1–S29, 2017.

Strawbridge WJ, Wallhagen MI: Simple tests compare well with a hand-held audiometer for hearing loss screening in primary care, *J Am Geriatr Soc* 65:2282–2284, 2017.

Sun G: Dealing with cerumen impaction, *Medscape Nurses,* 2017. https://www.medscape.com/viewarticle/875560_print. Accessed December 2017.

Wallhagen M, Strawbridge W: Hearing loss education for older adults in primary care clinics: benefits of a concise educational brochure, *Geriatr Nurs* 38(6):527–530, 2017.

Warren E, Grassley C: Over-the-counter hearing aids: the path forward, *JAMA Intern Med* 177(5):609–610, 2017.

13

Skin Care

Theris A. Touhy

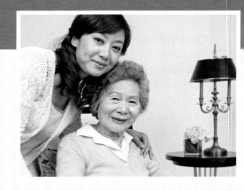

http://evolve.elsevier.com/Touhy/TwdHlthAging

A GRANDCHILD SPEAKS

An older woman and her little grandson, whose face was sprinkled with bright freckles, spent the day at the zoo. Lots of children were waiting in line to get their cheeks painted by a local artist who was decorating them with tiger paws.
"You've got so many freckles, there's no place to paint!" a girl in the line said to the little fellow.
Embarrassed, the little boy dropped his head. His grandmother knelt down next to him.
"I love your freckles. When I was a little girl I always wanted freckles," she said, while tracing her finger across the child's cheek. "Freckles are beautiful."
The boy looked up, "Really?"
"Of course," said the grandmother. "Why just name me one thing that's prettier than freckles?"
The little boy thought for a moment, peered intensely into his grandma's face, and softly whispered, "Wrinkles."

A STUDENT SPEAKS

My mother is always on to me to take care of my skin so that it will look good when I am older. Stay out of the tanning salon and the sun, wear sunscreen all the time, use moisturizer. It's hard to think that 50 years from now I might not have this beautiful skin anymore unless I take better care of it now. Mom keeps pointing to a magnet on her refrigerator: "Wrinkled was not one of the things I wanted to be when I was older."

Janine, age 19

AN OLDER ADULT SPEAKS

I have that white Irish skin and have really had a lot of problems ever since I was 40 with precancerous lesions and even a basal cell skin cancer or two. Of course, we didn't know about sunscreen when I was growing up and I remember lathering myself with baby oil and iodine to get a good tan (or a bad burn). I am pretty obsessive about going to the dermatologist every 3 months and staying out of the sun. A year ago she saw an area on my back that looked suspicious, so a biopsy was done. Turned out it was a melanoma and was removed by a plastic surgeon, who told me that I was lucky it was found or I would have been dead in
6 months. The area was not unusual looking at all—no change, no irritation, no irregular borders, no elevation—looked like nothing. Best advice I can give is to make the skin checks regular. It may save your life.

Bob, age 70

LEARNING OBJECTIVES

On completion of this chapter, the reader will be able to:
1. Identify age-related changes in the integument.
2. Identify skin problems commonly found in later life.
3. Identify preventive, maintenance, and restorative measures for skin health.
4. Identify risk factors for pressure injuries and design evidence-based interventions for prevention and treatment.

Gerontological nurses have an instrumental role in promoting the health of the skin of the persons who seek their care. The skin may often be overlooked when the focus is on management of disease or acute problems. However, skin problems can be challenging concerns, affecting health and compromising quality of life. Thorough assessment and intervention based on age-related evidence-based protocols is important to healthy aging and best practice gerontological nursing.

SKIN

The skin is the largest organ of the body and has at least seven physiological functions (Box 13.1). Exposure to heat, cold, water, trauma, friction, and pressure notwithstanding, the skin's function is to maintain a homeostatic environment. Healthy skin is durable, pliable, and strong enough to protect the body by absorbing, reflecting, cushioning, and restricting various substances and forces that might enter and alter its function, yet it is sensitive enough to relay subtle messages to the brain. When the integument malfunctions or is overwhelmed, discomfort, disfigurement, or death may ensue. However, the nurse can both promptly recognize and help to prevent many of the sources of danger to a person's skin in the promotion of the best possible health.

Many age-related changes in the skin are visible; similar changes in other organs of the body are not as readily observed. Although there are some changes related to the aging process, genetics and environmental factors (ultraviolet [UV] radiation, tobacco smoke, inflammatory responses, and gravity) contribute to these changes (McCance and Huether, 2014). Many skin problems are seen with aging, both in health and when compromised by illness or mobility limitations. Even though many worry about wrinkles and gray hair, the most common skin problems of aging are xerosis (dry skin), pruritus, seborrheic keratosis, herpes zoster (HZ), and cancer. Those who are immobilized or medically fragile are at risk for fungal infections and pressure injuries (PIs), both major threats to wellness. Table 13.1 provides an overview of skin changes related to aging.

BOX 13.1 Physiological Functions of the Skin

- Protects underlying structures
- Regulates body temperature
- Serves as a vehicle for sensation
- Stores fat
- Is a component of the metabolism of salt and water
- Is a site for two-way gas exchange
- Is a site for the production of vitamin D when exposed to sunlight

TABLE 13.1 Changes in the Integument Related to Aging.

CHANGES	EFFECTS
Skin	
Epidermis	
Melanocytes decrease	Lightening of overall skin tone; decreased protection against ultraviolet radiation
Keratinocytes smaller; regeneration slower	Slowed wound healing
Noncancerous pigmented spots (freckles, nevi) enlarge	Mostly cosmetic
Increased lentigine ("age" or "liver" spots) and seborrheic keratosis common	Mostly cosmetic (Fig. 13.2)
Dermatosis papulosa nigra, variant of keratosis in dark skin, increases	Clinically insignificant (Fig. 13.2)
Dermis	
20% loss of thickness	Skin more transparent and fragile; skin tears/bruising occur easily
Dermal blood vessels decrease	Skin pallor and cooler skin temperature; increased susceptibility to skin cancer; diminished dermal clearance, absorption, and immunological response
Cross-linking increases; collagen synthesis decreases	Skin "gives less" under stress and tears easily
Elastin fibers thicken and fragment	Loss of stretch and elasticity; "sagging" appearance
Decreased sebum production	Skin becomes drier; risk for cracking and xerosis increases
Hypodermis	
Shifting of subcutaneous fat; loss of subcutaneous tissue	Skinfolds on the back of the hand diminish even with substantial weight gain; more risk for injury as cushioning decreases; wrinkling and sagging of skin
Reduced efficiency of eccrine glands	Temperature regulation compromised; risk for hyperthermia and hypothermia; moisture evaporates quickly; skin is drier
Fewer Meissner's/Pacinian corpuscles	Diminished tactile sensitivity; increased susceptibility to injury
Decreased Langerhans cells	Reduces skin's immune response
Hair	
Diminished melanocytes; loss of hair follicles	50% of population have gray or partly gray hair
Other changes	Men experience hair loss in vertex, frontal, and temporal areas; by 60 years, 80% of men are substantially bald; less pronounced in women. Race, gender, sex-linked genes, and hormonal balance influence maximum amount hair one has and the changes that occur throughout life

TABLE 13.1 Changes in the Integument Related to Aging.—cont'd

CHANGES	EFFECTS
	Terminal hair can occur in face and chin area in women after menopause
	Amount of hair increases in ears, nose, eyebrows; axillary, extremity, and pubic hair diminishes or disappears
Nails	
Decreased circulation	Fingernails and toenails thicken and change in shape and color
	Nails become brittle, flat, or concave rather than convex; longitudinal striations; may appear yellow or grayish with poorly defined or absent lunulae; cuticle becomes thick and wide
	Onychogryphosis (thickening and distortion of nail plate) and fungal infection (onycholysis) common but not part of normal aging

COMMON SKIN PROBLEMS

Xerosis

Xerosis is extremely dry, cracked, and itchy skin. Xerosis is the most common skin problem experienced and may be linked to a dramatic age-associated decrease in the amount of epidermal filaggrin, a protein required for binding keratin filaments into macrofibrils. This leads to separation of dermal and epidermal surfaces, which compromises the nutrient transfer between the two layers of the skin. Xerosis occurs primarily in the extremities, especially the legs, but can also affect the face and the trunk. The thinner epidermis of older skin makes it less efficient, allowing more moisture to escape. Inadequate fluid intake worsens xerosis as the body will pull moisture from the skin in an attempt to combat systemic dehydration. Box 13.2 presents Tips for Best Practice in prevention and treatment of xerosis.

Pruritus

One of the consequences of xerosis is *pruritus*, that is, itchy skin. It is a symptom, not a diagnosis or disease, and is a threat to skin integrity because of the attempts to relieve it by scratching. It is aggravated by perfumed detergents, fabric softeners, heat, sudden temperature changes, pressure, vibration, electrical stimuli, sweating, restrictive clothing, fatigue, exercise, and anxiety. Medication side effects are another common cause of pruritus. Pruritus also may accompany systemic disorders such as chronic renal failure and biliary or hepatic disease. Subacute to chronic generalized pruritus that awakens the individual is an indication to look for secondary causes (especially lymphoma or hematological conditions) (Endo and Norman, 2014).

The gerontological nurse should always listen carefully to the patient's ideas of why the pruritus is occurring, and the patient's description of aggravating and relieving factors. If rehydration of the stratum corneum (outer layer of the skin) and other measures to prevent and treat xerosis are not sufficient to control itching, cool compresses or oatmeal or Epsom salt baths may be helpful. Failure to control the itching increases the risk for eczema, excoriations, cracks in the skin, inflammation, and infection arising from the usually linear excoriations resulting from scratching. The nurse should be alert to signs of infection.

Scabies

Scabies is a skin condition that causes intense itching, particularly at night. Scabies is caused by a tiny burrowing mite called *Sarcoptes scabiei.* Scabies is contagious and can be passed easily by an infested person to his or her household members, caregivers, or sexual partners. Scabies can spread easily through close physical contact in a family, childcare group, or school class. Scabies outbreaks have occurred among patients, visitors, and staff in institutions such as nursing homes and hospitals. These types of outbreaks are frequently the result of delayed diagnosis and treatment of crusted (Norwegian) scabies. Some immunocompromised, disabled, or debilitated persons are at risk for this form of scabies.

Individuals with crusted scabies have thick crusts of skin that contain large numbers of scabies mites and eggs. In addition to spreading through skin-to-skin contact, crusted scabies can transmit indirectly through contamination of clothing, linen, and furniture. Because the characteristic itching and rash of scabies can be absent in crusted scabies, there may be misdiagnosis and delayed or inadequate treatment and continued transmission. To diagnose scabies, a close skin examination is conducted to look for signs of mites, including their characteristic burrows. A scraping may be taken from an area of skin for microscopic examination to determine the presence of mites or their eggs.

BOX 13.2 Tips for Best Practice

Prevention and Treatment of Xerosis

Assessment
- Evaluate for dehydration, nutritional deficiencies, systemic diseases (diabetes mellitus, hypothyroidism, renal disease), and open lesions
- Determine precipitating and alleviating factors
- Evaluate current treatment and effectiveness

Interventions
- Maintain environment of 60% humidity
- Promote adequate fluid intake; skin can only be rehydrated with water
- Creams, lubricants, emollients should be applied to towel-patted dry, damp skin immediately after a bath; water-laden emulsions without perfumes or alcohol should be used
- Mineral oil or Vaseline is effective and more economical than commercial lotions and oils
- Use only tepid water for bathing; avoid long-duration baths; daily baths and showers may not be needed; advise sponge bathing
- Use super-fatted soaps or skin cleansers (Cetaphil, Dove, Caress soaps; Neutrogena and Oil of Olay bath washes); avoid deodorant soaps except in places such as axilla and groin
- In cases of extreme dryness, petroleum jelly can be applied to affected area before bed (can use cotton gloves and socks to cover hands/feet)

Scabies treatment involves eliminating the infestation with prescribed lotions and creams. Two or more applications, about a week apart, may be necessary, especially for crusted scabies. Treatment is usually provided to family members and other close contacts even if they show no signs of scabies infestation. Medication kills the mites, but itching may not stop for several weeks. Oral medications may be prescribed for individuals with altered immune systems, for those with crusted scabies, or for those who do not respond to prescription lotions and creams. All clothes and linen used at least three times before treatment should be washed in hot, soapy water and dried with high heat. Rooms used by the person with crusted scabies should be thoroughly cleaned and vacuumed (Centers for Disease Control and Prevention [CDC], 2017).

Purpura

Thinning of the dermis leads to increased fragility of the dermal capillaries and to easy rupture of blood vessels with minimal trauma. Extravasation of the blood into the surrounding tissue, commonly seen on the dorsal forearm and hands, is called *purpura*. Most cases are not related to a pathological condition. The incidence of purpura increases with age due to the normal changes in the skin. Persons who take blood thinners are especially prone to easily acquiring purpura. For those who find that they are prone to purpura, it is advisable to use protective garments—such as long-sleeved pants and shirts. Health care personnel must be advised to be gentle while providing care to persons with sensitive or easily traumatized skin.

Skin Tears

Skin tears (STs) are painful, acute, accidental wounds, perhaps more prevalent than PIs, and are largely preventable. Although STs are frequently caused by trauma, they are slow to heal and may become chronic wounds. If not managed properly, they can be susceptible to secondary wound infections. STs occur in individuals in all settings from long-term care to active individuals in the community but older adults are at highest risk. Physiological changes in the skin such as dermal and subcutaneous tissue loss and xerosis contribute to risk factors for STs in older adults. Older adults who are dependent on others for total care are at greatest risk for STs and independent ambulatory older adults are at second highest risk. The top causes of STs include equipment injury, patient transfers, falls, activities of daily living, and treatment and dressing removal. The literature pertaining to the prevalence and incidence of STs and risk factors is very limited. STs should be classified using the Adapted Payne-Martin Skin Tear Classification Tool 2 (Box 13.3) (LeBlanc et al, 2016).

Management of STs includes proper assessment of ST category, control of bleeding, cleansing with nontoxic solutions (normal saline or nonionic surfactant cleaners), use of appropriate dressings that provide moist wound healing, protection of periwound skin, management of exudate, prevention of infection, implementation of prevention protocols, and education. Skin flaps, if present, should not be removed but instead rolled back over the open, cleaned area. Steri-Strips can be very useful; suturing is not recommended (Cheung, 2017; LeBlanc et al, 2016).

BOX 13.3 Adapted Payne-Martin Skin Tear Classification Tool 2

- **Category 1A:** Linear type skin tear, epidermis and dermis pulled apart, without tissue loss
- **Category 1B:** Epidermal flap completely covers the dermis within 1 mm of the wound margin
- **Category 11A:** Scant tissue loss type (less than 25%) of the epidermal flap lost
- **Category 11B:** Greater than 25% of the epidermal flap lost
- **Category 111:** Epidermal flap absent

From Payne R, Martin M. The epidemiology and management of skin tears in older adults. *Ostomy Wound Manage* 26(1):26-37, 1990.

Prevention of STs is very important and needs attention by nurses in all settings. Bundled approaches to care need to include pressure injury (PI) prevention and fall prevention interventions, and bundled approaches for PIs and falls need to include ST prevention (LeBlanc and Baranoski, 2017). A Skin Tear Tool Kit (LeBlanc and Baranoski, 2013), dressing recommendations, and comprehensive information on assessment and prevention can be found on the International Skin Tear Advisory Panel website at www.skintears.org (Box 13.4). Box 13.5 presents tips for ST prevention and treatment.

Keratoses

There are two types of keratosis: seborrheic and actinic. *Actinic keratosis* is a precancerous lesion, and *seborrheic keratosis* is a benign growth that appears mainly on the trunk, the face, the neck, and the scalp as single or multiple lesions. One or more lesions are present on nearly all adults older than 65 years and are more common in men. An individual may have dozens of these benign lesions. Seborrheic keratosis is a waxy, raised

---

BOX 13.4 Resources for Best Practice
Pressure Ulcer Prevention and Treatment

Agency for Healthcare Research and Quality: Preventing pressure ulcers in hospitals: a toolkit for improving quality of care: https://www.ahrq.gov/professionals/systems/hospital/pressureulcertoolkit/putool3a.html; Safety program for nursing homes, On-Time Pressure Ulcer Prevention: https://www.ahrq.gov/professionals/systems/long-term-care/resources/ontime/pruprev/index.html

Hartford Institute for Geriatric Nursing: Braden Scale and video demonstrating use of Braden Scale; Nursing Standard of Practice Protocol: Pressure ulcer preventions and skin tear prevention

National Pressure Ulcer Advisory Panel (NPUAP) (www.npuap.org): International Pressure Ulcer Prevention Guidelines (available in 17 languages); Pressure Ulcer Scale for Healing (PUSH): PUSH Tool 3.0, Pressure Ulcer Healing Chart, Pressure Ulcer Prevention Points, Support Surface Standards Initiative, Pressure Ulcer Photos, and other educational materials on prevention and treatment also available online and via an application for iPhones, iPads, and Android devices

SkinTears.org: Skin Tears Tool Kit, State of the Science Consensus Statements, educational materials

Wound Source: Categories of wound-related devices and product information: www.woundsource.com

The VA Pressure Ulcer/Injury Resource app (VA PUR): The app is available on the Apple App Store and Google Play Store.

BOX 13.5 Tips for Best Practice

Skin Tears: Prevention and Treatment

Prevention

- Identify high-risk individuals. Risk factors include extremes of age; fragile skin; history of skin tears/falls; impaired activity, mobility, sensation, and cognition. Patients who are dependent are at greatest risk. Top causes of skin tears are equipment injury, patient transfers, activities of daily living, falls, and treatment and dressing removal.
- Have individual wear long sleeves or pants to protect extremities.
- Ensure adequate hydration and nutrition; provide a nutritional consultation.
- Lubricate skin with hypoallergenic moisturizer twice daily; apply to damp skin after bathing.
- Perform careful transfers; use a lift sheet to move and turn patients.
- Pad bed rails, wheelchair arms, leg supports, and furniture edges.
- Avoid use of adhesive products. Use nonadherent dressings and paper tape only as needed.
- Use gauze wrap, stockinettes, flexible netting, or other wraps to secure dressings.
- Use no-rinse, soapless bathing products and warm/tepid water for bathing.
- Caregivers need to keep nails short and not wear jewelry that can catch and contribute to skin tears.
- Implement fall prevention protocol.
- Educate patients, staff, and health care providers regarding prevention and management.

Treatment

- If skin tear occurs, assess and classify according to Payne-Martin classification system and assess size.
- Gently cleanse skin with normal saline.
- Air dry or pat dry carefully.
- Approximate skin tear flap if present; consider Steri-Strips; do not suture.
- Use nonadherent dressings.
- Use skin sealants to protect surrounding skin.
- Draw an arrow on the dressing to indicate direction of skin tear to minimize further injury during dressing removal; consider doing a wound tracing.
- Document assessment and treatment findings.

Data from LeBlanc K, Baranoski S: Skin tears: state of the science: consensus statements for the prevention, prediction, assessment and treatment of skin tears, *Adv Skin Wound Care* 24(Suppl 9):2, 2011.

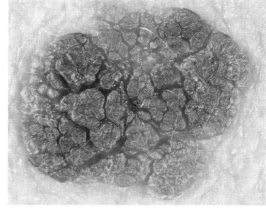

Fig. 13.1 Seborrheic Keratosis in an Older Adult. (From Habif TP: *Clinical dermatology: a color guide to diagnosis and therapy*, ed 5, St Louis, MO, 2010, Mosby.)

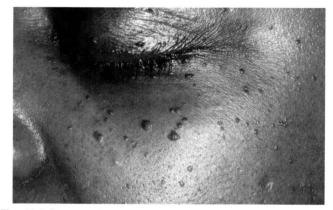

Fig. 13.2 Dermatosis Papulosa Nigra. (From Neville B, Damm DD, Allen CM, et al: *Oral and maxillofacial pathology*, ed 3, St Louis, MO, 2009, Saunders.)

lesion, flesh colored or pigmented in various sizes. The lesions have a "stuck-on" appearance, as if they could be scraped off. Seborrheic keratoses may be removed by a dermatologist for cosmetic reasons (Fig. 13.1). A variant seen in darkly pigmented persons occurs mostly on the face and appears as numerous small, dark, possibly tag-like lesions (Fig. 13.2).

Actinic keratosis is a precancerous lesion that is thought to be in the middle of the spectrum between photoaging changes and squamous cell carcinoma (Endo and Norman, 2014). It is directly related to years of overexposure to UV light. Risk factors are older age and fair complexion. It is found on the face, the lips, and the hands and forearms—areas of chronic sun exposure in everyday life. Actinic keratosis is characterized by rough, scaly, sandpaper-like patches, pink to reddish-brown on an erythematous base (Fig. 13.3). Lesions may be single or multiple; they may be painless or mildly tender. The person with actinic keratoses should be monitored by a dermatologist every 6 to 12 months

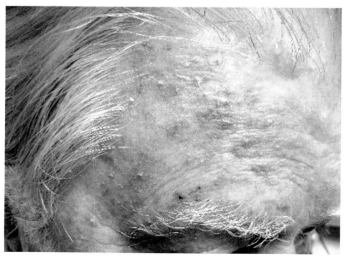

Fig. 13.3 Actinic Keratoses. (Courtesy Dr. Robert Norman.)

for any change in appearance of the lesions. Early recognition, treatment, and removal of these lesions are easy and important and may be combined with topical field therapy (Endo and Norman, 2014).

Herpes Zoster

HZ, or shingles, is a viral infection frequently seen in adults older than age 50, those who have medical conditions that compromise the immune system, or people who receive immunosuppressive drugs. About one out of every three people in the United States will develop HZ in their lifetime. HZ is caused by reactivation of latent varicella-zoster virus (VZV) within the sensory neurons of the dorsal root ganglion decades after initial VZV infection is established. More than 90% of the world's population is infected with this virus and about half of all cases occur in individuals 60 years or older (CDC, 2017).

HZ always occurs along a nerve pathway, or *dermatome*. The more dermatomes involved, the more serious the infection, especially if it involves the head. When the eye is affected it is always a medical emergency. Most HZ occurs in the thoracic region, but it can also occur in the trigeminal area and cervical, lumbar, and sacral areas. HZ vesicles never cross the midline. In most cases, the severity of the infection increases with age. It is important to differentiate HZ from herpes simplex. Herpes simplex does not occur in a dermatome pattern and is recurrent. The onset of HZ may be preceded by itching, tingling, or pain in the affected dermatome several days before the outbreak of the rash. During the healing process, clusters of papulovesicles develop along a nerve pathway. The lesions themselves eventually rupture, crust over, and resolve. Scarring may result, especially if scratching or poor hygiene leads to a secondary bacterial infection. HZ is infectious until it becomes crusty. HZ may be very painful and pruritic. Prompt treatment with the oral antiviral agents acyclovir, valacyclovir, and famciclovir may shorten the length and severity of the illness; however, to be effective, the medications must be started as soon as possible after the rash appears. Analgesics may help relieve pain. Wet compresses, calamine lotion, and colloidal oatmeal baths may help relieve itching.

Zoster vaccine (Zostavax) is recommended for all persons aged 60 years and older who have no contraindications, including persons who report a previous episode of zoster or who have chronic medical conditions (CDC, 2017). Older adults who are vaccinated may reduce their risk of acquiring HZ in half; and if they do get it, they are likely to have a milder case. *Healthy People 2020* includes a goal of increasing the percentage of adults who are vaccinated against zoster (shingles) in the overall goal of reducing or eliminating cases of vaccine-preventable diseases.

A common complication of HZ that is minimized for those who are immunized is postherpetic neuralgia (PHN), a chronic, often debilitating painful condition that can last months or even years. Older adults are more likely to have PHN and to have longer lasting and more severe pain. Another complication of HZ is eye involvement, which occurs in 10% to 25% of zoster episodes and can result in prolonged or permanent pain, facial scarring, and loss of vision. The pain of PHN has been difficult to control and can significantly affect quality of life. Treatment should include medical, psychological, complementary and alternative medicine options, and rehabilitation. The best evidence studies for medications indicate that the most effective are the tricyclic antidepressants, gabapentin and pregabalin, carbamazepine (for trigeminal neuralgia), opioids, tramadol, topical lidocaine patch, and duloxetine or venlafaxine. Relatively newer treatments for PHN include a high-concentration (8%) topical capsaicin patch, gastroretentive gabapentin, gabapentin enacarbil, and pregabalin in combination with lidocaine plaster, oxycodone, or transcutaneous electrical nerve stimulation (TENS) (Endo and Norman, 2014). Assessment and management of pain is discussed in Chapter 27.

Candidiasis *(Candida albicans)*

The fungus *Candida albicans* (referred to as "yeast") is present on the skin of healthy persons of any age. However, under certain circumstances and in the right environment, a fungal infection can develop. Persons who are obese or malnourished, are receiving antibiotic or steroid therapy, or have diabetes are at increased risk. *Candida* grows especially well in areas that are moist, warm, and dark, such as in skinfolds, in the axilla, in the groin area, and under pendulous breasts. It can also be found in the corners of the mouth associated with the chronic moisture of angular cheilitis. In the vagina it is also called a "yeast infection." If this is found in an older woman, it may mean that she has undiagnosed or poorly controlled diabetes.

Inside the mouth a *Candida* infection is referred to as "thrush" and is associated with poor hygiene and the immunocompromised individual, such as those who have long-term steroid use (e.g., because of chronic obstructive pulmonary disease), who are receiving chemotherapy, or who test positive for or are infected with human immunodeficiency virus (HIV) or have acquired immunodeficiency syndrome (AIDS). In the mouth, candidiasis appears as irregular, white, flat to slightly raised patches on an erythematous base that cannot be removed by scraping. The infection can extend down into the throat and cause swallowing to be painful. In severely immunocompromised persons the infection can extend down the entire gastrointestinal tract.

On the skin, *Candida* is usually maculopapular, glazed, and dark pink in persons with less pigmentation and grayish in persons with more pigmentation. If it is advanced, the central area may be completely red and/or dark and weeping with characteristic bright red and/or dark satellite lesions (distinct lesions a short distance from the center). At this point the skin may be edematous, itching, and burning.

The best approach to managing fungal infections is to prevent them, and the key to prevention is limiting the conditions that encourage fungal growth. Prevention is prioritized for persons who are obese, bedridden, incontinent, or diaphoretic (Box 13.6).

Photo Damage of the Skin

Although exposure to sunlight is necessary for the production of vitamin D, the sun is also the most common cause of skin damage and skin cancer. More than 90% of the visible changes

Candidiasis: Prevention and Treatment

- Identify high-risk individuals (e.g., obese, bedridden, incontinent, diaphoretic, immunocompromised) and limit conditions that encourage fungal growth.
- Provide adequate drying of target areas after bathing and prompt management of incontinent episodes. A hair dryer on the low setting can help dry hard-to-reach, vulnerable areas.
- A dry, folded washcloth or cotton sanitary pad can be placed under the breasts or between skinfolds to promote exposure to air and light.
- Use loose-fitting clothing and underwear; change clothing and bedding when damp.
- Avoid incontinent products that are tight or have plastic that touches the skin.
- Avoid use of cornstarch because it promotes growth of *Candida* organisms.
- Optimize nutrition and glycemic control.
- The goal of treatment is to eradicate the infection and may include the use of a prescribed antifungal medication for 7 to 14 days or until the infection is completely cleared. Antifungal preparations are available as powders, creams, and lotions. Powders are recommended because they trap moisture less than the others.

commonly attributed to skin aging are caused by the sun (Skin Cancer Foundation, 2017). With aging one accumulates years of sun exposure and the epidermis is thinner, significantly increasing the risk for older adults. The damage (photo or solar damage) comes from prolonged exposure to UV light from the environment or in tanning booths. Although the amount of sun-induced damage varies with skin type, genetics, and geographical location, much of the associated damage is preventable. Ideally, preventive measures begin in childhood, but clinical evidence has shown that some improvement can be achieved at any time by limiting sun exposure and using sunscreens regularly regardless of skin tones.

SKIN CANCERS
Facts and Figures
Each year in the United States more than 5.4 million cases of nonmelanoma skin cancer are treated in more than 3.3 million people. Cancer of the skin (including melanoma and nonmelanoma skin cancer) is the most common of all cancers. Skin cancer is a major public health problem and skin cancers in the United States, unlike many other cancers, continue to rise. One in five Americans will develop skin cancer in the course of a lifetime (Skin Cancer Foundation, 2017). Caucasian populations generally have a much higher risk of getting nonmelanoma or melanoma skin cancers than dark-skinned populations, but individuals of all skin colors should minimize sun exposure. Individuals with pale or freckled skin, fair or red hair, and blue eyes belong to the highest risk group. About 90% of nonmelanoma skin cancers are associated with exposure to UV radiation from the sun.

Recent research suggests that individuals who have a nonmelanoma skin cancer before their mid-20s have a high risk of developing cancers of the bladder, brain, breast, lung, pancreas, and stomach. With age, the risk for developing cancer decreased but remained higher compared with individuals who did not have nonmelanoma skin cancer when young (Ong et al, 2014). The exact number of basal and squamous cell cancers is not known for certain because they are not reported to cancer registries, but it is estimated that there are more than 2 million basal and squamous cell skin cancers found each year. Most of these are basal cell cancers. Squamous cell cancer is less common but rates are increasing. Most of these are curable; the type with the greatest potential to cause death is melanoma.

Basal Cell Carcinoma
Basal cell carcinoma is the most common malignant skin cancer. It occurs mainly in older age groups but is occurring more and more in younger persons. It is slow growing, and metastasis is rare. A basal cell lesion can be triggered by extensive sun exposure, especially burns, chronic irritation, and chronic ulceration of the skin. It is more prevalent in light-skinned persons. It usually begins as a pearly papule with prominent telangiectasias (blood vessels) or as a scar-like area with no history of trauma (Fig. 13.4). Basal cell carcinoma is also known to ulcerate. It may be indistinguishable from squamous cell carcinoma and is diagnosed by biopsy. Early detection and treatment are necessary to minimize disfigurement. Treatment is usually surgical with either simple excision or Mohs micrographic surgery (Endo and Norman, 2014).

Squamous Cell Carcinoma
Squamous cell carcinoma is the second most common skin cancer. However, it is aggressive and has a high incidence of metastasis if not identified and treated promptly. Major risk factors include sun exposure, fair skin, and immunosuppression. Individuals in their mid-60s who have been or are chronically exposed to the sun (e.g., persons who work outdoors or are athletes) are prime candidates for this type of cancer. Less common causes include chronic stasis ulcers, scars from injury, and exposure to chemical carcinogens, such as topical hydrocarbons, arsenic, and radiation (especially for individuals who received treatments for acne in the mid-twentieth century) (Endo and Norman, 2014).

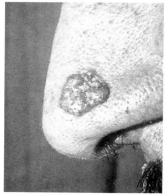

Fig. 13.4 **Basal Cell Carcinoma.** (Courtesy Gary Monheit, MD, University of Alabama at Birmingham School of Medicine.)

The lesion begins as a firm, irregular, fleshy, pink-colored nodule that becomes reddened and scaly, much like actinic keratosis, but it may increase rapidly in size. It may also be hard and wart-like with a gray top and horny texture, or it may be ulcerated and indurated with raised, defined borders (Fig. 13.5). Because it can appear so differently, it is often overlooked or thought to be insignificant. All persons, especially those who live in sunny climates, should be regularly screened by a dermatologist. Treatment depends on the size, histologic features, and patient preference and may include electrodesiccation and curettage, Mohs micrographic surgery, aggressive cryotherapy, or topical 5-fluorouracil (Endo and Norman, 2014). Once a person has been diagnosed with a squamous cell carcinoma, he or she needs to be routinely followed because the majority of recurrences are within the first few years.

Melanoma

Melanoma, a neoplasm of the melanocytes, affects the skin or, less commonly, the retina. Melanoma has a classical multicolor, raised appearance with an asymmetrical, irregular border. It may appear to be of any size, but the surface diameter is not necessarily reflective of the size beneath the surface, similar in concept to an iceberg. It is treatable if diagnosed early, before it has a chance to invade surrounding tissue. Melanoma accounts for less than 2% of skin cancer cases, but it causes most skin cancer deaths. Melanoma is highly curable if the cancer is detected in its earliest stages and treated promptly (Skin Cancer Foundation, 2017).

Incidence and Prevalence

The Skin Cancer Foundation (2017) estimates that about 87,110 new cases of melanoma were diagnosed in 2017. The number of new cases of melanoma in the United States has been increasing for at least 30 years. Overall, the lifetime risk of getting melanoma is about 1 in 50 for the white population, 1 in 1000 for

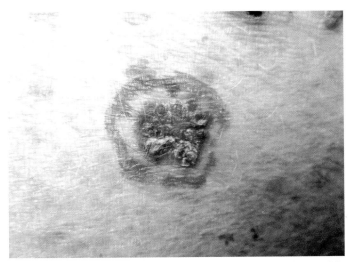

Fig. 13.5 Squamous Cell Carcinoma. (From Ham RJ, Sloane PD, Warshaw GA, et al: *Primary care geriatrics*, ed 6, Philadelphia, 2014, Saunders. Used with permission, University of Utah Department of Dermatology.)

black individuals, and 1 in 200 for the Hispanic population. Melanoma rates among middle-aged adults, especially women, have increased in the past 4 decades (Garrett et al, 2014). Men have a higher rate of melanoma than women and a person who has already had a melanoma has a higher risk of developing another one.

Risk Factors

Risk factors for melanoma include a personal history of melanoma; the presence of atypical, large, or numerous (more than 50) moles; sun sensitivity; history of excessive sun exposure and severe sunburns; use of tanning booths; natural blond or red hair color; diseases or treatments that suppress the immune system; and a history of skin cancer. Increasing age along with a history of sun exposure increases one's risk even further. The legs and backs of women and the backs of men are the most common sites of melanoma. Many studies have linked melanoma on the trunk, legs, and arms to frequent sunburns, especially in childhood. Blistering sunburns before the age of 18 years are thought to damage Langerhans cells, which affect the immune response of the skin and increase the risk for a later melanoma. Two-thirds of melanomas develop from preexisting moles; only one-third arise alone.

Indoor tanning. Although melanoma occurs more often in older adults, it is one of the most common cancers in people younger than 30 years. Exposure to indoor tanning, common in developed countries, is thought to be contributing to the increasing rates of melanoma and other skin cancers among younger individuals. Indoor tanning increases the risk of melanoma by 75% when use started before age 35 years. Indoor tanners are 2.5 times more likely to develop squamous cell cancer and 1.5 times more likely to develop basal cell cancer. In the United States, 35% of adults and 55% of college students have used indoor tanning devices. Worldwide, there are more skin cancer cases due to indoor tanning than there are lung cancer cases due to smoking (Skin Cancer Foundation, 2017). This is considered a major public health issue with many states limiting minors' access to tanning salons. Tanning devices have been reclassified by the Federal Drug Administration to Class II (moderate risk devices). *Healthy People 2020* includes objectives to reduce the proportion of adolescents and adults using indoor tanning devices.

PROMOTING HEALTHY AGING: IMPLICATIONS FOR GERONTOLOGICAL NURSING

Age-related skin changes, such as thinning and diminished numbers of melanocytes, significantly increase the risk for solar damage and subsequent skin cancer. The nurse has an active role in the prevention and early recognition of skin cancers. This role may include working with community awareness and education programs and screening clinics and providing direct care. By far the most important preventive nursing intervention is to provide education regarding skin cancer risk factors and adequate lifelong protective measures (Box 13.7).

Careful skin inspection is essential and the nurse is vigilant in observing skin for changes that require further evaluation.

BOX 13.7   Promoting Healthy Skin

Sun Protection
- Seek the shade.
- Do not burn.
- Avoid indoor tanning booths and sunlamps.
- Wear hats with a brim wide enough to shade face, ears, and neck, and clothing that adequately covers the arms, legs, and torso. Cover up with clothing, including a broad-brimmed hat and UV-blocking sunglasses.
- Use a broad-spectrum (UVA/UVB) sunscreen with an SPF of 30 or higher every day.
- Apply 1 ounce (2 tablespoons) of sunscreen to your entire body 30 minutes before going outdoors. Reapply every 2 hours or immediately after swimming or excessive sweating.
- Examine your skin head-to-toe every month.
- See your health care provider every year for a professional skin exam.

Modified from Skin Cancer Foundation: *Prevention guidelines.* http://www.skincancer.org/prevention/sun-protection/prevention-guidelines. Accessed March, 2019.

Patient education also includes teaching the individual how to examine his or her skin once a month to look for warning signs or any suspicious lesions. If the individual has a partner, partners can perform regular "checks" of each other's skin, watching for signs of change and the need to contact a primary care provider or dermatologist promptly. For the person with keratosis and multiple freckles (nevi), photographing the body parts may be a useful reference. The adage "when in doubt, get it checked" is an important one and regular screenings should be a part of the health care of all older adults. The "ABCDE" approach to assessing such potential lesions is used (Box 13.8).

PRESSURE INJURIES (PIs)

Aging carries a high risk for the development of PIs; 70% of PIs occur in older adults. PIs are recognized as one of the geriatric syndromes (Chapter 7), and *Healthy People 2020* has addressed this issue with a goal of reducing the rate of PI-related hospitalizations among older adults. Although prevention and treatment of PIs require an interprofessional approach, PIs are considered specifically a nurse-sensitive indicator by the U.S. National Database of Nursing Quality Indicators (Ayello et al, 2017) and a nurse-sensitive indicator for hospital-acquired

BOX 13.8   Danger Signs: Remember ABCDE

A   Asymmetry of a mole (one that is not regularly round or oval)
B   Border is irregular
C   Color variation (areas of black, brown, tan, blue, red, white, or a combination)
D   Diameter greater than the size of a pencil eraser (although early stages may be smaller)
E   Elevation and enlargement[a]

[a]Lesions that change, itch, bleed, or do not heal are also alarm signals.
From Skin Cancer Foundation: *Do you know your ABCDEs?*, 2018. https://www.skincancer.org/skin-cancer-information/melanoma/melanoma-warning-signs-and-images/do-you-know-your-abcdes. Accessed January 2018.

pressure injuries (HAPIs) (Al-Majid et al, 2017). Nurses play a key role in the prevention of PIs and selection of evidence-based treatment strategies.

Definition

The National Pressure Ulcer Advisory Panel (NPUAP) and the European Pressure Ulcer Advisory Panel (EPUAP) constitute an international collaboration convened to develop evidence-based recommendations to be used throughout the world to prevent and treat pressure-related injuries. In 2016 the NPUAP began using the term pressure injury to replace pressure ulcer to more accurately describe PIs to both intact and ulcerated skin. In addition to the change in terminology, Arabic numbers are now used in the names of the stages instead of Roman numerals. Stages have been more fully described, and two additional PI definitions have been added.

A PI is defined as "localized damage to the skin and/or underlying soft tissue usually over a bony prominence or related to a medical or other device. The injury can present as intact skin or an open ulcer and may be painful. The injury occurs as a result of intense pressure and/or prolonged pressure or pressure in combination with shear. The tolerance of soft tissue for pressure and shear may also be affected by microclimate, nutrition, perfusion, co-morbidities and condition of the soft tissue" (NPUAP, 2016).

Scope of the Problem

PIs cause pain, loss of function, extended length of hospitalization and long-term care stays, and increase in cost. Reported prevalence rates of HAPIs are as high as 38% in the acute care setting, 42% in critical care patients, 17% in home care, and 23% in long-term care. PIs are a major challenge worldwide and a major cause of morbidity, mortality, and health care burden globally (Ramundo et al, 2018). The epidemiology of PIs varies appreciably by clinical setting. Critically ill patients in the intensive care unit (ICU) are considered to be at the greatest risk for PI development as a result of high acuity and the multiple interventions and therapies they receive (Alderden et al, 2017).

HAPI rates have decreased across the United States. However, growing resources invested into the development and implementation of evidence-based prevention protocols, the rates of facility-acquired PIs are still much higher in many clinical areas across the globe, especially in high-risk populations such as older adults and critically ill patients (Balzer and Kottner, 2015; Rondinelli et al, 2018). Concern over the global problem of PIs had led the NPUAP to establish a Pressure Ulcer Registry, the first database of its type to allow clinicians to input cases of PIs in an effort to provide statistically significant rigorous analysis of the variables associated with the development of unavoidable PUs (NPUAP, 2014).

Cost and Regulatory Requirements

Treatment of PIs is costly in terms of both health care expenditure and patient suffering. In 2008, the Centers for Medicare and Medicaid Services (CMS) included HAPIs as one of the preventable adverse events (health care–acquired conditions

BOX 13.9 Avoidable and Unavoidable Pressure Injuries

Avoidable: Development of a pressure injury while the facility did not do one or more of the following:
- evaluate the resident's clinical condition and pressure ulcer risk factors
- define and implement interventions that are consistent with resident needs, resident goals, and recognized standards of practice
- monitor and evaluate the impact of the interventions; or revise the interventions as appropriate

Unavoidable: Development of a pressure injury even though the facility:
- evaluated the resident's clinical condition and pressure ulcer risk factors
- defined and implemented interventions that are consistent with resident needs and goals
- recognized standards of practice
- monitored and evaluated the impact of the interventions
- revised the approaches as appropriate

From Centers for Medicare and Medicaid Services: *CMS manual system.* Publication No. 100-07 State Operations. Baltimore, MD, 2004, Author.

[HACs]). The development of a stage/category 3 or 4 PI is considered a "never event" (preventable serious medical errors or adverse events that should never happen to a patient). Hospitals no longer receive additional reimbursement to care for a patient who has acquired PIs under the hospital's care, and this has the potential to greatly increase the financial strain for facilities that fail to rise to this challenge. In long-term care facilities, when PIs develop after admission and are identified as avoidable, civil monetary penalties can be assessed (Box 13.9).

Characteristics

PIs can develop anywhere on the body but are seen most frequently on the posterior aspects, especially the sacrum, the heels, and the greater trochanters. Secondary areas of breakdown include the lateral condyles of the knees and the ankles. The pinna of the ears, occiput, elbows, and scapulae are other areas subject to breakdown. The heel is particularly prone to the development of PIs due to its anatomy. It consists of skin overlying a cup-like shell of connective tissue that essentially forms a sealed compartment, creating a compartment of fat with comparatively low vascularity that is prone to ischemia. The shell of connective tissue and sealed compartment structure inhibit distribution of external pressure. Additionally, the small surface area of contact and little subcutaneous tissue lead to PI when pressure is exerted directly on bone (Ramundo et al, 2018).

⚡ SAFETY ALERT

Approximately 25% to 35% of pressure injuries are on heels. Those with peripheral vascular disease (PVD) are at high risk. Keep heels elevated off the bed with a pillow under calf or use heel suspension boots. Prophylactic multilayer foam dressings, in conjunction with a pressure injury prevention program, are recommended for prevention of pressure injuries on the heel (Ramundo et al, 2018).

Classification

The EPUAP and NPUAP classification of PIs is presented in Box 13.10. The following two additional PI definitions have also been added:

Medical Device–Related Pressure Injury: Medical device–related pressure injuries (MDRPIs) result from the use of devices designed and applied for diagnostic or therapeutic purposes. The resultant PI generally conforms to the pattern or shape

BOX 13.10 Pressure Injury Stages/Categories

Deep Tissue Pressure Injury (DTPI): Persistent Nonblanchable Deep Red, Maroon, or Purple Discoloration

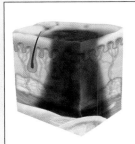
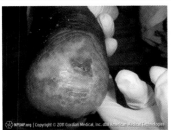

Heel, ethnic skin

Intact or nonintact skin with localized area of persistent nonblanchable deep red, maroon, or purple discoloration or epidermal separation revealing a dark wound bed or blood-filled blister. Pain and temperature change often precede skin color changes. Discoloration may appear differently in darkly pigmented skin. This injury results from intense and/or prolonged pressure and shear forces at the bone-muscle interface. The wound may evolve rapidly to reveal the actual extent of tissue injury or may resolve without tissue loss.

DTPI may evolve into a full thickness wound despite optimal care. If necrotic tissue, subcutaneous tissue, granulation tissue, fascia, muscle, or other underlying structures are visible, this indicates a full-thickness pressure injury (Unstageable,

Stage 3, or Stage 4). Do not use DTPI to describe vascular, traumatic, neuropathic, or dermatological conditions. If PI is on a mucosal membrane, document, but do not stage.

Stage 1 Pressure Injury: Nonblanchable Erythema of Intact Skin

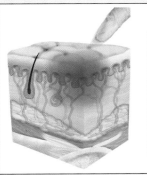
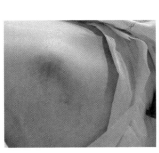

Intact skin with a localized area of nonblanchable erythema, which may appear differently in darkly pigmented skin. Presence of blanchable erythema or changes in sensation, temperature, or firmness may precede visual changes. Color changes do not include purple or maroon discoloration; these may indicate DTPI.

BOX 13.10   Pressure Injury Stages/Categories—cont'd

Stage 2 Pressure Injury: Partial-Thickness Skin Loss With Exposed Dermis

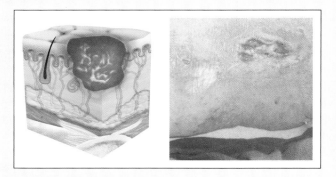

Partial-thickness loss of skin with exposed dermis. The wound bed is viable, pink or red, and moist, and may also present as an intact or ruptured serum-filled blister. Adipose (fat) is not visible and deeper tissues are not visible. Granulation tissue, slough, and eschar are not present. These injuries commonly result from adverse microclimate and shear in the skin over the pelvis and shear in the heels. This stage should not be used to describe moisture-associated skin damage (MASD) including incontinence-associated dermatitis (IAD), intertriginous dermatitis (ITD), medical adhesive–related skin injury (MARS), or traumatic wounds (skin tears, burns, abrasions).

Stage 3 Pressure Injury: Full-Thickness Skin Loss

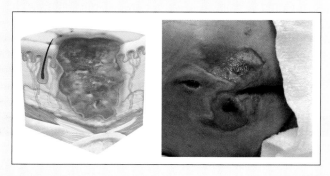

Full-thickness loss of skin, in which adipose (fat) is visible in the ulcer and granulation tissue and epibole (rolled wound edges) are often present. Slough and/or eschar may be visible. Undermining and tunneling may occur. Fascia,

muscle, tendon, ligament, cartilage, and/or bone are not exposed. If slough or eschar obscures the extent of tissue loss this is an Unstageable Pressure Injury.

Stage 4 Pressure Injury: Full-Thickness Skin and Tissue Loss

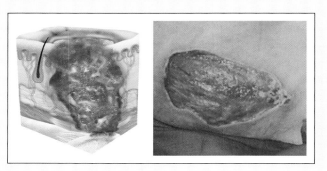

Full-thickness skin and tissue loss with exposed or directly palpable fascia, muscle, tendon, ligament, cartilage, or bone in the ulcer. Slough and/or eschar may be visible. Epibole (rolled edges), undermining, and/or tunneling often occur. Depth varies by anatomical location. If slough or eschar obscures the extent of tissue loss, this is an Unstageable Pressure Injury.

Unstageable Pressure Injury: Obscured Full-Thickness Skin and Tissue Loss

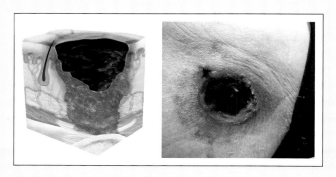

Full-thickness skin and tissue loss in which the extent of tissue damage within the ulcer cannot be confirmed because it is obscured by slough or eschar. If slough or eschar is removed, a Stage 3 or Stage 4 pressure ulcer will be revealed. Stable eschar (e.g., dry, adherent, intact without erythema or fluctuance) on an ischemic limb or the heels should not be removed.

From National Pressure Ulcer Advisory Panel (NPUAP): *National Pressure Ulcer Advisory Panel (NPUAP) announces a change in terminology from pressure ulcer to pressure injury and updates the stages of pressure injury,* 2016. Reprinted with permission of the NPUAP, 2016; National Pressure Ulcer Advisory Panel: *NPRAP Position Statement on Staging – 2017 Clarifications,* 2017. Reprinted with permission of the NPUAP, 2017. DTPI photo: From NPUAP. Stages 1–4 photos: From Cameron MH, Monroe L. *Physical rehabilitation for the physical therapist assistant,* St Louis, 2011, Saunders. Unstageable photo: From Ham RJ, Sloane PD, Warshaw GA, et al: *Primary care geriatrics,* ed 6, Philadelphia, 2014, Elsevier.

of the device. The injury should not be staged using the staging system.

Mucosal Membrane Pressure Injury: Mucosal membrane PI is found on mucous membranes with a history of a medical device in use at the location of the injury. Because of the anatomy of the tissue, these injuries cannot be staged.

PIs are always classified by the highest stage "achieved," and reverse staging is never used. This means that the wound is documented as the stage representing the maximal damage and depth

that has occurred. As the wound heals, it fills with granulation tissue composed of endothelial cells, fibroblasts, collagen, and an extracellular matrix. Muscle, subcutaneous fat, and dermis are not replaced. A stage 4 PI that is healing does not revert to stage 3 and then stage 2. It remains defined as a healing stage 4 PI.

Risk Factors

Many factors increase the risk of pressure injuries, including changes in the skin, comorbid illnesses, nutritional status,

BOX 13.11 Pressure Injury Risk Factors

Prolonged Pressure/Immobilization

Lying in bed or sitting in a chair or wheelchair without changing position or relieving pressure over an extended period

Lying for hours on hard x-ray and operating tables

Neurological disorders (coma, spinal cord injuries, cognitive impairment, or cerebrovascular disease)

Fractures or contractures

Debilitation: older adult in hospitals and nursing homes

Pain

Sedation

Shearing forces (moving by dragging on coarse bed sheets)

Disease/Tissue Factors

Impaired perfusion; ischemia

Fecal or urinary incontinence; prolonged exposure to moisture

Malnutrition, dehydration

Chronic diseases accompanied by anemia, edema, renal failure, malnutrition, peripheral vascular disease, or sepsis

Previous history of pressure injuries

Additional Risk Factors for the Critically Ill

Norepinephrine infusion

Acute Physiology and Chronic Health Evaluation (APACHE II) score

Anemia

Age older than 40 years

Multiple organ system disease or comorbid complications

Length of hospital stay

From McCance KL, Huether SE: *Pathophysiology*, ed 7, St Louis, 2014, Elsevier.

BOX 13.12 Key Elements of a Pressure Injury Prevention Program

- Skin assessment for all patients looking for pressure injury
- Daily risk assessment
- Daily skin inspection
- Moisture management
- Optimizing nutrition and hydration
- Minimizing pressure (posture changes)
- Pressure injury nursing care education
- Establishment of a wound care team
- Interdisciplinary cooperation

From Jin Y, Jin T, Lee S: Automated pressure injury risk assessment system incorporated into an electronic record system, *Nurs Res* 66(6):462–472, 2017.

frailty, surgical procedures (especially orthopedic/cardiac), cognitive deficits, incontinence, and reduced mobility (Box 13.11). A major risk factor is the combination of intensity and duration of pressure and tissue tolerance. Individuals confined to a bed or chair and who are unable to shift weight or reposition themselves at regular intervals are at high risk. Tissue tolerance, in addition to unrelieved pressure, contributes to the risk of a PI. Tissue tolerance is related to the ability of the tissue to distribute and compensate for pressure exerted over bony prominences. Factors that affect tissue tolerance include moisture, friction, shear force, nutritional status, age, sensory perception, and arterial pressure.

In darker-pigmented persons, redness and blanching may not be observed as early signs of skin damage. In dark skin, early signs of skin damage can manifest as a purplish color or appear like a bruise. It is important to observe for induration, darkening, change in color from surrounding skin, or a shadowed appearance of the skin. The affected skin area, when compared with adjacent tissues, may be firm, warmer, cooler, or painful. Improved assessment of dark skin for early signs of damage and increased attention to prevention of PIs before admission and during nursing home stays are important (Harms et al, 2014).

Prevention of Pressure Injuries

The importance of prevention of PIs has been frequently emphasized and is the key to treatment. Key elements of PI prevention are presented in Box 13.12. A comprehensive PI program that includes multiple interventions (care bundle) appears to be related to better outcomes. A bundle is composed of a set of evidence-based practices that when performed collectively and reliably have been shown to improve patient outcomes. Involvement of the patient and family may enhance the effectiveness of care bundles (Chaboyer et al, 2016; Gillespie et al, 20; Roberts et al, 2017). Core preventive strategies include risk assessment, skin assessment, nutritional assessment, repositioning, and appropriate support surfaces. Interventions that address limited mobility, compromised skin integrity, and nutritional support have been associated with improvements in PI rates (Gillespie et al, 2014). A recent quality improvement study reported that nurse practitioners assuming a leadership role as wound care consultants in acute care may be instrumental in decreasing HAPI rates (Irvin et al, 2017).

Systematic prevention programs have been shown to decrease HAPIs. Olsho and colleagues (2014) reported a 59% reduction in the monthly incidence of PIs in a nursing home with the use of the Agency for Healthcare Research and Quality [AHRQ] On-Time Pressure Ulcer Prevention Program (AHRQ, 2014) (Box 13.4). The focus of this project is on prevention and timely treatment of PIs in long-term care. Tools to document PI healing and treatments and reports to monitor the healing process are available. Despite recognition of its importance, PI prevention strategies are not consistently implemented and PIs continue to have a negative impact of patient outcomes and health care costs in a variety of care settings (Balzer and Kottner, 2015; Chaboyer et al, 2016).

Education programs on PI, both for practicing nurses and student nurses, are essential and should be a part of institutional and educational curricula (Garrigues et al, 2017). Research conducted in the United States and internationally in other countries has demonstrated that nurses, both wound certified and not, have limited levels of PI knowledge (Ayello et al, 2017). Miller et al. (2017) reported that nurses had greater knowledge of staging rather than prevention. Innovative approaches to education are important and may include "just in time" interactive educational methods, including mobile phone apps. The Department of Veterans Affairs (VA) has developed an innovative mobile app for veterans and caregivers working to prevent and treat PIs—the VA Pressure Ulcer/Injury Resource app (VA PUR) (Box 13.4). Continuing professional development for PI prevention and management needs to be interprofessional and include evidence-based educational material and strategies. Professional nursing checklists for competence and performance evaluations need to be implemented at all levels (novice to expert). Examples of competency checklists can be found in Ayello et al. (2017).

Consequences of Pressure Injuries

PIs are costly to treat and prolong recovery and extend rehabilitation. Complications include the need for grafting or amputation, sepsis, or even death and may lead to legal action by the individual or his or her representative against the caregiver. The personal impact of a PI on health and quality of life is also significant and not well understood or researched. Findings from a study exploring patients' perceptions of the impact of a PI and its treatment on health and quality of life suggest that PIs cause suffering, pain, discomfort, and distress that are not always recognized or adequately treated by nursing staff. PIs have a profound impact on the patients' lives—physically, socially, emotionally, and mentally (Spillsbury et al, 2007). Several patients' stories are presented in video format at https://vimeo.com/171515404.

Are Pressure Injuries Always Preventable?

PI development is a multicausal event. In the vast majority of cases, appropriate prevention and treatment interventions can prevent or minimize PI development. "However, in some cases, PIs are unavoidable because the magnitude and severity of risk are overwhelmingly high or preventive measures are either contraindicated or inadequate, given the magnitude and severity of risk" (Edsberg et al, 2014, p. 314). Some pressure injuries are unavoidable despite provision of evidence-based care by the health care team (NPUAP, 2017). Both the NPUAP (Edsberg et al, 2014) and the Wound, Ostomy, and Continence Nurses Society (WOCN Society) (Schmitt et al, 2017) have published statements on avoidable and unavoidable PIs. Clinical situations can severely impair efforts to prevent PIs. Some of these are preexisting deep tissue injury (DTI) (but no visible ulceration); immobility; hemodynamic instability; medical devices; compromised nutrition; and the patient who is nearing the end of life (Edsberg et al, 2014).

Skin failure is an emerging concept, particularly in the palliative care setting. "Skin is the largest organ of the body, and it fails like any other organ system" (Levine, 2017a, p. 201). Skin failure has been defined as "the state in which tissue tolerance is so compromised that cells can no longer survive in zones of physiological impairment that include hypoxia, local mechanical stress, impaired delivery of nutrients, and buildup of metabolic byproducts. This includes PIs, wounds that occur at life's end, and in the setting of multisystem organ failure" (Levine, 2017a). Skin failure can occur in the course of acute and chronic illness and at the end of life when the body is shutting down.

Skin failure at the end of life is not the same as PIs (Black et al, 2011). Preventing wound deterioration or healing may

not be realistic goals. The focus of wound management at the end of life is comfort and involves symptom control, stabilization of existing wounds, and prevention of additional wounds and infectious complications. If opportunity for wound healing is limited, maintenance of the wound in the present state may be the outcome. In some situations, palliative wounds may benefit from interventions such as surgical debridement or support surfaces even if the goal is not to heal the wound. The plan of care must be consistent with the patient and family goals and wishes. Further research is needed to fully understand the development of unavoidable PI in situations of high risk such as at the end of life (Levine, 2017a).

PROMOTING HEALTHY AGING: IMPLICATIONS FOR GERONTOLOGICAL NURSING

Nursing staff, as direct caregivers, are key team members who perform skin assessment, identify risk factors, and implement numerous preventive interventions. The nurse alerts the health care provider of the need for prescribed treatments, recommends treatments, and administers and evaluates the changing status of the wound(s) and adequacy of treatments.

Pressure Injury Risk Assessment

Skin assessments are performed on admission and whenever there is a change in the status of the patient (Box 13.13). In the nursing home, the MDS 3.0 provides an evidence-based assessment of skin integrity and PIs with accompanying care guidelines (Chapter 7). Assessment begins with a history, detailed head-to-toe skin examination, nutritional evaluation, and analysis of laboratory findings. Laboratory values that have been correlated with risk for the development and the poor healing of PIs include those that reflect anemia and poor nutritional status. Visual and tactile inspection of the entire skin surface with special attention to bony prominences is essential. The nurse looks for any interruption of skin integrity or other changes, including redness or *hyperemia*. Special attention must be given to the assessment of dark skin because tissue injury will appear differently in lighter skin. Assessment of pain related to the PI (dressing changes, turning) is important so that appropriate treatment can be given to relieve pain (Chapter 27).

If pressure is present, it should be relieved and the area reassessed in 1 hour. Pressure areas and surrounding tissue should be palpated for changes in temperature and tissue resilience. Blisters or pimples with or without hyperemia and scabs over

---

BOX 13.13 Guidelines for Skin Assessment

Acute care: On admission, reassess at least every 24 hours or sooner if patient's condition changes

Long-term care: On admission, weekly for 4 weeks, then quarterly and whenever resident's condition changes

Home care: On admission and at every nurse visit

Data from NPUAP: *Pressure ulcer prevention points,* 2007. http://www.npuap.org/wp-content/uploads/2012/03/PU_Prev_Points.pdf. Accessed January 2018.

weight-bearing areas in the absence of trauma should be considered suspect. Inspection is best accomplished in nonglare daylight or, if that is not possible, with focused lighting. Special attention should be directed to affected areas when an individual uses orthotic devices such as corsets, braces, prostheses, postural supports, splints, slings, or casts and to areas of skin around other devices such as endotracheal and tracheostomy tubes. MDRPIs result from the use of devices designed and applied for diagnostic purposes. On the skin, PIs tend to take on the shape of the device and should be staged using the NPUAP staging system (Box 13.10). There is little information available on the risks or frequency of device-related PIs and many times the skin condition is not labeled a PI. Box 13.14 presents a mnemonic for the prevention and treatment of MDRPIs (Delmore, 2017).

Early identification of risk status is critical so that timely interventions can be designed to address specific risk factors. The Braden Scale for Predicting Pressure Sore Risk, developed by nurses Barbara Braden and Nancy Bergstrom, is widely used and clinically validated. The Braden Scale is available online and used in most health care institutions (Murphree, 2017) (Box 13.4). This scale assesses the risk of PIs on the basis of a numerical scoring system of six risk factors: sensory perception, moisture, activity, mobility, nutrition, and friction/shear. Because the Braden Scale does not include all of the risk factors for PIs, it is recommended that it be used as an adjunct rather than in place of clinical judgment. A thorough patient history, to assess other risk factors such as age, medications, comorbidities (diabetes,

peripheral vascular disease), history of PIs, and other factors, is important to fully address the risk of PI development so that appropriate preventive interventions can be developed (Jull and Griffiths, 2010; Warner-Maron, 2015).

A systematic review found that formal PI risk assessment tools were not more effective than usual care (Chou, 2013). Some authors propose that Braden Scale subscale scores, rather than the cumulative score, should be the focus of prevention efforts (Alderden et al, 2017) (Research Highlights box).

RESEARCH HIGHLIGHTS

The purpose of the study was to examine the relationship between pressure injury development and the Braden Pressure Sore Risk subscale scores in a surgical intensive care unit (ICU) population and ascertain whether the risk represented by the subscale scores is different between younger and older patients. The authors note that there are no published studies examining pressure injury risk associated with Braden Scale subscores in older adults, even though older age is a critical risk factor for pressure injury development in ICU.

A retrospective review of electronic medical records of 6377 patients was conducted. Results reported that individuals with cumulative and subscale scores in the intermediate-risk levels had the highest likelihood of developing a pressure injury among all subscale categories *except* the friction/shear subscale. In this category, patients with the most severe scores were at markedly increased risk for pressure injury development. The interaction between age and Braden Scale scores and subscale scores, particularly the activity, moisture, sensory perception, and nutrition subscales, added an important dimension that should be considered a factor in care planning for prevention.

Mobility and moisture subscale scores were strongly associated with pressure injury development among older patients. Moisture management (continence programs) and increased activity are particularly important for older adults to prevent pressure injury. The authors postulate that patients with high Braden Scale scores on the Braden tool alerts nurses to apply maximal preventive interventions and that patients with lower (midrange) scores may not be considered in a high-risk group. Nurses need to carefully look at the subscale scores and include prevention interventions directed at risk in each area even if scores do not indicate high risk. While risk tool scores are important in designing prevention interventions, nursing assessment and clinical judgement must be ongoing.

Data from Alderden J, Cummins M, Pepper G et al: Midrange Braden subscale scores are associated with increased risk for pressure injury development among critical care patients. *J Wound Ostomy Continence Nurs* 44(5),420–428, 2017.

BOX 13.14 DEVICE Mnemonic for the Prevention of Medical Device-Related Pressure Injuries

D Determine that all medical devices
- are commercially manufactured for use in the clinical setting (not homemade)
- can be placed without making contact with prior or existing pressure injuries

E Evaluate all devices, every skin-device interface, and the surrounding skin at least twice daily, and more often in patients with localized or generalized edema

V Verify that all nursing staff have been taught how to correctly use and secure the medical devices and understand that mucosal MEDICAL device-related pressure injuries must be counted and tracked separately from skin pressure injuries

I Identify all medical devices on all patients, especially those most vulnerable to medical device-related injuries: critically ill patients, neonates, children, older adults, and bariatric patients

C Consider the following any time medical devices are in use:
- Does the patient still require use of the device—can it be rotated, repositioned, replaced or removed?
- Is the fit correct?
- Can a prophylactic dressing be used beneath the devices placed in high-risk areas (the nasal bridge, for example)?

E Educate all staff to look for objects that might be in the bed or chair under the patient

Used with permission by ©2017 Ayello EA, Delmore B: 2017. A version of this mnemonic was published in *Am J Nurs,* 117, 36–45.

Inadequate staffing and increased workload affect nurses' ability to perform comprehensive PI assessment. A PI risk assessment system that can reduce nurses' workload is needed. Nurse researchers in South Korea reported that an automated pressure injury risk assessment system (Auto-PIRAS), which assesses PI risk using available data and not requiring nurses to collect or input additional data, demonstrated similar predictive performance to Braden Scale assessments (Jin et al, 2017).

Interventions

The goal of prevention is to help maintain skin integrity against the various environmental, mechanical, and chemical assaults that are potential causes of breakdown. Nursing actions include eliminating friction and irritation to the skin, such as from shearing; reducing moisture so that tissues do not macerate; managing incontinence; enhancing mobility, and displacing body weight from prominent areas to facilitate circulation to the skin. The nurse should be familiar with the types of supportive surfaces so that the most effective products are used. The Support Surface Algorithm (SSA) is an evidence-based tool that helps determine a strong protocol for addressing PIs (Box 13.4). Use lifting devices to move the person rather than dragging the person during transfers and position changes. Use pillows or foam wedges so that skin surfaces do not touch and use devices that eliminate pressure on heels.

Repositioning is generally regarded as one of the most important and effective measures for preventing PI but there is no consensus on the frequency or type of repositioning most effective for individual patients. For some, 4-hour repositioning may be adequate while for others even hourly repositioning would not prevent PI. Historically, 2-hour turning has been recommended regardless of the individual need. Hampton (2017) argues that this recommendation originated from Florence Nightingale who recognized the importance of repositioning when caring for soldiers in the Crimean War. She did not stipulate the timing but it took 2 hours to work round the large ward from bed one and back to bed one. Hence the myth of 2-hourly turns was born.

Techniques for proper positioning include using a 30-degree side-lying position and avoiding head of bed elevation, as well as adequate support surfaces. Repositioning guidelines must also be followed when the patient is on a pressure-redistributing mattress. Continuous bedside pressure mapping (CBPM) devices (Fig. 13.6) enable caregivers and patients to visualize, assess, and monitor pressure points between the patient and the support surface. The pressure sensing map measures pressure from thousands of discrete points and the variations across the patient's body are depicted on a monitor using a color scheme to help visualize high (red) to low (blue) pressure

points. CBPM devices need further research but several studies reported improvement in PI prevention efforts (increased PI prevention activities and reduced interface pressure) (Hultin et al, 2017; Scott and Thurman, 2014). CBPM devices are considered an adjunct to PI prevention activities such as eliminating moisture; reducing pressure, shear, and friction; and improving nutrition.

Other important PI interventions include ensuring adequate fluid and food intake and providing PI prevention education programs to all levels of health care providers, patients, families, and caregivers.

> ⚡ **SAFETY ALERT**
> Individuals placed on pressure redistribution mattresses continue to need turning and repositioning according to an individualized schedule.

Consultation with the nutritional team is important. Nutritional intake should be monitored, along with the serum albumin, hematocrit, and hemoglobin levels. Caloric, protein, vitamin, and/or mineral supplementation can be considered if there is evidence of deficiencies of these nutrients. Routine use of higher than the recommended daily allowance of vitamin C and zinc for the prevention and/or treatment of PIs is not supported by evidence (Jamshed and Schneider, 2010). The nurse promotes nutritional health by ensuring that the person receives adequate assistance with eating and that dining time is a pleasant experience for the person (Chapter 14). PI prevention education programs need to be provided to all levels of health care providers, patients, families, and caregivers.

Pressure Injury Assessment

PIs are assessed with each dressing change and repeated on a weekly, biweekly, and as-needed basis. The purpose is to specifically and carefully evaluate the effectiveness of treatment.

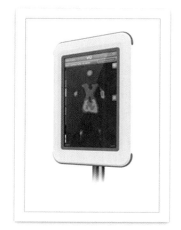
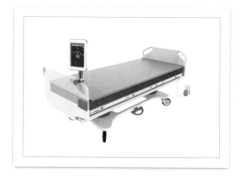

Fig. 13.6 Continuous Bedside Pressure Mapping (CBPM) Devices. (Used with permission from Wellsense, Inc.)

The PUSH tool (Pressure Ulcer Scale for Healing) (Box 13.4) provides a detailed form that covers all aspects of assessment but contains only three items and takes a short time to complete. Photographic documentation is highly recommended both at the onset of the problem and at intervals during treatment.

If there are no signs of healing from week to week or worsening of the wound is seen, then either the treatment is insufficient or the wound has become infected; in both cases, treatment must be changed. Determining the cause of the PI is important so that appropriate preventive measures can be implemented. The care team, in consultation with the individual and family, reviews the assessment and care plan and determines, if possible, if the underlying cause is reversible so that appropriate treatment decisions can be made to ensure patient comfort. Consultation with a wound care specialist is advisable for wounds that are extensive or nonhealing. Specialized nurses such as enterostomal therapists or nurse practitioners, who may work with wound centers or surgeons, provide consultation in nursing homes, offices, or clinics.

Pressure Injury Dressings

The type of dressing selected is based on careful assessment of the condition of the PI; the presence of granulation, necrotic tissue, and slough; the amount of drainage; the microbial status; and the quality of the surrounding skin. If the wound has necrotic tissue, it must be debrided. Debridement methods include mechanical (whirlpool, wet-to-dry); sharp (scalpel, scissors); enzymatic (collagenase); and autolytic (hydrocolloid, hydrogel). Wound cleansing should be done with nontoxic preparations; normal saline is recommended. Other principles are presented in Box 13.15. The NPUAP *Prevention and Treatment of Pressure Ulcers Clinical Practice Guidelines* (2017) provides guidance on selection of appropriate wound dressings based on wound characteristics. Box 13.16 presents general guidelines for PI dressings.

There are many PI products and devices available but little research evidence regarding whether particular wound dressings or topical treatments and devices have a beneficial impact on wound healing, even compared with basic dressings (Westby et al, 2017). Quality research is needed on the effectiveness of the most widely used dressings and should include time to healing and whether healing occurs. Cost-effectiveness should also be considered. Although further research is needed, the use of prophylactic multilayer silicone foam dressings, particularly on the heel and sacrum, can help in the prevention of PIs and shear and friction injuries and improve the microclimate of the skin. Prophylactic dressings must be considered an adjunct treatment to be used alongside standard pressure relieving measures (Al-Majid et al, 2017; Cornish, 2017; Padula, 2017; Ramundo et al, 2018).

Other general categories of wound care – related devices include compression therapy devices; off-weighting devices

BOX 13.15 Mnemonic for Pressure Injury Treatment: DIPAMOPI

D Debride
I   Identify and treat infection
P Pack dead space lightly
A Absorb excess exudate
M Maintain moist wound surface
O Open or excise closed wound edges
P Protect healing wound from infection/trauma
I   Insulate to maintain normal temperature

BOX 13.16 Factors to Consider in Selecting Pressure Injury Dressings

- Shallow, dry wounds with no/minimal exudate need hydrating dressings that add or trap moisture; very shallow wounds require cover dressing only (gels/transparent adhesive dressings, thin hydrocolloid, thin polyurethane foam, wound gel to add moisture).
- Shallow wounds with moderate to large exudate need dressings that absorb exudate, maintain moist surface, support autolysis if necrotic tissue present, protect and insulate, and protect surrounding tissue (hydrocolloids, semipermeable polyurethane foam, calcium alginates, silicone-type foam). Cover with an absorptive cover dressing.
- Deep wounds with moderate to large exudate require filling of dead space, absorption of exudate, maintenance of moist environment, support of autolysis if necrotic tissue present, protection, and insulation (copolymer starch, dextranomer beads, calcium alginates, foam cavity). Cover with gauze pad, abdominal dressing (ABD), transparent thin film, or polyurethane foam.

(off-loading); adjunctive therapies such as electrical stimulation and ultrasound and hyperbaric oxygen therapy (HBOT); negative pressure wound therapy (NPWT); and pressure redistribution surfaces (specialty beds, support surfaces). An evidence-based approach is recommended in the selection and prescription of equipment to prevent and manage wounds. Levine (2017b) comments that NPWT is an expensive cure-oriented treatment that is frequently overused in situations where treatment is hopeless. Health professionals need to consult reviews such as the Cochrane Review and clinical practice guidelines such as those from NPUAP when determining the most appropriate device or treatment (Krasner et al, 2017). Specific product information can also be found at www.woundsource.com (Box 13.4).

Provision of education to patients, families, and professional staff must also be included in any skin care program. Patient and family needs must be integrated into the plan of care. Teach the individual and his or her family about the normal healing process and keep them informed about progress (or lack of progress) toward healing, including signs and symptoms that should be brought to the professional's attention and education about any devices used.

KEY CONCEPTS

- The skin is the largest and most visible organ of the body; it has multiple roles in maintaining one's health.
- Maintaining adequate oral hydration and skin lubrication will reduce the incidence of xerosis and other skin problems.
- The best way to minimize the risk of skin cancer is to avoid prolonged sun exposure.
- The primary risk factors for PI development are immobility and reduced activity.
- Changes in the skin with age, comorbid illnesses, nutritional status, low body mass, shear, and friction also increase PI risk. Individuals at greatest risk include those who are confined to a bed or chair and unable to shift weight or reposition themselves.

- Structured protocols and prevention bundles should be present in all facilities and have been shown to reduce PI development.
- A PI is documented by stage, which reflects the greatest degree of tissue damage, and as it heals, reverse staging is not appropriate.
- A PI covered in dead tissue (eschar or slough) cannot be staged until it is debrided.
- Darkly pigmented skin will not display the "typical" erythema of a stage 1 PI or early DTI; therefore, close vigilance is necessary.

NURSING STUDY: SKIN CHANGES

James is an 84-year-old black male admitted to the hospital for surgical repair of a fractured right hip. He lives alone and his neighbors found him lying on his bathroom floor around 8 p.m. James told them he had been lying there since the afternoon but could not reach the phone to call for help and was unable to move. James has a history of hypertension and diabetes.

As the nurse is performing an assessment on the second postoperative day, he documents an area on James's right heel that is purplish in color and appears to be a bruise. The area is cooler to touch than the surrounding skin. There is no redness and there are no open areas; James denies any pain in the heel.

On the basis of the nursing study, develop a nursing care plan using the following procedure[a]:

- List the subjective data.
- List information that provides objective data.

- From these data, identify and state, using an accepted format, two nursing diagnoses you determine are most significant at this time.
- Determine and state outcome criteria for each diagnosis. These must reflect some alleviation of the problem identified in the nursing diagnosis and must be stated in concrete and measurable terms.
- Plan and state one or more interventions for each diagnosed problem. Provide specific documentation of the source used to determine the appropriate intervention.
- Evaluate the success of the intervention. Interventions must correlate directly with the stated outcome criteria to measure the outcome success.

[a]Students are advised to refer to their nursing diagnosis text and identify possible or potential problems.

CRITICAL THINKING QUESTIONS AND ACTIVITIES

1. What risk factors for PI are present in the nursing study presented above?
2. How does skin color affect the presentation of DTI?
3. What areas of the body are susceptible to PI development and why?
4. What education needs to be provided to the patient, staff, and family?
5. When James returns home, what interventions to enhance his safety would be appropriate?

RESEARCH QUESTIONS

1. What is the most effective strategy to inform younger people about the risk of skin cancer from sun and tanning bed exposure?
2. What is the knowledge level of older individuals about PI risk?
3. What are the major barriers identified by nursing staff to implementation of preventive interventions for PIs?
4. How effective are current patient education materials in enhancing knowledge of PI risk among racially and culturally diverse older individuals?

REFERENCES

Alderden J, Cummins MR, Pepper GA, et al: Midrange Braden subscale scores are associated with increased risk for pressure injury development among critical care patients, *J Wound Ostomy Continence Nurs* 44(5):420–428, 2017.

Al-Majid S, Vuncanon B, Carlson N, Rakovski C: The effect of offloading heels on sacral pressure, *AORN J* 106(3):194–200, 2017.

Agency for Healthcare Research and Quality (AHQR) Safety Program for Nursing Homes: *On-time pressure ulcer prevention*, Rockville, MD. Content last reviewed November 2014, Agency for Healthcare Research and Quality. http://www.ahrq.gov/professionals/systems/long-term-care/resources/ontime/pruprev/pruprev-intro.html. Accessed March 2019.

Ayello EA, Zulkowski K, Capezuti E, Jicman WH, Sibbald RG: Educating nurses in the United States about pressure injuries, *Adv Skin Wound Care* 30(2):83–94, 2017.

Balzer K, Kottner J: Evidence-based practices in pressure ulcer prevention: lost in implementation? *Int J Nurs Stud* 52(11):1655–1658, 2015.

Black JM, Edsberg LE, Baharestani MM, et al: Pressure ulcers: avoidable or unavoidable? Results of the National Pressure Ulcer Advisory Panel Consensus Conference, *Ostomy Wound Manage* 57(2):24–37, 2011.

Centers for Disease Control and Prevention: *Shingles (herpes zoster)*, 2017. https://www.cdc.gov/shingles/index.html. Accessed January 2018.

Centers for Medicare & Medicaid Services: *CMS manual system*, Publication No. 100-07 State Operations Manual, Baltimore, MD, 2004, Author.

Chaboyer W, Bucknall T, Webster J, et al: The effect of a patient centred care bundle intervention on pressure ulcer incidence (INTACT): a cluster randomised trial, *Int J Nurs Stud* 64:63–71, 2016.

Cheung C: Older adults, falls, and skin integrity, *Adv Skin Wound Care* 30(1):40–46, 2017.

Chou R: Pressure ulcer risk assessment and prevention, *Ann Intern Med* 159(1):28–38, 2013.

Cornish L: The use of prophylactic dressings in the prevention of pressure ulcers: a literature review, *Br J Community Nurs* 22 (Suppl 6):S26–S32, 2017.

Delmore BA, Ayello EA: Pressure injuries caused by medical devices and other objects: a clinical update, *Am J Nurs* 117(12):36–45, 2017.

Edsberg LE, Langemo D, Baharestani MM, Posthauer ME, Goldberg M: Unavoidable pressure injury: state of the science and consensus outcomes, *J Wound Ostomy Continence Nurs* 41(4):313–314, 2014.

Endo J, Norman R: Skin problems. In Ham R, Sloane P, Warshaw G, Potter J, Flaherty E, editors: *Ham's primary care geriatrics,* ed 6, Philadelphia, PA, 2014, Elsevier Saunders, pp 573–587.

Garrett C, Saavedra A, Reed K, et al: Increasing incidence of melanoma among middle-aged adults: an epidemiological study in Olmsted County, Minnesota, *Mayo Clin Proc* 89(1):52–59, 2014.

Garrigues LJ, Cartwright JC, Bliss DZ: Attitudes of nursing students about pressure injury prevention, *J Wound Ostomy Continence Nurs* 44(2):123–128, 2017.

Gillespie BM, Chaboyer W, Sykes M, O'Brien J, Brandis S: Development and pilot testing of a patient-participatory pressure ulcer prevention care bundle, *J Nurs Care Qual* 29(1):74–82, 2014.

Hampton S: Could lateral tilt mattresses be the answer to pressure ulcer prevention and management? *Br J Community Nurs* 22(Suppl 3):S6– S12, 2017.

Harms S, Bliss DZ, Garrard J, et al: Prevalence of pressure ulcers by race and ethnicity for older adults admitted to nursing homes, *J Gerontol Nurs* 40(3):20–26, 2014.

Hultin L, Olsson E, Carli C, Gunningberg L: Pressure mapping in elderly care: a tool to increase pressure injury knowledge and awareness among staff, *J Wound Ostomy Continence Nurs* 44(2):142–147, 2017.

Irvin C, Sedlak E, Walton C, Collier S, Bernhofer EI: Hospital-acquired pressure injuries: the significance of the advanced practice registered nurse's role in a community hospital, *J Am Assoc Nurse Pract* 29(4):203–208, 2017.

Jamshed N, Schneider E: Is the use of supplemental vitamin C and zinc for the prevention and treatment of pressure ulcers evidence-based? *Ann Longterm Care* 18:28–32, 2010.

Jin Y, Jin T, Lee SM: Automated pressure injury risk assessment system incorporated into an electronic health record system, *Nurs Res* 66(6):462–472, 2017.

Jull A, Griffiths P: Is pressure sore prevention a sensitive indicator of the quality of nursing care? A cautionary note, *Int J Nurs Stud* 47:531–533, 2010.

Krasner D, Sibbald R, Woo K, Norton L: Interprofessional perspectives on individualized wound device product selection, *Wound Source, White Paper,* 2017. http://www.woundsource.com/whitepaper/interprofessional-perspectives-individualized-wound-device-product-selection?page=show. Accessed January 2018.

LeBlanc K, Baranoski S: Skin tears: finally recognized, *Adv Skin Wound Care* 30(2):62–63, 2017.

LeBlanc K, Baranoski S, Christensen D, et al: The art of dressing selection: a consensus statement on skin tears and best practice, *Adv Skin Wound Care* 29(1):32–46, 2016.

LeBlanc K, Baranoski S, Christensen D, et al: International Skin Tear Advisory Panel: a tool kit to aid in the prevention, assessment, and treatment of skin tears using a Simplified Classification System©, *Adv Skin Wound Care* 26:459–476, 2013.

Levine JM: *Skin failure: a new paradigm*, GeriPal, 2017a. http://www.geripal.org/2017/10/skin-failure-new-paradigm.html. Accessed January 2018.

Levine JM: *Palliative wound care: a new frontier*, GeriPal, 2017b. http://www.geripal.org/2017/09/palliative-wound-care-new-frontier.html. Accessed January 2018.

McCance KL, Huether SE: Structure, function, and disorders of the integument. In McCance KL, Huether SE, editors: *Pathophysiology,* ed 7, St Louis, MO, 2014, Elsevier, pp 1616–1651.

Miller DM, Neelon L, Kish-Smith K, Whitney L, Burant CJ: Pressure injury knowledge in critical care nurses, *J Wound Ostomy Continence Nurs* 44(5):455–457, 2017.

Murphree RW: Impairments in skin integrity, *Nurs Clin North Am* 52:405–417, 2017.

National Pressure Ulcer Advisory Panel: *National Pressure Ulcer Advisory Panel (NPUAP) announces a change in terminology from pressure ulcer to pressure injury and updates the stages of pressure injury,* 2016. http://www.npuap.org/national-pressure-ulcer-advisory-panel-npuap-announces-a-change-in-terminology-from-pressure-ulcer-to-pressure-injury-and-updates-the-stages-of-pressure-injury/. Accessed January 2018.

National Pressure Ulcer Advisory Panel: *PUSH tool,* 2014. http://www.npuap.org/resources/educational-and-clinical-resources/push-tool/. Accessed January 2018.

National Pressure Ulcer Advisory Panel: *NPUAP position statement on staging—2017 clarifications,* 2017. http://www.npuap.org/wp-content/uploads/2012/01/NPUAP-Position-Statement-on-Staging-Jan-2017.pdf. Accessed January 2017.

Olsho LE, Spector WD, Williams CS, et al: Evaluation of AHRQ's on-time pressure ulcer prevention program: a facilitator-assisted clinical decision support intervention for nursing homes, *Med Care* 52(3):258–266, 2014.

Ong EL, Goldacre R, Hoang U, Sinclair R, Goldacre M: Subsequent primary malignancies in patients with nonmelanoma skin cancer in England: a national record-linkage study, *Cancer Epidemiol Biomarkers Prev* 23:490–498, 2014.

Padula WW: Effectiveness and value of prophylactic 5-layer foam sacral dressings to prevent hospital-acquired pressure injuries in acute care hospitals: an observational cohort study, *J Wound Ostomy Continence Nurs* 44(5):413–419, 2017.

Ramundo J, Pike C, Pittman J: Do prophylactic foam dressings reduce heel pressure injuries? *J Wound Ostomy Continence Nurs* 45(1):75–82, 2018.

Roberts S, Wallis M, McInnes E, et al: Patients' perceptions of a pressure ulcer prevention care bundle in hospital: a qualitative descriptive study to guide evidence-based practice, *Worldviews Evid Based Nurs* 14(5):385–393, 2017.

Rondinelli J, Zuniga S, Kipnis P, Kawar LN, Liu V, Escobar GJ: Hospital-acquired pressure injury: risk-adjusted comparisons in an integrated healthcare delivery system, *Nurs Res* 67(1):16–25, 2018.

Schmitt S, Andries MK, Ashmore PM, Brunette G, Judge K, Bonham PA: WOCN Society position paper: avoidable versus unavoidable pressure ulcers/injuries, *J Wound Ostomy Continence Nurs* 44(5):458–468, 2017.

Scott RG, Thurman KM: Visual feedback of continuous bedside pressure mapping to optimize effective patient repositioning, *Adv Wound Care* 3(5):376–382, 2014.

Skin Cancer Foundation: *Skin cancer facts & statistics,* 2017. https://www.skincancer.org/skin-cancer-information/skin-cancer-facts. Accessed January 2018.

Spilsbury K, Nelson A, Cullum N, Iglesias C, Nixon J, Mason S: Pressure ulcers and their treatment and effects on quality of life: hospital inpatient perspectives, *J Adv Nurs* 57:494–504, 2007.

Warner-Maron I: The risk of risk assessment: pressure ulcer assessment and the Braden Scale, *Ann Longterm Care* 23(5):23–27, 2015.

Westby MJ, Dumville JC, Soares MO, Stubbs N, Norman G: Dressings and topical agents for treating pressure ulcers, *Cochrane Database of Syst Rev,* 2017. http://www.cochrane.org/CD011947/WOUNDS_which-dressings-or-topical-agents-are-most-effective-healing-pressure-ulcers. Accessed January 2018.

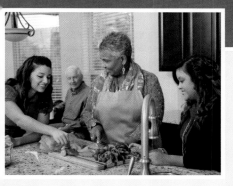

14

Nutrition

Theris A. Touhy

http://evolve.elsevier.com/Touhy/TwdHlthAging

A STUDENT SPEAKS

I work as a certified nursing assistant in a skilled nursing facility and I am responsible for feeding 10 residents at the dinner meal. I try to get them to eat but they eat very slowly and we only have a limited amount of time. Sometimes, I end up just mixing the food and getting them to take a few spoonfuls. The people with dementia need even more time and I know that they are not getting enough to eat. It makes me feel terrible and we need so much more help to do a good job.

Marcia, age 21

AN OLDER ADULT SPEAKS

If I do reach the point where I can no longer feed myself, I hope that the hands holding my fork belong to someone who has a feeling for who I am. I hope my helper will remember what she learns about me and that her awareness of me will grow from one encounter to another. Why should this make a difference? Yet I am certain that my experience of needing to be fed will be altered if it occurs in the context of my being truly known . . . I will want to know about the lives of the people I rely on, especially the one who holds my fork for me. If she would talk to me, if we could laugh together, I might even forget the chagrin of my useless hands. We would have a conversation, rather than a feeding.

From Lustbader W: Thoughts on the meaning of frailty, Generations 13:21–22, 1999.

LEARNING OBJECTIVES

On completion of this chapter, the reader will be able to:

1. Discuss nutritional requirements and factors affecting nutrition for older adults.
2. Delineate risk factors for undernutrition and identify strategies for management.
3. Describe a nutritional screening and assessment.
4. Identify evidence-based strategies to ensure adequate nutrition.
5. Describe special considerations in ensuring adequate nutrition for individuals experiencing hospitalization and institutionalization.
6. Discuss assessment and interventions for older adults with dysphagia.
7. Develop a plan of care to assist an older adult in developing and maintaining good nutritional status.

Adequate and affordable food supplies and improved nutrition are concerns worldwide with some differences between developed and developing countries. Although issues vary among different areas of the globe, nutrition as a major contributor to health is a significant concern for all nations. The link between healthy eating patterns and healthy aging is well documented. The quality and quantity of diet are important factors in preventing, delaying the onset of, and managing chronic illnesses associated with aging. About half of all American adults have one or more preventable diet-related chronic diseases, including cardiovascular disease, type 2 diabetes, and overweight and obesity (U.S. Department of Health and Human Services [USDHHS] and U.S. Department of Agriculture [USDA], 2015–2020).

Proper nutrition means that all of the essential nutrients (i.e., carbohydrates, fat, protein, vitamins, minerals, and water) are adequately supplied and used to maintain optimal health and wellness. Although some age-related changes in the gastrointestinal (GI) system do occur (Box 14.1), these changes are

BOX 14.1 Aging-Related Changes Affecting Nutrition

Taste

Individuals have varied levels of taste sensitivity that seem predetermined by genetics, constitution, and age variations

The number of taste cells decreases and the remaining cells atrophy as individuals age (beginning at age 40 to 60), but they can regenerate. Lag time in regeneration may contribute to diminished taste response

Mouth produces less saliva, which can affect sense of taste

Usually salty and sweet tastes lost first, followed by bitter and sour

Dentures, smoking, and medications can affect taste

Smell

Gradual decline in number of sensor cells that detect aromas and in nerves that carry signals to the brain and in olfactory bulb that processes them; less mucus produced in nose

Increase in odor threshold and decline in odor identification

Many factors affect smell: nasal sinus disease, injury to olfactory receptors through viral infections, damage from industrial work before proper safety standards/equipment in place, smoking, medications, periodontal disease/dental problems

Changes in smell associated with Alzheimer's and Parkinson's diseases

Smelling food while it is cooking and participation in preparation can stimulate appetite

Digestive System

Changes do not significantly affect function; digestive system remains adequate throughout life

Decreased gastric motility and volume and reductions in secretion of bicarbonate and gastric mucus caused by age-related gastric atrophy, which results in hypochlorhydria (insufficient hydrochloric acid)

Decreased production of intrinsic factor can lead to pernicious anemia if stomach is not able to use ingested B_{12} vitamins

Protective alkaline viscous mucus of stomach lost because of increase in stomach pH, making stomach more susceptible to *Helicobacter pylori* infection and peptic ulcer disease, particularly with use of nonsteroidal antiinflammatory drugs

Presbyesophagus (decrease in intensity of propulsive waves) may occur, forcing the lower end to dilate and may lead to digestive discomfort

Pathological processes seen with increasing frequency include gastroesophageal reflux disease (GERD) and hiatal hernia

Loss of smooth muscle in stomach delays emptying time, which may lead to anorexia or weight loss as a result of distention, meal-induced fullness, and premature satiety

Buccal Cavity

Teeth become worn, darker in color, prone to longitudinal cracks

Dentin becomes brittle and thick; pulp space decreases

Osteopenia of the facial bones and subtle changes to the connective tissues of the skin, sinuses, and oral cavity

Xerostomia (dry mouth) occurs in 30% of older individuals and can affect eating, swallowing, and speaking and lead to dental decay. More than 500 medications can affect salivary flow; artificial saliva preparations and adequate fluid intake can help

Regulation of Appetite

Appetite depends on physical activity, functional limitations, smell, taste, mood, socialization, comfort, medications, chronic illness, oral/dental problems

Individuals may be less hungry, fuller before meals, consume smaller meals, become more satiated following meal

Gastrointestinal hormones such as cholecystokinin (CCK) regulate satiety to varying degrees. With age, CCK is increased basally and following a meal and may have a more potent satiating effect. Disease states increase cytokine levels as a result of release by diseased tissues. Increase in CCK levels also occurs in malnutrition, which further decreases appetite

Endogenous opioid feeding and drinking drive may decline and contribute to decreased appetite and dehydration

Decreased stomach fundal compliance, decreased testosterone, and increased leptin and amylin also thought to contribute to decreased appetite

Ability to feed self/staff feeding techniques, and mealtime ambience also affect appetite

Body Composition

Increase in body fat, including visceral fat stores

Decrease in muscle mass

Body weight usually peaks fifth or sixth decade of life and remains stable until age 65 or 70, after which there is a slow decrease in body weight for remainder of life

rarely the primary factors in inadequate nutrition. Fulfillment of nutritional needs in older adults is more often affected by numerous other factors, including chronic disease, lifelong eating habits, ethnicity, socialization, income, transportation, housing, mood, food knowledge, functional impairments, health, and dentition.

This chapter discusses the dietary needs of older adults, the risk factors contributing to inadequate nutrition, and the effects of obesity, diseases, functional and cognitive impairments, and dysphagia on nutrition. Several conditions warrant further discussion because they are frequently encountered in older adults and are related to adequate diet and nutritional status. Dehydration and oral health are discussed in Chapter 15 and the effect of neurocognitive disorders on nutrition is discussed in Chapter 29. Readers are referred to a nutrition text for more comprehensive information on nutrition and aging and disease.

AGE-RELATED REQUIREMENTS

United States Dietary Guidelines

The *2015–2020 Dietary Guidelines for Americans*, published by the federal government, are designed to help individuals ages 2 years and older and their families consume a healthy, nutritionally adequate diet. The Guidelines are used in developing federal food, nutrition, and health programs and policies. Eating patterns and their food and nutrient characteristics are a focus of the newest Guideline. Five overarching Guidelines are provided that encourage healthy eating patterns, recognize that individuals will need to make shifts in their food and beverage choices to achieve a healthy pattern, and acknowledge that all segments of our society have a role to play in supporting healthy choices. The Guidelines provide an adaptable framework in which individuals can enjoy foods that meet their personal, cultural, and traditional preferences and fit within their budget (Box 14.2) (USDA and USDHHS, 2015–2020). *Healthy People 2020* also provides goals for nutrition (Healthy People 2020 box).

 HEALTHY PEOPLE 2020

Nutrition and Weight Status

- Promote health and reduce chronic disease through the consumption of healthful diets and achievement and maintenance of body weight.
- Increase the proportion of primary care physicians who regularly measure the body mass index in their adult patients.
- Increase the proportion of physician office visits made by adult patients who are obese that include counseling or education related to weight reduction, nutrition, or physical activity.
- Increase the proportion of adults who are at a healthy weight.
- Reduce household food insecurity and in so doing reduce hunger.

Data from U.S. Department of Health and Human Services, Office of Disease Prevention and Health Promotion: *Healthy People 2020*, 2012. http://www.healthypeople.gov/2020.

MyPlate for Older Adults

Choose MyPlate is a visual depiction of daily food intake. The USDA Human Nutrition Research Center on Aging at Tufts University provides a *MyPlate for Older Adults* emphasizing the nutritional needs of older adults in a framework based on the *2015–2020 Dietary Guidelines for Americans* (Fig. 14.1). The *MyPlate for Older Adults* depicts a colorful plate composed of approximately 50% fruits and vegetables; 25% grains, many of which are whole grains; and 25% protein-rich foods such as nuts, beans, fish, lean meat, poultry, and fat-free and low-fat dairy products such as milk, cheeses, and yogurts. Images of good sources of fluids, heart-healthy fats such as vegetable oils and soft margarines; and herbs and spices to be used in place of salt to lower sodium intake are also included (Tufts University, 2016).

Generally, older adults have lower energy requirements and need fewer calories because they may not be as active and metabolic rates decline. However, they still require the same or higher levels of nutrients for optimal health outcomes. The recommendations may need modification for individuals who have illnesses. The Dietary Approaches to Stop Hypertension (DASH) eating plan is a recommended eating plan to assist with maintenance of optimal weight and management of hypertension. This

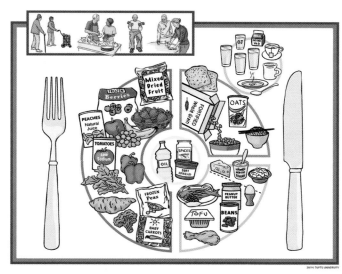

Fig. 14.1 MyPlate for Older Adults. (From the Jean Mayer USDA Human Nutrition Research Center on Aging, Tufts University: *MyPlate for older adults*, 2011. http://hnrca.tufts.edu/myplate/.)

plan consists of fruits, vegetables, whole grains, low-fat dairy products, poultry, fish, and restriction of salt intake.

The Mediterranean diet (MedDiet) has also been associated both with a lower incidence of chronic illness, weight gain, and impaired physical function and with improved cognition. This diet is characterized by a greater intake of fruits, vegetables, legumes, whole grains, and fish; a lower intake of red and processed meats; higher amounts of monosaturated fats, mostly provided by olive oil from Mediterranean countries; and lower amounts of saturated fats. The MIND (Mediterranean-DASH diet Intervention for Neurodegeneration Delay) combines the MedDiet with the DASH diet. In a large representative sample of older adults, greater adherence to the MedDiet and the MIND diet was independently associated with better cognitive function and lower risk of cognitive impairment. Further research and clinical trials are needed to understand the role of dietary patterns in cognitive aging and brain disease (McEvoy et al, 2017) (Box 14.3).

Other Dietary Recommendations

Fats

Similar to other age groups, older adults should limit intake of saturated fat and trans fatty acids. High-fat diets cause obesity and increase the risk of heart disease and cancer. Less than 10% of calories per day should come from saturated fats.

Protein

The current protein reference nutrient intake (RNI) is 0.8 g protein/kg body weight in healthy adults of all ages. However, emerging evidence-based studies suggest that an increased protein intake may be beneficial to fulfill the needs of vulnerable older adults, particularly those with chronic disease. Additionally, additional protein, calcium, and vitamin D are recommended to prevent bone loss and maintain existing bone density, thereby reducing the risk of falls and fractures (Chapter 26). Intakes above the RNI of certain nutrients, such as protein, vitamin D, and antioxidants, vitamin E, and selenium, are associated with beneficial effects on physical function and prevention of chronic diseases in older age (Baugreet et al, 2017). Older adults who are ill are the most likely segment of society to experience protein deficiency. Those with limitations affecting their ability to shop, cook, and consume food are also at risk for protein deficiency and malnutrition.

Fiber

Fiber is an important dietary component that some older adults do not consume in sufficient quantities. A daily intake of 25 g of fiber is recommended and must be combined with adequate amounts of fluid. Insufficient amounts of fiber in the diet, and insufficient fluids, contribute to constipation. Fiber is the indigestible material that gives plants their structure. It is abundant in raw fruits and vegetables and in unrefined grains and cereals (Box 14.4).

Vitamins and Minerals

Older adults who consume five servings of fruits and vegetables daily will obtain adequate intake of vitamins A, C, and E and also potassium. However, Americans of all ages eat less than half of the recommended amounts of fruits and vegetables. Vitamin B_{12} plays a key role in antiaging but 50% of adults over the age of 50 years are deficient. Vitamin B_{12} deficiency is a common and underrecognized condition (Hooshmand et al, 2016). After age 50, the stomach produces less gastric acid, which makes vitamin B_{12} absorption less efficient. Older adults should increase their intake of the crystalline form of vitamin B_{12} from fortified foods such as whole-grain breakfast cereals. Other food sources include salmon, tuna, grass-fed beef, sardines, eggs, and cottage cheese. Individuals who take proton pump inhibitors (e.g., Prilosec, Prevacid) show increased risk of vitamin B_{12} deficiency by as much as 65% when these medications are taken for 2 years. Individuals consuming a vegetarian diet and those with some form of weight-loss surgery are also more likely to be low in the vitamin.

OBESITY (OVERNUTRITION)

Most of the world's population live in countries where overweight and obesity kills more people than underweight. Every country, except for those in sub-Saharan Africa, faces alarming obesity rates that have risen 82% since 2000. In the United States, approximately 35% of adults over 60 years are obese, with a higher prevalence in women (38%) than men (32%) (Gretebeck et al, 2017). Since the 1990s, the prevalence of older adults who are obese has doubled. Overweight and obesity are associated with increased health care costs, functional impairments, disability, chronic disease, and nursing home admission. Obesity is a major risk factor for the most common disabling conditions—osteoarthritis, atherosclerosis, diabetes, and stroke (Kritchevsky, 2017).

The World Health Organisation (WHO) (2017) defines overweight and obesity as follows: overweight is a body mass index (BMI) greater than or equal to 25; obesity is a BMI greater than or equal to 30. However, there is no consensus about the best way to measure obesity in the older population. Normal changes in body composition may make BMI less

---

BOX 14.4 Tips for Best Practice

Teaching About Fiber in the Diet

Benefits of Fiber

- Facilitates absorption of water; helps control weight by delaying gastric emptying and providing feeling of fullness; improves glucose tolerance; prevents or reduces constipation, hemorrhoids, diverticulosis; reduces risk of heart disease; protects against cancer

Diet Tips to Add Fiber

- Best to get fiber from food rather than supplements because they do not contain essential nutrients found in high-fiber foods and anticancer benefits are questionable; the more refined or processed the food becomes, the lower the fiber content (e.g., apple with peel higher fiber than applesauce or juice)
- Increase consumption of fresh fruits and vegetables; eat dry beans, peas, and lentils; leave skin on fruits and vegetables; eat whole fruit rather than drink juice; eat whole-grain breads and cereals; add finely chopped veggies to pasta sauce, soups, and casseroles; add a cup of spinach or other leafy greens

to a smoothie (you will not taste the spinach at all but your drink will be green); sprinkle unsweetened bran on cereals or put in soups, meat loaf, or casseroles

- Some foods naturally high in fiber: large pear with skin (7 g); 1 cup fresh raspberries (8 g); 1/2 medium avocado (5 g); 1 oz almonds (3.5 g); 1/4 cup cooked black beans (7.5 g); 3 cups air-popped popcorn (3.6 g); 1 cup cooked pearled barley (6 g)

How Much Bran?

- Generally one to two tablespoons daily; begin with one teaspoon and increase gradually to avoid bloating, gas, diarrhea, other colon discomforts

How Much Fluid?

- 64 oz daily unless fluid restriction

accurate. Fat mass increases with age and lean mass decreases, BMI underestimates total adiposity. Additionally, most older adults also decline in height, resulting in overall overestimation of obesity.

Although there is strong evidence that obesity in younger people decreases life expectancy and has a negative effect on functionality and morbidity, less is known about the benefits and risks of obesity in older adults compared to children and adults. Older adults who are overweight or obese do not have the same risk of morbidity and mortality as younger individuals, particularly if obesity develops late in life. In what has been termed the *obesity paradox,* some research has found that for people who have survived to 70 years of age, mortality risk is lowest in those with a BMI classified as overweight (Kalish, 2016). Higher BMI is associated with an increased risk for osteoarthritis, diabetes, and disability but when weight gain occurs in late life, there is less time to impose metabolic and cardiovascular health risks. Obesity may protect against bone density loss and hip fracture and for frail older adults with severely decreased functional status, obesity may be regarded as a protective factor with regard to functionality and mortality (Kalish, 2016).

Further research is needed to understand how long-term intentional weight loss and associated shifts in body composition affect the onset of chronic disease (Bowman et al, 2017). Weight loss recommendations for older adults should be carefully considered on an individualized basis with attention to the weight history and medical conditions. A critical goal is to maintain or increase quality of life and physical function. Since weight loss is accompanied by a decline in free fat mass, activities to maintain muscle strength such as progressive resistance training, should be included in all weight loss plans for older adults. Maintaining a healthy weight throughout life can prevent many illnesses and functional limitations as a person grows older.

MALNUTRITION (UNDERNUTRITION)

Malnutrition is a recognized geriatric syndrome. The most common definition of malnutrition is too little or too much energy, protein, and nutrients, which can cause adverse effects on a person's body and its function and clinical outcomes. Malnutrition happens when a person has an imbalance between the nutrients they need and those that they receive and can result from overnutrition and undernutrition. The rising incidence of malnutrition among older adults has been documented in acute care, long-term care, and the community.

Hospital malnutrition is estimated to affect as many as one in two patients at admission, while many others develop malnutrition throughout hospitalization (Avelino-Silva and Jaluul, 2017). Up to 50% of older adult patients are malnourished when discharged from the hospital. Malnutrition is estimated to occur in up to 15% of community-dwelling older adults, 20% to 60% of hospitalized older adults, and 30% to 85% of those living in nursing homes. These figures are expected to rise dramatically in the next 30 years with the aging of the population. Those at greatest risk are older women, minorities, and people who are poor or live in rural areas. Being 75 years of age and older is an independent risk factor for poor nutrition (Crogan, 2017; Tilly, 2017). Malnutrition among older adults is clearly a serious challenge for health professionals in all settings.

Characteristics

The understanding of malnutrition is evolving, and research is ongoing. Malnutrition cannot be diagnosed based on a single marker or laboratory value. Characteristics have been identified to determine malnutrition (Mueller, 2015) (Box 14.5). Malnutrition is a complex syndrome that can develop following two primary trajectories. It can occur when the individual does not consume sufficient amounts of micronutrients (i.e., vitamins, minerals, phytochemicals) and macronutrients (i.e., protein, carbohydrates, fat, water) required to maintain organ function and healthy tissues. This type of malnutrition can occur from prolonged undernutrition or overnutrition. In contrast, inflammation-related malnutrition develops as a consequence of injury, surgery, or disease states that trigger inflammatory mediators that contribute to increased metabolic rate and impaired nutrient utilization (Cederholm et al, 2017; Mogensen and DiMaria-Ghalili, 2015). No single marker has been identified to diagnose adult malnutrition of any etiology.

Inflammation is increasingly identified as an important underlying factor that increases risk for malnutrition and a contributing factor to suboptimal responses to nutritional intervention and increased risk of mortality. Weight loss frequently occurs in both trajectories but weight alone is not an indicator of nutritional status. Individuals also experience malnutrition when they take in enough calories but miss important nutrients that affect their nutritional status (Tilly, 2017). Development of a consensus approach to identifying core attributes of malnutrition that consider ethnic/racial differences, and the presence of malnutrition among obese individuals, is being developed by an international guideline committee. Because there is a wide variation in approaches to the diagnosis of malnutrition, the international guideline committee will also propose criteria for identifying malnutrition (Cederholm et al, 2017).

Consequences

Malnutrition is a precursor to frailty and has serious consequences, including infections, pressure ulcers, anemia, hypotension, impaired cognition, sarcopenia (low muscle mass associated with aging), hip fractures, prolonged hospital stay, institutionalization, increased dependence, reduced quality of

---

BOX 14.5 Characteristics of Malnutrition

For a diagnosis of malnutrition, two or more of the following characteristics must be present:

- Insufficient energy intake
- Weight loss
- Loss of muscle mass
- Loss of subcutaneous fat
- Localized or generalized fluid accumulation that may mask weight loss
- Diminished functional status as measured by handgrip strength

life and increased morbidity and mortality (Tilly, 2017). Malnourished patients are twice as likely to develop pressure injuries and three times as likely to have infections. Almost half of the patients who fall during hospitalization are reported to be malnourished. Finally, older adults who are admitted to the hospital with malnutrition are more likely to have longer hospital stays and die before discharge (Avelino-Silva and Jaluul, 2017). Many factors contribute to the occurrence of malnutrition in older adults (Box 14.6)

FACTORS AFFECTING FULFILLMENT OF NUTRITIONAL NEEDS

Lifelong Eating Habits

The nutritional state of a person reflects the individual's dietary history and present food practices. "Foodways are defined as the eating habits and culinary practices of a people, region, or historical period" (Furman, 2014, p. 80). This includes unique eating patterns of various cultural and religious groups. Foodways influence food preferences, meal expectation, and nutritional intake. Eating habits do not always coincide with fulfillment of nutritional needs and may especially affect the ability and desire to consume food that is not consistent with individual foodways. The meaning of food and mealtimes, often established in childhood, "become more poignant with age" (Furman, 2014, p. 83). The Joint Commission and Centers for Medicare and Medicaid Services (CMS) (2014) specify assessment of dietary needs and restrictions in a patient safety tool (Box 14.7).

Lifelong habits of dieting or eating fad foods also echo through the later years. Individuals may fall prey to advertisements that claim specific foods can reverse aging or rid one of chronic conditions. Following the MyPlate for Older Adults (Fig. 14.1) is best for an ideal diet, with changes based on particular problems, such as hypercholesteremia. Individuals should be counseled to base their dietary decisions on valid research and consultation with their primary care provider. For the healthy individual, essential nutrients should be obtained from food sources rather than relying on dietary supplements.

Socialization

The fundamentally social aspect of eating has to do with sharing and the feeling of belonging that it provides. All of us use food as a means of giving and receiving love, friendship, or belonging. The presence of others during meals is a significant predictor of caloric intake. The meaning and enjoyment of eating can often be challenged as one ages, requires hospitalization or nursing home residence, or experiences chronic illnesses, depression, isolation, and functional limitations. Disinterest in food may also result from the effects of medication or disease processes. Misuse and abuse of alcohol are prevalent among older adults and are growing public health concerns. Excessive drinking interferes with nutrition. Drinking alcohol depletes the body of necessary nutrients and often replaces meals, thus making an individual susceptible to malnutrition (Chapter 28).

The elderly nutrition program, authorized under Title III of the Older Americans Act (OAA), is the largest national food and nutrition program specifically for older adults. Programs and services include congregate nutrition programs, home-delivered nutrition services (Meals-on-Wheels), and nutrition screening and education. The program is not means tested, and participants may make voluntary confidential contributions for meals. The OAA does require targeting services to those in greatest social and economic need. A large percentage of program participants are likely to be socioeconomically deprived,

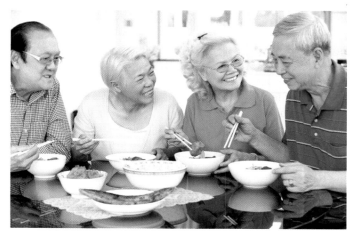

Older adults enjoying a meal together. (© iStock.com/monkeybusinessimages.)

minorities, living alone, and have disability or poor health. Home-delivered meals have been shown to be most effective in improving nutrition and other outcomes for older adults (Tilly, 2017). With the emphasis on community-based care rather than institutional care, expansion of nutrition services should be a priority.

Socioeconomic Deprivation

There is a strong relationship between poor nutrition and socioeconomic deprivation. Older adults are the fastest growing food insecure population in the United States, which means they are not sure where or how they will get their next meal. In 2016, 7.8% of all senior households were food insecure. Older adults are likely to be food insecure if they live in a southern state, have a disability, are younger than 69 years, live with a grandchild, and/or are African American or Hispanic (National Council on Aging, 2018). Individuals with low incomes may need to choose among fulfilling needs such as food, heat, telephone bills, medications, and health care visits. Some older people eat only once per day in an attempt to make their income last through the month.

The Supplemental Nutrition Assistance Program (SNAP), a program of the USDA, Food and Nutrition Services, offers nutrition assistance to eligible, socioeconomically deprived individuals and families, but older adults are less likely than any other age group to use food assistance programs. Three out of five older adults who qualify for SNAP do not participate. Some individuals may not see the benefit, and others, especially those who lived through the Great Depression, are very reluctant to accept "welfare" (Chapter 1). Low participation rates are also a result of barriers related to mobility and technology.

To enhance outreach to older adults, SNAP works with state agencies, nutrition educators, and neighborhood and faith-based organizations to assist those eligible for nutrition assistance to make informed decisions about applying for the program and accessing benefits. The National Council on Aging (NCOA), with support from the Walmart Foundation, has awarded over $2 million in grant funding to community-based organizations to assist older adults in applying for and enrolling in SNAP. NCOA's Benefits Checkup (Box 14.3) is a free online service to screen seniors with limited incomes for benefits.

Free food programs, such as donated commodities, are also available at distribution centers (food banks) for those with limited incomes. Although this is another valuable option, use of such programs is not always feasible. One takes a chance on the types of food available on any particular day or week; quantities distributed are frequently too large for the single older adult or the older couple to use or even carry from the distribution site; the site may be too far away or difficult to reach; and the time of food distribution may be inconvenient.

There are cafeterias and restaurants that provide special meal prices for older adults, but costs have risen with increases in food costs. The previous advantages of eating out have diminished. Yet many single older adults eat out for most meals. More older adults are eating at fast food restaurants that typically do not offer low-fat/low-salt menu items. Providing education about the nutritional content of fast food and other convenient ways to enhance healthy nutritional intake is important (Box 14.3).

Transportation

Available and easily accessible transportation may be limited for older adults. Many small, long-standing neighborhood food stores have been closed in the wake of the expansion of larger supermarkets, which are located in areas that serve a greater segment of the population. Small convenience stores may not have a selection of healthy foods. It may become difficult to walk to the market, to reach it by public transportation, or to carry a bag of groceries while using a cane or walker. Fear is apparent in older adults' consideration of transportation. They may fear walking in the street and being mugged, not being able to cross the street in the time it takes the traffic light to change, or being knocked down or falling as they walk in crowded streets. Despite reduced senior citizen bus fares, many older adults remain very fearful of attack when using public transportation. Functional impairments also make the use of public transportation difficult for others.

Transportation by taxicab or other transportation services may be unrealistic for an individual on a limited income, but sharing a taxicab with others who also need to shop may enable the older adult to go where food prices are cheaper and to take advantage of sale items. Senior citizen organizations in many parts of the United States have been helpful in providing older adults with van service to shopping areas. In housing complexes, it may be possible to schedule group trips to the supermarket. Many urban communities have multiple sources of transportation available, but the individual may be unaware of them. Resources in rural areas are more limited. It is important for nurses to be knowledgeable about transportation resources in the community.

In addition, many older adults, particularly widowed men, may have never learned to shop and prepare food. Often, individuals have to rely on others to shop for them, and this may be a cause of concern depending on the availability of support and the reluctance to be dependent on someone else, particularly family. For those who own a computer, shopping over the Internet and having groceries delivered offers advantages, although prices may be higher than those in the stores.

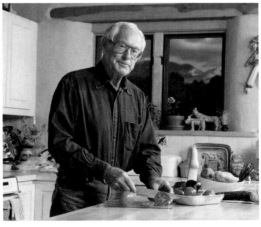

An older man preparing a meal. (Courtesy Corbis Images.)

Chronic Diseases and Conditions

Many chronic diseases and their sequelae pose nutritional challenges for older adults. Heart failure and chronic obstructive pulmonary disease (COPD) are associated with fatigue, increased energy expenditure, and decreased appetite. Dietary interventions for diabetes are essential but may also affect customary eating patterns and require lifestyle changes. Conditions of the teeth and dental problems also affect nutrition (Chapter 15). Functional and cognitive impairments associated with chronic disease interfere with the individual's ability to shop, cook, and eat independently. More detailed information on chronic illness can be found in Chapters 21 to 27.

The side effects of medications prescribed for chronic conditions may further impair nutritional status. There are clinically significant drug-nutrient interactions that result in nutrient loss, and evidence is accumulating that shows the use of nutritional supplements may counteract these possible drug-induced nutrient depletions. A thorough medication review is an essential component of nutritional assessment, and individuals should receive education about the effects of prescription medications, and herbals and supplements, on nutritional status (Chapter 9).

Chronic Conditions That Affect Nutrition

Although there are several physiological and functional changes in the gut associated with aging, the majority of the problems are the result of extrinsic factors. Polypharmacy, high-fat, high-volume meals, inactivity, and comorbid conditions are all aggravating factors. Some conditions that often affect nutritional intake, gastroesophageal reflux disease (GERD), diverticular disease, and dysphagia are discussed here.

Gastroesophageal reflux disease. GERD is a syndrome defined as mucosal damage from the movement of gastric contents backward from the stomach into the esophagus. It is the most common GI disorder affecting older adults. GERD is diagnosed empirically based on history and response to treatment. When the symptoms do not resolve with standard treatment, an endoscopy is indicated (Iannetti, 2017).

Etiology. The majority of GERD is caused by abnormalities of the lower esophageal sphincter (LES). When this muscle relaxes and allows reflux or is generally weak, GERD may occur. Risk factors include hiatal hernia, obesity, pregnancy, cigarette smoking, or inhaling second-hand smoke. People of all ages can develop GERD, some for unknown reasons.

Signs and symptoms. Although complaints of simple "heartburn" are often from dyspepsia, when other signs and symptoms are added it is a greater concern. The classic complaints indicative of GERD are heartburn plus regurgitation—a sensation of burning in the throat as partially digested food and stomach acid inappropriately return to the posterior oropharynx. Older adults more commonly have more atypical symptoms of persistent cough, exacerbations of asthma, laryngitis, and intermittent chest pain. Abdominal pain may occur within 1 hour of eating, and symptoms are worse when lying down with the added pressure of gravity on the LES. Consumption of alcohol before or during eating exacerbates the reflux.

Complications. Persistent symptoms may lead to esophagitis, peptic strictures, esophageal ulcers (with bleeding), and, most importantly, Barrett's esophagus, a precursor to cancer. The most serious complication is the development of pneumonia from the aspiration of stomach contents. Dental caries may be caused from chronic exposure to gastric acids.

Treatment. The management of GERD combines lifestyle changes with pharmacological preparations, used in a stepwise fashion. Lifestyle modifications include eating smaller meals; stopping eating 3 to 4 hours before bed; avoiding high-fat foods, alcohol, caffeine, and nicotine; and sleeping with the head of the bed elevated. Weight reduction and smoking cessation are helpful. These strategies alone may control the majority of symptoms when complications are not present. Pharmacological preparations begin with over-the-counter antacids, such as Tums and Rolaids, and progress to H_2 blockers, such as ranitidine (Zantac), and then proton pump inhibitors, such as lansoprazole (Prevacid). In severe cases of GERD, surgical tightening of the LES may be necessary. The nurse works with the older adult to identify situations that aggravate GERD symptoms (e.g., overeating, consuming alcohol at mealtime) and develop strategies to best deal with them. The nurse also teaches persons with GERD the alarm signs—the signs that should receive prompt evaluation by a health care provider (Box 14.8).

Diverticular disease. Diverticula are small herniations or saclike outpouchings of mucosa that extend through the muscle layers of the colon wall, almost exclusive of the sigmoid colon. They form at weak points in the colon wall, usually where arteries penetrate and provide nutrients to the mucosal layer. Usually less than 1 cm in diameter, diverticula have thin, compressible walls if empty or firm walls if full of fecal matter. The prevalence of diverticular disease increases with age. The risk factors for diverticular disease can be found in Box 14.9. Diverticulitis is an acute inflammatory complication of diverticulosis.

Etiology. Although the exact etiology of diverticular disease is unknown, it is thought to be the result of a low-fiber diet, especially one accompanied by increased intraabdominal pressure and chronic constipation. Smoking and obesity have

---

BOX 14.8 Warning Signs Suggesting Possible GERD Complication

- Anemia
- Anorexia
- Dysphagia
- Hematemesis
- Odynophagia
- Weight loss

GERD, Gastroesophageal reflux disease.

BOX 14.9 Risk Factors for Diverticular Disease

- Family history
- Personal history of gallbladder disease
- Low dietary intake of fiber
- Use of medications that slow fecal transit time
- Chronic constipation
- Obesity

been linked to diverticulitis and physical activity is associated with a decreased risk.

Signs and symptoms. The majority of persons with diverticulosis are completely asymptomatic, and the condition is found only when a barium enema, colonoscopy, or computed tomography (CT) scan is performed for some other reason. Persons with uncomplicated diverticulitis complain of abdominal pain, especially in the left-lower quadrant, and may have a fever and elevated white blood cell count, although the latter symptoms may be delayed or absent in the older adult. The physical assessment may be completely negative. Rectal bleeding is typically acute in onset, is painless, and stops spontaneously.

Complications. The complications of diverticulitis are rupture, abscess, stricture, or fistula. With any perforation, peritonitis is likely. Individuals with these complications may have an elevated pulse rate or are hypotensive; however, in the older adult, unexplained lethargy or confusion may be seen also or instead. A lower-left quadrant mass may be palpated. Complicated diverticulitis is always considered an emergency and requires hospitalization for treatment and possible surgical repair.

Treatment. For persons with diverticulosis, the goal is prevention of diverticulitis. High-fiber diets (25 to 30 g/day) have been cited in American, European, and Asian studies as protective against diverticulosis. In addition, persons should strive for intake of six to eight glasses of fluid per day, preferably with little caffeine.

Acute diverticulitis can be quite painful. The nurse works with the individual to find effective and safe comfort strategies that include pain medication and creative nonpharmacological approaches such as massage, hot or cold packs, stretching exercises, relaxation, music, or meditation techniques. Uncomplicated diverticulitis is treated with antibiotics and a clear liquid diet and is usually managed in the outpatient setting.

In the promotion of healthy aging, the nurse works with the older adult to analyze diet, fluid intake, and activity level to ensure adequate motility and minimal pressure within the GI tract. If the person is overweight or obese, weight loss will decrease intraabdominal pressure and decrease the risk for the development of new diverticula and exacerbations of GERD. The nurse works with the older adult to achieve lifestyle modifications and provide education regarding the appropriate use of medications, warning signs of potential problems, and the best response to the signs or symptoms. When working with an older adult in a cross-cultural setting, it is especially important for the nurse to communicate effectively and incorporate cultural expectations and habits (e.g., diet) into the plan of nursing care.

Dysphagia. Dysphagia, or difficulty swallowing, is a prevalent and growing concern in the older adult population. Swallowing is a complex process with some 50 pairs of muscles and many nerves working together to receive food into the mouth, prepare it, and move it from mouth to stomach. Normally, swallowing is a rapid and seamless act but involves several phases (Box 14.10). Dysphagia can occur secondary to deficits in any of the phases of swallowing. Any condition that weakens or damages the muscles and nerves used for swallowing may cause dysphagia. Examples include individuals with diseases of

---

BOX 14.10 Phases of Swallowing

1. Oral preparatory phase: food is chewed, mixed with saliva, and then formed into a softened mass (bolus) between the tongue and palate
2. Oral transit phase: the bolus is sent posteriorly toward the base of the tongue
3. Oro-pharyngeal phase: the bolus arrives at the base of the tongue and triggers the swallow reflex, which is automatic
4. Pharyngeal phase: the bolus travels down from the base of the tongue past the closed and elevated larynx and to the entrance of the esophagus. This is a continuation of the automatic swallow reflex.
5. Esophageal phase: the esophageal muscle relaxes to allow the bolus into the upper esophagus, from where it is passed downward by waves of muscle contraction through the lower esophageal sphincter and into the stomach.

---

the nervous system, such as amyotrophic lateral sclerosis (ALS) and Parkinson's disease (Chapter 23). Stroke or head injury may weaken or affect coordination of the swallowing muscles or limit sensation in the mouth and throat. Cerebrovascular accidents are the leading cause of neurological dysphagia and occurs in 51% to 73% of patients with stroke (Paik and Moberg-Wolff, 2017) (Chapter 22). In addition, cancer of the head, neck, or esophagus may cause swallowing problems. Memory loss and cognitive deficits may also make it difficult to chew or swallow (Box 14.11) (Chapter 29).

The most common type of dysphagia is otopharyngeal dysphagia (OD). OD is a highly prevalent but largely unrecognized health issue. Prevalence is highest in older adults with neurological conditions and increases with advancing age and frailty. Prevalence among independently living older adults 70 to 79 years is 16% and 33% in those over 80 years. Up to 47% of frail older adults hospitalized for acute illness suffer from OD and it affects more than 50% of nursing home residents. Data suggest that there is a large population of community and nursing home residents with a certain level of dysphagia at baseline which is worsened with acute illness, hospitalization, and increasing frailty (Finucane, 2017).

Dysphagia is a serious problem and has negative consequences, including severe distress during meals, aspiration with the consequence of chronic bronchial inflammation and aspiration pneumonia, weight loss, reduced food and fluid intake with the consequence of malnutrition and dehydration, and increased risk of death. Aspiration is the most profound and

---

BOX 14.11 Risk Factors for Dysphagia

- Cerebrovascular accident
- Parkinson disease
- Neuromuscular disorders (ALS, MS, myasthenia gravis)
- Dementia
- Head and neck cancer
- Traumatic brain injury
- Aspiration pneumonia
- Inadequate feeding technique
- Poor dentition

ALS, Amyotrophic lateral sclerosis; *MS,* multiple sclerosis.

dangerous problem for older adults experiencing dysphagia. The 30-day mortality rate from health care–associated aspiration pneumonia is 30%. Frail older adults with aspiration pneumonia have a significantly increased mortality within 30 days of hospital admission (Wirth et al, 2016).

ASSESSMENT

Screening assessment is important and serves to identify those patients with the greatest risk of dysphagia. It is important to obtain a careful history of the older adult's response to dysphagia and to observe the person during mealtime. Symptoms that alert the nurse to possible swallowing problems are presented in Box 14.12. If dysphagia is suspected, a comprehensive clinical assessment of swallowing and referral to a speech-language pathologist (SLP) are essential. A comprehensive exam includes a clinical swallowing evaluation, comprehensive medical history, physical exam of oral and motor function, and assessment of food intake. Instrumental assessment includes videofluoroscopy swallowing study (VFSS) and fiberoptic endoscopic evaluation of swallowing (FEES). Nothing-by-mouth (NPO) status should be maintained until the swallowing evaluation is completed.

Interventions

After the swallowing evaluation, a decision must be made about the person's potential for functional improvement of the swallowing disorder and the person's safety in swallowing liquid and solid food. The main goal of dysphagia therapy is to reduce morbidity and mortality associated with chest infections and poor nutritional status. Nurses work closely with speech therapy and the dietitian to implement interventions to prevent aspiration. Interventions include postural changes, such as chin tucks or head turns while swallowing, and modification of bolus volume, consistency, temperature, and rate of presentation. Diets may be modified in texture from pudding-like to nearly normal–textured solids. Liquids may range from spoon thick, to honey-like, nectar-like, and thin. Commercial thickeners and thickened products are also available. The evidence is not strong that texture-modified food and thickened liquids reduce the impact of dysphagia. Additionally, patients often do not prefer this kind of food, which may reduce nutritional intake.

Neuromuscular electrical stimulation has received clearance by the U.S. Food and Drug Administration for treatment of dysphagia. This therapy involves the administration of small electrical impulses to the swallowing muscles in the throat and is used in combination with traditional swallowing exercises. Research on the appropriate management of swallowing disorders in older adults, particularly during acute illness and in long-term care facilities, is very limited, and additional study is essential (Wirth et al, 2016). A protocol for preventing aspiration in older adults with dysphagia, and directions to access a video presentation of dysphagia, can be found in Box 14.3. Suggested interventions helpful in preventing aspiration during hand feeding are presented in Box 14.13.

A comprehensive assessment of swallowing problems and other factors that influence intake must be conducted before initiating severely restricted diet modifications or considering the use of feeding tubes, particularly in older adults with end-stage dementia or those at the end of life (Chapter 29). There is little evidence of a reduction in the risk of aspiration pneumonia with tube feeding in any group of adult patients and in fact, enteral nutrition is generally cited as a risk factor for aspiration pneumonia (Finucane, 2017). However, there may be certain

BOX 14.12 Symptoms of Dysphagia or Possible Aspiration

- Difficult, labored swallowing
- Drooling
- Copious oral secretions
- Coughing, choking at meals
- Holding or pocketing of food/medications in the mouth
- Difficulty moving food or liquid from mouth to throat
- Difficulty chewing
- Nasal voice or hoarseness
- Wet or gurgling voice
- Excessive throat clearing
- Food or liquid leaking from the nose
- Prolonged eating time
- Pain with swallowing
- Unusual head or neck posturing while swallowing
- Sensation of something stuck in the throat during swallowing; sensation of a lump in the throat
- Heartburn
- Chest pain
- Hiccups
- Weight loss
- Frequent respiratory tract infections, pneumonia

BOX 14.13 Tips for Best Practice

Preventing Aspiration in Patients With Dysphagia: Hand Feeding

- Provide a 30-minute rest period before meal consumption; a rested person will likely have less difficulty swallowing.
- The person should sit at 90 degrees during all oral (PO) intake.
- Maintain 90-degree positioning for at least 1 hour after PO intake.
- Adjust rate of feeding and size of bites to the person's tolerance; avoid rushed or forced feeding.
- Alternate solid and liquid boluses.
- Have the person swallow twice before the next mouthful.
- Stroke under chin downward to initiate swallowing.
- Follow speech therapist's recommendation for safe swallowing techniques and modified food consistency (may need thickened liquids, pureed foods).
- If facial weakness is present, place food on the nonimpaired side of the mouth.
- Avoid sedatives and hypnotics that may impair cough reflex and swallowing ability.
- Keep suction equipment ready at all times.
- Supervise all meals.
- Monitor temperature.
- Observe color of phlegm.
- Visually check the mouth for pocketing of food in cheeks.
- Check for food under dentures.
- Provide mouth care every 4 hours and before and after meals, including denture cleaning.

circumstances when providing temporary short-term tube feeding may be appropriate (e.g., individuals with stroke and resulting dysphagia and other conditions when it may be possible to resume oral nutrition at some point). Chapter 29 discusses feeding tubes in detail.

PROMOTING HEALTHY AGING: IMPLICATIONS FOR GERONTOLOGICAL NURSING

The role of nursing in nutrition assessment and intervention should be comprehensive and include attention to the process of eating and the entire ritual of meals and the assessment of nutritional status within the interprofessional team. Nurses are often the first to identify patients in need of nutrition intervention and are integral to encouraging nutritional intake from admission to discharge (Sauer et al, 2016). Comprehensive nutritional screening and assessment are essential in identifying older adults at risk for nutrition problems or who are malnourished. Evaluation of nutritional health can be difficult in the absence of severe malnutrition and older adults are less likely than younger people to show signs of malnutrition and nutrient malabsorption.

There is no historical, clinical, or laboratory parameter by itself that qualifies as a reliable and valid indicator of nutritional status, thus a comprehensive assessment is essential to reveal deficits (Mueller, 2015). Screening and assessment of concerns identified should be conducted within 24 hours of admission and periodically reassessed throughout the stay (Avelino-Silva and Jaluul, 2017). Nutrition risk screening using a validated tool such as the (Mini-Nutritional Assessment Short-Form [MNA-SF]) should be performed routinely and can be incorporated into annual health checks for those aged 75 years and older.

Nutritional Screening

Nutritional screening is the first step in identifying individuals who are at risk for malnutrition or have undetected malnutrition, and it determines the need for a more comprehensive

assessment and nutritional interventions. The screening is preliminary and is not to be viewed as a replacement to comprehensive assessment of the individual (Mueller, 2015). Nutrition screening performed by nurses in the first few hours of hospitalization or admission to a long-term care facility sets the stage for quality care. There are several screening tools specific to older individuals, and screening can be completed in any setting. The Nutrition Screening Initiative Checklist (Fig. 14.2) can be self-administered or completed by a family member or any member of the health care team.

The MNA-SF (Fig. 14.3) provides a simple, quick method of identifying older adults who are at risk of malnutrition. The Self-MNA is a simple tool designed to help older adults determine if they are getting the nutrition they need. The Self-MNA is available in English, Bulgarian, Danish, Finnish, German, Greek, Italian, Portuguese, Spanish, and Swedish (Box 14.3).

The Minimum Data Set 3.0 (MDS 3.0) (Chapter 7), used in long-term care facilities, is also a useful screening tool for nutritional risk. The MDS does not establish malnutrition but rather is a tool to generate a care plan (Mueller, 2015). The MDS includes assessment information that can be used to identify potential nutritional problems, risk factors, and the potential for improved function. Triggers for more thorough investigation of problems include weight loss, alterations in taste, medical therapies, prescription medications, hunger, parenteral or intravenous feedings, mechanically altered or therapeutic diets, percentage of food left uneaten, pressure ulcers, and edema.

Nutritional Assessment

When risk for malnutrition or malnutrition is detected, a comprehensive nutritional assessment is indicated and will provide the most conclusive data about a person's actual nutritional state. Interprofessional approaches are key to appropriate assessment and intervention and should involve medicine, nursing, dietary, physical, occupational and speech therapy, and social work. The collective results provide the data needed to

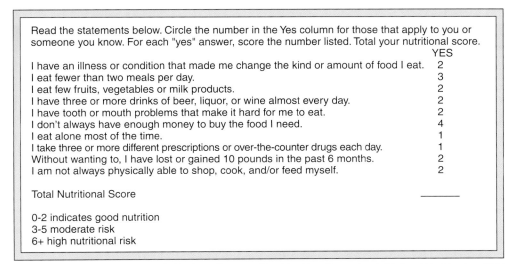

Read the statements below. Circle the number in the Yes column for those that apply to you or someone you know. For each "yes" answer, score the number listed. Total your nutritional score.

	YES
I have an illness or condition that made me change the kind or amount of food I eat.	2
I eat fewer than two meals per day.	3
I eat few fruits, vegetables or milk products.	2
I have three or more drinks of beer, liquor, or wine almost every day.	2
I have tooth or mouth problems that make it hard for me to eat.	2
I don't always have enough money to buy the food I need.	4
I eat alone most of the time.	1
I take three or more different prescriptions or over-the-counter drugs each day.	1
Without wanting to, I have lost or gained 10 pounds in the past 6 months.	2
I am not always physically able to shop, cook, and/or feed myself.	2

Total Nutritional Score   _____

0-2 indicates good nutrition
3-5 moderate risk
6+ high nutritional risk

Fig. 14.2 Nutrition Screening Initiative. (Courtesy The Nutrition Screening Initiative, Washington, DC.)

Mini Nutritional Assessment
MNA®

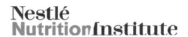

Last name:	First name:

Sex:	Age:	Weight, kg:	Height, cm:	Date:

Complete the screen by filling in the boxes with the appropriate numbers. Total the numbers for the final screening score.

Screening

A Has food intake declined over the past 3 months due to loss of appetite, digestive problems, chewing or swallowing difficulties?

0 = severe decrease in food intake
1 = moderate decrease in food intake
2 = no decrease in food intake ☐

B Weight loss during the last 3 months

0 = weight loss greater than 3 kg (6.6 lbs)
1 = does not know
2 = weight loss between 1 and 3 kg (2.2 and 6.6 lbs)
3 = no weight loss ☐

C Mobility

0 = bed or chair bound
1 = able to get out of bed / chair but does not go out
2 = goes out ☐

D Has suffered psychological stress or acute disease in the past 3 months?

0 = yes   2 = no ☐

E Neuropsychological problems

0 = severe dementia or depression
1 = mild dementia
2 = no psychological problems ☐

F1 Body Mass Index (BMI) (weight in kg) / (height in m)^2

0 = BMI less than 19
1 = BMI 19 to less than 21
2 = BMI 21 to less than 23
3 = BMI 23 or greater ☐

IF BMI IS NOT AVAILABLE, REPLACE QUESTION F1 WITH QUESTION F2.
DO NOT ANSWER QUESTION F2 IF QUESTION F1 IS ALREADY COMPLETED.

F2 Calf circumference (CC) in cm

0 = CC less than 31
3 = CC 31 or greater ☐

Screening score (max. 14 points)

12 - 14 points: Normal nutritional status
8 - 11 points: At risk of malnutrition
0 - 7 points: Malnourished ☐☐

References

1. Vellas B, Villars H, Abellan G, et al. Overview of the MNA® - Its History and Challenges. *J Nutr Health Aging.* 2006;**10**:456-465.
2. Rubenstein LZ, Harker JO, Salva A, Guigoz Y, Vellas B. Screening for Undernutrition in Geriatric Practice: Developing the Short-Form Mini Nutritional Assessment (MNA-SF). *J. Geront.* 2001; **56A**: M366-377
3. Guigoz Y. The Mini-Nutritional Assessment (MNA®) Review of the Literature - What does it tell us? *J Nutr Health Aging.* 2006; **10**:466-487.
4. Kaiser MJ, Bauer JM, Ramsch C, et al. Validation of the Mini Nutritional Assessment Short-Form (MNA®-SF): A practical tool for identification of nutritional status. *J Nutr Health Aging.* 2009; **13**:782-788.

® Société des Produits Nestlé, S.A., Vevey, Switzerland, Trademark Owners © Nestlé, 1994, Revision 2009. N67200 12/99 10M

For more information: www.mna-elderly.com

Fig. 14.3 Mini Nutritional Assessment (MNA). (From http://www.mna-elderly.com/forms/mini/mna_mini_english.pdf.)

identify the immediate and the potential nutritional problems so that plans for supervision, assistance, and education in the attainment of adequate nutrition can be implemented. Components of a nutrition assessment include interview, history, physical examination, anthropometric data, laboratory data, food/nutrient intake, and functional assessment. A summary is presented in Box 14.14. Explanations of several components are discussed in the following sections.

BOX 14.14 Components of Nutritional Assessment

Dietary History and Current Intake
- Food preferences and habits; meaning and significance of food to the individual; do they eat alone?
- Cultural or religious food habits
- Ability to obtain and prepare food including adequate finances to obtain nutritious food
- Social activities and normal patterns; meal frequency
- Control over food selection and choices
- Fluid intake
- Alcohol intake
- Special diet
- Vitamins/minerals/supplement use
- Chewing/swallowing problems
- Functional limitations that impair independence in eating
- Cognitive changes affecting appetite/ability to feed self
- Depression screen if indicated

History/Physical
- Chief complaint, medical history, chronic conditions, presence or absence of inflammation (fever, hypothermia, signs of systemic inflammatory response), usual weight and any loss or gain, fluid retention, loss of muscle/fat, oral health and dentition, medication use

Anthropometric Measurements
- Body mass index
- Height
- Current weight and usual adult weight
- Recent weight changes
- Skinfold measurements

Biochemical Analysis
- Complete blood count
- Protein status
- Lipid profile
- Electrolytes
- Blood urea nitrogen (BUN)/creatinine ratio

Food/Nutrient Intake
- Periods of inadequate intake (nothing-by-mouth [NPO] status)
- 24-hour or 3-day diet record

Functional Assessment
- Hand-grip strength
- Standard functional assessment (Chapter 7)

Adapted from Mathew M, Jacobs M: Malnutrition and feeding problems. In Ham R, Sloane P, Warshaw G, et al, editors: *Primary care geriatrics: a case-based approach*, ed 6, Philadelphia, 2014, Elsevier Saunders, p 318.

Food/Nutrient Intake

Frequently, a 24-hour diet recall compared with the MyPlate for Older Adults (Fig. 14.1) can provide an estimate of nutritional adequacy. When the individual cannot supply all of the requested information, it may be possible to obtain data from a family member or another source such as a shopping receipt. There will be times, however, when information will not be as complete as one would like, or the individual, too proud to admit that he or she is not eating, will furnish erroneous information. Even so, the nurse will be able to obtain additional data from the other three areas of the nutritional assessment.

Keeping a dietary record for 3 days is another assessment tool. This can be completed by the individual, family, or caregivers. The diet recall includes what foods were eaten, when food was eaten, and the amounts eaten. Computer analysis of the dietary records provides information on energy and vitamin and mineral intake. Printouts can provide the individual and the health care provider with a visual graph of the intake. Accurate completion of 3-day dietary records in hospitals and long-term care facilities can be problematic, and intake may be either underestimated or overestimated. Standardized observational protocols should be developed to ensure accuracy of oral intake documentation, and the adequacy and quality of feeding assistance during mealtimes. Nurses should ensure that direct caregivers are educated on the proper observation and documentation of intake and should closely monitor performance in this area.

Anthropomorphic Measurements

Anthropomorphic measurements provide significant data for the evaluation of nutritional status but are affected by the aging process. Height, weight, skinfold thickness, and muscle circumference are all affected by aging. Skeletal changes associated with bone disease, compromised integrity of the vertebral column, sarcopenia, and loss of subcutaneous fat all contribute to variation from normal standards that apply to younger adults (Mueller, 2015). The MNA-SF utilizes calf circumference for an anthropomorphic measurement (less than 31 cm indicative of at-risk category).

Weight/Height Considerations

Weight change (from usual) offers the most useful information on nutritional status and a detailed weight history should be obtained along with current weight. History should include a history of weight loss, if the weight loss was intentional or unintentional, and during what period it occurred. A history of anorexia is also important, and many older adults, especially women, have limited their weight throughout life. Debate continues in the quest to determine the appropriate weight charts for an older adult. Although weight alone does not indicate the adequacy of diet, unplanned fluctuations in weight are significant and should be evaluated.

Accurate weight patterns are sometimes difficult to obtain in long-term care settings. Procedures for weighing people should be established and followed consistently to obtain an accurate representation of weight changes. Weighing procedure should be supervised by licensed personnel, and changes should be reported immediately to the provider. One might meet correct weight values for height, but weight changes may be the result of fluid retention, edema, or ascites and merit investigation. A weight loss of

5% of usual body weight in 6 to 12 months is the most widely accepted definition for clinically important weight loss in older adults (DiMaria-Ghalili, 2014). In long-term care facilities, a loss of more than 5% of body weight in 1 month, more than 7.5% in 3 months, or more than 10% in 6 months is considered a significant indicator of poor nutrition and an MDS trigger.

Height should always be measured and never estimated or given by self-report. If the person cannot stand, an alternative way of measuring standing height is knee-height using special calipers. An alternative to knee-height measurements is a demispan measurement, which is half the total arm span. Measurement of BMI in older adults can be unreliable and does not provide the same clues to health status in older adults as it does in younger people. A BMI of less than 23 classifies an older adult (older than age 65) as underweight and may require nutrition intervention. Health risks associated with a BMI of 18.5 to 25 in younger populations may not apply for those older than age 65 (Chernoff, 2014; Sauer et al, 2016).

Biochemical Analysis/Measures of Visceral Protein

The relevance of laboratory tests of serum albumin, prealbumin, and transferrin, as indicators of malnutrition, is limited. These acute phase proteins do not consistently or predictability change with weight loss, calorie restriction, or negative nitrogen balance. They appear to better reflect severity of inflammatory response rather than poor nutritional status. Further investigation of the significance of low protein levels is needed (Avelino-Silva and Jaluul, 2017).

Interventions

Nurses hold a pivotal role in ensuring adequate nutrition to promote healthy aging. Inherent in the role is (1) assessment of the individual for issues related to performance at mealtimes; (2) modification of the environment to be pleasurable for eating; (3) supervision of eating; (4) provision of guidance and support to staff on feeding techniques that enhance intake and preserve dignity and independence; and (5) evaluation of outcomes (Amella and Aselage, 2012). Nurturing and nourishing have been described as the nurses' role in nutritional care (Jefferies et al, 2011) (Box 14.14). Collaboration with the interprofessional team (e.g., dietitian, pharmacist, social worker, occupational or speech therapist) is important in planning interventions.

For the community-dwelling older adult, nutrition education and problem solving with the older adult and family members or caregivers on how to best resolve the potential or actual nutritional deficit is important. Causes of poor nutrition are complex, and all of the factors emphasized in this chapter are important to assess when planning individualized interventions to ensure adequate nutrition for older adults. Box 14.3 presents resources to assist older adults in planning for good nutrition.

Older adults in hospitals and long-term care facilities are more likely to be admitted with malnutrition, be at high risk for malnutrition, and have disease conditions that contribute to malnutrition. Severely restricted diets, long periods of NPO status, and insufficient time and staff for feeding assistance also contribute to inadequate nutrition. Older adults with dementia are particularly at risk for weight loss and inadequate nutrition (Chapter 29).

Feeding Assistance

The incidence of eating disability in long-term care is high with estimates that 50% of all residents cannot eat independently. Inadequate staffing in long-term care facilities is associated with poor nutrition and hydration. In a classic study of feeding in long-term care, Kayser-Jones (1997) stated: "Certified nursing assistants (CNAs) have an impossible task trying to feed the number of people who need assistance" (p. 19). In a study by Simmons and colleagues (2001), 50% of residents significantly increased their oral food and fluid intake during mealtime when they received one-on-one feeding assistance. The time required to implement the feeding assistance (38 minutes) greatly exceeded the time nursing staff spent assisting residents in usual mealtime conditions (9 minutes).

In response to concerns about the lack of adequate assistance during mealtime in long-term care facilities, the CMS implemented a rule that allows feeding assistants with 8 hours of approved training to help residents with eating. Feeding assistants must be supervised by a registered nurse (RN) or licensed practical–vocational nurse (LPN-LVN). Family members may also be willing and able to assist at mealtimes and also provide a familiar social context for the patient. Assistance with meals in hospitals is also a concern and volunteer programs to address the unique needs of hospitalized patients have been reported (Buys et al, 2013). Further research is needed on the effectiveness of feeding assistance programs in hospital settings (Box 14.15).

BOX 14.15 Tips for Best Practice

Improving Nutritional Intake in Hospitals

- Assess nutritional and oral health status, including ability to eat and amount of assistance needed.
- Ensure proper fit and cleanliness of dentures and denture use.
- Provide oral hygiene, and allow the person to wash his or her hands before meals.
- Ensure environment is conducive to eating (remove objects such as urinals and bed pans; clear bedside tables). Ask yourself if you would want to eat the food in the environment in which it is presented.
- Position patient for safe eating (head of bed elevated or sit in a chair if possible).
- Stop nonessential clinical activity during meals (e.g., procedures, rounds, medication administration).
- Ensure that all nursing staff are aware of the patients who need assistance with eating and that adequate help is provided.
- Ensure that all necessary items are on the tray; prepare all food on the tray if needed; butter bread, open containers, provide straws, provide adaptive equipment as needed.
- Consider volunteers or family members to assist with eating and train and supervise.
- Administer medication for pain or nausea on a schedule that provides comfort at mealtime.
- Determine food preferences; provide for choices in food; include foods appropriate to cultural and religious customs.
- Accurately assess dietary intake using a validated method.
- Make dietary changes/referrals readily.
- Make food available 24 hours/day—provide snacks between meals and at night.
- Limit periods of nothing-by-mouth NPO status and provide food as soon as patient is able to eat.
- Consider liberalizing therapeutic diet if intake is inadequate; offer diet options/alternatives as indicated, including flavor enhancement.

From Furman E: The theory of compromised eating behavior, *Res Gerontol Nurs* 7(2):78–86, 2014.

The theory of compromised eating behavior, derived from a nursing study, suggests that the meaning of food and meals to older adults is challenged during hospitalization. As individuals age, traditional food and mealtimes become more meaningful. If food was not traditional in flavor or consistent with the older adult's acculturated foodways, the meaning of food and meal was compromised, thus influencing dietary intake. Strategies to enhance the meaning of food and mealtimes can improve the negative outcomes associated with undernutrition in the hospital setting (Research Highlights box).

Approaches to Enhancing Intake in Long-Term Care

In addition to adequate staff, many innovative and evidence-based ideas can improve nutritional intake in institutions. Many suggestions are found in the literature: home-like dining rooms; cafeteria-style service; refreshment stations with easy access to juices, water, and healthy snacks; kitchens on the nursing units; choice of mealtimes; finger foods; visually appealing pureed foods with texture and shape; music; touch.

Attention to the environment in which meals are served is important. It is not uncommon to hear over the public address system at mealtimes: "Feeder trays are ready." This reference to the need to feed those unable to feed themselves is, in itself, degrading and erases any trace of dignity the individual is trying to maintain in a controlled environment. It is not malicious intent by nurses or other caregivers but rather a habit of convenience. Feeding older adults who have difficulty eating can become mechanical and devoid of feeling. The feeding process becomes rapid, and if it bogs down and becomes too slow, the meal may be ended abruptly, depending on the time the caregiver has allotted for feeding the person. Any pleasure derived

through socialization and eating and any dignity that could be maintained are often absent (see "An Older Adult Speaks" at the beginning of this chapter). Other suggestions can be found in Box 14.16 and suggestions to improve intake for individuals with dementia are presented in Chapter 29.

Restrictive Diets and Caloric Supplements

The use of restrictive therapeutic diets for frail older adults in long-term care (low cholesterol, low salt, no concentrated sweets) often reduces food intake without significantly helping the clinical status of the individual (Pioneer Network and Rothschild Foundation, 2011). Dispensing a small amount of calorically dense oral nutritional supplement (2 calories/mL) during the routine medication pass may have a greater effect on weight gain than a traditional supplement (1.06 calories/mL) with or between meals. Small volumes of nutrient-dense supplement may have less of an effect on appetite and will enhance food intake during meals and snacks. This delivery method allows nurses to observe and document consumption. A growing

---

⑤ RESEARCH HIGHLIGHTS

Furman (2014) developed the Theory of Compromised Eating Behavior using grounded theory methodology. The study setting was a large, acute care hospital and participants included eight older adults and four health care providers. Interviews, mealtime observations, and document review were used to collect data. The following observations from the study can provide insights from patients that can be used to guide nurses in developing interventions to promote adequate intake in hospital settings:

"We have a meatloaf but it's turkey meatloaf and it's not really distinguished to me. It doesn't look like meatloaf to me either and these fancy dishes like shrimp Provencal. The menu describes it with these fancy descriptions. I think people are afraid to order it because they're not sure what it is."

"It depends where they leave the meal tray and how my bed goes. If my bed goes up a little maybe I can reach it or if it goes down a little, maybe I can reach it. If I can't, maybe I'll ask someone. If they come in I'll eat; if they don't I won't. I won't even look at it."

"An RN suggested that the patient try the soup. Yet, the nurse neglected to note that with his significant hand tremor, the patient would not be able to get the soup from tray to mouth without spilling. The nurse did not offer assistance nor did the patient ask for assistance. Total dietary intake for the meal consisted of a cracker, which the older adult struggled to access, in addition to sips of milk consumed during medication administration."

From Furman E: The theory of compromised eating behavior, *Res Gerontol Nurs* 7(2):78–86, 2014.

BOX 14.16 Tips for Best Practice

Improving Nutritional Intake in Long-Term Care

- Assess nutritional and oral health status.
- Assess ability to eat and amount of assistance needed.
- Serve meals with the person in a chair rather than in bed when possible.
- Provide analgesics and antiemetics on a schedule that provides comfort at mealtime.
- Determine food preferences; provide for choices in food; include foods appropriate to cultural and religious customs.
- Consider buffet-style dining, use of steam tables rather than meal delivery service from trays, café or bistro-type dining.
- Make food available 24 hours/day—provide snacks between meals and at night.
- Do not interrupt meals to administer medication if possible.
- Limit staff breaks to before and after mealtimes to ensure adequate staff are available to assist with meals.
- Walk around the dining area or the rooms at mealtime to determine if food is being eaten or if assistance is needed.
- Encourage family members to share the mealtimes for a heightened social situation.
- If caloric supplements are used, offer them between meals or with the medication pass.
- Ensure proper fit of dentures and denture use.
- Provide oral hygiene, and allow the person to wash his or her hands before meals.
- Have the person wear his or her glasses during meals.
- Sit while feeding the person who needs assistance, use touch, and carry on a social conversation.
- Provide soft music during the meal.
- Use small, round tables seating six to eight people. Consider using tablecloths and centerpieces.
- Seat people with like interests and abilities together, and encourage socialization.
- Involve in restorative dining programs.
- Make diets as liberal as possible depending on health status, especially for frail elders who are not consuming adequate amounts of food.
- Consider a referral to occupational therapist for individuals experiencing difficulties with eating.

body of evidence suggests that supplementation might improve outcomes of hospitalized patients, including length of stay, costs, and readmissions (Avelino-Silva and Jaluul, 2017).

Further studies and randomized clinical trials are needed to evaluate the effectiveness of nutritional supplementation. The American Geriatrics Society (2014) recommends avoiding high-calorie supplements for treatment of anorexia in older adults. Instead, recommendations are to optimize social supports, provide feeding assistance, and clarify patient goals and expectations. Unintentional weight loss is a common problem for medically ill or frail older adults. Although high-calorie supplements increase weight in older adults, there is no evidence that they affect other important clinical outcomes, such as quality of life, mood, functional status, or survival.

Pharmacological Therapy

The American Geriatrics Society (2014) does not recommend drugs that stimulate appetite (orexigenic drugs) to treat anorexia or malnutrition in older people. Use of drugs, such as megestrol acetate, results in minimum improvement in appetite and weight gain, no improvement in quality of life or survival, and increased risk of thrombotic events, fluid retention, and death. Systematic reviews of cannabinoids, dietary polyunsaturated fatty acids (DHA and EPA), thalidomide, and anabolic steroids have not identified adequate evidence for the efficacy and safety of these agents for weight gain. See Box 14.3 for an evidence-based protocol on assessment and management of mealtime difficulties.

Patient Education

Education should be provided on nutritional requirements for health, special diet modifications for chronic illness management, the effect of age-associated changes and medication on nutrition, and community resources to assist in maintaining adequate nutrition. Medicare covers nutrition therapy for select diseases, such as diabetes and kidney disease.

PROMOTING HEALTHY AGING: IMPLICATIONS FOR GERONTOLOGICAL NURSING

Maintenance of adequate nutritional health as a person ages is extremely complex. Knowledge of nutritional needs in later years and of the many factors contributing to inadequate nutrition is essential for the gerontological nurse and should be a part of every assessment of an older adult. Working with members of the interprofessional team in appropriate assessment and development of therapeutic interventions is a major nursing role in community, hospital, and long-term care settings. Use of evidence-based practice protocols is important in determining nursing interventions to support and enhance nutritional status.

Prevention of undernutrition and malnutrition and the maintenance of dietary needs and food are also ethical responsibilities. No older adult should be hungry or thirsty because he or she cannot shop, cook, buy and prepare food, or eat independently. Nor should any older adult have to suffer because of a lack of assistance with these activities in whatever setting the person may reside.

▮ KEY CONCEPTS

- Results of studies provide growing evidence that diet can affect longevity and, when combined with lifestyle changes, reduce disease risk.
- Many factors affect adequate nutrition in later life, including lifelong eating habits, income, age-associated changes, chronic illness, dentition, mood disorders, capacity for food preparation, and functional limitations.
- An escalating global epidemic of overweight and obesity—"globesity"—is a major public health concern in both developed and developing countries. In the United States, approximately 35% of adults over 60 years are obese, with a higher prevalence in women (38%) than men (32%) (Gretebeck et al, 2017).
- The rising incidence of malnutrition among older adults has been documented in acute care, long-term care, and the community and is expected to rise dramatically in the next 30 years. It is important to remember that overweight/obese individuals are also at risk for malnutrition.
- Malnutrition is a precursor to frailty and has serious consequences, including infections, pressure ulcers, anemia,

hypotension, impaired cognition, hip fractures, prolonged hospital stay, institutionalization, and increased morbidity and mortality.
- A comprehensive nutritional assessment is an essential component of the assessment of older adults.
- The role of nursing in nutrition assessment and intervention should be comprehensive and include attention to the process of eating and the entire ritual of meals, and the assessment of nutritional status within the interprofessional team.
- Making mealtimes pleasant and attractive for the older adult who is unable to eat unassisted is a nursing challenge; mealtimes must be made enjoyable, and adequate assistance must be provided.
- Dysphagia is a serious problem and has negative consequences, including weight loss, malnutrition, dehydration, aspiration pneumonia, and even death. Nurses must carefully assess risk factors for dysphagia, observe for signs and symptoms, refer for evaluation, and collaborate with SLPs on interventions to prevent aspiration.

NURSING STUDY: NUTRITION

Helen, 77 years old, had dieted all her life—or so it seemed. She often chided herself about it. "After all, at my age who cares if I'm too fat? I do. It depresses me when I gain weight and then I gain even more when I'm depressed." At 5 feet, 4 inches tall and 138 pounds, her weight was ideal for her height and age, but Helen, like so many women of her generation, had incorporated the image of women on TV who weighed 105 pounds as her ideal. She had achieved that weight for only a few weeks three or four times in her adult life. She had tried high-protein diets, celery and cottage cheese diets, fasting, commercially prepared diet foods, and numerous fad diets. She always discontinued the diets when she perceived any negative effects. She was invested in maintaining her general good health. Her most recent attempt at losing 30 pounds on an all-liquid diet had been unsuccessful and left her feeling constipated, weak, irritable, and mildly nauseated and experiencing heart palpitations. This really frightened her. Her physician criticized her regarding the liquid diet but seemed rather amused while reinforcing that her weight was "just perfect" for her age. In the discussion, the physician pointed out how fortunate she was that she was able to drive to the market, had sufficient money for food, and was able to eat anything with no dietary restrictions. Helen left his office feeling silly. She was an independent, intelligent woman; she had been a successful manager of a large financial office. Before her retirement 7 years ago, her work had consumed most of her energy. There had been no time for family, romance, or hobbies. Lately, she had immersed herself in reading the Harvard Classics as she had promised herself she would when she retired. Unfortunately, now that she had the time to read them, she was losing interest. She knew that she must begin to "pull herself together" and "be grateful for her blessings" just as the physician had said.

Based on the case study, develop a nursing care plan using the following procedure[a]:
- List Helen's comments that provide subjective data.
- List information that provides objective data.
- From these data, identify and state, using an accepted format, two nursing diagnoses you determine are most significant to Helen at this time. List two of Helen's strengths that you have identified from the data.
- Determine and state outcome criteria for each diagnosis. These must reflect some alleviation of the problem identified in the nursing diagnosis and must be stated in concrete and measurable terms.
- Plan and state one or more interventions for each diagnosed problem. Provide specific documentation of the source used to determine the appropriate intervention. Plan at least one intervention that incorporates Helen's existing strengths.
- Evaluate the success of the intervention. Interventions must correlate directly with the stated outcome criteria to measure the outcome success.

[a]Students are advised to refer to their nursing diagnosis text and identify possible or potential problems.

CRITICAL THINKING QUESTIONS AND ACTIVITIES

1. Discuss how you would counsel Helen regarding her weight.
2. If Helen insists on dieting, what diet would you recommend, considering her age and activity level?
3. What lifestyle changes would you suggest to Helen?
4. What are the specific health concerns that require attention in Helen's case?
5. What factors may be involved in Helen's preoccupation with her weight?
6. What are some of the reasons that fad diets are dangerous?

RESEARCH QUESTIONS

1. What are the dietary patterns of older men living alone?
2. What percentage of women and men older than age 60 are satisfied with their weight?
3. What factors influence older adults to implement dietary changes suggested by nurses, dietitians, or primary care providers?
4. What nursing interventions can enhance the nutritional intake of frail older adults residing in nursing facilities?
5. What is the level of knowledge about dysphagia among acute care and long-term care nurses?

REFERENCES

American Geriatrics Society: Feeding tubes in advanced dementia position statement. *J Am Geriatr Soc* 62(8):1590-1593, 2014. https://www.ncbi.nlm.nih.gov/pubmed/25039796.linical_guidelines_recommendations. Accessed March 2019.

American Geriatrics Society: *Choosing wisely: five things physicians and patients should question*, 2014. http://www.choosingwisely.org/american-geriatrics-society-releases-second-choosing-wisely-list-identifies-5-more-tests-and-treatments-that-older-patients-and-providers-should-question/. Accessed January 2018.

Avelino-Silva TJ, Jaluul O: Malnutrition in hospitalized older patients: management strategies to improve patient care and clinical outcomes, *Int J Geront* 11(2):56–61, 2017.

Baugreet S, Hamill RM, Kerry JP, McCarthy SN: Mitigating nutrition and health deficiencies in older adults: a role for food innovation? *J Food Sci* 82(4):848–855, 2017.

Bowman K, Delgado J, Henley WE, et al: Obesity in older people with and without conditions associated with weight loss: follow-up of 955,000 primary care patients, *J Gerontol A Biol Sci Med Sci* 72(2):203–209, 2017.

Buys DR, Flood KL, Real K, Chang M, Locher JL: Mealtime assistance for hospitalized older adults: a report on the SPOONS volunteer program. *J Gerontol Nur* 39(9):18–22, 2013.

Cederholm T, Jensen GL: To create a consensus on malnutrition diagnostic criteria: a report from the Global Leadership Initiative on Malnutrition (GLIM) meeting at the ESPEN Congress 2016, *Clin Nutr* 36:7–10, 2017.

Chernoff R: *Geriatric nutrition: the health professionals handbook,* ed 4, Burlington, MA, 2014, Jones and Bartlett Learning.

Crogan NL: Nutritional problems affecting older adults, *Nurs Clin North Am* 52:433–445, 2017.

Finucane TE: Questioning feeding tubes to treat dysphagia, *JAMA Intern Med* 177(3):443, 2017.

Furman E: The theory of compromised eating behavior, *Res Gerontol Nurs* 7(2):78–86, 2014.

Gretebeck KA, Sabatini LM, Black DR, Gretebeck RJ: Physical activity, functional ability, and obesity in older adults: a gender difference, *J Gerontol Nurs* 43(9):38–46, 2017.

Hooshmand B, Mangialasche F, Kalpouzos G, et al: Association of vitamin B_{12}, folate, and sulfur amino acids with brain magnetic resonance imaging measures in older adults: a longitudinal population-based study, *JAMA Psychiatry* 73(6):606–613, 2016.

Iannetti A: Updates on the management of GERD disease, *J Gastrointest Dig Syst* 7:523, 2017.

Kalish VB: Obesity in older adults, *Prim Care* 43(1):137–144, 2016.

Kayser-Jones J: Inadequate staffing at mealtime: implications for nursing and health policy, *J Gerontol Nurs* 23:14–21, 1997.

Kritchevsky SB: Taking obesity in older adults seriously, *J Gerontol A Biol Sci Med Sci* 73(1):57–58, 2017.

Lustbader W: Thoughts on the meaning of frailty, *Generations* 13:21, 1999.

McEvoy CT, Guyer H, Langa KM, Yaffe, K: Neuroprotective diets are associated with better cognitive function: the Health and Retirement Study, *J Am Geriatr Soc* 65:1857–1862, 2017.

Mogensen KM, DiMaria-Ghalili RA: Malnutrition in older adults, *Today's Dietician* 17(9):56, 2015.

Mueller CM: Nutrition assessment and older adults, *Top Clin Nutr* 30(1):94–102, 2015.

National Council on Aging: *SNAP and senior hunger facts,* 2018. https://www.ncoa.org/news/resources-for-reporters/get-the-facts/senior-hunger-facts/. Accessed January 2018.

Paik NJ, Moberg-Wolff A: *Dysphagia.* Medscape, 2017. https://emedicine.medscape.com/article/2212409-overview. Accessed January 2018.

Sauer AC, Alish CJ, Strausbaugh K, West K, Quatrara B: Nurses needed: identifying malnutrition in hospitalized older adults, *NursingPlus Open* 2:21–25, 2016.

Simmons SF, Osterweil D, Schnelle JF: Improving food intake in nursing home residents with feeding assistance: a staffing analysis, *J Gerontol A Biol Sci Med Sci* 56(12):M790–M794, 2001.

The Joint Commission: *Patient Safety Tool: Advancing effective communication, cultural competence and patient- and family-centered care: a roadmap for hospitals,* Oakbrook Terrace, IL, 2014, The Joint Commission.

Tilly J: *White Paper: Opportunities to improve nutrition for older adults and reduce risk of poor health outcomes,* 2017, National Resource Center on Nutrition and Aging. http://nutritionandaging.org/opportunities-to-improve-nutrition-for-older-adults-and-reduce-risk-of-poor-health-outcomes/. Accessed January 2018.

Tufts University: *MyPlate for Older Adults,* 2016. http://hnrca.tufts.edu/myplate/. Accessed January 2018.

U.S. Department of Health and Human Services and U.S. Department of Agriculture: *2015—2020 Dietary Guidelines for Americans,* ed 8, 2015-2020. https://health.gov/dietaryguidelines/2015/guidelines/. Accessed January 2018.

Wirth R, Dziewas R, Beck AM, et al: Oropharyngeal dysphagia in older adults—from pathophysiology to adequate intervention: a review and summary of an international expert meeting, *Clin Interv Aging* 11:189–208, 2016.

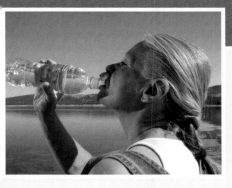

15

Hydration and Oral Care

Theris A. Touhy

http://evolve.elsevier.com/Touhy/TwdHlthAging

A STUDENT SPEAKS

I never thought that part of my nursing care was brushing someone's false teeth. I didn't even know my patient had false teeth until he asked me to help him take them out. Thank goodness he was able to tell me how to do it because I had no idea. He was really worried because he said the last time he was in the hospital, no one had taken them out for several days and he got a sore under them that was very painful. Together we got them out, cleaned, and back in with no problems. Made me realize how important the little things really are.

Jeff, age 22

AN OLDER ADULT SPEAKS

I know I don't drink enough water—coffee, yes; water, no. It's hard when you are in a wheelchair and only have one arm that works. This smart little student nurse really fixed me up. She gave me a plastic water bottle and attached it to my chair on my good side. Now wherever I go, the water goes.

Jack, age 84

LEARNING OBJECTIVES

On completion of this chapter, the reader will be able to:

1. Identify factors that influence hydration management in older adults.
2. Identify the components of hydration assessment.
3. Describe interventions for prevention and treatment of dehydration.
4. Demonstrate understanding of the relationship between oral health and disease.
5. Discuss common oral problems that can occur with aging and appropriate assessment and interventions.
6. Discuss interventions that promote good oral hygiene for older adults in a variety of settings.

HYDRATION MANAGEMENT

Hydration management is the promotion of an adequate fluid balance, which prevents complications resulting from abnormal or undesirable fluid levels. Water, an accessible and available commodity to almost all people, is often overlooked as an essential part of nutritional requirements. Water's function in the body includes thermoregulation, dilution of water-soluble medications, facilitation of renal and bowel function, and creation of requisite conditions for and maintenance of metabolic processes.

Daily needs for water can usually be met by functionally independent older adults through intake of fluids with meals and social drinks. However, a significant number of older adults (up to 85% of those 85 years of age and older) drink less than 1 liter of fluid per day. Older adults, with the exception of those requiring fluid restrictions, should consume at least 1500 mL of fluid per day. Maintenance of fluid balance (fluid intake equals fluid output) is essential to health, regardless of a person's age.

Age-related changes (Box 15.1 and Fig. 15.1), medication use, functional impairments, and comorbid medical and emotional illnesses place some older adults at risk for changes in fluid balance, especially dehydration. Hydration habits, as described by Mentes (2012), also influence how and why individuals consume liquids. Each group has different hydration habits that can guide assessment and interventions. Providing targeted interventions to those at greatest risk may decrease the prevalence of dehydration (Box 15.2).

Adapted from Mentes JC: Managing oral hydration. In Boltz M, Capezuti E, Fulmer T, et al, editors: *Evidence-based geriatric nursing protocols for best practice*, ed 4, New York, 2012, Springer, pp 419–438.

DEHYDRATION

Dehydration is considered a geriatric syndrome that is frequently associated with common diseases (e.g., diabetes, respiratory illness, heart failure) and frailty. It is often an unappreciated comorbid condition that exacerbates an underlying condition such as a urinary tract infection, respiratory tract infection, or worsening depression. Dehydration is a significant risk factor for delirium, thromboembolic complications, infections, kidney stones, constipation and obstipation, falls, medication toxicity, renal failure, seizure, electrolyte imbalance, hyperthermia, and delayed wound healing (McCrow et al, 2016; Mentes and Aronow, 2016).

Dehydration takes various forms (Box 15.3). Water-loss dehydration (hypertonic, hyperosmotic, or intracellular dehydration) is common in older adults and results from deficient fluid intake (Hooper et al, 2016). Although the prevalence of dehydration in older adults who are hospitalized has not been adequately

From Mentes JC: A typology of oral hydration, *J Gerontol Nurs* 32(1):13–19, 2006.

studied, rates of 10% to 45% have been reported. McCrow et al. (2016) reported a dehydration rate of 30% at admission to hospital. Dehydration is estimated to be present in half of long-term care residents. In the long-term care setting, difficulties in communication, mobility, and eating prevent many from accessing fluid independently and a recent study reported that the majority of residents are not even consuming 1500 mL of fluids per day (Namasivayam-MacDonald et al, 2018). A recent study reported that hydration levels in an assisted care facility for individuals

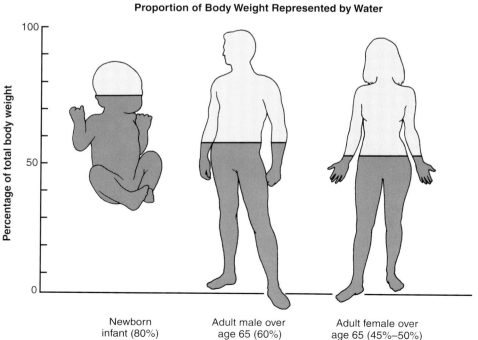

Proportion of Body Weight Represented by Water

Percentage of total body weight

- Newborn infant (80%)
- Adult male over age 65 (60%)
- Adult female over age 65 (45%–50%)

Fig. 15.1 Changes in Body Water Distribution with Age. (From Thibodeau GA, Patton KT: *Structure & function of the body*, ed 13, St Louis, 2008, Mosby.)

BOX 15.3 Types of Dehydration

- **Water-loss dehydration (hypertonic, hyperosmotic, intracellular):** Results from insufficient fluid intake, which leads to an elevation of serum osmolarity and a drop in extracellular fluid volume.
- **Volume depletion (hypovolemia) (salt loss, extracellular dehydration):** Results from excess fluid loss as occurs in vomiting/diarrhea, excessive bleeding, loss of plasma. Serum is depleted of both fluid and electrolytes. Fluid loss occurs more abruptly than water-loss dehydration. Serum osmolarity may remain stable or decrease slightly.

From Hooper L, Bunn D, Aldelhamid A, et al: Water-loss (intracellular) dehydration assessed using urinary tests: how well do they work? Diagnostic accuracy in older adults, *Am J Clin Nutr* 104:121–131, 2016.

with memory impairment were lower than comparison groups of nursing home residents (Gaspar et al, 2019).

Risk Factors for Dehydration

The presence of physical or emotional illness, surgery, trauma, frailty, or conditions of higher physiological demands increases the risk of dehydration. Older adults are particularly at risk for dehydration since their kidneys are less able to concentrate urine and some medications (diuretics) increase fluid excretion. However the main reason for dehydration is reduced fluid intake (Namasivayam-MacDonald et al, 2018). When the fluid balance of older adults is at risk, the limited capacity of homeostatic mechanisms becomes significant (Box 15.1 and Fig. 15.1). Box 15.4 presents risk factors for dehydration.

BOX 15.4 Risk Factors for Dehydration

Age-related changes
Medications: diuretics, laxatives, angiotensin-converting enzyme (ACE) inhibitors, psychotropics
Use of four or more medications
Functional deficits
Communication and comprehension problems
Oral problems
Dysphagia
Delirium
Dementia
Hospitalization
Low body weight
Diagnostic procedures requiring fasting
Requiring physical assistance at meals
Being female
Inadequate assistance with fluid/food intake
Diarrhea
Fever
Vomiting
Infections
Bleeding
Draining wounds
Artificial ventilation
Fluid restrictions
High environmental temperatures
Multiple comorbidities

PROMOTING HEALTHY AGING: IMPLICATIONS FOR GERONTOLOGICAL NURSING

Assessment

Prevention of dehydration is essential, but assessment is complex in older adults. Clinical signs may not appear until dehydration is advanced. Attention to risk factors for dehydration is very important. In addition, the Minimum Data Set (MDS) 3.0 (Chapter 7) assesses for dehydration/fluid maintenance. Education should be provided to older adults and their caregivers on the need for fluids and the signs and symptoms of dehydration. Acute situations such as vomiting, diarrhea, or febrile episodes should be identified quickly and treated. Assessment of hydration status must be conducted on admission to the hospital, particularly for those who are frail, and must be regularly monitored throughout their stay and at discharge (McCrow et al, 2016).

Signs/Symptoms of Dehydration

Typical signs of dehydration may not always be present in older adults and symptoms are often atypical. Skin turgor, assessed at the sternum and commonly included in the assessment of dehydration, is an unreliable marker in older adults because of the loss of subcutaneous tissue with aging. Dry mucous membranes in the mouth and nose, longitudinal furrows on the tongue, orthostasis, speech incoherence, rapid pulse rate, extremity weakness, dry axilla, and sunken eyes may indicate dehydration. However, the diagnosis of dehydration is biochemically proven.

Laboratory Tests

Serum osmolarity readings ≥300 mOsmol/L are indicative of dehydration in older adults (Hooper et al, 2016). Although most cases of dehydration have an elevated blood urea nitrogen (BUN) measurement, there are many other causes of an elevated BUN/creatinine ratio, so this test cannot be used alone to diagnose dehydration in older adults. Recent research reports that urinary measures reflecting hydration status in older adults (urine color, osmolarity, volume) should not be used because these measures are not sensitive or specific enough (Hooper et al, 2016). However, urine patterns and color should be observed for changes.

Interventions

Interventions are derived from a comprehensive assessment and consist of risk identification and hydration management (Box 15.5). Any older adult who has functional or cognitive impairments and is dependent on others for fluid intake is particularly at risk. Those who develop fever, diarrhea, vomiting, or a nonfebrile infection should be monitored closely by implementing intake and output records and providing additional fluids. NPO (nothing-by-mouth) requirements for diagnostic tests and surgical procedures should be as short as possible for older adults, and adequate fluids should be given once tests and procedures are completed. A 2-hour suspension of fluid intake is recommended for many procedures. Fluid intake needs to be monitored throughout a hospital stay and adequate assistance provided to maintain fluid intake.

Hydration management involves both acute and ongoing management of oral intake. Oral rehydration therapy is the first

BOX 15.5   Tips for Best Practice

Ongoing Management of Oral Intake: Long-Term Care

1. Calculate a daily fluid goal.
   - All older adults should have an individualized fluid goal determined by a documented standard for daily fluid intake. At least 1500 mL of fluid/day should be provided.
2. Compare current intake to fluid goal to evaluate hydration status.
3. Provide fluids consistently throughout the day.
   - Provide 75% to 80% of fluids at mealtimes and the remainder during non-mealtimes such as medication times.
   - Offer a variety of fluids and fluids that the person prefers.
   - Standardize the amount of fluid that is offered with medication administration (e.g., at least 6 oz).
4. Plan for at-risk individuals.
   - Have fluid rounds midmorning and midafternoon.
   - Provide two 8-oz glasses of fluid in the morning and evening.
   - Offer a "happy hour" or "tea time," when residents can gather for additional fluids and socialization.
   - Provide modified fluid containers based on resident's abilities—for example, lighter cups and glasses, weighted cups and glasses, plastic water bottles with straws (attach to wheelchairs, deliver with meals).
   - Make fluids accessible at all times and be sure residents can access them—for example, filled water pitchers, fluid stations, or beverage carts in congregate areas.
   - Allow adequate time and staff for eating or feeding. Meals can provide two-thirds of daily fluids.
   - Encourage family members to participate in feeding and offering fluids.
5. Perform fluid regulation and documentation.
   - Teach individuals, if possible, to use a urine color chart to monitor hydration status.
   - Document complete intake including hydration habits.
   - Know volumes of fluid containers to accurately calculate fluid consumption.
   - Frequency of documentation of fluid intake will vary among settings and is dependent on the individual's condition. In most settings, at least one accurate intake and output recording should be documented, including amount of fluid consumed, difficulties with consumption, and urine specific gravity and color.
   - For individuals who are not continent, teach caregivers to observe incontinent pads or briefs for amount and frequency of urine, color changes, and odor, and report variations from individual's normal pattern.

Adapted from Mentes JC: Managing oral hydration. In Boltz M, Capezuti E, Fulmer T, et al, editors: *Evidence-based geriatric nursing protocols for best practice*, New York, 2012, Springer, pp 419–438.

treatment approach for dehydration. Individuals with mild to moderate dehydration who can drink and do not have significant mental or physical compromise due to fluid loss may be able to replenish fluids orally. Water is considered the best fluid to offer, but other clear fluids may also be useful depending on the person's preference.

Rehydration Methods

Rehydration methods depend on the severity and the type of dehydration and may include intravenous or hypodermoclysis (HDC). A general rule is to replace 50% of the loss within the first 12 hours (or 1 L/day in afebrile individuals) or sufficient quantity to relieve tachycardia and hypotension. Further fluid replacement can be administered more slowly over a longer period of time. It is important to monitor for symptoms of overhydration (unexplained weight gain, pedal edema, neck vein distention, shortness of breath), especially in individuals with heart failure or renal disease. Individuals taking selective serotonin reuptake inhibitors (SSRIs) should have serum sodium levels and hydration status closely monitored due to risk for hyponatremia (Chapter 9). Increasing fluid intake may aggravate an evolving hyponatremia.

Hypodermoclysis

HDC (also known as clysis) is an infusion of isotonic fluids into the subcutaneous space. HDC is safe, easy to administer, and a useful alternative to intravenous administration for persons with mild to moderate dehydration, particularly those patients with altered mental status. HDC cannot be used in severe dehydration or for any situation requiring more than 3 L over 24 hours. Common sites of infusion are the lateral abdominal wall; the anterior or lateral aspects of the thighs; the infraclavicular region; and the back, usually the interscapular or subscapular regions with a fat fold at least 1 inch thick (Mei and Auerhahn, 2009). Normal saline (0.9%), half-normal saline (0.45%), 5% glucose in water infusion (D5W), or Ringer's solution can be used (Thomas et al, 2008).

HDC offers a wider range of infusion sites than traditional intravenous (IV) therapy and can be far less painful, especially when veins are difficult to find due to dehydration. IV access can also be difficult when older adults have mental status changes. HDC is considered a simple, safe, well-tolerated, and low-cost procedure but is little used. HDC can be administered in almost any setting, so hospital admissions may be avoided. Nurses have little knowledge of HDC as a fluid replacement therapy and there is need for more clinical studies to promote decision-making and guide clinical practice (Gomes et al, 2017; Smith, 2014). Other resources on hydration can be found in Box 15.5.

ORAL HEALTH

Orodental health is integral to general health. Orodental health is a basic need that is increasingly neglected with advanced age, debilitation, and limited mobility. Age-related changes in the oral cavity (Box 15.1), medical conditions, poor dental hygiene, and lack of dental care contribute to poor oral health. Older adults who are dependent on caregivers for bodily care assistance exhibit worse oral hygiene than those who are self-sufficient. Poor oral health is recognized as a risk factor for dehydration and malnutrition, and a number of systemic diseases, including pneumonia, joint infections, cardiovascular disease, and poor glycemic control in type 1 and type 2 diabetes. There has been an identified connection between poor oral health and mortality in a cohort of older adults (Kohli et al, 2016).

Poor oral health is an important public health issue and a growing burden to countries worldwide. Health disparities are evident across and within regions and result from living conditions and availability of oral health services. Tips for promotion of oral health are presented in Box 15.6. *Healthy People 2020* addresses oral health (Healthy People 2020 box).

BOX 15.6 Tips for Best Practice

Promoting Oral Health

Encourage annual dental exams, including individuals with dentures.

Brush and floss twice daily; use a fluoride dentifrice and mouthwash.

Ensure dentures fit well and are cleaned regularly.

Maintain adequate daily fluid intake (1500 mL).

Avoid tobacco.

Limit alcohol.

Eat a well-balanced diet.

Use an ultrasonic toothbrush (more effective in removing plaque).

Use a commercial floss handle for easier flossing.

Adapt toothbrush if manual dexterity impaired. Use a child's toothbrush or enlarge the handle of an adult-sized toothbrush by adding a foam grip or wrapping it with gauze or rubber bands to increase handle size.

If medications cause a dry mouth, ask your health care provider if there are other drugs that can be substituted. If dry mouth cannot be avoided, drink plenty of water, chew sugarless gum, avoid alcohol and tobacco.

HEALTHY PEOPLE 2020

Dental Health Goals for Older Adults

- Prevent and control oral and craniofacial diseases, conditions, and injuries, and improve access to preventive services and dental care.
- Reduce the proportion of adults with untreated dental decay.
- Reduce the proportion of older adults with untreated caries.
- Reduce the proportion of adults who have ever had a permanent tooth extracted because of dental caries or periodontal disease.
- Reduce the proportion of older adults 65 to 74 years of age who have lost all of their natural teeth.
- Reduce the proportion of adults 45 to 74 years of age with moderate or severe periodontitis.
- Increase the proportion of oral and pharyngeal cancers detected at the earliest stages.

Data from U.S. Department of Health and Human Services, Office of Disease Prevention and Health Promotion: *Healthy People 2020*, 2012. http://www.healthypeople.gov/2020.

Common Oral Problems

Xerostomia (Mouth Dryness)

Xerostomia and hyposalivation are present in approximately 30% of older adults and can affect eating, swallowing, and speaking and contribute to dental caries and periodontal disease. Adequate saliva is necessary for the beginning stage of digestion, helping to break down starches and fats. It also functions to clear the mouth of food debris and prevent overgrowth of oral microbes. The flow of saliva does not decrease with age, but medical conditions and medications affect salivary flow (Becerra, 2017). More than 400 medications have a side effect of hyposalivation including antihypertensives, antidepressants, antihistamines, antipsychotics, diuretics, and antiparkinson agents.

Treatment of xerostomia. A review of all medications is important, and if medication side effects are contributing to dry mouth, medications may be changed or altered. Affected individuals should practice good oral hygiene practices and have regular dental care to screen for decay. Consumption of adequate water intake and avoidance of alcohol and caffeine are recommended. Over-the-counter saliva substitutes (Oral Balance Gel, MouthKote) and salivary stimulants such as Biotene, Xylitol gum, and sugarless candy can be helpful.

Oral Cancer

Oral cancers occur more with age. The median age at diagnosis is 61 years; men are affected twice as often as women. It is much more common in Hungary and France than in the United States and much less common in Mexico and Japan. The 5-year survival rate is 60% and has not changed significantly since the late 1960s. This is largely the result of late identification of the disease. There are several types of oral cancer but around 90% are squamous cell carcinomas. Historically, the majority of individuals are over the age of 40 years at the time of discovery; however, the incidence is increasing in those under this age. Exact causes are becoming clearer in peer reviewed research and include the human papilloma virus 16 and the use of "smoke-less" chewing or spit tobacco. In a younger age group, including those who have never used any tobacco products, human papilloma virus may be replacing tobacco as the primary causative agent. This virus is sexually transmitted between partners and is also responsible for more than 90% of all cervical cancers. Risk factors are listed in Box 15.7.

Early detection is essential, but more than 60% of oral cancers are not diagnosed until an advanced stage. Early signs and symptoms may be subtle and not recognized by the individual or health care provider. Common areas for oral cancer to develop are the tongue, tonsils and oropharynx, the gums and floor of the mouth. Oral examinations can assist in early identification and treatment. All persons, especially those older than 50 years of age, with or without dentures, should have oral examinations on a regular basis. A new initiative from the Oral Cancer Foundation *Check Your Mouth* (www.checkyourmouth.org) is built around an interactive website designed to help individuals learn to self-discover suspicious tissue changes in their own mouths (Box 15.8). Box 15.9 presents common signs

BOX 15.7 Risk Factors for Oral Cancer

Tobacco, including smokeless tobacco

Alcohol

Human papilloma virus 16

Genetic susceptibility

BOX 15.8 Resources for Best Practice

Oral Cancer Foundation: Check Your Mouth (www.checkyourmouth.org)—interactive website to assist individuals in self-screening for oral cancer/oral changes.

Smiles for Life: http://www.smilesforlifeoralhealth.org/buildcontent.aspx?tut=555&pagekey=62948&cbreceipt=0: National curriculum to help primary care clinicians integrate oral health care into care of patients

The Hartford Institute for Geriatric Nursing (Consultgeri.org): Nursing Standard of Practice Protocols: Hydration management; Oral care; The Kayser-Jones Brief Oral Health Status Examination (BOHSE)

University of Alabama at Birmingham School of Medicine: Video of techniques for providing mouth care to individuals with dementia: http://www.uab.edu/medicine/alzheimers/care-resistant-behavior

BOX 15.9 Signs and Symptoms of Oral and Throat Cancer

- Swelling or thickening, lumps or bumps, or rough spots or eroded areas on the lips, gums, or other areas inside the mouth
- Velvety white, red, or speckled patches in the mouth
- Persistent sores on the face, neck, or mouth that bleed easily
- Unexplained bleeding in the mouth
- Unexplained numbness or pain or tenderness in any area of the face, mouth, neck, or tongue
- Soreness in the back of the throat; a persistent feeling that something is caught in the throat
- Difficulty chewing or swallowing, speaking, or moving the jaw or tongue
- Hoarseness, chronic sore throat, or changes in the voice
- Dramatic weight loss
- Lump or swelling in the neck
- Severe pain in one ear—with a normal eardrum
- Pain around the teeth; loosening of the teeth
- Swelling or pain in the jaw; difficulty moving the jaw

and symptoms of oral cancer. Once diagnosed, therapy options are based on diagnosis and staging and include surgery, radiation, and chemotherapy. If detected early, these cancers can almost always be treated successfully. Individuals with treated oral cancer will need to have follow-up exams for the rest of their lives, since another cancer can develop later in the mouth, lung, throat, or other areas (Oral Cancer Foundation, 2018).

Oral Care

Nearly one-third of individuals older than age 65 have untreated tooth decay. Nearly one in five adults 65 years and older have lost all of their teeth (edentulous), primarily as a result of periodontitis, which occurs in about 68% of those in this age group (CDC, 2016). There has been a dramatic reduction in the prevalence of tooth loss as knowledge increases and more people use fluorides, improve nutrition, engage in new oral hygiene practices, and take advantage of improved dental health care. However, many individuals may not have had the advantages of new preventive treatment, and those with functional and cognitive limitations may be unable to perform oral hygiene.

Access to dental care for older adults may be limited and cost prohibitive. In the existing health care system, dental care is a low priority. Medicare does not provide any coverage for oral health care services, and few Americans 75 years of age or older have private dental insurance. Medicaid coverage for dental varies from state to state, but funding has decreased and coverage can be limited. Older adults have fewer dentist visits than any other age group. Those with the poorest oral health are those who are economically disadvantaged and lack insurance. Being disabled, homebound, or institutionalized increases the risk of poor oral health. Access to dentists in long-term care facilities is very limited and many are unwilling to provide care in these facilities (Jablonski et al, 2017). If a long-term care resident needs dental care, it requires transportation to a dentist's office which is not only costly, but many times not possible because of the individual's condition. In many undeveloped

countries, there is a shortage of trained dental professionals. Dental care is nonexistent except that provided by groups such as medical and dental ministries from other countries.

PROMOTING HEALTHY AGING: IMPLICATIONS FOR GERONTOLOGICAL NURSING

Assessment

Good oral hygiene and timely assessment of oral health are nursing responsibilities. Oral care is "oral infection control" (Jablonski-Jaudon et al, 2016, p. 15). The relationship between poor oral health and systemic infections, such as pneumonia, is well documented (Jablonski et al, 2017). In addition, examination of the mouth can serve as an early warning system for some diseases and lead to early diagnosis and treatment. Assessment of the mouth, teeth, and oral cavity is an essential part of health assessment (Chapter 7) and especially important when an individual is hospitalized or in a long-term care facility. An oral exam should be included as part of a general medical exam in primary care (Becerra, 2017). The MDS 3.0 requires information obtained from an oral assessment. Federal regulations mandate an annual examination for residents of long-term care facilities. Although the oral examination is best performed by a dentist, nurses in health care settings can provide oral health screenings using an instrument such as the Kayser-Jones Brief Oral Health Status Examination (BOHSE) (Box 15.8).

Interventions

Nurses may be involved in promoting oral health through teaching individuals or caregivers recommended interventions, screening for oral disease, and making dental referrals, or by providing, supervising, and evaluating oral care in hospitals and long-term care facilities. Box 15.10 presents information on providing oral hygiene.

Dentures

Older adults and those who may care for them should be taught proper care of dentures and oral tissue to prevent odor, stain, plaque buildup, and oral infections. All nursing staff should be knowledgeable about care of dentures (Box 15.11). Dentures are very personal and expensive possessions and the utmost care should be taken when handling, cleaning, and storing dentures, especially in hospitals and long-term care facilities. It is not uncommon to hear that dentures were lost, broken, or mixed up with those of others, or not removed and cleaned during a hospital or nursing home stay. Dentures should be marked, and many states require all newly made dentures to contain the client's identification. Denture marking kits are easily available and provide a simple, efficient, and permanent means of marking dentures.

Broken or damaged dentures and dentures that no longer fit because of weight loss or changes in the oral cavity are a common problem for older adults. Many older adults believe that there is no longer a need for oral care once they have dentures, but regular professional attention is important. Rebasing of dentures is a technique to improve the fit of dentures. Ill-fitting dentures or dentures that are not cleaned contribute

BOX 15.10 Tips for Best Practice

Providing Oral Care

1. Explain all actions to the individual; use gestures and demonstration as needed; cue and prompt to encourage as much self-care performance as possible.
2. If the individual is in bed, elevate his or her head by raising the bed or propping it with pillows, and have the individual turn his or her head to face you. Place a clean towel across the chest and under the chin, and place a basin under the chin.
3. If the individual is sitting in a stationary chair or wheelchair, stand behind the individual and stabilize his or her head by placing one hand under the chin and resting the head against your body. Place a towel across the chest and over the shoulders.
4. The basin can be kept handy in the individual's lap or on a table placed in front of or at the side of the patient. A wheelchair may be positioned in front of the sink.
5. If the individual's lips are dry or cracked, apply a light coating of petroleum jelly or use lip balm.
6. Inspect the oral cavity to identify teeth in ill repair, pain, lesions, or inflammation.
7. Brush and floss the individual's teeth (use an electric toothbrush if possible, with sulcular brushing). It may be helpful to retract the lips and cheek with a tongue blade or fingers to see the area that is being cleaned. Use a mouth prop as needed if the individual cannot hold his or her mouth open. If manual flossing is too difficult, use a floss holder or interproximal brush to clean the proximal surfaces between the teeth. Use a dentifrice containing fluoride. Brush the tongue.
8. Provide the conscious individual with fluoride rinses or other rinses as indicated by the dentist or hygienist.

BOX 15.11 Tips for Best Practice

Providing Denture Care

1. Remove dentures or ask individual to remove dentures. Observe ability to remove dentures.
2. Inspect oral cavity.
3. Rinse denture or dentures after each meal to remove soft debris. Do not use toothpaste on dentures because it abrades denture surfaces.
4. Once each day, preferably before retiring, remove denture and brush thoroughly.
   a. Although an ordinary soft toothbrush is adequate, a specially designed denture brush may clean more effectively. (CAUTION: Acrylic denture material is softer than natural teeth and may be damaged by being brushed with very firm bristles.)
   b. Brush denture over a sink lined with a facecloth and half-filled with water. This will prevent breakage if the denture is dropped.
   c. Hold the denture securely in one hand, but do not squeeze. Hold the brush in the other hand. It is not essential to use a denture paste, particularly if dentures are soaked before being brushed to soften debris. Never use a commercial tooth powder because it is abrasive and may damage the denture materials. Plain water, mild soap, or sodium bicarbonate may be used.
   d. When cleaning a removable partial denture, great care must be taken to remove plaque from the curved metal clasps that hook around the teeth. This can be done with a regular toothbrush or with a specially designed clasp brush.
5. After brushing, rinse denture thoroughly; then place it in a denture-cleaning solution and allow it to soak overnight or for at least a few hours. (NOTE: Acrylic denture material must be kept wet at all times to prevent cracking or warping.) In the morning, remove denture from the cleaning solution and rinse it thoroughly before inserting it into the mouth. Use denture paste if necessary to secure dentures.
6. Dentures should be worn constantly except at night (to allow relief of compression on the gums) and replaced in the mouth in the morning.

to oral problems (lesions, stomatitis) and to poor nutrition and reduced enjoyment of food.

Oral Hygiene in Hospitals and Long-Term Care

Oral care is an often neglected part of daily nursing care and should receive the same priority as other kinds of care. Illness, acute care situations, and functional and cognitive impairments make the provision of oral care difficult. Factors contributing to less than adequate oral care include inadequate knowledge of how to provide care, lack of appropriate supplies, inadequate training and staffing, and lack of oral care protocols. When the person is unable to carry out his or her dental/oral regimen, it is the responsibility of the caregiver to provide oral care.

In the acute care setting, good oral care is crucial to the prevention of ventilator-associated pneumonia (VAP), one of the most common hospital-acquired infections and a leading cause of morbidity and mortality in intensive care units (ICUs). Attention to oral care is essential in all settings but often not consistently implemented. In an observational study of oral hygiene care interventions provided by nurses to older adults in postacute hospital settings, oral hygiene care was supported in just over one-third of encounters. Denture care was inconsistently performed; also, nurses did not encourage adequate self-care of natural teeth by patients and infrequently moisturized tissues (Coker et al, 2017). Mouth care may be perceived as a comfort measure rather than a critical component of infection control (Research Highlights box).

RESEARCH HIGHLIGHTS

The purpose of the study was to report on the actual oral hygiene interventions nurses were observed to provide to patients in postacute hospital settings during their evening rounds. Five hospital sites in Southern Ontario were utilized. Twenty-five registered nurses and registered practical nurses were shadowed during their evening care. Observations were recorded and then categorized during data analysis. In addition to observation, nurses were engaged in conversation and these conversations were audiotaped with consent.

Practices observed were inconsistent with existing evidence in practice guidelines. The most notable exceptions related to the frequency and timing of oral hygiene care, caring for patients with dentures, cleaning the oral cavity, and keeping tissues moist. Little more than a third of patients were supported to complete their oral care. Rinsing with mouthwash was rarely done and the hospital-supplied mouthwash was not antibacterial and would have been ineffective. Practice guideline recommendation for twice daily oral care was not met. The study of adequate and feasible oral hygiene interventions is urgently needed.

From Coker SE, Ploeg J, Kaasalainen S, Carter N: Observations of oral hygiene care interventions provided by nurses to hospitalized older adults, *Geriatr Nurs* 38(1):17–21, 2017.

Individuals residing in long-term care facilities are particularly vulnerable to problems with oral care as a result of functional and cognitive impairments. A large number are dependent on staff for the provision of oral hygiene. Older adults with dementia often resist caregiving activities associated with mouth care. Care-resistant behavior (CRB) is one of the primary reasons for the omission of mouth care (Hoben et al, 2017; Jablonski-Jaudon et al, 2016). Long-term care residents with dementia who exhibit CRBs are three times more likely to have more tooth decay than those who allow mouth care.

Nurse researcher Rita Jablonski has researched CRBs and developed the MOUTh intervention (*Managing Oral Hygiene Using Threat reduction strategies*) to prevent and minimize CRBs to provide mouth care to older adults with dementia. Components include (1) an evidence-based mouth care protocol; (2) recognition of CRBs; and (3) strategies designed to lower the perception of mouth care as a threatening, scary, or assaultive activity. Strategies include approach, establishing rapport, avoiding elderspeak (Chapter 6), gestures/pantomime, cueing, and chaining (initiating the action with the expectation that the individual will take over). For a link to a video demonstrating techniques, see Box 15.8. Techniques may have applicability to other activities that trigger CRB, such as bathing (Chapter 29) (Jablonsk-Jaudoni et al, 2016).

The use of therapeutic rinses (e.g., chlorhexidine) that are broad-spectrum antimicrobial agents has been shown to help control plaque and reduce VAP by 40% (Erickson, 2016). These can be used in conjunction with brushing or instead of brushing in those unable to tolerate brushing. A correlation between tongue coating and aspiration pneumonia risk points to the benefit of including tongue cleaning as part of mouth care (Erickson, 2016).

Many long-term care institutions have implemented programs, such as special training of nursing assistants for dental care teams, dental care champions, providing visits from mobile dentistry units on a routine basis, or using dental students to perform oral screening and cleaning of teeth (Kohli et al, 2017). An important nursing role in all health care settings is to assist in the development of oral care protocols, staff education, and monitoring of oral health care. Caregivers of older adults at home who require oral care also need education about the importance of oral care and techniques for providing oral care.

Other Considerations in Oral Hygiene Provision

Tube feeding is associated with significant pathologic colonization of the mouth, greater than that observed in people who received oral feeding. Individuals with dysphagia (Chapter 14) often receive inadequate mouth care and experience poor oral health (Jablonski et al, 2017). Recommendations are that individuals receiving tube feeding should have their teeth brushed twice a day but techniques and safety have not been determined (Huang et al, 2017). In hospitals, nurses routinely provide mouth care to patients unable to swallow using toothbrushes connected to wall suction. In a pilot study, Jablonski et al. (2017) examined the effectiveness of using soft toothbrushes dipped in alcohol-free mouthwash for individuals with dysphagia in long-term care settings without access to suction equipment. The protocol resulted in improved oral hygiene without aspiration. Research into the oral hygiene status of non–oral feeding patients and optimal and safe oral care interventions for individuals with dysphagia and tube feeding is needed, especially in long-term care and home settings (Ohno et al, 2017). Foam swabs are available to provide oral hygiene but do not remove plaque as well as toothbrushes. Foam swabs may be used to clean the oral mucosa of an edentulous older adult.

> ⚡ **SAFETY ALERT**
>
> Lemon glycerin swabs should never be used for oral care. In combination with decreased salivary flow and xerostomia, they inhibit salivary production, causing dry mouth and promoting bacterial growth (Booker et al, 2013).

▌ KEY CONCEPTS

- Age-related changes, medication use, functional impairments, and comorbid medical and emotional illnesses place some older adults at risk for changes in fluid balance, especially dehydration.
- In older adults, dehydration most often develops as a result of disease, age-related changes, and/or the effects of medication; dehydration is not primarily due to lack of access to water. Dehydration is considered a geriatric syndrome that is frequently associated with common diseases (e.g., diabetes, respiratory illness, heart failure) and declining stages of the frail older adult.
- Prevention of dehydration is essential, but assessment is complex in older adults. Clinical signs may not appear until dehydration is advanced and signs and symptoms may be nonspecific, making prevention and early identification important.

- Age-related changes in the oral cavity, medical conditions, poor dental hygiene, and lack of dental care contribute to poor oral health. Poor oral health is a risk factor for dehydration and malnutrition, and a number of systemic diseases, including pneumonia, joint infections, cardiovascular disease, and poor glycemic control in type 1 and type 2 diabetes.
- Good oral hygiene and timely assessment of oral health are essentials of nursing care.
- Nurses may be involved in promoting oral health by teaching individuals or caregivers recommended interventions, by screening for oral disease and making dental referrals, or by providing, supervising, and evaluating oral care in hospitals and long-term care facilities.

NURSING STUDY: HYDRATION STATUS

Violet Barnes is an 87-year-old woman who resides in a skilled nursing facility. Her diagnoses include dementia, hypertension, and diabetes. She is able to walk and feed herself with assistance. She knows her name and responds to conversation appropriately, although she is not oriented to time or place. Two days ago she underwent a colonoscopy on an outpatient basis in the hospital for a suspected mass in the large intestine. She was maintained nothing-by-mouth (NPO) for 12 hours before the procedure and returned to the skilled facility following the procedure. Since she has returned, she has become very lethargic and not able to respond to familiar caregivers. She is refusing any food or fluids offered. She has had four episodes of diarrhea and her stool is being tested for *C. difficile.*

On the basis of the nursing study, develop a nursing care plan using the following procedure[a]:

- List information that provides objective data.
- From the data, identify and state, using an accepted format, two nursing diagnoses you determine are most significant to Violet at this time. List two of Violet's strengths that you have identified from the data.

- Determine and state outcome criteria for each diagnosis. These must reflect some alleviation of the problem identified in the nursing diagnosis and must be stated in concrete and measurable terms.
- Plan and state one or more interventions for each diagnosed problem. Provide specific documentation of the source used to determine the appropriate intervention. Plan at least one intervention that incorporates Violet's existing strengths.
- Evaluate the success of the intervention. Interventions must correlate directly with the stated outcome criteria to measure the outcome success.

[a]Students are advised to refer to their nursing diagnosis text and identify possible or potential problems.

CRITICAL THINKING QUESTIONS AND ACTIVITIES

1. What risk factors for Violet's condition are present in nursing study above?
2. What preventive interventions by nursing would have been appropriate?
3. What are your suggestions for enhancing fluid intake for individuals with dementia residing in skilled nursing facilities?

RESEARCH QUESTIONS

1. What is the knowledge level of older adults about oral health practices?
2. What factors influence adequate dental care among older adults?
3. What strategies are most helpful in enhancing fluid intake of older adults in long-term care facilities?
4. What are the barriers to adequate oral care for older adults in hospitals and long-term care facilities?
5. What content related to oral health is included in your nursing education program?

REFERENCES

Becerra K: Oral health in older patients: a job for primary care, *Medscape* 2017. https://www.medscape.com/viewarticle/881460/. Accessed February 2018.

Centers for Disease Control and Prevention: *Facts about older adult oral health,* 2016. https://www.cdc.gov/oralhealth/basics/adult-oral-health/adult_older.htm. Accessed February 2018.

Coker E, Ploeg J, Kaasalainen S, Carter N: Observations of oral hygiene care interventions provided by nurses to hospitalized older people, *Geriatr Nurs* 38(1):17–21, 2017.

Erickson LE: The mouth-body connection, *Generations* 40(3), 2016. https://www.asaging.org/blog/mouth%E2%88%92body-connection. Accessed March 2019.

Gaspar P, Scherb C, Rivera-Mariana F: Hydration status of assisted living memory care residents. *J Gerontol Nurs* 45(4):21–28, 2019.

Gomes NS, DaSilva A, Zago L: Nursing knowledge and practices regarding subcutaneous fluid administration, *Rev Bras Enferm* 70(5), 2017. http://www.scielo.br/scielo.php?pid=S0034-71672017000501096&script=sci_arttext. Accessed January 2018.

Hooper L, Bunn DK, Abdelhamid A, et al: Water-loss (intracellular) dehydration assessed using urinary tests: how well do they work? Diagnostic accuracy in older people, *Am J Clin Nutr* 104:121–131, 2016.

Huang S, Chiou C, Liu H: Risk factors for aspiration pneumonia related to improper oral hygiene behavior in community dysphagia persons with nasogastric tube feeding, *J Dent Sci* 12(4):375–381, 2017.

Jablonski-Jaudon RA, Kolanowski AM, Winstead V, Jones-Townsend C, Azuero A: Maturation of the MOUTh intervention: from reducing threat to relationship-centered care, *J Gerontol Nurs* 42(3):15–23, 2016.

Jablonski RA, Winstead V, Azuero A, et al: Feasibility of providing safe mouth care and collecting oral and fecal microbiome samples from nursing home residents with dysphagia: proof of concept study, *J Gerontol Nurs* 43(9):9–15, 2017.

Kohli R, Nelson S, Ulrich S, Finch T, Hall K, Schwarz E: Dental care practices and oral health training for professional caregivers in long-term care facilities: an interdisciplinary approach to address oral health disparities, *Geriatr Nurs* 38(4):296–301, 2017.

McCrow J, Morton M, Travers C, Harvey K, Eeles E: Associations between dehydration, cognitive impairment, and frailty in older hospitalized patients: an exploratory study, *J Gerontol Nurs* 42(5):19–27, 2016.

Mei A, Auerhahn C: Hypodermoclysis: maintaining hydration in the frail older adult, *Ann Long-term Care* 17:28–30, 2009.

Mentes JC: Managing oral hydration. In Boltz M, Capezuti E, Fulmer T, editors: *Evidence-based geriatric nursing protocols for best practice,* ed 4, New York, NY, 2012, Springer, pp 419–438.

Mentes JC, Aronow H: Comparing older adults presenting with dehydration as a primary diagnosis versus a secondary diagnosis in the emergency department, *J Aging Res Clin Pract* 5(4):181–186, 2016.

Namasivayam-MacDonald AM, Slaughter SE, Morrison J, et al: Inadequate fluid intake in long term care residents: prevalence and determinants, *Geriatr Nurs* 39:330–335, 2018.

Ohno T, Heshiki Y, Kogure M, Sumi Y, Miura H: Comparison of oral assessment results between non-oral and oral feeding patients: a preliminary study, *J Gerontol Nurs* 43(4):23–28, 2017.

Smith LS: Hypodermoclysis with older adults, *Nursing* 44(12):66, 2014.

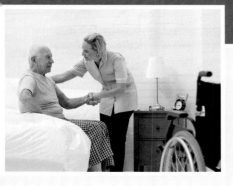

16

Elimination

Theris A. Touhy

http://evolve.elsevier.com/Touhy/TwdHlthAging

A STUDENT SPEAKS

My grandmother doesn't like to go out shopping with me anymore. She says she has to go to the bathroom all the time and can't walk fast enough to get to the bathrooms in the mall. She won't wear a protective garment or a pad because she says they smell. I hope I learn something in this class that will help her.

Molly, 20 years old

OLDER ADULTS SPEAK

"Being incontinent is like being a bad kid or a big baby."
"There's nothing that can be done. Well, I don't think there is anything else but a diaper."
"Sometimes I have to wet my bed before they get here, you know, and they are all busy and I have to wait for somebody."
"I do something that is very wrong. I try not to drink too much. How can you drink a lot, you would be soaked all the time?"

Comments from participants in a study of living with urinary incontinence in long-term care (MacDonald and Butler, 2007)

A NURSE SPEAKS

Urinary incontinence is a preventable and treatable condition and yet continence remains undervalued and UI remains underassessed. Even though UI is a basic nursing issue, nurses are not claiming it as one.

Comment from nurse in expert continence care (Mason et al, 2003, p. 3)

LEARNING OBJECTIVES

On completion of this chapter, the student will be able to:

1. Identify age-related changes and other contributing factors affecting bowel and bladder elimination.
2. Identify appropriate assessment of bowel and bladder function.
3. Explain the types of urinary incontinence and their causes.
4. Identify risk factors for accidental bowel leakage and describe appropriate nursing interventions.
5. Use evidence-based protocols in the assessment and development of interventions to promote bowel and bladder health.

The body must remove waste products of metabolism to sustain healthy function, but bladder and bowel activity are fraught with social implications. Bladder and bowel function in later life, although normally only slightly altered by the physiological changes of age (Box 16.1), can contribute to problems severe enough to interfere with the ability to continue independent living and can seriously threaten the body's capacity to function and to survive. The effects of uncontrolled bladder and bowel action are a threat to the person's independence and well-being.

Elimination is a private matter, not publicized socially. In most cultures, children are taught early to deal with their own body waste. Deviations from this may be socially unacceptable and can lead to chastisement, ostracism, and

BOX 16.1 Age-Related Changes in the Renal and Urological Systems

Kidneys

Decreased size and function begins in fourth decade; kidney is 20% to 30% smaller by end of eighth decade

Decrease in renal blood flow and glomerular filtration rate (GFR) (less pronounced in healthy individuals)

Diverticula of renal tubules in distal portion of nephron

Glucose reabsorption decreases (more glucose in the urine)

Decline in renal activation of vitamin D decreases intestinal absorption of calcium; more vitamin D is needed to counteract diminishing renal function

Ability to concentrate urine decreases; hyperkalemia more common; sudden large changes in pH or fluid load can quickly lead to hypervolemia or hypovolemia. These changes cause a high risk for adverse events if individual is exposed to changes in environment (high temperatures, renal-toxic medications) or to functional restrictions that limit ability to obtain adequate fluids

Ureters, Bladder, Urethra

Less tone and elasticity

Loss of bladder holding capacity

Total bladder capacity decreases to 300 mL from 600 mL

Urge to void occurs at lower bladder volume (160 to 300 mL)

Weakened contractions during emptying, which can lead to postvoid residual and increased risk for bladder infection

More urine produced at night; may be due to changes in circadian rhythm, output, medications, or be indicator of sleep apnea

Increased collagen content, changes in gap junctions, increased space between myocytes, and changes in sensitivity of sensory afferents, all of which may contribute to involuntary bladder contractions and overactive bladder symptoms

From Gibson W, Wagg A: New horizons: urinary incontinence in older adults, *Age Ageing* 43:167–163, 2014; McCance K, Huether S: *Pathophysiology*, ed 7, St Louis, 2014, Elsevier.

BOX 16.2 Normal Bladder Elimination

• Normal bladder function requires an intact brain and spinal cord, competent lower urinary tract function, the motivation to maintain continence, the functional ability to use a toilet, and an environment that facilitates the process.

• A full bladder increases pressure and signals the spinal cord and the brainstem center of the desire to micturate. Social training then dictates whether micturition should be addressed or should be postponed until there is an appropriate opportunity to locate toilet facilities.

• When the bladder contents reach 500 mL or more, the pressure is such that it becomes more difficult to control the urge to void. As volume increases, emptying the bladder becomes an uncontrollable act.

BOX 16.3 Promoting a Healthy Bladder

• Drink 8 to 10 glasses of water a day before 8 PM.
• Eliminate or reduce the use of coffee, tea, brown cola, and alcohol, particularly before bedtime.
• Empty bladder completely before and after meals and at bedtime.
• Urinate whenever the urge arises; never ignore it.
• Limit the use of sleeping pills, sedatives, and alcohol because they decrease sensation to urinate.
• Make sure toilet is nearby with a clear path to it and good lighting, especially at night. Consider a grab bar or a raised toilet seat if there is difficulty getting on and off the toilet.
• Maintain ideal body weight.
• Get regular physical exercise.
• Avoid smoking.
• Seek professional treatment for complaints of burning, urgency, pain, blood in urine, or difficulties maintaining continence.

social withdrawal. Nurses are in a key position to implement evidence-based assessment and interventions to enhance continence and improve function, independence, and quality of life.

AGE-RELATED CHANGES IN THE RENAL AND UROLOGICAL SYSTEMS

The renal system is responsible for excreting toxins, regulating water and salts, and maintaining the acid-base balance in the blood. The kidneys, the primary organs in the renal system, are highly vascular. They produce the hormone *erythropoietin*, which stimulates the bone marrow to produce red blood cells, and the enzyme *renin*, which helps regulate blood pressure. In aging there are both anatomical and functional changes. The age-related loss of nephrons, kidney mass, and ability to concentrate urine ordinarily leads to little change in the body's ability to regulate its body fluids and the ability to maintain adequate fluid homeostasis under usual circumstances. Renal disease or urinary tract obstruction can amplify age-related declines in function. Changes that may contribute to urinary incontinence, nocturia, and increase in frequency of urination, but UI

should never be considered a normal part of aging. Box 16.2 describes the process of normal bladder elimination and Box 16.3 describes promotion of a healthy bladder.

URINARY INCONTINENCE

Urinary incontinence (UI) is the complaint of involuntary loss of urine sufficient to be a problem. UI is an important yet neglected geriatric syndrome. UI is a stigmatized, underreported, underdiagnosed, undertreated condition that is erroneously thought to be part of normal aging. Less than half of older adults with UI bring up this problem to their health care provider (Hsu et al, 2016). On average, women wait 6.5 years from the first time they experience symptoms until they obtain a diagnosis for their bladder control problems. Instead, they try to cope with the condition on their own, with variable success. Older individuals are less likely to receive evidence-based care for UI complaints than younger people (Gibson and Wagg, 2014; Wilde et al, 2014).

Individuals may not seek treatment for UI because they are embarrassed to talk about the problem or think that it is a normal part of aging. They may be unaware that successful treatments are available. Men may be unlikely to report UI to their primary care provider because they feel it is a woman's disease. Older adults want more information about bladder control, and nurses must take the lead in implementing approaches to continence promotion and public health education about UI. Nurses are intimately involved in providing personal hygiene care and it is essential that they assume a leading role in assessing and managing UI. Yet, nursing staff tend to view UI as an inconvenience rather than a condition requiring assessment and treatment.

Research has identified nurses' negative attitudes toward the older adult population, lack of knowledge about UI, inadequate assessment, diagnosis, or proper documentation of the condition, and limited use of evidence-based interventions for UI. In a recent study in the acute care setting, nurses were often unaware of UI assessment tools, designed their own assessment tool, or used assessment tools that were not validated for use with older adults. The most common strategies to manage UI were adult incontinence pads and adult briefs; assessment was infrequently performed (Colborne and Dahlke, 2017).

Without an adequate knowledge base of continence care and use of evidence-based practice guidelines, nursing care will continue to consist of only containment strategies, such as the use of pads and briefs, to manage UI. Often, these are used out of convenience, nursing habit, and patient preference, or due to lack of time (Colborne and Dahlke, 2017). Nurses in all practice settings who care for older adults should be prepared to assess data that relate to urine control and implement nursing interventions that promote continence. There is a growing role for nurses in continence care, and advanced training and certification are available through specialty organizations such as the Society of Urologic Nurses and Associates and the Wound, Ostomy and Continence Nurses Society (Holtzer-Goor, 2015; Spencer et al, 2017).

UI Facts and Figures

Inconsistencies with definitions and measurements, underreporting, and underassessment make definitive statistics on prevalence and incidence of UI problematic. However, because of the high prevalence and chronic but preventable nature of UI, it is most appropriately considered a public health problem. UI affects millions of adults worldwide with increasing incidence in older adults. Over 25 million individuals in the United States live with bladder leakage (National Association for Continence, 2017). UI is more common in women than men by a ratio of two to one. More than 50% of women and 25% of men aged 65 years and older, not residing in health care facilities or institutions, reported symptoms of UI of varying severities. Approximately 50% of men and women over the age of 65 years living in residential care facilities reported UI and another 50% reported both fecal incontinence and UI (Searcy, 2017). UI is more prevalent than diabetes, Alzheimer's disease, and many other chronic conditions that have prompted more attention and treatment. The direct medical costs of UI are similar to those of coronary heart disease and higher than the costs of diabetes (Holtzer-Goor et al, 2015).

BOX 16.4 Risk Factors for Urinary Incontinence

- Age
- Immobility, functional limitations
- Diminished cognitive capacity (dementia, delirium)
- Medications (those with anticholinergic properties, diuretics)
- Smoking
- High caffeine intake
- Low fluid intake
- Obesity
- Constipation, fecal impaction
- Pregnancy, vaginal delivery, episiotomy, forceps birth, large baby
- Environmental barriers
- High-impact physical exercise
- Diabetes, stroke, Parkinson's disease, multiple sclerosis, spinal cord injury
- Hysterectomy
- Pelvic muscle weakness, pelvic organ prolapse
- Childhood nocturnal enuresis
- Prostate surgery
- Estrogen deficiency
- Arthritis and/or back problems
- Malnutrition
- Depression
- Hearing or visual impairments

Risk Factors for UI

UI is often the result of multiple risk factors (Box 16.4). Physiological, pathological, and functional changes can result in a loss of continence. "The maintenance of continence is dependent not only on a functional lower urinary tract and pelvic floor, but also on sufficient cognition to interpret the desire to void and locate a toilet, adequate mobility and dexterity to manipulate clothing and allow safe and effective walking to the toilet, and an appropriate environment in which to allow this" (Gibson and Wagg, 2014, p. 168).

Older adults with dementia are at high risk for UI. Dementia does not cause UI but affects the ability of the person to recognize the urge to void and find a bathroom. Mobility problems and dependency in transfers are better predictors of continence status than dementia, suggesting that persons with dementia may have the potential to remain continent as long as they are mobile. Drugs that increase urinary output and sedatives, tranquilizers, and hypnotics, which produce drowsiness, confusion, or limited mobility, promote incontinence by dulling the transmission of the desire to urinate.

Consequences of UI

UI affects quality of life and has physical, psychosocial, and economic consequences. UI is identified as a marker of frailty in community-dwelling older adults. UI is more common and more severe in older adults and associated with sequelae not seen in younger people, such as increased risk of falls, fractures, hospitalization, and admission to long-term care. UI affects self-esteem and increases the risk for

BOX 16.5   Dignity in Continence Care Framework Approaches

- Provide empathic continence care
- Support personhood in dementia
- Utilize therapeutic communication
- Establish authentic partnerships
- Acknowledge stigma and social taboos
- Perform foundational continence assessment

TABLE 16.1   Types and Symptoms of Urinary Incontinence.

Type	Symptoms
Stress	Loss of small amount of urine with activities that increase intraabdominal pressure (coughing, sneezing, exercising, lifting, bending) More common in women but can occur in men after prostate surgery/treatment Postvoid residual (PVR) low
Urge	Loss of moderate to large amount of urine before getting to toilet; inability to suppress need to urinate Frequency and nocturia may be present PVR low May be associated with overactive bladder (OAB) characterized by urinary frequency (>8 voids/24 hour), nocturia, urgency, with or without urinary incontinence (UI). About half of individuals with OAB have urge UI
Overflow	Nearly constant urine loss (dribbling), hesitancy in starting urine, slow urine stream, passing small volumes of urine, feeling of incomplete bladder emptying; may be urge, stress, or mixed UI with high residuals PVR high
Functional	Lower urinary tract intact but individual unable to reach toilet due to environmental barriers, physical limitations, cognitive impairment, lack of assistance, difficulty managing belts, zippers, getting a dress up and undergarments down, or sitting on a toilet May occur with other types of UI; more common in individuals who are institutionalized
Mixed	Combination of more than one UI problem; usually stress and urge

depression, anxiety, loss of dignity and autonomy, social isolation, falls, skin breakdown, and avoidance of sexual activity (Ostaszkiewicz, 2017). Older adults with UI experience a loss of independence and self-confidence and feelings of shame and embarrassment. In a survey of hospitalized older adults, 67% considered bladder and bowel incontinence to be a state the same as, or worse than, death. "Despite the value individuals place on being continent, many nurses do not consider incontinence to be a clinically important issue" (Ostaszkiewicz, 2017, p. 11).

The psychosocial impact of UI affects the individual and family and professional caregivers. An important nursing role is to provide education to caregivers about UI and strategies to assist in practical and effective management. The provision of continence care to a dependent individual or an individual with cognitive impairment can be challenging and cause significant distress for both caregivers and care recipients. Continence care is frequently a trigger for agitation or aggression in individuals with cognitive impairment who may perceive intimate personal care interventions as frightening (Chapter 29). Ostaszkiewicz (2017) suggests that this can result in coercive or abusive care and proposes a model of relationship between elder abuse, incontinence, and care dependence. Box 16.5 presents the Dignity in Continence Care Framework to guide practice in continence care with individuals with dementia.

Types of UI

Incontinence is classified as either *transient* (acute) or *established* (chronic). *Transient* incontinence has a sudden onset, is present for 6 months or less, and is usually caused by treatable factors such as urinary tract infections (UTIs), delirium, constipation and stool impaction, and increased urine production caused by metabolic conditions such as hyperglycemia and hypercalcemia. Hospitalized older adults are at risk of developing transient UI and may also be at risk of being discharged without resolution of the condition. Use of medications such as diuretics, anticholinergic agents, antidepressants, sedatives, hypnotics, calcium channel blockers, and α-adrenergic agonists and blockers can also lead to transient UI. *Established* UI may have either a sudden or a gradual onset and is categorized into the following types: (1) stress, (2) urge, (3) overflow, (4) functional UI, and (5) mixed UI (Table 16.1).

PROMOTING HEALTHY AGING: IMPLICATIONS FOR GERONTOLOGICAL NURSING

Assessment

A case-finding question about bladder and bowel problems is recommended as part of all interactions between older adults and clinicians (Shaw and Wagg, 2016). Health care personnel must begin to change their thinking about incontinence and acknowledge that incontinence can be cured in about 80% of individuals (National Association for Continence, 2017). If it cannot be cured, it can be treated to minimize its detrimental effects. In frail older adults, interventions will improve UI in most cases but complete continence may not be a realistic goal (Engberg and Li, 2017). Nurses are often the ones to identify UI, but neither nurses nor physicians have been particularly aggressive in its management.

Assessment of UI is multidimensional and targeted to identify continence patterns, alterations in continence, and contributing factors. If the individual is being admitted to a hospital, home care agency, or skilled nursing facility, it is important to document the presence or absence of UI, past continence patterns, the presence or absence of an indwelling urinary catheter, and the reasons for the catheter

BOX 16.6 Tips for Best Practice

Continence Assessment

Screening Questions
"Have you ever leaked urine/water? If yes, how much does it bother you?"
"Do you ever leak urine/water on the way to the bathroom?"
"Do you ever use pads, tissue, or cloth in your underwear to catch urine/water?"
"Do you dribble urine/water most of the time?"
"Do you have any burning, hesitancy, or pain with urination?"

Screening Instruments
Urogenital Distress Inventory—6
Incontinence Impact Questionnaire Male Urinary Distress Inventory
Bladder (Voiding) Diary
Kept for 3 to 7 days by the individual or caregiver (Fig. 16.1)
Voiding record for even 1 day can be helpful

Patterns of Fluid Intake
Usual fluid intake over 24 hours
Types of fluids and time consumed
Decreased or increased urine output

Bowel Patterns
Frequency, consistency, straining
Use of laxatives

Exploration of Symptoms of Urinary Incontinence (UI)
When did UI start?
What have you done to manage the problem?
How often does it occur?
What things make it better or worse?
How severe is it?
Presence of voiding symptoms: hesitancy, straining, slow stream, intermittency, spraying
RED FLAGS: Hematuria, pain on urination

Focused History (Medical, Neurological, Gynecological, Genitourinary)
Review past health history: possible contributing factors to UI, pertinent diagnoses (heart failure, stroke, diabetes mellitus, multiple sclerosis, Parkinson's disease)

Medication Review
Review all medications including over-the-counter (OTC) with focus on diuretics, anticholinergics, psychotropics, α-adrenergic blockers, α-adrenergic agonists, calcium channel blockers
Review use of alcohol

Focused Assessment
Screen for depression
Cognitive, functional

Observe Individual Using the Toilet
Ability to reach a toilet and use it, time it takes to reach the toilet, finger dexterity for clothing manipulation; character of the urine (color, odor, sediment); difficulty starting or stopping urinary stream.

Physical Examination
Abdominal, rectal, genital: Assess for suprapubic distention indicative of urinary retention
Observe for signs of perineal irritation, itching, burning, lesions, discharge, tenderness, thin and pale genital tissues (atrophic vaginitis), dyspareunia, pelvic organ prolapse
Check for fecal impaction, tenderness

Other Tests That May Be Ordered
Urinalysis; culture and sensitivity if clinically significant systemic or urinary symptoms
If indicated, postvoid residual (PVR) (bladder sonography or catheterization) 16 minutes or less postvoid

Adapted from Shaw C, Wagg A: Urinary incontinence in older adults, *Med Older Adults* 45:1, 2016.

if present. In the long-term care setting, the Minimum Data Set (MDS) 3.0 (Chapter 7) provides an evidence-based overview of the assessment, treatment, and evaluation of bladder continence based on the Centers for Medicare and Medicaid Services (CMS) guidelines. Residents should be assessed on admission and whenever there is a change in cognition, physical ability, or urinary tract function. An environmental assessment including the accessibility of bathrooms, the adequacy of room lighting, the availability of assistance, and the use of aids such as raised toilet seats or commodes is also important.

For individuals with UI, the nurse collaborates with the interprofessional team to (1) determine if UI is transient or established (or both); (2) determine the type of UI; and (3) identify and document possible etiologies of the UI, including a review of risk factors (Spencer et al, 2017). Additional assessment is presented in Box 16.6. Box 16.7 provides information on a video of a nurse conducting an assessment for transient UI. More extensive examinations are considered after the initial findings are assessed.

Individuals who do not fit a simple pattern for UI should be referred promptly for urodynamic assessment.

Interventions

Nursing interventions focus primarily on the appropriate assessment of continence, teaching about treatments, and implementation and evaluation of supportive and therapeutic modalities to promote and restore continence and to prevent incontinence-related complications, such as skin breakdown. The nurse should share appropriate resources and explain clinical information and differences in treatment choices (Box 16.8).

Lifestyle interventions. Several lifestyle factors have been associated with either the development or the exacerbation of UI. These include increased fluid intake, weight reduction, smoking cessation, bowel management, avoiding caffeine and alcohol (if identified as causative factors), and physical activity (Research Highlights box). Research has shown that women with stress UI who undergo a 5% to 10% weight loss experience a positive impact on UI symptoms.

BOX 16.7   Resources for Best Practice

Catheterout.org: Protocols, Educational tools, Toolkit

Centers for Disease Control and Prevention: Guideline for prevention of catheter-associated urinary tract infections, 2017

Continence Produce Advisor (https://www.continenceproductadvisor.org/): Impartial advice for continence product users and health care professionals

Hartford Institute for Geriatric Nursing (consultgeri.org): Try This Series: Urinary incontinence assessment in older adults. Part 1: Transient Incontinence (includes link to video of assessment), Part 2: Persistent Incontinence; Prevention of catheter-associated urinary tract infection

International Continence Society—Educational materials, product guide, research, advocacy

National Association for Continence (NAC)—Comprehensive site for information for caregivers, professional clinicians, and individuals on UI and FI. Includes educational materials, product guide, advocacy, bowel and bladder diaries, OAB treatment tracker.

National Institute of Diabetes and Digestive and Kidney Disease (NIDDK): The NIDDK Bowel Control Awareness Campaign

Safe Care Campaign: Preventing health care and community associated infections: urinary tract infections

Simon Foundation for Continence: Educational materials, resources and products. Stool diary and Bristol Form Stool Scale

FI, Fecal incontinence; *OAB,* overactive bladder; *UI,* urinary incontinence.

BOX 16.8   Tips for Best Practice

Teaching About Urinary Incontinence Interventions

- Use therapeutic communication skills and a positive and supportive attitude to help individuals overcome any embarrassment about urinary incontinence (UI).
- Teach about the range of interventions available for management of UI.
- Share helpful resources for continence management.
- Share techniques found useful by others.
- Collaborate with the individual to help him or her choose the most appropriate and acceptable intervention based on needs.
- Assist individual to develop a detailed, realistic action plan and set goals.
- Determine an evaluation plan to assess the effectiveness of interventions.
- Review progress, identify any barriers to implementation, set alternative goals, or select alternate treatments if indicated.
- Consider using various teaching formats: face-to-face counseling, small-group sessions, computer-based continence promotion systems, informative written materials.
- Make teaching collaborative and interactive.
- Reinforce effort and persistence.

From Wilde M, Bliss D, Booth J, et al: Self-management of urinary and fecal incontinence, *Am J Nurs* 114(2):38–45, 2014.

This is most likely due to the effects of reduced abdominal weight, intraabdominal pressure, and intravesicular pressure (Wilde et al, 2014). The benefits of weight loss in frail older adults is more complex (Chapter 14). Good diabetic control to manage the hyperglycemic symptoms of osmotic diureses and constipation management are also important (Shaw and Wagg, 2016).

⚡ RESEARCH HIGHLIGHTS

Dancing to Treat Urinary Incontinence

The study evaluated the feasibility of using a combination of pelvic floor muscle exercises and virtual reality rehabilitation to treat mixed urinary incontinence (UI) in older women. The virtual reality program was one that involved dancing. Evaluation was done through a bladder diary, pad test, patient-reported symptoms, and quality of life and satisfaction questionnaire. Results indicated that the frequency and quantity of urine leakage decreased and the patient-reported symptoms and quality of life improved significantly. About 91% of the participants were very satisfied with the treatment. Further exploration of this type of combination therapy should be evaluated through further randomized controlled studies. The program was acceptable, efficient, and satisfying for the participants, encouraging exercise and social enjoyment while improving UI.

From Elliott V, de Bruin E, Dumoulin C: Virtual reality rehabilitation as a treatment approach for older women with mixed UI: a feasibility study, *Neurourol Urodyn* 34(3):236–243, 2015.

Environmental Interventions: Promotion of Continence Friendly Environment

Environmental, functional, and cognitive assessments are important to determine factors that may affect the individual's ability to use the toilet in public settings, at home, and in hospital and institutional settings. Observing the individual using the toilet should be included in any assessment of UI. If the individual is in a hospital or institution, occupational therapists can be helpful in these assessments and provide suggestions and equipment for improved abilities (e.g., elevated toilet seat, grab bars).

Accessibility to toilets and the availability of toileting assistance in a timely manner are identified risk factors in frail older adults, particularly those who are institutionalized. Toileting aids such as grab bars, raised toilet seats, toilet visibility, signage, and images may be effective in older adults with cognitive impairment or visual-perceptual deficits. For those who are not able to toilet independently, the availability of timely toileting assistance is critical to all other interventions for UI (Engberg and Li, 2017). In all settings, nurses play a key role in arranging the environment to facilitate toilet use and assist the individual to maintain or return to continence.

Behavioral Interventions

Behavioral techniques, such as scheduled (timed) voiding, prompted voiding (PV), habit retraining, bladder retraining, and pelvic floor muscle exercises (PFMEs), are recommended as first-line treatment of UI. Because UI in older adults can have multiple precipitating factors, a single intervention may not be adequate and more complex, multicomponent interventions may be required (Gibson and Wagg, 2014). Behavioral interventions have a good basis in research and can be implemented by nurses without extensive and expensive evaluation. Selection of a modality and interventions will depend on a comprehensive assessment, the type of incontinence and its underlying cause, and whether the outcome is to cure or to minimize the extent and complications of the incontinence. Interventions that have proved useful for UI among community-dwelling, robust older adults should also be implemented with those in long-term care settings, especially frail older adults (Shaw and Wagg, 2016).

Scheduled (timed) voiding. Scheduled (timed) voiding is used to treat urge and functional UI in both cognitively intact and cognitively impaired older adults. The individual uses the toilet at fixed intervals, such as every 4 hours. The schedule or timing of voiding can be based on common voiding patterns (voiding on arising, before and after meals, midmorning, midafternoon, and bedtime).

Pelvic floor muscle exercises. PFMEs, also called Kegel exercises, involve repeated voluntary pelvic floor muscle contraction. The targeted muscle is the pubococcygeal muscle, which forms the support for the pelvis and surrounds the vagina, the urethra, and the rectum. The goal of the repetitive contractions is to strengthen the muscle and decrease UI episodes. PFMEs are recommended for stress, urge, and mixed UI in older women and have also been shown to be helpful for men who have undergone prostatectomy. PFMEs can also be used to avoid an incontinence episode associated with urge UI (Shaw and Wagg, 2016).

Biofeedback may improve PFME teaching and outcomes, but further research is needed. Medicare covers biofeedback for individuals who do not improve after 4 weeks of a trial of PFMEs (DeBeau, 2014). Recent reports of a study evaluating an app with instructions for PFMEs for treating stress UI suggest that it may be a feasible way to deliver high-quality care in a cost-effective manner to large groups of individuals (Sjöström et al, 2017). Box 16.9 presents a protocol for PFMEs. Although there are some frail individuals and individuals in long-term care settings who may benefit from PFMEs and are capable of learning and practicing, the numbers may be insufficient to justify an emphasis on this approach in this setting.

Vaginal weight training was introduced in Europe as an alternative for women who have difficulty identifying the pelvic floor muscles. Graded-weight vaginal balls or cones are worn for two 16-minute periods each day or are used in addition to PFMEs. When the weighted cone is placed in the vagina, the pelvic floor muscle contractions keep it from slipping out. Although this technique involves less time and is more easily taught than PFMEs, difficulty inserting the cones and discomfort have been noted as deterrents to use.

Habit retraining. The individual's voiding pattern is identified, usually by means of a voiding diary (Fig. 16.1). A schedule is then devised so that the individual uses the toilet to avoid UI episodes identified from the diary.

Bladder retraining. Bladder retraining aims to increase the time interval between the urge to void and voiding. This method is appropriate for individuals with urge UI who are cognitively intact and independent in toileting or after removal of an indwelling catheter. Bladder retraining involves frequent voluntary voiding to keep bladder volume low and suppression of the urge to void using PFMEs, distraction, or relaxation techniques. When the individual feels the urge to urinate, he or she uses the urge control techniques. After the urge subsides, the

---

BOX 16.9 Pelvic Floor Muscle Training Exercises

Purpose

Prevent the involuntary loss of urine by strengthening the muscles under the uterus, bladder, and bowel.

Who Should Perform These Exercises?

Men and women who have problems with urine leakage or bowel control.

Identifying Pelvic Floor Muscles

When urinating, start to go and then stop. Feel the muscles in your vagina, bladder, or anus get tight and move up. These are the pelvic floor muscles. If you feel them tighten, you have done the exercise right.

If you are still not sure you are tightening the right muscle, keep in mind that all the muscles of the pelvic floor relax and contract at the same time. Because these muscles control the bladder, rectum, and vagina, the following tips may help:

Women: Inset a finger into your vagina. Tighten the muscles as if you are holding your urine; then let go. You should feel the muscles tighten and move up or down. These are the same muscles you would tighten if you were trying to prevent yourself from passing gas.

Men: Insert a finger into your rectum. Tighten the muscles as if you were holding your urine; then let go. You should feel the muscles tighten and move up and down. These are the same muscles you would tighten if you were trying to prevent yourself from passing gas.

NOTE: Nurses can teach correct muscle identification when performing a rectal or vaginal exam.

Pelvic Floor Muscle Exercises (PFME) Routine

1. Begin by emptying your bladder.
2. You can lie down, stand up, or sit in a chair.
3. Tighten the pelvic floor muscles and hold for a count of 10.
4. Relax the muscles completely for a count of 10.
5. Do 10 repetitions, 3 to 5 times a day.
6. Breathe deeply and relax your body when doing the exercises.
7. It is very important to keep the abdomen, buttocks, and thigh muscles relaxed when doing PFME.
8. After 4 to 6 weeks, most people see some improvement but it may take as long as 3 months. The regimen should be continued for 12 weeks.
9. After a few weeks, you can also try doing a single PFME contraction at times when you are likely to leak.

From U.S. National Library of Medicine, NIH National Institutes of Health: Pelvic floor muscle training exercises, *Medline Plus*, 2018. http://www.nlm.nih.gov/medlineplus/ency/article/003975.htm. Accessed February 2018.

---

individual walks at a normal pace to the toilet. The initial toileting frequency is every 2 hours and is progressively lengthened to 4 hours, depending on tolerance over the course of days or weeks.

Prompted voiding. PV is a technique that combines scheduled voiding with monitoring, prompting, and verbal reinforcement. The objective of PV is to increase self-initiated voiding and decrease the number of episodes of UI. The person is assisted to the toilet at predetermined times during waking hours if he or she requests it and receives positive feedback if he or she voids successfully. PV is associated with modest short-term improvement in daytime UI in individuals residing in long-term care settings (Lai and Wan, 2017).

Bladder Diary ("Uro-Log")

Complete one form for each day for 4 days before your appointment with a health care provider. In order to keep the most accurate diary possible, you'll want to keep it with you at all times and write down the events as they happen. Take the completed forms with you to your appointment.

Your Name: _____

Date: _____

Time	Fluids		Foods		Did you urinate?		Accidents			
	What kind?	How much?	What kind?	How much?	How many times?	How much? (sm, med, lg)	Leakage How much? (sm, med, lg)	Did you feel an urge to urinate?		What were you doing at the time? Sneezing, exercising, etc.
Sample	Coffee	1 cup	Toast	1 slice	✓✓	med	sm	Yes	No	Running
6-7 a.m.								Yes	No	
7-8 a.m.								Yes	No	
8-9 a.m.								Yes	No	
9-10 a.m.								Yes	No	
10-11 a.m.								Yes	No	
11-12 noon								Yes	No	
12-1 p.m.								Yes	No	
1-2 p.m.								Yes	No	
2-3 p.m.								Yes	No	
3-4 p.m.								Yes	No	
4-5 p.m.								Yes	No	
5-6 p.m.								Yes	No	
6-7 p.m.								Yes	No	
7-8 p.m.								Yes	No	
8-9 p.m.								Yes	No	

Fig. 16.1 Bladder Diary. (Provided by the National Association for Continence; 1-800-BLADDER; www.nafc.org.)

Newly admitted individuals to long-term care facilities who are incontinent (and able to use the toilet) should receive a 3- to 5-day trial of PV or other toileting programs. The trial can be helpful in demonstrating responsiveness to toileting and determining patterns of and symptoms associated with the incontinence (Box 16.10). PV is also combined with functional intervention training in which direct care givers incorporate strengthening exercises into toileting routines (Shaw and Wagg, 2016).

Special considerations in long-term care settings. Continence programs in long-term care facilities are required by CMS regulations. Monitoring and documentation of continence status in relation to implemented continence care is a *quality of care indicator* in this setting. Despite a growing body of evidence suggesting that toileting programs can be successful in long-term care, they are difficult to sustain (Liu and Wan, 2017). Barriers to implementation and continuation of toileting programs include inadequate staffing, lack of knowledge about UI and existing evidence-based protocols, and insufficient professional staff. Successful implementation of continence programs requires a systems-based approach with consideration of individual, group, organizational, and environmental level factors.

Other Interventions

Urinary catheters

Intermittent catheterization. Intermittent catheterization may be used in people with urinary retention related to a weak detrusor muscle (e.g., diabetic neuropathy), those with a blockage

of the urethra (e.g., benign prostatic hypertrophy [BPH]), or those with reflux incontinence related to a spinal cord injury. The goal is to maintain 300 mL or less of urine in the bladder. Most of the research on intermittent catheterization has been conducted with children or young adults with spinal cord injuries, but it may be useful for older adults who are able to self-catheterize. It provides an important alternative to indwelling catheterization.

Indwelling catheters. Indwelling catheter use is not appropriate in any setting for long-term management (more than 30 days) except in the following clinical conditions:

- Acute urinary retention or bladder outlet obstruction
- Need for accurate measurements of urinary output in critically ill patients
- Perioperative use for selected surgical procedures: urological or other surgery on contiguous structures of the genitourinary tract; anticipated prolonged surgery duration (should be removed in postanesthesia unit); patients anticipated to receive large-volume infusions or diuretics during surgery; need for intraoperative monitoring of urinary output
- To assist in healing of open sacral or perineal wounds in incontinent patients
- Patient requires prolonged immobilization (e.g., potentially unstable thoracic or lumbar spine, multiple traumatic injuries such as pelvic fractures)
- To improve comfort for end-of-life care if needed (Gould et al, 2017)

BOX 16.10 Prompted Voiding Protocol: Long-Term Care

1. Contact resident every 2 hours from 8 AM to 9 PM (or the resident's usual bedtime).
2. Focus attention on voiding by asking if the resident is wet or dry.
3. Ask a second time if the resident does not respond.
4. Check clothes and bedding to determine if wet or dry. Give feedback on whether response was correct or incorrect.
5. Whether wet or dry, ask if the resident would like to use toilet or urinal.

If the resident says **YES:**

Offer assistance.

Record results on bladder record.

Praise for appropriate toileting.

If the resident says **NO:**

Repeat the question once or twice.

If wet and declines to use the toilet, change him or her.

Inform the resident you will be back in 2 hours and request that the resident try to delay voiding until then.

If there has been no attempt to void in the past 2 to 3 hours, repeat the request to use the toilet at least twice more before leaving.

1. Offer fluids.
2. For nighttime management, use either modified prompted voiding schedule, toilet when awake, or use padding, depending on individual's sleep pattern and preferences.
3. If the individual who has been responding well has an increase in incontinence frequency despite adequate staff implementation of the protocol, further evaluation for reversible factors is indicated.

From Joseph Ouslander, MD, In person communication, February 2016.

Regulatory standards in nursing homes follow these same guidelines, and the use of indwelling catheters must be justified on the basis of medical conditions and failure of other efforts to maintain continence. In hospitals, the use of indwelling catheters is often unjustified, and they are used inappropriately or left in place too long. Approximately 25% of hospitalized patients have a urinary catheter at some time during their hospitalization. Hospitalized older adults are more likely to have urinary catheters placed without indication, of which 44% to 54% have been shown to have been improperly used. Those with more care needs, cognitive impairment, and pressure injuries are at higher risk of catheter placement (Hu et al, 2017). Reasons for this include (1) convenience to manage UI; (2) lack of knowledge of risks associated with use and alternative treatments; (3) providers not tracking continued use; and (4) lack of valid continence assessment tools for older adults. Misuse of catheterization should be considered a medical error.

External catheters. External catheters (condom catheters) are sometimes used in males who are incontinent and cannot be toileted. Long-term use of external catheters can lead to fungal skin infections, penile skin maceration, edema, fissures, contact burns from urea, UTIs, and septicemia. The catheter should be removed and replaced daily, and the penis cleaned, dried, and aired to prevent irritation, maceration, and the development of skin breakdown. If the catheter is not sized appropriately and applied and monitored correctly, strangulation of the penile shaft can occur.

Absorbent products. Some individuals prefer to use absorbent products in addition to toileting interventions to maintain "social continence," and a wide variety of products are available (Box 16.7). Disposable types are available in several sizes, determined by hip and waist measurements, or as one size made to fit all. Many of these undergarments now look like regular underwear and you even see them in stylish television commercials. Nurses should avoid the use of the word diaper since it is infantilizing and demeaning to older adults—the word brief is preferred. It is important that individuals are counseled to purchase proper continence products that will wick moisture away from the skin. These products are costly but they protect skin integrity. Women may tend to use menstrual pads but these do not absorb significant amounts of fluid.

Pharmacological Interventions

Medications are not considered first-line treatment but can be considered in combination with behavioral strategies in some cases. Pharmacological treatment (anticholinergic, antimuscarinic agents) may be indicated for urge UI and overactive bladder (OAB). These include oxybutynin (Oxytrol, Ditropan, Ditropan XL), tolterodine (Detrol, Detrol LA), trospium chloride (Sanctura), darifenacin (Enablex), fesoterodine (Toviaz), and solifenacin (VESIcare). Oxytrol for Women is the first FDA-approved over-the-counter (OTC) treatment for OAB. It is available in patch form, which is applied to the skin every 4 days. All of these medications have similar efficacy in reducing urge UI frequency, and the choice of medication depends on avoidance of adverse drug effects, drug-drug and drug-disease interactions, dosing frequency, titration range, and cost (DeBeau, 2014). However, oxybutynin should be avoided in older adults and is associated with an increased likelihood of cognitive impairment (Engberg and Li, 2017). β_3-Agonists (mirabegron) are a new class of medications for urge UI and OAB. They should not be used in individuals with severe uncontrolled hypertension, hepatic insufficiency, or bladder obstruction from BPH, or in those taking antimuscarinic agents. These medications can also raise digoxin levels (DeBeau, 2014).

Dosages of medications for urge UI and OAB should be started low and titrated with careful attention to side effects and drug interactions. A trial of 4 to 8 weeks is adequate and recommended. If one medication is not effective, another may be tried. Undesirable side effects of anticholinergic medications such as dry mouth and eyes, constipation, and cognitive impairment are problematic. People with narrow-angle glaucoma cannot use these medications, and they should not be combined with cholinesterase inhibitors. These medications can be especially problematic for those with cognitive impairment.

None of these medications have been evaluated in frail older adults and should only be considered after all potentially remediable comorbid conditions/factors are evaluated and addressed and there has been an appropriate trial of behavioral and lifestyle interventions. With cautious use, there may be some benefit in pharmacological management of symptom control

(Shaw and Wagg, 2016). Drug treatment should generally be avoided in individuals who make no attempt to toilet when assisted, become agitated when toileted, or are so cognitively and functionally impaired that there is no prospect for meaningful benefit (Engberg and Li, 2017).

Surgical Interventions

There are numerous surgical treatments for urge and stress UI available for individuals when they are referred to a specialist. These include in-office urethral bulking agents, surgical placements of urethral slings and bladder neck suspensions for stress UI, and intradetrusor botulinum toxin injection. For individuals with urge UI associated with OAB who have not responded to conservative or pharmacological therapies, sacral neuromodulation (SNM) may be recommended. SNM stimulates the sacral nerve root to control urination and can be an office-based 12 week treatment or a surgical implantation of a sacral neuromodulator system. Surgical SNM includes implantation of the Medtronic Interstim Therapy device, FDA-approved for bladder dysfunction, including UI and fecal incontinence, and has shown efficacy for decreasing symptoms of UI.

Outflow obstruction incontinence secondary to prostatic hypertrophy is generally corrected by prostatectomy. Sphincter dysfunction resulting from nerve damage following surgical trauma or radical perineal procedures is 70% to 90% repairable through sphincter implantation. There is limited evidence on surgical treatments for UI in frail older adults; however, age alone is not a contraindication to surgical treatment (Engberg and Li, 2017; Searcy, 2017; Shaw and Wagg, 2016).

Nonsurgical Devices

There are a variety of intravaginal or intraurethral devices to relieve stress UI. These include intravaginal support devices, pessaries, external occlusive devices, and urethral plugs for women. For men, there are foam penile clamps. The pessary, used primarily to prevent uterine prolapse, is a device that is fitted into the vagina and exerts pressure to elevate the urethrovesical junction of the pelvic floor. The individual is taught to insert and remove the pessary, much like inserting and removing a diaphragm used for contraception. The pessary is removed weekly or monthly for cleaning with soap and water and then reinserted. Adverse effects include vaginal infection, low back pain, and vaginal mucosal erosion. Another concern is the danger of forgetting to remove the pessary. Several of the resources in Box 16.7 provide detailed information on these devices but an evaluation of the stress UI by the health care provider should be conducted to determine if these devices would be helpful.

URINARY TRACT INFECTIONS (UTIs)

UTIs are the most common cause of bacterial sepsis in older adults and are 10 times more common in women than in men. The clinical spectrum of UTIs ranges from asymptomatic and recurrent UTIs to sepsis associated with UTI requiring hospitalization. There is significant disagreement in clinical practice as to what constitutes a UTI and overdiagnosis of UTI is a significant

problem in the older adult population. Assessment and appropriate treatment of UTIs in older adults, particularly long-term care residents, are complex. Cognitively impaired individuals may not be able to report symptoms and nurses often rely on nonspecific signs and symptoms (lack of appetite, change in behavior) as indicators of UTI. It is widely believed that UTI in older adults can manifest atypically but there is little evidence that nonspecific symptoms, when present in isolation, are reliable indicators of UTI (Crnich et al, 2017; Kitsler et al, 2017). The presence of nonspecific signs/symptoms in the absence of fever or urinary tract symptoms should trigger consideration of noninfectious conditions rather than a UTI.

Asymptomatic bacteriuria is transient and considered benign in older women. Significant bacteriuria and urinary symptoms are common, often occur together, and generally resolve spontaneously in noncatheterized, medically stable adults without structural or functional urinary tract abnormalities. Neither is linked strongly to serious urinary tract disease or to a likelihood of benefit from antibiotic treatment (Finucane, 2017). The American Geriatrics Society recommends that antimicrobials should not be used to treat bacteriuria in older adults unless specific urinary tract symptoms are present (American Geriatrics Society, 2014). However, antibiotic treatment is common even though more than half of the antibiotics initiated for suspected UTIs are unnecessary or inappropriate (Crinch et al, 2017).

Screening urine cultures should also not be performed in individuals who are asymptomatic. As many as half of all positive urine cultures should be considered false positives for the presence of a UTI (Kistler et al, 2017). The diagnosis of symptomatic UTI is made when the patient has both clinical features (painful urination, lower abdominal pain/tenderness, blood in urine, new or worsening urinary urgency or frequency, incontinence, and fever) and laboratory evidence of a UTI. Treatment is with antibiotics selected by identifying the pathogen, knowing local resistance rates, and considering adverse effects.

Catheter-Associated Urinary Tract Infections

Catheter-associated urinary tract infections (CAUTIs) refer to UTIs that occur in a patient with an indwelling catheter or within 48 hours of catheter removal. CAUTIs are one of the most common health care–associated infections (HAI) (CDC, 2018). CAUTIs are the leading cause of secondary bloodstream infections and were among the first hospital-acquired conditions (HACs) targeted for nonpayment by Medicare in 2008 (Timmons et al, 2017). They have also been further targeted as a "never event" and a hospital national safety goal (The Joint Commission, 2018). One of the goals of *Healthy People 2020* is to prevent, reduce, and ultimately eliminate HAIs. Implementation of evidence-based guidelines, catheter reminders, stop orders, nurse-initiated removal protocols, using proven guidelines to prevent CAUTIs, education of staff, patients, and families about CAUTI prevention and symptoms of a UTI, and a urinary catheter bundle can decrease CAUTIs in both acute and long-term care settings (Mody et al, 2017; Safdar et al, 2016; Saint et al, 2016). Box 16.11 presents Tips for Best Practice for prevention of CAUTI.

BOX 16.11 Tips for Best Practice

Prevention of CAUTI Using the ABCDE Approach

A Adherence to general infection control principles (hand hygiene, surveillance, aseptic catheter insertion, proper maintenance of a sterile, closed, unobstructed drainage system, and education)

B Be sure to use protocol in place to avoid unnecessary catherizations

C Condom catheters or other alternatives to an indwelling catheter such as intermittent catheterization should be considered in appropriate patients

D Do not use the indwelling catheter unless you must. Do not use antimicrobial catheters. Do not irrigate catheters unless obstruction is anticipated (e.g., as might occur with bleeding after prostatic or bladder surgery). Do not clean the periurethral area with antiseptics (cleansing of the meatal surface during daily bathing or showering is appropriate)

E Early removal of the catheter using a reminder or nurse-initiated removal protocol

CAUTI, Catheter-associated urinary tract infection.
From Centers for Disease Control and Prevention: *Healthcare-associated infections (HAI) progress report,* 2016. http://www.cdc.gov/hai/progress-report/index.html. Accessed February 2018.

⚡ SAFETY ALERT

Long-term catheter use increases the risk of recurrent urinary tract infections leading to urosepsis, urethral damage in men, urethritis, or fistula formation. Catheter-associated urinary tract infection is one of the most common health care–associated infection in the United States, and Medicare no longer reimburses hospitals for this infection. Indwelling catheters should be inserted only for appropriate conditions and must be removed as soon as possible, and alternatives should be investigated (e.g., condom catheters, intermittent catheterization, toileting programs).

BOWEL ELIMINATION

Bowel function of the older adult, although normally only slightly altered by the physiological changes of age (Box 16.12), can be a source of concern and a potentially serious problem, especially for the older adult who is functionally impaired. Normal elimination should be an easy passage of feces, without undue straining or a feeling of incomplete evacuation or defecation. The urge to defecate occurs when the distended walls of the sigmoid and the rectum, which are filled with feces, stimulate pressure receptors to relax the sphincters for the

BOX 16.12 Age-Related Changes in the Bowel

Small Intestine
Villi become broader, shorter, and less functional; blood flow decreases Proteins, fats, minerals (including calcium), vitamins (especially vitamin B_{12}), and carbohydrates (especially lactose) are absorbed more slowly and in lesser amounts

Large Intestine
Slowed peristalsis, blunted response to rectal filling, increased collagen deposition leading to dysmotility, fibro-fatty degeneration, and increased thickness of the internal anal sphincter

BOX 16.13 Rome III Criteria for Defining Chronic Functional Constipation in Adults

Two or more of the following for at least 12 weeks in the preceding 12 months:
- Straining with defecation more than 25% of the time
- Lumpy or hard stools more than 25% of the time
- Sensation of incomplete emptying more than 25% of the time
- Manual maneuvers used to facilitate emptying in more than 25% of defecations (digital evacuation or support of the pelvic floor)
- Fewer than three bowel movements per week

expulsion of feces through the anus. Evacuation of feces is accomplished by relaxation of the sphincters and contraction of the diaphragm and abdominal muscles, which raises the intraabdominal pressure.

Constipation

Constipation is defined as a reduction in the frequency of stool or difficulty in formation or passage of stool. The Rome Criteria outline the operational definitions of constipation and should be used as a guide to diagnosis (Box 16.13). Constipation is one of the most common gastrointestinal complaints encountered in clinical practice in all settings. Many individuals, both the lay public and health care professionals, may view constipation as a minor problem or nuisance. However, it is associated with impaired quality of life, significant health care costs, and a large economic burden. Constipation can also have very serious consequences including fecal impaction, bowel obstruction, cognitive dysfunction, delirium, falls, and increased morbidity and mortality. Individuals with chronic constipation are also at greater risk for developing colorectal cancer and benign colorectal neoplasms (Guérin et al, 2014).

Constipation is a common complaint and challenge for older adults. Constipation is associated with female gender and increasing age. In individuals 65 years of age or older in the community, the prevalence is 25% for women and 16% for men. In those over the age of 84 years, the rate increases to 34% for women and 26% for men. In long-term care residents, the prevalence is as high as 80% and between 50% and 74% use laxatives (Blekken et al, 2016; Schuster et al, 2015).

Constipation is a symptom, not a disease. It is a reflection of poor habits, delayed response to the colonic reflex, and many chronic illnesses—both physical and psychological—and a common side effect of medication. Diet and activity level play a significant role in constipation. Constipation and other changes in bowel habits can also signal more serious underlying problems, such as colonic dysmotility or colon cancer. Thorough assessment is important, and these complaints should not be blamed on age alone. It is important to note that alterations in cognitive status, incontinence, increased temperature, poor appetite, or unexplained falls may be the only clinical symptoms of constipation in the cognitively impaired or frail older adult.

Fecal Impaction

Fecal impaction is a major complication of constipation. It is especially common in incapacitated and institutionalized older adults and those who require narcotic medications (e.g., end-of-life care). Symptoms of fecal impaction include malaise, loss of appetite, abdominal bloating/pain, nausea, vomiting, urinary retention, elevated temperature, incontinence of bladder or bowel, leaking of stool, alterations in cognitive status, fissures, hemorrhoids, and intestinal obstruction. Unrecognized, unattended, or neglected constipation eventually leads to fecal impaction. Digital rectal examination for impacted stool and abdominal x-rays will confirm the presence of impacted stool. Continued obstruction by a fecal mass may eventually impair sensation, leading to the need for larger stool volume to stimulate the urge to defecate, which contributes to megacolon.

Paradoxical diarrhea, caused by leakage of fecal material around the impacted mass, may occur. Reports of diarrhea in older adults must be thoroughly assessed before the use of antidiarrheal medications, which further complicate the problem of fecal impaction. Stool analysis for *Clostridium difficile* toxin should be ordered in patients who develop new-onset diarrhea, especially for those who live in a communal setting or have been recently hospitalized.

Removal of a fecal impaction is at times worse than the misery of the condition. Management of fecal impaction requires the digital removal of the hard, compacted stool from the rectum with use of lubrication containing lidocaine jelly. In general, this is preceded by an oil-retention enema to soften the feces in preparation for manual removal. Use of suppositories is not effective because their action is blocked by the amount and size of the stool in the rectum. Suppositories do not facilitate the removal of stool in the sigmoid, which may continue to ooze once the rectum is emptied. Several sessions or days may be necessary to totally cleanse the sigmoid colon and rectum of impacted feces. Once this is achieved, attention should be directed to planning a regimen that includes adequate fluid intake, increased dietary fiber, administration of medications if needed, and many of the suggestions presented later in the chapter for prevention of constipation. Protocols and policies for removal of a fecal impaction should be in place in all facilities.

For patients who are hospitalized or residing in long-term care settings, accurate bowel records are essential; unfortunately, they are often overlooked or inaccurately completed. Education about the importance of bowel function and the accurate reporting of size, consistency, and frequency of bowel movements should be provided to all direct care providers. This is especially important for frail or cognitively impaired older adults to prevent fecal impaction, a serious and often dangerous condition for older adults.

PROMOTING HEALTHY AGING: IMPLICATIONS FOR GERONTOLOGICAL NURSING

Assessment

Assessment and management of bowel function are important nursing responsibilities. The precipitants and causes of constipation must be included in the evaluation of bowel function. A review of these factors will also determine whether the individual is at risk for altered bowel function and if any of the known risks are modifiable. Recognizing constipation can be a challenge because there may be a significant disconnect between the individual's definition of constipation and those of clinicians (Box 16.13). Constipation has different meanings to different people. Assessment begins with clarification of what the person means by constipation and discussion of the criteria for the diagnosis.

It is important to obtain a bowel history including usual patterns, frequency of bowel movements, size, consistency, any changes, and occurrence of straining and hard stools. However, recall of bowel frequency has been shown to be unreliable in establishing the presence of constipation. Having the individual keep a bowel diary (Box 16.7) and using the Bristol Stool Form Scale (Lewis and Heaton, 1997), which provides a visual description of stool appearance, will be more accurate. Assessment data are presented in Box 16.14.

Interventions

The first intervention is to examine the medications the person is taking and eliminate those that are constipation producing, preferably changing to medications that do not carry that side effect. Medications are the leading cause of constipation, and almost any drug can cause it.

Nonpharmacological Interventions

Nonpharmacological interventions for constipation that have been implemented and evaluated are as follows: (1) fluid and diet related, (2) physical activity, (3) environmental manipulation, (4) toileting regimen, and (5) a combination of these. Fluid intake of at least 1.5 liters per day, unless contraindicated, is the cornerstone of constipation therapy, with fluids coming mainly from water. A gradual increase in fiber intake, either as supplements or incorporated into the diet, is generally recommended. Fiber helps stools become bulkier and softer and move through the body more quickly. This will produce easier and more regular bowel movements. High fiber intake is not recommended for individuals who are immobile or do not consume at least 1.5 liters of fluid per day. The importance of dietary fiber to adequate nutrition and bowel function is discussed in Chapter 14.

Physical activity. Physical activity is important as an intervention to stimulate colon motility and bowel evacuation. Daily walking for 20 to 30 minutes, if tolerated, is helpful, especially after a meal. Pelvic tilt exercises and range-of-motion (passive or active) exercises are beneficial for those who are less mobile or who are bedridden. Exercise and physical activity are discussed in Chapter 18.

Positioning. The squatting or sitting position, if the individual is able to assume it, facilitates bowel function. A similar position may be obtained by leaning forward and applying firm pressure to the lower abdomen or by placing the feet on a stool. Rocking back and forth while sitting solidly on the toilet may facilitate stool movement. Massaging the abdomen or rectum may also help stimulate the bowel.

Toileting regimen. Establishing a routine for toileting promotes or normalizes bowel function (bowel retraining). The gastrocolic reflex occurs after breakfast or supper and may be enhanced by a warm drink. Given privacy and ample time (a minimum of 10 minutes), many will have a daily bowel

BOX 16.14 Tips for Best Practice
Assessment of Constipation

Sample Questions
- What is your usual bowel pattern?
- How many minutes did you sit on the bedpan or toilet before you had your bowel movement?
- How much did you have to strain before you had your bowel movement?
- Do you think you are constipated? If yes, why do you think so?
- Have you had any abdominal pain, nausea, vomiting, weight loss, blood in your bowel movement, or rectal pain?
- Have you had any bowel or rectal surgery?
- What type of physical activity do you engage in and how often?

Review of Food and Fluid Intake
Medication Review
- Include over-the-counter (OTC), herbal preparations, supplements

Psychosocial History
- With attention to depression, anxiety, and stress management

Review of Concurrent Medical Conditions
Other Measures
- Bowel diary
- Bristol Stool Form Survey

Focused Physical Examination
- Abdominal exam to detect masses, distention, tenderness, high-pitched or absent bowel sounds
- If these abnormalities are present, primary care provider should be contacted
- Rectal exam, following institutional policy, to identify painful anal disorders such as hemorrhoids or fissures, rectal prolapse, stool presence in the vault, strictures, masses, anal reflex

Other Tests as Indicated
- Complete blood count, fasting glucose, chemistry panel, thyroid studies
- Flexible sigmoidoscopy, colonoscopy, computed tomography scan, abdominal x-ray

From McKay S, Fravel M, Scanlon C: Management of constipation, *J Gerontol Nurs* 38(7):9–16, 2014.

movement. However, any urge to defecate should be followed by a trip to the bathroom. Older adults dependent on others to meet toileting needs should be assisted to maintain normal routines and provided opportunities for routine toilet use. Box 16.15 presents a bowel training program.

Pharmacological Interventions

When changes in diet and lifestyle are not effective, the use of laxatives is considered. Use of these medications, both prescribed and OTC, is high. The extensive use of laxatives among older adults in the United States can be considered a cultural habit. During earlier times, weekly doses of rhubarb, cascara, castor oil, and other types of laxatives were consumed and believed by many to promote health. The belief that cleaning out the colon and having a daily bowel movement is paramount to maintaining good health still persists in some groups. Providing information about normal bowel function, definition of constipation, and lifestyle modifications can assist in promoting healthy bowel habits without the use of laxatives.

Older adults receiving opiates need to have a constipation prevention program in place because these drugs delay gastric emptying and decrease peristalsis. Correction of constipation associated with opiate use requires senna or an osmotic laxative to overcome the strong opioid effect. Stool softeners and bulking agents alone are inadequate. Laxatives commonly used in chronic constipation are presented in Table 16.2.

Enemas. Enemas of any type should be reserved for situations in which other methods produce no response or when it is known that there is an impaction. Enemas should not be used on a regular basis. A normal saline or tap water enema (500 to 1000 mL) at a temperature of 105°F is the best choice. Sodium citrate enemas are another safe choice. Soapsuds and phosphate enemas irritate the rectal mucosa and should not be used. Oil retention enemas are used for refractory constipation and in the treatment of fecal impaction.

BOX 16.15 Tips for Best Practice
Bowel Training Program

1. Obtain a bowel history and establish a schedule for the bowel training program that is normal and comfortable for the patient and conforms to his or her lifestyle.
2. Ensure adequate fiber and fluid intake (normalize stool consistency).
   a. Fiber
      i. Add high-fiber foods to diet (dried fruit, dried beans, vegetables, and wheat products).
      ii. Suggest adding one to three tablespoons of bran or Metamucil to the diet once or twice each day. (Titrate dosage on the basis of response.)
   b. Fluid
      i. Consume 2 to 3 liters daily (unless contraindicated).
      ii. Four ounces of prune, fig, or pear juice (or a warm fluid) may be given daily as a stimulus (e.g., 30 to 60 minutes before the established time for defecation).
3. Encourage an exercise program.
   a. Pelvic tilt, modified sit-ups for abdominal strength
   b. Walking for general muscle tone and cardiovascular system
   c. More vigorous program if appropriate
4. Establish a regular time for the bowel movement.
   a. Established time depends on patient's schedule.
   b. Best times are 20 to 40 minutes after regularly scheduled meals, when the gastrocolic reflex is active.
   c. Attempts at evacuation should be made daily within 15 minutes of the established time and whenever the patient senses rectal distention.
   d. Instruct patient about normal posture for defecation. (The patient normally sits on the toilet or bedside commode; for the patient who is unable to get out of bed, the left side-lying position is best.)
   e. Instruct the patient to contract the abdominal muscles and "bear down."
   f. Have the patient lean forward to increase the intraabdominal pressure by use of compression against the thighs.
   g. Stimulate the anorectal reflex and rectal emptying if necessary.
5. Insert a rectal suppository or mini-enema into the rectum 15 to 30 minutes before the scheduled bowel movement, placing the suppository against the bowel wall, or insert a gloved, lubricated finger into the anal canal and gently dilate the anal sphincter.

TABLE 16.2 Types of Laxatives: Actions, Use, Side Effects.

Types of Laxatives	Actions, Use, Side Effects
Bulk-forming (e.g., psyllium, methylcellulose)	Usually first-line agents due to low cost and few adverse effects Do not use in presence of obstruction or compromised peristaltic activity Use with caution in frail older adults, bedbound individuals, those with swallowing problems Must be taken with adequate fluid intake to avoid obstruction in esophagus, stomach, intestines Can cause abdominal distention and flatulence
Emollients and lubricants (e.g., docusate sodium, mineral oil)	Increase moisture content of stool Insufficient evidence to recommend docusate for prevention or treatment of constipation; may alleviate straining in selected patients who undergo rectal surgery or had myocardial infarction Use with caution in frail older adults who may not have the strength to "push" when having a bowel movement since soft stool can accumulate in rectal vault The emollient laxative mineral oil should be avoided because of the risk of lipoid aspiration pneumonia
Osmotic laxatives (e.g., milk of magnesia [MOM], lactulose, sorbitol, polyethylene glycol [PEG], MiraLax)	Cause water retention in the colon Avoid MOM in individuals with renal insufficiency since use can lead to hypermagnesemia or hyperphosphatemia Lactulose and sorbitol can cause diarrhea, abdominal cramping, and flatulence MiraLax associated with less bloating and flatulence These medications can be added if bulk laxatives are ineffective
Stimulant laxatives (e.g., senna, bisacodyl)	Stimulate colorectal motor activity May cause cramping and electrolyte or fluid losses but when used appropriately, they are a safe and effective option, especially in those with opioid-induced constipation
Chloride channel stimulating (lubiprostone [Amitiza])	Stimulate ileal secretion and increase fecal water Generally safe, well tolerated, and effective in older adults with chronic constipation Side effects include nausea, diarrhea, headaches Expense of these medications may limit use except in individuals for whom other medications have failed or who have demonstrated intolerance to other agents

From McKay S, Fravel M, Scanlon C: Management of constipation, *J Gerontol Nurs* 38(7):9–16, 2014; Schuster B, Kosar L, Kamrul R: Constipation in older adults, *Can Fam Physician* 6(12):152–158, 2015.

⚡ SAFETY ALERT

Sodium phosphate enemas (e.g., Fleets) should not be used in older adults because they may lead to severe metabolic disorders associated with high mortality and morbidity.

BOX 16.16 Natural Laxative Recipes

Beverley-Travis Natural Laxative Mixture
Ingredients
1 cup raisins
1 cup pitted prunes
1 cup figs
1 cup dates
1 cup currants
1 cup prune concentrate

Directions
Combine contents in grinder or blender to a thickened consistency. Store in refrigerator between uses.

Dosage
Administer 2 tablespoons (tbs) twice a day (once in the morning and once in the evening). May increase or decrease according to the frequency of bowel movements.

Nutritional Composition
Each 2-tbs dose contains the following:
61 calories
137 mg of potassium
8 mg of sodium
11.9 g of sugar
0.5 g of protein
1.4 g of fiber

Power Pudding
Ingredients
1 cup wheat bran
1 cup applesauce
1 cup prune juice

Directions
Mix and store in refrigerator. Start with administration of 1 tbs/day. Increase slowly until desired effect is achieved and no disagreeable symptoms occur.

Alternative Treatments

Combinations of natural fiber, fruit juices, and natural laxative mixtures are often recommended in clinical practice, and some studies have found an increase in bowel frequency and a decrease in laxative use when these mixtures are used (Box 16.16). Although research is still limited, many modalities of complementary and alternative medicine, such as probiotic bacteria, traditional herbal medicines, biofeedback, and massage, are also used to treat constipation.

ACCIDENTAL BOWEL LEAKAGE/FECAL INCONTINENCE

Fecal incontinence (FI) is defined as the recurrent involuntary loss of feces, which is defined by the frequency of episodes (such as daily or weekly episode counts) and by the consistency of the feces (solid, liquid, or mucus) (AHRQ, 2016). Estimates of prevalence vary but in general, range between

1.4% and 18%. In women over 45 years of age, nearly 20% have FI at least once a year and 9.5% have at least 1 episode/month. Higher prevalence rates are found among individuals with diabetes, irritable bowel syndrome, stroke, multiple sclerosis, and spinal cord injury. Among older adults in long-term care facilities, FI may affect up to 50% and is a frequent reason for transfer to a nursing home (Buswell et al, 2017; Paquette et al, 2015).

Often FI is associated with UI, and up to 50% to 70% of individuals with UI also carry the diagnosis of FI. FI can be transient (episodes of diarrhea, acute illness, fecal impaction) or persistent. Fecal incontinence, like UI, has devastating social ramifications for the individuals and families who experience it. UI and FI share similar contributing factors, including damage to the pelvic floor as a result of surgery or trauma, neurological disorders, functional impairment, immobility, and dementia.

Bowel continence and defecation depend on coordination of sensory and motor innervation of the rectum and anal sphincters. Conditions or deficits that alter any of these factors may result in fecal incontinence. The etiology may be multifactorial and risk factors include pregnancy, diabetes, previous anorectal surgery, UI, smoking, obesity, limited physical activity, white race, and neurological disease. Sphincter damage from obstetric injury, particularly among multiparous women, those with prolonged labor, or those who had instrument-assisted deliveries, increases FI risk. Injury from obstetrical trauma is often delayed in onset, and many women do not manifest symptoms until after the age of 50 years (Paquette et al, 2015).

PROMOTING HEALTHY AGING: IMPLICATIONS FOR GERONTOLOGICAL NURSING

Assessment

An important point in assessment is the term that is chosen to describe FI. In a large study of female patients, "accidental bowel leakage" was preferred over FI (Brown et al, 2012; Paquette et al, 2015). Assessment should include a complete client history as in UI (see Box 16.6) and investigation into stool consistency and frequency, use of laxatives or enemas, surgical and obstetrical history, medications, effect of FI on quality of life, focused physical examination with attention to the gastrointestinal system, and a bowel record. A digital rectal examination should be performed to identify any presence of a mass, impaction, or occult blood.

Interventions

Nursing interventions are aimed at managing and/or restoring bowel continence. Dietary and medical management are recommended as first-line management for FI. Therapies similar to those used to treat UI such as environmental manipulation (access to toilet), dietary alterations, habit training schedules, PFMEs, improving transfer and ambulation ability, sphincter training exercises, biofeedback, medications, and/or surgery to

BOX 16.17 Tips for Best Practice
Interventions for Accidental Bowel Leakage

- Use therapeutic communication skills and a positive and supportive attitude to help individuals overcome any embarrassment.
- Use the term accidental bowel leakage rather than fecal incontinence.
- Emphasize the importance of thorough evaluation.
- Teach about the range of interventions available for management.
- Share helpful resources for continence management.
- Have individual keep a bowel diary and identify triggers. For example, if eating a meal or drinking a cup of coffee stimulates defecation, use the toilet at a given time after the trigger event. Have a regular toileting routine.
- Encourage being prepared. Schedule outings, appointments, exercise routines around anticipated bowel patterns; suggest keeping a change of underwear, clothing, and toileting supplies with them when out; use an absorbent pad and have bags to dispose of pad if soiled; deodorant sprays for odor; wear darker clothing when away from home so that if soiling occurs, it will be less noticeable; scan environment when out for toilet locations.
- Avoid greasy and flatus-producing foods, dairy products, fruits with edible seeds, acidic citrus fruits, nuts, spicy foods, and other foods that trigger leakage. Bake or broil foods instead of frying; eat meals at regular times; eat after public events to reduce likelihood of leakage.

From Wilde M, Bliss D, Booth J, et al: Self-management of urinary and fecal incontinence, *Am J Nurs* 114(2):38–45, 2014.

correct underlying defects are effective. Studies have shown that 22% to 54% of individuals can have improvement in FI with formal counseling from a specialist regarding dietary habits, fluid management, bowel routines, and changes to medications (Paquette et al, 2015). Providing resources and educational information is important and will help in self-management (see Box 16.7). Other interventions are presented in Box 16.17.

Pharmacological interventions may include the use of antidiarrheal medications and fiber therapy. Biofeedback may also be recommended and there are some surgical options that can be considered if conservative interventions are not successful. SNM may also be considered as a first-line surgical option and has been shown to reduce the frequency of FI episodes. SNM is thought to modulate rectal sensation by activating or deactivating chemical mediating receptors, stimulating the afferent pathway, and changing brain activity relevant to the continent mechanism. Injection of bulking agents into the anal canal has been reported to reduce FI but guidelines suggest a weak recommendation for this treatment based on moderate-quality evidence (Paquette et al, 2015). Further study is needed on these types of treatments.

The effectiveness of interventions in fecal incontinence will be self-evident but will take time. As in the treatment of UI, goals must be realistic. It cannot be stated too often or too strongly that the nurse must always provide immaculate skin care to persons with incontinence, because self-esteem and skin integrity depend on it.

KEY CONCEPTS

- UI is not a part of normal aging. It is a symptom of an underlying problem and requires thorough assessment.
- UI can be minimized or cured, and there are many therapeutic modalities available for treatment that nurses can implement.
- Nonpharmacological treatments (PFMEs, PV, bladder training, timed voiding, lifestyle modifications) are first-line treatments for UI.
- Asymptomatic bacteriuria is common in older women and does not need treatment.

- Indwelling catheter use is not appropriate in any setting for long-term management (more than 30 days) except in certain clinical conditions. Proper insertion, care, and timely removal of indwelling catheters can reduce the number of CAUTIs.
- Health promotion teaching, identification of risk factors, comprehensive assessment of UI, education of formal and informal caregivers, and use of evidence-based interventions are basic continence competencies for nurses.

NURSING STUDY: CONTINENCE

Helen is an 80-year-old woman who lives in her own apartment in an assisted living residence. Helen is the mother of four adult children, whom she sees often, and enjoys family activities. She is independent in all of her activities of daily living and walks with a cane. She has osteoarthritis of her knees and although she walks slowly, she is able to get around without any difficulty. Helen is 5 feet, 2 inches tall and weighs 150 pounds. She takes an antihypertensive medication and a diuretic. She has come to see the nurse practitioner in the on-site clinic for an annual physical examination. While the nurse practitioner is obtaining Helen's health history, he asks Helen if she has any problems with control of her urine such as leaking or not getting to the bathroom before she loses urine. Helen replies: "Sometimes I do have some leaking of urine because I can't get to the bathroom quickly enough, so I wear a pad. It also sometimes happens when I cough or sneeze but I don't think at my age there is much that can be done about that."

Based on the nursing study, develop a nursing care plan using the following procedure[a]:

- List Helen's comments that provide subjective data.
- List information that provides objective data.

- From these data, identify and state, using an accepted format, two nursing diagnoses you determine are most significant to Helen at this time. List two of Helen's strengths that you have identified from the data.
- Determine and state outcome criteria for each diagnosis. These criteria must reflect some alleviation of the problem identified in the nursing diagnosis and must be stated in concrete and measurable terms.
- Plan and state one or more interventions for each diagnosed problem. Provide specific documentation of the source used to determine the appropriate intervention. Plan at least one intervention that incorporates Helen's existing strengths.
- Evaluate the success of the intervention. Interventions must correlate directly with the stated outcome criteria to measure the outcome success.

[a]Students are advised to refer to their nursing diagnosis text and identify possible or potential problems.

CRITICAL THINKING QUESTIONS AND ACTIVITIES

1. What are the risk factors for UI in this situation?
2. What should be included in a more comprehensive assessment of Helen's stated problems with urine control?
3. What type of UI do you think Helen is experiencing?
4. What type of behavioral interventions might be helpful for Helen so that she has better urine control?
5. What health teaching would you provide to Helen related to urinary problems of older women?
6. What resources would you suggest for Helen to help her be more informed about her urine control concerns and how to manage them?

NURSING STUDY: CONSTIPATION

Stella, at age 78, has never had problems with her bowel movements. They have been regular—each morning about an hour after breakfast. In fact, she hardly thought about them because they had been so regular. While hospitalized for podiatric surgery last year, she never regained her usual pattern of bowel function. She was greatly distressed by this because it had been a symbol to her of her good health. Admittedly, she did not move about as much now, or as well, and had begun to use a cane. And she had heard that pain medications sometimes make one constipated, so she tried to use them sparingly despite the pain. She tried to reestablish her pattern of having a bowel movement every morning after breakfast but with little success. She now began to worry about constipation and to use laxatives. She thought, "This constipation really upsets me. I just don't feel like myself if I don't have a bowel movement every day."

On the basis of the nursing study, develop a nursing care plan using the following procedure[a]:

- List Stella's comments that provide subjective data.
- List information that provides objective data.

- From these data, identify and state, using an accepted format, two nursing diagnoses you determine are most significant to Stella at this time. List two of Stella's strengths that you have identified from the data.
- Determine and state outcome criteria for each diagnosis. These criteria must reflect some alleviation of the problem identified in the nursing diagnosis and must be stated in concrete and measurable terms.
- Plan and state one or more interventions for each diagnosed problem. Provide specific documentation of the source used to determine the appropriate intervention. Plan at least one intervention that incorporates Stella's existing strengths.
- Evaluate the success of the intervention. Interventions must correlate directly with the stated outcome criteria to measure the outcome success.

[a]Students are advised to refer to their nursing diagnosis text and identify possible or potential problems.

CRITICAL THINKING QUESTIONS AND ACTIVITIES

1. What information will you need to obtain from Stella to help her determine the causes of her constipation?
2. What advice will you give Stella regarding the use of laxatives?
3. What dietary changes will you suggest to her, and how will you do this to encourage modifications?
4. What information regarding the relationships of medications to constipation will be useful to Stella?

RESEARCH QUESTIONS

1. Do childhood toilet training experiences and beliefs about elimination affect one's elimination functions later in life? How do these experiences vary across different cultures?
2. What is the knowledge level of graduating nursing students and practicing nurses in UI care?
3. What factors are associated with effective implementation and maintenance of PV programs in long-term care?
4. What are some of the reasons individuals do not seek professional help for incontinence concerns?
5. What types of techniques do individuals use to manage their incontinence problems and what is their level of satisfaction with the techniques?
6. How are decisions made by community-living individuals about the types of incontinence products to buy?
7. What are the specific concerns of older adults related to constipation?
8. What is the knowledge level of young, middle-aged, and older individuals about normal bowel function?

REFERENCES

Agency for Healthcare Quality and Research: *Treatments for fecal incontinence: current state of the evidence,* 2016. https://effectivehealthcare.ahrq.gov/topics/fecal-incontinence/research. Accessed February 2018.

American Geriatrics Society Choosing Wisely Workgroup: American Geriatrics Society identifies another five things that healthcare providers and patients should question, *J Am Geriatr Soc* 62(5): 950–960, 2014.

Blekken LE, Nakrem S, Vinsnes AG, et al: Constipation and laxative use among nursing home patients: prevalence and associations derived from the Resident Assessment Instrument for Long-Term Care Facilities (interRAI LTCF), *Gastroenterol Res Pract* 1215746, 2016. https://www.hindawi.com/journals/grp/2016/1215746/. Accessed February 2018.

Brown HW, Wexner SD, Segall MM, Brezoczky KL, Lukacz ES: Accidental bowel leakage in the mature women's health study, *Int J Clin Pract* 66(11):1101–1108, 2012.

Buswell M, Goodman C, Roe B, et al: What works to improve and manage fecal incontinence in care home residents with dementia: a realist synthesis of the evidence, *J Am Med Dir Assoc* 18(9): 752–760.el, 2017.

Centers for Disease Control and Prevention: *Healthcare-associated infections (HAI) progress report, 2016,* 2018. http://www.cdc.gov/hai/progress-report/index.html. Accessed February 2018.

Colborne M, Dahlke S: Nurses' perceptions and management of urinary incontinence in hospitalized older adults, *An Integr Rev J Gerontol Nurs* 43(10):46–55, 2017.

Crnich CJ, Jump RL, Nace DA: Improving management of urinary tract infections in older adults: a paradigm shift or therapeutic nihilism? *J Am Geriatr Soc* 65:1661–1663, 2017.

DeBeau C: Urinary incontinence. In Ham R, Sloane R, Warshaw G, editors: *Primary care geriatrics,* ed 6, Philadelphia, PA, 2014, Elsevier Saunders, pp 269–280.

Engberg S, Li H: Urinary incontinence in frail older adults, *Urologic Nurs* 37(3):119–124, 2017.

Finucane TE: "Urinary tract infection"—requiem for a heavyweight, *J Am Geriatr Soc* 65:1650–1655, 2017.

Gibson W, Wagg A: New horizons in urinary incontinence in older adults, *Age Ageing* 43:157–163, 2014.

Guérin A, Mody R, Fok B, et al: Risk of developing colorectal cancer and benign colorectal neoplasm in patients with chronic constipation, *Aliment Pharmacol Ther* 40(1):83–92, 2014.

Holtzer-Goor KM, Gaultney JG, van Houten P, et al: Cost-effectiveness of including a nurse specialist in the treatment of urinary incontinence in primary care in the Netherlands, *PLoS One* 10(10):e0138225, 2015.

Hsu A, Suskind A, Huang AJ: Urinary incontinence among older adults. In Lindquist L, editor: *New directions in geriatric medicine,* 2016, Springer, New York, pp 49–69.

Kitsler CE, Zimmerman S, Scales K, et al: The antibiotic prescribing pathway for presumed urinary tract infections in nursing home residents, *J Am Geriatr Soc* 65:1719–1725, 2017.

Lewis SJ, Heaton KW: Stool form scale as a useful guide to intestinal transit time, *Scand J Gastroenterol* 32:920–924, 1997.

Lai CKY, Wan X: Using prompted voiding to manage urinary incontinence in nursing homes: can it be sustained? *J Am Med Dir Assoc* 18(6):509–514, 2017.

MacDonald DG, Butler L: Silent no more: elderly women's stories of living with urinary incontinence in long-term care, *J Gerontol Nurs* 33:14–20, 2007.

Mason DJ, Newman DK, Palmer MH: Changing UI practice, *Am J Nurs* 103:129, 2003.

Mody L, Greene MT, Meddings J, et al: A national implementation program to prevent catheter-associated urinary tract infection in nursing home residents, *JAMA Intern Med* 177(8):1154–1162, 2017.

National Association for Continence: *urinary incontinence overview, facts and statistics* 2017. https://www.nafc.org/urinary-incontinence/. Accessed February 2018.

Ostaszkiewicz J: A conceptual model of the risk of elder abuse posed by incontinence and care dependence, *Int J Older People Nurs* 13(2):e12182, 2017.

Paquette IM, Varma MG, Kaiser AM, Steele SR, Rafferty JF: The American Society of Colon and Rectal Surgeons clinical practice guideline for the treatment of fecal incontinence, *Dis Colon Rectum,* 58:623–636, 2015.

Safdar N, Codispoti N, Purvis S, Knobloch MJ: Patient perspectives on indwelling catheter use in the hospital, *Am J Infect Control* 44(3):e23–e24, 2016.

Schuster BG, Kosar L, Kamrul R: Constipation in older adults: stepwise approach to keep things moving, *Can Fam Physician* 61(2):152–158, 2015.

Searcy JAR: Geriatric urinary incontinence, *Nurs Clin North Am* 52:447–455, 2017.

Shaw C, Wagg A: Urinary incontinence in older adults, *Med Older Adults* 45(1), 2016. doi:10.1016/j.mpmed.2016.10.001.

Sjöström M, Lindholm L, Samuelsson E: Mobile app for treatment of stress urinary incontinence: a cost-effectiveness analysis, *J Med Int Res* 19(5):e154, 2017.

Spencer M, McManus K, Sabourin J: Incontinence in older adults: the role of the geriatric multidisciplinary team, *BC Med J* 59(2): 99–105, 2017.

The Joint Commission: *Hospital National Patient Safety Goals,* 2018. https://www.jointcommission.org/assets/1/6/2018_HAP_NPSG_goals_final.pdf. Accessed February 2018.

Timmons B, Vess J, Conner B: Nurse-driven protocol to reduce indwelling catheter time: a health care improvement initiative, *J Nurs Care Qual,* 32(2):104–107, 2017.

Wilde MH, Bliss DZ, Booth J, Cheater FM, Tannenbaum C: Self-management of urinary and fecal incontinence, *Am J Nurs* 114(2): 38–45, 2014.

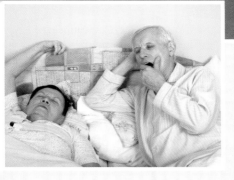

17

Sleep

Lenny Chiang-Hanisko and Theris A. Touhy

http://evolve.elsevier.com/Touhy/TwdHlthAging

A STUDENT SPEAKS

I am so stressed and tired all the time in this nursing program. The workload is so intense there is never enough time to sleep. When I have any time, I would go to bed at 7 p.m. and sleep until 11 in the morning if I could. When will I ever feel rested and not tired?

Marybeth, 22 years old

AN OLDER ADULT SPEAKS

The years have changed my sleep patterns. Bedtime rituals take longer. Nature wakens me two or three times a night for trips to the bathroom. Sleep returns at once unless my mind turns on and it gets launched on a needless project. The earlier remedies are called on to slow down the activities, or the next day is a disaster. My 90-year-old aunt, who slept very little and lightly and lay awake many nights, said she went to the bathroom several times just for something to do instead of just lying there.

Ricarda, 80 years old

LEARNING OBJECTIVES

On completion of this chapter, the reader will be able to:
1. Identify age-related changes that affect sleep.
2. Describe the signs, symptoms, treatment, and nursing interventions for sleep disorders: insomnia, obstructive sleep apnea, Willis-Ekbom disease (restless legs syndrome—RLS), rapid eye movement sleep behavior disorder, circadian rhythm sleep disorder.
3. Use evidence-based protocols in assessment and development of nursing interventions for sleep.
4. Educate individuals/families/health care staff about sleep disorders and sleep hygiene measures.

Sleep occupies one-third of our lives and is a vital function that affects cognition and performance. Research into the physiology of sleep suggests that the restorative function of sleep may be a consequence of the enhanced removal of potentially neurotoxic waste products that accumulate in the awake central nervous system. Sleep is a barometer of health, and sleep assessment and interventions for sleep concerns should receive as much attention as other vital signs. There is increasing awareness of the relationship between sleep problems and health outcomes, including premature mortality, osteoporosis, cardiovascular disease, diabetes, metabolic disease, impaired cognition and physical function, anxiety and depression, pain, and decreased quality of life (Jike et al, 2018; Silva et al, 2016).

Insufficient sleep is a public health epidemic and the Centers for Disease Control and Prevention (CDC, 2018) has called for continued public health surveillance of sleep quality, duration, behaviors, and disorders to monitor for sleep difficulties and their health impact. Sleep problems also constitute a global epidemic, affecting up to 45% of the world's population. Gender differences exist in sleep disturbances and may be more common in women and older adults (Theorell-Haglöw et al, 2018; World Association of Sleep Medicine, 2018). Sleep problems are projected to increase in both low- and high-income countries, as the proportion of older adults and the prevalence of obesity increase across the world (Matricciani et al, 2017; Senaratna et al, 2017). Because of the public health burden of chronic sleep loss and sleep disorders, and the low awareness of poor sleep health, *Healthy People 2020* includes sleep health as a special topic area. Goals for adults are presented in the Healthy People 2020 box.

 HEALTHY PEOPLE 2020

Sleep Health

Goals
- Increase public knowledge of how adequate sleep and treatment of sleep disorders improve health, productivity, wellness, quality of life, and safety on roads and in the workplace.
- Increase the proportion of persons with symptoms of obstructive sleep apnea who seek medical evaluation.
- Increase the proportion of adults who get sufficient sleep.

Data from U.S. Department of Health and Human Services, Office of Disease Prevention and Health Promotion: *Healthy People 2020,* 2018. https://www.healthypeople.gov/2020/topics-objectives/topic/sleep-health/objectives

BIORHYTHM AND SLEEP

Our lives proceed in a series of rhythms that influence and regulate physiological function, chemical concentrations, performance, behavioral responses, moods, and the ability to adapt. It is clear that body temperature, pulse rate, blood pressure, and hormonal levels change significantly and predictably in a circadian rhythm. Circadian rhythms are linked to the 24-hour day by time cues (zeitgebers), the most important of which is the light-dark cycle. Biorhythms vary between individuals, and age-related changes in biorhythms (circadian rhythms) are relevant to health and the process of aging. With aging, there is a reduction in the amplitude of all circadian endogenous responses (e.g., body temperature, pulse rate, blood pressure, hormonal levels).

The most important biorhythm is the circadian sleep-wake rhythm. As people age, the natural circadian rhythm may become less responsive to external stimuli, such as changes in light during the course of the day. In addition, the endogenous changes in the production of melatonin are diminished, resulting in less sleep efficacy and further disruption of restorative sleep (Saccomano, 2014). Genetic research is investigating pathways linking sleep, circadian rhythm, metabolism, functioning, and disease, and genome-wide determinants of sleep duration (Mukherjee, 2018).

SLEEP AND AGING

The predictable pattern of normal sleep is called **sleep architecture.** The body progresses through the five stages of the normal sleep pattern consisting of **rapid eye movement (REM)** sleep and **non–rapid eye movement (NREM)** sleep. Sleep structure is shown in Box 17.1. Most of the changes in sleep architecture in healthy adults begin between the ages of 40 and 60 years. The age-related changes include less time spent in stages 3 and 4 sleep (slow wave sleep) and more time spent awake or in stage 1 sleep. The changes contribute to fragmented sleep and early

---

BOX 17.1   The Stages of Sleep

Non–Rapid Eye Movement (NREM)
- 75% of night
- As we begin to fall asleep, we enter NREM sleep, which is composed of stages 1–4

N1 (Formerly Stage 1)
- Between being awake and falling asleep
- Light sleep

N2 (Formerly Stage 2)
- Onset of sleep
- Becoming disengaged from surroundings
- Breathing and heart rate are regular
- Body temperature drops (so sleeping in a cool room is helpful)

N3 (Formerly Stages 3 and 4)
- Deepest and most restorative sleep
- Blood pressure drops
- Breathing becomes slower
- Muscles are relaxed
- Blood supply to muscles increases
- Tissue growth and repair occurs
- Energy is restored
- Hormones are released, such as: growth hormone, essential for growth and development, including muscle development

Rapid Eye Movement (REM)
- 25% of night
- First occurs about 90 minutes after falling asleep and recurs about every 90 minutes, getting longer later in the night
- Provides energy to brain and body
- Supports daytime performance
- Brain is active and dreams occur
- Eyes dart back and forth
- Body becomes immobile and relaxed, as muscles are turned off

Adapted from National Sleep Foundation: *What happens when you sleep?* https://sleepfoundation.org/how-sleep-works/what-happens-when-you-sleep. Accessed May 20, 2018.

---

awakening (Suzuki et al, 2017). Time spent in REM sleep also declines with age, and transitions between stages 1 and 2 are more common. REM sleep is seen as important for older adults since it is a time for the brain to replenish neurotransmitters essential for remembering, learning, and problem solving. Declines in stages 3 and 4 sleep begin between 20 and 30 years of age and are nearly complete by the age of 50 to 60 years. In adults over 90 years, stages 3 and 4 may disappear completely (Xiong, 2017).

Research suggests that the deterioration of a cluster of neurons associated with regulating sleep patterns, the ventrolateral preoptic nucleus, may be responsible for sleep decline in aging. The more neurons that are lost, the more difficult it is for the person to sleep. For individuals with dementia, the link between the loss of neurons is greater and causes more problems with sleep (Petrovsky et al, 2018). The changes that occur in sleep with aging are summarized in Box 17.2.

BOX 17.2 Age-Related Sleep Changes

- More time spent in bed awake before falling asleep
- Total sleep time and sleep efficiency are reduced
- Awakenings are frequent, increasing after age 50 years (>30 min of wake-fulness after sleep onset in >50% of older subjects)
- Daytime napping
- Changes in circadian rhythm (early to bed, early to rise)
- Sleep is subjectively and objectively lighter (more stage 1, little stage 4, more disruptions)
- Rapid eye movement (REM) sleep is short, less intense, and more evenly distributed
- Frequency of abnormal breathing events is increased
- Frequency of leg movements during sleep is increased

Adapted from Saccomano S: Sleep disorders in older adults, *J Gerontol Nurs* 40(3):38–45, 2014.

⚡ SAFETY ALERT

Poor sleep is not an inevitable consequence of aging but rather an indicator of health status and calls for investigation.

BOX 17.3 Risk Factors for Sleep Disturbances in Older Adults

Physical Health
- Age-related changes in sleep architecture
- Comorbidities (cardiovascular disease, diabetes, pulmonary disease, musculoskeletal disorders), CNS disorders (Parkinson's disease, seizure disorder, dementia), GI disorders (hiatal hernia, GERD, PUD), urinary disorders (incontinence, BPH)
- Pain
- Polypharmacy
- Lack of exercise
- Excessive napping
- Sleep disorders (apnea, restless legs syndrome, periodic leg movement, rapid eye movement behavior disorder, alcohol, smoking)

Psychological Condition
- Depression, anxiety, delirium, psychosis
- Life stressors/response to stress
- Sleep-related beliefs
- Sleep habits (daily sleep/activity cycle, napping)
- Loneliness
- Loss of partner
- Poor sleep hygiene

Physical Environment
- Environmental noises, institutional routines
- Caregiving for a dependent older adult
- Limited exposure to sunlight
- New environment

BPH, Benign prostatic hyperplasia; *CNS*, central nervous system; *GERD*, gastroesophageal reflux disease; *GI*, gastrointestinal; *PUD*, peptic ulcer disease.
Adapted from Teodorescu M: Sleep disruptions and insomnia in older adults, *Consultant* 54(3):166–173, 2014.

Older adults with good general health, positive moods, and engagement in more active lifestyles and meaningful activities report better sleep and fewer sleep complaints. Results of a large study (155,877 participants) that explored the prevalence of sleep-related complaints across age groups found that on average, older adults reported sleeping better than younger adults (Varrasse et al, 2015). Sleep complaints are usually linked to other health problems and sleep disorders (Rodriguez et al, 2015).

SLEEP DISORDERS

Insomnia

Insomnia is the most common sleep disorder worldwide (Bhaskar et al, 2016). The American Academy of Sleep Medicine defines insomnia as the subjective perception of difficulty with sleep initiation, duration, consolidation, or quality that results in some form of daytime impairment (Matheson and Hainer, 2017). The diagnosis of insomnia requires that the person has difficulty falling asleep for at least 1 month and that impairment in daytime functioning results from difficulty sleeping.

Insomnia is classified as either primary or comorbid. Primary insomnia implies that no other cause of sleep disturbance has been identified. Comorbid insomnia is more common and is associated with psychiatric and medical disorders, medications, and primary sleep disorders, such as obstructive sleep apnea (OSA) or restless legs syndrome (RLS). Comorbid insomnia does not suggest that these conditions cause insomnia but that insomnia and the other conditions co-occur and each may require attention and treatment (Bhaskar et al, 2016; Winkelman, 2015).

More than half of older adults suffer from insomnia and sleep complaints are generally higher in women than in men (Suzuki et al, 2017). Chronic insomnia is a significant risk factor for cognitive decline in men. Insomnia is also associated with an increased risk of cardiovascular-related and all-cause mortality

as well as a predictor of long-term care placement (Suzuki et al, 2017). The number of insomnia symptoms is associated with an increased risk of falls in older adults, and the use of sleeping medications, irrespective of insomnia symptoms, further increases fall risk (Chen et al, 2017) (Chapters 19 and 28).

There are many influencing factors for insomnia including physiological, psychological, and environmental (Box 17.3). Prescription and nonprescription medications and alcohol create sleep disturbances (Box 17.4). The times of day that medications are given can also contribute to sleep problems—for example, a diuretic given before bedtime or sedating medication given in the morning.

Insomnia and Alzheimer's Disease

Sleep disruption affects approximately 60% to 70% of older adults with dementia and varies by dementia subtype. Individuals with Lewy body dementia and Parkinson's dementia have the highest prevalence of sleep disruption (90%) and 25% to 60% of individuals with Alzheimer's disease have sleep disruptions or abnormal circadian rhythms. Multiple factors contribute to sleep disruption in dementia, including degenerative changes in the suprachiasmatic nuclei (SCN) of the hypothalamus, which generates the circadian rhythm, psychiatric and medical comorbidities, and physiological changes associated

---

BOX 17.4   Medications Affecting Sleep

Antiarrhythmics
Antihypertensives (beta-blockers, clonidine, reserpine, methyldopa)
Anticholinergics
Corticosteroids
Diuretics
Levodopa
Medications containing alcohol (cough, cold, flu)
Medications containing caffeine (headaches, pain)
Nicotine replacement products
Opiates
Phenytoin
Sedating antihistamines (cold, allergy)
Selective serotonin reuptake inhibitors (SSRIs)
Sympathomimetic stimulants (attention deficit disorder)
Theophylline
Thyroid hormone

---

with aging (Scales et al, 2018). Additionally, decreased exposure to daytime light and increased exposure to nighttime noise and light contributes to disrupted sleep. Sleep disruption is associated with increased neuropsychiatric symptoms, functional decline, morbidity, and mortality. Sleep disruption is a major predictor of institutionalization and caregiver burden. Caregivers of individuals with dementia also experience poor sleep quality, and this influences caregiver stress and health problems (Leggett et al, 2018; Petrovsky et al, 2018).

PROMOTING HEALTHY AGING: IMPLICATIONS FOR GERONTOLOGICAL NURSING

Assessment

Sleep habits should be reviewed with older adults in all settings. Many people do not seek treatment for insomnia and may blame poor sleep on the aging process. Nurses are in an excellent position to assess sleep and suggest interventions to improve the quality of the older adult's sleep. "No other group of health care providers watch more people sleep than nurses, and sleep disorders can affect all aspects of health and illness" (Dean et al, 2016, p. 438).

Assessment for sleep disorders and awareness of contributing factors to poor sleep (pain, chronic illness, medications, alcohol use, depression, anxiety) are important. The nurse should learn how well the person sleeps at home, how many times the person is awakened at night, what time the person retires, and what rituals occur at bedtime. Rituals include bedtime snacks, watching television, listening to music, or reading—activities whose execution is crucial to the individual's ability to fall asleep. Complete sleep assessment data are presented in Box 17.5.

The sleep diary or log is also an important part of assessment (Box 17.6). This information will provide an accurate account of the person's sleep problem and help identify the sleep disturbance. A period of 2 to 4 weeks is needed to obtain a clear picture of the sleep problem. A self-rating scale, the Pittsburgh Sleep Quality Index (PSQI), can be used to measure the quality and patterns of sleep in the older adult, and daytime sleepiness can be assessed with the Epworth Sleepiness Scale, both recommended by the Hartford Institute for Geriatric

---

BOX 17.5   Tips for Best Practice
Assessment of Sleep Disturbances

Basic Sleep History Questions
- Where do you sleep at night (bed, couch, recliner chair)?
- Do you have any difficulty falling asleep?
- What do you do at night before you go to bed?
- Are you having any difficulty sleeping until morning?
- Are you having difficulty sleeping throughout the night?
- How often do you awaken and how long are you awake? What prevents you from falling back to sleep?
- Have you or someone else ever noticed that you snore loudly or stop breathing in your sleep?
- Do you find yourself falling asleep during the day when you do not want to?

Follow-Up Questions
- What time do you usually go to bed? Fall asleep?
- What prevents you from falling asleep?
- Do your legs kick or jump around while you sleep?
- Are you outside in natural light most days?
- Do you have any pain, discomfort, or shortness of breath during the night?
- What type of exercise do you get during the day?

Additional Assessment
- Individual's bed partner, family member, or caregiver can also be asked to provide information
- Review intake of alcohol, nicotine, caffeine, and medications
- Review risk factors (obesity, arthritis, poorly controlled illnesses)
- Review of depressive symptoms; weight loss; sadness, or recent losses
- Review involvement in social activities
- Review functional status/activities of daily living (ADL)/instrumental activities of daily living (IADL) performance

Objective Measures
- Sleep diary (keep for 24 hours daily for 2 to 4 weeks)
- Self-rating of sleep scales—Pittsburgh Sleep Quality Index; Epworth Sleepiness Scale; Insomnia Severity Scale
- On a scale of 1 to 10 (10 the highest), how would you rate your sleep?

Adapted from Dean GE, Klimpt ML, Morris JL, Chasens ER: Protocol: excessive sleepiness. In Boltz M, Capezuti E, Fulmer T, Zwicker D editors: *Evidence-based geriatric nursing protocols for best practice*, New York, 2016, Springer, pp. 431–441.

BOX 17.6   Sleep Diary

Instructions: Record the following for 2 to 4 weeks. Should be completed by the person or the caregiver if the person is unable. Record when you:
- Go to bed
- Go to sleep
- Wake up
- Get out of bed
- Take naps
- Exercise
- Consume alcohol
- Consume caffeinated beverages

From Centers for Disease Control and Prevention: *What should I do if I can't sleep?* 2013. https://www.cdc.gov/sleep/about_sleep/cant_sleep.html. Accessed May 20, 2018.

Hartford Institute for Geriatric Nursing: Try This, General Assessment Series: Epworth Sleepiness Scale and Pittsburg Sleep Quality Index: https://consultgeri.org/try-this/general-assessment/issue-6.2; https://consultgeri.org/try-this/general-assessment/issue-6.1.pdf.

Qaseem A, Owens D, Dallas P, et al: *Management of obstructive sleep apnea in adults: a clinical practice guideline from the American College of Physicians.* https://www.ncbi.nlm.nih.gov/pubmed/24061345.

Restless Legs Syndrome Foundation: *RLS symptom diary.* https://www.rls.org/file/symptom-diary.pdf. Accessed May 20, 2018.

Nursing (Box 17.7). The Epworth Sleepiness Scale helps to distinguish between the average amount of sleep and problems with sleep deprivation that require intervention (Kendzerska et al, 2014; Yaremchuk, 2018) (Box 17.7). The Insomnia Severity Index (ISI) is another tool to measure insomnia severity. Objective measures include polysomnography conducted in sleep laboratories, including electroencephalograms (EEGs), electromyograms (EMGs), wrist actigraphy, and direct observations.

Interventions
Nonpharmacological Treatment
Interventions begin after a thorough sleep history has been recorded and, if possible, a sleep log obtained. Management is directed at identifiable causes. Nonpharmacological interventions are considered first-line treatment for insomnia. Education should be provided on changes in sleep architecture with aging and the importance of attention to sleep hygiene principles to promote good sleep habits.

Cognitive behavioral therapy for insomnia is a multidimensional approach combining psychological and behavioral therapies that include healthy sleep habits, relaxation techniques, and interventions (Box 17.8). A combination of approaches is most effective, and these interventions have been reported to be an effective and practical treatment for chronic insomnia in older adults (Anderson, 2018; Haynes et al, 2018). Computerized

cognitive behavioral therapy is associated with improved sleep and a higher adherence rate than traditional face-to-face therapy sessions (Xiong and Hategan, 2017). Cognitive training programs (Chapter 5) may improve sleep quality and cognitive performance. Tai chi quigong (TCQ), a less complex form of tai chi movements, can be considered a useful nonpharmacological approach for sleep complaints for individuals with cognitive impairment (Chan et al, 2016) (Research Highlights box).

RESEARCH HIGHLIGHTS

More than a quarter of older adults with cognitive impairment experience sleep disturbances such as day-night sleep pattern reversals, frequent night-time awakening, and daytime sleep. The purpose of this pilot study was to evaluate the preliminary effects of tai chi quigong (TCQ) on improving the nighttime sleep quality of older adults with cognitive impairment. TCQ was chosen because it involves repetition of easy-to-follow movements and is recommended over traditional tai chi practice for individuals with dementia. A randomized controlled trial with two groups was conducted with 53 older community-living older adults. The intervention group received TCQ training in two 60-minute sessions each week for 2 months. The control group was advised to maintain their usual activities. Sleep quality was measured by the Chinese Pittsburgh Sleep Quality Index, quality of life measured by Short-form 12, and cognitive functions measured by Mini-Mental State Examination (MMSE) and a memory inventory. The TCQ participants reported better sleep quality (sleep duration, sleep efficiency) and a better quality of life (mental health component) than the control group. Further studies are needed but as a low intensity exercise, TCQ is an appropriate intervention for older adults with cognitive impairment.

Chan A, Yu D, Choi K et al: Tai chi quigong as a means to improve night-time sleep quality among older adults with cognitive impairment, *Clin Interv Aging* 11:1277–1286, 2016.

Sleep in hospitals and nursing homes. In hospital and institutional settings, promotion of a good sleep environment is important. Studies have shown that as many as 22% to 61% of hospitalized patients experience impaired sleep (Dean et al, 2016). A multidisciplinary approach to identify sources of noise and light, such as equipment and staff interactions, could result

BOX 17.8 Interventions for Insomnia

Healthy Sleep Habits
- Keep a consistent sleep schedule. Get up at the same time every day, even on weekends or during vacations.
- Set a bedtime that is early enough to get at least 7 hours of sleep.
- Don't go to bed unless sleepy.
- If you don't fall asleep after 20 minutes, get out of bed.
- Establish a relaxing bedtime routine.
- Use bed only for sleep and sex.
- Make bedroom quiet and relaxing. Keep the room at a comfortable, cool temperature.
- Limit exposure to bright light in the evenings.
- Turn off electronic devices at least 30 minutes before bedtime.
- Don't eat a large meal before bedtime. If hungry at night, eat a light, healthy snack.
- Exercise regularly and maintain a healthy diet.
- Avoid caffeine, alcohol, and tobacco in the late afternoon or evening.

- Reduce fluid intake before bedtime.
- Limit or avoid daytime napping.

Relaxation Techniques
- Diaphragmatic breathing
- Progressive relaxation
- White noise or music
- Guided imagery
- Stretching
- Yoga or tai chi

Interventions
- Cue circadian rhythm by connecting with environmental signals (light exposure, meals, activity, medications).
- Maintain stable daytime routines with meals, activity, and medications.
- Increase duration and intensity of bright light or sunlight exposure during the day.
- Melatonin 1 to 2 hours before bedtime may be helpful.

Adapted from American Academy of Sleep Medicine: *Healthy sleep habits*, 2017. http://www.sleepeducation.org/essentials-in-sleep/healthy-sleep-habits. Accessed May 20, 2018.

BOX 17.9   Tips for Best Practice

Suggestions to Promote Sleep When Hospitalized or in a Nursing Home

- Allow individual to stay out of bed and out of the room for as long as possible before bed.
- Provide 30 minutes or more of sunlight exposure in a comfortable outdoor location.
- Provide low-level physical activity three times a day.
- Keep noise level at a minimum, speak in hushed tones, do no use overhead paging, reduce light in hallways and resident rooms.
- Institute a sleep improvement protocol—"do not disturb" times, soft music, relaxation, massage, aromatherapy, sleep masks, headphones, allowing patients to shut doors. Consider having a kit that can be taken to bedside with music, aromatherapy.
- Perform necessary care (e.g., turning, changing) when the individual is awake rather than awakening the individual between the hours of 10:00 p.m. and 6:00 a.m.
- Limit intake of caffeine and other fluids in excess before bedtime.
- Provide a light snack or warm beverage before bedtime.
- Discontinue invasive treatments when possible (Foley catheters, percutaneous gastrostomy tubes, intravenous lines).
- Encourage and assist to the bathroom before bed and as needed.
- Give pain medication before bedtime for patients with pain.
- Institute the same time for resident to arise and get out of bed every morning.
- Maintain comfortable temperature in room; provide blankets as needed.
- Provide meaningful activities (individualized and group) during the daytime.

in modification without compromising safety and quality of patient care (Box 17.9). Sleep deprivation due to noise can potentially exacerbate delirium. Noise from monitoring equipment alarms and infusion devices and the ringing from telephones cause an elevation of heart rate (Grossman et al, 2017; McGough et al, 2018; Ye and Richards, 2018). Efforts to allow sufficient time before interruptions, such as checking for incontinence or doing routine tasks, are important to promote a full sleep cycle of 90 minutes.

In institutions, there is often limited communication between night and day staff, and a lack of emphasis on the importance of sleep patterns. Night shift staff have the opportunity to assess sleep patterns and implement appropriate interventions to enhance sleep. Fillary and colleagues (2015) offer comprehensive suggestions for night staff, including the development of overnight care plans. Passive music therapy given at bedtime was found to increase sleep quality among a group of older adults residing in nursing homes (Sarikaya and Oguz, 2016). A recent study found that a nurse-led sleep program improved the sleep quality and reduced depressive symptomatology in cognitively intact nursing home residents. The program utilized comprehensive assessment of the sleep experience, sleep hygiene, simple lifestyle recommendations, and stimulus control, as well as sleep restriction. Components were integrated with motivational interviewing techniques, and participants were actively involved in the process (Dolu and Nahcivan, 2019). Further research is needed on the sleep problems of older adults in the community and in acute and long-term care settings.

Pharmacological Treatment

The use of over-the-counter (OTC) sleep aids, as well as the use of prescription sedative and hypnotic medications, is increasing in the United States. Individuals over the age of 60 years receive 33% of all hypnotic prescriptions, although they constitute only 14% of the population. The American Geriatrics Society (AGS) Beers Criteria (2015) strongly suggests avoiding any type of benzodiazepine for the treatment of insomnia since it is associated with adverse outcomes including motor vehicle accidents, impaired cognition, and falls (Markota et al, 2016; Maust et al, 2016; Schroeck et al, 2016). Adverse reactions to these medications are also increasing. Use of narcotic pain medications and sedatives and the use of alcohol, in combination with these medications and other prescribed medications, is a growing concern (Chapter 28). Individuals should be educated on the proper use of medications, their side effects, and their interactions with alcohol and other prescription drugs. Pharmacological treatments for sleep disorders may be used in combination with behavioral interventions but must be managed with caution in older adults (Albert et al, 2017). In long-term care settings, there are specific regulatory guidelines on the use of hypnotics, including appropriate prescribing and tapering and discontinuation of use.

⚡ SAFETY ALERT

Benzodiazepines or other sedative-hypnotics should not be used in older adults as a first choice of treatment for insomnia (American Geriatrics Society, 2015).

OTC drugs such as diphenhydramine, found in many OTC sleep products such as Tylenol PM, are often thought to be relatively harmless but should be avoided because of antihistaminic and anticholinergic side effects. Other OTC sleep aid preparations contain ingredients such as kava kava, valerian root, melatonin, chamomile, and tryptophan. Because these ingredients are not regulated, information and outcomes of efficacy may not be known (Chapter 10). Endogenous nocturnal melatonin, a major loop for circadian rhythm, may have decreased levels in older adults. Melatonin, taken 1 to 2 hours before bedtime, may replicate the natural secretion pattern of melatonin and lead to improvements in the circadian regulation of the sleep-wake cycle.

Routine use of OTC medications for sleep may delay appropriate assessment and treatment of contributing medical or psychological conditions, identification of sleep disorders, and appropriate counseling and treatment. The individual should report use of all OTC drugs to his or her health care provider since they may interact with other medications.

Benzodiazepine receptor agonists, such as zolpidem (Ambien), eszopiclone (Lunesta), and zaleplon (Sonata), are considered benzodiazepine-like in their action because they induce sleep easily. They can have detrimental effects, causing changes in mental status (delirium), memory loss, falls and fractures, daytime drowsiness, and increased risk for motor vehicle accidents, with only minimal improvement in sleep latency and duration (American Geriatrics Society, 2014). Zolpidem is the medication most often implicated in emergency department visits for adverse drug events in adults (Hampton et al, 2014).

Assessment of sleep problems should be conducted before medication use. Nonpharmacological interventions are first-line treatment. If sleeping medications are used, they should be taken immediately before bedtime because of their rapid action. Short-term use (2 to 3 weeks, never more than 90 days) is recommended.

The U.S. Food and Drug Administration (FDA, 2019) has added a black box warning on patient medication guides and prescription information for insomnia drugs such as zolpidem, zaleplon, and eszopiclone, calling attention to side effects that can lead to serious injury or death. Rare but serious incidents have occurred when users of these medications experienced complex sleep behaviors: sleepwalking, sleep driving, and engaging in other activities when not fully awake. Rozerem (Ramelteon), a melatonin agonist, has modest effectiveness and few side effects and is not habit forming. It is indicated for insomnia characterized by difficulty with sleep onset. Suvorexant is the first orexin receptor antagonist approved for the treatment of insomnia. The orexin system regulates the sleep arousal cycle that promotes wakefulness. Side effects are similar to the benzodiazepine receptor agonists and it is thought to have moderate potential for addiction. Given its high cost and addictive potential, it is not recommended as a first-line treatment for insomnia (Matheson and Hainer, 2017).

Box 17.10 presents health teaching guidelines about sleeping medications.

BOX 17.10 Tips for Best Practice

Use of Sleeping Medications

Provide health education on:
1. Normal changes in sleep patterns with age
2. Importance of appropriate assessment of sleep problems before any medications are used
3. Nonpharmacological treatment of sleeping problems as first-line treatment (sleep hygiene, stimulus control, sleep restriction, relaxation techniques)
4. Avoiding over-the-counter (OTC) medications that contain diphenhydramine, which can have side effects of confusion, blurred vision, constipation, falls
5. Adverse effects of sleep medications, even OTC medications; include problems with daily function, changes in mental status, possibility of motor vehicle accidents, increase in daytime drowsiness, and increased risk of falls with only minimal improvement in sleep
6. Avoiding benzodiazepines (flurazepam, triazolam, temazepam) for sleep due to long-acting sedation effects
7. If sleeping medications are prescribed, the benzodiazepine receptor agonists (zolpidem, eszopiclone, zaleplon) or ramelteon are preferred; given at the lowest possible dose for short-term use only (2 to 3 weeks, never longer than 90 days). Medications for sleep should be taken immediately before bedtime
8. Avoiding the use of alcohol, narcotic pain relieving medications, and antianxiety medications if taking sleeping medications
9. Reviewing all medications, including OTC, with health care provider for interactions with sleeping medications
10. Using caution the day after taking sleeping medications, particularly with driving and activities that require full alertness; accidents are common

BOX 17.11 Abbreviations for Sleep Disorders

Sleep disordered breathing (SDB)
Obstructive sleep apnea (OSA)
Restless legs syndrome/Willis-Ekbom disease (RLS/WED)
Rapid eye movement sleep behavior disorder (RBD)
Circadian rhythm sleep disorder (CRSD)
Advanced sleep phase disorder (ASPD)
Irregular sleep-wake disorder (ISWD)

Sleep Disordered Breathing and Sleep Apnea

Sleep disordered breathing (SDB) affects approximately 25% of older individuals (more men than women), and the most common form is OSA (Box 17.11). In long-term care facilities, the prevalence of OSA has been estimated to be as high as 70%. Untreated obstructive sleep apnes (OSA) is related to heart failure, cardiac dysrhythmias, stroke, type 2 diabetes, osteoporosis, and even death (Kapur et al, 2017). Older adults with OSA demonstrate significant cognitive decline compared with younger people with the same disease severity (Leng et al, 2017). The diagnosis of OSA is often delayed in older adults and symptoms are blamed on age (McMillan and Morrell, 2016).

Age-related decline in the activity of the upper airway muscles, resulting in compromised pharyngeal patency, predisposes older adults to OSA. A high body mass index (BMI) and large neck circumference have been identified as risk factors for OSA but are not as significant in older adults (Martin and Alessi, 2014). Other risk factors are presented in Box 17.12. Symptoms of sleep apnea include loud periodic snoring, gasping and choking on awakenings, unusual nighttime activity such as sitting upright or falling out of bed, morning headache, unexplained daytime sleepiness, poor memory and intellectual functioning, and irritability and personality change. If the person has a sleeping partner, it is often the partner who reports the nighttime symptoms. If there is a sleeping partner, he or she may move to another room to sleep because of the disturbance to his or her own rest.

BOX 17.12 Risk Factors for Obstructive Sleep Apnea

- Increasing age
- Increased neck circumference (not as significant in older adults)
- Male gender
- Anatomical abnormalities of the upper airway
- Upper airway resistance and/or obstruction
- Family history
- Excess weight
- Use of alcohol, sedatives, or tranquilizers
- Smoking
- Hypertension

PROMOTING HEALTHY AGING: IMPLICATIONS FOR GERONTOLOGICAL NURSING

Assessment

The individual with SDB may present with complaints of insomnia or daytime sleepiness, and insomnia should be assessed as discussed previously, including the use of screening instruments such as the Epworth Sleepiness Scale (Box 17.7). Assessment of symptoms of OSA and information from the sleeping partner, if present, are obtained. A medication review is always indicated when investigating sleep complaints. The upper airway, including the nasal and pharyngeal airways, should be examined for anatomical obstruction, tumors, or cysts. Comorbid conditions such as heart failure and diabetes should be assessed and managed appropriately.

If OSA is suspected, a referral for a sleep study should be made. A sleep study or polysomnogram is a multiple-component test that electronically transmits and records specific physical activities during sleep. The data obtained are analyzed by a qualified physician to determine whether or not the person has a sleep disorder. In most cases, sleep studies take place in a sleep lab specially set up for the test and are monitored by a technician, but they can also be conducted at home. Recognition of OSA in older adults may be more difficult because there may not be a sleeping partner to report symptoms. If presenting symptoms suggest the disorder, a tape recorder can be placed at the bedside to record snoring and breathing sounds during the night.

Interventions

Therapy will depend on the severity and type of sleep apnea, and the presence of comorbid illnesses. Treatment of sleep apnea may involve avoidance of alcohol and sedative-hypnotic medications, cessation of smoking, avoidance of supine sleep positions, and weight loss. The use of hypnotics can exacerbate OSA (Xiong and Hategan, 2017). There should be risk counseling about impaired judgment from sleeplessness and the possibility of accidents when driving.

Continuous positive airway pressure (CPAP) is recommended as the initial therapy for OSA and generally can reverse this condition quickly with the appropriate titration of devices (Downey et al, 2018). The CPAP device delivers pressurized air through tubing to a nasal mask or nasal pillows, which are fitted around the head. The pressurized air acts as an airway splint and gently opens the individual's throat and breathing passages, allowing the individual to breathe normally, but only through the nose. Teaching should be provided about the effects of untreated OSA and the need for treatment emphasized. A stepwise approach during the initiation of therapy and continued monitoring can foster better use of CPAP or prevent discontinuation of therapy. CPAP nonadherence is a major challenge with estimates indicating about half of individuals either discontinue the therapy or are not adherent (use for less than 4 hours per night) (Jacobsen et al, 2017; Nadal et al, 2018).

Mandibular advancement devices are recommended as an alternative treatment for individuals who prefer this type of device or experience adverse effects with CPAP. However, this treatment has a weak recommendation with low-quality evidence. These appliances also require a stable dentition and may be problematic for individuals with dentures or extensive tooth loss (Dean et al, 2016).

Restless Legs Syndrome/Willis-Ekbom Disease

Restless legs syndrome/Willis-Ekbom disease (RLS/WED) is a neurological movement disorder of the limbs that is often associated with a sleep complaint. Individuals with RLS/WED have an uncontrollable need to move the legs, often accompanied by discomfort in the legs. Other symptoms include paresthesias; creeping sensations; crawling sensations; tingling, cramping, and burning sensations; pain; or even indescribable sensations. RLS/WED has a circadian rhythm, with the intensity of the symptoms becoming worse at night and improving toward the morning. Symptoms may be temporarily relieved by movement.

An estimated 7% to 10% of adults in North America and Europe have the disease. The disorder is familial in about 50% of individuals, and several predisposing genes have been identified through genome-wide association studies (Suzuki et al, 2017). RLS/WED is less common in Asian populations. Incidence is about twice as high in women, and while the disease may begin at any age (including childhood), many individuals who are severely affected are middle-aged or older. Symptoms become more frequent and last longer with age (National Institute of Neurological Disorders and Stroke [NINDS], 2017).

In most cases, RLS/WED is a primary idiopathic disorder but it also can be associated with underlying medical disorders including iron deficiency, end-stage renal disease (especially in individuals requiring dialysis), diabetes, and pregnancy. Antidepressants, antihypertensives, and neuroleptic medications can aggravate RLS/WED symptoms. Increased BMI, caffeine use, alcohol or tobacco use, sleep deprivation, and sedentary lifestyle may also be contributing factors. Other contributing factors under study include iron metabolism and neurotransmitter dysfunctions involving dopamine and glutamate (NINDS, 2017).

Diagnosis of RLS/WED is based on symptoms and a sleep study may be indicated. Possible contributing conditions should be evaluated and all individuals with symptoms should be tested for iron deficiency with a complete iron panel. If iron stores are low, iron replacement is needed. Medication treatment should only start when symptoms have a significant impact on quality of life in terms of frequency and severity; intermittent treatment might be considered in intermediate cases. Medications used include levodopa, benzodiazepines, or low-potency opioids. The chronic persistent form of the disorder may be treated with nonergot dopamine agonists (pramipexole, ropinirole, rotigotine patch) or with gabapentin, gabapentin enacarbil, and pregabalin (Garcia-Borreguero et al, 2016).

Nonpharmacological therapy includes stretching of the lower extremities, mild to moderate physical activity, hot baths, massage, acupressure, relaxation techniques, and avoidance of caffeine, alcohol, and tobacco. Individuals should be encouraged to keep a symptom diary for 7 to 14 days to identify triggers and aid in diagnosis. The Restless Legs Syndrome Foundation provides a symptom diary on their website (Box 17.7).

Rapid Eye Movement Sleep Behavior Disorder

REM sleep behavior disorder (RBD) is characterized by loss of voluntary muscle atonia during REM sleep associated with complex behavior while dreaming. Individuals report elaborate enactment of their dreams, often with violent content, during sleep. This may include violent behaviors, such as punching and kicking, with the potential for injury of both the individual and the bed partner. The mean age at emergence of RBD is 60 years and it is more common in males. (National Sleep Foundation, 2018; Suzuki et al, 2017).

The chronic form is usually idiopathic or associated with Parkinson's disease and dementia with Lewy bodies and 80% to 90% of individuals with RBD eventually develop a neurodegenerative disorder. The acute form of the disorder can be caused by toxic-metabolic abnormalities, drug or alcohol withdrawal, and medications (tricyclic antidepressants, monoamine oxidase inhibitors, cholinergic agents, and selective serotonin reuptake inhibitors [SSRIs]). Diagnosis is based on history, symptoms, and a sleep study to test for the key features of the disorder. Clonazepam curtails or eliminates the disorder about 90% of the time but side effects of daytime sleepiness and dizziness are of concern in older adults. If clonazepam is not effective, some antidepressants or melatonin may reduce the behaviors. A safe environment in the bedroom should be provided (Suzuki et al, 2017).

Circadian Rhythm Sleep Disorders

In circadian rhythm sleep disorders (CRSDs) relatively normal sleep occurs at abnormal times. Two clinical presentations are seen: advanced sleep phase disorder (ASPD) and irregular sleep-wake disorder (ISWD). In ASPD, the individual begins and ends sleep at unusually early times (e.g., going to bed as early as 6 or 7 p.m. and waking up between 2 and 5 a.m.). Not all individuals with an advanced sleep phase have ASPD. If they are not bothered by their sleep phases and have no functional impairment, we may just consider them "morning" people. In ISWD, sleep is dispersed across the 24-hour day in bouts of irregular length. Factors contributing to these disorders are age-related changes in sleep and circadian rhythm regulation combined with decreased levels of light exposure and activity.

A combination of good sleep hygiene practices and methods to delay the timing of sleep and wake times is recommended as treatment for ASPD. Bright light therapy is designed to promote the synchronization of circadian rhythms with environmental light-dark cycles through stimulation of the SCN (Scales et al, 2018). Bright light therapy is a reasonably low cost treatment that, unlike medication usage, does not generally result in residual effects and tolerance. It should be noted that older adults may be less sensitive to light due to age-related changes that may influence the effectiveness of light therapy (Kim and Duffy, 2018).

In ISWD, the individual may obtain enough sleep over the 24-hour period, but time asleep is broken into at least three different periods of variable length. Erratic napping occurs during the day, and nighttime sleep is severely fragmented and shortened. Chronic insomnia and/or daytime sleepiness are present. ISWD is most commonly encountered in individuals with dementia, particularly those who are institutionalized. Box 17.8 provides suggested interventions.

▮ KEY CONCEPTS

- Sleep is a barometer of health and can be considered one of the vital signs.
- Sleep problems constitute a global epidemic affecting up to 50% of the world's population.
- In addition to age-related changes in sleep architecture, many chronic conditions interfere with quality and quantity of sleep in older adults. Complaints of sleep difficulties should be thoroughly investigated and not attributed to age.
- Nonpharmacological interventions (sleep hygiene, sleep restriction measures, stimulus control, circadian interventions, relaxation techniques) are first-line treatments for sleep problems.
- Benzodiazepines or other sedative-hypnotics should not be used in older adults as a first choice of treatment for insomnia.
- All sleeping medications, including OTC, have adverse effects that include daytime drowsiness, changes in mental status, and increased likelihood of falls.
- If sleeping medications are prescribed, benzodiazepine receptor agonists are preferred and should be given at the lowest possible dose and used only short term (2 to 3 weeks, never more than 90 days).
- SDB affects approximately 25% of older individuals (more men than women), and the most common form is OSA.
- Untreated OSA is related to heart failure, cardiac dysrhythmias, stroke, type 2 diabetes, and even death.

NURSING STUDY: REST AND SLEEP

Gerald, 80 years old, had a sleeping disorder and was tired most of the day and lonely at night. His wife of 45 years had recently moved into her sewing room, where she slept on the couch at night because she could no longer cope with his loud snoring. He sometimes even seemed to stop breathing, which kept her awake watching his abdomen rise and fall, or not. Sometimes he would awaken suddenly, gasping for air. However, Gerald had tolerated it because he thought nothing could be done for it. Because it had become a threat to his marriage, he became motivated to investigate possible solutions. Gerald said to his nurse clinician, "This isn't anything, but it upsets my wife." Although he did not admit it, he was also worried because he was beginning to feel rather weak and listless during the day.

Continued

NURSING STUDY: REST AND SLEEP—cont'd

When he had consulted the clinic nurse, Gerald was diagnosed with obstructive sleep apnea. He found that some very practical means of dealing with this problem of sleep apnea were available, and if these were not effective, the nurse had reassured him that additional medical interventions could be helpful.

On the basis of the nursing study, develop a nursing care plan using the following procedure[a]:

- List Gerald's comments that provide subjective data.
- List information that provides objective data.
- From these data, identify and state, using an accepted format, two nursing diagnoses you determine are most significant to Gerald at this time. List two of Gerald's strengths that you have identified from the data.

- Determine and state outcome criteria for each diagnosis. These must reflect some alleviation of the problem identified in the nursing diagnosis and must be stated in concrete and measurable terms.
- Plan and state one or more interventions for each diagnosed problem. Provide specific documentation of the source used to determine the appropriate intervention. Plan at least one intervention that incorporates Gerald's existing strengths.
- Evaluate the success of the intervention. Interventions must correlate directly with the stated outcome criteria to measure the outcome success.

[a]Students are advised to refer to their nursing diagnosis text and identify possible or potential problems.

CRITICAL THINKING QUESTIONS AND ACTIVITIES

1. What lifestyle factors may be increasing Gerald's episodes of sleep apnea?
2. In what circumstances is sleep apnea particularly dangerous to health?
3. Compose a list of 10 questions you would ask Gerald to obtain a clear picture of factors contributing to his sleep apnea. Discuss the rationale behind each.

4. List some of the common methods for dealing with this problem that Gerald's nurse may have given to him.

RESEARCH QUESTIONS

1. Does better management of chronic disease improve sleep quality?
2. Does improving sleep quality have a favorable effect on the course of chronic illness?
3. What is the average time of the total sleep cycle as experienced by a healthy individual older than 70 years?
4. What type of exercise is effective for improved sleep?

5. Which nonpharmacological interventions are most effective for sleep and for what type of individual?
6. What are the concerns of caregivers of persons with dementia as they relate to sleep?
7. How do nurses in hospitals and nursing homes evaluate sleep quality for their patients/residents?

REFERENCES

Albert SM, Roth T, Toscani M, Vitiello MV, Zee P: Sleep health and appropriate use of OTC sleep aids in older adults-recommendations of a Gerontological Society of America workgroup, *Gerontologist* 57(2):163–170, 2017.

American Geriatrics Society Choosing Wisely Group: American Geriatrics Society identifies another five things that healthcare providers and patients should question, *J Am Geriatr Soc* 62(5): 950–960, 2014.

American Geriatrics Society 2015 Beers Criteria Update Expert Panel: American Geriatrics Society 2015 updated Beers criteria for potentially inappropriate medication use in older adults, *J Am Geriatr Soc* 63(11):2227–2246, 2015.

Anderson KN: Insomnia and cognitive behavioural therapy—how to assess your patient and why it should be a standard part of care, *J Thorac Dis* 10(Suppl 1):S94–S102, 2018.

Centers for Disease Control and Prevention (CDC): *CDC declares sleep disorders a public health epidemic,* 2018. https://www.sleepdr. com/the-sleep-blog/cdc-declares-sleep-disorders-a-public-health-epidemic/. Accessed May 20, 2018.

Chan AW, Yu DD, Choi KC, Lee DT, Sit JW, Chan HY: Tai chi qigong as a means to improve night-time sleep quality among older adults with cognitive impairment: a pilot randomized controlled trial, *Clin Interv Aging* 11:1277–1286, 2016.

Chen TY, Lee S, Buxton OM: A greater extent of insomnia symptoms and physician-recommended sleep medication use predict fall risk in community-dwelling older adults, *Sleep* 40(11), 2017. https://academic.oup.com/sleep/article/40/11/zsx142/4159943. Accessed June 2018.

Dean G, Klimpt M, Morris J, et al: Excessive sleepiness. In Boltz M, Capezuti E, Fulmer T, Zwicker D, editors: *Evidence-based geriatric nursing protocols for best practice,* ed 5, New York, 2016, Springer, pp 431–441.

Doku, I, Nahcivan N. Impact of a nurse-led sleep programme on the sleep quality and depressive symptomatology among older adults in nursing homes: a non-randomised controlled study, *Int J Older People Nurs* 14:e12215, 2019.

Downey R, Mosenifar Z, Gold P, et al: Obstructive sleep apnea (OSA) treatment and management, *Medscape,* January 9, 2018. https://emedicine.medscape.com/article/295807-treatment. Accessed June 2018.

Fillary J, Chaplin H, Jones G, Thompson A, Holme A, Wilson P: Noise at night in hospital general wards: a mapping of the literature, *Br J Nurs* 24(10):536–540, 2015.

Garcia-Borreguero D, Silber MH, Winkelman JW, et al: Guidelines for the first-line treatment of restless legs syndrome/Willis-Ekbom disease, prevention and treatment of dopaminergic augmentation: a combined task force of the IRLSSG, EURLSSG, and the RLS-foundation, *Sleep Med* 21:1–11, 2016.

Grossman MN, Anderson SL, Worku A, et al: Awakenings? Patient and hospital staff perceptions of nighttime disruptions and their effect on patient sleep, *J Clin Sleep Med* 13(2):301–306, 2017.

Hampton LM, Daubresse M, Chang HY, Alexander GC, Budnitz DS: Emergency department visits by adults for psychiatric medication adverse effects, *JAMA Psychiatry* 79(9):1006–1014, 2014.

Haynes J, Talbert M, Fox S, Close E: Cognitive behavioral therapy in the treatment of insomnia, *South Med J* 111(2):75–80, 2018.

Jacobsen AR, Eriksen F, Hansen RW, et al: Determinants for adherence to continuous positive airway pressure therapy in obstructive sleep apnea, *PLoS One* 12(12):e0189614, 2017.

Jike M, Itani O, Watanabe N, Buysse DJ, Kaneita Y: Long sleep duration and health outcomes: a systematic review, meta-analysis and meta-regression, *Sleep Med Rev* 39:25–36, 2018.

Kapur VK, Auckley DH, Chowdhuri S, et al: Clinical practice guideline for diagnostic testing for adult obstructive sleep apnea: an American Academy of sleep medicine clinical practice guideline, *J Clin Sleep Med* 13(3):479–504, 2017.

Kendzerska TB, Smith PM, Brignardello-Petersen R, Leung RS, Tomlinson GA: Evaluation of the measurement properties of the Epworth sleepiness scale: a systematic review, *Sleep Med Rev* 18(4):321–331, 2014.

Kim JH, Duffy JF: Circadian rhythm sleep-wake disorders in older adults, *Sleep Med Clin* 13(1):39–50, 2018. doi:10.1016/j.jsmc.2017.09.004.

Leggett A, Polenick CA, Maust DT, et al: "What hath night to do with sleep?" The caregiving context and dementia caregivers' nighttime awakenings, *Clin Gerontol* 41(2):158–166, 2018.

Leng Y, McEvoy CT, Allen IE, Yaffe K: Association of sleep-disordered breathing with cognitive function and risk of cognitive impairment: a systematic review and meta-analysis, *JAMA Neurol* 74(10):1237–1245, 2017.

Markota M, Rummans TA, Bostwick JM, Lapid MI: Benzodiazepine use in older adults: dangers, management, and alternative therapies, *Mayo Clin Proc* 91(11):1632–1639, 2016.

Martin J, Alessi C: Sleep disorders. In Ham R, Sloane P, Warshaw G, et al, editors: *Primary care geriatrics*, ed 6, Philadelphia, 2014, Elsevier Saunders, pp 343–352.

Matheson E, Hainer BL: Insomnia: pharmacologic therapy, *Am Fam Physician* 96(1):29–35, 2017. https://www.aafp.org/afp/2017/0701/p29.html. Accessed June 2018.

Matricciani L, Bin YS, Lallukka T, et al: Past, present, and future: trends in sleep duration and implications for public health, *Sleep Health* 3(5):317–323, 2017.

Maust DT, Kales HC, Wiechers IR, Blow FC, Olfson M: No end in sight: benzodiazepine use among older adults in the United States, *J Am Geriatr Soc* 64(12):2546–2553, 2016.

McGough NNH, Keane T, Uppal A, et al: Noise reduction in progressive care units, *J Nurs Care Qual* 33(2):166–172, 2018.

McMillan A, Morrell MJ: Sleep disordered breathing at the extremes of age: the elderly, *Breathe (Sheff)* 12(1):50–60, 2016.

Mukherjee S, Saxena R, Palmer LJ: The genetics of obstructive sleep apnoea, *Respirology* 23:18–27, 2018.

Nadal N, de Batlle J, Barbé F, et al: Predictors of CPAP compliance in different clinical settings: primary care versus sleep unit, *Sleep & Breath* 22(1):157–163, 2018.

National Institute of Neurological Disorders and Stroke: *Restless legs syndrome fact sheet*, 2017. https://www.ninds.nih.gov/Disorders/Patient-Caregiver-Education/Fact-Sheets/Restless-Legs-Syndrome-Fact-Sheet. Accessed May 20, 2018.

National Sleep Foundation: *REM behavior disorder and sleep*, 2018. https://sleepfoundation.org/sleep-disorders-problems/rem-behavior-disorder. Accessed May 20, 2018.

Petrovsky DV, McPhillips MV, Li J, Brody A, Caffeé L, Hodgson NA: Sleep disruption and quality of life in persons with dementia: a state-of-the-art review, *Geriatr Nurs* 39(6):640–645, 2018.

Restless Legs Syndrome Foundation: *RLS symptom diary*, 2018. https://www.rls.org/file/symptom-diary.pdf. Accessed May 20, 2018.

Rodriguez JC, Dzierzewski JM, Alessi CA: Sleep problems in the elderly, *Med Clin North Am* 99(2):431–439, 2015.

Sarikaya A, Oguz S: Effect of passive music therapy on sleep quality in elderly nursing home residents, *J Psychiatr Nurs* 7(2):55060, 2016.

Scales K, Zimmerman S, Miller SJ: Evidence-based nonpharmacological practice to address behavioral and psychological symptoms of dementia, *Gerontologist* 58(Suppl 1):S88–S102, 2018.

Schroeck JL, Ford J, Conway EL, et al: Review of safety and efficacy of sleep medicines in older adults, *Clin Ther* 38(11):2340–2372, 2016.

Senaratna CV, Perret JL, Lodge CJ, et al: Prevalence of obstructive sleep apnea in the general population: a systematic review, *Sleep Med Rev* 34:70–81, 2017.

Silva AA, de Mello RG, Schaan CW, Fuchs FD, Redline S, Fuchs SC: Sleep duration and mortality in the elderly: a systematic review with meta-analysis, *BMJ Open* 6:e008119, 2016.

Suzuki K, Miyamoto M, Hirata K: Sleep disorders in the elderly: diagnosis and management, *J Gen Fam Med* 18(2):61–71, 2017.

Theorell-Haglöw J, Miller CB, Bartlett DJ, Yee BJ, Openshaw HD, Grunstein RR: Gender differences in obstructive sleep apnoea, insomnia and restless legs syndrome in adults—what do we know? A clinical update, *Sleep Med Rev* 38:28–38, 2018.

U.S. Food and Drug Administration: *FDA adds boxed warning for risk of serious injuries caused by sleepwalking with certain prescription insomnia medications*. https://www.fda.gov/drugs/drug-safety-and-availability/fda-adds-boxed-warning-risk-serious-injuries-caused-sleepwalking-certain-prescription-insomnia. Accessed May 2019.

Varrasse M, Li J, Gooneratne N: Exercise and sleep in community-dwelling older adults, *Curr Sleep Med Rep* 1(4):232–240, 2015.

Winkelman JW: Clinical Practice. Insomnia disorder, *N Engl J Med* 373(15):1437–1444, 2015.

World Association of Sleep Medicine: *World Sleep Day*, 2018. http://worldsleepday.org. Accessed May 20, 2018.

Xiong G, Hategan A: Geriatric sleep disorder, *Medscape*, December 21, 2017. https://emedicine.medscape.com/article/292498-overview?pa=FoKIu4vX0dMcRVgVjSVTmYLaTejRnqVqku9xeP7q1BqUA5zw3fPxKTv30G3JQT0e8SIvl8zjYv73GUyW5rsbWA%3D%3D. Accessed June 2018.

Ye L, Richards KC: Sleep and long-term care, *Sleep Med Clin* 13(1):117–125, 2018.

18

Physical Activity and Exercise

Theris A. Touhy

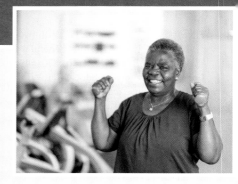

http://evolve.elsevier.com/Touhy/TwdHlthAging

A STUDENT SPEAKS

I work in a local gym on the weekends and, over the last several years, I have been amazed at the number of older adults who work out. We even have an older gentleman on staff who is a trainer. Some of them are really fit and look like they have been "gym rats" their whole life. Others take it a bit easier, but they come a couple of times a week to lift weights or walk on the treadmill. There are also a few people recovering from knee replacements who do their exercises at the gym. I hope I can stay fit when I get old.

Jeff, age 20

AN OLDER ADULT SPEAKS

I am 82 years young. My girlfriends and I have had a walking club for 15 years. Coffee first and then our one mile walk down to the park. Now we are trying something new and are going to a yoga class at the local senior center. We've got our mats and our tights and are really enjoying ourselves. Of course, the lunch afterward is nice as well. My grandson thinks it's funny, but you should see the moves we are learning!

Peggy, age 74

LEARNING OBJECTIVES

On completion of this chapter, the reader will be able to:

1. Describe the relationship between physical activity and health.
2. Describe the guidelines for physical activity for older adults.
3. Identify components of assessment and screening to determine appropriate physical activity interventions and exercise programs.
4. Identify appropriate exercise regimens for older adults and strategies to enhance adherence.
5. Discuss ways to incorporate physical activity into daily life.
6. Discuss adaptations for individuals with chronic illness, mobility limitations, and cognitive impairment.
7. Develop a plan of care to improve the activity level of an older adult.

Physical activity is defined as any bodily movement produced by skeletal muscle that requires energy expenditure. This includes exercise and other activities such as playing, working, active transportation (walking, running, biking), household chores, and recreational activities. Exercise is a subcategory of physical fitness that is planned, structured, repetitive, and purposeful in the sense that improvement or maintenance of one or more components of physical fitness is the objective.

Few factors contribute as much to health in aging as being physically active. The adage "use it or lose it" certainly applies to muscles and physical fitness. Regular physical activity throughout life is essential for healthy aging. Physical activity enhances health and functional status while also decreasing the number of chronic illnesses and functional limitations often assumed to be a part of growing older (Lee et al, 2017). Moderate physical activity may be beneficial for neurometabolic function and assist in combating Alzheimer's-related changes in midlife (Dougherty et al, 2017) (Box 18.1). The frail health and loss of function we associate with aging are, in large part, due to physical inactivity. "Reduced physical mobility and immobility contribute to the development of geriatric syndromes (pressure injuries, urinary incontinence, falls, functional decline, and delirium)" (Gray-Miceli, 2017, p. 471).

PHYSICAL ACTIVITY AND AGING

Despite a large body of evidence about the benefits of physical activity to maintain and improve function, only 16% of older adults meet the national guideline recommendations for physical activity. With advancing age (75 years and older) participation is even lower with only 9% of men and 6% of women meeting the recommended guidelines (Taylor, 2014). For women, patterns of physical activity have been reported to decline between ages 55 and 64, and again at age 75 and older. These may be prime times to enhance education on the benefits of physical activity for women as they age. The levels of physical activity among older adults have not improved over the past decade in the United States. Increasing physical activity for people of all ages is a global concern in both developed and developing countries. Physical inactivity is identified as a leading risk factor for global mortality (hypertension, smoking, high blood glucose level, physical inactivity, obesity).

Worldwide, it is important for governments and policy makers to initiate actions to create environments that encourage lifelong physical activity. There are a number of global and national guidelines for physical activity, although physical activity among older adults has attracted less interest and research (Box 18.2). *Healthy People 2020* goals for physical activity can be found in the Healthy People 2020 box.

♥ HEALTHY PEOPLE 2020

Physical Activity

- Reduce the proportion of adults who engage in no leisure-time physical activity.
- Increase the proportion of adults who engage in aerobic physical activity of at least moderate intensity for at least 150 minutes/week, or 75 minutes/week of vigorous intensity, or an equivalent combination.

Physical activity is important for all older adults, not just active healthy older adults. Even a small amount of time (at least 30 minutes of moderate activity several days a week) can improve health. Studies have found that increasing physical activity improves health outcomes in individuals with chronic illnesses (regardless of severity) and in those with functional impairment.

Increasing evidence suggests that high-quality exercise programs are central to older adults who are either frail or sarcopenic (Morley, 2016). Exercise training appears to improve brain health or lower the risk of dementia and may also improve the ability to perform activities of daily living (ADLs) in individuals with dementia and consequently reduce caregiver burden (Ding et al, 2018; Lee et al, 2017). Results of a recent study suggest that multimodal exercise that includes physical and cognitive stimulation improved several cognitive abilities and physical fitness components of nursing home residents (Marmeleira et al, 2018). Strength training interventions seem most important for functional improvement, but further research is needed to determine the type of exercise necessary to maintain or improve functional ability in frail older adults.

Regardless of age or situation, the older adult can find some activity suitable for his or her condition. Reducing sedentary time, independent of physical activity, has cardiovascular, metabolic, and functional benefits in older adults. Any amount of exercise is better than being sedentary and even a little activity is better than none (Jefferis et al, 2018). Recent research results report that older adults with lower-extremity arthritis, who engaged in just 45 minutes of moderate-intensity activity, such as brisk walking, per week, were 80% more likely to maintain or improve their physical functioning than those who exercised for under 45 minutes weekly (Dunlop et al, 2017; Lee et al, 2017). It is important to keep older adults moving any way possible for as long as possible (Box 18.3).

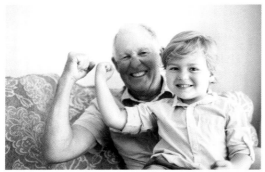

Physical activity is important for all older adults. (©iStock.com/ Squaredpixels.)

BOX 18.3 Ways to Keep Fit During Aging

- After four unsuccessful attempts, Diana Nyad, 64 years old, became the first person to swim from Cuba to Florida without the use of a shark cage.
- Nellie, 83 years old, began swimming to ease the discomfort resulting both from a short left arm, the residual effect of poliomyelitis, and from a frozen left shoulder. She became an award-winning synchronized swimmer with 20 gold medals, 12 blue ribbons, and 13 trophies to her credit. Nellie continued to exercise this way despite the need to wear cataract goggles.
- James, 72 years old, was taking 40 mg of Lipitor daily for his high cholesterol level and lisinopril 40 mg for hypertension. He was a self-proclaimed couch potato. He joined Silver Sneakers, a program through his Medicare Advantage Plan, and started going to the gym. After a year of walking on the treadmill for 30 minutes three times a week and lifting weights, his cholesterol level and blood pressure value approached normal limits. His medications were reduced and he was 10 pounds lighter. Even his 14-year-old grandson admired his biceps.
- Em, an 86-year-old nursing home resident, jogged every morning in place for about 5 minutes and then briskly walked around outside the facility. Although she had occasional lapses of memory, she was vital, erect, and interested in life around her.

PROMOTING HEALTHY AGING: IMPLICATIONS FOR GERONTOLOGICAL NURSING

Assessment

Assessment of function and mobility are components of a health assessment for older adults. Exercise counseling should be provided as part of this assessment. For individuals 65 years of age and older, if they are relatively fit and have no limiting health conditions, initiation of a moderate intensity exercise program is safe and does not require any type of cardiac screening (Lee et al, 2017). The consensus is that there is minimal cardiovascular risk to engaging in physical activity and a much greater risk in maintaining a sedentary lifestyle. Individuals with specific health conditions, such as cardiovascular disease and diabetes, may need to take extra precautions and seek medical advice before beginning an exercise program (CDC, 2015). Frail individuals will need more comprehensive assessment to adapt exercise recommendations to their abilities and ensure benefit without compromising safety.

SCREENING

Interventions

The Centers for Disease Control and Prevention (CDC) "Growing Stronger" program materials are very useful to help determine a safe exercise program and provide detailed information about appropriate exercises and precautions (Box 18.2). The nurse should be knowledgeable about recommended physical activity guidelines, educate individuals about the importance of exercise and physical activity, and provide suggestions on ways to incorporate exercise into daily routines. Many older adults mistakenly believe that they are too old to begin a fitness program. Older adults are less likely to receive exercise counseling from their primary care providers than younger individuals. Research has noted that health care providers value the benefits of physical activity but have inadequate knowledge of specific recommendations. Giving specific advice about the type and frequency of exercise is important (CDC, 2015; Lee et al, 2017). Nurses can also design and lead exercise and physical activity programs for groups of older adults in the community or in long-term care.

Physical Activity Guidelines

Guidelines for physical activity for adults 65 years of age or older who are generally fit and have no limiting health conditions are presented in Box 18.4. Recommendations for all adults include participation in 30 minutes of moderate-intensity for 5 or more days of the week. People do not have to be active for 30 minutes at a time but can accumulate 30 minutes over 24 hours. As little as 10 minutes of exercise has health benefits and three 10-minute bouts of activity have the same fitness effects as one 30-minute bout (Table 18.1). Extremely frail individuals may not be able to engage in aerobic activities and should begin with strength and balance training before participating in as little as 5 minutes of aerobic training.

BOX 18.4 Exercise Guidelines

Older Adults Need at Least:
- 2 hours and 30 minutes (150 minutes) of moderate-intensity aerobic activity (e.g., brisk walking, swimming, bicycling) every week **and**
- Muscle-strengthening activities on two or more days that work all major muscle groups (legs, hips, abdomen, chest, shoulders, and arms)

  Additionally: Stretching (flexibility) and balance exercises (particularly for older adults at risk of falls) are also recommended. Yoga and tai chi exercises have been shown to be of benefit to older adults in terms of improving flexibility and balance and reducing pain and enhancing psychological well-being (Miller and Taylor-Piliae, 2014). Tai chi can be adapted for level of function and mobility status. Home-based balance-training exercise programs are also available.

From Centers for Disease Control and Prevention: *How much physical activity do older adults need?* 2015. https://www.cdc.gov/physicalactivity/ basics/adults/index.htm. Accessed February 2018.

TABLE 18.1 Guidelines for Teaching About Exercise.

Exercise	Description	Benefits	Intensity	Frequency	Examples
Moderate-intensity aerobic activity	Continuous movement involving large muscle groups that is sustained for a minimum of 10 min; should make your heart beat faster	Improves cardiovascular functioning, strengthens heart muscle, decreases blood glucose and triglycerides, increases HDL, improves mood	On a 10-point scale, where sitting is 0 and working as hard as you can is 10, moderate-intensity aerobic activity is a 5 or 6. You will be able to talk but not sing the words to your favorite song	30 min, 5 days/wk Perform for at least 10 min at a time	Biking, swimming and other water-based activities, dancing, brisk walking, lifestyle activities that incorporate large muscle groups (pushing a lawn mower, climbing stairs)
Muscle-strengthening activities	Activities that involve moving or lifting some type of resistance and work all major muscle groups (legs, hips, back, abdomen, chest, shoulders, arms)	Increases muscle strength, prevents sarcopenia, reduces fall risk, improves balance, modifies risk factors for cardiovascular disease and type 2 diabetes	To gain health benefits, muscle-strengthening activities need to be done to the point at which it is difficult to do another repetition without help. A repetition is one complete movement of an activity such as lifting a weight. An effort should be made to do 8–12 repetitions (one set) per activity or continue until it would be difficult to do another repetition without help	2 days/wk, but not consecutive days to allow muscles to recover between sessions	Lifting weights, calisthenics, working with resistance bands, Pilates, exercises that use the body's own weight for resistance (push-ups, sit-ups), heavy gardening (digging, shoveling), washing windows/floors
Stretching (flexibility)	A therapeutic maneuver designed to elongate shortened soft tissue structures and increase flexibility	Facilitates ROM around joints, prevents injury	Stretch muscle groups but not past the point of resistance or pain	At least 2 days/wk	Yoga, ROM exercises
Balance exercises	Movements that improve the ability to maintain control of the body over the base of support to avoid falling	Improves lower body strength, improves balance, helps prevent falls	Safety precautions are essential (holding on to a chair, working with another person)	Can be incorporated into regularly scheduled strength exercises. Older adults at risk of falling should do balance training for 3 or more days /week	Tai chi, yoga, exercises such as standing on one foot, walking heel to toe or backward or sideways, leg raises, hip extensions (can be done holding on to a chair), standing up from a sitting position without using your hands

HDL, High-density lipoprotein; *ROM*, range of motion.
Data from Centers for Disease Control and Prevention: *How much physical activity do older adults need?* 2015. https://www.cdc.gov/physicalactivity/basics/adults/index.htm. Accessed February 2018.

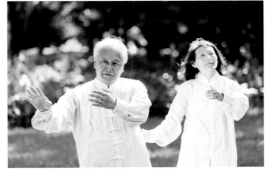
Tai chi can improve flexibility and balance. (©iStock.com/Kali Nine LLC.)

Incorporating Physical Activity Into Lifestyle

One does not have to invest in expensive gym equipment or gym memberships to incorporate the recommended physical activity guidelines into his or her daily routine. Hand weights (or use cans of food as weights), a chair, and an exercise mat can easily get the individual started (Fig. 18.1). Individuals may also be able to integrate activity into daily life rather than doing a specific exercise. Examples include walking, golfing, tennis, biking, raking leaves, yard work/gardening, dancing, washing windows or floors, washing and waxing the car, and swimming and water-based exercises. The Wii game system offers other possibilities for exercise at all levels and is increasingly used by older adults in their own homes and in senior living facilities to encourage physical activity, improve balance, and provide enjoyable entertainment.

The benefits of group exercise in terms of social and emotional health have been reported, and the socialization provided may be important for individuals who live alone or do not have social networks (Brach et al, 2017; Komatsu et al, 2017; McCaffrey et al, 2017). Some older adults prefer to exercise at home, but guidance and motivation are necessary

Be #Fit4Function with *Go4Life*®

Exercise and be active every day so you can keep doing what's most important to you.

Practice all 4 types of exercise fo the most benefits.

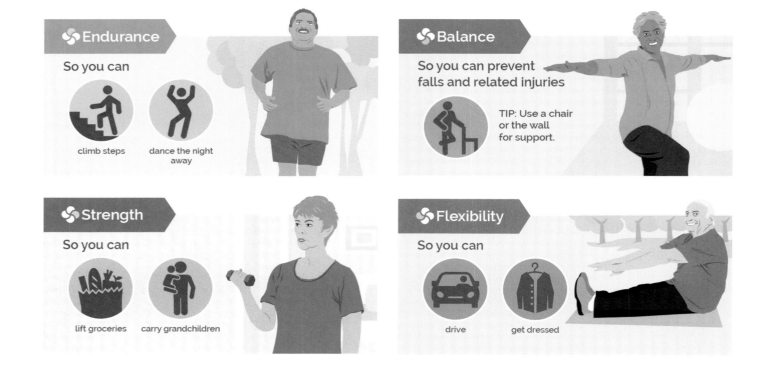

Endurance
So you can
- climb steps
- dance the night away

Balance
So you can prevent falls and related injuries
TIP: Use a chair or the wall for support.

Strength
So you can
- lift groceries
- carry grandchildren

Flexibility
So you can
- drive
- get dressed

Visit go4life.nia.nih.gov and be #Fit4Function.

Get exercise ideas, motivational tips, and more from *Go4Life*®, an exercise and physical activity campaign for older adults from the National Institute on Aging at NIH.

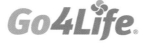

Fig. 18.1 Practice All 4 Types of Exercises for the Most Benefits. (Image courtesy of the National Institute on Aging/National Institutes of Health.)

and has not been adequate in home-based exercise programs. Electronic tablets and smartphones that use mobile Internet are being evaluated for home-based exercise programs to stimulate adherence. Instructions via video, motivational contact with a coach, and the use of body-worn sensors to measure physical activity have been evaluated as ways to measure daily physical activity and support individually tailored stimulation of physical activity. Motivational contact with a coach seems to be especially important for adherence (Geraedts et al, 2017).

Maintaining motivation to adhere to a program of physical activity often presents challenges for older adults. Making exercise programming enjoyable is recommended as a strategy to improve commitment and adherence to exercise activities. Results of a study of an innovative program incorporating playful simulated laughter into a moderate-intensity strength, balance, and flexibility physical activity program (LaughActive) for older adults reported significant improvements in aerobic endurance, mental health, and motivation to exercise. Over 96% of the participants found laughter to be a welcome addition to their traditional exercise program (Greene et al, 2017). Dancing is another enjoyable activity to promote physical and cognitive function and socialization. Dancing was compared to endurance training in a recent study (Rehfeld et al, 2017) and was found to improve reaction time and working memory. In comparison, it was only dancing that led to improvement in posture and balance.

Resistance exercise programs have higher rates of adherence than aerobic exercise programs among older adults. The high prevalence of joint diseases, such as osteoarthritis (OA), may hamper successful performance of aerobic exercises that cause joint impact. Chair yoga, a gentle form of yoga practiced sitting in a chair or standing while holding on to the chair for support, is well suited for older adults with OA who cannot participate in traditional yoga or standing exercises (Park et al, 2017) (Research Highlights box). Muscle-strengthening exercises without weight bearing also provide more joint stability for individuals with lower extremity OA. Swimming is a low-risk activity that provides aerobic benefit, and water-based exercises are particularly beneficial for individuals with arthritis or other mobility limitations.

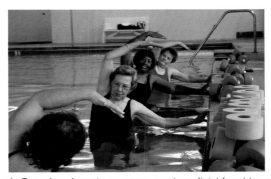

Aquatic Exercise. Aquatic programs are beneficial for older adults with mobility and joint problems. They improve circulation, muscle strength, and endurance and provide socialization and relaxation. (©iStock.com/ftwitty.)

There are many excellent resources available that provide instructions, tips, pictures, videos, and stories from individuals who have embarked on fitness regimens. The National Center on Health, Physical Activity and Disability (Box 18.2) provides many suggestions for adaptation of exercises for individuals with mobility limitations. Box 18.5 provides helpful tips that nurses can use for encouraging individuals to adopt physical activity. Box 18.6 presents safety precautions.

RESEARCH HIGHLIGHTS

An interprofessional team of social work, nursing, and medicine conducted a study to determine the effects of *Sit 'N' Fit Chair Yoga*, compared to a health education program (HEP), on pain and physical function in older adults with lower extremity osteoarthritis (OA) who could not participate in standing exercise. The chair yoga program was designed for older adults who are unable to participate in standing yoga or other exercise programs due to weakness, fatigue, or fear of falling. The chair yoga program includes breathing, centering and relaxation, yoga posture to stretch and flex muscles and joints in the lower and upper body, and meditation and focusing on inner peace.

The study was a two-arm randomized controlled trial with 106 community-dwelling older adults. Participants attended either chair yoga or HEP twice weekly in 45 minute sessions for 8 weeks. Pain, pain interference, balance, gait speed, fatigue, and functional ability were measured at baseline, after 4 weeks of intervention, at the end of the 8 week intervention, and postintervention (1 and 3 months). The 8-week chair yoga program was associated with reduction in pain, pain interference, and fatigue, and improvement in gait speed, but only the effects on pain interference were sustained 3 months postintervention. Chair yoga may be a promising nonpharmacological intervention to improve physical function in older adults who are unable to participate in regular exercise programs.

From Park J, McCaffrey R, Newman D et al: A pilot randomized controlled trial of the effects of chair yoga on pain and physical function among community-dwelling older adults with lower extremity arthritis, *JAGS* 65:592–597, 2017.

Many senior living communities and skilled nursing facilities (SNFs) provide gym equipment for residents. The Silver Sneakers program, the nation's leading exercise program for active community-dwelling older adults, is a membership benefit through some of the Medicare Advantage plans. Local community centers often provide exercise programs for older adults, and many gyms in the United States have reduced-cost memberships for individuals older than 65 years of age. Some have trainers on staff with expertise in exercises appropriate for older individuals. The nurse can share resources in the community, and communities should be encouraged to provide accessible and affordable options for physical activity.

Special Considerations

The benefits of physical activity extend to the more physically frail older adult, those who are nonambulatory or experience cognitive impairment, and those residing in assisted living facilities (ALFs) or SNFs. In fact, these individuals may benefit most from an exercise program in terms of function and quality of life (Box 18.7). Nursing home residents should be involved in an exercise program two to three times per week (Morley, 2016). There are many creative and enjoyable ideas for enhancing physical activity such as using lower extremity cycling equipment, marching in place, tossing a ball, stretching, using resistive bands (Chen et al, 2016), group exercises (Kocic et al, 2018), and doing chair yoga.

Individuals with cognitive impairment are often not included in physical activity programs. Results of research suggest that older adults with cognitive impairment who participate in exercise programs may improve strength and endurance, mood and behavior, cognitive function, and ability to perform ADLs.

BOX 18.5 Tips for Best Practice

Physical Activity/Exercise Participation

- Provide appropriate screening before beginning an exercise program.
- Assess functional abilities and discuss how exercise can enhance function.
- Provide information about the benefits of exercise, emphasizing short-term benefits such as sleeping better, improved walking ability, decreasing fall risk.
- Clarify the misconceptions associated with exercise (fatigue, injury).
- Assess barriers to exercise and provide tips on how to overcome.
- Provide an "exercise prescription" that specifies what exercises and how often the person should exercise.
- Collaborate with the individual to set short- and long-term goals that are specific, achievable, and match perceived needs, health, cognitive abilities, culture, gender, and interests.
- Encourage individual to keep a journal or diary to reflect experience and progress.
- Provide choices about types of exercises, and design the program so that the person can do it at home or elsewhere.
- Refer to community resources for physical fitness (e.g., YMCA, mall walking).
- Group-based programs and exercising with a buddy may be more successful.

- Try to make the program fun and entertaining (walking with favorite music, socializing with friends).
- Discuss potential exercise side effects and any symptoms that should be reported.
- Provide safety tips and situations that may require medical attention (Box 18.6).
- Share stories about the benefits of your own personal exercise program and those of older adults (Box 18.2).
- Provide ongoing support and follow up on progress; support from experts and family and peers is a significant factor in encouraging continued participation.
- Begin with low-intensity physical activity for sedentary individuals.
- Initiate low-intensity activities in short sessions (less than 10 minutes), and include warm-up and cool-down components with active stretching.
- Progression from low to moderate intensity is important to obtain maximal benefits, but activity level changes should be instituted gradually.
- Teach the importance of warming up and cooling down.
- Encourage use of proper, well-fitted footwear.
- Lifestyle activities (e.g., raking, gardening) can build endurance when performed for at least 10 minutes.

BOX 18.6 Tips for Best Practice

Exercise Safety

- Always wear comfortable, loose-fitting clothing and appropriate shoes for your activity.
- Warm up: Perform a low- to moderate-intensity warm up for 5–10 minutes.
- Drink water before, during, and after your exercise session.
- When exercising outdoors, evaluate your surroundings for safety: traffic, pavement condition, weather, and strangers.
- Wear clothes made of fabrics that absorb sweat and remove it from your skin.
- Never wear rubber or plastic suits. These could hold the sweat on your skin and make your body overheat.
- Wear sunscreen when you exercise outdoors.

Stop Exercising Right Away if You:
- Have pain or pressure in your chest, neck, shoulder, or arm.
- Feel dizzy or sick.
- Break out in a cold sweat.
- Have muscle cramps.
- Feel acute (not just achy) pain in your joints, feet, ankles, or legs.
- Have trouble breathing. Slow down; you should be able to talk while exercising without gasping for breath.

Times Exercise Should Not Be Done
- Avoid hard exercise for 2 hours after a big meal. (A leisurely walk around the block would be fine.)
- Do not exercise when you have a fever and/or viral infection accompanied by muscle aches.
- Do not exercise if your systolic blood pressure is greater than 200 mm Hg and your diastolic blood pressure is greater than 100 mm Hg.
- Do not exercise if your resting heart rate is greater than 120 beats/min.
- Do not exercise if you have a joint that you are using to exercise (such as a knee or an ankle) that is red and warm and painful.
- If you have osteoporosis, always avoid stretches that flex your spine or cause you to bend at the waist, and avoid making jerky, rapid movements.
- Stop exercising if you experience severe pain or swelling in a joint. Discomfort that persists should always be evaluated.
- Do not exercise if you have a new symptom that has not been evaluated by your health care provider, such as pain in your chest, abdomen, or a joint; swelling in an arm, leg, or joint; difficulty catching your breath at rest; or a fluttering feeling in your chest.

BOX 18.7 Positive Effects of Exercise in Long-Term Care

- Reduce frailty
- Enhance walking speed
- Improve function
- Decrease hospitalization
- Improve mobility
- Decrease falls
- Enhance cognition
- Decrease agitation
- Decrease dysphoria
- Enhance sleep
- Decrease sleep apnea
- Enhance quality of life

From Morley J: High-quality exercise programs are an essential component of nursing home care, *JAMDA* 17:373–375, 2016.

Elements of successful exercise interventions with individuals with dementia include individualized approaches, caregiver involvement, strength-training interventions, one-component exercises, and enjoyable activities (Forbes et al, 2015; Rodriguez-Larrad et al, 2017; Schwenk et al, 2014). While further research is needed to understand the level and intensity of exercise that is beneficial for each type of dementia, exercise should be a component of the plan of care (Box 18.2).

Maintaining Function Across Care Settings

Even though the focus in hospitals is on acute illness management, there is growing awareness of the need to also focus on functional status, especially in older adults. Hospitalization is associated with significantly greater loss of total, lean, and fat mass strength in older adults. Individuals older than age

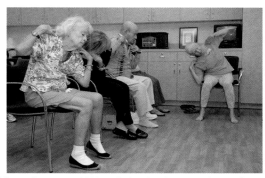

Yoga. Ninety-five-year-old Vera Paley leads yoga class. (Courtesy the Louis and Anne Green Memory and Wellness Center of the Christine E. Lynn College of Nursing at Florida Atlantic University.)

> ### BOX 18.8 Tips for Best Practice
> #### Function-Focused Care in Acute Care
>
> - Ask or encourage the individual to move in bed and give the person time to move rather than moving the person yourself.
> - Give step-by-step cues on how to move in bed (e.g., "put your right hand on the rail and pull yourself over onto your left side").
> - Ask or encourage the individual to transfer and wait for the individual to move rather than transferring the individual yourself or automatically using lift equipment (use of assistive equipment depends on mobility and cognitive status).
> - Give step-by-step cues and use gestures/demonstration on how to transfer safely (e.g., "plant feet firmly on the floor and slide to the edge of the chair").
> - Ask or encourage the individual to walk or independently propel wheelchair and give the person time to perform the activity rather than doing it yourself.
> - Give step-by-step cues and use gestures/demonstration (e.g., "move your left foot forward; now move your right foot").
> - Assist, ask, and/or encourage use of assistive devices; provide instruction on use and ensure that device is available and appropriate.

85 experience the most functional decline with hospitalization. The onset of functional decline can occur in a matter of days and may start preadmission and continue after discharge, depending on the individual's condition and comorbid problems (Gray-Miceli, 2017). Bedrest, restricted activity/low mobility, and the tendency for staff to perform ADL care rather than encouraging self-care all contribute to functional decline. Generally, older hospitalized medical patients spend at least 83% of their acute care stay in bed and engage in only 2.4 minutes of moderate level activity (Resnick et al, 2016a).

Evidence demonstrates that nurses insufficiently promote mobility in older adults admitted to medical inpatient hospital units. Nurses need increased knowledge and awareness of older hospitalized adults' mobility needs and older adults also need increased knowledge of the significance of mobility during hospitalization (Dermody and Kovach, 2017). Recommendations for reducing functional decline during hospitalization include structured exercise, progressive resistance strength training, and walking programs in coordination with rehabilitation. Outcomes of early mobility to prevent functional decline include lower hospital costs, fewer delirium days, and improved functional independence (Fraser et al, 2015).

Function-Focused Care

Function-focused care (FFC) is a comprehensive, systems-level approach that prioritizes the preservation and restoration of functional capacity. FFC teaches nurses to evaluate older adults' underlying capability with regard to function and physical activity and integrate functional and physical activities into all care interactions (Box 18.8). The FFC approach can be used across settings of care to maintain and improve functional abilities in older adults. Nurse researcher Barbara Resnick and her colleagues have conducted numerous studies evaluating the use of FFC care in improving function and physical activity in older adults in hospitals, assisted living residences, and SNFs (Gray-Miceli, 2017; Resnick et al 2016a, 2016b). A family-centered, function-focused care intervention (Fam-FCC) incorporates an educational empowerment model for family caregivers that focuses on improving function during and after an acute care hospitalization. Outcomes of the Fam-FCC include fewer 30-day hospital readmissions, less delirium severity, improved ADL performance, less decrease in walking ability, and an increase in preparedness for caregiving and less anxiety among family caregivers (Boltz et al, 2015). Box 18.2 includes information on FCC.

▌ KEY CONCEPTS

- Few factors contribute as much to health in aging as being physically active.
- Physical activity enhances health and functional status while also decreasing the number of chronic illnesses and functional limitations often assumed to be a part of growing older.
- Despite a large body of evidence about the benefits of physical activity to maintain and improve function, physical activity levels of older adults remain low and have not improved over the past decade.

- Components of a health assessment for older adults include assessment of function and mobility. Exercise counseling should be provided as a part of that assessment.
- The benefits of physical activity extend to the more physically frail older adult, those who are nonambulatory or experience cognitive impairment, and those residing in ALFs or SNFs. In fact, these individuals may benefit most from an exercise program in terms of function and quality of life.

NURSING STUDY: EXERCISE AND ACTIVITY

Tom, 75 years old, had lost his wife, Ella, a year ago and had been feeling down and tired much of each day. He had retired at age 70 from his job as a housing contractor and had spent much of his time with Ella. They had been married for 50 years. He now sometimes seemed to sit in front of the television most of the day without actually remembering what it was that he had seen. Many of the couple's friends had moved away or relocated to retirement settings, and other than his daughter, who lived about 45 minutes from his house, Tom rarely saw anyone anymore. He had lived like this for nearly a year, and it had become his daily pattern of life. Tom took the initiative after a suggestion from his daughter to go to the local senior citizen center. He went and had lunch there nearly every day. At one point he was asked if he would allow a nursing student to spend time with him during her semester in a gerontology course. He agreed. In the course of her assessment, she (and he) found that his activity level was nearly completely sedentary. She gave Tom information about the ramifications of such a sedentary life. She pointed out that the center had an exercise class every day between 10.00 a.m. and 12 noon. Because he came every day (except Saturday and Sunday) for lunch, it seemed a good thing to do. Tom said to his nursing student, "This isn't anything I am really interested in doing, but I will give it a try." Though he did not admit it, he was also worried because he usually felt weak and listless during the day after his lunch. When he did attend the first class, he found that there were basic exercises and more advanced ones for older adults who had participated regularly for 6 months. He found after a few weeks that he was enjoying the social aspect of the exercise, if not the exercise itself. After nearly a year of fairly regular participation, Tom began playing golf with some of the men from the center. Once he attended a dance.

On the basis of the nursing study, develop a nursing care plan for the nursing student using the following procedure[a]:
- List Tom's comments that provide subjective data.
- List information that provides objective data.
- From these data identify and state, using an accepted format, two nursing diagnoses you determine are most significant to Tom at this time. List two of Tom's strengths that you have identified from these data.
- Determine and state outcome criteria for each diagnosis. These must reflect some alleviation of the problem identified in the nursing diagnosis and must be stated in concrete and measurable terms.
- Plan and state one or more interventions for each diagnosed problem. Provide specific documentation of the source used to determine the appropriate intervention. Plan at least one intervention that incorporates Tom's existing strengths.
- Evaluate the success of the intervention. Interventions must correlate directly with the stated outcome criteria to measure the outcome success.

[a]Students are advised to refer to their nursing diagnosis text and identify possible or potential problems.

CRITICAL THINKING QUESTIONS AND ACTIVITIES

1. In the nursing study above, what lifestyle factors developed by Tom after his wife's death had become dangerous to his health?
2. Compose a list of 10 questions you would ask Tom to obtain a clear picture of factors contributing to his activity level. Discuss the rationale behind each.
3. List some of the common methods for motivating Tom that his nursing student may have used.
4. Describe the level of activity that should be Tom's starting point and discuss symptoms he might expect as he increases his activity level.

RESEARCH QUESTIONS

1. What activities and exercises are most useful in maintaining mobility in older adults?
2. What factors increase adherence to an exercise program among community-dwelling older adults?
3. What are the benefits of group exercise programs?
4. What factors in the institutional environment induce immobility?
5. What are some creative ways to implement exercise in the long-term care setting?
6. How does the design of an exercise program differ for individuals with cognitive impairment?

REFERENCES

Boltz M, Chippendale T, Resnick B, Galvin JE: Testing family-centered, function-focused care in hospitalized persons with dementia, *Neurodegener Dis Manag* 5(3):203–215, 2015.

Brach JS, Perera S, Gilmore S, et al: Effectiveness of a timing and coordination group exercise program to improve mobility in community-dwelling older adults: a randomized clinical trial, *JAMA Intern Med* 177(10):1437–1444, 2017.

Centers for Disease Control and Prevention: *How much physical activity do older adults need?* 2015. https://www.cdc.gov/physicalactivity/basics/adults/index.htm. Accessed February 2018.

Chen KM, Li CH, Huang HT, Cheng YY: Feasible modalities and long-term effects of elastic band exercises in nursing home older adults in wheelchairs: a cluster randomized controlled trial, *Int J Nurs* Stud 55:4–14, 2016.

Ding K, Tarumi T, Zhu DC, et al: Cardiorespiratory fitness and white matter neuronal fiber integrity in mild cognitive impairment, *J Alzheimers Dis* 61(2):729–739, 2018.

Dermody G, Kovach CR: Nurses' experience with and perception of barriers to promoting mobility in hospitalized older adults: a descriptive study, *J Gerontol Nurs* 43(11):22–29, 2017.

Dougherty RJ, Schultz SA, Kirby TK, et al: Moderate physical activity is associated with cerebral glucose metabolism in adults at risk for Alzheimer's disease, *J Alzheimers Dis* 58(4): 1089–1097, 2017.

Dunlop DD, Song J, Lee J, et al: Physical activity minimum threshold predicting improved function in adults with lower-extremity symptoms, *Arthritis Care Res (Hoboken)* 69(4):475–483, 2017.

Forbes D, Forbes SC, Blake CM, Thiessen EJ, Forbes S: Exercise programs for people with dementia, *Cochrane Database Syst Rev* (4):CD006489, 2015.

Fraser D, Spiva L, Forman W, Hallen C: Original research: implementation of an early mobility program in an ICU, *Am J Nurs* 115(12):49–58, 2015.

Geraedts HA, Zijlstra W, Zhang W, et al: A home-based exercise program driven by tablet application and mobility monitoring for frail older adults: feasibility and practical implications, *Prev Chronic Dis* 14:E12, 2017.

Gray-Miceli D: Impaired mobility and functional decline in older adults: evidence to facilitate a practice change, *Nurs Clin North Am* 52:469–487, 2017.

Greene CM, Morgan JC, Traywick LS, Mingo CA: Evaluation of a laughter-based exercise program on health and self-efficacy for exercise, *Gerontologist* 57(6):1051–1061, 2017.

Jefferis BJ, Parsons TJ, Sartini C, et al: Objectively measured physical activity, sedentary behavior and all-cause mortality in older men: does volume of activity matter more than pattern of accumulation? *Br J Sports Med* 2018 Feb 12. [Epub ahead of print] doi:10.1136/bjsports-2017-098733.

Kocic M, Stojanovic Z, Nikolic D, et al: The effectiveness of group Otago exercise program on physical function in nursing home residents older than 65 years: a randomized controlled trial, *Arch Gerontol Geriatr* 75:112–118, 2018.

Komatsu H, Yagasaki K, Saito Y, Oguma Y: Regular group exercise contributes to balanced health in older adults in Japan: a qualitative study, *BMC Geriatr* 17:190, 2017.

Lee PG, Jackson EA, Richardson CR: Exercise prescription in older adults, *Am Fam Physician* 95(7):425–432, 2017.

Marmeleira J, Galhardas L, Raimundo A: Exercise merging physical and cognitive stimulation improves physical fitness and cognitive functioning in older nursing home residents: a pilot study, *Geriatr Nurs* 39:303–309, 2018.

McCaffrey R, Park J, Newman D: Chair yoga: feasibility and sustainability study with older community-dwelling adults with osteoarthritis, *Holist Nurs Pract* 31(3):148–157, 2017.

Morley JE: High-quality exercise programs are an essential component of nursing home care, *J Am Med Dir Assoc* 17:373–375, 2016.

Park J, McCaffrey R, Newman D, Liehr P, Ouslander JG: A pilot randomized controlled trial of the effects of chair yoga on pain and physical function among community-dwelling older adults with lower extremity osteoarthritis, *J Am Geriatr Soc* 65:592–597, 2017.

Rehfeld K, Müller P, Aye N, et al: Dancing or fitness sport? The effects of two training programs on hippocampal plasticity and balance abilities in healthy seniors, *Front Hum Neurosci* 11:305, 2017.

Resnick B, Wells C, Galik E, et al: Feasibility and efficacy of function-focused care for orthopedic trauma patients, *J Trauma Nurs* 23(3): 144–155, 2016a.

Resnick B, Galik E, Vigne E, Carew AP: Dissemination and implementation of function focused care for assisted living, *Health Educ Behav* 43(3):296–304, 2016b.

Rodriguez-Larrad A, Arrieta H, Rezola C, et al: Effectiveness of a multicomponent exercise program in the attenuation of frailty in long-term nursing home residents: study protocol for a randomized clinical controlled trial, *BMC Geriatr* 17:60, 2017.

Schwenk M, Dutzi I, Englert S, et al: An intensive exercise program improves motor performance in patients with dementia: translational model of geriatric rehabilitation, *J Alzheimers Dis* 39(3):487–498, 2014.

Taylor D: Physical activity is medicine for older adults, *Postgrad Med J* 90:26–32, 2014.

19

Falls and Fall Risk Reduction

Theris A. Touhy

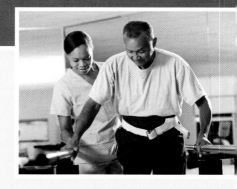

http://evolve.elsevier.com/Touhy/TwdHlthAging

A STUDENT SPEAKS

The thought of needing someone to help me shower and dress and transfer me from a chair to bed requires more acceptance than I have ever had to muster. I'm very good at making the best out of a bad situation, but somehow adapting to something like never walking again cannot be equated with a "bad situation." It is permanent, and it is the sacrifice of my precious independence. I was born on Independence Day! Thinking about these things overwhelms me with sadness.

Holiday, age 22

AN OLDER ADULT SPEAKS

I hate to have the family see me like this. You know, I was a military man. I took pride in the way I marched . . . or just stood at attention. I never imagined a time when I wouldn't be able to walk without assistance.

Jerry, age 78

LEARNING OBJECTIVES

On completion of this chapter, the reader will be able to:

1. Discuss the effects of impaired mobility on general function and quality of life.
2. Identify risk factors for impaired mobility.
3. Identify factors that increase vulnerability to falls.
4. Describe assessment measures to determine gait and walking stability.
5. List several interventions to reduce fall risks and identify those at high risk.
6. Describe the effects of restraints, and identify alternative safety interventions.
7. Develop a plan of care for an older adult at risk for falls.

This chapter focuses on the importance of maintaining maximal mobility; assessing gait, mobility, and fall risk factors; implementing fall risk–reduction interventions; providing restraint-free care; and implementing interventions that are useful when mobility is impaired.

MOBILITY AND AGING

Mobility is the capacity one has for movement within the personally available microcosm and macrocosm. This includes abilities such as moving oneself by turning over in bed, transferring from lying to sitting and from sitting to standing, walking, using assistive devices, or accessing transportation within the community environment. In infancy, moving about is the major mode of learning and interacting with the environment. Throughout life, movement remains a significant means of personal contact, sensation, exploration, pleasure, and control. Retaining pride and maintaining dignity, self-care, independence, social contacts, and activity are all needs identified as important to older adults, and all are facilitated by mobility. Mobility is intimately linked to health status and quality of life and healthy aging (Freedman et al, 2017).

Mobility and comparative degrees of agility are based on muscle strength, flexibility, postural stability, vibratory sensation, cognition, and perceptions of stability. Aging produces changes in muscles and joints (Chapter 26). Individuals who maintain regular physical activity and good health habits throughout life may have fewer of these changes (Chapter 18). Prenatal and postnatal development of muscle fibers and muscle growth during puberty may also have critical effects on musculoskeletal aging.

Gait and mobility impairments are not an inevitable consequence of aging, but often a result of chronic diseases or past or recent trauma. Mobility and gait impairments are caused by diseases ed impairments across many organ systems. For some older adults, osteoporosis, Parkinson's disease, strokes, and arthritic conditions markedly affect movement and functional capacities. Mobility may be limited by paresthesias; hemiplegia; neuromotor disturbances; fractures; foot, knee, and hip problems; and respiratory diseases and other illnesses that deplete one's energy. All these conditions are likely to occur more frequently and have more devastating effects as one ages. Many older adults have some of these impairments, with women significantly outnumbering men in this respect (Chapter 21).

Difficulties in mobility are often the first sign of functional decline and may indicate that an individual could benefit from preventive actions. Impairment of mobility is an early predictor of physical disability and is associated with poor outcomes such as falling, loss of independence, depression, decreased quality of life, institutionalization, and death (Bergland et al, 2017). Approximately one-third of noninstitutionalized older adults have trouble walking or require assistance from another person or equipment to ambulate. For those older than age 85 years, the prevalence of these limitations is even higher (Federal Interagency Forum on Aging, 2016). Individuals residing in nursing homes have even higher rates of mobility impairment. Maintenance of mobility and function is an essential component of best practice gerontological nursing and is effective in preventing falls, unnecessary decline, and loss of independence.

FALLS

Falls are defined as any sudden drop from one surface to a lower surface with or without injury. Falls are one of the most important geriatric syndromes and the leading cause of morbidity and mortality for older adults. Falls are the most common adverse event in health care facilities and the leading cause of injury-related emergency department (ED) visits and injury-related deaths in older adults. Of particular concern, rates of fall-related ED visits and hospitalizations are increasing (de Vries et al, 2018; Phelan et al, 2017). Each year, about one-third of adults aged 65 years or older, and half of those aged 80 years and older, will fall. More than half of those will fall more than once (Pirker and Katzenschlager, 2017; Taylor-Piliae, 2017). Nearly half of all falls result in injury, of which 10% are serious. About 3% to 20% of hospital inpatients fall at least once during their hospitalization (Quigley et al, 2016). Between 50% and 75% of nursing home residents fall annually, twice the rate of community-dwelling older adults, and these falls result in more serious complications than other falls (CDC, 2017; Gray-Miceli et al, 2016). Nearly 50% of hospital admissions and most nursing home placements are a direct result of fall-related injuries such as hip fractures, upper limb injuries, and traumatic brain injuries (Jackson, 2016; Taylor-Piliae et al, 2017). Estimates are that up to two-thirds of falls may be preventable (Gray-Miceli et al, 2016).

Falls are a significant public health problem. Various national studies from across the globe have demonstrated increasing fall-related incidence of injury and this can be expected to increase substantially with the aging of the population (Taylor-Piliae et al, 2017) (Fig. 19.1). Worldwide, falls are the second leading cause of accidental or unintentional injury deaths (Box 19.1). *Healthy People 2020* includes several goals related to falls (Healthy People 2020 box).

 HEALTHY PEOPLE 2020

Falls, Fall Prevention, Injury

- Reduce the rate of emergency department visits due to falls among older adults.
- Reduce fatal and nonfatal injuries.
- Reduce hospitalizations for nonfatal injuries.
- Reduce fatal and nonfatal traumatic brain injuries.

Data from U.S. Department of Health and Human Services, Office of Disease Prevention and Health Promotion: *Healthy People 2020,* 2012. http://www.healthypeople.gov/2020.

⚡ **SAFETY ALERT**

The Quality and Safety Education for Nurses (QSEN) project has developed quality and safety measures for nursing and proposed targets for the knowledge, skills, and attitudes to be developed in nursing prelicensure and graduate programs. Education on falls and fall risk reduction is an important consideration in the QSEN safety competency, which addresses the need to minimize risk of harm to patients and providers through both system effectiveness and individual performance. Safe and effective transfer techniques are an important component of safety measures.

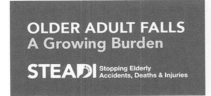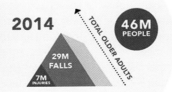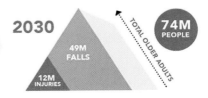

Fig. 19.1 Older Adults Falls: A Growing Burden. (From Centers for Disease Control and Prevention: *STEADI Stopping Elderly Accidents, Deaths & Injuries,* 2017. https://www.cdc.gov/steadi/materials.html. Accessed February 2018.)

Consequences of Falls

Hip Fractures

More than 95% of hip fractures among older adults are caused by falling, usually by falling sideways. Hip fractures are associated with considerable morbidity and mortality. The likelihood of recovery to prefracture level of function is less than 50% regardless of the individual's previous level of function. Returning to a high level of function is particularly low in those older than age 85, with multiple comorbid conditions, or dementia. Morbidity and mortality are high, with approximately 10% of patients dying within 1 month, 30% at 1 year, and 80% at 8 years following hip fracture. This excess mortality persists for 10 years after the fracture and is higher in men. White women have significantly higher hip fracture rates than black women due to a higher incidence of osteoporotic changes (CDC, 2017; Riemen and Hutchison, 2016; Tang et al, 2017).

Traumatic Brain Injury

Traumatic brain injury (TBI) is associated with almost half of all admissions for major trauma in older adults. Older adults (75 years of age and older) have the highest rates of TBI-related hospitalization and death. Advancing age negatively affects the outcome after TBI, even with relatively minor head injuries. TBI has been called the "silent epidemic" (CDC, 2016). Falls are the leading cause of TBI for older adults.

Factors that place the older adult at greater risk for TBI include the presence of comorbid conditions, use of antiplatelet and anticoagulant medications, and changes in the brain with age. Preinjury use of antiplatelet and anticoagulant medications is especially problematic with head trauma and increases the risk of traumatic intracranial hemorrhage and premature disability and death (Nishijima et al, 2017). Brain changes with age, although clinically insignificant, do increase the risk of TBIs and especially subdural hematomas, which are much more common in older adults. There is a decreased adherence of the dura mater to the skull, increased fragility of bridging cerebral veins, and increases in the subarachnoid space and atrophy of

the brain, which create more space within the cranial vault for blood to accumulate before symptoms appear. Falls are the leading cause of TBI, but older adults may experience TBI with seemingly more minor incidents (e.g., sharp turns or jarring movement of the head). Some patients may not even remember the incident. TBIs have been associated with an earlier age of dementia onset and increasing the risk of Parkinson's disease (Gardner et al, 2018; Schaffert et al, 2018).

In cases of moderate to severe TBI, there will be cognitive and physical sequelae obvious at the time of injury or shortly afterward that will require emergency treatment. However, older adults who experience a minor incident with seemingly lesser trauma to the head often present with more insidious and delayed symptom onset. Because of changes in the aging brain, there is an increased risk for slowly expanding subdural hematomas. TBIs are often missed or misdiagnosed among older adults. If clinicians do not have information on the usual cognitive status of the older adult, manifestations of TBI are often misinterpreted as signs of dementia, which can lead to inaccurate prognoses and limit implementation of appropriate treatment (Hawley et al, 2017).

Health professionals should have a high suspicion of TBI in an older adult who falls and strikes the head or experiences even a more minor event, such as sudden twisting of the head. For older adults who are receiving warfarin and experience minor head injury with a negative computed tomography (CT) scan, a protocol of 24-hour observation followed by a second CT scan is recommended. Box 19.2 presents signs and symptoms of TBI.

Fallophobia

Even if a fall does not result in injury, falls contribute to a loss of confidence that leads to reduced physical activity, increased dependency, and social withdrawal. Fear of falling (fallophobia) may restrict an individual's life space (area in which an individual performs activities). Fear of falling is an important predictor of general functional decline and a risk factor for future falls. Assessing the presence of fallophobia and referring for further assessment and management are important in all settings. Nursing staff may also contribute to fear of falling in their patients by telling them not to get up by themselves or by using restrictive devices to keep them from independently moving. This further decreases mobility, safety, and function and increases fall risk. More appropriate responses include the use of function-focused care (FCC) (Chapter 18). FCC is an approach that teaches nurses to evaluate older adults' underlying capability with regard to function and physical activity and integrate functional and physical activities into all care interactions to promote independence, self-care, safety, and function.

The presence of fallophobia should be assessed in older adults as part of fall risk-reduction interventions. It is important to listen to the story of the individual's experience related to falling and the personal impact the fall experience has had on their life. In collaboration with the older adult, the nurse can more effectively design individualized interventions to enhance independence, mobility, safety, and reduce fall risk. It is important to explore the personal accounts of older adults in research about falls and other experiences but there exists little research in this area (Gray-Miceli, 2017).

BOX 19.2 Signs and Symptoms of Traumatic Brain Injury in Older Adults[a]

Symptoms of Mild Traumatic Brain Injury (TBI)
- Low-grade headache that will not dissipate
- Having more trouble than usual remembering things, paying attention or concentrating, organizing daily tasks, or making decisions and solving problems
- Slowness in thinking, speaking, acting, or reading
- Getting lost or easily confused
- Feeling tired all of the time, lack of energy or motivation
- Change in sleep pattern (sleeping much longer than usual, having trouble sleeping)
- Loss of balance, feeling light-headed or dizzy
- Increased sensitivity to sounds, lights, distractions
- Blurred vision or eyes that tire easily
- Loss of sense of taste or smell
- Ringing in the ears
- Change in sexual drive
- Mood changes (feeling sad, anxious, listless, or becoming easily irritated or angry for little or no reason)

Symptoms of Moderate to Severe TBI
- Severe headache that gets worse or does not disappear
- Repeated vomiting or nausea
- Seizures
- Inability to wake from sleep
- Dilation of one or both pupils
- Slurred speech
- Weakness or numbness in the arms or legs
- Loss of coordination
- Increased confusion, restlessness, or agitation

[a]Older adults taking blood thinners should be seen immediately by a health care provider if they have a bump or blow to the head, even if they do not have any of the symptoms listed here.

FALL RISK FACTORS

Falls are a symptom of a problem and are rarely benign in older adults. The etiology of falls is multifactorial and the result of a convergence of risk factors across biological and behavioral aspects of the individual and factors in their environment. Episodes of acute illness or exacerbations of chronic illness are times of high fall risk and falls may indicate impending illness (Taylor-Piliae et al, 2017). New onset delirium is a common cause of falls (Morley, 2017). Deanna Gray-Miceli and colleagues (2010, 2016) developed seven types of fall classifications based on research in nursing homes (Box 19.3).

⚡ SAFETY ALERT

A history of falls is a significant risk factor and individuals who have fallen have three times the risk of falling again and being injured compared with persons who did not fall in the past year. Recurrent falls are often the result of the same underlying cause but can also be an indication of disease progression (e.g., heart failure, Parkinson's disease) or a new acute problem (e.g., infection, dehydration) (Rubenstein and Dillard, 2014; Taylor-Piliae et al, 2017).

BOX 19.3 Fall Classifications

- Falls due to acute events such as orthostatic hypotension, loss of balance, syncope
- Falls due to chronic events such as chronic dizziness or lower extremity weakness
- Falls due to medications
- Falls due to environmental mishaps
- Falls due to equipment malfunction
- Falls due to poor safety awareness
- Falls due to poor patient judgment

From Gray-Miceli D, deCordova P, Crane G, Quigley P, Ratcliffe S: Nursing home registered nurses' and licensed practical nurses' knowledge of causes of falls, *J Nurs Care Qual* 31(2):153–160, 2016.

Individual risk factors can be categorized as either intrinsic or extrinsic (Box 19.4). Intrinsic risk factors are unique to each individual and are associated with factors such as reduced vision and hearing, unsteady gait, cognitive impairment, acute and chronic illnesses, and effects of medications. Extrinsic risk factors are external to the individual and related to the physical environment and include lack of support equipment for bathtubs and toilets, height of beds, condition of floors, poor lighting, inappropriate footwear, and improper use of assistive devices.

Falls in the young-old and the more healthy old occur more frequently because of external reasons; however, with increasing age and comorbid conditions, internal and locomotor

BOX 19.4 Common Fall Risk Factors for Older Adults

Conditions (Intrinsic)
- Sedative and alcohol use, psychoactive medications, opioids, diuretics, anticholinergics, antidepressants, antihypertensives, anticoagulants, bowel preparations
- Four or more medications
- Previous falls and fractures
- Female, 80 years of age or older
- Acute and recent illness; recent hospitalization
- Cognitive impairment (delirium, dementia)
- Chronic pain
- Abnormalities of gait and balance
- Unsteadiness, dizziness, syncope
- Foot problems
- Depression, anxiety
- Decreased vision or hearing
- Wearing multifocal glasses while walking
- Fear of falling
- Orthostatic hypotension
- Postprandial drop in blood pressure
- Sleep disorders
- Functional limitations in self-care activities; inability to complete activities of daily living without assistance
- Inability to rise from a chair without using the arms
- Slow walking speed
- Wheelchair-bound

Continued

BOX 19.4 Common Fall Risk Factors for Older Adults—cont'd

Situations (Extrinsic)

- Urinary incontinence, urgency, nocturia
- Recent relocation, unfamiliarity with new environment
- Inadequate response to transfer and toileting needs
- Improper use of assistive devices
- Inadequate or missing safety rails, particularly in bathroom
- Poorly designed or unstable furniture
- Slippery or uneven surfaces
- Glossy, highly waxed floors
- Inadequate visual support (glare, low wattage bulbs, lack of nightlights)
- General clutter
- Inappropriate footwear/clothing
- Pets that inadvertently trip an individual
- Electrical cords
- Loose carpeting
- Stairs that do not have weight-bearing handrails
- Throw rugs
- Inability to reach personal items, lack of access to call bell or inability to use it
- Side rails, restraints

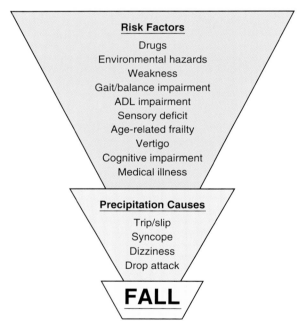

Fig. 19.2 Multifactorial Nature of Falls. *ADL,* Activities of daily living. (From Ham RJ, Sloane PD, Warshaw GA, et al: *Primary care geriatrics,* ed 6, Philadelphia, 2014, Elsevier Saunders.)

reasons become increasingly prevalent as factors contributing to falls. The risk of falling increases as the number of risk factors increases. Most falls occur from a combination of intrinsic and extrinsic factors that combine at a certain point in time (Fig. 19.2). Community-dwelling older adults may fall for different reasons than individuals living in long-term care. Environmental factors (indoors and outdoors) may bring a higher risk for falls when combined with current health conditions. Falls in health care settings are more often related to the health status of the individual and the change in their environment (Kruschke and Butcher, 2017). Inadequate staffing in health care settings is also a factor that may increase fall risk if patients attempt to get up for bathroom use or get out of bed because help is not readily available. Impaired cognition affects safety awareness and also increases fall risk. Other factors may also influence risk for falls including stressful life events such as illness, accidents, death of spouse/partner or close relatives or friends, loss of pet, financial trouble, a move or change in residence, or giving up an important hobby (Fink et al, 2014).

Gait Disorders

The prevalence of gait disorders increases from 10% in individuals aged 60 to 69 years to more than 60% in community-dwelling individuals over the age of 80 years. Gait disorders are associated with a threefold increase in fall risk. Marked gait disorders are not normally a consequence of aging alone but are more likely indicative of an underlying pathological condition. Arthritis of the knee may result in ligamentous weakness and instability, causing the legs to give way or collapse. Diabetes, dementia, Parkinson's disease, stroke, alcoholism, and vitamin B deficiencies may cause neurological damage and resultant gait problems (Pirker and Katzenschlager, 2017). Gait deformities affect walking and balance. Fall assessments need to include assessment using tools such as the Timed Up & Go (TUG) and 30-Second Chair Stand (Figs. 19.3 and 19.4).

Foot Deformities

Foot deformities and ill-fitting footwear also contribute to gait problems and potential for falls. Care of the feet is an important aspect of mobility, comfort, and a stable gait and is often neglected. Little attention is given to one's feet until they interfere with walking and moving and ultimately the ability to remain independent. Foot problems are often unrecognized and untreated, leading to considerable dysfunction. Older adults may consider foot problems and foot pain to be part of aging rather than a treatable medical condition (Menz, 2016).

As we age, feet are subjected to a lifetime of stress and may not be able to continue to adapt, and inflammatory changes in bone and soft tissue can occur. Foot problems are present in a large number of older adults and may include foot pain, nail fungus, dry skin, corns and calluses, bunions, neuropathy (Fig. 19.5). Some older adults are unable to walk comfortably, or at all, because of neglect of corns, bunions, and overgrown nails. Other causes of problems may be traced to loss of fat cushioning and resilience with aging, diabetes, ill-fitting shoes, poor arch support, excessively repetitive weight-bearing activities, obesity, or uneven distribution of weight on the feet. Table 19.1 presents common foot problems.

Foot health and function may reflect systemic disease or give early clues to physical illness. Sudden or gradual changes in the condition of the nails or the skin of the feet or the appearance of recurring infections may be precursors of more serious health

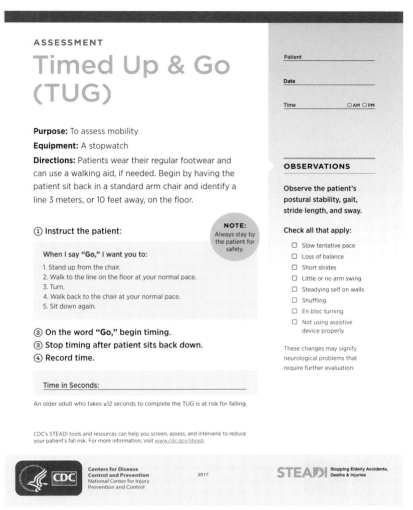

Fig. 19.3 Timed Up & Go (TUG). (From Centers for Disease Control and Prevention: https://www.cdc.gov/steadi/pdf/TUG_Test-print.pdf. Accessed April 2019.)

problems. Rheumatological disorders such as the various forms of arthritis can also affect the feet. Gout occurs most often in the joint of the great toe but is a systemic disease. Both diabetes and peripheral vascular disease (PVD) commonly cause problems in the lower extremities that can quickly become life-threatening (Chapter 24).

PROMOTING HEALTHY AGING: IMPLICATIONS FOR GERONTOLOGICAL NURSING

Care of the foot takes a team approach, including the individual, the nurse, the podiatrist, and the primary health care provider. Nursing care of the individual with foot problems should be directed toward providing optimal comfort and function, removing possible mechanical irritants, and decreasing the likelihood of infection. The nurse has the important function of assessing the feet for clues of functional ability and their owner's well-being (Box 19.5). Difficulty cutting toenails is common in older adults since it requires

joint flexibility, manual dexterity, and visual acuity and nurses often care for toenails. Appropriate cutting of toenails is important and safety precautions are essential (Fig. 19.6). Nurses can identify potential and actual problems and make referral to or seek assistance as needed from the primary care provider or podiatrist for any changes in the feet. Regular podiatry treatment can maintain or improve foot health in older adults. There is evidence that nursing staff lack confidence in managing foot problems but providing education has been shown to be effective in improving foot care knowledge and practices (Menz, 2016) (Box 19.6).

Orthostatic and Postprandial Hypotension

Declines in depth perception, proprioception, and normotensive response to postural changes are important factors that contribute to falls (Finucane et al, 2017). Clinically significant orthostatic hypotension (OH) is a common clinical finding in frail older adults and has been reported to be present in up to 50% of older adults in nursing homes.

ASSESSMENT

30-Second Chair Stand

Purpose: To test leg strength and endurance

Equipment: A chair with a straight back without arm rests (seat 17" high), and a stopwatch.

NOTE: Stand next to the patient for safety.

① Instruct the patient:

1. Sit in the middle of the chair.
2. Place your hands on the opposite shoulder crossed, at the wrists.
3. Keep your feet flat on the floor.
4. Keep your back straight, and keep your arms against your chest.
5. On "**Go,**" rise to a full standing position, then sit back down again.
6. Repeat this for 30 seconds.

② On the word "**Go,**" begin timing.

If the patient must use his/her arms to stand, stop the test. Record "0" for the number and score.

③ Count the number of times the patient comes to a full standing position in 30 seconds.

If the patient is over halfway to a standing position when 30 seconds have elapsed, count it as a stand.

④ Record the number of times the patient stands in 30 seconds.

Number: _____   Score: _____

Patient _____

Date _____

Time _____ ☐ AM ☐ PM

SCORING

Chair Stand Below Average Scores

AGE	MEN	WOMEN
60-64	< 14	< 12
65-69	< 12	< 11
70-74	< 12	< 10
75-79	< 11	< 10
80-84	< 10	< 9
85-89	< 8	< 8
90-94	< 7	< 4

A below average score indicates a risk for falls.

CDC's STEADI tools and resources can help you screen, assess, and intervene to reduce your patient's fall risk. For more information, visit www.cdc.gov/steadi

Centers for Disease Control and Prevention
National Center for Injury Prevention and Control

2017

STEADI Stopping Elderly Accidents, Deaths & Injuries

Fig. 19.4 30-Second Chair Stand (STEADI). (From Centers for Disease Control and Prevention: https://www.cdc.gov/steadi/pdf/STEADI-Assessment-30Sec-508.pdf. Accessed April 2019.)

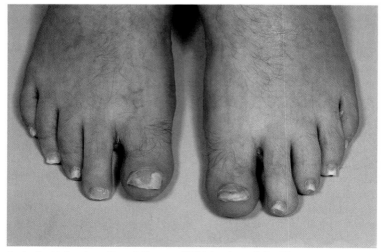

Fig. 19.5 Onycholysis, Yellowing, Crumbling, and Thickening of the Toenails. (From Bolognia J, Jorizzo JL, Rapini RP, editors: *Dermatology*, ed 2, St Louis, 2007, Mosby.)

TABLE 19.1 Common Foot Problems.

Foot Problem	Prevention/Treatment
Corns/calluses: Growths of compacted skin that occur as a result of prolonged pressure, usually from ill-fitting, tight shoes. Corns are cone-shaped and develop on the top of toe joints or between opposing surfaces of the toes from prolonged squeezing. Once formed, corns will cause pain. Unless friction and pressure are relieved, will continue to enlarge and cause increasing pain	Over-the-counter preparations may remove temporarily but may burn surrounding tissue and should not be used by diabetics or those with neurological impairment or poor circulation. For individuals with diabetes mellitus or peripheral vascular disease, foot care should be performed by a nurse with expertise in foot care, a doctor, or a podiatrist. **DO NOT** use razor blades, pocket knives, or scissors to remove corns/calluses Padding and protecting the area is the best practice (oval corn pads, gel pads, moleskin, lamb's wool, with a hole cut in the center for the corn) Daily lubrication of the feet; shoes with proper fit
Bunions: Bony deformities that develop from over the medial aspect of the joint of the great toe or at the lateral aspect of the fifth metatarsal head (little toe) Occur from long-standing squeezing of first and second toes; may be a hereditary factor	May be treated with corticosteroid injections and antiinflammatory pain medications. Surgery is also an option Use custom-made shoe(s) that provide(s) forefront space (e.g., running shoes)
Hammer toes: A permanently flexed toe with a clawlike appearance resulting from muscle imbalance and pressure from big toe slanting toward second toe; the toe contracts, leaving a bulge on top of the joint. Result of ill-fitting shoes and often seen in conjunction with bunions	Professional orthotics or specially designed protective devices; properly fitting, nonconstricting shoes and/or surgical intervention
Fungal infections: May affect skin of feet **(tinea pedis)** and nails. Nail fungus (*onychomycosis*) is most common nail disorder. Nail plate degenerates with color changes to yellow or brown and opaque, brittleness, and thickening of nail (Fig. 19.3). Fine powdery collection of fungus forms under center of the nail, separating the layers and pushing it up, causing the sides of the nail to dig into the skin like an ingrown toenail	Wash hands after handling the feet. Culturing is the only way to diagnose; cure difficult to impossible due to limited circulation to the nails. Several oral medications available but expensive and of limited effectiveness; potentially toxic to liver and heart. Photodynamic therapy (PDT) may be helpful For **tinea pedis** keep areas between the toes clean and dry and regularly exposed to sun and air. Topical antifungal powders are usual treatment. If diabetic, glycemic control important

BOX 19.5 Tips for Best Practice

Foot Assessment

Observation of Mobility
- Gait
- Use of assistive devices
- Footwear type and pattern of wear

Past Medical History
- Neuropathies
- Musculoskeletal limitations
- Peripheral vascular disease
- Vision problems
- History of falls
- Pain affecting movement

Bilateral Assessment
- Color
- Circulation and warmth
- Pulses
- Structural deformities
- Skin lesions
- Lower-extremity edema
- Evidence of scratching
- Abrasions and other lesions
- Rash or excessive dryness
- Condition and color of toenails

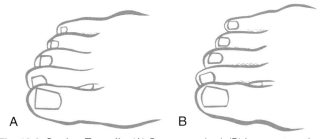

Fig. 19.6 Cutting Toenails. (A) Correct method. (B) Incorrect method.

Approximately one-third of falls are due to syncope and this may be higher in residents with Alzheimer's disease so there is a need to monitor orthostasis and postprandial hypotension (PPH) (Morley, 2017). The detection of OH is of clinical importance to fall prevention because OH is treatable. However, questions remain about the physiological basis of loss of balance or dizziness which may be treatable. Dr. Deanna Gray-Miceli, noted nurse researcher and falls expert, is conducting innovative research on detection of OH proactively to prevent recurrent falls by identifying pattern changes. Dr. Gray-Miceli describes her research in the Research Highlights box.

BOX 19.6   Tips for Best Practice

Care of the Feet

- Comprehensive annual foot examination for all persons with diabetes mellitus (DM) including identification of risk factors for ulcers and amputations, test for loss of protective sensation, assessment of pedal pulses
- Care of toenails: trimmed after bath or shower when softened or soak 20 to 30 minutes before cutting; clip straight across and even with top of toe, edges filed slightly to remove sharpness but not to the point of rounding (Fig. 19.6)
- Diabetic foot care done only by podiatrist or registered nurse (RN) with expertise; persons with DM or peripheral vascular disease (PVD) should not have pedicures from commercial establishments.
- Ingrown toenails are a fragment of nail that pierces the skin at the edge of the nail; may be due to hypertrophy of the nail with onychomycosis, improper cutting, pressure on toes from tight hosiery or shoes. Should be treated by podiatrist due to risk of infection. Temporary relief can be provided by inserting a small piece of cotton under affected nail corner.

- Counsel individual about proper footwear. Shoes should cover, protect, and stabilize the foot and provide maximal toe space. Feet increase in size with age and one foot is usually larger than the other. Shoes should be fitted to the largest foot and purchased in the afternoon when feet may be larger. Velcro closures are helpful for those with limited finger dexterity. Closed back shoes of low heel height and high surface contact may reduce risk of falls. Rubber-soled shoe such as sneakers may increase risk of stumbling while walking and may promote too much "sway" and affect balance if person not accustomed to shoes of this kind.
- Orthotic and orthopedic shoes may be indicated for certain foot problems. Medicare Part B covers one pair of therapeutic shoes and inserts as durable medical equipment (DME) for individuals with DM.

RESEARCH HIGHLIGHTS

Older Adults With Symptomatic Falls: Thoughts for Advancing Science and Improving Care

Older adults with symptoms such as loss of balance (LOB) or dizziness with standing are at risk for falls. Professional nurses caring for these individuals avert falls by standing by their side, offering arm-in-arm assistance or instructing the older adult to sit down until further assessment takes place. While this evidence-based intervention continues to take precedence as best practice for safe mobility, questions remain about the physiological basis of loss of balance or dizziness which may be treatable. For instance, was the older adult's loss of balance related to misfooting[1] or a drop in blood pressure with standing[2]? These questions remain unanswered without a focused assessment of the older adult at the time of their occurrence. The shortage of staff, few trained specialists in geriatric nursing,[3] and limited use of technology in long-term care settings to detect and monitor these symptoms create missed opportunities for preventing falls and improving delivery of appropriate health care.

The use of continuous monitoring of motion and balance can help professional nurses and care providers to understand some details about the physiological basis of loss of balance or dizziness symptoms, especially in practice settings like long-term care where upward of 60% of residents are falling repeatedly. LOB frequently occurs during the transition from sit to stand, often due to a drop in blood pressure. To develop interventions against this occurrence, a database of physiological and biomechanical parameters of related to balance in the older adult population is needed.

Our project evaluates bodily biomechanics and blood pressures in a sample of older adults while performing typical activities, such as sit-to-stand and walking. Dynamic and kinematical parameters were registered as indices of balance, using wearable inertial sensors (inertial measurement units [IMUs]). Enrolled older adults wore these small portable IMU sensors at several sites

on their torso while older adult's blood pressure was assessed and recorded during sit to stand maneuvers. Biomechanical engineers examined the relationships between blood pressure and biomechanics during the controlled physical maneuvers.

LOB is potentially reversible, but interventions are complicated and have not been widely used, in part because patients can be cognitively impaired, making communication of symptoms experienced difficult. Methods to quantify and document balance though force plate balance machines are cumbersome to implement and not always reimbursable by Medicare. So, precisely because of the high incidence of cognitive impairment and memory loss in older adult populations who reside in long-term care institutions where fall incidence is highest, early detection of impending or worsening impairments to balance is critical. Development of a streamlined system to quantitate balance on a large scale has the potential to proactively prevent recurrent falls by identifying pattern changes.

References

1. Gray-Miceli D: Part I. Falls in the environment: faulty footwear or footing? Interdisciplinary case-based perspectives. *Ann Long-Term Care* 18(4):32–36, 2010.
2. Gray-Miceli D, Ratcliffe, SJ, Liu, S et al: Orthostatic hypotension in elderly nursing home residents who fall: are they dizzy? *Clin Nurs Res* 21(1):64–78, 2012.
3. Mion LC: Care provision for older adults: who will provide? *Online J Issues Nurs* 8(2):4, 2003. www.nursingworld.org/MainMenuCategories/ANAMarketplace/ANAPeriodicals/OJIN/TableofContents/Volume82003/No2May2003/CareProvisionforOlderAdults.aspx. Accessed May 2018.

OH is considered a decrease of 20 mm Hg (or more) in systolic pressure and/or a decrease of 10 mm Hg (or more) in diastolic pressure with position change from lying or sitting to standing. Assessment of OH in everyday nursing practice is often overlooked or assessed inaccurately and needs to be included as a competency in nursing education and practice (Box 19.7). However, there is considerable variability in the

recommendations by clinical experts regarding the timing and position of blood pressure measurements, and further research is needed (Lipsitz, 2017). Box 19.8 presents a protocol for care of individuals with OH in nursing homes.

PPH is associated with increased risk of syncope and falls. PPH occurs after ingestion of a carbohydrate meal and may be related to the release of a vasodilatory peptide, but research is

BOX 19.7 Measuring Orthostatic Blood Pressure

- Orthostatic hypotension is more common in the morning, and therefore assessment should occur then.
- Have the individual lie down for 5 minutes.
- Measure the blood pressure and pulse rate in both arms. Use the arm with the higher blood pressure for measurements following position change.
- Have the individual stand (use safety precautions as needed). If unable to stand, measure blood pressure sitting with feet hanging.
- Take the blood pressure immediately after standing and ask about dizziness.
- Repeat blood pressure and pulse rate measurements after standing for 3 minutes and ask about dizziness.
- A drop in BP of ≥20 mm Hg or in diastolic BP of ≥10 mm Hg or experiencing light-headedness, dizziness, or loss of balance is considered abnormal.

From Momeyer M: Orthostatic hypotension in older adults with dementia, *J Gerontol Nurs* 40(6):22–29, 2014.

BOX 19.8 Tips for Best Practice

Care of Individuals in Nursing Homes With Orthostatic Hypotension

- Keep head of bed elevated 30 degrees at all times.
- Avoid rapid changes in position, especially in the morning. When transferring out of bed, have individual sit up gradually and dangle feet on side of bed for a few minutes. After assisting to standing position, support for a few minutes before walking.
- Wear compression stockings during the daytime (thigh or knee high). Put on in the morning before getting out of bed; remove at night.
- Have individual sit for 20 minutes following a meal.
- Delay physical activity from morning to afternoon or evening when blood pressure is naturally higher.
- Encourage sitting after any type of exercise.
- Avoid standing up too quickly after toileting.
- Encourage adequate fluid intake.
- Encourage dorsiflexion of feet several times before standing.
- Encourage crossing and uncrossing of legs when sitting.
- If orthostatic hypotension (OH) is present, provide assistance with ambulation
- Educate the individual/family about OH

From Momeyer M: Orthostatic hypotension in older adults with dementia, *J Gerontol Nurs* 40(6):22–29, 2014.

needed on the epidemiology and pathophysiology of PPH. PPH is usually asymptomatic and may be overlooked. Patients with neurological disease and diabetes have a higher frequency of PPH. Lifestyle interventions such as increasing water intake before eating or eating smaller more frequent meals may be important, but further research is needed. Older individuals with risk factors should be cautioned against sudden rising from sitting or supine positions, particularly after eating. Assessment of OH should be conducted after a fall, particularly if related to a meal (Krbot Skorić et al, 2017).

Cognitive Impairment

Older adults with cognitive impairment are at double the risk of falling compared to age-matched individuals, with reports of 60% to 80% falling within a year of diagnosis of dementia.

A twofold increased fall risk is present even in mild impairment (Peach et al, 2017). Cognition plays a crucial role in control of gait, and individuals with cognitive impairment may have an altered gait pattern. Other factors such as medications (neuroleptics), visual acuity, functional impairments, falls history, insight, memory, and behavior contribute to the complex mix of risk factors for falls in this population. There is little research on fall prevention programs for individuals with cognitive impairment, but combined cognitive and physical interventions have been reported to improve balance, functional mobility, and gait speed in individuals with mild cognitive impairment. Further research is needed to determine the most appropriate fall risk-reduction programs for the different stages of dementia (Lach et al, 2017). Fall risk assessments should include more specific cognitive risk factors, and cognitive assessment measures need to be more frequently conducted with individuals at risk for falls (Booth et al, 2015, 2016).

Vision and Hearing

Vision and hearing impairment have been associated with falls and should be assessed in older adults and corrected to the extent possible (Chapters 11 and 12). Poor visual acuity, reduced contrast sensitivity, decreased visual field, cataracts, and use of nonmiotic glaucoma medications have all been associated with falls. There is little research on interventions for either vision or hearing problems and falls and fractures (Gopinath et al, 2016; Gupta et al, 2017).

Medications

Medications implicated in increasing fall risk include those causing potentially dangerous side effects including drowsiness, mental confusion, problems with balance, loss of urinary control, and sudden drops in blood pressure with standing. These include antidepressants, antihypertensives, diuretics, some analgesics, sedative-hypnotics, and psychotropic medications. The association between psychotropic medications and falls is well established (Chen et al, 2017; de Vries et al, 2018). Antidepressant use is also associated with an increased risk of hip fracture among older adults (Torvinen-Kiiskinen et al, 2017).

The literature on cardiovascular medications as potential fall-risk–increasing drugs is conflicting and needs further research. In a systematic meta-analysis (de Vries et al, 2018), loop diuretics and digitalis were consistently associated with increased fall risk. Additionally, the initiation of cardiovascular drugs showed an association with increased risk of falling. When cardiovascular drugs are prescribed, beginning with a smaller dose, increasing the dose slowly, monitoring response, and fall prevention teaching are important.

Medication review is an evidence-based strategy for reducing falls among older adults. Attention to medications should become a key focus of public health educational efforts and fall prevention in all settings (Phelan et al, 2017). All medications, including over-the-counter (OTC) and herbal medications, should be reviewed and limited to those that are absolutely essential. The addition of any new medication should trigger a fall risk evaluation (Musich et al, 2017). Psychotropic prescribing should be carefully considered, initiated at low doses, and monitored closely. If these medications are being used, patient teaching should be provided related to fall risk, fall prevention interventions, appropriate dosing, and use of other medications, such as benzodiazepines, and alcohol use (Chapter 28). Chapter 9 discusses geropharmacology and Chapter 29 discusses the use of these medications and alternative approaches for behavioral symptoms that may occur in individuals with dementia.

PROMOTING HEALTHY AGING: IMPLICATIONS FOR GERONTOLOGICAL NURSING

Screening and Assessment

The American Geriatrics Society/British Geriatrics Society *Clinical Practice Guideline: Prevention of Falls in Older Persons* (2010) recommends that fall risk assessment be an integral part of primary health care for the older adult. All older adults should be asked whether they have fallen in the past year and whether they experience difficulties with walking or balance. In addition, ask about falls that did not result in an injury and the circumstances of a near-fall, mishap, or misstep because this may provide important information for prevention of future falls. Older adults may be reluctant to share information about falls for fear of losing independence, so the nurse must use judgment and empathy in eliciting information about falls, assuring the individual that there are many modifiable factors to increase safety and help maintain independence.

The intensity of the assessment will vary with the target population:

- Low-risk community-dwelling individuals should be asked at least once a year about fall occurrence and circumstances.

- Individuals who report a single fall should be evaluated for mobility impairment and unsteadiness using a simple observational test (Figs. 19.3 and 19.4), with those who demonstrate mobility problems or unsteadiness being referred for further assessment.

- High-risk populations (individuals who have had multiple falls in the past year, have abnormalities of gait and/or balance, have received medical attention related to a fall, or reside in a nursing home) should undergo a more comprehensive and detailed assessment.

- Comprehensive fall assessments include the following components: history of falls, medical history, complete physical examination (including vision and hearing), medication review (including alcohol/other drugs), functional assessment, cognitive assessment, gait, balance, and mobility, muscle strength, pain assessment, heart rate and rhythm, postural hypotension, feet and footwear, continence assessment, depression screening, cardiovascular assessment, skin assessment, sleep assessment, nutrition assessment (Kruschke, 2017) (Chapter 7) (Fig. 19.7).

Screening and Assessment in Hospital/Long-Term Care

Individuals admitted to acute or long-term care settings should have an initial fall assessment on admission, after any change in condition, and at regular intervals during their stay. Assessment is an ongoing process that includes multiple and continual types of assessment, reassessment, and evaluation following a fall or intervention to reduce the risk of a fall. An interprofessional team (physician or nurse practitioner, nurse, risk manager, physical and occupational therapists, and other designated

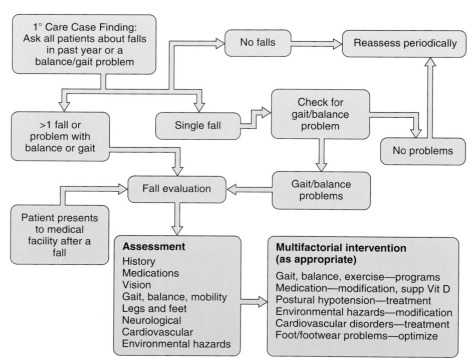

Fig. 19.7 American Geriatrics Society Fall Assessment and Prevention Algorithm. (From Ham RJ, Sloane PD, Warshaw GA, et al: *Primary care geriatrics,* ed 6, Philadelphia, 2014, Elsevier Saunders. Adapted from Kenny RA, Rubenstein LZ, Tinetti ME, et al: AGS/BGS clinical practice guideline: prevention of falls in older persons, *J Am Geriatr Soc* 59:148–157, 2011.)

staff) should be involved in planning care on the basis of find-ings from an individualized assessment. Nurses bring expert knowledge of patient activities, abilities, and needs from a 24-hours-per-day, 7-days-per-week perspective to help the team implement the most appropriate interventions and evalu-ate outcomes.

Fall Risk Assessment Instruments

The following key questions can be asked during assessment and can alert clinicians to fall risk and the need for more follow up: (1) Have you fallen in the past year? (2) Do you feel unsteady when standing or walking? (3) Are you worried about falling? Red flag risk factors such as osteoporosis, mobility problems, or anticoagulant therapy also alert the clinician of the need for further assessment. A patient self-assessment screening tool is available from the STEADI (*Stopping Elderly Accidents, Deaths, and Injuries*) program (CDC, 2017) (Box 19.9).

Fall risk assessment instruments are still commonly included in fall prevention interventions; instruments that are utilized need to be reliable and valid and nurses need to use them judi-ciously. Often, these instruments are completed in a routine manner and risk factors are not identified or may not be known because of lack of assessment and knowledge of the individual's history. A fall risk score is not adequate assessment to prevent falls. To be able to prevent a fall, it is important to know why someone is at risk for falls, the individual's actual fall and injury risk factors, identifying the factors that are modifiable and those that are not, treating modifiable factors, and helping pa-tients compensate for those that are not modifiable. This infor-mation is obtained from comprehensive fall risk assessments. Additional research is needed to develop valid, reliable instru-ments to differentiate levels of fall risk in various settings.

The National Center for Patient Safety recommends the Morse Falls Scale, but not for use in long-term care. The Performance-Oriented Mobility Assessment (Tinetti, 1986) is a well-validated tool. The Hendrich II Fall Risk Model (Hendrich et al, 2003) which also includes a modified Get Up and Go test, is recommended by the Hartford Foundation for Geriatric Nursing (Box 19.9). This instrument has been vali-dated with skilled nursing and rehabilitation populations and is also easy to use in the outpatient setting. In the skilled nursing facility, the Minimum Data Set (MDS 3.0) includes information about history of falls and hip fractures and an assessment of balance during transitions and walking (moving from seated to standing, walking, turning around, moving on and off toilet, and transfers between bed and chair or wheelchair) (Chapter 7).

Postfall Assessment

Postfall assessment (PFA) is an integral component of fall prevention programs in institutional settings. It is important to identify underlying causes of falls and risk factors, and the PFA is a way of critically examining each fall. The purpose of the PFA is to identify the clinical status of the individual, verify and treat injuries, identify underlying causes of the fall when possible, and assist in implementing appropriate indi-vidualized risk-reduction interventions. Incomplete analysis of the reasons for a fall can result in repeated incidents. If the patient cannot tell you about the circumstances of the fall, information should be obtained from staff or witnesses. Stan-dard "incident report" forms do not provide adequate PFA information.

Conducting a postfall huddle (after action review) as soon as possible after a fall is recommended for PFA. Staff at all levels should be involved, as well as the patient, to discuss the

BOX 19.10   Postfall Assessment Suggestions

Initiate emergency measures as indicated.

History
- Description of the fall from the individual or witness
- Individual's opinion of the cause of the fall
- Circumstances of the fall (trip or slip)
- Person's activity at the time of the fall
- Presence of comorbid conditions, such as a previous stroke, Parkinson's disease, osteoporosis, seizure disorder, sensory deficit, joint abnormalities, depression, cardiac disease
- Medication review
- Associated symptoms, such as chest pain, palpitations, light-headedness, vertigo, loss of balance, fainting, weakness, confusion, incontinence, or dyspnea
- Time of day and location of the fall
- Presence of acute illness

Physical Examination
- Vital signs: postural blood pressure changes, fever, or hypothermia
- Head and neck: visual impairment, hearing impairment, nystagmus, bruit
- Heart: arrhythmia or valvular dysfunction
- Neurological signs: altered mental status, focal deficits, peripheral neuropathy, muscle weakness, rigidity or tremor, impaired balance
- Musculoskeletal signs: arthritic changes, range of motion (ROM), podiatric deformities or problems, swelling, redness or bruises, abrasions, pain on movement, shortening and external rotation of lower extremities

Functional Assessment
- Functional gait and balance: observe resident rising from chair, walking, turning, and sitting down
- Balance test, mobility, use of assistive devices or personal assistance, extent of ambulation, restraint use, prosthetic equipment
- Activities of daily living: bathing, dressing, transferring, toileting

Environmental Assessment
- Staffing patterns, unsafe practice in transferring, delay in response to call light
- Faulty equipment
- Use of bed, chair alarm
- Call light within reach
- Wheelchair, bed locked
- Adequate supervision
- Clutter, walking paths not clear
- Dim lighting
- Glare
- Uneven flooring
- Wet, slippery floors
- Poorly fitted seating devices
- Inappropriate footwear
- Inappropriate eyewear

fall—what happened, how it happened, why it happened, how the outcome could be avoided the next time, what is the follow-up plan. Other components to be addressed in PFA are presented in Box 19.10. The Department of Veterans Affairs National Center for Patient Safety provides comprehensive information about fall assessment, fall risk reduction, policies and procedures, and includes a postfall huddle guide. For falls that happen outside the hospital or skilled nursing facility, individuals can complete the "Story of Your Falls" (Box 19.9) to provide PFA information.

Interventions

Nurses play a major role in fall prevention but fall prevention is a shared responsibility of all health care providers caring for older adults. Across settings of care, fall prevention programs incorporating multifactorial and interprofessonal approaches, aimed at multiple risk factors contributing to falls, are the most effective (Gray-Miceli et al, 2017; Isaranuwatchai et al, 2017; Jackson, 2017). The focus of the program may differ according to the setting (community, hospital, home, long-term care) (Kruschke, 2017).

Engaging older adults in teaching about fall prevention is especially important during the transition from hospital to home. Transitional care programs need to be tailored for fall risk and prevention. Yet a recent study reported that "despite the availability of evidence-based patient and provider resources, these resources are not being routinely used to engage older adults in fall prevention" (Shuman et al, 2019, p. 28). Home-bound or semi-homebound older adults are another population at risk for falls and are 50% more likely to

experience a fall than non-homebound individuals. Impaired balance was the strongest predictor for falls in this population, followed by problems moving around in the home. Assessment of these risk factors is very important when nurses are caring for older adults in the home setting so that tailored fall prevention programs can be implemented (Zhao et al, 2018).

Choosing the most appropriate interventions to reduce the risk of falls depends on appropriate assessment at various intervals depending on the person's changing condition and tailoring interventions to individual cognitive function, language, and health literacy. A one-size-fits-all approach is not effective. Further research is needed to determine the type, frequency, and timing of interventions best suited for specific populations. The majority of research on fall-risk reduction interventions has been conducted with community-dwelling older adults and there is a need for more research on effective interventions in acute and long-term care settings. CDC's STEADI program provides excellent free materials on fall assessment and prevention for health care providers and older adults (Box 19.9).

Best Practice Fall Risk Reduction in Acute and Long-Term Care

Fall risk-reduction programs in hospitals and long-term care settings should be designed to meet organizational needs and to match patient population needs and clinical realities of the staff. A system-level quality improvement approach, including educational programs for staff, has been reported to decrease fall rates in hospitals and nursing homes (Dykes et al, 2017; Gray-Miceli et al, 2016, 2017; Quigley et al, 2016).

BOX 19.11   Suggested Components of Fall Risk–Reduction Interventions

- Adaptation or modification of the home environment
- Withdrawal or minimization of psychoactive medications
- Withdrawal or minimization of other medications
- Detection and prevention of delirium
- Management of orthostatic hypotension
- Continence programs such as prompted voiding
- Management of foot problems and footwear
- Exercise, particularly balance, strength, and gait training
- Staff and patient education

From American Geriatrics Society/British Geriatrics Society: *2010 AGS/BGS clinical practice guideline: Prevention of falls in older persons, Summary of recommendations*, 2010. https://geriatricscareonline.org/application/content/products/CL014/html/CL014_BOOK001.html. Accessed March 2018.

Suggested components of fall prevention programs are presented in Box 19.11.

Some examples of effective programs in acute care settings include Acute Care of the Elderly units (ACE), Nurses Improving Care for Healthsystem Elders (NICHE), and the Geriatric Resource Nurse (GRN) model. The Hospital Elder Life Program (HELP) is another valuable resource in fall prevention in the hospital (Chapter 2). Innovative programs in nursing homes include the Visiting Angels and neighborhood watch teams. In the Visiting Angels program, alert residents visit and converse with cognitively impaired residents in the late afternoon and evening when fall risk starts to rise. Neighborhood watch teams involve the evening and night staff in morning reviews of any fall or incident that happened during the night. The optimal bundle of interventions is not established but suggested components are presented in Box 19.12.

Best Practice Fall Risk Reduction in the Community

Group and home-based exercise programs, along with home safety interventions, reduced the rate of falls and risk of falling in community-dwelling older adults. Vision screening, medication reduction, assessment of cardiovascular syncope and postural hypotension, providing hip protectors and other assistive devices, and education on falls and fall prevention also have been associated with decreased fall risk (Taylor-Pilae et al, 2017). Home-based tai chi chuan (TCC) has been shown to reduce falls and improve physical performance among older adults in community settings more than conventional lower extremity exercise training (Hwang et al, 2016; Li et al, 2016).

Environmental Modifications

Among community-living older adults, falls are more likely to occur during activities of daily living but occur most frequently when the individual is transferring or changing physical positions (sitting to standing, using a bathtub/shower, or walking downstairs). Environmental modifications alone have not been shown to reduce falls, but when included as part of a multifactorial program, they may be of benefit in risk reduction. A home safety assessment and home modification interventions are effective in reducing the rates of falls, especially for individuals at high risk of falling and those with visual impairments. However, referrals for home safety assessment are not consistently done in primary care (Phelan et al, 2016). A recent survey of community-living older adults found that approximately one-half reported never seeing a home safety checklist, an accessible and easy tool for older adults to complete (Lack and Noimontree, 2018). As part of the STEADI program, the CDC provides a comprehensive home fall prevention checklist that can be used by older adults and clinicians (Box 19.9).

In institutional settings, the patient care environment should be assessed routinely for extrinsic factors that may contribute to falls and corrective action taken. About 50% to 70% of falls in hospitals occur while transferring between bed/chair; and 10% to 20% occur in bathrooms (Quigley et al, 2016). Patients should be able to access the bathroom or be provided with a bedside commode, routine assistance to toilet, and programs such as prompted voiding (Chapter 16). Dual stiffness flooring which incorporates a layer of compressible material meant to cushion falls can reduce fractures in nursing homes (Morley, 2017). Important areas to check for safety are presented in Box 19.13.

BOX 19.12   System-Level Interventions for Fall Prevention in Acute Care

- Nurse Champions
- Use of advanced practice nurse consultation
- Teach Backs (all patients and families receive education about their fall and injury risks)
- Comfort Care and Safety Rounds
- Safety Huddle Postfall
- Interventions to Reduce Trauma/Protective Bundles (patients with risk factors for serious injury such as osteoporosis, anticoagulant use, history of head injury, or falls are automatically placed on high-risk fall precautions and interventions to reduce risk of serious injury; bundles may include interventions such as bedside mat on floor at side of bed, height-adjustable bed, helmet use, hip protectors, comfort and safety rounds)
- Interprofessional teams

BOX 19.13   Environmental Safety Check

- Outdoor grounds and indoor floor surfaces checked for spills, wet areas, and unevenness
- Hallways, doorways have clear paths free of clutter, equipment
- Proper illumination and functioning of lights, including night lights
- Tabletops, furniture, and beds are sturdy and in good repair
- Grab rails and nonskid appliqués or mats are in place in the bathroom (toilet and shower)
- Appropriate shoe wear is available and used
- Adaptive aids are available, work properly, and are in good repair
- Bed rails do not collapse when used for transitioning or support
- Bed wheels lock
- Patient gowns/clothing does not cause tripping
- IV poles are sturdy if used during ambulation and tubing does not cause tripping

Assistive Devices

Research on multifactorial interventions including the use of assistive devices has demonstrated benefits in fall risk reduction. Many devices are available that are designed for specific conditions and limitations. Physical therapists provide training on use of assistive devices, and nurses can supervise correct use. Improper use of these devices can lead to increased fall risk (Box 19.14). Creative solutions for fall prevention have been implemented in nursing homes in the United Kingdom and involve the use of walkers. The Pimp My Zimmer campaign ("zimmer" is UK term for walkers) was begun by staff in a nursing home. Residents were falling, especially those with dementia, because they would forget to use their walker or pick up the wrong walker, which was not adjusted for their height. With the help of staff and children in the area, the residents decorated their walkers—the fancier the better. In addition to being fun and making life more enjoyable, the intervention also decreased falls. In one care home, schoolchildren came in and helped the residents decorate their walkers (http://www.wales.nhs.uk/sitesplus/866/news/47028).

For the community-dwelling individual, Medicare may cover up to 80% of the cost of assistive devices with a written prescription. New technologies such as "smart canes" that assess gait and fall risk or that "talk" and provide feedback to the user, sensors that detect when falls have occurred or when risk of falling is increasing, and other developing assistive technologies hold the potential to significantly improve functional ability, safety, and independence for older adults (Muchna et al, 2017) (Chapter 20).

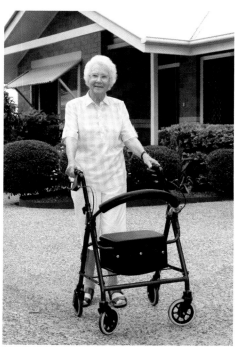

Maintaining ambulation and safety with appropriate assistive devices. (©iStock.com/pamspix.)

BOX 19.14 Tips for Best Practice

Use of Assistive Devices

Cane Use

- Place your cane firmly on the ground before you take a step, and do not place it too far ahead of you. Put all of your weight on your unaffected leg, and then move the cane and your affected leg at a comfortable distance forward. With your weight supported on both the cane and your affected leg, step through with your unaffected leg.
- Wear low-heeled, nonskid shoes. Best to have the individual wear the kind of shoes he or she is accustomed to wearing, and consideration should be given to properly fit orthotic shoes as appropriate.
- When using a cane on stairs, step up with the unaffected leg and down with the affected leg. Use the cane as support when lifting the affected leg. Bring the cane up to the step just reached before climbing another step. When descending, place the cane on the next step down, move the affected leg down, and then move the unaffected leg down.
- Every assistive device must be adjusted to individual height; the top of the cane should align with the crease of the wrist.
- Choose a size and shape of cane handle that fits comfortably in the palm; like a tight shoe, it will be a constant irritant if it is not properly fitted.
- Cane tips are most secure when they are flat at the bottom and have a series of rings. Replace tips frequently because they wear out, and a worn tip is insecure.

Walker Use

- When using a walker, stand upright and lift or roll the walker with both hands a step's length ahead of you. Lean slightly forward, and hold the arms of the walker for support. Step toward it with the affected leg and then bring the unaffected leg forward.
- Do not climb stairs with a walker.

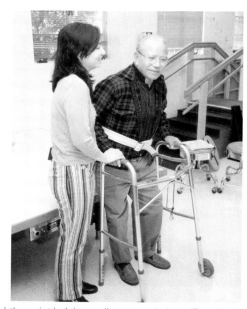

A physical therapist helping a client to ambulate. (From Ignatavicius DD, Workman ML: *Medical-surgical nursing: patient-centered collaborative care*, ed 6, St Louis, 2010, Saunders.)

Safe Patient Handling

Lifting, transferring, and repositioning patients are the most common tasks that lead to injury for health care staff and patients in hospital and nursing home environments. Handling and moving patients offers multiple challenges because of variations in size, physical abilities, cognitive function, level of cooperation, and changes in condition. Evidence-based practices for safe patient handling include: (1) use of patient handling equipment/devices; (2) patient-care ergonomic assessment protocols; (3) no lift policies; (4) training on proper use of patient handling equipment/devices; and (5) patient lift teams. Examples of helpful equipment are ceiling- and floor-based dependent lifts, sit-to-stand assists, ambulation aids, motorized hospital beds, powered shower chairs, and friction-reducing devices (American Nurses Association, 2013; Campo et al, 2013). Key aspects of patient assessment to improve safety for patients and staff are presented in Box 19.15.

Wheelchairs

Wheelchairs are a necessary adjunct at some level of immobility and for some individuals, but they are overused in nursing homes, with up to 80% of residents spending time sitting in a wheelchair every day. Often, the individual is not assessed for therapeutic treatment and restorative ambulation programs to improve mobility and function. Improperly maintained or ill-fitting wheelchairs can cause pressure ulcers, skin tears, bruises and abrasions, and nerve impingement, and contribute to falls in nursing homes. It is important that a professional evaluate the wheelchair for proper fit and provide training on proper use, and evaluate the resident for more appropriate mobility and seating devices and ambulation programs. There are many new assistive devices that could replace wheelchairs, such as small walkers with wheels and seats.

All nursing homes need to implement programs that promote ambulation and improve function. Brief walks and repeated chair stands four times a day improved walking and endurance in frail, deconditioned, cognitively impaired nursing home residents. If the individual is unable to ambulate without assistance, he or she should be seated in a comfortable chair with frequent repositioning and wheelchairs should be used for transport only. Electric scooters and wheelchairs may also be appropriate for some residents, but instruction on safe use is necessary. At one Veterans Affairs medical center, the physical therapists held driving classes to teach safety with these devices.

The GROW initiative (Getting Residents Out of Wheelchairs) (Box 19.9) was conceived by a group of health professionals to lobby against the overuse of wheelchairs in nursing homes. The program advocates for increased ambulation whenever possible and decreasing the use of wheelchairs when regular chairs could be used for stationary seating.

Osteoporosis Treatment/Vitamin D Supplementation

Practice guidelines recommend calcium and vitamin D supplements for older adults with osteoporosis to prevent fractures. Evidence of the association between calcium, vitamin D, or combined calcium and vitamin D supplements and fracture risk has not reached consistent conclusions. A recent meta-analysis reported that calcium, calcium plus vitamin D, and vitamin D supplementation were not significantly associated with a lower incidence of hip, nonvertebral, vertebral, or total fractures in community-dwelling older adults. There is evidence that these supplements may lower fracture risk for individuals living in residential institutions because of their poorer mobility, infrequent sun exposure, and poorer diet. However, findings do not support the routine use of these supplements in community-dwelling older adults (Zhao et al, 2017) (Chapter 26).

Hip Protectors

The use of hip protectors for prevention of hip fractures in high-risk individuals may be considered. There is some evidence that they may be protective when used in individuals who are at risk for hip fracture, but further research is needed to determine their effectiveness (Quigley et al, 2016). Compliance has been a concern related to the ease of application and removing them quickly enough for toileting, but newer designs that are more attractive and practical may assist with compliance issues.

Alarms/Motion Sensors/Staff Observation

Alarms, either personal or chair/bed, are often used in fall risk-reduction programs. Alarms were designed to be early warning systems and there has been no research to support their effectiveness in prevention of a fall. Use of alarms may increase patient agitation, especially in cognitively impaired individuals. Silent alarms, visual or auditory monitoring systems, motion detectors, and physical staff presence may be more effective. Continuous video monitoring has been demonstrated as an effective intervention to significantly reduce the incidence of patient falls and the likelihood of injury if the patient does experience a fall. Motion sensors inside patient rooms may be another viable, cost-efficient, unobtrusive solution to prevent and detect falls (Potter et al, 2017; Rantz et al, 2015; Sand-Jecklin et al, 2016). One of the most effective methods used in fall prevention is every 1 to 2 hour rounding to assess patient needs (Jackson, 2016). The use of sitters is very costly and is not effective in preventing falls.

RESTRAINTS AND SIDE RAILS

Definition and History

A physical restraint is defined as any manual method, physical or mechanical device, material, or equipment that immobilizes or reduces the ability of a patient to move his or her arms, legs, body, or head freely. Restraints include vests, belts, mittens, bedrails, geriatric chairs, and other devices. A chemical restraint is the use of a medication that is not a standard treatment or dosage for the individual's condition as a restriction to manage behavior or restrict freedom of movement. Historically, restraints and side rails have been used for the "protection" of the patient and for the security of the patient and staff. Originally, restraints were used to control the behavior of individuals with mental illness considered to be dangerous to themselves or others (Evans and Strumpf, 1989).

Research over the past 30 years by nurses such as Lois Evans, Neville Strumpf, and Elizabeth Capezuti has shown that the practice of physical restraint is ineffective and hazardous. The use of physical restraints in long-term care settings was effectively addressed almost 30 years ago through nursing home reform legislation, resulting in a major reduction of physical restraint use in these facilities. Physical restraint use is part of public reporting for nursing homes through the Centers for Medicare and Medicaid Services (CMS) Nursing Home Compare website and a critical quality indicator. Restraints are a nurse-sensitive indicator. The Joint Commission and the CMS have focused on restraint reduction strategies in acute care over the past 15 to 20 years but the use still remains a concern, particularly in intensive care units (ICUs).

Consequences of Restraints

Physical restraints, intended to prevent injury, do not protect patients from falling, wandering, or removing tubes and other medical devices. Physical restraints may actually exacerbate many of the problems for which they are used and can cause serious injury and death, and emotional and physical problems. Physical restraints are associated with higher death rates, injurious falls, nosocomial infections, incontinence, contractures, pressure ulcers, agitation, and depression. Although prevention of falls is most frequently cited as the primary reason for using restraints, restraints do not prevent serious injury and may even increase the risk of injury and death. Injuries occur as a result of the patient attempting to remove the restraint or attempting to get out of bed while restrained.

The use of restraints is a great source of physical and psychological distress to older adults and may intensify agitation and contribute to depression. Side rails may be seen as a barrier rather than a reminder of the need to request assistance with transfers. And, for some older adults, especially those with a history of trauma (such as that induced by war, rape, or domestic violence), side rails may cause fear and agitation and a feeling of being jailed or caged (Box 19.16).

Side Rails

Side rails are no longer viewed as simply attachments to a patient's bed but are considered restraints with all the accompanying concerns just discussed. Side rails are now defined as restraints or restrictive devices when used to impede a person's ability to voluntarily get out of bed when the person cannot lower them by themselves. Restrictive side

---

BOX 19.16 Being Restrained

"I felt like a dog and cried all night. It hurt me to have to be tied up. I felt like I was nobody, that I was dirt. It makes me cry to talk about it. The hospital is worse than a jail."

"I don't remember misbehaving, but I may have been deranged from all the pills they gave me. Normally, I am spirited, but I am also good and obedient. Nevertheless, the nurse tied me down, like Jesus on the cross, by bandaging both wrists and ankles. . . . It felt awful, I hurt and I worried. Callers, including men friends, saw me like that and thought I lost something. I lost a little personal prestige. I was embarrassed, like a child placed in a corner for being bad. I had been important . . . and to be tied down in bed took a big toll. . . . I haven't forgotten the pain and the indignity of being tied."

---

rail use is defined as two full-length or four half-length raised side rails. If the patient uses a half- or quarter-length upper side rail to assist in getting in and out of bed, it is not considered a restraint. The proper use of side rails can be considered a means of assisting in-bed movement and getting in and out of bed (Morse et al, 2015). Side rails manufactured for use on hospital beds have been redesigned and are no longer a threat to patient entrapment but use of outmoded designs and incorrect assembly continue to be a concern. The CMS require nursing homes to conduct individualized assessments of residents, provide alternatives, or clearly document the need for restrictive side rails.

Restraint-Free Care

Restraint-free care is now the standard of practice and an indicator of quality care in all health care settings, although transition to that standard is still in progress, particularly in acute care settings. Physical restraint use in acute care is now predominantly in ICUs, particularly for patients with medical devices and those with delirium. Physical restraint is more likely to be used in ICUs because nurses fear tube dislodgement related to greater frequency of invasive lines and mechanical ventilation. However, physical restraints are not effective in preventing unplanned endotracheal extubation and increase its risk threefold (Hall et al, 2018). Daily evaluation of the necessity of medical devices (intravenous lines, nasogastric tubes, catheters, endotracheal tubes), and securing or camouflaging (hiding) the device, is important (Box 19.17). Both the American Geriatrics Society and the American Board of Internal Medicine recommend that physical restraints should not be used to manage behavioral symptoms of hospitalized older adults with delirium (American Geriatrics Society, 2014). Further research is needed in ICU settings to determine the best strategies to manage delirium (Chapter 29).

Implementing best practice nursing in fall risk reduction and restraint-free care is a complex clinical decision-making process and calls for recognition, assessment, and intervention for physical and psychosocial concerns contributing to patient safety, knowledge of restraint alternatives, interdisciplinary teamwork, and institutional commitment. Nursing staff can benefit from educational

BOX 19.17 Tips for Best Practice

Dealing With Tubes, Lines, and Other Medical Devices

- First question: "Is the device really necessary?" Remove it as soon as possible.
- Preoperative teaching about the device: allowing the person to see the tubes may be effective in decreasing anxiety about devices.
- Use guided exploration and a mirror to help the patient understand what devices are in place and why.
- Provide comfort care to the site—oral and nasal care, anchoring of tubing, topical anesthetic on site.
- Indwelling catheters should be used only if the patient needs intensive output monitoring or has an obstruction.
- Weigh risks and benefits of restraint versus therapy: alternatives available—for example, replace intravenous (IV) tubing with saline lock, deliver medications intramuscularly (IM), consider intermittent IV administration or hypodermoclysis.
- Use camouflage: clothing or elastic sleeves, temporary air splint (occupational therapy can be helpful), skin sleeves to prevent IV tube dislodgement.
- Use mitts instead of wrist restraints; use roll belts instead of vest restraints.

- Use diversional activity aprons (zipping-unzipping, threading exercises, dials and knobs), busy box, therapeutic activity kit, twiddle (activity) muff.
- Hide lines by placing them in an unobtrusive place; hang IV bags behind the patient's line of vision, have patient wear long sleeves or double surgical gowns with cuffs to prevent access.
- Nasogastric (NG) tubes—replace with percutaneous endoscopic gastrostomy (PEG) tube if necessary but obtain comprehensive speech therapy swallowing evaluation. If NG tube is used, use as small a lumen as possible to minimize irritation; consider taping with occlusive dressings.
- Cover the PEG tube or abdominal incisions and other tubes with an abdominal binder and/or sweat pants.
- For men with indwelling catheters—shave area just above pubis, and tape catheter to pubis. *Never* secure catheter to leg (causes discomfort and can cause a fistula). Run tubing around back and down leg to a leg bag. Patient should wear underpants and pajama pants.
- Remove restraints while working with the patient.
- Use a modified soft collar for tracheostomy protection.

programs focused on correcting misperceptions related to physical restraint application and the use of alternatives (Hall et al, 2017). The use of advanced practice nurse consultation in implementing alternatives to restraints has been most effective. Important areas of focus derived from research on advanced practice nurse consultations are presented in Box 19.18. Many of the suggestions on safety and fall risk reduction in this chapter can be used to promote a safe and restraint-free environment. Fall risk reduction and alternative strategies to restraints are presented in Box 19.19.

BOX 19.18 Suggestions From Advanced Practice Nursing Consultation on Restraint-Free Fall Prevention Interventions

- Compensating for memory loss (e.g., improving behavior, anticipating needs, providing visual and physical cues)
- Improving impaired mobility; reducing injury potential
- Evaluating nocturia/incontinence; reducing sleep disturbances
- Implementing restraint-free fall prevention interventions based on conducting careful individualized assessments; what works for one individual may not necessarily be effective for another
- Careful medication review

BOX 19.19 Tips for Best Practice

Fall Risk Reduction and Restraint Alternatives

Assessment
- Work with the interdisciplinary team; nurses cannot manage these complicated challenges alone.
- Perform fall risk screening; gait, balance, and mobility assessment; and multifactorial assessment as indicated.
- Individualize the patient's plan of care based on risk factors and condition.
- Assess ambulation ability; refer to physical therapy for walking and/or strengthening programs.
- Check for postural hypotension
- Use a behavior log to track when the person is trying to get up and/or when he or she seems agitated.
- Assess for delirium/dementia.
- Assess vision and hearing. If the person wears glasses, hearing aid, or dentures, ensure that the assistive devices are worn.
- Assess continence status.
- Assess for pain and ensure that pain is well managed.
- Involve family and all staff in fall risk–reduction education and activities.
- Inform all staff of fall risk, and put fall risk and fall risk-reduction interventions on care plan.
- Use identification bracelet or door sign to indicate patients at risk for falling.
- Use red socks with treads to identify patients at risk.

Patient Room
- Evaluate the patient's ability to transfer in and out of bed and adjust height of bed for safety.
- Use a concave mattress.
- Use bed boundary markers to mark the edges of the bed, such as mattress bumpers, rolled blanket, or "swimming noodles" under sheets.
- If the person is (or has been married), line the spouse's side of the bed with pillows or bolsters.
- Place a soft floor mat or a mattress by the bed to cushion any falls.
- Use a water mattress to reduce movement to the edge of the bed.
- Remove wheels from the bed.
- Clear the floor of debris or excessive furniture; make sure it is not wet or slippery.
- Place nonskid strips on the floor next to the bed; ensure that floors are nonskid.
- Place a call bell within reach, and make sure the patient can use it—attach the call bell to the patient's garment or obtain an adapted call device.
- Have a purse (empty or without harmful items or important papers or money) in the bed with the person, if a woman.
- Ensure all personal items are within reach.
- Have ambulation devices within reach, and make sure the patient knows how to use them properly.

Continued

BOX 19.19   Tips for Best Practice—cont'd

Fall Risk Reduction and Restraint Alternatives

- Provide a trapeze or patient assist handles (transfer bars) to enhance mobility in bed.
- If the person is able, he or she should walk at every opportunity possible. If the patient walked in or could walk before hospitalization, make every effort to keep the patient walking during hospitalization.
- Do frequent bed checks, especially during the evening and at night.
- Be especially alert for falls at change-of-shift times.
- Understand that very few people spend all day in bed; activity is necessary.
- Provide diversional activities (catalogs, puzzles, therapeutic activity kit) (http://consultgerirn.org/uploads/File/trythis/try_this_d4.pdf).
- Know sleeping patterns—if the person is usually up during the night, get him or her up in a chair and keep at nursing station or involve in activities.

Bathroom
- Establish toileting plan, and take the person to the bathroom frequently.
- Have the person use a bedside commode.
- Make sure the person knows the location of the bathroom—leave the door open so that he or she can see the toilet, put a picture of a toilet on the door; clear the path to the bathroom; provide night lights; paint the door frame around the toilet and the light switch with luminous paint; put

a light inside the toilet bowl; put glow-in-the dark footprints going from bed to toilet door.
- Provide grab bars in the bathroom and shower; provide a shower chair with suction bottom.
- Provide an elevated toilet seat.
- Have the person wear clothing that is easy to pull down for toileting.

On the Unit
- Assess for environmental hazards.
- Keep the person in a supervised area or room within view of the nurses' station.
- Have the person sit in a reclining chair, chair with a deep seat, bean bag chair, rocker—keep close to nurses' station in the chair.
- Consider occupational therapy evaluation for seating devices.
- Provide a supervised area and meaningful activities.
- Provide hip protectors, helmets, and arm pads for high-risk individuals.
- Investigate the Hospital Elder Life Program (HELP) and consider implementing (http://www.hospitalelderlifeprogram.org/public/public-main.ph.).
- Provide a restraint management cart with alternative restraint products arranged in order of least restrictive measures.

KEY CONCEPTS

- Mobility provides opportunities for exercise, exploration, and pleasure and is the crux of maintaining independence.
- As one ages, illnesses and changes in bones, muscles, and ligaments affect balance and gait and increase instability. Gait and mobility impairments are not an inevitable consequence of aging, but often a result of chronic diseases or remote or recent trauma.
- Impairment of mobility is an early predictor of physical disability and associated with poor outcomes such as falling, loss of independence, depression, decreased quality of life, institutionalization, and death.
- Falls are one of the most important geriatric syndromes and the leading cause of morbidity and mortality for individuals older than 65 years of age.
- The risk of falling increases with the number of risk factors. Most falls occur from a combination of intrinsic and extrinsic factors that unite at a certain point in time.

- Fall risk assessments identify risk factors but do not provide information on why someone is at risk or what the actual risk factors are. Comprehensive assessments are essential for fall prevention efforts and the development of individualized interventions.
- Postfall assessments (PFAs) must be used to identify multifactorial, complex fall and injury risk factors in those who have fallen.
- Physical restraints, intended to prevent injury, do not protect patients from falling, wandering, or removing tubes and other medical devices. Physical restraints may actually exacerbate many of the problems for which they are used and can cause serious injury and death, and emotional and physical problems.
- Restraint free care is the standard of practice in all settings, and knowledge of restraint alternatives and safety measures is essential for nurses.

NURSING STUDY: FALL RISK REDUCTION

Jim is an 80-year-old World War II veteran who has resided in the skilled nursing facility for 2 years. His diagnoses include Alzheimer's disease, hypertension, and depression. Medications include an antihypertensive drug and an antidepressant. He is able to walk but has an unsteady gait and requires assistance. Due to his cognitive status, he often attempts to ambulate alone and today was found on the floor in the bathroom. No injuries were immediately apparent, and he says he is fine. His partner of 30 years is requesting that restraints be applied to prevent him from suffering injuries from falling.

On the basis of the nursing study, develop a nursing care plan using the following procedure[a]:
- List information that provides objective data.
- Discuss the assessment that needs to be completed related to Jim's fall.

- From these data, identify and state, using an accepted format, two nursing diagnoses you determine are most significant to Jim at this time.
- Determine and state outcome criteria for each diagnosis. These must reflect some alleviation of the problem identified in the nursing diagnosis and must be stated in concrete and measurable terms.
- Plan and state one or more interventions for each diagnosed problem. Provide specific documentation of the source used to determine the appropriate intervention.
- Evaluate the success of the intervention. Interventions must correlate directly with the stated outcome criteria to measure the outcome success.

[a]Students are advised to refer to their nursing diagnosis text and identify possible or potential problems.

CRITICAL THINKING QUESTIONS AND ACTIVITIES

1. What risk factors for falls are present in the nursing study presented above?
2. What interventions are appropriate to ensure safety?
3. How would you respond to the partner's request for the use of restraints?

RESEARCH QUESTIONS

1. What types of gait disorders trigger falls and in what situations?
2. How does cognitive impairment influence risk of falls?
3. What are the psychological reactions of older adults to the use of assistive devices for ambulation?
4. What factors among community-dwelling older adults are most hazardous for mobility?
5. What are the major reasons individuals are restrained in ICUs and what interventions are most effective in decreasing restraint use in this setting?

REFERENCES

Alexander N: Balance, gait and mobility. In Ham R, Sloane R, Warshaw G, et al, editors: *Primary care geriatrics*, ed 6, Philadelphia, PA, 2014, Elsevier Saunders, pp 227–234.

American Geriatrics Society: American Geriatrics Society identifies another five things that healthcare providers and patients should question, *J Am Geriatr Soc* 62(5):950–960, 2014.

American Geriatrics Society/British Geriatrics Society: *2010 AGS/BGS clinical practice guideline: prevention of falls in older persons, summary of recommendations*, 2010. https://geriatricscareonline.org/ProductAbstract/updated-american-geriatrics-societybritish-geriatrics-society-clinical-practice-guideline-for-prevention-of-falls-in-older-persons-and-recommendations/CL014. Accessed April 2019.

American Nurses Association: *Safe patient handling and mobility: interprofessional national standards across the care continuum*, 2013. https://www.nursingworld.org/~498de8/globalassets/practiceandpolicy/work-environment/health—safety/ana-sphmcover__finalapproved.pdf. Accessed April 2019.

Bergland A, Jørgensen L, Emaus N, Strand BH: Mobility as a predictor of all-cause mortality in older men and women: 11.8 year follow-up in the Tromsø study, *BMC Health Serv Res* 17(1):22, 2017.

Booth V, Hood V, Kearney F: Interventions incorporating physical and cognitive elements to reduce falls risk in cognitively impaired older adults: a systematic review, *JBI Database System Rev Implement Rep* 14(5):110–135, 2016.

Booth V, Logan R, Harwood R, Hood V: Falls prevention interventions in older adults with cognitive impairment: a systematic review of reviews, *Int J Ther Rehabil* 22(6):289–296, 2015.

Campo M, Shiyko MP, Margulis H, Darragh AR: Effect of a safe patient handling program on rehabilitation outcomes, *Arch Phys Med Rehabil* 94(1):17–22, 2013.

Centers for Disease Control and Prevention (CDC): *Important facts about falls*, 2017. https://www.cdc.gov/homeandrecreationalsafety/falls/adultfalls.html. Accessed February 2018.

Chen TY, Lee S, Buxton OM: A greater extent of insomnia symptoms and physician-recommended sleep medication use predict fall risk in community-dwelling older adults, *Sleep* 40(11), 2017.

de Vries M, Seppala LJ, Daams JG, et al: Fall-risk-increasing drugs: a systematic review and meta-analysis: I. Cardiovascular drugs, *J Am Med Dir Assoc* 19(4):371.e1–371.e9, 2018.

Dykes PC, Duckworth M, Cunningham S, et al: Pilot testing fall TIPS (Tailoring Interventions for Patient Safety): a patient-centered fall prevention toolkit, *Jt Comm J Qual Patient Saf* 43(8):403–413, 2017.

Federal Interagency Forum on Aging-Related Statistics: *Older Americans 2016: key indicators of well-being*, Washington, DC, 2016, US Government Printing Office.

Fink HA, Kuskowski MA, Marshall LM: Association of stressful life events with incident falls and fractures in older men: the osteoporotic fractures in men (MrOS) study, *Age Ageing* 43:103–108, 2014.

Finucane C, O'Connell MD, Donoghue O, Richardson K, Savva GM, Kenny RA: Impaired orthostatic blood pressure recovery is associated with unexplained and injurious falls, *J Am Geriatr Soc* 65:474–482, 2017.

Freedman VA, Carr D, Cornman JC, Lucas RE: Aging, mobility impairments and subjective wellbeing, *Disabil Health J* 10:525–531, 2017.

Gardner RC, Byers AL, Barnes DE, Li Y, Boscardin J, Yaffe K: Mild TBI and risk of Parkinson disease: a chronic effects of neurotrauma consortium study, *Neurology* 90(20):e1771–e1779, 2018.

Gopinath B, McMahon CM, Burlutsky G, Mitchell P: Hearing and vision impairment and the 5-year incidence of falls in older adults, *Age Ageing* 45(3):409–414, 2016.

Gray-Miceli D: Impaired mobility and functional decline in older adults: evidence to facilitate a practice change, *Nurs Clin North Am* 52:469–487, 2017.

Gray-Miceli D, de Cordova PB, Crane GL, Quigley P, Ratcliffe SJ: Nursing home registered nurses' and licensed practical nurses' knowledge of causes of falls, *J Nurs Care Qual* 31(2):153–160, 2016.

Gray-Miceli D, Mazzia L, Crane G: Advanced practice nurse-led statewide collaborative to reduce falls in hospitals, *J Nurs Care Qual* 32(2):120–125, 2017.

Gray-Miceli D, Ratcliffe SJ, Johnson J: Use of a postfall assessment tool to prevent falls, *West J Nurs Res* 32(7):932–948, 2010.

Gupta P, Aravindhan A, Gand ATL, et al: Association between the severity of diabetic retinopathy and falls in an Asian population with diabetes: the Singapore epidemiology of eye diseases study, *JAMA Ophthalmol* 135(12):1410–1416, 2017.

Hall DK, Zimbro KS, Maduro RS, Petrovitch D, Ver Schneider P, Morgan M: Impact of a restraint management bundle on restraint use in an intensive care unit, *J Nurs Care Qual* 33(2):143–148, 2018.

Hwang HF, Chen SJ, Lee-Hsieh J, Chien DK, Chen CY, Lin MR: Effects of home-based tai chi and lower extremity training and self-practice on falls and functional outcomes in older fallers from the emergency department-a randomized controlled trial, *J Am Geriatr Soc* 64(3):518–525, 2016.

Isaranuwatchai W, Perdrizet J, Markle-Reid M, Hoch JS: Cost-effectiveness analysis of a multifactorial fall prevention intervention in older home care clients at risk for falling, *BMC Geriatr* 17:199, 2017.

Jackson KM: Improving nursing home falls management program by enhancing standard of care with collaborative care multi-interventional protocol focused on fall prevention, *J Nurs Educ Pract* 6(6):84–95, 2016.

Krbot Skorić M, Crnošija L, Habek M, Pavelić A: Postprandial hypotension in neurological disorders: systematic review and meta-analysis, *Clin Auton Res* 27(4):263–271, 2017.

Kruschke C, Butcher HK: Evidence-based practice guideline: fall prevention for older adults, *J Gerontol Nurs* 43(11):15–21, 2017.

Lach HW, Harrison BE, Phongphanngam S: Falls and fall prevention in older adults with early-stage dementia: an integrative review, *Res Gerontol Nurs* 10(3):139–148, 2017.

Lach HW, Noimontree W: Fall prevention among community-dwelling older adults: current guidelines and older adult responses, *J Gerontol Nurs* 44(9):21–29, 2018.

Li F, Harmer P, Fitzgerald K: Implementing an evidence-based fall prevention intervention in community senior centers, *Am J Public Health* 106(11):2026–2031, 2016.

Lipsitz LA: Orthostatic hypotension and falls, *J Am Geriatr Soc* 65: 470–471, 2017.

Menz HB: Chronic foot pain in older people, *Maturitas* 91:110–114, 2016.

Morley JE: The future of long-term care, *J Am Med Dir Assoc* 18:1–7, 2017.

Morse JM, Gervais P, Pooler C, Merryweather A, Doig AK, Bloswick D: The safety of hospital beds: ingress, egress, and in-bed mobility, *Glob Qual Nurs Res* 2:2333393615575321, 2015.

Muchna A, Najafi B, Wendel CS, Schwenk M, Armstrong DG, Mohler J: Foot problems in older adults: associations with incident falls, frailty syndrome, and sensor-derived gait, balance, and physical activity measures, *J Am Podiatr Med Assoc* 108(2):126–139, 2018.

Musich S, Wang SS, Ruiz J, Hawkins K, Wicker E: Falls-related drug use and risk of falls among older adults: a study in a US Medicare population, *Drugs Aging* 34:555–565, 2017.

Nelson A, Baptiste AS: Evidence-based practices for safe patient handling and movement, *Online J Issues Nurs* 9(3):4, 2004. http://www.seiu1991.org/files/2013/07/Audrey_Nelson_Safe_Patient_Handling.pdf. Accessed March 2018.

Nishijima DK, Gaona SD, Waechter T, et al: Out-of-hospital triage of older adults with head injury: a retrospective study of the effect of adding "anticoagulation or antiplatelet medication use" as a criterion, *Ann Emerg Med* 70(2):127–138.e6, 2017.

Peach T, Pollock K, van der Wardt V, das Nair R, Logan P, Harwood RH: Attitudes of older people with mild dementia and mild cognitive impairment and their relatives about falls risk and prevention: a qualitative study, *PLoS One* 12(5):e0177530, 2017.

Phelan EA, Aerts S, Dowler D, Eckstrom E, Casey CM: Adoption of evidence-based fall prevention practices in primary care for older adults with a history of falls, *Front Public Health* 4:190, 2016.

Pirker W, Katzenschlager R: Gait disorders in adults and the elderly: a clinical guide, *Wien Klin Wochenschr* 129(3-4):81–95, 2017.

Potter P, Allen K, Costantinou E, et al: Evaluation of sensor technology to detect fall risk and prevent falls in acute care, *Jt Comm J Qual Patient Saf* 43(8):414–421, 2017.

Quigley PA, Barnett SD, Bulat T, Friedman Y: Reducing falls and fall-related injuries in medical-surgical units: one-year multi-hospital falls collaborative, *J Nurs Care Qual* 31(2):139–145, 2016.

Rantz M, Skubic M, Abbott C, et al: Automated in-home fall risk assessment and detection sensor system for elders, *Gerontologist* 55(Suppl 1):S78–S87, 2015.

Riemen AH, Hutchison JD: The multidisciplinary management of hip fractures in older patients, *Orthop Trauma* 30(2):117–122, 2016.

Rubenstein L, Dillard D: Falls. In Ham R, Sloane P, Warshaw G, et al, editors: *Primary care geriatrics*, ed 6, Philadelphia, PA, 2014, Elsevier Saunders, pp 235–242.

Sand-Jecklin K, Johnson JR, Tylka S: Protecting patient safety: can video monitoring prevent falls in high-risk patient populations? *J Nurs Care Qual* 31(2):131–138, 2016.

Schaffert J, LoBue C, White CL, et al: Traumatic brain injury history is associated with an earlier age of dementia onset in autopsy-confirmed Alzheimer's disease, *Neuropsychology* 32(4):410–416, 2018.

Shuman CJ, Montie M, Hoffman GJ, et al: Older adults' perceptions of their fall risk and prevention strategies after transitioning from hospital to home, *J Gerontol Nurs* 45(1):23–30, 2019.

Tang VL, Sudore R, Cenzer IS, et al: Rates of recovery to pre-fracture function in older persons with hip fracture: an observational study, *J Gen Intern Med* 32(2):153–158, 2017.

Taylor-Piliae RE, Peterson R, Mohler MJ: Clinical and community strategies to prevent falls and fall-related injuries among community-dwelling older adults, *Nurs Clin North Am* 52:489–497, 2017.

Tinetti ME: Performance-oriented assessment of mobility problems in elderly patients, *J Am Geriatr Soc* 34(2):119–126, 1986.

Torvinen-Kiiskinen S, Tolppanen AM, Koponen M, et al: Antidepressant use and risk of hip fractures among community-dwelling persons with and without Alzheimer's disease, *Int J Geriatr Psychiatry* 32:e107–e115, 2017.

Zhao JG, Zeng XT, Wang J, Liu L: Association between calcium or vitamin D supplementation and fracture incidence in community-dwelling older adults: a systematic review and meta-analysis, *JAMA* 318(24):2466–2482, 2017.

Zhao YL, Alderden J, Lind BK, Kim H: A comprehensive assessment of risk factors for falls in community-dwelling older adults, *J Gerontol Nurs* 44(10):40–48, 2018.

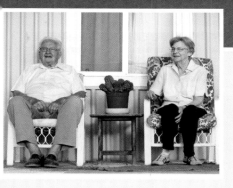

20

Safety and Security

Theris A. Touhy

http://evolve.elsevier.com/Touhy/TwdHlthAging

A STUDENT SPEAKS

During the community nursing experience my client decided to stay in her own home in spite of being barely able to shuffle around. A community program provided a homemaker for a few hours daily. She had to rely on the goodwill of neighbors when the budget for those services was discontinued. She wants so much to remain in her own home. I worry about her but don't know what I should do.

Jennifer, age 24

AN OLDER ADULT SPEAKS

I have been in my home for 50 years and widowed for 25 of those 50. The upkeep on my home is expensive and my resources are limited. I'm hoping I can manage to remain here, but I need some modifications to make it safe and I really don't know how to go about getting assistance to make the necessary changes.

Esther, age 79

LEARNING OBJECTIVES

On completion of this chapter, the reader will be able to:

1. Identify interactions of intrapersonal, interpersonal, geographical, economic, and health factors that influence environmental safety and security for older adults.
2. Discuss the effects of declining health, reduced mobility, isolation, and unpredictable life situations on the older adult's perception of security.
3. Explain the underlying vulnerability of older adults to effects of extreme temperatures, and identify actions to prevent and treat hypothermia and hyperthermia.
4. Define strategies and programs designed to prevent, detect, or alleviate crimes against older adults.
5. Discuss fire prevention and safety for older adults.
6. Consider the impact of available transportation and driving in relation to independence.
7. Discuss the use of assistive technologies to promote self-care, safety, and independence.
8. Identify the components of an elder-friendly community to enhance the ability to age in place.

ENVIRONMENTAL SAFETY

A safe environment is one in which one is capable, with reasonable caution, of carrying out activities of daily living (ADLs) and instrumental activities of daily living (IADLs), and the activities that enrich one's life, without fear of attack, accident, or imposed interference. Vulnerability to environmental risks increases as people become less physically or cognitively able to recognize or cope with real or potential hazards.

This chapter discusses the influence of changing health and disability on safety and security. Included are vulnerability to temperature extremes, natural disasters, crime, fire safety, driving safety, and the role of assistive technology in enhancing independence and the ability to live safely at home. Elder-friendly communities that foster aging in place and promote safety and security are also discussed.

HOME SAFETY

Awareness and assessment of home safety is an important component of preventing accidents and injury for older adults. Home safety assessments must be multifaceted and individualized to the areas of identified risks. They are particularly important for the older adult who is at risk for falls and home safety assessments by occupational therapists are recommended in evidence-based protocols for fall risk reduction (Chapter 19). The Home Safety Self-Assessment Tool (HSSAT) is an online tool that has been shown to increase knowledge of safety and assist older adults and their caregivers to develop home safety plans (Horowitz et al, 2016) (Box 20.1). Education about home safety is an important component of comprehensive assessment of older adults.

CRIMES AGAINST OLDER ADULTS

Risks and Vulnerability

Older individuals share many of the same fears about violent crime held by the rest of the population, but they may feel more vulnerable because of frailness or disability. Living alone, being lonely, and having sensory, mobility, and memory impairments may make older adults more susceptible to crime. Property crime is the most common crime against individuals age 65 years and older. Older adults are more likely to be victims of consumer fraud and scams that include telemarketing fraud,

email scams, and undelivered services. Older adults also experience rising problems with identity theft. Cybercrime is any criminal activity in which a computer (or networked device) is targeted or used. Every year, cybercriminals steal approximately $40 billion from vulnerable older adults in the United States. Resources for protection from crime can be found in Boxes 20.1 to 20.3. Nurses can be instrumental in reducing fear of crime and assisting older adults in exploring ways they may protect themselves and feel more secure.

Fraudulent Schemes Against Older Adults

Fraud against older adults ranges from solicitations from seemingly worthwhile charities to requests for a cash deposit to win a nonexistent prize. Increasingly common is a phone call from someone posing as a grandchild who requests money for an emergency. Trusting persons may be fooled into giving money to pen pals, Internet acquaintances, phony religious causes, or

BOX 20.3 Protection Against Fraud/Cybercrime

- No one should come to your house uninvited.
- No one can ask for personal information during his or her marketing activities.
- All Internal Revenue Service (IRS) employees carry identification and are required to show it to taxpayers when visiting a home or office.
- No check should ever be made payable to an IRS employee. Checks for federal taxes should be made payable to the Internal Revenue Service, not IRS; spelling out the full name makes it more difficult for criminals to alter the check.
- Keep personal information safe, including your Medicare number, and do not provide any information about bank accounts or credit cards to marketers.
- Legitimate Medicare drug plans will not ask for payment over the telephone or Internet and must send a bill to the beneficiary for the monthly premium.
- Avoid shopping online.
- Have computers and Internet checked for malware and protected frequently.
- Visit known and trustworthy websites and avoid unfamiliar websites.
- Avoid opening emails from unknown senders or clicking on links in email.
- Avoid making charitable contributions over the telephone.

BOX 20.4 Tips for Best Practice

Preventing Fires and Burns

- Do not smoke in bed or when sleepy.
- When cooking, do not wear loose-fitting clothing (e.g., bathrobes, nightgowns, pajamas).
- Set thermostats for water heater or faucets so that the water does not become too hot.
- Install a portable hand fire extinguisher in the kitchen.
- Keep access to outside door(s) unobstructed.
- Identify emergency exits in public buildings.
- If you consider entering a boarding or foster home, check to see that it has smoke detectors, a sprinkler system, and fire extinguishers.
- Wear clothing that is nonflammable or treated with a permanent fire-retardant finish.
- Use several electrical outlets rather than overloading one outlet.

new acquaintances who "need help." Attractive prices of fraudulent door-to-door contractors, who offer services the individual cannot perform, may entice a substantial cash outlay.

According to the Internal Revenue Service (IRS), every year impersonators swindle vulnerable taxpayers out of thousands of dollars by posing as IRS agents. Older adults are often targets of these frauds. Scams may involve announcements that they have won a large cash sweepstakes that requires payment of taxes before the prize is delivered. Other IRS impersonators have called on widows or widowers to pay the "back taxes" owed by their deceased spouse. These abuses often go unpunished because the individual waits too long to report the fraud or feels embarrassed over the mistake.

Medical fraud is another serious type of fraud that affects older adults on a national scale. Medical supplies and equipment delivered to homes by various suppliers have either been grossly overpriced or charged for but never received by the client. Scams to defraud Medicare beneficiaries for the Medicare Part D benefit have also been reported. Callers ask for bank information and use the account numbers to electronically withdraw money for a Medicare card and drug plan that is not legitimate. The Centers for Medicare and Medicaid Services (CMS) has offices to inform Medicare and Medicaid beneficiaries of ways to avoid fraud and also provides toll-free numbers to report suspected fraud. National agencies have combined forces to bring about reform.

FIRE SAFETY FOR OLDER ADULTS

Older adults are more threatened with death or injury by fire than any other age group. Fire-related death rates are three times higher in people older than 80 years than in the rest of the population (National Hispanic Council on Aging, 2017). The risk of injury during a fire is greater if medication, illness, mobility, and sensory impairments slow response time or

decision-making and if help is not available to contain the fire and help the person escape.

A number of factors predispose the older adult to fire injuries. In home-dwelling older adults, economic or climatic conditions may promote the use of ill-kept heating devices. Attempts to cook over an open flame while wearing loose-fitting clothing or inability to manage spattering grease from a frying pan can often start a fire from which the individual cannot escape. Failing vision can contribute to a person setting a cook-top burner, heating pad, or hot plate at too high a temperature, resulting in fire or thermal injury. Those living in apartment dwellings are often at the mercy of inadequate repair and safety measures and the careless behaviors of others. Many individuals living in their own homes cannot afford home repairs, placing them at risk for fire.

Most fires occur at home during the night, and deaths are attributed to smoke injury more often than burns. Smoking materials are the most common sources of residential fires. Plastic articles and other synthetics can produce noxious fumes that are deadly, particularly to individuals with preexisting respiratory disorders. Specific fire prevention guidelines for older adults appear in Box 20.4 and Box 20.1 presents fire safety resources.

VULNERABILITY TO ENVIRONMENTAL TEMPERATURES

Extreme weather events such as heat waves, cold spells, floods, storms, and droughts are increasing across the globe. These extreme events are an emerging environmental health concern and potentially affect the health status of millions of people around the globe. Many individuals are exposed to temperature extremes in their own dwellings. Environmental temperature extremes impose a serious risk to older adults with declining physical health. Heat-related and cold-related deaths increase with age, particularly for those aged 75 years and over (Berko et al, 2014). Preventive measures require attentiveness to impending climate changes and protective alternatives. Early intervention in extreme temperature exposure is crucial because excessively high or low body temperatures further impair thermoregulatory function and can be lethal.

Thermoregulation

Neurosensory changes in thermoregulation delay or diminish the individual's awareness of temperature changes and may impair behavioral and thermoregulatory response to dangerously high or low environmental temperatures. These changes vary widely among individuals and are related more to general health than to age. Additionally, many drugs affect thermoregulation by affecting the ability to vasoconstrict or vasodilate, both of which are thermoregulatory mechanisms. Other drugs inhibit neuromuscular activity (a significant source of kinetic heat production), suppress metabolic heat generation, or dull awareness (tranquilizers, pain medications). Alcohol inhibits thermoregulatory function by affecting vasomotor responses in either hot or cold weather.

Economic, behavioral, and environmental factors may combine to create a dangerous thermal environment in which older adults are subjected to temperature extremes from which they cannot escape or that they cannot change. Caregivers and family members should be aware that individuals are vulnerable to temperature extremes if they are unable to shiver, sweat, control blood supply to the skin, take in sufficient liquids, move about, add or remove clothing, adjust bedcovers, or adjust the room temperature. A temperature that may be comfortable for a young and active person may be too cold or too warm for a frail older adult.

Economic conditions often play a role in determining whether an older adult living in the community can afford air conditioning or adequate heating. Local governments and communities must coordinate response strategies to protect the older adult. Strategies may include providing fans and opportunities to spend part of the day in air-conditioned buildings and identification of high-risk individuals.

Temperature Monitoring in Older Adults

Diminished thermoregulatory responses and abnormalities in both the production and the response to endogenous pyrogens may contribute to differences in fever responses between older and younger patients in response to an infection. Up to one-third of older adults with acute infections may present without a robust febrile response, leading to delays in diagnosis and appropriate treatment, and increased morbidity and mortality. Careful attention to temperature monitoring in older adults is very important, and often this technical task is not given adequate consideration by professional nurses.

> ### ⚡ SAFETY ALERT
>
> Because of thermoregulatory changes, up to one-third of older adults with acute infections may present without a febrile response. Additionally, baseline temperatures in frail older adults may be lower than the expected 98.6°F. If the baseline temperature is 97°F, a temperature of 98°F is a 1°F elevation and may be significant.
>
> Temperatures reaching or exceeding 100.9°F are very serious in older adults and are more likely to be associated with serious bacterial or viral infections. Careful attention to temperature monitoring in older adults is very important and can prevent morbidity and mortality. Accurate measurement and reporting of body temperature require professional nursing supervision.

Hyperthermia

When body temperature increases above normal ranges because of environmental or metabolic heat loads, a clinical condition called heat illness, or *hyperthermia*, develops (Table 20.1). Administration

TABLE 20.1   Heat Syndromes.

Illness	Symptoms	Treatment
Heat fatigue	Pale, sweaty skin that is still cool and moist to the touch, weakness, exhaustion Core temperature stays normal because individual can sweat	Oral hydration with electrolyte replacement Cooler, less humid environment Rest
Heat syncope	Syncope or dizziness after exercising in the heat, sweating Has lost fluids and electrolytes Pale, sweaty, weak pulse, elevated heart rate, body temperature still normal	Oral hydration with electrolyte replacement Cooler, less humid environment Rest
Heat cramps	Muscle cramps, still sweating Pulse and blood pressure elevated May need emergency care	Cool environment Oral liquids and IV saline Rest
Heat exhaustion	Can be life threatening Thirsty but altered mental status (dizzy, confused, weak), cool and clammy, tachycardia, nausea Core temperature slightly elevated Emergency treatment	Cool environment Oral liquids and IV saline Rest
Heat stroke	Fatal if neglected Body temperature rises quickly and out of control (often 104°F) Individual is hot and dry, confused, combative, delirious, and then comatose Tachycardia, hypotension, hyperventilation End-organ damage; acute renal failure, and hypercoagulation states occur	Need emergency room treatment Start by fanning patient and using tepid water sprays, aiming to cool slowly Call EMS Complex medical emergency; if untreated, can cause death Cool as rapidly as possible; consider IV infusions

EMS, Emergency medical services; *IV*, intravenous.
Modified from Hogan T, Rios-Alba T: Emergency care. In Ham R, Sloane PD, Warshaw GA, et al, editors: *Primary care geriatrics: a case-based approach*, Philadelphia, 2014, Elsevier, pp 177–192.

BOX 20.5   Tips for Best Practice

Preventing Hyperthermia

- Drink 2 to 3 L of cool fluid daily.
- Minimize exertion, especially during the warmest times of the day.
- Stay in air-conditioned places, or use fans when possible.
- Wear hats and loose clothing of natural fibers when outside; remove most clothing when indoors.
- Take tepid baths or showers.
- Apply cold wet compresses, or immerse the hands and feet in cool water.
- Evaluate medications for risk of hyperthermia.
- Avoid alcohol.

BOX 20.6   Factors That Increase the Risk of Hypothermia in Older Adults

Thermoregulatory Impairment
Failure to vasoconstrict promptly or sufficiently on exposure to cold
Failure to sense cold
Failure to respond behaviorally to protect oneself against cold
Diminished or absent shivering to generate heat
Failure of metabolic rate to rise in response to cold

Conditions That Decrease Heat Production
Hypothyroidism, hypopituitarism, hypoglycemia, anemia, malnutrition, starvation
Immobility or decreased activity (e.g., stroke, paralysis, parkinsonism, dementia, arthritis, fractured hip, coma)
Thinning hair, baldness
Diabetic ketoacidosis

Conditions That Increase Heat Loss
Open wounds, generalized inflammatory skin conditions, burns

Conditions That Impair Central or Peripheral Control of Thermoregulation
Stroke, brain tumor, Wernicke's encephalopathy, subarachnoid hemorrhage
Uremia, neuropathy (e.g., diabetes, alcoholism)
Acute illnesses (e.g., pneumonia, sepsis, myocardial infarction, congestive heart failure, pulmonary embolism, pancreatitis)

Drugs That Interfere With Thermoregulation
Tranquilizers (e.g., phenothiazines); sedative-hypnotics (e.g., barbiturates, benzodiazepines); antidepressants (e.g., tricyclics); vasoactive drugs (e.g., vasodilators); alcohol (causes superficial vasodilation; may interfere with carbohydrate metabolism and judgment); others (e.g., methyldopa, lithium, morphine)

---

of diuretics and low intake of fluids exacerbate fluid loss and can precipitate the onset of hyperthermia in hot weather. Hyperthermia is a temperature-related illness and is classified as a medical emergency. Annually, there are numerous deaths among older adults from temperature extremes; therefore prevention and education are very important nursing responsibilities.

Although most of these problems occur in the home among individuals who do not have air conditioning to use during temperature extremes, older adults with multiple physical problems residing in institutions may be especially vulnerable to temperature changes. Individuals with cardiovascular disease, diabetes, or peripheral vascular disease and those taking certain medications (anticholinergics, antihistamines, diuretics, beta-blockers, antidepressants, antiparkinsonian drugs) are at risk. Interventions to prevent hyperthermia when ambient temperature exceeds 90°F (32°C) are presented in Box 20.5.

Hypothermia

More than half of all hypothermia-related deaths happen in individuals over age 65 (University of Maryland, 2018). Hypothermia is produced by exposure to cold environmental temperatures and is defined as a core temperature of less than 95°F (35°C). Hypothermia is a medical emergency requiring comprehensive assessment of neurological activity, oxygenation, renal function, and fluid and electrolyte balance. When exposed to cold temperatures, healthy individuals conserve heat by vasoconstriction of superficial vessels, shunting circulation away from the skin where most heat is lost. Heat is generated by shivering and increased muscle activity, and a rise in oxygen consumption occurs to meet aerobic muscle requirements. Under normal circumstances, heat is produced in sufficient quantities by cellular metabolism of food, friction produced by contracting muscles, and the flow of blood.

Paralyzed or immobile individuals lack the ability to generate significant heat by muscle activity and become cold even in normal room temperatures. Individuals who are emaciated and have poor nutrition lack insulation and fuel for metabolic heat-generating processes, so they may be mildly hypothermic. Circulatory, cardiac, respiratory, or musculoskeletal impairments affect either the response to or the function of thermoregulatory mechanisms. Other risk factors include excessive alcohol use, exhaustion, poor nutrition, inadequate housing, and the use of sedatives, anxiolytics, phenothiazines, and tricyclic antidepressants (Box 20.6).

Older adults with some degree of thermoregulatory impairment, when exposed to cold temperatures, are at high risk for hypothermia if they undergo surgery, are injured in a fall or accident, or are lost or left unattended in a cool place. The more severe the impairment or prolonged the exposure, the less able the thermoregulatory responses are to defend against heat loss. Unfortunately, a dulling of awareness accompanies hypothermia, and individuals experiencing the condition rarely recognize the problem or seek assistance. For the very old and frail, environmental temperatures less than 65°F (18°C) may cause a serious drop in core body temperature to 95°F (35°C).

All body systems are affected by hypothermia, although the most deadly consequences involve cardiac arrhythmias and suppression of respiratory function. Correctly conducted rewarming is the key to good management, and the guiding principle is to warm the core before the periphery and raise the core temperature 0.5°C to 2°C per hour. Heating blankets and specially designed heating vests are used in addition to warm humidified air by mask, warm intravenous boluses, and other measures depending on the severity of the hypothermia.

Detecting hypothermia among community-dwelling older adults is sometimes difficult because, unlike in the clinical setting, no one is measuring body temperature. For individuals exposed to low temperatures in the home or the environment, confusion and disorientation may be the first overt signs. As

BOX 20.7   Tips for Best Practice

Preventing Cold Discomfort and Development of Accidental Hypothermia in Frail Older Adults

- Maintain a comfortably warm ambient temperature no lower than 68°F. Many frail older adults will require much higher temperatures.
- Provide generous quantities of clothing and bedcovers. Layer clothing and bedcovers for best insulation. Be careful not to judge your patient's needs by how you feel working in a warm environment.
- Provide a head covering whenever possible—in bed, out of bed, and particularly out-of-doors.
- Cover patients well when in bed or bathing. The standard—a light bath blanket over a naked body—is not enough protection for frail older adults.
- Cover patients with heavy blankets for transfer to and from showers; dry quickly and thoroughly before leaving shower room; cover head with a dry towel or hood while wet. Shower rooms and bathrooms should have warming lights.
- Dry wet hair quickly with warm air from an electric dryer. Never allow the hair of frail older adults to air-dry.
- Use absorbent pads for individuals with UI who are unable to ambulate to toilet rather than allowing urine to wet large areas of clothing, sheets, and bedcovers.
- Provide as much exercise as possible to generate heat from muscle activity.
- Provide hot, high-protein meals and bedtime snacks to add heat and sustain heat production throughout the day and as far into the night as possible.

judgment becomes clouded, an individual may remove clothing or fail to seek shelter, and hypothermia can progress to profound levels. For this reason, regular contact with home-dwelling older adults during cold weather is crucial. For those with preexisting alterations in thermoregulatory ability, this surveillance should include even mildly cool weather. Because heating costs are high in the United States, the Department of Health and Human Services provides funds to help low-income families pay their heating bills. Specific interventions to prevent hypothermia are shown in Box 20.7.

PROMOTING HEALTHY AGING: IMPLICATIONS FOR GERONTOLOGICAL NURSING

Recognition of clinical signs and severity of hypothermia and hyperthermia is an important nursing responsibility. Nurses are responsible for keeping frail older adults in environments with appropriate temperatures for comfort and prevention of problems. It is important to closely monitor body temperature and pay particular attention to lower or higher than normal readings compared with the person's baseline. The potential risk of hypothermia and its associated cardiorespiratory and metabolic exertion make prevention important and early recognition vital. Nurses must advocate for resources in the community to ensure appropriate temperatures in the homes of older adults and surveillance when temperature changes occur.

VULNERABILITY TO NATURAL DISASTERS

Natural disasters such as hurricanes, tornadoes, floods, wildfires, and earthquakes claim the lives of many individuals worldwide each year. In addition, human-made or human-generated disasters include chemical, biological, radiological, and nuclear terrorism and food and water contamination. Older adults are at great risk during and after disasters and have the highest casualty rate during disaster events when compared with all other age groups (Malik et al, 2018). Many older adults can't easily evacuate because they don't drive, are physically unable, or may refuse. Older adults at most risk include, but are not limited to, those who depend on others for daily functioning; the medically frail; those with limited mobility; those who are socially isolated or live alone; and those who are cognitively impaired or institutionalized. A 2014 survey found that 15% of the sample used medical devices requiring externally supplied electricity so power interruptions pose concerns for this group (Al-Rousan et al, 2014). The older and poorer the individual, the more likely he or she is to be isolated and vulnerable. Older adults may be less likely to seek formal or informal help during disasters or may be unable to do this independently. Nursing facility residents compose a particularly vulnerable group due to their frailty, and facilities are required to have disaster plans in place.

Adopting tailored disaster preparedness plans that address the general and emergency health needs for older adults is a worldwide concern. Families caring for older adults need to have individualized emergency plans. Public health prevention planning and programs are needed to identify older adults at increased risk in the event of disasters and address their needs. Communities need to enhance preparedness and information networks among organization and agencies that serve older adults (Shih et al, 2018). Gerontological nurses can assist in the development of these plans and educate fellow professionals and community agencies about the special needs of older adults. Nurses can also provide educational programs and outreach on disaster preparedness to older adults. Box 20.1 presents resources for emergency and disaster preparedness for special populations, including older adults.

TRANSPORTATION SAFETY

Available transportation is a critical link in the ability of older adults to remain independent and functional. The lack of accessible transportation may contribute to other problems, such as social withdrawal, poor nutrition, depressive symptoms, and health decline. Urban buses and subways can be physically hazardous and often dangerous. Rural and suburban areas may not have accessible transportation systems, making transportation by car essential. Even walking can be dangerous and older adults are more likely to be injured or killed as pedestrians than as car drivers. Suggested pedestrian improvements include raised pavement markings, median islands, larger street signs with bigger lettering, increased time for pedestrian crossings, and lowered speed limits.

A "crisis in mobility" exists for many older adults because of the lack of an automobile, an inability to drive, limited access to public transportation, health factors, geographical location, and economic considerations. County, state, or federally subsidized transportation is provided in certain areas to assist individuals in reaching social services, nutrition sites, health services, emergency care, recreational centers, day care programs, physical and vocational rehabilitation centers, grocery stores, and library services. Some senior centers and assisted living facilities also offer transportation services. Although transportation can often be found for special needs, it is virtually impossible to locate transportation for pleasure or recreation and many of these services are restricted to individuals with serious physical or mental impairments. Ride-sharing services such as Uber and Lyft can assist in providing more transportation options, but some older adults may not be able to afford these services or may not feel safe using them. Some of these transportation services are offering special services for individuals who need more assistance such as wheelchair accessible vehicles or a driver trained to provide additional assistance (Andruszkiewicz and Fike, 2015–2016).

Adequate, affordable, and convenient transportation services are essential to health and quality of life and the ability to age in place. Assessment of older adults needs to include transportation needs. Referrals to local social service and aging organizations, such as Area Agencies on Aging, can be made to assist in obtaining information on transportation resources and financial assistance for services.

Driving

Older adults' driving is a critical public health issue. Driving is one of the IADLs for most older adults because it is essential to obtaining necessary resources. Currently, almost half of drivers on the road are over the age of 65 years with substantial increases predicted in the next 30 years (Wiese and Wolff, 2016). For many older adults, alternate transportation is not available and, consequently, they may continue driving beyond the time when it is safe. Driving is a highly complex activity that requires a variety of visual, motor, and cognitive skills. Age alone is not a good indicator of driving safety, but health conditions, sensory functioning, road design and traffic, and weather conditions contribute to increasing concern with driving safety as individuals age (Edwards et al, 2017; Liddle et al, 2017).

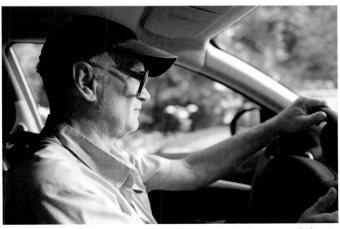

Driving is the preferred means of travel for older adults. (©iStock.com/danr13.)

BOX 20.8 **Adaptations for Safer Driving**

- Wider rear-view mirrors
- Pedal extensions
- Less complicated, larger, and legible instrument panels
- Electronic detectors in front and back that signal when the car is getting too close to other cars, drifting into another lane, or likely to hit center dividers or other highway infrastructure
- Technology that facilitates left turns by alerting drivers when it is safe to make the turn
- Better protection on doors
- Booster cushions for shorter-stature drivers
- "Smart" driving assistants (under development) that automatically plan a safe driving route based on the person's driving habits
- GPS devices

Modified from Dugan E, Lee C: Biopsychosocial risk factors for driving cessation: findings from the Health and Retirement Study, *J Aging Health* 25:1313–1328, 2013.

Driving Safety

Older drivers typically drive fewer miles than younger drivers and tend to drive less at night, during adverse weather conditions, or in congested areas. Generally, they choose familiar routes, and fewer older drivers speed or drive after drinking alcohol than drivers of other ages. However, when compared with younger age groups, older adults have more accidents per mile driven. Driving fatalities increase with age and the risk of death for drivers 85 years or older is ninefold greater in a crash than it is for drivers 69 years or younger (Roe et al, 2017). Improving the safety of cars through new design and adaptations should be considered for older drivers to enhance safety (Box 20.8).

The legal regulations regarding driver's license renewal in older drivers and the responsibility of medical practitioners to identify unsafe drivers vary among states and countries. Driver's license renewal procedures may include accelerated renewal cycles, renewal in person rather than electronically or by mail, and vision and road tests. The issues of driving in the older adult population are the subject of a great deal of public discussion. Many older drivers and their families struggle with issues related to continued safety in driving and when and how to tell older adults that their driving safety is a concern (Box 20.9).

Driving and Dementia

Driving is one of the largest ethical issues associated with dementia. Dementia, even in the early stages, can impair the cognitive and functional skills required for safe driving. There is at least a twofold greater risk of crashes for drivers with dementia when compared to age-matched individuals without dementia (Wiese and Wolff, 2016). Many individuals early in the course of dementia are still able to pass a driving performance test, so a diagnosis of dementia should not be the sole justification for revocation of a driver's license. However, a recent study found that declines in driving performance likely precede problems with thinking, memory, or cognition in individuals in the later stages of preclinical Alzheimer's disease (Roe et al, 2017). Discussions about driving safety should begin when dementia

BOX 20.9 Tips for Best Practice

Driving Safety

- Include the person in all discussions about driving safety.
- Encourage the individual to conduct a self-assessment of driving abilities.
- Assess vision and hearing and ensure appropriate use of corrective lenses and hearing devices.
- Evaluate medical conditions that may interfere with driving ability (arthritis, Parkinson's disease, dementia, stroke) and ensure appropriate treatment, and adaptations that may be necessary to enhance driving safety.
- Discuss the impact of medical conditions and sensory impairments on driving safety.
- Suggest vehicle adaptations and older adult driving assessment programs if indicated.
- Encourage the individual to modify driving habits, such as not driving on unfamiliar roads, during rush hour, at dusk or at night, in inclement weather, or in heavy traffic.
- Avoid risky spots like ramps and left turns.
- Advise individual to limit night driving.
- Discuss strategies to decrease the need to drive including arranging for home-delivered groceries, prescriptions, and meals; having personal services provided in the home; asking a caregiver to obtain needed supplies or act as a copilot; and exploring community resources for transportation.
- Ask the family to have the family lawyer discuss with the individual the financial and legal implications of a crash or injury.

From National Institute on Aging: *More safe driving tips*, 2016. https://www.nia.nih.gov/health/older-drivers. Accessed March 2018.

BOX 20.10 Action Strategies Used to Bring About Driving Cessation

Imposed Type	Involved Type
Report person to division of motor vehicles for possible license suspension	All family members and individual meet, discuss the situation, and come to a mutual agreement of the problem
Use of deception or threats such as false keys, disabling the car, saying car was stolen	Dialogue is ongoing from the earliest signs of cognitive impairment about the eventuality of the need to stop driving
Attempts to order or control, such as provider writing a prescription, commands from children to stop driving	Arrangements are made for alternative transportation plans that are available when needed and acceptable to the individual

From Jett K, Tappen R, Rosselli M: Imposed versus involved: different strategies to effect driving cessation in cognitively impaired older adults, *Geriatr Nurs* 26:111–116, 2005.

is diagnosed and driving evaluations should be conducted every 6 months or as needed as the disease progresses.

Many states have implemented the Silver Alert system. Similar to Amber Alerts for missing children, the Silver Alert is designed to create a widespread lookout for older adults who have wandered from their surroundings while driving a car. Silver Alert features a public notification system to broadcast information about missing persons, especially older adults with Alzheimer's disease or other mental disabilities, in order to aid in their return. Silver Alert uses a wide array of media outlets, such as commercial radio stations, television stations, and cable television, to broadcast information about missing persons. Silver Alert also uses message signs on roadways to alert motorists to be on the lookout for missing older adults and provides the car's make, model, and license plate number.

Driving Cessation

Relinquishing the mobility and independence afforded by driving one's own car has many psychological ramifications and inconveniences. Giving up driving is a major loss for an older adult both in terms of independence and pleasure as well as in feelings of competence and self-worth. The health consequences of driving cessation include social isolation, health problems, institutionalization, higher mortality, and an approximately doubled risk of depression (Davis and Ohman, 2017). Women are more likely than men to stop driving for less pressing reasons than health, and at a younger age. Older men seem to place more value on the ability to drive, and on owning a car, than

older women. Therefore, one can expect more stress involved with the decision not to drive for older men.

Planning for driving cessation should occur for all older adults before their mobility situations become urgent. Health care providers should encourage open discussion of issues related to driving with the older adult and his or her family and should identify impairments that affect safe driving, correct them when possible, and offer alternatives for transportation. Forty percent of individuals aged 50 years or older believed that their primary care provider could best determine their driving ability. But health care providers often feel unprepared to identify unfit drivers and may benefit from education about driving in dementia so they have the skills needed to counsel patients and families (Arms, 2016; Davis and Ohman, 2017).

Voluntarily giving up a driver's license, rather than having it revoked, is associated with more positive outcomes. Specialized driving cessation support groups aimed at the transition from driver to nondriver may also be beneficial in decreasing the negative outcomes associated with this decision. "Family members require support and education about how to give feedback on driving safety in a way that ensures the message is carefully timed, received as well as possible, and supports relationships" (Liddle et al, 2017). Strategies helpful in counseling on driving cessation derived from research with individuals with dementia are presented in (Box 20.10).

PROMOTING HEALTHY AGING: IMPLICATIONS FOR GERONTOLOGICAL NURSING

Assessments of functional capacities often neglect driving ability. Assessment should include evaluation of whether an individual can drive, feels safe driving, and has a driver's license. A mnemonic, SAFE DRIVE, addresses key components in screening older drivers (Box 20.11). The National Institute on Aging (2015) provides a self-assessment of driving (Box 20.12). and the American Automobile Association also provides an

BOX 20.11 Safe Driving

S	Safety record	D	Drugs
A	Attention skills	R	Reaction time
F	Family report	I	Intellectual impairment
E	Ethanol use	V	Vision and visuospatial function
		E	Executive functions

BOX 20.12 Questions to Ask in Self-Assessment of Unsafe Driving Risk

- Do cars or people walking appear out of nowhere?
- Do I get distracted while driving?
- Do people blow their horn often at me?
- Do I forget where I am or how to get somewhere even in an often-traveled area?
- Do I have trouble staying in my lane?
- Do I have trouble moving my foot between the gas and brake pedals, or do I sometimes confuse the two?
- Am I driving less these days because I'm not as sure about my driving as I used to be?
- Have my family, friends, or my doctor said they're worried about my driving?
- Have I been pulled over by the police about my driving or received two or more driving citations in the past 12 months?
- Have I had some accidents, even if they were only "fender benders"?

From National Institute on Aging: *Older drivers*, 2016. https://www.nia.nih.gov/health/older-drivers. Accessed March 2018.

interactive driving evaluation available on-line or in DVD format (Box 20.1). These kinds of tools can be effective in raising awareness of threats to driving fitness.

There is no gold standard for determining driving competency, but driving evaluations are offered by driver rehabilitation specialists through local hospitals and rehabilitation centers and private or university-based driving assessment programs. Components of a thorough driving examination include a history and physical, vision and hearing evaluation, cognitive assessment, and a road test (Wiese and Wolff, 2016). Some programs that evaluate driving ability may use a standardized computer driving simulation. The local Alzheimer's Association and Area Agency on Aging can assist in locating driving evaluation sites. State Departments of Motor Vehicles (DMVs) also conduct performance-based road tests. Box 20.9 presents tips for driving safety. There is a lack of resources for driving evaluations and the evaluation

is also very expensive and not covered by Medicare or insurance. More research is needed to address driving safety in older adults. Nurse researcher and public health nursing expert Dr. Lisa Wiese discusses implications for research and nursing practice to enhance driving safety (Research Highlights box).

RESEARCH HIGHLIGHTS

"But I'm a good driver; I have never had a car accident and have been driving for over 60 years" is a phrase I hear often while interviewing patients referred to the nurse-managed memory and wellness center for a driving evaluation. Our clients often come to us because a family member or friend has observed an increase in unsafe driving behaviors, or a police officer has written a temporary driver's license suspension. Several states also have a mechanism for anonymous reporting of unsafe driving, after which the individual will receive written notice of a mandatory driving evaluation.

Prior to my work at the memory and wellness center with older drivers, I was not aware of the myriad challenges for older adults and their families associated with driving, particularly when the individual is experiencing cognitive decline. I saw this as a public health nursing opportunity and researched the topic for a manuscript for *Public Health Nursing*. In this Research Highlights box, I offer suggestions for nursing practice, education, and research to address this important public health concern.

Assessing for Risk of Unsafe Driving

Nurses are well positioned during outpatient visits or inpatient stays to identify older adults who are at risk for unsafe driving behavior. Some questions to ask the individual are presented in Box 20.12. Family members can also be asked about unsafe driving.

Assessment of the functional skills needed for safe driving includes hearing and vision screening, medication review, and physical assessment, including active range of motion tests. For example, to determine if the individual can look over their shoulder adequately prior to changing lanes, ask the individual to turn their head and identify an object the nurse is holding ten feet behind. Observing the individual attempting to walk 10 feet and return within 7 seconds can reveal deficits in strength and general mobility. These assessments can help to identify weaknesses that would impair a person's ability to drive or to quickly exit the car.

A brief assessment for memory loss is also important. All nurses who care for older adults need to know how to conduct a brief cognitive screen, such as the *Mini-Cog* (Chapter 7), which can identify if memory changes are significant enough to warrant further in-depth evaluation.

Nursing Interventions to Assist Older Drivers and Their Families

Nurses can empower older adult drivers by teaching them about health promoting behaviors that will minimize driving errors (Box 20.9). If a family member or friend has observed a pattern of unsafe driving behaviors, the nurse can share key phrases for starting a conversation regarding driving concerns such as "Driving on the roads today is so much more difficult than it used to be," "That was a close call today while driving to the ____; I worry about your safety," and "Did you speak with your doctor about the effects of your recent medications on driving?" Having a calm conversation is vital to protecting the older adult's dignity.

For families facing a dementia diagnosis, the Alzheimer's Association's Dementia and Driving Resource Center website contains examples of helpful communication techniques and short video role-plays of talking about driving cessation. For many older adults, giving up driving is a major loss, and the emotional and physical consequences can be significant. A key component of successful management of driving cessation is the support group, where all family members can express their frustrations, and also learn about effective techniques for coping with challenges. Memory and wellness centers, including adult day programs, and senior centers, may offer support groups as a component of driving cessation programs. Otherwise, as a nurse, you can

Continued

answer the call for this vital service and initiate a driving cessation support group in your community.

Educating Nursing Students About Driving Safety

Older adults and their families look to health care providers for information and guidance on these issues, but there has been little emphasis in health professional curricula on driving safety. Many providers do not feel qualified to identify unfit drivers. Nurses can play a significant role in enhancing the safety of older drivers. Nursing education programs should include content on driving safety, functional assessment of older drivers, driving cessation programs, and community transportation resources.

Increasing Road Safety Through Nursing Research

Despite the growing challenges associated with driving safety in older adults, there is a lack of research on the effectiveness of interventions to improve safety, address driving cessation, and educate health professionals on the issue. Nursing research can contribute to the development and testing of effective interventions.

There are no validated protocols to evaluate driving safety. Development of an empirically validated screening process to assess driving safety is essential. A program to conduct a brief functional driving skills assessment as part of the vision test at the yearly checkup could be tested for effectiveness.

Another pilot project would be to train staff at the local Division of Motor Vehicles to conduct brief memory screens and refer those who are unsuccessful to their provider prior to issuing the license. Would this screening process be effective in decreasing the number of fatalities associated with older adult driving?

Questions to be researched related to evaluation of the effectiveness of driving safety programs and driving support groups may include the following:

- Do older adults who attend driving safety/accident prevention programs have fewer accidents or voluntarily "retire" their driver's license?
- Are there fewer incidents of "Silver Alerts" as a result of participation in these preventive activities?
- What is the impact of new "driver assist" features (e.g., warning systems, forward collision, lane-departures) on reducing the number of accidents?

More work needs to be done on the effects experienced by older adults who lose their driving privileges. What are the health consequences (depression, earlier dementia, other costly chronic illnesses) experienced by older adults who lose their driving privileges? What are the most effective ways to therapeutically communicate concerns about unsafe driving and driving cessation to decrease emotional upset? Most importantly, we need to discover and disseminate ways that communities can support with dignity their older residents who can no longer drive and reduce the risk of deleterious effects of isolation and loss of independence.

Adapted from Wiese L, Wolff L: Supporting safety in the older adult driver: a public health nursing opportunity, *Public Health Nurs* 33(5): 460–471, 2016.

EMERGING TECHNOLOGIES TO ENHANCE SAFETY OF OLDER ADULTS

Advancements in all types of technology hold promise for improving quality of life, decreasing the need for personal care, and enhancing independence and the ability to live safely at home and age in place. The costs of nursing home and assisted living are driving sales and innovation in the technology market. A growing concern related to the increasing number of older adults is the lack of both family and paid caregivers (Chapter 34). Emerging technologies will play a larger role in ensuring care for older adults in the future (Chi and Demiris, 2017). "Existing and emerging solutions are opening the door for a new era of 'tech-enabled caregiving' with the potential to make life better for caregivers and older adults" (Andruszkiewicz and Fike, 2015–2016, p. 64).

Assistive technology is any device or system that allows a person to perform a task independently or that makes the task easier and safer to perform. Assistive technology is decreasing the number of older adults who depend on others for personal care in ADLs and presents cost-effective alternatives to human services and institutionalization. Gerotechnology is the term used to describe assistive technologies for older adults and these technologies are expected to significantly influence how we live in the future. Health care technologies, robotics, telemedicine, mobility and ADL aids, and environmental control systems (smart houses/intelligent homes) are some examples of assistive technology.

Telehealth

Telehealth (telemedicine) is the use of technologies to enable clinicians to remotely diagnose, monitor, and treat patients. Telehealth offers exciting possibilities for managing medical problems in the home or other setting, reducing health care costs, and promoting self-management of illness, particularly in rural and underserved areas. A number of studies have reported that telehealth technology improves patient outcomes and decreases hospital readmissions and health care costs (Marchibroda, 2015). Telehealth can also be effective for delivering interventions designed for family caregivers (Chi and Demiris, 2017). The number of telehealth programs is increasing worldwide, and these programs offer exciting possibilities for nurses, particularly advanced practice nurses.

Smart Homes

There are many exciting technologies being developed to support monitoring and management of older adults' health and homes and to support aging in place and remote caregiving. Remote monitoring via in-home sensors allows caregivers to passively track daily behavior and be notified about deviations from daily routines. Newly evolving smart-home systems include a combination of home-control applications (e.g., appliances, lighting, security systems) and safety, health, wellness, and social connectivity technologies that can simultaneously and continuously monitor environmental conditions, daily activity patterns, vital signs, movement patterns, sleep patterns, medication adherence, and fall-detection (Czaja, 2015). The

MEDCottage (granny-pod) is an interesting example of a smart home. The MEDCottage provides a family communication center that allows telemetry, environmental control, and dynamic interaction to off-site caregivers through smart and robotic technology. Technology inside the home includes monitoring of the person's vital signs and safety, medication reminders, and adaptive devices. The MEDCottage can be purchased or leased and temporarily placed on the caregiver's family property (http://www.medcottage.com/).

Motion and pressure sensors may be useful in the homes of older adults with cognitive impairment. These sensors can detect movement and the absence of movement. If there has been no movement for a period of time, a monitoring system is activated and a plan of action initiated depending on the person's response or lack of response. Pressure sensors can be used under the mattress and can turn on bedside lights when the individual gets out of bed and activate an alarm if he or she does not return to bed in a specified period of time. Sensors placed in entry doors or GPS watches or pendants can detect if a person leaves the home, and their location, and can send messages to caregivers. SmartSoles, shoe insoles with an embedded GPS device, are being developed and may be an aid to locate individuals with dementia who wander from their home.

In hospitals and long-term care facilities, devices such as wireless pendants that track people's movements, load cells built into beds that create an alert when individuals get out of bed, and monitor weight and sleep patterns, and bed lifts that allow individuals to go from lying down to standing up with the push of a button are being used. Wheelchair technology that enables the user to go down stairs, move to an upright position, be reminded to change positions to alleviate pressure, or use mechanical arms to change a light bulb or get things out of the refrigerator are other developing technologies.

Robots

Robotic technology for health care is more advanced in Europe and Japan than in the United States at this time, but we can expect to see increased development and use of robotics in nursing. Already developed are robots that can help lift both individuals and objects, remind patients to take their medicine or administer the medication, check a person's vital signs, provide help in the event of a fall, and assist with baths and meals. A child-sized therapist robot on wheels with a human-like torso is being developed for use in homes and long-term care facilities to assist with the high level of attention individuals with dementia require for safety and function. Humanoid nurse robots are being developed and will soon be a reality in clinical practice (Tanioka et al, 2017). Many ethical issues have been raised about the use of robots, and nurses will play an important role in ensuring that technological competence is balanced with caring to enhance the well-being of the individual (Beuscher et al, 2017).

As the baby boomers and future generations age, comfort with technology will be increased, and people will seek options for better, safer, and more independence in ways not yet imagined.

At this time, many of the assistive technologies can be cost prohibitive, but with advances in development they may be more accessible and affordable for more people. Issues of privacy and data sharing need consideration and training and support for proper use of devices and application are important. Many technologies were initially designed to serve the rich and young, and later adopted for older adults without a great deal of input. Many systems are complex and difficult to use, especially for individuals with limited technology and health literacy skills. "Nurses can play essential roles in designing future research to improve the design and use of mobile and connected health technologies and researching their effects on older adults' health outcomes and ability to age in place. Nurses are also in a prime position to lead interprofessional teams of engineers, computer scientists, physicians, informaticians and other health professionals and partner with patients and their families to design, develop and implement technology in a holistic manner" (Wang, 2018, p. 4). Research is needed on assistive technologies that are user friendly and nurses need to be aware of available technology to improve safety (Czaja, 2015).

AGING IN PLACE

Developing elder-friendly communities and providing increasing opportunities to age in place can lead to enhanced health and well-being. Aging in place is the ability to live in one's own home and community safely, independently, and comfortably, regardless of age, income, or ability level. Many state and local governments are assessing the community and designing interventions to enhance the ability of older adults to remain in their homes and familiar environments. These interventions range from adequate transportation systems to home modifications and universal design standards for barrier-free housing.

Components of an elder-friendly community include the following: (1) addresses basic needs; (2) optimizes physical health and well-being; (3) maximizes independence for the frail and disabled; and (4) provides social and civic engagement. Fig. 20.1 presents elements of an elder-friendly community. Efforts to create physical and social urban environments that promote healthy and active aging and a good quality of life are occurring worldwide. The World Health Organization (WHO) Global Network of Age-Friendly Cities and Communities helps cities and communities become more supportive of older adults by addressing their needs across eight dimensions: the built environment, transportation, housing, social participation, respect and social inclusion, civic participation and employment, communication, and community support and health services (WHO, 2018).

A majority of older midlife and older adults want to age in place and want to stay in their own homes or, if that is not possible, stay in their communities as they grow older. However, for many older adults, the ability to find affordable, physically accessible, and well-located homes in their community is a

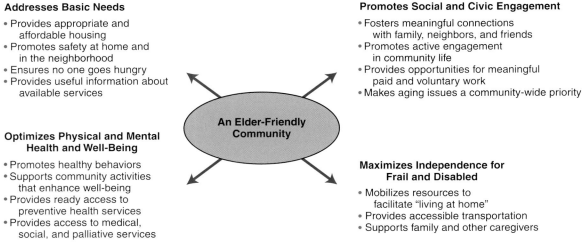

Addresses Basic Needs

- Provides appropriate and affordable housing
- Promotes safety at home and in the neighborhood
- Ensures no one goes hungry
- Provides useful information about available services

Optimizes Physical and Mental Health and Well-Being

- Promotes healthy behaviors
- Supports community activities that enhance well-being
- Provides ready access to preventive health services
- Provides access to medical, social, and palliative services

An Elder-Friendly Community

Promotes Social and Civic Engagement

- Fosters meaningful connections with family, neighbors, and friends
- Promotes active engagement in community life
- Provides opportunities for meaningful paid and voluntary work
- Makes aging issues a community-wide priority

Maximizes Independence for Frail and Disabled

- Mobilizes resources to facilitate "living at home"
- Provides accessible transportation
- Supports family and other caregivers

Fig. 20.1 Essential Elements of an Elder-Friendly Community. (From AdvantAge Initiative, Center for Home Care Policy and Research, Visiting Nurse Service of New York.)

significant challenge. Only 1% of US housing units have all five components of what are known as "universal design" features: no-step entry; single floor living; extra-wide doorways and halls; accessible electric controls and switches, and level-style doors and faucet handles. Remodeling an existing home to install these accessibility features is expensive and many cannot afford to remodel. There is also a lack of affordable and accessible rental units and federally subsidized housing for older renters. The racial and ethnic diversity of the growing number of older adults in the United States also has significant implications. "Faced with lifelong discrimination, many minority groups have lower rates of home ownership, lower median incomes, and fewer assets—factors that significantly constrain their housing choices in old age" (Gonyea and Melekis, 2018, p. 50). New models of housing for older adults are growing across the country and hold promise to help to address the crisis in housing and support aging in place.

Aging in Community Models

Naturally Occurring Retirement Communities (NORCs) are neighborhoods or buildings in which a large segment of the residents are older adults. They are not purpose-built senior housing or retirement communities but are places where community residents have aged in place and where they intend to spend the rest of their lives. NORCs provide a range of health and social services for the residents, and individual assessments of risk, coordination of nonprofessional services, and referrals and follow up.

The Village model is another community program that aids in successful aging in neighborhoods. You can join an existing village in your area or create your own village with neighbors. The prototype village is Beacon Hill in Boston. Beacon Hill is an independent, self-governing, not-for-profit organization run by volunteers and paid staff who coordinate access to affordable services for older adults in their communities. Services include transportation, health and wellness programs, home repair,

social and education activities and trips, and discounts on goods and services.

Cohousing communities, a concept that originated in Denmark, are another growing option that older adults may find appealing. Most of the cohousing projects are intergenerational, but some also are designed specifically for individuals 50 years of age and older. Cohousing is a type of intentional, collaborative housing in which residents actively participate in the design and operation of their neighborhoods. Communities are usually designed as attached or single-family homes along one or more pedestrian streets or clustered around a central courtyard. There is a common house where residents can gather and share a common meal or socialize. Community members work together to care for the common property. In most cases, cohousing communities are started by prospective residents, who often partner with a developer to design and finance the project. Some are started by architects and developers who then organize a group of future residents to buy into the project.

Shared housing among adult children and their older relatives has become a choice for many because of cultural preferences or need. The sharing may relieve the economic burdens of maintaining a home after widowhood or retirement on a fixed income. Chapter 34 discusses multigenerational housing. Another model of shared housing is that of opening up one's personal home to others. Older adults often live in houses that were purchased in their young adult years and find that as they age, much of the space may be underused. Sharing a house can be easily implemented by locating, screening, and matching older adults looking for houses to share with those who have them. The National Shared Housing Resource Center has established subgroups nationally to assist individuals interested in home sharing.

As the baby boomers age, we can expect to see more innovative housing movements that create successful opportunities for healthy aging in the community and provide a range of options for older adults beyond what is available now. Box 20.1 presents some resources for aging in the community.

KEY CONCEPTS

- Thermoregulatory changes, chronic illness, and medications may predispose the older adult to hypothermia and hyperthermia. Careful attention must be paid to temperature monitoring and provision of adequate heating and cooling in weather extremes.
- Transportation for older adults is critical to their physical, psychological, and social health.
- Neighborhoods change over the years, and long-term dwellers may find themselves in dangerous or crime-ridden areas as they age.
- Older adults are often targets of fraud and deception.

- Reducing fire hazards is essential to feelings of security.
- Driving safety for older adults is an important issue, and health care professionals must be knowledgeable about assessment, safety interventions, and transportation resources.
- Technology advances hold promise for improving quality of life, decreasing need for personal care assistance, and enhancing independence and the ability to live safely.
- Efforts to make communities more elder friendly are under way across the globe. New and innovative ideas for aging in the community will continue to change living options for older adults.

NURSING STUDY: CHANGING LIFE SITUATIONS AND ENVIRONMENTAL VULNERABILITY

Ethel had lived in one home for all her married life, but when her husband died her children worried about her safety, being alone in a big home. They feared she could fall and lie undiscovered to die of hypothermia, the deteriorating neighborhood was no longer considered safe, and she could no longer drive and was limited in her ability to get around. They convinced her to move to a community in Phoenix near them.

They were able to find a suitable apartment that she could afford. For a while they visited her each week, but each visit became more depressing for them as she continually talked about her old home, old friends, old furniture, old priest—everything old. Their visits became less frequent. She called them faithfully each morning but detected their urge to get off the phone and on with their lives. One morning she called her daughter Gladys and said, "I'm so sick! Yesterday I walked outside and I swear I saw my friend Rose from the old neighborhood getting on the bus, but she didn't see me. I was so disappointed but managed to make it home, then couldn't find the key to my apartment so finally had to call 911 for help. They were really irritated with me when I said I had lost my key. I want to go back to Detroit. I know how things work there." After a family conclave, Ethel's family found a nice place in assisted living for Ethel and they were relieved. Ethel said, "I don't know where I am anymore. Seems I bounce

around like a rubber ball." She seldom left her room except for meals, and soon she needed meals brought to her. Last week she wandered out and, when found, had suffered a serious case of heat stroke.

Based on the nursing study, develop a nursing care plan using the following procedure[a]:

- List Ethel's comments that provide subjective data.
- List information that provides objective data.
- From these data, identify and state, using an accepted format, two nursing diagnoses you determine are most significant to Ethel at this time. List two of Ethel's strengths that you have identified from the data.
- Determine and state outcome criteria for each diagnosis. These must reflect some alleviation of the problem identified in the nursing diagnosis and must be stated in concrete and measurable terms.
- Plan and state one or more interventions for each diagnosed problem. Provide specific documentation of the source used to determine the appropriate intervention. Plan at least one intervention that incorporates Ethel's existing strengths.
- Evaluate the success of the intervention. Interventions must correlate directly with the stated outcome criteria to measure the outcome success.

[a]Students are advised to refer to their nursing diagnosis text and identify possible or potential problems.

CRITICAL THINKING QUESTIONS AND ACTIVITIES

1. What alternatives could you suggest to Ethel's family as they decide on the best living situation for her?
2. How could Ethel's family have involved her in the decision making about her living situations?
3. Locate low-cost housing in your area, and assess for convenience and safety.
4. What type of support does your community provide to assist older adults to safely age in place?
5. What crimes against older adults are of concern in your community?
6. List several aspects of your environment that are important to you, and discuss their significance.
7. Discuss housing options that would be suitable and feasible for you if you were unable to get around without the assistance of a walker.
8. What are your city's and state's plans for disaster preparedness for disabled and older adults living in the community and in institutions?
9. Compare your community to the characteristics of an elder-friendly community described in the chapter.
10. Survey the homes of older adults you are serving in your clinical practice for the presence or absence of safety features.
11. Discuss how you would assist your parents in making a decision regarding a change in living situations if they become increasingly disabled and unable to care for themselves.

RESEARCH QUESTIONS

1. What criminal activities are of most concern to older adults?
2. What home safety factors are the most frequent causes of concern for older adults?
3. What is the geographical distribution and incidence of hypothermia and hyperthermia in the United States?
4. What are the most frequent causes of fires among older adults?
5. What do older adults fear most in their environment?
6. What are the barriers to the use of assistive technology in institutions and personal homes?

REFERENCES

Al-Rousan TM, Rubenstein LM, Wallace RB: Preparedness for natural disasters among older US adults: a nationwide survey, *Am J Public Health* 104(3):506–511, 2014.

Andruszkiewicz G, Fike, K: Emerging technology trends and products: how tech innovations are easing the burden of family caregiving, *Generations* 39(4):64–68, 2015–2016.

Berko J, Ingram DD, Saha S, Parker JD: Deaths attributed to heat, cold, and other weather events in the United States: 2006-2010, *Natl Health Stat Report* (76):1–15, 2014.

Beuscher LM, Fan J, Sarkar N, et al: Socially assistive robots: measuring older adults' perceptions, *J Gerontol Nurs* 43(12):35–43, 2017.

Byszewski A, Power B, Lee L, Rhee GG, Parson B, Molnar F: Driving and dementia: workshop module on communicating cessation to drive, *Can Geriatr J* 20(4):241–245, 2017.

Chi NC, Demiris G: The roles of telehealth tools in supporting family caregivers, *J Gerontol Nurs* 43(2):3–5. 2017.

Czaja SJ: Can technology empower older adults to manage their health? *Generations J Am Soc Aging* 39(1):46–51, 2015.

Davis RL, Ohman JM: Driving in early-stage Alzheimer's disease: an integrative review of the literature, *Res Gerontol Nurs* 10(2): 86–100, 2017.

Edwards JD, Lister JJ, Lin FR, Andel R, Brown L, Wood JM: Association of hearing impairment and subsequent driving mobility in older adults, *Gerontologist* 57(4):767–775, 2017.

Gonyea J, Melekis K: Women's housing challenges in later life: the importance of a gender lens, *Generations, J Am Soc Aging* 41(4): 45–52, 2017–2018.

Horowitz BP, Almonte T, Vasil A: Use of the home safety self-assessment tool (HSSAT) within community health education to improve home safety, *Occup Ther Health Care* 30(4):356–372, 2016.

Jett K, Tappen RM, Rosselli M: Imposed versus involved: different strategies to effect driving cessation in cognitively impaired older adults, *Geriatr Nurs* 26:111–116, 2005.

Liddle J, Gustafsson L, Mitchell G, Pachana NA: A difficult journey: reflections on driving and driving cessation from a team of clinical researchers, *Gerontologist* 57(1):82–88, 2017.

Malik S, Lee DC, Doran KM, et al: Vulnerability of older adults in disasters: emergency department utilization by geriatric patients after Hurricane Sandy, *Disaster Med Public Health Prep*, 12(2):184–193, 2018. doi:10.1017/dmp.2017.44.

Marchibroda JM: New technologies hold great promise for allowing older adults to age in place, *Generations* 39(1):52–54, 2015.

Munanga A: Cybercrime: a new and growing problem for older adults. *J Gerontol Nurs* 45(2), 3-5, 2019.

National Hispanic Council on Aging: *Home fire safety for older adults,* 2017. http://www.nhcoa.org/home-fire-safety-for-older-adults/. Accessed March 2018.

Roe CM, Babulal GM, Head DM, et al: Preclinical Alzheimer's disease and longitudinal driving decline, *Alzheimers Dement (N Y)* 3(1):74–82, 2017.

Shih RA, Acosta JD, Chen EK, et al: *Improving disaster resilience among older adults*, Rand Corporation Research Report, 2018. https://www.rand.org/pubs/research_reports/RR2313.html. Accessed March 2018.

Tanioka T, Yasuhara Y, Osaka K et al: *Nursing robots: robotic technology and human caring for the elderly,* Okayama City, Japan, 2017, Fukuro Shuppan Publishing.

Wang J: Mobile and connected health technologies for older adults aging in place, *J Gerontol Nurs* 44(6):3–5, 2018.

Wiese LK, Wolff L: Supporting safety in the older adult driver: a public health nursing opportunity, *Public Health Nurs* 33(5):460–471, 2016.

World Health Organization: *Global network for age-friendly cities and communities,* 2018. https://extranet.who.int/agefriendlyworld/who-network/. Accessed March 2018.

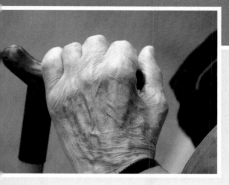

21

Living Well With Chronic Illness

Kathleen Jett

http://evolve.elsevier.com/Touhy/TwdHlthAging

AN OLDER ADULT SPEAKS

If I'd known I was going to live this long, I'd have taken better care of myself.

Eubie Blake, on his 100th birthday

LEARNING OBJECTIVES

On completion of this chapter, the reader will be able to:

1. Identify the most common chronic disorders of late life.
2. Describe the concept of frailty and explain how it applies to chronic disease.
3. Describe a conceptual model that may be useful for guiding the nurse in the development of strategies to promote healthy aging regardless of limitations in function.
4. Construct nursing interventions that are consistent with the Chronic Illness Trajectory.
5. Propose strategies to reduce chronic disease in the global community.

Chronic illnesses are those that are persistent regardless of treatment. Their onset may be insidious and identified only during a health screening. Chronic diseases are not always obvious and may not interfere with the person's daily life until late in the disease.

Noncommunicable disease kills 41 million people each year, 36 million of whom are over 69 years of age (WHO, 2018). Heart disease, cancer, and diabetes are the leading causes of death and disability in the United States. Six out of 10 adults have at least one chronic condition and 4 in 10 have at least two (Fig. 21.1). The most common chronic diseases in the United States are heart disease, stroke, cancer, diabetes, obesity, chronic lung disease, Alzheimer's disease, chronic kidney disease, and osteoarthritis (CDC, 2019).

In a younger adult the initial signs of a pending chronic disease may be identified early enough to prevent later problems. For example, control of one's blood pressure may prevent the development of heart disease. In older adults a chronic disease may not be diagnosed until some amount of end-organ damage has already occurred. For example, irreversible diabetic retinopathy may be found during an annual eye exam, indicating that diabetes has been present long enough to have already caused permanent damage.

If a diagnosis does not occur until late in the disease process, the major goal is tertiary prevention, to remediate to the extent possible rather than cure. The goals include minimizing complications, delaying the associated mortality, and optimizing health-related quality of life while attending to the person as a holistic being (Chapter 1).

For today's older adult with a preexisting chronic disease, the importance is its effect on function. The effect may be as little as an inconvenience or as great as an impairment of one's ability to live independently. When superimposed on the normal changes with aging, the likelihood of the person developing frailty and needing assistance in daily living increases over time.

The relationship between chronic disease, aging, and lifestyle is complex. Many diseases have been viewed as intrinsic to aging. Although chronic diseases are not normal parts of aging, the number of persons with them is growing rapidly worldwide; no country can avoid this burgeoning problem. We know now that many chronic diseases could be eliminated through preventive strategies, especially when started at a young age. If the major lifestyle risk factors are eliminated (Box 21.1), all of which are within control of the individual, a significant amount of disease could be prevented. Understanding which preventive strategies are the most effective is becoming clearer as organizations such as the National Institutes of Health invest heavily in related research.

As discussed in Chapter 1, the US Department of Health and Human Services has developed multiple strategies to attempt to reduce the incidence of chronic disease and publishes their

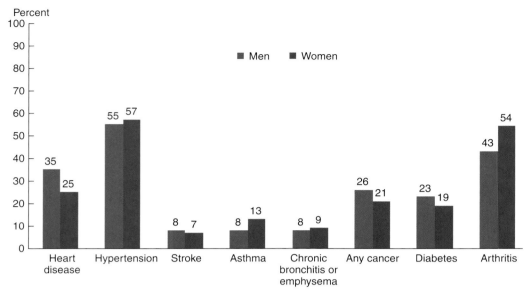

NOTE: Data are based on a 2-year average from 2013–2014. See Appendix B for the definition of race and Hispanic origin in the National Health Interview Survey.
Reference population: These data refer to the civilian noninstitutionalized population.
SOURCE: Centers for Disease Control and Prevention, National Center for Health Statistics, National Health Interview Survey.

Fig. 21.1 Chronic Health Conditions Among the Population Age 65 and Older, by Sex, 2013–2014.
(Redrawn from Federal Interagency Forum on Aging-Related Statistics: *Older Americans 2016: key indicators of well-being*, Washington, DC, 2016, U.S. Government Printing Office.)

BOX 21.1 Major Global Lifestyle Risk Factors for the Development of Chronic Disease

Tobacco use	Physical inactivity
Unhealthy diet	Alcohol abuse

From World Health Organization (WHO): *10 facts on noncommunicable diseases*, 2018. http://www.who.int/features/factfiles/noncommunicable_diseases/en/. Accessed July 2018.

BOX 21.2 Resources for Best Practice

World Health Organization: *10 Facts on noncommunicable diseases*, http://www.who.int/features/factfiles/noncommunicable_diseases/en.

World Health Organization: *Chronic disease and health promotion*, http://www.who.int/chp/en.

Healthy People: *Older adults*, http://www.healthypeople.gov/2020/topics-objectives/topic/older-adult.

Centers for Disease Control and Prevention: www.cdc.gov (search "frailty" and "chronic disease")

National Institute of Aging: http://www.nia.nih.go. Research focuses on the increased risk and severity of health problems as people age.

---

progress in the document *Healthy People 2020* (USDHHS, 2018). Important strategies to help a person prevent or live healthily with chronic diseases are engaging in physical activity, reducing obesity, stopping smoking, and taking medications as prescribed. The World Health Organization (WHO) has developed a global action plan identifying multiple targets and indicators that assist countries to set national goals and policies addressing the prevention and optimal management of chronic diseases. These cover a wide range of topics and are similar to many of those found in *Healthy People 2020* (WHO, 2017) (Box 21.2).

Any consideration of chronic disease in later life leads to multiple questions. How is it that some persons develop many of the "chronic diseases of old age" and others do not? As the understanding of genomics develops, will the line between aging and chronic conditions become more blurred or clearer? We have learned that most lung diseases in late life are the result of life choices earlier in life, such as smoking, yet as one ages, so does the susceptibility to pneumonia, even for the nonsmoker. With the introduction of antiretroviral therapy in the 1990s, persons with human immunodeficiency virus (HIV) are living longer than they ever had before. An HIV diagnosis no longer means imminent death; it has become a chronic disease instead.

How will this new "collection" of diseases affect aging persons with HIV and society?

A MODEL FOR CHRONIC ILLNESS

Although there are many conceptual models from which chronic illness can be viewed, the trajectory model has long aided health care providers to understand the realities of chronic illness and its effect on individuals (Corbin and Strauss, 1992; Lubkin and Larsen, 2012; Strauss and Glaser, 1975). Using this model, chronic illness is viewed from a life course perspective or along a trajectory—on a health and wellness continuum (Chapter 1).

The chronic illness trajectory (Table 21.1) represents nine phases along which a person moves back and forth, up and down. These are (1) pretrajectory, (2) trajectory onset, (3) stable, (4) unstable, (5) acute, (6) crisis, (7) comeback, (8) downward, and (9) dying.

TABLE 21.1   Chronic Illness Trajectory.

Phase	Definition
1. Pretrajectory	Before the illness course occurs, the preventive phase, no signs or symptoms present
2. Trajectory onset	Signs and symptoms are present to some extent, includes diagnostic period
3. Stable	Controlled illness course/symptoms
4. Unstable	Illness course/symptoms not controlled by regimen but not requiring or desiring hospitalization
5. Acute	Active illness or complications that require hospitalization for management
6. Crisis	Life-threatening situation; acute threat to self-identity
7. Comeback	While this is much less likely to occur along the trajectory of those who are frail, this is a period of temporary remission from the crisis
8. Downward	Progressive decline in physical/mental status characterized by increasing disability/symptoms
9. Dying	Immediate weeks, days, hours preceding death

During the pretrajectory phase (#1) preventive practices are used to prevent the development of a chronic disease to the extent possible. Healthy aging includes behaviors such as eating a heart healthy diet to prevent hypertension. The nurse advocates for health-promoting activities with individuals and in the community.

At the beginning of the trajectory phase (#2), initial signs of illnesses appear, and diagnoses are made. In the stable phase (#3), the chronic condition is present and while not curable, it can be *controlled* so that the person has few, if any, symptoms and is able to maintain a high quality of life. This stability is due in large part to secondary prevention and multiple factors. It is also the result of a combination of factors, including high-quality nursing and personal care for the person residing in a care setting such as an assisted living facility or nursing home. The person is receiving high-quality medical care provided by nurse practitioners and high-quality nursing from the gerontological nurse and staff. For those with more complex chronic diseases, control requires coordination among members of the health care team, often with the nurse coordinating this care.

During periods of unstable disease exacerbations (#4), one or more of the dimensions which define the individual are stressed. In the aging adult this is a particularly precarious stage because the uncontrollable chronic disease is superimposed on reduced physiological reserve and other normal changes of aging. In some cases, the chronic diseases lead to frailty, at which time further deterioration of health is likely. For the older adult who is already frail, a previously controlled health condition can rapidly become acute or life threatening. The nurse is instrumental in ensuring that prompt care is delivered in a manner that maximizes the chances that the person can return to the highest level of wellness possible. If care is delayed for those who are frail, it may not be possible to stop the overall downward trend.

In the acute phase (#5), severe and unrelieved symptoms or disease complications are present. But every effort is made to stop the escalating symptoms in the frail older adult and the development of geriatric syndromes and enable the person to return to some level of stability if possible. Should this phase be reached, the nurse may be the one to inform the person and his or her family that a complete return to the trajectory phase (#2) may not be possible, but every effort will be made to control any distressing symptoms and to keep the person comfortable. For those who are very ill with multiple comorbidities, this phase may be bypassed, and the person may proceed directly from the unstable phase (#4) to the crisis phase (#6).

In the crisis phase (#6), major complications of a chronic disease become critical and life-threatening. It may be triggered by an event such as an acute myocardial infarction (AMI) or a fracture as a result of the imbalance associated with Parkinson's disease. The nurse provides or facilitates immediate emergency care but only to the point that had been expressed by the person in an advance directive or by a health care proxy at the time of the incident. Nurses caring for ill and especially frail patients need to know the content of their advance directives and understand their wishes in order to respond appropriately in a life-threatening situation.

Although less likely in frail older adults, the person may be able to restore equilibrium (#7) or a somewhat steady state for some period of time. The older one becomes, the more chronic diseases accumulate and the less likely the person will ever return to a period when symptoms are not noticeable. This is important in conversations about resuscitative efforts in frail persons or those with multiple chronic conditions. The final downward phase (#9) is that which ends in death (Lubkin and Larsen, 2012). During this phase the nurse has a significant opportunity, responsibility, and privilege to provide comfort at the end of life; of reassuring those who are dying; and then of ensuring that the dying patient continues to receive the highest quality nursing and medical care possible (Chapter 35).

During acute exacerbations of chronic diseases, hospitalization may be necessary, followed by active rehabilitation at home or at designated rehabilitation centers/skilled nursing facilities, such as those found in high-income countries. Once the disease has stabilized the person may return to full function or to partial function. If the limitations become chronic, physical, functional, or cognitive assistance will likely be needed. Informal help may be available with a move to the home of a friend or family member. Others may have the resources to hire the formal help of professional caregivers. Still others move to institutional settings such as assisted living facilities, nursing homes, or group homes. Unfortunately, options in the United States are highly dependent on personal financial resources; there are solutions for the very poor and the wealthy but are tenuous at best for near-poor and middle-income individuals and families.

The shape and stability of the trajectory are influenced by the combined efforts, attitudes, and beliefs held by the person, family members, and significant others. Gerontological nurses have the opportunity to promote healthy aging at any point on the trajectory. The person's perceptions of both needs met and functional limitations are paramount to predicting movement along the illness trajectory (Corbin and Strauss, 1992).

FRAILTY, AGING, AND CHRONIC DISEASE

The association between age and chronic disease and the development of frailty remains unclear. However, there is an international consensus in the meaning of frailty as "a multi-dimensional syndrome characterized by decreased reserves and diminished resistance to stressors" (Cesari et al, 2014). The more frail one is, the faster one proceeds along the Chronic Illness Trajectory, the less likely one can move backward toward stability, and the greater the risk for death at any time the person becomes unstable. Medical and social diagnoses leading to frailty may never be found (primary frailty). At other times, it is related to the downward progression of a specific chronic disease (secondary frailty) consistent with the downward slope of the chronic disease trajectory.

The phenotype of frailty designed by Fried and colleagues in 2001 is still recognized. The formal diagnosis is based on the evaluation of at least three of the following: unintentional weight loss, self-reported exhaustion, muscle weakness, slow walking speed, and low activity (Fried et al, 2001).

Sarcopenia has also been found to be associated with frailty (Box 21.3). With a multifactorial pathogenesis, it is an expression of age-related changes, neuromuscular function, and muscle protein turnover. Sarcopenia is associated with adverse health outcomes during exacerbation of chronic diseases, such as that at trajectory phase 4 and above (Liguori et al, 2018).

In much of the geriatric literature, the signs leading to frailty are referred to as "geriatric syndromes." Together, they significantly increase the vulnerability to any challenge to the physical, cognitive, or emotional state of health; it becomes more difficult to maintain independence. In other words, the normal age-related decreases in reserve capacity are exacerbated, sometimes to the point that compensation is not possible. Of note is that there is not necessarily a diagnosis in the usual sense of the word, but rather the report or observation of problems that cannot be explained by other means.

The number of frail older adults is increasing at an alarming rate. In a meta-analysis of 5447 older adults, 19.1% were found to be physically frail (Verlaan et al, 2017). A burgeoning population

---

BOX 21.3   Tips for Best Practice

Assessing Frailty

Frailty is loosely defined as evidence of three of the following: unexplained weight loss, self-reported exhaustion, weak grip strength, slow walking speed, and low activity.

It is better to ask the patient specifically about each one of these symptoms. Many people consider the signs as "just a normal part of aging."

BOX 21.4   Nurses' Role in Caring for Persons With Chronic Disease

- Assessing the older person and his or her family strengths and challenges
- Teaching related to healthy lifestyle modifications, preservation of energy, and self-care strategies
- Encouraging the reduction of modifiable risk factors
- Counseling the individual in the development of reasonable expectations of self
- Providing access to resources when possible
- Referring appropriately and when needed
- Organizing and leading interdisciplinary case conferences and team meetings
- Facilitating advance care planning and palliative care when appropriate

---

drives the need to actively address wellness in aging to prevent both chronic disease and the development of frailty in future generations.

Working with older adults who are either frail or are living with chronic illnesses means that the gerontological nurse has the opportunity to decrease both the morbidity and the mortality of older adults (Box 21.4). The next several chapters provide basic information on the most common chronic conditions the gerontological nurse will encounter in persons as they age in today's society. Strategies will be proposed to promote healthy aging regardless of the limitations with which one lives. We do not cover all possible conditions, nor do we provide a comprehensive medical management of these disorders. However, certain disorders are encountered frequently enough in late life to merit special attention.

KEY CONCEPTS

- The nation's goals include increasing the span of healthy life. The challenge to this goal is to help persons find ways to promote healthy aging in the presence of chronic disease.
- The effects of chronic illness range from mild to life-limiting, with each person responding to unique circumstances in a highly individualized manner.
- Coping with chronic illness can be a physical, psychological, and spiritual challenge.
- The Chronic Illness Trajectory is a useful framework to facilitate understanding chronic illness and designing nursing interventions to promote healthy aging.

- The goals of promoting healthy aging include minimizing risk for disease and frailty, and in the presence of either, alleviating symptoms, delaying or avoiding the development of complications including end-organ damage, and maximizing function and quality of life. It also includes providing comfort to the dying.
- The gerontological nurse has the potential to serve as a leader in the promotion of health and the prevention of disease at all phases along the trajectory.

REFERENCES

Cesari M, Gambassi G, van Kan GA, Vellas B: The frailty phenotype and the frailty index: different instruments for different purposes, *Age Ageing* 43(1):10–12, 2014.

Corbin JM, Strauss A: A nursing model for chronic illness management based upon the trajectory framework. In Woog P, editor: *The chronic illness framework: the Corbin and Strauss nursing model,* New York, 1992, Springer.

Centers for Disease Control and Prevention (CDC): *About chronic disease,* 2019. https://www.cdc.gov/chronicdisease/about/index.htm. Accessed March 2019.

Fried LP, Tangen CM, Walston J, et al: Frailty in older adults: evidence for a phenotype, *J Gerontol A Biol Sci Med Sci* 56(3):M146–M156, 2001.

Liguori I, Russo G, Coscia V, et al: Orthostatic hypotension in the elderly: a marker of clinical frailty? *J Am Med Dir Assoc* 19(9): 779–785, 2018.

Lubkin I, Larsen PD: *Chronic illness: impact and intervention,* ed 8, Burlington, MA, 2012, Jones & Bartlett.

Strauss A, Glaser B: *Chronic illness and the quality of life,* St Louis, MO, 1975, Mosby.

U.S. Department of Health and Human Services (USDHHS): *Healthy People 2020,* 2018. http://www.healthypeople.gov. Accessed July 2018.

Verlaan S, Ligthart-Melis GC, Wijers SLJ, Cederholm T, Maier AB, de van der Schueren MAE: High prevalence of physical frailty among community-dwelling malnourished older adults—a systematic review and meta-analysis, *J Am Med Dir Assoc* 18(5):374–382, 2017.

World Health Organization (WHO): *10 facts on ageing and the life course,* 2017. http://www.who.int/features/factfiles/ageing/en/. Accessed July 2018.

World Health Organization (WHO): *Noncommunicable diseases,* 2018. http://www.who.int/news-room/fact-sheets/detail/noncommunicable-diseases. Accessed July 2018.

22

Cardiovascular and Cerebrovascular Health and Wellness

Kathleen Jett

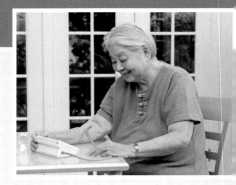

http://evolve.elsevier.com/Touhy/TwdHlthAging

A STUDENT SPEAKS

I thought all hearts sounded the same, but after gaining a little more experience I started hearing all sorts of differences.

Helen, a 19-year-old nursing student

AN OLDER ADULT SPEAKS

I had always been very active and healthy and then slowly I started feeling more and more tired. I just thought it was due to growing older but found out that my heart was no longer beating as it should.

Isabelle, age 86

LEARNING OBJECTIVES

On completion of this chapter, the reader will be able to:

1. Describe the normal changes in the aging cardiovascular system.
2. Identify the most common cardiovascular disorders seen in later life.
3. Describe how the presentation of these disorders in older adults differs from that seen in younger adults.
4. Suggest interventions to promote healthy aging in the face of cerebrovascular disease regardless of the stage of illness.

The cardiovascular system, composed of the heart and blood vessels, is the vehicle through which oxygenated nutrient-rich blood is transported throughout the body and metabolic waste is carried to the excretory organs. There are several age-related changes in the system, but these have little or no effect on the day-to-day lives of healthy older adults. However, by the time one is in later life, the lifestyle choices made earlier, such as smoking, coupled with these normal changes, result in a very high rate of cardiovascular disease (CVD). Both the prevalence and the incidence of CVD are so high that they are often mistaken as normal parts of aging and referred to as a disease of old age. While cardiovascular changes frequently occur, CVD is not always inevitable.

THE AGING HEART

One normal change to the aging heart muscle is the progressive decline in cardiac reserve. That is, it takes longer for the heart to accelerate to meet a sudden demand for oxygen and longer to return to its resting state. This becomes quite significant when an increased cardiac response is needed in the presence of a physical or mental challenge such as acute emotional distress, infection, fluid or blood loss, or tachycardia. The associated increased pulse rate seen under these circumstances in younger adults is less likely to occur in older adults, and the recognition of a psychological or physiological crisis may be delayed. Even a person with a presumably healthy heart may not be able to maintain heart function during stress, and failure can occur suddenly. In the presence of preexisting disease, this age-related change has the potential to increase both morbidity and mortality when it is not possible for the already damaged heart to suddenly work harder.

In normal aging, the heart valves separating the chambers thicken and stiffen because of lipid deposits and collagen cross-linking. In many cases the valves no longer close completely. A murmur is the sound of the backflow of blood through such a valve. A *mild systolic murmur* (between S_1 and S_2) is an expected finding in the older adult. If the nurse auscultates a systolic murmur in an asymptomatic older adult, questions should be asked. Quite unlike a younger adult, most older adults will say, "Oh, yes, I have had that for years." If this is not the case, the person is referred to a cardiologist. If the new finding is accompanied by any signs or symptoms of cardiovascular distress, it is a medical emergency. *Diastolic murmurs* (heard between S_2 and S_1) are always indicative of a serious problem in cardiac hemodynamics and these persons are followed closely by a cardiologist. The nurse's ability to monitor this fragile condition is an essential skill in geriatrics and a means to work with the patient and the family to achieve the highest health-related quality of life possible.

CARDIOVASCULAR DISEASE

In the United States, one of every four deaths is related to heart disease, that is, about 610,000 deaths a year. Coronary heart disease (CHD) is the most common type, killing 370,000 people a year. The first sign is often an acute myocardial infarction (AMI) or heart attack. Each year 735,000 people have an AMI, 525,000 of these are the first for the person and 210,000 will have had at least one previously (CDC, 2017a). Research has found that the risk factors for CVD are universal. They include those that the person cannot control, those in full control of the person, and those suspected to have an influence (Fig. 22.1). Among those that cannot be controlled are genetic factors (Khera et al, 2016).

CVD derives from damage to the blood vessels or to the heart itself. Hypertension (HTN), CHD, heart failure (HF), atrial fibrillation (AF), and peripheral and cerebral vascular disorders (strokes) in older adults are summarized in this chapter. For more detailed examinations of these conditions, the reader is referred to geriatric medicine and nursing texts that are disease based.

Hypertension

HTN is the most common chronic CVD encountered by the gerontological nurse. It occurs in 75 million people in the United States, or one out of every three persons, the majority of whom are African American and men; only about 50% of those with HTN have it under control, increasing one's risk for heart disease, HF, and stroke (CDC, 2016a, 2019; NHLBI, 2017a). The most common pattern for older adults is what is referred to as isolated systolic HTN with a drop in diastolic blood pressure (DBP) over time (Aronow, 2017).

The American College of Cardiology and the National Heart, Lung, and Blood Institute work to provide both the professional and lay community with the best, evidence-based information about the treatment and prevention of HTN (CDC, 2014). The guidelines are drawn from the results of a number of well-known studies, including the long-standing Framingham Study, the European Working Party on High Blood Pressure in the Elderly (EWPHE), Hypertension in the Very Elderly Trial (HYVET), Systolic Hypertension in the Elderly Program (SHEP), and the Systolic Hypertension in Europe (Syst-Eur) Trial (NHLBI, 2013).

Signs and Symptoms

Most persons with HTN are asymptomatic, and diagnoses are made only during a routine health screening or after the manifestation of a disease that has developed because of long-standing uncontrolled HTN. Some people complain of a headache, "bad blood," light-headedness, a "swimmy head," or a "full head." These and other phrases are culture-based idioms and the nurse must first determine if the person believes that the symptoms are from an elevated or lowered blood pressure. Upon blood pressure (BP) measurement, the person may be normotensive, hypotensive, or hypertensive.

Diagnosis

The past guidelines for the diagnosis of high blood pressure categorized stage 1, 2, and 3 with a goal of "normal" BP or less than 140/90 mm Hg and less than 160/90 mm Hg for persons older than age 65 (Whelton et al, 2018).

New guidelines from the American Heart Association, American College of Cardiology, and others recommend that a target systolic blood pressure (SBP) and DBP be no greater than 120/80 mm Hg for all persons, including those at least 65 years of age. However, health care providers such as nurse practitioners are expected to work with the individual older adult to determine what "numbers" are best for him or her while considering the risk for heart disease, comorbidities, and expected longevity. An SBP over 180 mm Hg and/or a DBP over 120 mm Hg in the presence of target organ damage is always a hypertensive emergency (Whelton et al, 2018)

Diagnosis requires two measurements. A second set is done at a different time for the diagnosis to be confirmed. Out of office and self-monitoring measurements are recommended for both diagnosis and decision making about medication use and dosage changes, especially any time "white coat syndrome" is suspected or known (Whelton et al, 2018). It is very important that any home device used is reliable and the person's technique is accurate (Box 22.1).

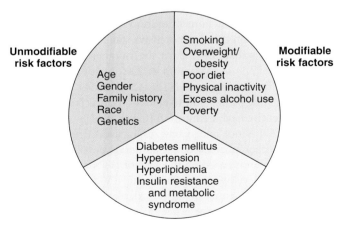

Unmodifiable risk factors
Age
Gender
Family history
Race
Genetics

Smoking
Overweight/ obesity
Poor diet
Physical inactivity
Excess alcohol use
Poverty
Modifiable risk factors

Diabetes mellitus
Hypertension
Hyperlipidemia
Insulin resistance
and metabolic
syndrome

Treatable risk factors

Fig. 22.1 Risk Factors for Coronary Heart Disease. (From Whelton PK, Carey R M, Aronow WS, et al: 2017 ACC/AHA/AAPA/ABC/ACPM/AGA/APhA/ASH/ASPC/NMA/PCNA Guideline for the prevention, detection, evaluation, and management of high blood pressure in adults A report of the American College of Cardiology/American Heart Association task force on clinical practice guidelines. American College of Cardiology, May 7, 2018. http://www.acc.org/latest-in-cardiology/ten-points-to-remember/2017/11/09/11/41/2017-guideline-for-high-blood-pressure-in-adults. Accessed April 2019.)

Etiology

The exact cause of primary HTN cannot be determined in most persons. Risk factors include smoking, diabetes, dyslipidemia, excessive weight, low fitness, unhealthy diet, psychosocial stress, and sleep apnea (Whelton et al, 2018). The normal changes in the aging vascular system (p. 287), coupled with lifelong habits are the factors most likely to account for the increased incidence of SBP with aging (CDC, 2016a). Secondary HTN can be caused by several conditions including chronic kidney disease, obstructive sleep apnea, and several medications such as non-steroidal antiinflammatories, decongestants, and caffeine (Whelton et al, 2018).

Complications

While many of the complications of HTN are preventable, there is a very low level of adequate control of BP (Healthy People 2020 A box). The percentages of those with diagnosed HTN increases for those 75 years and over (66.7% men and 78.5% women) (CDC, 2016b). The complications of uncontrolled HTN are many, most notably increased rates of strokes, AMIs, and coronary artery disease (CAD) (Box 22.2). Finally, while still controversial, in recent years there has been more and more discussion of the relationship between cognitive functioning and BP. If too high, small vessel clots can lead to vascular dementia. If the BP is too low then the already compromised brain will suffer from the reduced circulation (Foster-Dingley et al, 2015; Meissner, 2016).

 HEALTHY PEOPLE 2020 A

Hypertension

Goal
- Reduce the proportion of adults with hypertension.

Baseline
- 29.9% of adults aged 18 years and older had high blood pressure/hypertension in 2005 to 2008 (age adjusted to the year 2000 standard population).

Target
- 26.9% of those older than 18 years of age by 2020.

Data from U.S. Department of Health and Human Services, Office of Disease Prevention and Health Promotion: *Healthy People 2020*, 2018. https://www.healthypeople.gov/2020/topics-objectives/topic/heart-disease-and-stroke/objectives. Accessed March 2018.

Adapted from Potter J, Myint P: Hypertension. In Fillit HM, Rockwood K, Young J, editors: *Brocklehurst's textbook of geriatric medicine and gerontology*, Philadelphia, 2016, Elsevier, pp 295–306.

TABLE 22.1   Relationship Between Lifestyle Change and Reduction in Systolic Blood Pressure.

Lifestyle Change	Approximate Reduction in SBP
Reduce weight	Decrease of 5–20 mm Hg per 20 lb loss
Adopt DASH diet	Decrease of 8–14 mm Hg
Lower sodium intake	Decrease of 2–8 mm Hg
Increase physical activity	Decrease of 4–9 mm Hg
Limit alcohol intake	Decrease of 2–4 mm Hg

DASH, Dietary Approaches to Stop Hypertension; *SBP*, systolic blood pressure.

Treatment

Nonpharmacological interventions that promote a healthy lifestyle have been found to be highly effective in reducing BP and, in doing so, minimize or even prevent long-term complications. There is considerable evidence regarding the influence of diet and obesity on blood pressure. Healthy eating habits, especially the Dietary Approaches to Stop Hypertension (DASH) or Mediterranean diets, have been found to irrefutably lower blood pressure. Even modest reductions in sodium intake and body weight may return a person to a normotensive state, reduce the risk for other CVD or stroke, or reduce the number of medications needed (Table 22.1). A maximum of 2300 mg of sodium is recommended for those without HTN (CDC, 2014). If the person can read, teaching people how to read food labels is an important part of preventive health education (Chapter 14).

When HTN is not adequately responsive to nonpharmacological approaches, pharmacological interventions may be necessary. The decision is based on the level of HTN and a calculated 10-year risk of developing atherosclerotic CVD (http://tools.acc.org/ASCVD-Risk-Estimator-Plus/#!/calculate/estimate/).

It is not uncommon for a person to require three different types of antihypertensives to obtain control. Additionally, which medications are prescribed is highly dependent on concurrent medical conditions. The most common medications the gerontological nurse will work with are calcium channel blockers (CCBs), thiazide diuretics, beta-blockers, angiotensin-converting enzyme inhibitors (ACEs), or angiotensin receptor blockers (ARBs). The ACE and the ARB cannot be used together due to the risk of hyperkalemia. There are three types of CCB. The CCB dihydropyridines (e.g., nifedipine) cause edema

BOX 22.3 Tips for Best Practice

Controlling Hypertension

With few exceptions the nurse promotes healthy aging by helping people maintain their blood pressure within an acceptable range. For those with late- or end-stage illness such as dementia, the range of acceptable blood pressures is broader.

BOX 22.4 Signs of Potential Exacerbation of Illness in an Older Adult With Coronary Heart Disease

- Light-headedness or dizziness
- Disturbances in gait and balance
- Loss of appetite or unexplained loss of weight
- Inability to concentrate or shortened attention span
- Changes in personality or mood
- Changes in grooming habits
- Unusual patterns in urination or defecation
- Vague discomfort, frequent bouts of anxiety
- Excessive fatigue, vague pain
- Withdrawal from usual sources of pleasure

and the nondihydropyridines are associated with bradycardia and heart block. Thiazide and loop diuretics ("water pills") are used most often. The latter group (e.g., furosemide) is potassium wasting so it must be given either with a potassium-sparing medication such as an ACE or with potassium supplementation. According to the American College of Cardiology, the diuretic chlorthalidone is preferred because of a long half-life and proven reduction of CVD risk. Finally, beta-blockers area frequently prescribed to older adults due to the high rate of CAD. The nurse must watch for bradycardia with this group of medications (Whelton et al, 2018).

A prescribing provider, such as a nurse practitioner, should do everything possible to minimize the number of medications taken by older adults to reduce polypharmacy and to keep the regimen simple with once-daily dosing (Chapter 9). Due to the high risk for orthostatic hypotension and related falls, the lowest dose is initially prescribed and the gerontological nurse checks the person's BP frequently to assess for medication side effects and the need for a dose adjustment. By reducing or eliminating modifiable risk factors, HTN can often be controlled or prevented, leading to healthier aging (Box 22.3).

Coronary Heart Disease

The heart is dependent on the coronary arteries for the oxygen and nutrients it needs to survive. Although not a normal change of aging, the incidence of CHD rises significantly with age and is the most common form of heart disease. CHD is referred to as atherosclerosis, hardening of the arteries, coronary artery disease (CAD), or ischemic heart disease.

About 610,000 persons die of heart disease each year in the United States; 370,000 of these die of CAD. Heart disease is the number one cause of death among non-Hispanic blacks/whites (23.8% each). It is second to cancer among American Indians/ Alaskan Natives (18.4%) and Asian/Pacific Islanders (22.2%). Every year 735,000 Americans will have an AMI, and for 210,000 of them it is not their first. Someone will have a heart attack every 40 seconds (CDC, 2017b).

Signs and Symptoms

The major symptoms of CAD in older adults are exertional shortness of breath (dyspnea) and unexplained fatigue, identical to those symptoms that are seen in many other health problems common in late life (Box 22.4). However, angina from ischemia is usually less severe in later life, shorter in duration, and described as postprandial epigastric pain or as pain in the back or shoulders rather than the jaw or chest (Aronow, 2017). These symptoms may be misdiagnosed as arthritis, muscular back pain, or reflux. If anginal, symptoms may worsen over

time, increase in frequency, intensity, or duration, and occur with less and less provocation (unstable angina). Cardiac death as the first sign of CAD increases with age (Aronow, 2017). Unstable angina is associated with arrhythmias, tachycardia, and ventricular fibrillation.

If an older adult has an AMI there may be no anticipatory symptoms at all, referred to as a "silent MI." The classic symptoms such as sudden gripping chest pain with radiation to arm and chin may not be present or they may be completely atypical, such as an unexplained fall or an acute change in mental status (Table 22.2). AMIs without the classic symptoms rarely occur in younger adults. However, younger adults may have no symptoms of early CAD and may not know they have it until suffering an AMI.

Diagnosis

The diagnosis of CAD in the older adult may be incidental to another examination that includes a resting electrocardiogram (ECG) (e.g., during an annual Wellness Visit covered by Medicare) or during the evaluation of another problem that is found to be the result of end-organ damage, such as AF. If abnormalities are found on the ECG, interventions can begin immediately (e.g., smoking cessation, weight loss) before damage progresses or to reverse the existing damage.

TABLE 22.2 Key Differences in the Signs of Typical Cardiac-Related "Chest Pain" (Angina) in a Younger Adult Compared With Atypical Signs More Common in an Older Adult.

Symptom	Classic	Atypical
Chest pain	Present	Absent
Radiations of pain to arm or jaw	Often present	Absent
Sweating	Often present	Absent
Dyspnea	Often present	May be only symptom
Fatigue	Often present	May be only symptom

Adapted from Taffet GF: Coronary artery disease and atrial fibrillation. In Ham RJ, Sloane PD, Warshaw GA, et al, editors: *Primary care geriatrics: a case-based approach*, Philadelphia, 2014, Elsevier, pp 395–405.

Noninvasive diagnostic measures include a stress test and cardiac serum markers (e.g., CK-MB and troponins) and invasive tests include cardiac catheterization. Definitive testing may not always be appropriate, such as in those who are very frail with limited life expectancies, when the focus of care is on optimizing quality of life and healthy aging (Chapter 35). If a person is suspected of having an AMI, a definitive diagnosis requires the documentation of changes in biochemical markers within 24 to 72 hours of the event (Bashore et al, 2017) (Chapter 8). Life-saving measures can be initiated if they are consistent with the patient's expressed or pre-expressed wishes.

Etiology

The Cardiovascular Health Study, the SHEP study, and others have clearly identified the risk factors for CAD (Fig. 22.1). Any of these exacerbate the changes in the blood vessels that occur with aging. The walls of the arteries, pliable in youth, thicken and stiffen; there are changes in lipid, cholesterol, and phospholipid metabolism. This may result in the formation of plaques that adhere to vessel walls and ultimately occlude the vessel or cause a spasm in the pericardium when the heart is stressed. Once this occurs, the capacity for oxygenation of the surrounding heart tissue is reduced and will ultimately lead to tissue death (necrosis).

Complications

The most important complication of CAD is the AMI because of either acute or long-term cardiac anoxia. Approximately 15% of those who have a heart attack will die from it immediately or soon thereafter (CDC, 2017b). The event may be triggered by a situation in which there is a sudden need for myocardial oxygen and the body cannot respond adequately. This may be part of a normal change of aging or from a sudden occlusion of an artery from a blood clot or plaque attempting to pass through a narrowed vessel. Even if the person recovers, an AMI can cause from a small to extensive amount of damage to the heart muscle. If it is witnessed and resuscitation is desired (the person is a "code") and promptly initiated, both the morbidity and the mortality of the person are significantly decreased.

In chronic CHD/CAD the body attempts to compensate for the damage through a process called remodeling in which the heart enlarges and changes shape. This remodeling eventually leads to a decrease in cardiac pumping efficiency and the gradual onset of other cardiomyopathies.

Treatment

Both nonpharmacological and pharmacological approaches are usually necessary to treat the person with CAD. Nonpharmacological features of treatment emphasize addressing all reversible factors. Pharmacological interventions usually include a combination of aspirin, clopidogrel (Plavix), and nitrates (isosorbide). Beta-blockers (e.g., metoprolol, atenolol) and ACE inhibitors have been found to prolong life following an AMI. CCBs can only be used with caution (Reuben et al, 2017). During acute events additional treatment is needed, usually sublingual or aerosol nitroglycerin. Pharmacological interventions are geared toward minimizing morbidity and mortality and promoting health-related quality of life, including palliative care when appropriate.

Atrial Fibrillation

AF is the most common cardiac dysrhythmia and caused by disorganized electrical impulses to the atria. On assessment it is heard and felt as an irregular pulse. The irregularity may have a pattern or be completely random (paroxysmal); it may occur once, intermittently, or persistently. While it may occur in younger adults, it has a high incidence and prevalence in older adults and increases with each decade; approximately 10% of those over 80 years of age have AF (Cole and Zimmerman, 2017).

Signs and Symptoms

In many cases, AF itself is completely asymptomatic and is only identified at the time of a stroke or by the nurse or other practitioner as part of a thorough auscultation of the heart and cardiovascular assessment. If symptoms occur, they are vague, such as fatigue, and since the person usually already has other underlying chronic diseases, this is difficult to attribute specifically to the AF. The fatigue may be attributed to "old age" or the onset of frailty. Occasionally people report the sensation of "palpations" and intermittent shortness of breath, or nonspecific chest pain, especially if the fibrillation is paroxysmal (Box 22.5).

Diagnosis

AF is the only common arrhythmia in which ventricular rate is rapid and the rhythm is irregular at the time of diagnosis. It may be associated with recurrent falls, episodes of syncope, "dizzy spells," and worsening of HF. It may be acute (lasting <48 hours) or chronic. The frequency of the irregularity can be evaluated by a 24-hour Holter monitor. An ECG may confirm persistent AF but may miss that which is paroxysmal.

Etiology

AF can be the end-result of diabetes, sleep apnea, thyroid disorders, alcohol abuse, several cardiomyopathies, including CHD and HTN, and a number of other conditions. It also may be related to the use of beta-blockers (Bashore et al, 2017). More than half of the incidence of AF is related to inadequate control of modifiable risk factors, identical to those associated with CAD (Fig. 22.1). It is associated with a heightened risk for dementia and stroke-related mortality; however, in each case the rates are highly variable (Alonso and Arenas de Larriva, 2016).

BOX 22.5   Sometimes I Can Feel the Palpitations

Ruth is a 75-year-old active and energetic woman with paroxysmal atrial fibrillation. Because of this condition, she takes anticoagulants—that is, she takes medication to prevent her blood from clotting and to decrease her risk of having a stroke. Most of the time Ruth's heart beats regularly and at other times it does not. When it does not, she has a sense of "chest palpitations" but they have never given her "problems." One day Ruth's heart seems to be beating much more than usual. She checked it and it was at least 180 beats per minute, it was highly irregular, and she was not feeling well. She called for an ambulance and was taken immediately to the hospital where she was stabilized and then sent home.

Complications

Because the pulsations of the heart in AF are irregular, there is always a risk for pooling of blood in the atria when the time between the beats is prolonged. This pooling increases the risk for the development of emboli. The most serious complication of an AF is a stroke if emboli should leave the heart and travel to the brain (Bashore et al, 2017). If the fibrillation causes persistent tachycardia as a compensating mechanism, then significant hypotension, myocardial ischemia, and other cardiomyopathies can develop.

Treatment

Treatment for AF is to correct precipitating causes, control heart rate (<110 beats/min), and antithrombotic therapy. In some cases, a person is a candidate for cardiac ablation. In 2014, the American College of Cardiology/American Heart Association provided detailed guidelines for the management of AF (January et al, 2014). This includes the use of the CHA2DS2-VASc Risk Score (easily available on the Internet, e.g., https://www.mdcalc.com/cha2ds2-vasc-score-atrial-fibrillation-stroke-risk) in assessing individual stroke risk and determining the appropriateness of initiating antithrombotic therapy (Lane and Lip, 2012; Li et al, 2018). In the outpatient setting, including in long-term care facilities, rate control is usually achieved using beta-blockers, but bradycardia is a potential side effect. Patients can be taught to monitor their pulses. For the person at a low risk for a stroke, aspirin along with clopidogrel (Plavix) is used. For those with any higher risk, even for intermittent AF, lifelong anticoagulation therapy remains the gold standard.

The anticoagulant warfarin has long been the gold standard for the reduction of risk for stroke (Cole and Zimmerman, 2017). It can be used in persons with both nonvalvular and valvular (e.g., artificial heart valve) disease. However, it has a very narrow therapeutic window and must be monitored closely and regularly to ensure that the level of anticoagulation is within an appropriate range (via INR) (Chapter 8). There is always a heightened risk of bleeding. Vitamin K is the antidote and can quickly inactivate the effects of warfarin. It interacts with most antibiotics and many dietary supplements and herbal products (Chapters 9 and 10); when these are taken, even closer monitoring is necessary and temporary reductions in the dose of warfarin may be necessary.

Several newer anticoagulants, the direct-acting oral anticoagulants (DOACs), are available. They do not require monitoring, making these more acceptable to some. Two of these (dabigatran and apixaban) are associated with less risk for intracranial bleeding than warfarin (Bashore et al, 2017). Rivaroxaban has a similar bleeding profile to warfarin. A person who is taking any of the DOACs should be directed to promptly seek emergency support with any obvious bleeding or the potential of bleeding (e.g., following trauma to the head following a fall). A reversal agent for dabigatran was approved in October 2017.

Nurses have important roles in helping patients understand the dangers and benefits of anticoagulation therapy, the impact of medication/food/herb/nutritional supplement interactions (Chapters 9 and 10), the need for strict adherence, and the effect of high and low vitamin K diets on coagulation when taking warfarin. Nurses often perform point-of-care warfarin monitoring, and advanced practice nurses adjust doses as needed. Nurses are often involved in the conversations regarding the risk/benefit ratio of continuing anticoagulation therapy for the person at risk for falling or with a history of falling.

Heart Failure

HF is a general term used to describe a buildup of fluid in the lungs, liver, gastrointestinal tract, and arms and legs due to the heart's inability to either fill with enough blood or pump hard enough to meet the body's needs. It develops over time and affects the right side of the heart, left side, or both at the same time. While it is quite common in the United States, it is not a normal part of aging. In 2016 it was reported that 5.7 million adults had HF and about half of those who develop HF die within 5 years (CDC, 2016c). In a study of 8532 persons hospitalized for HF, the majority of these were African Americans (51%,) followed by Hispanic (29%), white (18%), and Asian (3.3%) (Durstenfeld et al, 2016). The incidence of HF increases with age (Healthy People 2020 B box).

 HEALTHY PEOPLE 2020 B

Hospitalizations for Heart Failure

Goal
- Reduce hospitalizations of older adults with heart failure as the principal diagnosis.

Ages 65–74
Baseline
- 9.8 hospitalizations for heart failure per 1000 people aged 65 to 74 years occurred in 2007.

Target
- No more than 8.8 hospitalizations per 1000 people aged 65 to 74 years will occur by 2020.

Ages 75–84
Baseline
- 22.4 hospitalizations for heart failure per 1000 people aged 75 to 84 years occurred in 2007.

Target
- No more than 20.2 hospitalizations per 1000 people aged 75 to 84 years will occur by 2020.

Ages 85+
Baseline
- 42.9 hospitalizations for heart failure per 1000 people aged 85 years and older occurred in 2007.

Target
- No more than 38.6 hospitalizations per 1000 people aged 85 and older will occur by 2020.

Data from U.S. Department of Health and Human Services, Office of Disease Prevention and Health Promotion: *Healthy People 2020*, 2018. https://www.healthypeople.gov/2020/topics-objectives/topic/heart-disease-and-stroke/objectives. Accessed March 2018.

BOX 22.6 Classic and Atypical Signs of Heart Failure in Older Adults

Classic (Noncerebral)	Atypical	Atypical (Cerebral)
Dyspnea	Chronic cough	Falls
Orthopnea	Insomnia	Anorexia, dyspnea
Paroxysmal nocturnal	Weight loss	Behavioral disturbances
Peripheral edema	Nausea	Decreased functional status
Unexplained weight gain	Nocturia	
Weakness	Syncope	
Poor exercise tolerance		
Abdominal pain		
Fatigue		

From Ham RJ, Sloane PD, Warshaw GA, et al: *Primary care geriatrics*, ed 6, Philadelphia, 2014, Elsevier.

Clinical HF is categorized as systolic failure, diastolic failure, or both. End-stage HF and acute HF are known as congestive heart failure (CHF). The extent of illness is in proportion to the person's ejection fraction, or the amount of blood leaving the ventricle with each pulsation.

CHF can appear quickly in persons with underlying CAD, especially those who have already had at least one AMI, and more slowly in persons with long-standing HTN. Accurately attributing the signs and symptoms reported by the patient to HF is complicated in the older adult because any one of these symptoms can also be caused by other chronic diseases, geriatric syndromes, or commonly prescribed medications. The signs and symptoms are often atypical in the older adult (Box 22.6). HF symptoms are ranked by their effect on function and activity.

Left-Sided Failure

Left-sided failure is a weakening of the left side of the heart. In left ventricular (LV) systolic dysfunction the weakened ventricle cannot pump adequately and blood flows backward into the organs, causing fluids to build-up in the lungs and/or edema in other parts of the body. In the presence of LV *diastolic dysfunction*, the heart is unable to relax enough to allow adequate diastolic function, yet the ejection fraction remains 50% or higher and persons may be only minimally symptomatic in day-to-day life. Symptoms may only occur when the heart is stressed (i.e., when there is a need to increase stroke volume).

Right-Sided Failure

Long-standing left-sided failure will eventually also cause right-sided failure. The ejection fraction is 40% or less, and the person is always symptomatic, may be very ill, and has a poor prognosis. The typical chronic illness trajectory is one of steady decline.

Signs and Symptoms

Early in left-sided failure, the only symptom may be shortness of breath, especially on exertion (dyspnea on exertion [DOE]). However, it will eventually progress to orthopnea, paroxysmal nocturnal dyspnea, and dyspnea at rest (Bowker et al, 2013). It is

common for the person to find ways to compensate for declining cardiac function without realizing it. For example, a person slowly reduces their activity level saying they are "not so fit anymore," "just not feeling right," or have a case of "the dwindles," all of which the person may attribute to advancing age. It is much more likely to be a pathological condition that may benefit from treatment. The typical chronic illness trajectory of a person with left-sided failure is periods of minimal symptoms interspersed with exacerbations of illness, often leading to hospitalizations for stabilization until this is no longer possible or the repeated hospitalizations are no longer desired.

The predominant signs and symptoms of right-sided failure are breathlessness, fatigue and malaise, dependent edema, sleep problems, and hepatic congestion (Inamdar and Inamdar, 2016). Changes in edema can be notable and the nurse works with the person to weigh himself or herself at the same time every day and look for a gain of 3 to 5 pounds as an indicator of cardiac compromise and the need to contact the health care provider for medication adjustment or hospitalization.

Etiology

HF is the end-organ damage from preexisting conditions, especially diabetes, HTN, and CAD. To compensate for the damage, the heart, especially the ventricles, enlarge and dilate. The enlargement decreases heart muscle function as the walls are remodeled and weakened. Eventually, the heart cannot compensate for the lost stroke volume and evidence of failure appears.

Secondary causes of HF include drug and alcohol abuse, uncontrolled hyperthyroidism, and valvular heart disease. Persons with CHD who have already had extensive damage have a very high risk of developing HF. Its onset can be acute—often within the first few hours or days after a myocardial infarction, but even a moderate amount of muscle damage will lead to eventual HF.

Diagnosis

The diagnosis of early HF in older adults can be very difficult. All other diseases with similar signs and symptoms must be ruled out, such as thyroid disturbances and uncontrolled AF. While the working diagnosis is often made empirically, there are many false-positives. Measurement of brain natriuretic peptide (BNP) and NT-proBNP is potentially useful in differentiating shortness of breath due to HF with that caused by other conditions (Chapter 8) (Bashore et al, 2013). Biomarkers are also used to measure the severity of the disease.

Complications

As the severity increases and HF advances into intermittent or chronic HF, the pulse pressure narrows, and signs of impaired tissue perfusion develop, such as cool skin and central or peripheral cyanosis. Diminished cognition, perhaps to the point of delirium, is common. Recurrent hospitalization is usually required until the point is reached when only palliative care is possible or desired. An episode of syncope, ventricular tachycardia, or uncontrolled fibrillation should be regarded as a harbinger of sudden death. Increased jugular venous pressure is the most reliable way to determine the prognosis. A transplant is the only cure but rarely appropriate for persons in later life due to the number of preexisting comorbidities (Inamdar and Inamdar, 2016).

Treatment

Treatment of HF begins with optimal treatment of the underlying cause(s). The goals are to prevent more damage, control symptoms, and increase health-related quality of life to the extent possible through lifestyle changes, medications, and ongoing health monitoring. The nurse works with the person to find ways to follow a medical treatment plan, improve eating habits (DASH diet), attain a healthy weight, increase physical activity, and stop smoking and stay away from others who smoke. For those with advanced disease, the nurse can work with the person to minimize fatigue and teaches the person how to recognize signs and symptoms indicating the early or pending onset of acute HF. Nurses work with persons and their significant others to determine their wishes related to medical crises and their desire for aggressive measures, such as hospitalization, intubation, and resuscitation (NHLBI, 2017b). For those with CHF, treatment is one of palliative care (Chapter 35). Pharmacological interventions and goals are based on the level of symptoms as recommended by the American Heart Association; levels range from A (asymptomatic) to D (refractory) (Box 22.7).

THE AGING PERIPHERAL VASCULAR SYSTEM

The younger heart propels oxygen-rich blood through highly elastic and flexible arteries that expand and contract depending on the body's need for oxygen. Deoxygenated blood returns to the heart by way of the veins, propelled by contractions of the surrounding muscles. The blood is prevented from moving backward (by the pull of gravity) by a series of valves. Several of the same age-related changes seen in the skin and muscles affect the blood vessels.

The most significant age-related changes in the arteries are reduced elasticity and narrowing. Elastin fibers fray, split, straighten, and fragment. For those without CVD or diabetes, there is little change in blood flow to the coronary arteries or brain. However, perfusion of other tissues and organs is reduced and can be significant in relation to medication metabolism and excretion, and fluid and electrolyte balance (Chapter 9). The veins become stretched and the valves less efficient. Pooling of the blood leads to increased venous pressure and edema develops more quickly.

PERIPHERAL VASCULAR DISEASE

Peripheral vascular disease (PVD) is that in which there is partial or complete occlusion of the veins or arteries. The two major types of PVD are chronic venous insufficiency (CVI) and peripheral arterial disease (PAD). The reported incidence and prevalence of each disorder vary widely, but overall, they increase with age (Rapp et al, 2013; Robertson et al, 2008, 2013).

BOX 22.7 Classification of Heart Failure by the American College of Cardiologists Combined With That of the New York Heart Association[a]

Stage A
- High risk but no symptoms or structural disorder (e.g., CAD, HTN)

Class 1 Mild
- *No evidence of symptoms at rest or during activity*

Stage B
- No symptoms but with structural disorder (e.g., LVH, hx MI)

Class 2 Mild
- *Ordinary activities result in fatigue, palpitation, or dyspnea*

Stage C
- Current or past symptoms and structural disorder
- Especially dyspnea from LVSD

Class 3 Moderate
- *Less than ordinary activities cause symptoms*

Stage D
- End-stage disease
- Symptomatic at rest despite optimal treatment

Class 4 Severe
- *Symptoms at rest, any activity increases discomfort*

[a]Text in italics is from the New York Heart Association.
CAD, Coronary artery disease; *HTN,* hypertension; *hx,* history; *LVH,* left ventricular hypertrophy; *LVSD,* left ventricular systolic dysfunction; *MI,* myocardial infarction.
From Yancy CW, Jessup V (chair and vice chair.). 2017 ACC/AHA/HFSA focused update of the 2013 guideline for the management of heart failure, *Circulation* 137(12):2018; American Heart Association: *Classes of heart failure,* 2018. http://www.heart.org/HEARTORG/Conditions/HeartFailure/AboutHeartFailure/Classes-of-Heart-Failure_UCM_306328_Article.jsp. Accessed March 2018.

Signs and Symptoms

The major signs and symptoms of CVI and PAD are pain, changes to the skin, and wounds that do not heal. Early complaints of CVI may include numbness or tingling in the affected extremity or mild edema with standing. The reverse blood flow through the incompetent valves results in increased hydrostatic pressure, and pain is present when the extremity is dependent and during ambulation. There is pooling of blood from venous stasis, and the affected limb has a dark erythema in lighter skinned people and a dull gray appearance in more darkly pigmented persons.

Over time, long-standing stasis of blood leads to the deposition of hemosiderin, giving the skin a speckled brown appearance, especially in the lower calf. Varicosities of the superficial veins are obvious. Dependent edema, dermatitis, venous stasis ulcers, and firm induration are common.

In contrast, PAD reduces the blood flowing into a limb, and the early symptom is pain when the limb is elevated. It is classically described as an ache, numbness, or squeezing sensation, especially in the arch of the foot and toes but also in the calf,

TABLE 22.3 Comparison of Arterial and Venous Insufficiency of the Lower Extremities.

Characteristics	Arterial	Venous
Pain	Pain with elevation of lower extremities Pain initially relieved when legs become dependent Pain returns when walking short distances (claudication) but is relieved by rest (legs still dependent)	Deep ache, relieved by elevation Deep muscle pain with acute deep vein thrombosis
Pulses	Absent or weak	Normal
Skin	Thin, shiny, dry skin Thickened toenails Absence of hair growth Cool Pallor with elevation Rubor with dependency	Firm ("brawny") edema Reddish brown discoloration (hyperpigmentation) Evidence of healed ulcers Presence of varicose veins Progressive edema Dark erythema with acute deep vein thrombosis
Ulcer location	Between toes or at tips of toes Metatarsal or phalangeal heads Heels, sides, or soles of feet Lateral malleolus Pretibial area	Medial malleolus
Ulcer characteristics	Well-defined edges Necrotic tissue Deep, pale base Nonbleeding	Uneven edges Ruddy granulation tissue Superficial Bleeding

thigh, or buttocks. The pain may be instantly relieved when the limb is moved to a dependent position, when gravity pulls the blood into the ischemic limb. While temporarily relieved, pain returns with exertion as the tissue demands more oxygen and is relieved again by rest. This is referred to as intermittent claudication. When elevated, the extremity may be pale and cool, consistent with ischemia, and red or purple with dependency (Reuben et al, 2017). See Table 22.3 which assists in the differentiation of these two very different disorders.

Etiology

Most of the changes to both the arteries and the veins are attributable to CVD, especially HTN and the development of plaques, superimposed on normal age-related changes. Both CVI and PAD are significantly exacerbated by a history of smoking. CVI usually begins with a deep vein thrombosis (DVT); others are the result of varicose veins, leg trauma, or surgery which damage the venous valves resulting in venous HTN. Obesity is a complicating factor (Owens et al, 2017). PAD is an atherosclerotic disease with circulation compromised by fatty plaques.

Diagnosis

PVD may be completely asymptomatic early in the disease, making prompt diagnosis difficult and delayed treatment decreasing the ability to prevent complications. Multiple conditions common in late life can have some of the same signs and symptoms. For example, both heart disease and many medications can cause lymphedema—as does CVI. The gerontological nurse may be the first one to notice the symptoms or hear the concerns from the older adult leading to a diagnosis, especially in the inpatient or other institutional setting. Diagnosis of all the vascular disorders discussed here begins with a good history, physical examination, and review of symptoms (Chapter 7). While the type of problem appears evident, confirmatory testing includes an ankle-brachial index (ABI), Doppler and duplex ultrasound, magnetic resonance angiogram (MRA), or a computed tomography (CT) angiogram (Reuben et al, 2017).

Complications

Chronic intense pain from PAD and wounds that do not heal are serious complications of PAD. When ischemia is present long enough the surrounding tissue deteriorates, and skin ulcers develop with or without trauma. If an ulcer is not found or treated early enough, infection may develop to the point of gangrene, necessitating amputation to save the part of the limb above the lesion.

As most CVI is caused from DVT, the most serious complication is the development of a pulmonary embolism (PE). A PE should be suspected anytime the person has recently had a DVT, or is at risk for one, and complains of sudden shortness of breath and has a low oxygen saturation rate. A PE will be confirmed with a chest x-ray or magnetic resonance imaging (MRI), but even the suspicion of one should be treated as a potential medical emergency. Both DVT and PE require hospitalization to resolve the clots.

In CVI, nonhealing venous ulcers may develop, as well as edema and chronic pain from the reduced circulation, especially when standing. Darkened reddish-brown pigmentation (hemosiderin) often appears on the lower legs. This darkening is caused by the breakdown of blood hemoglobin when the iron normally inside red blood cells seeps into the skin.

Treatment

CVI and PAD are end-organ diseases. Consequently, treatment and prevention are tied to addressing the modifiable risk factors of the original disorders but there are also specific strategies that can be used to reduce the risk of PVD. The nurse has a major role in working with persons to adopt day-to-day preventive care strategies. For example, the nurse can encourage weight reduction to decrease the pressure on the veins from obesity, smoking cessation, control of diabetes and HTN, and a healthy diet (Zhang and Melander, 2014).

For persons with *arterial* insufficiency, exercise rehabilitation and protection of the skin are paramount. Exercise rehabilitation includes establishing a walking program to slowly and steadily increase the pain-free walking distance. The person is asked to walk until maximal tolerable pain occurs, rest, and then continue.

Daily skin inspection and protection against the effects of pressure, friction, shear, and maceration are essential for the early detection and prevention of wounds. Nothing should be done to limit circulation to the affected limb. Wearing restrictive clothing and using compression stockings are contraindicated. Medications are prescribed for persons with PAD antiplatelet agents (e.g., aspirin). Angioplasty or the insertion of a stent may be necessary (Reuben, 2017).

Although the person with chronic *vascular* insufficiency will need intermittent courses of diuretics for severe edema, the mainstay of management is the use of customized, fitted, *graduated* compression stockings. The hose can facilitate wound healing, reduce venous dermatitis, control sclerotic changes, and counteract excessive venous pressure. In addition to compression stockings, other devices that have been found useful to improve venous return include Unna boots (or equivalent), pneumatic compression pumps, and orthotic devices. Elevation of the legs above the heart for 30 minutes three to four times a day can reduce edema and improve skin microcirculation.

The DVT of CVI is the formation of a thrombus on the vein wall, most often near a valve (Johanning, 2014). It may be asymptomatic early in the disease. However, when the DVT progresses to the point where it completely occludes the vein, the person will have acute pain. Most often the thrombus will be treated with anticoagulants. Once the acute clot is resolved the person will have postembolic syndrome due to irreversible damage to the vessel wall, increasing the risk for another DVT. The person may require anticoagulation treatment that is extended or even for a lifetime (Owens et al, 2017).

In the management of PVD-related ulcers special care must be taken to ensure that venous stasis ulcers and arterial ulcers are differentiated and treated appropriately. Because of the potentially limb-threatening nature of these ulcers, it is recommended that the nurse consult with colleagues who are wound care specialists to develop the most appropriate treatment plans. The nurse is usually the leader in planning and implementing patient education related to skin care (Table 22.4).

NEUROLOGICAL/CEREBROVASCULAR DISORDERS

The neurological disorders that may also be discussed from a cerebrovascular perspective include transient ischemic attack (TIA), ischemic stroke, and both subarachnoid and subdural hemorrhagic strokes. All are characterized by acute-onset neurological changes from anoxic damage to the brain. Both morbidity and mortality are dependent on the type of event and the time between onset and treatment. Because the immediate neurological deficits appear at the same time, but the treatment and prognoses of ischemic and hemorrhagic events are dramatically different, an urgent and accurate diagnosis is essential. Only when the cause is known can appropriate therapy be implemented. All strokes are medical emergencies.

TABLE 22.4 Promoting Healthy Aging for the Person With Peripheral Vascular Disease.

Give Legs a Rest

Elevate the feet above heart level while sleeping, while sitting, and several times a day.

Change Positions Frequently

Avoid activities that require standing or sitting with feet dangling for long periods.

Give Legs Support (as Directed Only)

As directed (chronic venous insufficiency [CVI] only), wear professionally made graduated compression from ankles to knees.

Replace hose as needed to maintain usefulness.

Hose on in a.m. and off in p.m.

Take Care of the Skin

Examine feet daily, including the soles, sides, and between the toes.

Wash lower legs and feet regularly with mild soap and water.

Use moisturizing cream and emollients after washing.

Do **not** use lanolin or petroleum-based creams when wearing support hose made with latex.

Avoid activities that can injure the legs or feet.

Monitor legs for skin changes:
Persistent edema
Discoloration
Dryness and/or itching

Stroke is a leading cause of death and disability in the United States. Worldwide, 17 million people die of CVD each year, especially of AMI and stroke; two-fifths of these are related to smoking (WHO, 2018). In the United States, someone dies every 4 minutes from a stroke: 140,000 people a year, most of whom are older than 65 years of age. One of the goals of *Healthy People 2020* is to reduce this number from the baseline of 43.5 deaths per 100,000 persons in 2007 to 34.8 in 2020 (ODPHP, 2018).

There are notable racial, ethnic, and geographical differences. Between the ages of 45 and 54 black men and women die of strokes three times more often than their white counterparts. This disparity decreases at the age of 85 when the rate is the same for all (Howard et al, 2016). The U.S. death rates are highest in the 11 "stroke belt" states of the Southeast and lowest in the Northeast and Southwest. African Americans are twice as likely as whites to have a first stroke and die from this. While overall the death rate from a stroke has decreased, it has increased for persons who self-identify as Hispanic (CDC, 2017c).

The most common type of stroke is ischemic (87%), one in which there is a blockage of blood from getting to the brain (CDC, 2017c). A TIA is a partial blockage which resolves quickly and usually completely. A hemorrhagic stroke occurs when an artery in the brain leaks or ruptures. Most of the risk factors for strokes are those of any of the other CVDs.

Signs and Symptoms

The signs and symptoms of neurological events are a large part of both the ultimate diagnosis and the prognosis. The most common symptom of an ischemic stroke is sudden weakness, tingling, and other neurological deficits consistent with the area of the brain affected, most often on one side of the body. The whole side may be affected or just a part, such as the side of the face or unilateral arm (Aminoff and Douglas, 2017).

The symptoms of TIAs are those of ischemic strokes but transient, as little as 1 to 5 minutes or several hours and can vary greatly. In most cases they appear to resolve completely on their own. The signs often resolve before the person is even seen by a health care provider. Instead, the person reports, "I think I had a small stroke last week."

Hemorrhagic strokes are both sudden and explosive and often preceded by "the worst headache of my life." There are more focal neurological changes, a more depressed level of consciousness, and a potential for seizures. Like the ischemic stroke, the types of neurological deficits indicate the parts of the brain affected but are usually much broader. They include alterations in motor, sensory, and visual function; coordination; cognition; and language. Nausea and vomiting suggest increased cerebral edema. Loss of consciousness indicates a very poor prognosis (Aminoff and Vania, 2017).

Etiology

Strokes, formerly referred to as cerebrovascular events, are the result of a partial or complete occlusion in blood vessels, and therefore oxygenation, to the brain. Because of the anoxia, brain tissues die quickly. *One minute of brain ischemia can kill 2 million nerve cells and 14 billion synapses!*

The main causes of ischemic strokes are arterial disease, cardioembolism, hematological disorders, and hypoperfusion. Arterial disease in the form of arteriosclerosis is probably most common (Fig. 22.2). Cardioembolism is caused by an arrhythmia such as AF, frequently seen in CHD. Hematological causes include coagulation disorders and hyperviscosity syndromes. Hypoperfusion can occur from dehydration, hypotension (including overtreatment of HTN), cardiac arrest, or syncope. The blockage is complete in the ischemic stroke and will persist until it is removed or dissolved. Even though the TIA is also an ischemic event, the blockage is only partial; it lasts only a few minutes to several hours and resolves on its own.

In a subarachnoid hemorrhagic stroke, a vessel ruptures within the brain and quickly fills a space between the dura and the subarachnoid mater with blood. The rupture is usually at the site of an embolus. If the person is also receiving anticoagulant medications, the bleeding will be more rapid (Aminoff and Douglas, 2017). The most common cause is an aneurysm. The most important contributing factors for the incidence of

spontaneous intracerebral hemorrhagic stroke in older adults are HTN, the use of anticoagulants (iatrogenic strokes), acute inflammatory illness, contusions (e.g., from falls), and central cerebral thrombi.

Diagnosis and Treatment

There are several classic signs of a potential stroke (Box 22.8). When these signs are present, a stroke is presumed until proven otherwise. Diagnosis includes the analysis of the presenting signs as a clue to the type of stroke and moves quickly to a CT scan or an MRI whenever possible, to differentiate the hemorrhagic from the ischemic stroke. It is imperative that first the type of stroke be determined immediately and later the cause of the stroke be determined to prevent a succession of these events whenever possible. The initial treatment of a confirmed ischemic stroke is the administration of recombinant tissue plasminogen activator (rtPA) within 3 hours of the event to dissolve the clot (Aminoff and Douglas, 2017).

Since the TIA is self-limiting, treatment revolves around the prevention of a subsequent stroke through the adoption of any of the preventive measures discussed in this chapter or in Chapter 1 (e.g., smoking cessation or never smoking).

A very small intracerebral hemorrhage may resolve on its own. If caught early enough, surgery may be helpful to stop the bleeding in a subarachnoid hemorrhage; there are no alternative treatments and the prognosis is very poor. If the person survives the first several hours, the goal is palliative care for the patient and support for the family. The escalating potential of any stroke as one ages increases the responsibility of the gerontological nurse to ensure that the person's wishes regarding resuscitation in such circumstances are known.

Complications

In an ischemic stroke, the occlusion is complete; but in some cases, the occlusion is reversible with prompt treatment. Even so, the resultant damage may be permanent. The greater the occlusion and the longer time before treatment, the greater amount of damage to the brain. Rehabilitation (third level prevention) will be necessary for any chance of restoring full function or functioning to the degree possible. While these services are available in high-income countries, they are not always available to all in lower-income countries. Although not all persons with TIAs have strokes, more than one-third who do not get treatment have a major stroke within 1 year and 10% to 15% have one within 3 months (CDC, 2017c). First-line pharmacological treatment for both a TIA and a stroke is daily

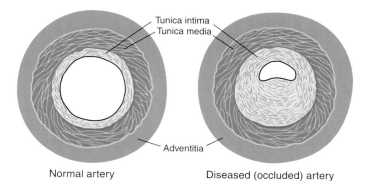

Fig. 22.2 Arteriosclerosis. (From Huether SE, McCance KL: *Understanding pathophysiology*, ed 5, St Louis, 2012, Mosby.)

Normal artery   Diseased (occluded) artery

Tunica intima
Tunica media
Adventitia

> **BOX 22.8   Quick Assessment of the Person Who May Be Having a Stroke**
>
> If you think someone may be having a stroke, act FAST and do the following simple test:
> **F** Face: Ask the person to smile. Does one side of the face droop?
> **A** Arms: Ask the person to raise both arms. Does one arm drift downward?
> **S** Speech: Ask the person to repeat a simple phrase. Is the person's speech slurred or strange?
> **T** Time: If you observe any of these signs, call 9-1-1 immediately.

aspirin (81 to 325 mg) (Reuben et al, 2017). In older adults, enteric coated ASA is recommended. For those who cannot dependably swallow pills, chewable aspirin is available.

For those few who have survived a hemorrhagic stroke, brain edema is a problem and could result in obstructive hydrocephalus. The long-term effects of a stroke include depression, paralysis and hemiparesis, and dysarthria, dysphagia and aphasias, depending on type, extent, and area affected (Hackett et al, 2014). Whenever paralysis results, the development of spasticity in the affected limb(s) is a risk. Spasticity can lead to contractures if it is not managed. Iatrogenic-type complications include DVT in a flaccid lower limb, contractures, aspiration pneumonia, or urinary tract infections. The person with a period of unresponsiveness is unlikely to survive (Moran et al, 2017).

PROMOTING HEALTHY AGING: IMPLICATIONS FOR GERONTOLOGICAL NURSING: CARDIOVASCULAR DISEASE

Due to the prevalence and incidence of cardiovascular and cerebrovascular diseases, the role of the nurse is broad and complex. First and foremost is prevention—in individual encounters with persons in every setting; as family members, colleagues, or neighbors; and in the community at large (Chapter 1). The nurse conducts expert assessments for the early detection of both CVDs and their exacerbations.

Assessment

The gerontological nurse participates in the accurate assessment of the person in wellness and disease. In advanced practice, the nurse may have the additional responsibility of providing evidence-based pharmacological interventions.

Review of Symptoms

The cardiovascular and cerebrovascular assessments begin with the subjective review of symptoms. This should include the onset, location (for pain), duration, characteristics, alleviating and aggravating factors, and all measures taken to relieve them (e.g., prescribed medications, fasting, herbal and over-the-counter products, prayer). Symptoms of particular importance in the cardiovascular assessment include dyspnea, strength, fall history, dizziness, changes in usual functioning, and other signs and symptoms discussed throughout this chapter.

Observation

The nurse can make informed observations: ease of movement, skin color and evidence of hemosiderin deposition, presence or absence of varicosities, presence or absence of wounds and their location, and presence of edema. If the person's heart is markedly enlarged, pulsations may be visible and there will be a left shift of the point of maximum impact. While assessment for jugular venous pressure is standard in a complete assessment, this is not always possible or appropriate in the older adult due to difficulty in assuming the needed recumbent position and to changes of the neck tissue that lead to inaccurate readings.

While the finding of an absence of lower extremity (LE) hair is important in a younger adult, this is not a significant finding in later life due to the increasing loss of body hair in the normal course of aging. If a DVT is suspected, the assessment of a comparative measurement of calf circumference is necessary (Owens et al, 2017). If any signs of a TIA or stroke are observed the nurse contacts emergency medical services unless there is an advance directive not to.

Palpation

The nurse examines the skin for temperature and degree of edema if present. Edema is assessed as firm or pitting and the degree of pitting. A small amount of pitting is a normal change of aging when the legs have been dependent for an extended period but is not expected to be present after the legs have been elevated, such as after sleep.

It is important to attempt to palpate the pulses. Peripheral pulses are palpated for presence or absence, equality, and quality. They include the femoral, popliteal, posterior tibial, and dorsalis pedis. There are several reasons that a pulse may not be easily palpable, especially in the presence of edema; other measures of circulatory health must be used in this case. Unless the limb has acute ischemia, it is not that there is no pulse but that the pulse is not palpable. Testing of capillary refill time (should be <3 seconds) becomes even more important when pulses are not palpable. Unless the skin is broken, the nurse must make a judgment whether to wear gloves, especially for the assessment of temperature.

Auscultation

Auscultation is the most detailed aspect of assessment of the cardiovascular system. Auscultation often begins with laying the stethoscope lightly on the carotid arteries for a sign of bruits or a "swishing" sound. It is important to auscultate the heart for 30 to 60 seconds to determine if any irregularities are heard. It is ideal to be able to auscultate all four areas (aortic, pulmonic, tricuspid, and mitral) of the heart, with the length of time in each area dependent on what is heard. For example, if a murmur or irregular rhythm is detected in the aortic area, then 60 seconds would be a reasonable time to auscultate; if the nurse auscultates for less time, the irregularity may be missed. In the older woman the first three areas are often easier to auscultate than in a younger woman because of the age-related increased laxity of the breast tissue. Due to changes in the rib cage and spine, auscultation of the mitral area may not be possible. In someone with cardiac enlargement, the point of maximal impulse (PMI) will be found more lateral than where it is in the younger adult. The quality, rate, and rhythm of the pulsations of the carefully auscultated heart are evaluated. Murmurs are heard most often in the aortic and less so in pulmonic areas. An occasional ectopic beat may be heard and is usually insignificant. The rhythm may be irregularly irregular (IRIR) or regularly irregularly (RIR) in those with AF.

If the person is being seen in the outpatient setting with minimal or no symptoms of active heart disease or has significant positioning problems, such as from orthopedic deformities, assessment may need to take place in the sitting position.

While it is ideal to auscultate on exposed skin, this may not be possible for a number of reasons. In that case, listening through one thin layer of a smoothed cotton fabric (no synthetics) may be adequate for the nurse with experience and advanced skills. In a symptomatic person or a person who has any positive findings, skin to stethoscope contact is required.

The assessment includes the practice of both preventive measures and those that are in the presence of disease or disease progression, such as smoking status, level of ongoing emotional distress, current intensity of exercise (and changes in this ability), and diet. Unless the person is nearing the end of life, the importance of diabetes control is an essential point of preventive education (Chapter 24).

Despite the normal age-related changes, the healthy older heart and blood vessels continue to sustain adequate function for everyday life. At the same time, the gerontological nurse must recognize that the increased heart rate expected in a younger person who is physiologically, psychologically, or emotionally distressed is not usually found in the older adult. Additionally, due to the high rate of heart disease in today's population older than 60 or 65 years of age, the gerontological nurse must be alert to signs of rapid decompensation of both the well and the fragile older adult.

Intervention: The Nurse as Advocate

In addition to the nursing interventions discussed throughout this chapter, the role of an advocate will advance healthy aging for persons with CVD and cerebrovascular disease and for those at risk for these diseases by promoting preventive activities and ensuring that early signs and symptoms of both disease states and exacerbations are promptly addressed. Primary prevention includes promoting smoking cessation, healthy eating, exercise, and maintaining an appropriate body weight (Chapter 1). Secondary prevention includes doing everything possible to control the conditions already present (e.g., HTN). These activities cannot be overstated and can improve health-related quality of life and in many cases slow the progression of the chronic diseases (Box 22.9). The nurse advocate is involved in introducing evidence-based programs to communities (Box 22.10). The nurse can volunteer in mobile clinics and work with the many people who have cardiovascular health problems, including older adults with more advanced disease. The nurse identifies those older adults at high risk for stroke. The nurse advocate serves as a healthy role model.

In the long-term care setting, the nurse is the key health care provider to promote healthy aging and to advocate and secure appropriate interventions for the older adult who is dependent on others. The nurse alerts the resident's nurse practitioner or physician about observed changes including atypical signs and symptoms and indicators of iatrogenesis. The provider is then responsible for the prescriptive interventions that are consistent

---

BOX 22.9 Nursing Interventions to Promote Healthy Aging for Persons With Heart Disease

1. Activities: pacing and tolerance
2. Exercise: strategizing adherence to prescribed program
3. Medications: timing, side effects, evaluation of effectiveness, obstacles to adherence
4. Disease self-management: signs and symptoms of exacerbation; intake, output; weight management; when to call for help and who to call with questions or questions interpreting laboratory values; diet
5. Diet: low cholesterol, fat, and sodium
6. Fluid restriction if necessary
7. Help person develop strategies to maintain:
   a. Blood pressure ≤150/90 mm Hg
8. Help the person maintain individually tailored cholesterol and triglycerides control
9. Optimal control of diabetes as appropriate

BOX 22.10 Resources for Best Practice

Promoting Healthy Hearts

United States Department of Health and Human Services (USDHHS): *Million hearts: the initiative*, 2012. http://millionhearts.hhs.goc

Centers for Disease Control and Prevention (CDC): *WISEWOMAN*, 2013a. http://www.cdc.gov/wisewoman.

Dietary Approaches to Stop Hypertension (DASH) Diet: https://www.nhlbi.nih.gov/health-topics/dash-eating-plan

---

BOX 22.11 Use of Statin Therapy in Older Adults

Five different guidelines for the use of statins in the treatment of high cholesterol were produced between 2012 and 2017 in Europe and the United States. While they vary greatly, they were all in agreement in treating all of those with diabetes and a 10-year (or more) risk for a major cardiovascular event. The decision to initiate the use of statins in persons at least 75 years of age is considerably less clear. While prevention is very important so is attention to polypharmacy in those who are frail and with multiple comorbid conditions, all of which can make statin use more dangerous.

From Mortensen MB, Falk E: Primary prevention with statins in the elderly, *J Am Coll Cardiol* 71:85–94, 2017.

---

both with the latest evidence-based practice and with the patient's and family's wishes and advance directives (Box 22.11).

The nurse advocate listens carefully to the stories that are being told and is often the first to identify the progression of CVD, such as both slow and sudden decompensation of the older adult, and the prevention of these. The nurse counters the expectation that problems that have been evaluated are not attributed to "just getting older."

KEY CONCEPTS

- Cardiovascular diseases (CVDs) are the leading cause of death and a frequent cause of disability in the older adult.

- The presentation of many CVDs or nuances of these in older adults differ from those in younger adults (e.g., the "silent MI").

- The goals of promoting healthy aging include minimizing risk for disease and, in the presence of disease, alleviating symptoms, delaying or avoiding the development of complications including end-organ damage, and maximizing function and quality of life.
- The gerontological nurse is involved with the assessment of persons with CVD in daily practice.

- The gerontological nurse has the potential to serve as a leader in the promotion of health and the prevention of CVD and in the improvement of the lives of those with CVD.
- Embolic and hemorrhagic strokes must be differentiated before treatment can be initiated.

NURSING STUDY: ADHERING TO MRS. LEWIS'S WISHES

Mrs. Lewis is an 85-year-old widowed woman with three sons and a daughter. Although her husband was not of the Jewish faith, she raised her children in the practices and traditions in which she had been raised. None of her children live nearby, but she does have a very close friend from her synagogue who has been at her side during a long and difficult battle with CHF. She has been admitted to the subacute unit in the skilled nursing home where you are employed. Her prognosis is very poor, and death is imminent. She has a do-not-resuscitate (DNR) order in place and a living will designating her friend as her decision maker. Between breaths she tells you that most of the time in the last 2 months she has been in the hospital and has been told there was nothing left to do but to allow a natural death. She is adamant that under no circumstances should she be returned to the hospital.

- What is the priority of care for Mrs. Lewis if you are the registered nurse assigned to provide care to her?

- What are your priorities if you are an advanced practice nurse providing "medical" care to her?
- After you have thought about Mrs. Lewis's situation, discuss with a classmate how you would feel about caring for her. Could you care for her and respect her wishes?
- What symptoms do you expect she will develop in the hours or days between her admission and her death? What are your responsibilities related to them?
- Is Mrs. Lewis' decision consistent with her faith?

CRITICAL THINKING QUESTIONS AND ACTIVITIES

1. A patient's family member disagrees with the wishes of the patient. What is the role of the nurse? (See also Chapter 31.)
2. In a discussion with other students, describe your personal feelings about caring for someone who declines treatment.
3. In this same discussion, consider how you might reconcile personal feelings and professional responsibilities if they differ.

RESEARCH QUESTIONS

1. Are there any rituals or customs that are expected at the time nearing death or at the time of death in the Jewish faith?
2. Is a person with heart disease ever considered eligible for hospice services, and if so, under what circumstance?

REFERENCES

Alonso A, Arenas de Larriva AP: Atrial fibrillation, cognitive decline, and dementia, *Eur Cardiol* 11(1):49–53, 2016.

Aminoff MJ, Douglas VJ: Nervous system disorders. In Papadakis MA, McPhee SJ, editors: *2017 Current medical diagnosis and treatment*, New York, 2017, McGraw-Hill Lange, pp 977–1049.

Aronow WS: Diagnosis and management of coronary artery disease. In Fillit H, Rockwood K, Young J, editors: *Brocklehurst's textbook of geriatric medicine*, ed 8, Philadelphia PA, 2017, Elsevier, pp 278–287.

Bashore TM, Granger CB, Jackson KP, et al: Heart disease In Papadakis MA, McPhee SJ, editors: *2017 Current medical diagnosis and treatment*, New York, 2017, McGraw-Hill Lange, pp 322–428.

Centers for Disease Control and Prevention (CDC): *Preventing high blood pressure: healthy living habits*, 2014. https://www.cdc.gov/bloodpressure/healthy_living.htm. Accessed March 2018.

Centers for Disease Control and Prevention (CDC): *High blood pressure facts*, 2016a. https://www.cdc.gov/bloodpressure/facts.htm. Accessed March 2018.

Centers for Disease Control and Prevention (CDC): *Health, United States, 2016*, 2016b. https://www.cdc.gov/nchs/data/hus/hus16.pdf#053. Accessed March 2018.

Centers for Disease Control and Prevention (CDC): *Heart failure fact sheet*, 2016c. https://www.cdc.gov/dhdsp/data_statistics/fact_sheets/fs_heart_failure.htm. Accessed March 2018.

Centers for Disease Control and Prevention (CDC): *Heart disease facts*, 2017a. https://www.cdc.gov/heartdisease/facts.htm. Accessed March 2018.

Centers for Disease Control and Prevention (CDC): *Know the signs and symptoms of a heart attack*, 2017b. https://www.cdc.gov/dhdsp/data_statistics/fact_sheets/fs_heartattack.htm. Accessed March 2018.

Centers for Disease Control and Prevention (CDC): *Stroke facts*, 2017c. https://www.cdc.gov/stroke/facts.htm. Accessed March 2018.

Cole CS, Zimmerman R: Anticoagulant options in atrial fibrillation: when new treatments become standard practice, *Nurse Pract* 42(12):29–35, 2017.

Hackett ML, Köhler S, O'Brien, JT, Mead GE: Neuropsychiatric outcomes of stroke, *Lancet Neurol* 13(5):525–534, 2014.

Howard G, Moy CS, Howard VJ, et al: Where to focus efforts to reduce the black-white disparity in stroke mortality: incidence versus case fatality? *Stroke* 47(7):1893–1898, 2016.

Inamdar AA, Inamdar AC: Heart failure: diagnosis, management and utilization, *J Clin Med* 5(7):E62, 2016.

January CT, Wann S, Alpert JS, et al: 2014 AHA/ACC/HRS guideline for the management of patients with atrial fibrillation: executive summary, *JACC* 64(21):2246–2280, 2014.

Johanning JM: Peripheral vascular disease. In Ham RJ, Sloane PD, Warshaw GA, et al, editors: *Primary care geriatrics: a case-based approach,* ed 6, Philadelphia, 2014, Elsevier, pp 413–421.

Khera AV, Emdin CA, Drake I, et al: Genetic risk, adherence to a healthy lifestyle, and coronary disease, *N Engl J Med* 375: 2349–2358, 2016.

Lane DA, Lip GY: Use of the CHA(2)DS(2)-VASc and HAS-BLED scores to aid decision making for thromboprophylaxis in nonvalvular atrial fibrillation, *Circulation* 126:860–865, 2012.

Li Y, Wang J, Lv L, Xu C, Liu H: Usefulness of the $CHADS_2$ and R_2CHADS_2 scores for prognostic stratification in patients with coronary artery disease, *Clin Interv Aging* 13:565–571, 2018.

Meissner A: Hypertension and the brain: a risk factor for more than heart disease, *Cerebrovasc Dis* 42(3-4):255–262, 2016.

Moran C, Phan TG, Srikanth VK: Stroke: clinical presentation, management, and organization of services. In Fillit HM, Rockwood K, Young J, editors: *Brocklehurst's textbook of geriatric medicine and gerontology,* ed 8, Philadelphia, 2017, Elsevier, pp 483–490.

National Heart, Lung, and Blood Institute (NHLBI): *Managing blood pressure in adults: A systematic evidence review panel from the blood pressure expert panel,* 2013. https://www.nhlbi.nih.gov/sites/default/files/media/docs/blood-pressure-in-adults.pdf. Accessed March 2018.

National Heart, Lung, and Blood Institute (NHLBI): *Sex and race disparities in high blood pressure emerge early in life,* 2017a. https://www.nhlbi.nih.gov/news/2017/sex-and-race-disparities-high-blood-pressure-emerge-early-life. Accessed March 2018.

National Heart, Lung, and Blood Institute (NHLBI): *Heart failure,* 2017b. https://www.nhlbi.nih.gov/health-topics/heart-failure. Accessed March 2018.

Owens CD, Gaspar WJ, Johnson MD: Blood vessel & lymphatic disorders. In Papadakis MA, McPhee SJ, editors: *2017 Current medical diagnosis and treatment,* New York, 2017, McGraw-Hill Lange, pp 472–498.

Reuben DB, Herr KA, Pacala JT, et al: *Geriatrics at your fingertips,* ed 19, New York, NY, 2017, American Geriatric Society.

Robertson L, Evans C, Fowkes FG: Epidemiology of chronic venous disease, *Phlebology* 23(3):103–111, 2008.

Robertson L, Lee AJ, Evans CJ, et al: Incidence of chronic venous disease in the Edinburgh Vein Study, *J Vasc Surg Venous Lymphat Disord* 1:59–67, 2013.

Whelton PK, Carey RM, Aronow WS, et al. 2017 ACC/AHA/AAPA/ABC/ACPM/AGA/APhA/ASH/ASPC/NMA/PCNA guideline for the prevention, detection, evaluation, and management of high blood pressure in adults, *Hypertension* 71(6):e13–e114, 2018.

World Health Organization (WHO): *The atlas of heart disease and stroke,* 2018. http://www.who.int/cardiovascular_diseases/resources/atlas/en/. Accessed March 2018.

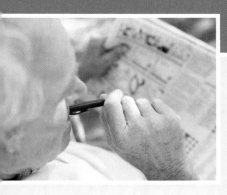

Neurodegenerative Disorders

Kathleen Jett*

http://evolve.elsevier.com/Touhy/TwdHlthAging

A STUDENT SPEAKS

It is so frustrating taking care of someone who has Parkinson's disease. Some of them just never seem to smile and seem so depressed. I try to be extra cheerful, but it just doesn't seem to make any difference!

Helen, age 20

AN OLDER ADULT SPEAKS

I always kept active and healthy. I had lots of friends and we had lots of fun together. Now it seems like I am just fading away!

Ruth, age 82

LEARNING OBJECTIVES

On completion of this chapter, the reader will be able to:

1. Differentiate Parkinson's disease from the neurodegenerative disorders due to Alzheimer's disease and the presence of Lewy bodies.
2. Describe the signs and symptoms that suggest the need for neurocognitive testing.
3. Identify the key aspects of the evaluation of the person with signs of cognitive limitations.
4. Identify the key characteristics of Parkinson's disease.
5. Describe the definitive test for the presence of Parkinson's disease.
6. Describe the recent genomic advances in an understanding of the mechanisms of neurodegenerative disorders.
7. Differentiate the key pharmacological interventions and their efficacy in Parkinson's disease and the neurocognitive disorders due to Alzheimer's disease and the presence of Lewy bodies.
8. Describe the nurse's role in the promotion of healthy aging in persons with neurodegenerative disorders.

Neurodegenerative disorders are seen in older adults more than any other age group. All are terminal conditions and characterized by a progressive decline in function. The declines may be barely noticeable in the beginning, with slight exacerbations and remissions, but the ultimate trajectory is always a downward slope. The impairments become so severe that the person cannot even meet his or her most basic self-care needs. However, there are interventions available to promote the healthiest aging possible for both the older adult and significant others while the diseases progress. The three neurodegenerative disorders addressed in this chapter are the movement disorder Parkinson's disease (PD), Alzheimer's disease (AD), and Lewy body dementia (LBD). There are several neurocognitive disorders (NCDs) of importance that are not necessarily terminal conditions, but they are beyond what is possible in this text (Box 23.1).

In the fifth edition of the *Diagnostic and Statistical Manual of Mental Health Disorders* (American Psychiatric Association [APA], 2013), the term "dementia" was replaced with the phrase "neuro*cognitive* disorder (NCD)." However, "dementia" is still what is heard most often in clinical settings and situations.

Although they rarely occur to persons younger than the age of 60, NCDs are not normal parts of aging (Box 23.2). The most common forms are AD and LBD. Both are characterized by progressive impairments in memory, thinking, language, judgment, and behavior. A distinct difference in the two is that persons with LBD will eventually also develop motor symptoms, and the use of traditional (typical) antipsychotics (e.g., Haldol) is always contraindicated. A small group of those with PD will develop dementia late in their illness (PDD).

NCDs are the major causes of disability and dependence worldwide. According to the World Health Organization, about 50 million people worldwide are affected by one of the dementias. Ten million more people are affected each year. By 2030 it

**Special thanks to Madertric Woods, MSN, GNP-BC, for reviewing this chapter.

is expected that the number will increase to 82 million and to 152 million by 2050. Sixty percent of those with one or more types of dementia live in low- and middle-income countries (Chapter 1) (WHO, 2017).

DIAGNOSIS

The evaluation leading to a diagnosis of a presumed neurodegenerative disorder is initiated by the person, significant other, or a health care provider, when changes are noted in comparison to a prior state, especially memory or physical stability, such as balance or tremors. All signs are insidious in onset, delaying diagnosis. People with an undiagnosed dementia may remark that they are having a "senior moment," when it may be something far more serious than the very slight memory loss of normal aging. Those with undiagnosed PD may remark that they are just "slowing down."

The diagnostic process begins with the assessment of all potentially reversible causes for the changes (Box 23.3). If a reversible cause is not found, or the signs remain after treatment, a more expanded, comprehensive exam is necessary to make a diagnosis and establish a baseline. This will include all the components described in Chapter 7, tests of gait and balance (Chapter 19), and a detailed neurological and psychological examination, using highly reliable and sensitive screening instruments (see https://www.alz.org/health-care-professionals/cognitive-tests-patient-assessment.asp#cognitive_screening).

The evaluation of people with signs or symptoms of neurodegenerative disorders increases in complexity when the person has other confounding chronic diseases, is very frail, or has

sensory limitations. For those living in low- or middle-income countries, expert care, including treatment of reversible conditions, may not be possible.

PARKINSON'S DISEASE

PD was first described by James Parkinson in 1817. It affects 10 million people worldwide. In the United States, about 1 million people have PD and about 60,000 more are diagnosed each year. It affects 50% more men than women and most people are diagnosed in later life (Parkinson's foundation, n.d.a). Persons of all races and ethnicities throughout the world are affected; however, several studies have found a higher prevalence in high-income countries (Khandelwal and Kaufer, 2014).

Diagnosis

The symptoms that initiate the diagnostic process in PD are often asymmetrical resting tremor, especially in the arm or hand, or unexplained falls. Due to the medical complexity of many in late life, the diagnosis of PD can be very difficult; accuracy may be as low as 76% (Meara, 2017). It is necessary to depend on the presence or absence of classic signs and symptoms during a thorough health history and physical exam. The accuracy of a diagnosis is improved through a "challenge test"—when symptoms improve dramatically after the administration of the medication levodopa (Vasta et al, 2017). Early falls, poor response to levodopa, symmetry of motor symptoms, lack of tremor, and early autonomic dysfunction are characteristic of atypical parkinsonism or several other movement disorders (Box 23.4).

Etiology

PD is the result of a deficiency of the neurotransmitter dopamine in the substantia nigra, a reduction of dopamine receptors, loss of nerve endings that produce norepinephrine (the chemical that controls many autonomic functions), and the accumulation of Lewy bodies, especially in the basal ganglia (NIA, 2017a). The severity of the illness is associated with the degree of neuron loss. About 50% of the dopamine-producing neurons are lost by the time a person becomes overtly symptomatic (NIEHS, 2017).

There are several factors which appear to increase and decrease one's risk for the development of PD (Box 23.5). Inherited PD is rare, only an estimated 10% to 15%, with any one individual at increased risk if a first-degree relative (e.g., parent) has been affected; all others are referred to as "sporadic" (Parkinson's foundation, n.d.b).

Signs and Symptoms

The four core signs of PD are *resting tremor* (hands, arms, legs, jaw, face), *muscular rigidity, bradykinesia,* and *asymmetrical*

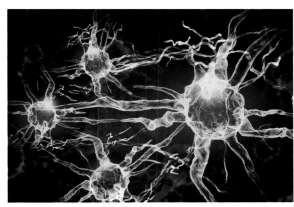

Neurons. (©iStock.com/Sergey Nivens.)

BOX 23.5 Risk Factors for the Development of Parkinson's Disease

Male
Increasing age
Having a close relative with Parkinson's
Exposure to toxins
Repeated head trauma

onset (Box 23.6). Resting tremor is the first sign in 70% of those with PD. When present, tremors are asymmetrical and rhythmic, are of low amplitude, and disappear briefly during voluntary movement. The arm and hand are most commonly affected—the leg, foot, and head less often. They are not present during sleep but increase with stress and anxiety.

Rigidity can be assessed with passive range of motion. Instead of smooth movement, it is "cogwheel" in nature—that is, movement alternates with resistance. Severe muscle cramps may occur in the toes or hands due to lack of free and regular movement. Bradykinesia affects the person's ability to perform fine motor tasks. This early sign may have the most effect on the person's ability to independently perform day-to-day self-care functions.

As muscle rigidity and bradykinesia worsen, all of the striated muscles in the extremities, trunk, and ocular areas will ultimately be affected, including the muscles of mastication (chewing), deglutition (swallowing), and articulation (speaking). In the later stages, the person blinks infrequently and the face shows little animation, including that of emotion (masked facies).

Several other motor symptoms are of special importance in relation to independent functioning and safety. Downward gaze becomes more difficult, and there is an involuntary flexion of the head and neck, a stooped posture, and postural instability.

BOX 23.6 Core Signs of Parkinson's Disease

Resting tremor	Asymmetrical onset
Bradykinesia	Impaired balance and coordination
Rigidity	

BOX 23.7 Other Symptoms Experienced by People With Parkinson's Disease

Frequent changes in body temperature	Sexual dysfunction
Unstable blood pressure	Urinary incontinence
Dizziness	Constipation
Fainting	A poor sense of smell
Frequent falls	Sialorrhea (drooling)
Sensitivity to heat and cold	Micrographia (small handwriting)

The characteristic gait consists of very short steps and minimal arm movements (festination). Initiating and restarting movement is difficult (freezing) later in the disease, but once it starts the person moves forward with small steps and a forward lean, increasing the person's risk for falling (Chapter 19). Turning is difficult and may require many steps. If the person is off balance, correction is very slow. There are many other symptoms that are of importance to persons with PD, all of which decrease their quality of life (Box 23.7).

PD can also present with nonmotor symptoms. The nonmotor symptoms can be categorized as neuropsychiatric (mood changes, depression, apathy), autonomic (constipation, sexual dysfunction), sleep (insomnia, vivid dreams, excessive daytime sleepiness), and sensory (pain, burning, numbness, loss of smell).

Symptoms and their intensity vary from person to person; some become severely disabled early in the disease and others experience only minor motor disturbances until much later. However, the number of symptoms and the degree to which they will affect a person's life and function will always increase over time.

Treatment

Currently there is no cure for PD, but when the symptoms are such that they interfere with the person's functioning, pharmacological interventions are initiated, sometimes providing dramatic relief. Drug therapy focuses on replacing or mimicking dopamine or slowing its breakdown.

The first-line medication is levodopa; it is especially effective in reducing bradykinesia and rigidity. Crossing the blood-brain barrier, it is converted to dopamine in the basal ganglia and therefore increases the amount of dopamine in the brain and inhibits hyperactive cholinergic activity. Carbidopa is usually added to the levodopa to minimize side effects and limit peripheral breakdown of the levodopa. To maximize effectiveness, levodopa/carbidopa must be taken on an empty stomach (30 to 60 minutes before or 45 to 60 minutes after a meal) and must be given at the same time daily. Although it can be highly and rapidly effective, it has a number of side effects and drug interactions. Efficacy decreases with long-term use and higher doses are needed more often, increasing the side effects, such as the risk for hallucinations. Dopamine agonists such as pramipexole and ropinirole are sometimes used early in the disease or concurrently with levodopa/carbidopa. These are usually prescribed and monitored by a neurologist.

When medications no longer provide relief from disabling symptoms, some persons elect surgical interventions. A new treatment involves inserting a small tube directly into the small intestine so that a formulation of carbidopa/levodopa can be directly instilled. In deep brain stimulation (DBS), small electrodes are implanted in the brain and stimulate the brain in such a way to stop many of the movement-related symptoms (NIA, 2017a). The latter is rarely done in older adults and then only in the severest of cases in younger adults. They only address the symptoms that improved on levodopa. It is highly unlikely that these would be appropriate for persons with other serious chronic conditions as is the case with many older adults. Caring for persons with PD requires a combination of pharmacological and nonpharmacological approaches. Early nonpharmacological approaches include gait training and muscle strengthening.

ALZHEIMER'S DISEASE

AD was first described by Dr. Alois Alzheimer in 1906. The incidence increases dramatically with age—from 3% of those 65 to 74 years of age, 17% in persons 75 to 84 years old, and 32% of those 85 and older. Two-thirds of these are women. This has not been found to be associated with biological or social differences, but "survivor bias" (i.e., there are just more women in later life) (AA, 2018a).

AD is the sixth leading cause of death overall, and 1 in 10—or 5.8 million—Americans 65 years of age or older has AD. It is projected that 15 million Americans will have AD by 2050 (AA, 2019a). It is expected that the actual number of persons diagnosed will escalate as they take advantage of the free annual wellness visit now available through the Affordable Care Act, where cognitive screening is part of the overall assessment (Chapter 30).

The Alzheimer's Association and the National Institute of Aging have developed guidelines wherein three stages of AD are described: (1) preclinical disease, (2) mild cognitive impairment (MCI) due to Alzheimer's, and (3) AD. In the preclinical period, biological/neurological changes are under way but the person has no symptoms yet. Persons with MCI have mild but noticeable changes in memory and thinking that can be measured but do not disturb the person's day-to-day life yet (AA, 2018b).

Researchers have found distinct ethnic and racial differences among persons with dementia. According to the Alzheimer's Association reports, older Latinos and Latinas as are about one and a half times more likely to develop AD and other dementias than whites, while African Americans are twice as likely as whites (2019b). It may be that African Americans more often carry the *APOE* ε4 gene which increases the risk for AD, but this is not yet confirmed (Barnes and Bennett, 2014; Sinha et al, 2018). Research has become increasingly intense in the past 30 years, fueled by the anticipation of the influx of the aging baby boomers into later life (Chapter 1). Of particular interest has been to find a means to prevent and more adequately treat this terminal condition. See Chapter 5 for a discussion of promoting brain health while aging.

Etiology

Through advances in genomic science, we now know the influence of the specific genes in the development of an NCD due to AD. Less than 5% of all persons have what is referred to as "early onset" or familial Alzheimer's disease (FAD) that is diagnosed between 30 and 60 years of age. FAD is thought to be caused by a single gene mutation on one of three chromosomes: 21, 14, or 1. The mutations result in the development of abnormal amyloid precursor proteins, presenilin 1 or presenilin 2. A child whose mother or father carries a genetic factor for FAD has a 50/50 chance of developing FAD (AA, 2018c).

Most AD is diagnosed in persons older than age 60, likely due to several factors including genetic risk. Everyone inherits at least one copy of the *APOE* gene found on chromosome 19. There are three forms: ε2, ε3, and ε4. *APOE* ε3 is the most common (50% to 90% of all persons) and believed to be a neutral factor, neither increasing nor decreasing one's risk. The inheritance of *APOE* ε2 appears to have a protective influence, decreasing one's risk, while ε4 appears to increase the risk (AA, 2018c; NIA, 2015).

Persons with neurocognitive dementia due to AD also have an increased number of beta-amyloid proteins (plaques) outside the neurons and an accumulation of abnormal tau proteins inside the neurons (neurofibrillary tangles). Both damage the cortical areas of the brain. As a result, the number of synapses that normally connect the neurons decreases, and the neurons are deprived of nutrients, malfunction, and eventually die. More and more brain cells die as the number of beta-amyloid and tau proteins increases. The initial memory loss seen in all persons with AD is the result of damage to the part of the brain where memories are stored.

Symptoms

The initial symptom of AD is memory loss, specifically the ability to remember new information. As time goes on, additional signs and symptoms develop. Depression and other mental health issues are common at some time in the illness. They may go unrecognized and untreated, but the person should be monitored for these and treated appropriately and promptly should they be found. Detailed information about the symptoms associated with early to end-stage AD can be found in the document "The Global Deterioration Scale" by geriatrician Barry Reisberg and colleagues (Table 23.1). This provides an excellent tool when providing anticipatory guidance to both the individual and the future caregivers. As can be seen, functional decline correlates with cognitive decline.

Diagnosis

A diagnosis of AD requires the following: (1) there has been a decline from a previous level of functioning; (2) the onset was insidious; and (3) there has been gradual regression in cognitive abilities. Of important note is that the changes are "greater than expected for the person's age and educational background," and these changes can be documented with standardized neuropsychological testing.

When available, a magnetic resonance imaging (MRI) or a functional positron emission tomography (PET) scan is done. When the results are combined with the presence of specific proteins in the cerebrospinal fluid, a fairly reliable diagnosis can be made (AA, 2018d).

TABLE 23.1   The Global Deterioration Scale.

Diagnosis	Stage	Signs and Symptoms
No dementia	Stage 1: no cognitive decline	In this stage the person functions normally, has no memory loss, and is mentally healthy. People with no dementia would be considered to be in stage 1.
No dementia	Stage 2: very mild cognitive decline	This stage is used to describe normal forgetfulness associated with aging—for example, forgetfulness of names and where familiar objects were left. Symptoms are not evident to loved ones or the physician.
No dementia	Stage 3: mild cognitive decline	This stage includes increased forgetfulness, slight difficulty concentrating, and decreased work performance. People may get lost more often or have difficulty finding the right words. At this stage, a person's loved ones will begin to notice a cognitive decline. Average duration: 7 years before onset of dementia.
Early stage	Stage 4: moderate cognitive decline	This stage includes difficulty concentrating, decreased memory of recent events, and difficulties managing finances or traveling alone to new locations. People have trouble completing complex tasks efficiently or accurately and may be in denial about their symptoms. They may also start withdrawing from family or friends because socialization becomes difficult. At this stage a physician can detect clear cognitive problems during a patient interview and exam. Average duration: 2 years.
Midstage	Stage 5: moderately severe cognitive decline	People in this stage have major memory deficiencies and need some assistance to complete their daily activities (e.g., dressing, bathing, preparing meals). Memory loss is more prominent and may include major relevant aspects of current lives—for example, people may not remember their address or phone number and may not know the time or day or where they are. Average duration: 1.5 years.
Midstage	Stage 6: severe cognitive decline (middle dementia)	People in stage 6 require extensive assistance to carry out daily activities. They start to forget names of close family members and have little memory of recent events. Many people can remember only some details of earlier life. They also have difficulty counting down from 10 and finishing tasks. Incontinence (loss of bladder or bowel control) is a problem in this stage. Ability to speak declines. Personality changes, such as delusions (believing something to be true that is not), compulsions (repeating a simple behavior, such as cleaning), or anxiety and agitation may occur. Average duration: 2.5 years.
Late stage	Stage 7: very severe cognitive decline (late dementia)	People in this stage have essentially no ability to speak or communicate. They require assistance with most activities (e.g., using the toilet, eating). They often lose psychomotor skills—for example, the ability to walk. Average duration: 1.5–2.5 years.

From Reisberg B, Ferris SH, de Leon MJ, et al: The Global Deterioration Scale for assessment of primary degenerative dementia. *Am J Psychiatry* 139, 1136–1139, 1982. Copyright ©1983 Barry Reisberg, MD. Reproduced with permission.

Pharmacological Treatment

Because cure is not possible, pharmacological therapy for those with AD is aimed at slowing cognitive decline and thereby increasing the potential to help persons continue to function to the best of their ability longer and therefore maximize their quality of life and that of their loved ones. The effectiveness of the medications varies from person to person.

First-line treatment for AD continues to be cholinesterase inhibitors (CIs). Begun as soon as the person is diagnosed, they may not only help slow the speed of cognitive decline but also help control any behavioral difficulties the person may be having because of the brain damage (AA, 2018c).

The CIs work by blocking the breakdown of acetylcholine, a chemical believed to be important for memory and thinking. The most common side effects of the CIs are nausea and diarrhea. Donepezil (Aricept) can be used at all stages; galantamine (Razadyne) and rivastigmine (Exelon) are indicated for mild to moderate neurocognitive decline. The medication memantine (Namenda) acts on the brain chemical glutamate, which is involved with learning and memory. It is used by those with moderate to severe disease and almost always with one of the drugs just mentioned, especially donepezil.

As the disease progresses, it is not uncommon for persons to develop other symptoms that may be hard to manage without medications. Especially troublesome are depression, aggression, restlessness, sleeplessness, and hallucinations. Any number of medications may be tried, all of which must be used with caution. These include antidepressants, sleep aids, and anticonvulsants when all else fails or when the person or others are in potential danger due to their behavior. Antipsychotics are only indicated for those who develop a psychosis related to their dementia (NIA, 2018).

As with any medications, a trial to determine both effectiveness and ability of the person to tolerate side effects should be done at repeated intervals. It is important to note that these medications are not curative and once stopped the decline that "would have been" may be quickly seen.

LEWY BODY DEMENTIA

What are referred to as the dementias with Lewy bodies were named by Dr. Friederich Lewy in 1912. He discovered a new type of abnormal proteins in the brain neurons of persons with PD, both those with and without an accompanying neurocognitive decline. Persons with dementias who have Lewy bodies either have LBD (without PD) or dementia associated with Parkinson's disease (PDD). LBD is a rare progressive brain disorder wherein the abnormal proteins build up in the areas of the brain that control behavior, cognition, and movement. It affects about 1 million people ages 50 and over in the United States (NIA, 2017b). It is second in prevalence to that of AD and often confused with PDD but distinctly different in chronology of symptomatology. In PDD, movement disorders always precede cognitive changes (if they occur at all), and in LBD the cognitive changes always precede movement disorders, which *will* occur. Men are affected slightly more than women with an increasing incidence with age. The prevalence is estimated to be approximately 1.3 million Americans but thought to be highly underdiagnosed.

Signs and Symptoms

Although some memory may stay intact, the person with LBD will develop severe loss of the ability to think, especially problem solving and using language and numerical concepts. A common symptom is fluctuating attention and alertness—that is, periods of time when the flow of ideas is illogical interspersed with periods of clarity. Unlike AD, about 80% of persons with LBD hallucinate (NIA, 2017c). These may lead to delusions and paranoia. Factors contributing to psychiatric disturbances include misidentifying objects and visuospatial problems, such as in judging distance or depth.

Disordered sleep is a problem specific to persons with LBD and may appear long before other signs become obvious to anyone other than the sleep partner. Most of the time "asleep" is spent in the REM stage (Chapter 17) in which the person actively dreams and may talk in his or her sleep, thrash about, and even fall out of bed (NIA, 2017c). Restless legs syndrome may occur during nighttime sleep, and there may be a significantly increased need for daytime naps. Problems in mood occur, like those with PD: depression, apathy, anxiety, and agitation. Some of the conditions we refer to as "geriatric syndromes" occur as the disease advances. They are the result of damage to the part of the brain controlling the autonomic nervous system (Box 23.8). Clear differentiation between cognitive declines due to PD and those due to LBD is necessary to avoid inadvertent but life-threatening treatment.

Etiology

In normal healthy brains alpha-synuclein proteins help neurons communicate with one another at their synapse. However, Lewy bodies are abnormal spherical protein aggregates found within neurons in persons with both dementia and PD. Alpha-synuclein is highly expressed within these bodies, which can displace other cellular structures and may contribute to cell death (NIA, 2017a). In LBD these proteins are found in the brainstem, midbrain, olfactory bulb, neocortex, and several other locations. The progression of this disease leads to significant deficits in neurotransmitter production along the cholinergic and dopaminergic pathways. An acetylcholine deficit leads primarily to cognitive dysfunction, and the deficit in dopamine production is responsible for the motor dysfunction that appears as the disease advances. Although mutations have been identified that are associated with the risk for developing PDD, neither familial nor

---

BOX 23.9 Features Considered With a Diagnosis of Lewy Body Dementia

Central Feature	Progressive Deficits in Attention and Executive Function (Dementia)
Core features	Fluctuating cognitive ability
	Variations in attention and alertness
	Recurrent visual hallucinations, detailed
	Parkinsonian symptoms
Suggestive features	Disordered sleep (may be many years ahead of other symptoms)
	Significant sensitivity to first-generation neuroleptics
	Low dopamine update in the basal ganglia
Supportive features	Repeated falls and syncope
	Transient, unexplained loss of consciousness
	Autonomic dysfunction (Box 23.8)
	Hallucinations of other senses
	Visuospatial abnormalities

Lewy Body Dementia Association: *Symptoms: Lewy body dementia symptoms and diagnostic criteria*, 2016c. https://www.lbda.org/go/symptoms-0. Accessed April 2018.

lifestyle factors have been found to influence the development of LBD. Based on our knowledge at this time, the etiology of this disease is unknown (NIA, 2017d; Vigneswara et al, 2013).

Diagnosis

The diagnostic evaluation includes all the other testing discussed in this chapter, including a physical exam, detailed neurological exams, and neuropsychological and mental status evaluations. When possible, an MRI or computed tomography (CT) scan is done, as it is with AD. If there is no other explanation for the signs and symptoms, a determination is made of "possible" or "probable" LBD based on the presentation of the core features (Box 23.9). A diagnosis of probable LBD is made when dementia is present with two or more core features or dementia and one core feature with one or more suggestive features. A diagnosis of possible LBD is made if the person has dementia and one core feature or dementia and one or more suggestive features (LBDA, 2016c). A conclusive diagnosis can only be made through a brain autopsy (LBDA, 2016a).

Pharmacological Treatment

Over time, persons with LBD have a wide range of symptoms resulting in changes to the priority of treatment. CIs are often used as they are in AD. If severe, movement problems may be treated with levodopa as they are in PD. However, as levodopa alone has many side effects, including hallucinations, it can only be used with great caution. If an antipsychotic is needed for hallucinations that are disruptive or upsetting, one of the new medications may be used, such as quetiapine (Seroquel) (LBDA, 2016b).

BOX 23.8 Autonomic Signs and Symptoms of Lewy Body Dementia

Frequent falls	Unexplained loss of consciousness
Syncope	Incontinence
Orthostatic hypotension	Eating disorder/risk for aspiration

⚡ SAFETY ALERT

Typical antipsychotics (e.g., Haldol) can never be used in persons with neurocognitive disorder (NCD) due to Lewy bodies because of the very high rate of irreversible side effects and possible death.

BOX 23.10 Potential Complications of Those With Neurodegenerative Disorders

Pneumonia
Pressure ulcers
Abuse or neglect from excess burden to caregiver
Untreated pain
Unable to report symptoms of another health problem
Unable to follow any prescribed treatment plan
Injuries from falls
Untreated depression
Malnutrition or dehydration

Complications

LBD can last from 2 to 20 years with an average of 5 to 7 years (NIA, 2017b). For patients in the late stages of neurodegenerative diseases, complications are consistent with any person in later life who is medically fragile (Box 23.10). Complications include pressure ulcers, pneumonia, dysphagia, aspiration, and other problems associated with geriatric frailty. Undernutrition and weight loss occur even with adequate caloric consumption. Weight loss is an indication that the terminal stage is approaching. Behavioral disturbances can be frightening and at times dangerous to the person affected and to those in the immediate environment. These are brought about by the extent of and location of brain damage and side effects of medications.

PROMOTING HEALTHY AGING: IMPLICATIONS FOR GERONTOLOGICAL NURSING

Everyone, especially those with strong family histories of neurodegenerative disorders, would like to find ways to prevent them. Unfortunately, at this time this is not possible. For those with PD and the NCDs due to AD, LBD, and PDD, factors have been proposed that may somewhat decrease the risk (Box 23.11). It is of special note that research related to the effect of preventive strategies is still inconclusive.

Most of the potentially preventive strategies and nonpharmacological interventions to promote healthy aging in persons with neurodegenerative disorders involve the nurse working with the individual and those who are either already providing

BOX 23.11 Tips for Best Practice

Decreasing Risk for Neurocognitive Disorders

- Maintain blood pressure within normal limits
- Keep cholesterol at healthy levels
- Maintain healthy body weight
- Have a regular sleep/wake schedule
- Avoid excess alcohol
- Hemoglobin $A_{1c} \leq 7\%$
- Aspirin (81 mg enteric coated) for persons with risk for heart disease and without contraindications
- Maintain optimal control of heart failure
- Stop smoking or never start
- Exercise
- Maintain mental health and stimulation

care or will be doing so. Early comprehensive health, fall risk, and gait assessments are important to help the caregivers and nursing staff provide the highest quality and most empowering care possible. The assessment is repeated periodically to monitor changes and make modifications to the plan of care as needed. In the skilled nursing setting periodic reassessments are done through the Resident Assessment Instrument (RAI) process (Chapter 7); however, it is just as important in the outpatient setting. This information guides the discussions around end-of-life care, including legal preparation when the point of cognitive incapacity is reached (Chapter 31).

To prepare those with PD for anticipated changes in muscular flexibility, early training in relaxation such as modified yoga or Zen techniques and exercises may be helpful. Tai chi has been found to increase balance skills (Gao et al, 2014; Li et al, 2014; Pickut et al, 2013).

Persons with neurodegenerative disorders eventually experience changes in roles and may avoid social situations due to the accompanying signs and symptoms. For those with PD, tremors may produce embarrassing movements such as spilling food when eating in public. Drooling, a common problem with those with PD, is a socially unacceptable "behavior" in most societies. The expressionless face, slowed movement, and soft, monotone speech or aphasias may give the impression of apathy, depression, and disinterest and therefore others are discouraged from continuing long-time relationships. A sensitive nurse is aware that the visible symptoms produce an undesired façade that may hide an alert and responsive individual who wishes to interact but is trapped in a body or brain that no longer cooperates.

Nowhere in the care of others is a skilled and caring multidisciplinary team more essential than in the care of persons with neurodegenerative disorders. It includes a nurse; a neurologist; a physiatrist; speech, occupational, and physical therapists; an ophthalmologist; a rehabilitation specialist; a psychologist; a movement disorders' specialist; and the hospice team. It also may include a spiritual advisor or indigenous healer. It always includes the person's significant other(s), who will be involved in day-to-day life at some point in time. Ideally it includes a physician and a nurse practitioner working as a primary care team.

Occupational therapists can assist with teaching the person how to use adaptive equipment, such as weighted utensils, non-slip dinnerware, and other self-care aids. Speech therapy is beneficial for dysarthria and dysphagia; patients can be taught facial exercises and swallowing techniques to lower the risk for aspiration-related pneumonia and weight loss.

The nurse has an active role in prevention of complications. The nurse works to prevent skin breakdown and falls and identifies exacerbation of confusion or function, which may indicate the development of a treatable condition such as an infection. The nurse is alert for problems with sleep and depression as the disease progresses.

Treatment focuses on relieving symptoms with medication, increasing functional ability, preventing excess disability, and decreasing the risk of injury. In caring for persons with neurodegenerative disorders, regular pain assessments and appropriate management are essential (Chapter 27). In PD, rigidity, contractures, and dystonia may cause a considerable amount of pain. There is also a recognized but not well-understood central-pain syndrome associated with the disease itself. Persons with any of the NCDs may not be able to verbally express their pain but nonetheless experience it as anyone else would under the same circumstances. The nurse is aware of this and uses alternative means to observe for potential pain (Chapter 27).

Persons with neurodegenerative disorders watch their own decline over time, challenging self-esteem. The nurse can direct the person and care partners to formal programs in stress management or group support and urge them to attempt to maintain former relationships (Chapters 29 and 34).

The key factors in the care of those with neurodegenerative disorders are (1) appropriate use of available nonpharmacological and pharmacological interventions, (2) prompt treatment of all reversible conditions (e.g., infections), and (3) coordination between all care providers, including family members or partners. Pharmaceutical management of PD is customized for each individual.

Considering the current inability to enact a cure for any of the neurodegenerative disorders, the goals of care are to maximize quality of life, promote self-esteem, and maintain independent function for as long as possible. The goal of treatment is to preserve self-esteem, retain self-care abilities, and prevent complications.

KEY CONCEPTS

- Neurodegenerative conditions are those that have a downward trajectory and for which there is no cure. The conditions discussed in this chapter are limited to AD, LBD and PDD, and PD.
- Some persons with PD also develop late-stage cognitive disorders.
- The diagnostic process for any of these conditions is extensive and complex.
- A key difference in LBD and PD is timing of symptoms. LBD begins with cognitive declines and movement disorders develop later. PD is a movement disorder that may or may not lead to cognitive declines. Both are classified as Lewy body disorders.

- At least some of the genes associated with AD have been identified.
- The signal characteristics of PD include a resting tremor and bradykinesia.
- Treatment of each condition must be individually tailored and will change over time.
- The nurse has a key role in monitoring changes that indicate increased risk for poor outcomes and in developing interventions to maximize quality of life and healthy aging at all points along the wellness continuum.

NURSING STUDY: "IT IS SO HARD TO WATCH ... HE WAS LOST TO ME SO LONG AGO!"

Helen's husband, Sam, had been slowly dying over a period of about 5 years from Alzheimer's disease. As it progressed, he began to have what are called "behavioral disturbances." He lashed out at those around him one moment and was affectionate the next. This was especially painful for his wife. During brief moments of lucidity, he would kiss her and tell her how much he loved her, but moments later would physically hurt her in some way. Most of the time he was completely disoriented, and the nurses caring for him charted Sam as "disoriented × 4" (person, place, time, and situation). After a long and steady decline in cognitive and functional ability, one day he simply stopped eating and

drinking and he began to fail rapidly. We all knew that death was imminent. His wife carefully shared that while she was glad for him that he would soon no longer suffer, she whispered, "and it will also bring an end to my suffering, is that terrible to think that??? He was lost to me so long ago ..."

- What are the subjective and objective data found in the case study?
- If you were one of the nurses caring for Sam, how would your plan of care change over time?
- If you were Helen, what would be the hardest part of your husband's illness?
- What strengths has Helen brought to the situation?

CRITICAL THINKING QUESTIONS AND ACTIVITIES

1. Have a classroom discussion about resources in the community that would be particularly helpful for persons with neurodegenerative disorders and the persons who care for them.

2. Discuss or write a paper about the skills the nurse must have to be able to provide expert care to persons with NCDs of any kind.

RESEARCH QUESTIONS

1. What is the average life expectancy of someone with AD?
2. Are there parts of the country that have unusually high or low rates of neurodegenerative conditions? What are the areas of the country and what might be the cause of this variation?

3. Has any genomic progress been made in understanding any of the other neurodegenerative disorders that are not addressed in this chapter?

REFERENCES

Alzheimer's Association (AA). *2018 Alzheimer's disease facts and figures*, 2018a. https://www.alz.org/media/Documents/facts-and-figures-2018-r.pdf. Accessed April 2019.

Alzheimer's Association (AA): *New diagnostic criteria and guidelines for Alzheimer's disease*, 2018b. https://www.alz.org/research/diagnostic_criteria/.

Alzheimer's Association (AA): *The search for Alzheimer's causes and risk factors*, 2018c. https://www.alz.org/research/science/alzheimers_disease_causes.asp#genetics.

Alzheimer's Association (AA): *What we know today about Alzheimer's disease*, 2018d. https://www.alz.org/research/science/alzheimers_disease_treatments.asp.

Alzheimer's Association (AA). *Facts and figures*, 2019a. https://alz.org/alzheimers-dementia/facts-figures. Accessed April 2019.

Alzheimer's Association (AA). *Causes and risk factors*, 2019b. https://alz.org/alzheimers-dementia/what-is-alzheimers/causes-and-risk-factors. Accessed April 2019.

American Psychiatric Association (APA): *Diagnostic and statistical manual of mental disorders*, ed 5, Arlington, VA, 2013, American Psychiatric Association Publishing.

Barnes LL, Bennett DA: Alzheimer's disease in African Americans: risk factors and challenges for the future, *Health Aff (Millwood)* 33(4):580–586, 2014.

Gao Q, Leung A, Yang Y, et al: Effects of tai chi on balance and fall prevention in Parkinson's disease: a randomized controlled trial, *Clin Rehabil* 28(8):748–753, 2014.

Khandelwal C, Kaufer DI: Alzheimer's disease and other dementias. In Ham RJ, Sloane D, Warshaw GA, et al, editors: *Primary care geriatrics: a case-based approach*, ed 6, Philadelphia, PA, 2014, Elsevier, pp 201–213.

Lewy Body Dementia Association (LBDA): *Diagnosis*, 2016a. https://www.lbda.org/go/diagnosis-0.

Lewy Body Dementia Association (LBDA): *Treatment*, 2016b. https://www.lbda.org/go/treatment-0.

Lewy Body Dementia Association (LBDA): *Symptoms: lewy body dementia symptoms and diagnostic criteria*, 2016c. https://www.lbda.org/go/symptoms-0.

Li F, Harmer P, Liu Y, et al: A randomized controlled trial of patient-reported outcomes with tai chi exercise in Parkinson's disease, *Mov Disord* 29(4):539–545, 2014.

Meara J: Parkinsonism and other movement disorders. In Fillit HM, Rockwood K, Young J, editors: *Brocklehurst's Textbook of geriatric medicine and gerontology*, ed 8, Philadelphia, PA, 2017, Elsevier, pp 510–518.

National Institute of Environmental Health Sciences (NIEHS): *Parkinson's disease*, 2017. http://www.niehs.nih.gov/health/topics/conditions/parkinson.

National Institute on Aging (NIA): *Alzheimer's disease genetics fact sheet*, 2015. http://www.nia.nih.gov/alzheimers/publication/alzheimers-disease-genetics-fact-sheet#genetics.

National Institute on Aging (NIA): *Parkinson's disease*, 2017a. https://www.nia.nih.gov/health/parkinsons-disease.

National Institute on Aging (NIA): *What is Lewy body dementia?* 2017b. https://www.nia.nih.gov/health/what-lewy-body-dementia.

National Institute on Aging (NIA): *Symptoms of lewy body dementia*, 2017c. https://www.nia.nih.gov/health/symptoms-lewy-body-dementia.

National Institute on Aging (NIA): *What causes Lewy Body dementia?* 2017d. https://www.nia.nih.gov/health/what-causes-lewy-body-dementia.

National Institute on Aging (NIA): *How is Alzheimer's disease treated?* 2018. https://www.nia.nih.gov/health/how-alzheimers-disease-treated.

Parkinson's Foundation: *Statistics*, n.d.a. http://parkinson.org/Understanding-Parkinsons/Causes-and-Statistics/Statistics.

Parkinson's Foundation: *Genetic factors*, n.d.b. http://parkinson.org/Understanding-Parkinsons/Causes-and-Statistics/Genetic-Factors.

Pickut BA, Van Hecke W, Kerckhofs E, et al: Mindfulness based intervention in Parkinson's disease leads to structural brain changes on MRI: a randomized controlled longitudinal trial, *Clin Neurol Neurosurg* 115(12):2419–2425, 2013.

Sinha N, Berg CN, Tustison NJ, et al. APOE ε4 status in healthy older African Americans is associated with deficits in pattern separation and hippocampal hyperactivation, *Neurobiol Aging* 69:221–229, 2018.

Vigneswara V, Cass S, Wayne D, Bolt EL, Ray DE, Carter WG: Molecular ageing of alpha- and beta-synucleins: protein damage and repair mechanisms, *PLoS One* 8(4):e61442, 2013.

Vasta R, Nicoletti A, Mostile G, et al: Side effects induced by the acute levodopa challenge in Parkinson's disease and atypical parkinsonisms, *PLoS One* 12(2):e0172145, 2017.

World Health Organization (WHO): *Media centre: dementia*, 2017. http://www.who.int/mediacentre/factsheets/fs362/en/.

24

Endocrine and Immune Disorders

Kathleen Jett

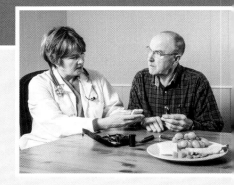

http://evolve.elsevier.com/Touhy/TwdHlthAging

A STUDENT SPEAKS

The immune system is so complex and affects so many other systems it is difficult to grasp. However, I see now how important my understanding is in order to provide the highest quality of care I can.

Tamara, age 30, a nurse practitioner student

AN OLDER ADULT SPEAKS

I had been wondering why I was so tired. I just could not get enough sleep. I went to my primary care provider, who did a bunch of tests and discovered I had a problem with my thyroid gland. Now that it is being treated, I cannot believe how much better I feel. Just like my old self again.

Ruth, age 72

LEARNING OBJECTIVES

On completion of this chapter, the reader will be able to:

1. Discuss the effects of the aging immune system on the body's ability to respond to potential infectious agents.
2. Discuss common conditions that may be related to changes in the aging immune system.
3. Determine how diabetes is different in older adults compared with those who are younger.
4. Describe the nurse's response to the older adult with fluctuations in glycemic levels.
5. Identify the most common pharmacological agents used to treat diabetes and explain how their use may differ in older adults.
6. Differentiate between the two major types of thyroid disorders.
7. Describe how the signs and symptoms of thyroid disorders differ in younger adults compared with older adults.
8. Describe the nurse's role in advancing healthy aging in persons with immune and endocrine disorders.

THE IMMUNE SYSTEM

The immune system functions to protect the host (the human body) from invasion by foreign substances and organisms through the activity of lymphocytes, particularly T and B cells. T cells scan the body for invading substances such as infections and contribute to the body's immunity. While the total number of circulating T cells does not change with aging, the relative proportion of the types of cells does; the thymus, where T cells mature, may be only 15% of the size in late life that it was in midlife (Rote, 2014).

B cells secrete antibodies in response to the presence of antigens such as infectious agents and other foreign substances. In aging, this function decreases, resulting in a reduced ability to produce antibodies. For example, there is a decreased ability to develop adequate immunity after an infection or even after an immunization such as that for influenza.

At the same time, there is an increase in the number of circulating autoantibodies, resulting in B cells becoming less sensitive to self-antigens; that is, they are less able to differentiate self-cells from non–self-cells. Although their effect is not well understood, there is an increase in the number of immunoglobulins leading to a decrease in innate immunity and increase in common autoimmune responses, hence autoimmune disorders are much more likely to occur in later life (Box 24.1). These changes are referred to as *immunosenescence* (Chapter 3). Being alert for signs and symptoms of autoimmune disorders is probably as important as prevention and protection from infection for the older adult (Box 24.2).

BOX 24.1 Tips for Best Practice

Reduced Immune Response

Early studies found that oral temperature norms in healthy older adults were significantly lower in women older than age 80 compared with younger women. Older men consistently had an even lower temperature than women of comparable age. The old-old may have a temperature of 96.8°F, with an average range of 95°F to 97°F. By tympanic membrane thermometer, the temperature may be 96°F. These findings emphasize the need to carefully evaluate the basal temperature of older adults and recognize that even low-grade fevers (99°F) in the older adult may signify serious illness. Due to age-related delayed immune response, a lack of fever (temperature greater than 98.6°F) cannot be used to rule out an infection.

From Stengel GB: Oral temperatures in the elderly, *Gerontologist* 23:306, 1983 (special issue).

BOX 24.2 The Aging Immune System and Immune Disorders

Diabetes
Insulin resistance
Hypothyroidism (chronic autoimmune thyroiditis)
Pernicious anemia
Renal insufficiency
Environmental allergies

THE ENDOCRINE SYSTEM

The endocrine system works with multiple body organs through the release of hormones to regulate and integrate body activities. Hormones are responsible for, and control, reproduction, growth and development, maintenance of homeostasis, response to stress, nutrient balance, cell metabolism, and energy balance. The primary glands of the endocrine system are the pituitary, thyroid, parathyroid, adrenal, pineal, and thymus. The pancreas, ovaries, and testes are not glands, but they contain endocrine tissue. Except for the ovaries, age-related changes in the endocrine system are thought to be very mild and most likely due to the autoimmunity described in the previous section.

The complex interrelationships between the components of the system and the number of concurrent chronic conditions (including frailty) make it almost impossible to specifically attribute any endocrine disease to the aging process itself. As with most other biological systems, the signs and symptoms of a problem are often subtle and nonspecific, especially in the older adult. Endocrine disorders are common in later life but may only become known during a routine screening, laboratory testing, or the evaluation for another problem such as confusion or an unexplained fall. In this chapter, diabetes and thyroid disturbances as seen in the older adult are addressed.

Diabetes Mellitus

There are two main types of diabetes mellitus (DM): type 1 and type 2. Over 25 million adults aged at least 65 in the United States have diabetes; 20.8 million have been diagnosed and 4.4 million are undiagnosed (CDC, 2017). Type 1 is the result of absolute insulin deficiency due to the autoimmune destruction of beta-cells in the pancreas. Historically, most people with type 1 have not lived to late life.

Type 2 diabetes is a combination of *relative* insulin deficiency combined with insulin resistance. It is the most common type of DM seen in older adults. Genetics, epigenetics, lifestyle, and aging are all significant contributing factors. While a number of proteins are thought to be associated with DM, the largest risk factor is thought to be the presence of the gene *TCF7L2*. There is also a very strong family association; the more family members with DM, the greater the risk. Part of this is likely related to familial obesity, either with genetic influence or that of lifestyle and diet (Haddad et al, 2017). About one in three Americans have "prediabetes," in which the person's blood glucose is high but not to the point of diabetes.

Due to the high prevalence and incidence of DM in older adults, diagnostic tests are done when clinical signs and symptoms are present. The US Preventive Services Task Force (USP-STF) recommends that screening for abnormal blood glucose and type 2 diabetes is part of cardiovascular (CV) risk assessment for all obese or overweight adults age 40 to 70 (USPSTF, 2015). Three-year intervals between screenings are recommended (Ngo-Metzger and Owens, 2016).

There is a wide variation in the prevalence of DM among ethnic/racial groups and subgroups (Table 24.1). In the United States, American Indians/Alaskan Natives have the highest rate of diabetes of all other groups. This is influenced by the high prevalence of DM in the Pima Indians of the Southwest (Schulz and Chaudhari, 2015). Another group at high risk is veterans who have been exposed to Agent Orange and other herbicides during military service in Vietnam and the Korean War, all of whom are now in late life (Box 24.3). In 2014, 422 million people worldwide had diabetes; 90% of those with diabetes around the world have type 2, attributed to obesity and physical inactivity (WHO, 2017). Eighty percent of those with DM live in low- and middle-income countries. The number of persons who die from the consequences of hyperglycemia is expected to double between 2005 and 2030.

TABLE 24.1 Diabetes by Race/Ethnicity.

Race/Ethnicity	Percentage Diagnosed With Diabetes
Non-Hispanic whites	7.2
Asian Americans	8.0
Chinese	4.3
Filipinos	8.9
Asian Indians	11.2
Other Asian Americans	8.5
Hispanics	12.1
Central and South Americans	8.5
Cubans	9.0
Mexican Americans	13.8
Puerto Ricans	12.0
Non-Hispanic blacks	12.7
American Indians/Alaskan Natives	15.1

From American Diabetes Association: *Statistics about diabetes*, 2018. http://www.diabetes.org/diabetes-basics/statistics. Accessed April 2018.

Signs and Symptoms

The classic signs of both DM type 1 and DM type 2 are polyuria, polyphagia, and polydipsia (the three "Ps"). However, in late life, polyuria does not occur as often due to normal age-related increases in the renal threshold for glucose. Instead, the older adult may develop urinary incontinence or find that it has worsened. Polydipsia (excessive thirst) is not present as often due to a normal age-related reduced thirst reflex. Polyphagia (excessive hunger) is reduced by age-related decreased appetite. Unplanned weight loss may occur instead of weight gain. Fatigue is common. Women may present with recurrent candidiasis as the first sign. Due to the absence or delayed signs and symptoms, the person may be found obtunded in a hyperglycemic-hyperosmolar nonketotic coma before an initial diagnosis is made (ADA, 2018). The older adult with DM should be screened regularly for the development of signs of complications that are more likely to occur in this population (Box 24.4).

Complications

The risk for the development of complications in older adults with DM type 2 is compounded by the presence of multiple comorbid diseases and disorders. Although the same types of macro- and microvascular complications occur in both older and younger adults, the risk of heart disease is two to four times higher and the life expectancy is up to 10 years shorter (NIDDK, 2017). Prolonged periods of hyperglycemia lead to glycosylation of proteins and the production of by-products, which, in turn, cause tissue damage. Functional declines are more likely unless proactive measures are taken to promote wellness (Box 24.5). Diabetes is associated with a high rate of depression, and those who are depressed have a higher mortality rate.

Too often a diagnosis is not made until evidence of end-organ damage becomes visible (Box 24.6). Cardiovascular disease

BOX 24.4 Complications of Diabetes More Common in Older Adults

Dry eyes	Anorexia
Dry mouth	Dehydration
Confusion	Delirium
Incontinence	Nausea
Weight loss	Delayed wound healing

From Razzaque I, Morley JE, Nau KC, et al: Diabetes mellitus. In Ham RJ, Sloane PD, Warshaw GA, et al, editors: *Primary care geriatrics: a case-based approach*, Philadelphia, 2014, Elsevier, pp 431–439.

BOX 24.5 Functional Disability Associated With Diabetes

Mobility impairment	Muscle weakness
Falls	Fatigue
Incontinence	Weight loss
Cognitive impairments	

BOX 24.6 Signs of End-Organ Damage in Diabetes

Decreased visual acuity	Heart disease
Paresthesia	Stroke
Neuropathy	Periodontal disease

From Razzaque I, Morley JE, Nau KC, et al: Diabetes mellitus. In Ham RJ, Sloane PD, Warshaw GA, et al, editors: *Primary care geriatrics: a case-based approach*, Philadelphia, 2014, Elsevier, pp 431–439.

(CVD) (Chapter 22) is the most common cause of death among people with diabetes (IDF, n.d.). The combined macrovascular and microvascular complications cause nerve damage ranging from peripheral neuropathy to gastroparesis to sexual dysfunction. It is the leading cause of neuropathy, blindness, amputation, and kidney failure (IDF, n.d.). Impotence in men results from reduced vascular flow, neuropathy, and uncontrolled circulating blood glucose levels. Sexual dysfunction is two to five times greater in this group than in the general population.

Persons with DM commonly have problems with their lower extremities, which can have a considerable impact on function. Warning signs of problems include cold feet, neuropathic burning, tingling, hypersensitivity, and numbness. Infections are common and difficult to treat. Both the infections and the necessary antibiotics often result in unstable glucose control.

Several of the geriatric syndromes are highly associated with DM and contribute to excess morbidity and mortality compared with other conditions. The particular syndromes include cognitive impairment, depression, polypharmacy, incontinence, persistent pain, and falls.

Hypoglycemia (blood glucose level <60 mg/dL) can occur from many causes, such as unusually intense exercise, alcohol intake, or medication mismanagement. Signs in the older adult include tachycardia, palpitations, diaphoresis, tremors, pallor, and anxiety. Later symptoms may include headache, dizziness, fatigue, irritability, confusion, hunger, visual changes, seizures, and coma. Immediate care involves giving the patient glucose either orally if conscious, or intravenously if unconscious.

Subjective hyperglycemia in older adults is harder to detect than in a younger adult because there is a higher tolerance for elevated levels of circulating glucose. It is not uncommon to find persons with fasting glucose levels of 200 to 600 mg/dL or higher. This level of unrecognized hyperglycemia increases the risk for hyperosmolar hyperglycemic nonketotic coma. This is life threatening to persons who are otherwise medically frail and should be considered in any older adult with diabetes who is difficult to arouse. This is always a medical emergency.

PROMOTING HEALTHY AGING: IMPLICATIONS FOR GERONTOLOGICAL NURSING

The gerontological nurse has a major role in promoting healthy aging in people with diabetes. Ideally, the nurse helps the person move toward the goals of *Healthy People 2020* and ensures that the standards of diabetic care are obtained (see http://clinical.diabetesjournals.org/content/36/1/14). The focus is on prevention, early identification, and delay of complications for as long as possible. Prevention includes identifying those persons at greatest risk (e.g., obese or with a positive family history), encouraging regular exercise, and maintaining excellent control of other chronic conditions.

Although glycemic control is important, more emphasis in late life is now on the prevention and treatment of CVD. Research has indicated that it may take 8 years of glycemic control before benefits are seen, while the benefits of better control of blood pressure and lipid levels are seen as early as 2 to 3 years. Promoting CV health has the potential to be the most efficacious in the minimization of complications in persons with DM (Box 24.7). At the same time, it has been found (ACCORD trial) that intensive glycemic therapy for those at risk for CVD may increase mortality (McCulloch and Munshi, 2018). At all times, interventions must be considered in the context of the life expectancy and cost/benefit ratio for the individual.

 HEALTHY PEOPLE 2020

Goals Related to Diabetes

Reduce annual number of new cases.
Reduce death rate.
Reduce number of lower extremity amputations.
Improve glycemic control.
Improve lipid control.
Increase the proportion of persons with controlled hypertension.
Increase the number of persons with at least annual dental, foot, and dilated eye exams.
Increase the proportion of persons with at least biannual glycosylated hemoglobin measurement.
Increase the proportion of persons who obtain an annual microalbumin measurement.
Perform self-monitoring blood glucose measurement at least twice a day.
Receive formal diabetes education.
Increase the number of persons who have been diagnosed.
Increase preventive measures in persons at high risk.

From U.S. Department of Health and Human Services, Office of Disease Prevention and Health Promotion: *Healthy People 2020: Diabetes*, 2018. https://www.healthypeople.gov/2020/topics-objectives/topic/diabetes/objectives. Accessed April 2018.

BOX 24.7   Minimizing Cardiovascular Risk in Persons With Diabetes

Maintain a healthy diet
Exercise regularly
Maintain target blood pressure (BP) (<130/80 to 140/90 mm Hg)[a]
No smoking or exposure to smoke
Maintain target Hgb A1C
Attain and maintain acceptable cholesterol and triglyceride levels

[a]Identified goal varies by organization at this time.

Screening for DM is important for early identification of prediabetes or diabetes. Nurses participate in screenings at community health fairs and in clinical settings. Nurses also participate in community education about the need for early diagnosis, glycemic control, and prompt treatment of complications. Some nurses choose to develop an expertise in working with those who have diabetes and become certified diabetes educators and clinicians.

Assessment

Health promotion for older adults with DM begins with a comprehensive geriatric assessment (Chapter 7). It also includes the assessment of painless neuropathy and requires a careful neurological examination with an emphasis on sensation and history of functioning. Clinical guidelines suggest that the best means of testing neurological and sensory intactness is the use of the Semmes-Weinstein type monofilament. The measurements of height, weight, and waist circumference are used to calculate the body mass index (BMI) (Chapter 18); however, for the very old, BMI measurement is less useful because of the age-related replacement of muscle mass with adipose tissue. Physical assessment includes a careful inspection of the feet, skin, and mouth for signs of injury or the presence of lesions.

Use of herbal products (Chapters 9 and 10) and nutritional supplements, over-the-counter and prescription drugs, and alcohol and tobacco are all components of the assessment of someone with diabetes. All have a direct or indirect effect on renal, circulatory, neurological, and nutritional health.

Due to the high prevalence of depression, the assessment includes a screen for this at the time of diagnosis, at intervals thereafter, or at any time depression is suspected by the health care provider (e.g., nurse) or reported by the patient (Chapters 7 and 28). The nurse uses the results of the assessment to work with the older adult and significant others to develop the plan of care related to both pharmacological and nonpharmacological approaches to everyday life. The regular assessment of mood and coping ensures that timely and effective interventions are initiated when needed.

Management

Promoting healthy aging in the person with diabetes requires an array of interventions and an interdisciplinary team working together. This includes ancillary nursing staff and licensed nurses, nutritionists, pharmacists, podiatrists, ophthalmologists, physicians, nurse practitioners, certified diabetes educators, and counselors working in collaboration with the patient and his or her family/significant others in culturally appropriate ways (Chapter 4). The nurse often serves as team leader, educator, care provider, supporter, and guide. If the person's disease is difficult to control, endocrinologists are involved, and as complications develop, more specialists are utilized, such as nephrologists, cardiologists, and wound care specialists. Nurses are expected to advocate for older adults and encourage them to expect and receive quality care to prevent the devastating end-results of poor management.

While the goals of minimizing hyperglycemia and controlling risk factors are potentially the same at any age, life expectancy and comorbid conditions can change the focus of care. If the person is frail, prevention of hypoglycemia, hypotension, and drug interactions is especially important. If there is not a consistent caregiver or one who has obtained the necessary diabetes education on behalf of, or with, the older adult, diabetes control may be impossible.

The glycated hemoglobin test (Hgb A1C) is the best measure of ongoing glycemic control in many people. However, it is not reliable in some persons with specific ancestry, a number of conditions more common in late life, and in those who have had DM for a longer time (Box 24.8). While the Hgb A1C goal in younger persons is less than 5.7%, in later life, patient characteristics and life expectancy influence the target (ADA, 2018) (Table 24.2).

Pharmacological management. Care of the older adult with DM requires that the bedside or community nurse develop a knowledge base of the commonly used pharmacological interventions. These include the antiglycemics and preventive (cardiac) adjuvant therapy, such as angiotensin-converting enzyme (ACE) inhibitors and aspirin. All have demonstrated to improve outcomes. The primary care advanced practice nurse is expected to have expertise in the spectrum of pharmacological approaches to assist persons in the appropriate management of their disease and its complications.

Several medications have implications for use or lack of safety in older adults. Metformin (Glucophage) is commonly prescribed as first-line therapy; it does not cause hypoglycemia or weight gain. However, it is contraindicated in persons with advanced renal disease and must be used with caution in those with reduced hepatic function or congestive heart failure due to the greater risk of lactic acidosis. Thiazolidinediones can only be used with great caution, especially in those with heart failure or at risk for falls. Due to the very high risk for hypoglycemia, sulfonylureas must be used with caution, if at all (ADA, 2018). Incretin-based therapies can be very expensive and, if injectable, require the same skills as insulin (see next).

⚡ SAFETY ALERT
Do Not Use

> The sulfonylurea glyburide is contraindicated for use with older adults. A long half-life results in a very high risk for prolonged hypoglycemia (ADA, 2018).

Insulin is used when all other strategies have failed to maintain the glycemic goals for that person. There are long-acting preparations (e.g., Lantus), but they cannot be used until the required daily total dose is determined. This is done using shorter acting preparations until this is known. "Sliding-scale" adjustments are not recommended (AGS, 2015). The use of insulin requires manual dexterity in the person or caregiver to ensure that glucose levels are monitored and that doses are administered correctly and at the correct times. Prefilled syringes can be obtained and therefore could be used by someone with visual limitations; however, the cost of these is often prohibitive.

Nonpharmacological management. The cornerstones of nonpharmacological management of DM are nutrition, exercise, and self-care.

BOX 24.8 Variations in Hgb A1C

For people of African, Mediterranean, or Southeast Asian heritage the Hgb A1C can be highly unreliable due to the possibility of the presence of a variant of hemoglobin that cannot be accurately tested by the Hgb A1C.

From National Institute of Diabetes and Digestive and Kidney Diseases (NIDDK): *Diabetes tests and diagnosis*, 2016. https://www.niddk.nih.gov/health-information/diabetes/overview/tests-diagnosis. Accessed April 2018.

TABLE 24.2 Diabetes Treatment Goals in Consideration of Health Status.

Patient Health	Potential A1C (%) in Consideration of Burden and Risk	Fasting or Preprandial Glucose (Mg/Dl)	Bedtime Glucose (Mg/Dl)	Blood Pressure (Mm Hg)	Use of Statin	Rationale
Healthy, few coexisting conditions	<7.5	90–130	90–150	<140/90	Unless contraindicated	Longer life expectancy
Complex/intermediate coexisting illnesses with activities of daily living (ADL) impairments or mild to moderate cognitive impairments	<8.0	90–150	100–180	<140/90	Unless contraindicated	Intermediate life expectancy with high treatment burden
Very complex, poor health, long-term care or end-stage, ADL impairments, moderate to severe cognitive impairment	<8.5	100–180	110–200	<150/90	Consider benefit	Limited life expectancy, uncertain benefit

Data from American Diabetes Association: Older adults: standards of medical care in diabetes 2018–2019. *Diabetes Care* 42(Suppl 1): S139–S147, 2019.

BOX 24.9 Evidence-Based Practice: Dietary Supplements and Diabetes

There is weak evidence that chromium may help control blood sugar and that alpha-lipoic acid may be helpful for diabetic neuropathy. There is insufficient evidence to support a beneficial effect of other supplements at this time. Patients should always check a reputable source prior to starting a supplement and the nurse should be very well informed before making any suggestions.

National Center for Complementary and Integrative Health (NCCIH): *Diabetes and dietary supplements.* https://nccih.nih.gov/health/diabetes/supplements. Accessed April 2019.

Nutrition. Adequate and appropriate nutrition is a key factor in healthy living and aging with DM. An initial nutrition assessment with a 24-hour recall will provide some clues to the patient's dietary habits, intake, and style of eating (Chapter 14) (Box 24.9). It is part of the nurse's responsibility to learn if appropriate food is accessible, including necessary funds and a means of food preparation. The nurse works with the individual to identify culturally specific foods that can be translated into a "diabetic diet."

Helping people who have developed eating patterns over a lifetime is always challenging. If the older adult is from an ethnic group different from that of the nurse, the nurse will need to learn more about the usual ingredients and methods of food preparation to be able to give reasonable instructions related to adjustments for diets optimal for living with DM. Meal planning with a diabetes specialist is a covered service under Medicare (Table 24.3) (Chapter 30) (CMS, 2016). Healthy eating rather than weight loss is recommended since the latter has been shown to increase mortality among older persons with diabetes (Razzaque et al, 2014).

Exercise. Exercise improves tissue sensitivity to insulin and promotes cardiac health. Walking is an inexpensive and beneficial way to exercise; however, it needs to be done in a safe location, which cannot be assumed to be in the person's neighborhood (Chapter 18). A more intensive exercise program, such as aerobics, should not be started until the health care provider has been consulted. Those who have limited mobility can do chair exercises or, if possible, use exercise machines that enable sitting and holding on to something for support. If the person is using insulin, exercise needs to be done on a regular rather than an erratic basis, and blood glucose level must be checked before and after to avoid, or respond promptly to, hypoglycemia.

Self-care. Due to the complexity of DM in late life, maximum wellness is difficult to achieve without considerable self-care skills. The nurse is often the professional who is responsible for working with the older adult in developing such skills (Box 24.10).

Self-management essentials for diabetes include knowing the signs of hypoglycemia and hyperglycemia and the actions to take if these complications arise. An identification

TABLE 24.3 Medicare Coverage for Supplies and Services for Those With Diabetes.

Supply/Service	Frequency	Cost
Screening (laboratory)	Twice a year for those at risk	No cost
Diabetes Self-Management Training (DSMT)	One-time teaching of decreasing risks or managing diabetes	20% of approved amount after deductible met
Equipment needed for home glucose monitoring	Some restrictions to amount of quarterly supplies	20% of Medicare-approved amount after annual deductible
Foot exams and treatment	Every 6 months for those with peripheral neuropathy	20% of Medicare-approved amount after annual deductible
Glaucoma testing	Annually	20% of Medicare-approved amount after annual deductible
Insulin	As needed	Per prescription plan
Medical nutrition services	Initial assessment and one follow up	No cost
Therapeutic shoes or inserts	For those with severe diabetic foot disease	20% of Medicare-approved amount after annual deductible

For more information and details, see Centers for Medicare and Medicaid Services (CMS): *Your Medicare coverage,* 2016. https://www.medicare.gov/coverage/diabetes-supplies-and-services.html. Accessed April 2018.

BOX 24.10 Self-Care Skills Needed for the Person With Diabetes

Glucose Self-Monitoring
Obtaining a blood sample correctly
Using the glucose monitoring equipment correctly
Troubleshooting when results indicate an error
Recording the values from the machine
Understanding the timing and frequency of self-monitoring
Understanding what to do with the results

Medication Self-Administration: Insulin
Selecting appropriate injection site
Using correct technique for injections
Disposing of used needles and syringes correctly
Storing and transporting insulin correctly

Oral Medication Use
Knowing drug, dose, timing, and side effects
Knowing drug-drug and drug-food interactions
Recognizing side effects and knowing when to report

Foot Care and Examination
Selecting and using appropriate and safe footwear

Handling Sick Days
Recognizing the signs and symptoms of both hyperglycemia and hypoglycemia
Knowing what to do in response to symptoms

bracelet is recommended because delirium may be a manifestation of low blood glucose level and misinterpreted as dementia, delaying treatment. Self-care also includes preventive care practices for the heart, eyes, kidneys, and feet. Nurses support patients in obtaining the needed services. Annual diabetes self-management training and a number of other diabetes-specific services are available through Medicare (Table 24.3). A large number of resources are available about diabetes on the website for the National Institute of Diabetes and Digestive and Kidney Diseases (https://www.niddk.nih.gov/health-information/diabetes). This site provides links to a multitude of other sites, including those specific to ethnic and racial groups and in a variety of languages.

Implications for the Frail and Those Living in Residential Care Settings

Many of those who are frail also have DM. They may be dependent on others for various self-care activities. This may include meal preparation, assistance with exercise, or even help with physical movement of any kind. In a residential care setting such as a nursing home or assisted living facility, the nurse assesses the person for signs of hypoglycemia and hyperglycemia and evidence of complications. The nurse ensures that the standards of care for the person with DM are met. The nurse monitors the effect and side effects of diet, exercise, and medication use. The nurse administers or supervises the safe administration of medications.

In the home care setting the nurse works with the individual if he or she is capable, and if not, the nurse identifies the caregiver(s) who are providing the support and care for the person. In this case, the caregiver is the *de facto* nurse with the support of professionals in providers' offices or home health staff.

Thyroid Disease

There are significant age-related changes in thyroid anatomy and function. The gland undergoes progressive fibrosis and atrophy. This makes it more difficult to palpate than in a younger person (Ajish and Jayakumar, 2012). All thyroid dysfunction and disorders increase with aging, especially in women. While several of the symptoms mirror those of other nonthyroid conditions, screening for thyroid disease should always be a component of the primary health care assessment of older adults, especially for persons with depression, anxiety, cognitive disorders, or CVDs. Unfortunately, diagnosis may be delayed or never made because many of the signs and symptoms are incorrectly attributed to normal aging, another disorder, a geriatric syndrome, or side effects of medications. A fully functioning thyroid gland (or its replacement) is necessary to maintain life.

Thyroid diseases are diagnosed by the clinical presentation combined with laboratory findings of the total and free triiodothyronine (T_3) levels, the free thyroxine (T_4) levels, and the concentration of thyroid-stimulating hormone (TSH). However, the accuracy of the laboratory findings is easily affected by laboratory errors, acute illness and frailty, concurrent

TABLE 24.4 Examples of Factors Affecting Laboratory Testing of Thyroid Functioning

Test	Increased Result	Depressed Result
TSH	Potassium iodide and lithium, laboratory error, autoimmune disease, strenuous exercise, acute sleep deprivation	Severe illness, aspirin, dopamine, heparin, and steroids
T_3	Estrogen and methadone	Anabolic steroids, androgens, phenytoin, naproxen, propranolol, reserpine, and salicylates
T_4	Estrogen, methadone, and clofibrate	Anabolic steroids, androgens, lithium, phenytoin, and propranolol (see T_3)

TSH, Thyroid-stimulating hormone; *T_3*, triiodothyronine; *T_4*, thyroxine. From Chernecky CC, Berger BJ: *Laboratory tests and diagnostic procedures*, ed 6, St Louis, 2013, Elsevier; Fitzgerald PA: Endocrine disorders. In Papadakis MA, McPhee SJ, editors: *Current medical diagnosis and treatment 2013*, New York, 2013, McGraw-Hill, pp 1093–1191.

environmental conditions, and drug intake, making an accurate diagnosis difficult at times (Table 24.4).

Hypothyroidism

Hypothyroidism, insidious in onset, is thought to be most often caused by chronic autoimmune thyroiditis (Hashimoto's disease). It can also occur following treatment of hyperthyroidism, accompanying hypothalamic disorders, or the use of medications, especially amiodarone and lithium (Reuben et al, 2017). The TSH level is elevated (>7.5 units/mL in persons over 80), and the T_3 and T_4 are low as the pituitary gland tries to stimulate the underfunctioning thyroid gland. It is important to always note that while there are a number of signs and symptoms of hypothyroidism, they are more subtle or vague in older adults and may be very different from those seen in younger adults (Box 24.11). The signs are often evaluated for other causes with consideration of possible hypothyroidism as a "rule out."

⚡ SAFETY ALERT

Amiodarone is an antiarrhythmic agent. It has many contraindications but is still in use. It is associated with multiple toxicities including thyroid disease. All persons taking amiodarone must be monitored regularly for both hyperthyroidism and hypothyroidism (AGS, 2015).

Thyroid hormone replacement is usually in the form of the medication levothyroxine. Treatment with levothyroxine is not

---

BOX 24.11 Symptoms of Hypothyroidism in Older Adults

- Fatigue
- Weakness
- Depression
- Dry skin
- Mental slowness
- Drowsiness
- Constipation

innocuous, especially for women. Side effects include decreased bone mass and increased risk of heart disease. The older adult is very sensitive to exogenous thyroid hormones. Oral replacement should begin with 25 mcg of levothyroxine, or 12.5 mcg in persons with preexisting heart disease. The dose is adjusted every 4 to 6 weeks until stabilized and then in most cases is monitored annually (Reuben et al, 2017).

Myxedema coma is a serious complication of untreated hypothyroidism in the older patient. Rapid replacement of the missing thyroxine is not possible due to risk of drug toxicity. Even with the best treatment, death may ensue. Many of those who are very ill and hospitalized may have an elevation in TSH level that is transient. If the illness resolves, many will return to a euthyroid state.

Subclinical hypothyroidism. Subclinical hypothyroidism is defined as a normal serum T_4 level and a somewhat elevated TSH level (7.5 to 10 units/mL). There is controversy regarding the treatment of subclinical hypothyroidism in older adults who are otherwise asymptomatic. Only a small percentage of persons have been found to convert to true hypothyroidism.

Hyperthyroidism

Hyperthyroidism it is an overproduction of thyroid hormones. It is much less common than hypothyroidism but associated with a high cardiac mortality and morbidity (Ajish and Jayakumar, 2012). It is most often caused by the autoimmune disorder Graves' disease, but also can be caused from a toxic nodule, a multinodular goiter, or several medications, especially the iodine-containing amiodarone (Reuben et al, 2017). The onset of hyperthyroidism may be quite abrupt.

The manifestations of hyperthyroidism are often atypical in later life. Instead of heat intolerance, tremor, or nervousness the older adult is more likely to have depression, weight loss, dyspnea, unexplained atrial fibrillation, heart failure, or even confusion. The presence of any of the geriatric syndromes such as constipation, anorexia, or muscle weakness and other vague complaints may also be noted. However, on further examination the causative factor in any of these complaints may be hyperthyroidism. In later life, a condition known as apathetic thyrotoxicosis, rarely seen in younger persons, may occur in which usual hyperkinetic activity is replaced with slowed movement and depressed affect.

Diagnosis is made through a physical exam and laboratory testing. Primary hyperthyroidism is indicated by a low TSH and an elevated T_4. Subclinical disease is diagnosed with a low TSH and T_4 and T_3 that are within normal limits. Persons

with symptoms of heart disease are usually treated. Treatment includes antithyroid medications or ablative therapy.

PROMOTING HEALTHY AGING: IMPLICATIONS FOR GERONTOLOGICAL NURSING

As advocates, nurses can ensure that a thyroid screening test be done anytime there is a possibility of concern. The nurse caring for frail older adults can be attentive to the possibility that the person who is diagnosed with anxiety, dementia, or depression may instead have a thyroid disturbance. All persons suspected of having a depressive disorder must be checked for hypothyroidism (Demartini et al, 2013).

Although the nurse may understand that little can be done to prevent thyroid disturbances in late life, organizations such as the Monterey Bay Aquarium have launched campaigns to inform consumers of the iodine and mercury levels found in seafood (www.seafoodwatch.org) because of their association with thyroid disease.

The nurse may be instrumental in working with the person and family to understand both the seriousness of the problem and the need for very careful adherence to the prescribed regimen (Box 24.12). If the older adult is hospitalized for acute management, the life-threatening nature of both the disorder and the treatment can be made clear so that advanced planning can be done that will account for all possible outcomes.

The management of hypothyroidism is one of careful pharmacological replacement and, in the case of hyperthyroidism, one of surgical or chemical ablation followed by hormone replacement—both with the medication levothyroxine. The nurse works with the person and significant others in the correct self-administration of medications and in the appropriate timing of monitoring blood levels of the TSH and signs or symptoms indicating an exacerbation of the illness (Box 24.11).

BOX 24.12 Tips for Best Practice
Specific Instructions for Administration

Levothyroxine must always be taken on an empty stomach. Either early in the morning, at least 30 to 60 minutes before a meal or 4 hours after the last meal. It must be taken with a full glass of water to ensure it does not begin to dissolve in the esophagus. It cannot be taken within 4 hours of anything containing a mineral, such as calcium (including fortified orange juice), antacids or iron supplements. It is always dosed in micrograms and care must be taken that it is not confused with milligrams.

KEY CONCEPTS

- Although there are relatively few age-related changes in the immune system, the decreased ability to mount a defense against antigens increases the risk for infections.
- With aging, there is an increase in autoimmunity leading to an increase in autoimmune disorders.
- The majority of diabetes cases seen worldwide among older adults is type 2.

- The prevalence of diabetes increases with age.
- While the incidence of hyperthyroidism in late life is rare, hypothyroidism is seen with increasing frequency, especially among older women.
- There is a strong association between thyroid disease and heart disease. A person with either should be screened for the other on a regular basis.

- Undiagnosed or inadequately treated and monitored thyroid disorders can be life threatening.
- The nurse plays an active role in the early detection of auto-immune disorders and infections.

- The nurse facilitates the person's receipt of evidence-based standards of care and the utilization of benefits available to the person to help control and treat endocrine diseases.

NURSING STUDY: "THERE IS NOTHING WRONG WITH ME. I AM JUST A LITTLE TIRED!"

Ms. P., an 82-year-old single woman, lives in a life-care community in her own apartment and has the reassurance of knowing her medical and functional needs will be taken care of, regardless of the extent of these needs. She is at present independent. She has been gaining weight steadily since she moved into the community and attributes that to the fact that she eats much better now that she joins others in the congregate dining room for meals. She has heart failure, mild arthritis, and diabetes which she manages with diet, exercise, and oral medications. Although she says she feels fine, lately she has noticed some increased fatigue and that her toes are cold and somewhat numb. The great toe on her left foot seems to be discolored. Because of the lack of feeling, she often walks around her apartment barefoot because it seems to increase the sensation in her

feet. She has not needed to use the health care center and goes to the clinic only to pick up her medication. Her niece stopped by last week to see her and called the clinic and spoke with the nurse. The niece reported that her aunt seemed a little confused and lethargic. The niece accompanied Ms. P. to the clinic, where the nurses checked her blood pressure and blood sugar and found them to be 170/80 mm Hg and 280 mg/dL, respectively. Ms. P. said, "Oh, I don't think it is anything to worry about! I am just a little tired."
- Of all of Ms. P.'s symptoms and signs, which one should the nurse be most concerned about related to her long-term health?
- Of all of the symptoms that Ms. P. reports, which one should the nurse be most concerned about related to Ms. P.'s ability to live alone?

CRITICAL THINKING QUESTIONS AND ACTIVITIES

1. What commonly held beliefs about aging would lead a person to believe that the changes in his or her health did not warrant seeking health care?
2. You are assigned to teach a patient the basics of diabetes care. You have one day to do this before the person is discharged home. When you walk in the room and begin talking with

the person you find out that she is from a culture completely different from yours. How will you begin?
3. Expanding on the question above, discuss with a classmate how you would approach the same situation when you find out that your patient is responsible for cooking for the whole family.

RESEARCH QUESTIONS

1. Is there any information that explains the differences in the incidence and prevalence of diabetes in various ethnic groups?

2. What types of nutritional food supplements are used by persons with diabetes?

REFERENCES

Ajish TP, Jayakumar RV: Geriatric thyroidology: an update, *Indian J Endocrinol Metab* 16(4):542–547, 2012.
American Diabetes Association (ADA): *Hyperosmolar hyperglycemic nonketotic syndrome (HHNS)*, 2018. www.diabetes.org/living-with-diabetes/complications/hyperosmolar-hyperglycemic.html. Accessed April 2018.
American Geriatrics Society (AGS): American Geriatrics Society 2015 updated Beers Criteria for potentially inappropriate medication use in older adults, *J Am Geriatr Soc* 63(11):2227–2246, 2015.
Centers for Disease Control and Prevention (CDC): *National diabetes statistics report*, 2017. https://www.cdc.gov/diabetes/data/statistics/statistics-report.html.
Centers for Medicare and Medicaid (CMS): *Medicare's coverage of diabetes supplies and services*, 2016. www.medicare.gov/pubs/pdf/11022-Medicare-Diabetes-Coverage.pdf. Accessed April 2018.
Demartini B, Ranieri R, Masu A, Selle V, Scarone S, Gambini O: Depressive symptoms and major depressive disorder in patients affected by subclinical hypothyroidism: a cross-sectional study, *J Nerv Ment Dis* 202(8):603–607, 2013.
Haddad SA, Palmer JR, Lunetta KL, Ng MC, Ruiz-Narváez EA: A novel TCF7L2 type 2 diabetes SNP identified from fine mapping in African American women, *PLOS One* 12(3):e0172577, 2017.

https://journals.plos.org/plosone/article?id=10.1371/journal.pone.0172577. Accessed April 2019.
National Institute of Diabetes and Digestive and Kidney Diseases (NIDDK): *Diabetes, heart disease, and stroke*, 2017. https://www.niddk.nih.gov/health-information/diabetes/overview/preventing-problems/heart-disease-stroke. Accessed April 2018.
Ngo-Metzger Q, Owings J: Screening for abnormal blood glucose and type 2 diabetes mellitus, *Am Fam Physician* 93(12):1025–1026, 2016.
Razzaque I, Morley JE, Nau, KC, et al: Diabetes mellitus. In Ham RJ, Sloane PD, Warshaw GA, et al, editors: *Primary care geriatrics: a case-based approach*, ed 6, Philadelphia, PA, 2014, Elsevier, pp 431–439.
Rote NS: Adaptive immunity. In McCance KL, Huether SE, editors: *Pathophysiology: the biological basis for disease in adults and children*, ed 7, St Louis, MO, 2014, Elsevier, pp 224–261.
Schulz LO, Chaudhari LS: High-risk populations: the Pimas of Arizona and Mexico, *Curr Obes Rep* 4(1):92–98, 2015.
US Preventive Services Task Force (USPSTF): *Screening for abnormal blood glucose and type 2 diabetes mellitus*, 2015. https://www.uspreventiveservicestaskforce.org/Page/Document/UpdateSummaryFinal/screening-for-abnormal-blood-glucose-and-type-2-diabetes. Accessed April 2018.
World Health Organization (WHO): *Diabetes*, 2017. http://www.who.int/mediacentre/factsheets/fs312/en/. Accessed April 2018.

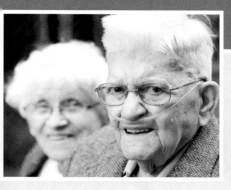

25

Respiratory Health and Illness

Kathleen Jett

http://evolve.elsevier.com/Touhy/TwdHlthAging

A STUDENT SPEAKS

Sometimes I must take care of someone who smokes. When they return from the smoking area the smell is so strong I can hardly stand getting close to them.

La'Shawn, age 18

AN OLDER ADULT SPEAKS

I have smoked since I was 12 or 13. I started coughing a little now and then when I was in my 40s. Now that I am in my 50s, it seems like I can't ever catch my breath. They say it is something called COPD. I don't quite understand that and what it has to do with my cigarettes. I certainly could not give them up after all these years!

Helen, age 56

LEARNING OBJECTIVES

On the completion of this chapter, the reader will be able to:

1. Describe the normal changes with aging that affect the respiratory system and discuss how these affect the goal of achieving healthy aging.

2. Identify the most important factors influencing respiratory health.

3. Develop strategies to promote respiratory health.

The respiratory system is the vehicle for gas exchange, especially the transfer of oxygen into and the release of carbon dioxide out of the blood. Respiration depends on cardiac health, musculoskeletal structures, and the nervous system for full function. Although there are a number of age-related changes, they are insignificant when one is free of respiratory disorders, cardiovascular illnesses, or musculoskeletal deformities of the chest. Like all other systems, there is a reduced capacity to respond to sudden changes, and when confronted with a sudden demand for increased oxygen or exposed to noxious or infectious agents, a respiratory deficit may become evident and can quickly become life-threatening. The most common chronic diseases of the respiratory system seen late in life are chronic obstructive pulmonary disease (COPD) and asthma. The most common and life-threatening acute condition is pneumonia.

NORMAL AGE-RELATED CHANGES

There are several age-related changes in the pulmonary system, all of which increase a person's risk for disability and infection. These include loss of elastic recoil due to stiffening of the chest wall and an increase in resistance to airflow. Because of these changes, auscultation of slight bibasilar atelectasis is common due to incomplete lung expansion (Table 25.1). Total lung capacity is not altered, but instead redistributed. Residual capacity increases with the diminished inspiratory and expiratory muscle strength of the thorax (Fig. 25.1). Age-related changes lead to more effort required for movement of the diaphragm. If skeletal defects such as kyphoscoliosis or arthritic costovertebral joints occur in the presence of normal age-related changes, the chest cavity can be significantly reduced. Among the most significant age-related changes are lowered efficiency of gas exchange and reduced ability to handle secretions. The cilia, which normally act as brushes to repel foreign substances or propel mucus out of the trachea, become less responsive and less effective. Compounded by a diminished cough reflex and immune response, there is a high risk for infections such as bronchitis and pneumonia. When impairments such as dysarthria, dysphagia, or decreased esophageal motility are superimposed, the risk for infection such as aspiration pneumonia increases even further. Overall, the changes are especially dangerous for those who have limited mobility, who have

TABLE 25.1 Normal Changes With Aging and Potentially Serious Consequences at the Time of Illness.	
Change	**Potential Consequence**
Ossification of the costal cartilage, less compliant rib cage	Potential for less expansion such as when exercising or when increased respirations are needed
Loss of elastin attachment in the alveolar walls	Collapse of the small airways and uneven alveolar ventilation, trapping air and increasing dead space, decreasing vital capacity, and decreasing expiratory flow
Chemoreceptor function is altered or blunted at the peripheral and central chemoreceptor sites	Compensatory responses to hypercapnia and hypoxia are decreased while perception of dyspnea is intact or even enhanced. This response is independent of mechanical lung changes and is attributed to alterations in the neuromuscular drive to breathe. Compensatory responses may be significantly hindered in situations of stress

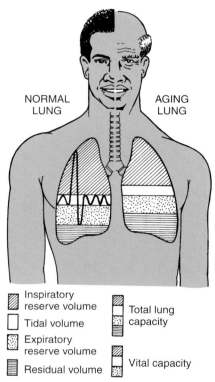

NORMAL LUNG   AGING LUNG

- ▨ Inspiratory reserve volume
- ☐ Tidal volume
- ▦ Expiratory reserve volume
- ▤ Residual volume
- ▨ Total lung capacity
- ☐ Vital capacity

Fig. 25.1 Changes in Lung Volume With Aging. (From McCance KL, Huether SE: *Pathophysiology: the biologic basis for disease in adults and children,* ed 7, St Louis, 2014, Mosby.)

changes to the oropharyngeal muscles due to injury such as stroke or chronic disease such as Parkinson disease, or who already have chronic pulmonary disorders.

PULMONARY DISORDERS

Normal age-related changes increase the risk for pulmonary problems, and when they occur, the mortality rate is higher in older adults than in younger adults. While the incidence of lung cancer increases significantly in later life, so does the presence of COPD. Asthma may be part of long-term COPD or a late-onset disease alone. In this chapter the diseases that make up COPD (formerly referred to separately as emphysema or chronic bronchitis) and asthma are addressed.

Chronic Obstructive Pulmonary Disease

COPD is characterized by a persistent and irreversible reduction in airflow. Each year 3.17 million people worldwide die from COPD, and it is expected to become the third most common cause of death worldwide by 2020 (WHO, 2016). In the United States it is already number three, behind ischemic heart disease and stroke. There is significant geographic variation, with the associated death rate highest in Mississippi, Arkansas, Kentucky, and West Virginia (CDC, 2017a). Approximately 15.7 million adults and 10% of those at least 65 years of age have COPD in the United States, with approximately 50% of those with low pulmonary function not aware they already have it (CDC, 2017b; Reuben et al, 2017).

COPD is the one noninfectious chronic disease that is increasing in prevalence despite the efforts to combat it. This is attributed to the rise in the number of women who are affected as a direct result of smoking and exposure to toxic fumes during indoor cooking.

The diagnosis of COPD is primarily made based on a careful evaluation of signs and symptoms and the elimination of cardiac causes. Spirometry confirms and quantifies the amount of airflow restriction. This measurement can then be used to monitor the progression of the disease. Measurement of the diffusing capacity for carbon monoxide may help differentiate the subtypes of emphysema and chronic bronchitis. Chronic or recurrent bronchitis is diagnosed clinically by a productive cough for 3 months in 2 consecutive years or 6 months in 1 year (Chesnutt and Prendergast, 2017).

Etiology

The airway obstruction of COPD is caused from inhalation of toxins and pollutants earlier in life, such as dust, chemicals, and especially tobacco smoke, either directly or indirectly from second-hand smoke. This inhalation exposure causes airway and lung destruction. Additional factors influence the likelihood that someone with such exposure will develop COPD (Box 25.1).

An inherited deficiency of α_1-antitrypsin may cause COPD. It is estimated that 161 million persons worldwide have at least one gene that could lead to increased risk for pulmonary disease (Genetics Home Reference, 2018).

Some persons with COPD have irritation of the lung tissues resulting in ongoing or intermittent symptoms. The airflow

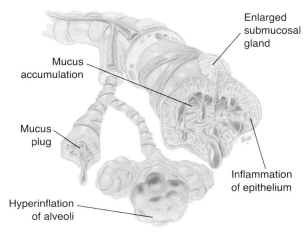

Fig. 25.2 Chronic Bronchitis. Inflammation and thickening of mucous membrane with accumulation of mucus and pus leading to obstruction characterized by productive cough. (From McCance KL, Huether SE: *Pathophysiology: the biologic basis for disease in adults and children*, ed 7, St Louis, 2014, Mosby. Modified from Des Jardins T, Burton GG: *Clinical manifestations and assessment of respiratory disease*, ed 3, St Louis, 1995, Mosby.)

obstruction in chronic bronchitis is caused by a combination of thickening and inflammation of bronchial walls, hypertrophy of mucous glands, constriction of smooth muscle, and production of excess mucus, all of which cause lumen compromise, stimulated by exposure to toxins, including both viruses and bacteria (Fig. 25.2) (Chesnutt and Prendergast, 2017).

Signs and Symptoms

COPD has a long asymptomatic stage; overt symptoms may not appear until 40 to 50 years of age when partial lung function has already been irretrievably lost. The most common symptoms are a sense of breathlessness, a chronic cough, dyspnea on exertion, and increased mucus production. Many also have wheezing (Reuben et al, 2017; WHO, 2016). Later signs include prolonged expiration with pursed-lip breathing, barrel chest, hyperresonance on percussion, fingernail clubbing, use of accessory muscles for breathing, and either pink (emphysema dominant) or pale lips or nail beds (bronchitis predominant) (Chesnutt and Prendergast, 2017).

In advanced disease, cyanosis, evidence of right-sided heart failure, and peripheral edema are present. In older adults, a high level of fatigue is found, and this in turn significantly decreases functional status (Reuben et al, 2017).

Complications

COPD is a progressively debilitating condition characterized by exacerbations and remissions in symptoms. When advanced, there is damage to the terminal bronchiole and destruction of the alveolar wall (Chesnutt and Prendergast, 2017).

Exacerbations are seen as worsening of the baseline signs, symptoms, and function; they may be insidious or acute and are characterized by significant worsening of dyspnea and increasing volume and changes in sputum color. Spirometry results of less than 150 mL, worsening orthopnea, paroxysmal nocturnal dyspnea, and respiration rate greater than 30 breaths/min signal an emergent exacerbation. These have numerous inciting factors, including viral or bacterial infections, or exposure to toxins such as air pollution or other environmental exposures, and changes in the weather. Exacerbations must be differentiated from congestive heart failure, arrhythmias, a pulmonary embolism, cor pulmonale, and pneumonia, so that the appropriate response can be initiated. A spontaneous pneumothorax can occur (rarely). Hospitalizations are frequent (Healthy People 2020 A box).

♥ HEALTHY PEOPLE 2020 A

COPD Hospitalizations

Goal
Reduce hospitalizations for chronic obstructive pulmonary disease (COPD)

Baseline
112.2 hospitalizations for COPD per 10,000 adults aged 65 years and older occurred in 2010

Target
50.1 hospitalizations per 10,000 by 2020

Data from U.S. Department of Health and Human Services: *Healthy People 2020*, Office of Disease Prevention and Health Promotion, 2018. https://www.healthypeople.gov/2020/data/disparities/summary/Chart/5167/4.

COPD significantly impairs the person's quality of life (Box 25.2). Exacerbations frequently precipitate the need for changes in medications or hospitalization with respiratory support. Pneumonia is a frequent and serious complication. Invasive endotracheal intubation may be needed for patients with respiratory acidosis that progresses despite therapy or for those with impaired consciousness. In the older adult, sudden altered mental status may indicate acute hypoxemia or hypercapnia. Although the acute phase (Chapter 21) of an exacerbation is usually resolved in 10 days to 2 weeks, lung function may take 4 to 6 weeks to return to baseline, if ever. In the advanced stages the prognosis is very poor. Seventy-five percent of COPD-related deaths are attributed to cigarette use (CDC, 2011) (Healthy People 2020 B box).

HEALTHY PEOPLE 2020 B
COPD Deaths

Goal
Reduce deaths from chronic obstructive pulmonary disease (COPD) among adults

Baseline
261.4 COPD deaths per 100,000 adults aged 65 years and older occurred in 2016

Target
102.6 deaths per 100,000 by 2020

Data from U.S. Department of Health and Human Services: *Healthy People 2020*, Office of Disease Prevention and Health Promotion, 2018. https://www.healthypeople.gov/2020/data/disparities/summary/Chart/5166/4.

BOX 25.2 Complications and Effects of Living With COPD

Mobility limitations
Early disability/inability to work
Need for special equipment such as supplemental oxygen
Limitations in social activities
Increased risk for memory loss or confusion
Increased risk for depression
Increased number of comorbid chronic conditions (e.g., heart disease, arthritis, diabetes, stroke)
Frequent emergency room visits and hospitalizations

From Centers for Disease Control and Prevention: *Chronic obstructive pulmonary disease (COPD)*, 2017. Available at: https://www.cdc.gov/copd/index.html. Accessed May 2018.

Asthma

Asthma is an inflammatory airway disease affecting about 235 million people (all ages) worldwide with most deaths occurring in low- and middle-income countries (WHO, 2017). It is closely linked to allergic mechanisms and viral or bacterial infections. It may be chronic or intermittent following exposure to triggers (Box 25.3). Asthma is characterized by variable and reoccurring airway hyperresponsiveness, bronchoconstriction, and inflammation (Chesnutt and Prendergast, 2017). Approximately 5% to 10% of older adults have asthma but compose two-thirds of all related deaths. Fifty percent also have COPD (Reuben et al, 2017).

Asthma is both underdiagnosed and undertreated in older adults. Instead, the symptoms are attributed to normal changes with aging or cardiovascular disease or are simply labeled "COPD." The person with asthma may have developed a tolerance to the bronchorestriction and minimizes the reports of symptoms, despite the respiratory compromise that is present.

There is still a significant gap in knowledge in this area, complicated by the number of comorbid conditions and socioeconomic factors involved in its presentation and treatment. It is recognized that there are at least two asthma phenotypes in later life: long-standing and late onset. Those who have had asthma for many years have more severe airflow obstruction with less reversibility than those with late-onset asthma.

BOX 25.3 Triggers for the Development of Asthma or Onset of Asthmatic Episode

Tobacco smoke
Dust mites
Outdoor air pollution/allergens
Cockroach allergen
Pets
Mold
Chemical irritants: smoke from burning grass or wood
Upper respiratory tract infections
Strong odors
Cold air
Gastroesophageal reflux disease (GERD)
Nonsteroidal antiinflammatory drugs (NSAIDS) (e.g., Advil)
Beta-blockers

Adapted from World Health Organization: *Asthma: key facts*, 2017. http://www.who.int/news-room/fact-sheets/detail/asthma. Accessed May 2018.

Asthma and its treatment are staged from mild to severe based on the frequency of symptoms—from dyspnea only with activity to dyspnea at rest. Clinically significant asthma is present when the forced expiratory volume (FEV-1) increases by 12% or 200 mL in the first second after inhaling a bronchodilator such as albuterol (Chesnutt and Prendergast, 2017). Reducing the number of older adults with asthma and decreasing the number of related hospitalizations and deaths are part of the U.S. plan to improve health by 2020 (ODPHP, 2018) (Healthy People 2020 C and D boxes).

 HEALTHY PEOPLE 2020 C
Asthma Hospitalizations

Goal
Reduce hospitalizations for asthma among adults aged 65 years and older

Baseline
25.5 hospitalizations for asthma per 10,000 adults aged 65 years and older occurred in 2010

Target
20.1 hospitalizations per 10,000 by 2020

Data from U.S. Department of Health and Human Services: *Healthy People 2020*, Office of Disease Prevention and Health Promotion, 2018. https://www.healthypeople.gov/2020/data-search/Search-the-Data#objid=5173.

 HEALTHY PEOPLE 2020 D
Asthma Deaths

Goal
Reduce asthma deaths among adults aged 65 years and older

Baseline
86.8 asthma deaths per million adults aged 65 years and older occurred in 2016

Target
21.5 deaths per million by 2020

Data from U.S. Department of Health and Human Services: *Healthy People 2020*, Office of Disease Prevention and Health Promotion, 2018. https://www.healthypeople.gov/2020/data/disparities/summary/Chart/5165/4.

Etiology

The development of asthma is influenced by genetics, environment, and lifestyle. The strongest risk factor for the development of asthma is exposure to inhaled substances and particles that provoke an allergic reaction in the form of airway inflammation (Barnes, 2018; WHO, 2017).

After a susceptible person is exposed to an antigen, a cascade of reactions occurs with immediate, late, and recurrent effects. These reactions not only have effects on airway smooth muscle and mucus secretion but also recruit the participation of monocytes, lymphocytes, neutrophils, and eosinophils into the cells lining the airways. Repeated exposure either potentiates the person's inflammatory response or desensitizes the person to the antigens to which he or she has become susceptible.

Signs and Symptoms

The classic presentation of asthma is one of recurrent episodes of wheezing, dyspnea on exertion, shortness of breath, and chest tightness. A dry cough may be dominant in older adults and confused with that seen in heart failure, COPD, gastroesophageal reflux disease (GERD), or chronic aspiration (Reuben et al, 2017). The cough may sound identical to that caused by nonsteroidal antiinflammatories, angiotensin-converting enzyme (ACE) inhibitors, or beta-blockers. The wheezing is characteristically limited to expiratory respirations and may increase in intensity during cold weather, exercise, and sleep. The latter condition often causes paroxysmal nocturnal dyspnea.

The tolerance of symptoms varies greatly from one person to another. For those with mild to moderate disease, there are often periods of asymptomatic remission. Asthmatic symptoms are usually worse at night or in the early morning hours but may begin any time following exposure to a trigger (Box 25.3). The frequency of symptoms provides a reliable measure of a person's need for, and response to, therapy. In younger adults, day-to-day variations of respiratory function can be measured by home peak (expiratory) flow meters (PFMs). However, readings are less reliable in older adults due to normal age-related decreases in peak flow (Reuben et al, 2017).

Complications

Asthma can interfere with quality of life and acute or severe exacerbations may require repeated hospitalizations. Those older than 65 have the highest asthma-related death rate of all age groups (ODPHP, 2018). When asthma is long-standing, untreated, or undertreated, structural changes to the airway occur (remodeling), such as thickening of the airway wall and bronchial fibrosis. Those with obstructive sleep apnea (OSA) are more at risk for asthma and, in turn, those with asthma are more at risk for OSA (Kong et al, 2017). When a person has asthma, he or she is at significantly higher risk for lower respiratory tract infections (e.g., pneumonia) and prolonged associated debility.

PROMOTING HEALTHY AGING: IMPLICATIONS FOR GERONTOLOGICAL NURSING

As with most chronic conditions, a team approach is needed to maximize the quality of life and functional capacity for persons with respiratory disorders. The core team may include the nurse, a pulmonologist, and a pharmacist. It may also include an occupational therapist to help the person adapt to declining function. A respiratory therapist can work with the person to maximize exercise and activity capacity and minimize disability. The gerontological nurse works with a person with asthma and COPD and his or her significant others to understand the illness and both the pharmacological and nonpharmacological self-management strategies.

Management of respiratory disorders in late life is often complicated by the presence of other chronic disorders and side effects from the necessary medications. Caring for persons with respiratory disorders requires complex nursing skills (Box 25.4). For chronically ill patients who exhibit frequent exacerbations or whose diseases have left them significantly deteriorated, carefully planned advance care directives are recommended. This planning should include a discussion of how long rehospitalizations are to be continued and the conditions under which intubation is desired, especially for the patient with end-stage COPD.

The goals of health promotion when working with the person with COPD or asthma include optimizing pulmonary function, controlling cough and wheezing, maximizing functional status, avoiding triggers, promptly recognizing exacerbations, and knowing when to seek care. Each of these goals may be more difficult to attain for older adults with comorbid conditions, especially cardiovascular disorders, which frequent accompany COPD. For those who are very frail or cognitively impaired, the promotion of respiratory health is the responsibility of the nurse and other caregivers.

Viral infections are very common in older adults, especially in those with respiratory compromise. The viral infection can rapidly become acute bacterial bronchitis or pneumonia.

BOX 25.4 Tips for Best Practice

Caring for the Person With COPD

Emotional Support
Accept/encourage expression of emotions.
Be an active listener.
Be cognizant of conversational dyspnea; do not interrupt or cut off conversations.

Education
Teach breathing techniques:
- pursed-lip breathing
- diaphragmatic breathing
- cascade coughing (series)

Teach postural drainage.
Teach about medications: what, why, frequency, amount, side effects, and what to do if side effects occur.
Teach use and care of inhalers and spacers and equipment.
Teach signs and symptoms of respiratory tract infection.
Teach about sexual activity:
- Sexual function improves with rest.
- Schedule sex around best breathing time of day.
- Use prescribed bronchodilators 20 to 30 minutes before sex.
- Use positions that do not require pressure on the chest or support of the arms.

COPD, Chronic obstructive pulmonary disease.

Age-related decrease in immune response may delay diagnosis, hence treatment. The classic symptoms of new pulmonary infiltrates on chest x-ray, elevated white blood cell (WBC) count, and fever may not initially be present. However, a drop in oxygen saturation, purulent sputum, a sudden increase in the volume of expectorant, or unusual dyspnea can suddenly become life-threatening in an older adult. Antibiotics are usually indicated in frail older adults when the *strong possibility* of pneumonia or an acute exacerbation of bronchitis is suspected; to wait for the appearance of the signs and symptoms seen in younger adults can put the person at great risk.

COPD is a disorder characterized by breathlessness. The Modified British Medical Research Questionnaire may be used in the qualitative aspect of the assessment: patients are asked to rate their level of dyspnea from "I only get breathless with strenuous exercise" to "I am too breathless to leave the house," or "I am breathless when dressing or undressing." This is always used in combination with the qualitative measurement of peak flow using spirometry (GOLD, 2018). In treatment, medications must augment lifestyle changes (Box 25.5).

An evidence-based practice guide for the assessment and management of asthma is used broadly (Box 25.6). Using such a standardized assessment allows both the registered nurse and the advanced practice nurse (APN) to work with the person in very specific ways to maximize quality of life. For the person with only intermittent "asthma attacks" only a "rescue inhaler" may be necessary. These contain short-acting bronchodilators (e.g., albuterol) to enable air to move in and out of the lungs easily. If exacerbation of the disease occurs more often, medications

such as inhaled corticosteroids and long-acting β_2-agonists are added. Inhaled medications may be taken a number of ways, including metered-dose inhalers (MDIs), home electric nebulizers, and dry-powder inhalers. There are also long-acting oral medications, such as Singulair, that may be an effective alternative for some. Several devices are available to facilitate effective drug administration, such as spacers for helping persons with hand limitations to manage medication cylinders. All of these require manual dexterity to some extent and the cognitive ability to follow directions. The nurse helps determine which of these devices has the greatest chance to be used successfully and works with the caregivers to help the person who would benefit from their use. In the long-term case setting the nurse directly oversees the use of all inhalers and nebulizers. The person must rinse his or her mouth out thoroughly after inhaled steroids are used to minimize the risk of a *Candida* infection.

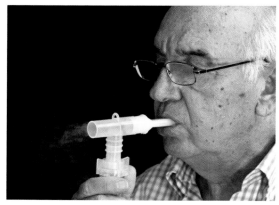

Older adult using a nebulizer device. (©iStock.com/Juanmonino.)

Nurses actively promote healthy aging through prevention of respiratory problems. This means primary prevention by promoting or conducting smoking cessation programs and participating in community efforts to administer vaccinations, especially those against influenza (annual) and pneumonia (Prevnar and Pneumovax) (Box 25.7). There is no Medicare copay or deductible for these.

Primary prevention includes political activism with industry leaders and environmental agencies to advocate for clean air and water. In occupational settings, the nurse can contribute to the health of the coworkers by promoting healthy work environments and, in some cases, monitoring patients, residents, and employees

---

BOX 25.5 Examples of Medications That May Be Taken by Someone With COPD

Bronchodilators (long and short acting)
β_2-Agonists (long and short acting)
Antimuscarinics
Methylxanthines
Leukotriene modifiers
Anticholinergics[a]
Inhaled corticosteroids
Combined products
Antiinfectives (especially macrolides)

[a]Use with caution.

BOX 25.6 Key Factors Considered in the Assessment of an Older Adults With Asthma

Frequency of symptoms[a]
Nighttime awakenings[a]
Frequency of need for "rescue inhaler"[a]
Forced expiratory volume/forced vital capacity (FEV1/FVC)[b]
Respiratory rate
Functional limitations due to respiratory status
Ability and accuracy of using medication delivery devices

[a]Weekly.
[b]Noting that this is less accurate due to normal age-related changes.

BOX 25.7 Promoting Healthy Lungs

Primary Prevention
- Obtain pneumonia immunizations.
- Obtain annual influenza immunization.
- Avoid exposure to smoke and pollutants.
- Do not smoke.
- Avoid persons with respiratory illnesses.
- Seek prompt treatment of respiratory tract infections.
- Wash hands frequently.

for exposure to, and adequate treatment of, any of the respiratory disorders, especially infections. In doing so, the nurse can decrease the prevalence of respiratory diseases and their associated morbidity and mortality in older adults. At all times, the nurse is instrumental in facilitating palliative care when appropriate.

The nurse advances self-care when teaching the person how to avoid triggers, be alert to exacerbations, use at-home PFMs to monitor disease, and know when to use "rescue inhalers" for quick, short-term use. The person should be taught that rescue medications should never be used regularly, and that long-acting medications can never be used in acute situations. If rescue medications are needed on a regular basis, a reevaluation of the plan of care is needed to improve control of chronic symptoms. Nurses can work with individuals to identify what triggers their COPD exacerbations and to learn how to respond to these and, in doing so, promote healthy aging.

KEY CONCEPTS

- Two important normal changes with aging in the respiratory system are the decreased effectiveness of gas exchange and the reduced ability to handle secretions.
- COPD is almost exclusively the result of long-term exposure to tobacco smoke.
- Chronic bronchitis is characterized by repeated infections.
- Although asthma affects persons of all ages, those with the highest mortality rate are older women.
- The nurse can have a large impact on the quality of life for the older adult with respiratory problems and his or her family members.

- The nurse helps the person learn to monitor symptoms and their effect on function and educates the person about the appropriate use of medications, oxygen, exercise, and the avoidance of triggers.
- The nurse encourages the person with respiratory disorders to remain as active as possible for as long as possible and to function as fully as possible within the limitations of his or her disease.

NURSING STUDY: HAS MRS. CHU BEEN UNDIAGNOSED?

One of your assigned patients in the acute care hospital where you are working is being prepared for an elective hip replacement due to long-standing arthritis. In your assessment, you find that Mrs. Chu seems to become slightly short of breath when she is speaking. This had been attributed to her advanced age and heart disease, even though her heart disease is well controlled at the time. As you gently proceed in your assessment she admits that she has a cough that seems to "come and go a lot" and that she is no longer doing many of the things she used to do because she is easily fatigued. When you inquire, she tells you that she was a heavy smoker "but that was many years ago."

- What is your nursing priority in caring for Mrs. Chu at this time?
- Discuss with another student two nursing diagnoses that can be drawn from this case.
- Develop a nursing intervention for the diagnoses and then compare them with another student's interventions.

CRITICAL THINKING QUESTIONS AND ACTIVITIES

1. Are end-of-life topics appropriate when caring for someone with COPD?
2. Think about the last place you either worked as a nurse or were assigned to as part of your nursing studies. Discuss any strategies that were used in the facility to minimize the development of respiratory illnesses among patients.
3. What additional strategies would you recommend?

RESEARCH QUESTIONS

1. What are three key reasons that asthma is undiagnosed in older adults?
2. Which chronic diseases are some of those that are the most undertreated?
3. Are there any changes with aging that have a direct effect on the development of respiratory disorders?
4. Explore reliable sources to determine if older adults are subject to the development of iatrogenic respiratory tract infections while in an acute care setting. (HINT: The AHRQ and CDC websites might be good places to start.) If so, to what extent are older adults affected?

REFERENCES

Barnes KC: *Genetics of asthma*, UpToDate, 2018. https://www.uptodate.com/contents/genetics-of-asthma#H17.

Centers for Disease Control and Prevention (CDC): *Public health strategic framework for COPD prevention*, 2011. https://www.cdc.gov/copd/pdfs/framework_for_copd_prevention.pdf.

Centers for Disease Control and Prevention (CDC): *Chronic obstructive pulmonary disease (COPD)*, 2017a. https://www.cdc.gov/dotw/copd/.

Centers for Disease Control and Prevention (CDC): *Chronic obstructive pulmonary disease (COPD)*, 2017b. https://www.cdc.gov/copd/index.html.

Chesnutt MS, Prendergast TJ: Pulmonary disorders. In Papadakis MA, McPhee SJ, editors: *Current medical diagnosis and treatment*, New York, NY, 2017, McGraw-Hill Lance, pp 241–321.

Genetics Home Reference: *Alpha-1 antitrypsin deficiency,* 2018. https://ghr.nlm.nih.gov/condition/alpha-1-antitrypsin-deficiency#inheritance.

Global Initiative for Chronic Obstructive Lung Disease (GOLD): *Pocket guide to COPD diagnosis, management, and prevention: a guide for health care professionals,* 2018. www.goldcopd.org.

Kong DL, Qin Z, Shen H, et al: Association of obstructive sleep apnea with asthma: a meta-analysis, *Sci Rep* 7(1):4088, 2017.

Office of Disease Prevention and Health Promotion (ODPHP): *Respiratory diseases,* 2018. https://www.healthypeople.gov/2020/topics-objectives/topic/respiratory-diseases/objectives.

Reuben DB, Herr KA, Pacala JT: *Geriatrics at your fingertips,* New York, NY, 2017, American Geriatric Society.

World Health Organization (WHO): *Chronic obstructive pulmonary disease (COPD),* 2016. http://www.who.int/en/news-room/fact-sheets/detail/chronic-obstructive-pulmonary-disease-(copd).

World Health Organization (WHO): *Asthma: key facts,* 2017. http://www.who.int/news-room/fact-sheets/detail/asthma.

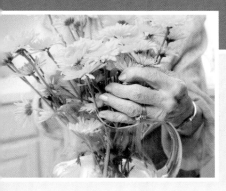

26

Common Musculoskeletal Concerns

Kathleen Jett

http://evolve.elsevier.com/Touhy/TwdHlthAging

A STUDENT SPEAKS

I thought that if you were 75 you would be all crippled up and could not do anything anymore, but some of the older people I have gotten to know are still playing tennis and hiking. They say their hands and feet hurt afterward, but that is not going to keep them down!

Rebecca, 19-year-old nurse

AN OLDER ADULT SPEAKS

These old bones just aren't what they used to be. I sound like a rocker just a creakin' away.

Jesse, age 92

LEARNING OBJECTIVES

On completion of this chapter, the reader will be able to:

1. Identify the normal changes in the aging musculoskeletal system that have the potential for the greatest effect on functional status.
2. Describe a "frailty fracture" and explain its relationship to osteoporosis.
3. Differentiate the signs and symptoms of osteoarthritis, rheumatoid arthritis, and gout as manifested in older adults.
4. Describe the key aspects of promoting musculoskeletal health while aging.
5. Describe the key areas of patient education related to both nonpharmacological and pharmacological approaches for the treatment of common musculoskeletal disorders.

A functioning musculoskeletal system is necessary for the body's movement in space, responses to environmental forces, and the maintenance of posture and activity level. Full function is needed to independently meet the activities of daily living (ADLs) (Chapter 7). Although none of the age-related changes are life-threatening, any can affect one's ability to remain independent, to be comfortable, and to maintain an acceptable quality of life. As the changes become visible to self and others, they have the further potential to affect the individual's self-esteem.

STRUCTURE AND POSTURE

Changes in stature and posture are two of the obvious outward signs of aging (Fig. 26.1). They occur gradually and are caused by multiple changes involving skeletal, muscular, and subcutaneous and fat tissue. Vertebral disks become thinner as a result of gravity and dehydration; spontaneous spinal fractures may occur causing shortening of the trunk. The more height lost, the more the likelihood of osteoporosis (OP). A stooped,

slightly forward-bent posture is common and may be accompanied by slightly flexed hips and knees. To maintain eye contact, it may be necessary to extend the head slightly, which makes it appear that the person is jutting forward. These changes occur primarily because of age-related bone calcium loss and atrophic cartilage and muscle.

Bones

Bones are composed of constantly changing organic tissue and inorganic products, especially minerals. The minerals, especially calcium, are in a constant state of flux. They are resorbed from the bloodstream and sent back into renewed bone. Bone mineral density (BMD) peaks at about the age of 20. The ability to achieve peak mass is influenced by nutrition, hormonal and genetic factors, and weight-bearing exercises. Without exercise, premature bone loss will occur (Roberts et al, 2016).

With aging, bone renewal cannot keep pace with resorption and the bones become brittle and fracture more easily. Reduced BMD is four times more common in older women than

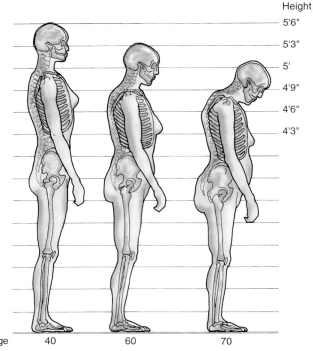

Fig. 26.1 Age-Related Changes in the Spine as a Result of Bone Loss. (From Ignatavicius DD, Workman ML: *Medical-surgical nursing: patient-centered collaborative care*, ed 6, Philadelphia, 2010, Saunders.

in men, but is present in all persons as they age, regardless of ethnicity or race. Women may lose up to 50% of their cortical bone mass by the time they are 70 years old, the extent of which is dependent on several factors (Crowther-Radulewicz, 2014). In men, reduced BMD is primarily due to prolonged steroid use. Excessive loss of BMD leads to *osteopenia* or *osteoporosis (OP)*.

Joints, Tendons, and Ligaments

The tendons and ligaments in and around joints are bands of connective tissue that bind the bones to each other and make movement possible. Cartilage is a fibrous tissue that lines the joints and supports specific body parts, such as the ears and nose. While the ears and nose enlarge (especially in men), age-related deterioration in articular cartilage results from biochemical changes: increases in the levels of transglutaminase and calcium pyrophosphates. Cellular cross-linkage affects the cartilage, ligaments, and tendons. As joints dry, movement is less fluid. Pain may result if these changes progress to the extent where bone rubs on bone, as in the case of arthritis.

Muscles

The three types of muscles are smooth, skeletal, and cardiac. Smooth muscles are responsible for the contractibility of hollow organs such as the blood vessels. Skeletal muscles, primarily under voluntary control, are essential for movement, posture, and heat production. After the age of 50 there is a gradual loss of muscle bulk and strength. These changes are referred to as *sarcopenia* and are seen almost exclusively in the skeletal muscle. Accelerated loss occurs with inactivity and deconditioning.

MUSCULOSKELETAL DISORDERS

The most common musculoskeletal disorders in later life are OP, osteoarthritis (OA), rheumatoid arthritis (RA), and gout. Pseudogout and polymyalgia rheumatica are significant but occur much less often. Pain or problems with function associated with these and other musculoskeletal problems are among the most common reasons older adults seek medical care, and the second most common cause of disability. One-third to one-half of those with musculoskeletal conditions also have other illnesses, especially depression (WHO, 2018). In this chapter we address OP, OA, RA, and gout.

Osteoporosis

OP is the most common metabolic bone disease and characterized by bone fragility. While it can affect persons at all ages and in all ethnic and racial groups, those at highest risk are postmenopausal white (Caucasian) women (Box 26.1). It is estimated that 200 million people worldwide have OP (Sözen et al, 2017). It is anticipated that by 2020 approximately 12.3 Americans at least 50 years of age will have OP. The prevalence increases dramatically with age; from 5.1% of those 50 to 59 years old to 26.2% of those 80 years and older (USPSTF, 2017). BMD declines rapidly in women after menopause and in anyone who takes steroids for an extended period of time.

OP is diagnosed either following a fragility fracture (Box 26.2) or through the results of a dual-energy x-ray absorptiometry (DEXA) scan of the femoral neck and spine (Fig. 26.2). The DEXA scan (also referred to as DXA), where available, is still considered the gold standard in the diagnosis of OP and osteopenia. The results of the scan yields a score indicating the individual's BMD in comparison to a healthy (young) reference group. *Osteopenia*, or a moderate amount of decreased BMD,

---

BOX 26.1   Major Risk Factors for Osteoporosis

Whites and Asians at highest risk
Low body weight (<117 lb)
Family history of osteoporosis
Estrogen deficiency
Inadequate calcium and vitamin D intake
Lack of weight-bearing activities
Excess alcohol use (>1 drink/day for women and >2 for men)
Smoking/exposure to tobacco smoke
Eating disorders

BOX 26.2   Fragility Fractures

Fragility fractures are those resulting from forces that would not normally cause a fracture, such as that of the hip or wrist from a fall from standing height or from activities such as coughing, sneezing, or abrupt movement. Nontraumatic vertebral fractures are also considered the result of injury to frail bones.

From Wilson HD: Osteoporosis. In Ham RJ, Sloane PD, Warshaw GA, et al, editors: *Primary care geriatrics: a case-based approach*, ed 6, Philadelphia, 2014, Elsevier.

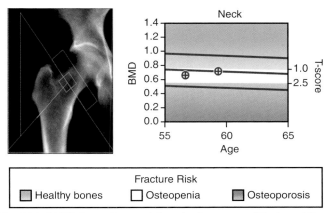

Fig. 26.2 DEXA Scan: Determining the Presence of Reduced Bone Mineral Density *(BMD)*. T-score = −1.4 = osteopenia. (Radiograph from Colledge NR, Walker BR, Ralston SH: *Davidson's principles and practice of medicine*, ed 21, London, 2010, Elsevier.)

is diagnosed if a "T-score" is between −1 and −2.5 standard deviations from the norm, and *osteoporosis*, or a significant amount of loss of bone density, is diagnosed if the T-score is greater than −2.5 standard deviations from the norm (Reuben et al, 2017). The greatest concern related to reduced BMD is a significantly increased risk for potentially life-threatening fractures (Chapter 19).

The U.S. Preventive Services Task Force (USPSTF) recommends that all women at least 65 years old be screened for OP to allow them to take proactive preventive measures and receive treatment as appropriate. It is also recommended that women younger than 65 be screened if they postmenopausal and are at increased risk for OP based on a formal clinical risk tool such as the Fracture Risk Assessment Tool (FRAX). There is insufficient evidence to make a recommendation for or against screening in men (USPSTF, 2018). Medicare covers the cost of an initial screening and repeat scans at 24-month intervals if the person is diagnosed with OP or osteopenia and receiving treatment or otherwise at increased risk. There is no deductible or copay for this service (Medicare, n.d.).

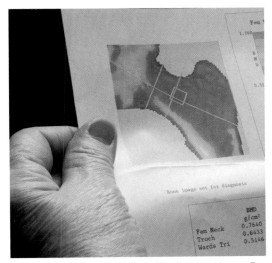

A DEXA Scan of Right "Hip," Specifically the Upper Femur and Acetabulum. (©iStock.com/kgerakis.)

Etiology

OP is the result of a gradual loss of cortical (outer shell) and trabecular bone (inner spongy meshwork) and microarchitectural deterioration. While family history is a predictor, primary OP is a very common and near normal change in aging women, particularly in postmenopausal women who do not take hormone replacement therapy. Secondary OP occurs in up to 30% of women with the diagnosis and 50% of men.

Signs and Symptoms

OP is a silent condition and a person may have neither symptoms nor a diagnosis until a fracture occurs. A subtle sign suggestive of reduced BMD is the loss of height of more than 3 cm (Fig. 26.1). The nurse may be the one to identify the changes to the spine or realize that the person had a fracture or unexplained back pain, a sign of a vertebral fracture, but has not received a medical diagnosis. Without a diagnosis the person does not have access to the full treatments that are available.

Complications

The most serious health consequence of OP is the morbidity and mortality resulting from an OP-related fall. The most common sites for such fractures are hips, vertebra, wrist, and pelvis. Hip fractures lead to a high degree of morbidity and premature mortality (Chapter 19). Many people suffer another fracture, require long-term care, or never walk unassisted again. Wrist fractures can result in severe limitations in self-care. The FRAX noted earlier is a computerized calculator for the determination of the 10-year probability of a fracture using a combination of risk factors and T-score. It is available in many formats including applications for tablets and iPhones (http://www.shef.ac.uk/FRAX/).

Vertebral compression fractures are common in older women. They can occur from anything from a fall to a sneeze. While most are asymptomatic they can also result in intense pain, disability, or even pneumonia. The person may not attribute back pain to a potentially pathological process and instead accept it as a "normal change of aging." Tenderness may be found along the spine at the area of the fracture. Treatment usually includes aggressive pain management to allow early mobilization. If not contraindicated nonsteroidal anti-inflammatory drugs (NSAIDs) may provide the analgesia needed, but due to the intensity of pain, the short-term use of narcotics is usually necessary. Epidural injections, bracing, and physical therapy may be helpful. When pain is still uncontrolled, surgical procedures may be attempted (McCarthy and Davis, 2016).

Arthritis

Arthritis is an umbrella term for over 100 diseases and conditions affecting the joints and surrounding tissues. Fifty-four million (22.7%) adults in the United States are affected; the majority of these are women (CDC, 2017). The prevalence of arthritis and the type and activity limitations vary by race/ethnicity but always increase with age. It affects forty-one million non-Hispanic whites and considerable fewer persons from other racial or ethnic groups (Table 26.1).

TABLE 26.1   Prevalence of Arthritis by Race/Ethnicity.

Race/Ethnicity	Prevalence
Asian/Pacific Islander	11.8%
Hispanic	15.4%
Non-Hispanic black	22.2%
Non-Hispanic white	22.6%
American Indian/Alaskan native	24.4%
Multiracial/other	25.2%

From Centers for Disease Control and Prevention: *Health disparities statistics*, 2017. https://www.cdc.gov/arthritis/data_statistics/disparities. htm. Accessed May 2018.

TABLE 26.2   Prevalence of Activity Limitation Among Adults by Race/Ethnicity.

Race/Ethnicity	Prevalence
Asian/Pacific Islander	37.6%
Non-Hispanic white	40.1%
Hispanic	44.3%
Non-Hispanic black	48.6%
Multiracial/other	50.5%
American Indian/Alaskan native	51.6%

From Centers for Disease Control and Prevention: *Health disparities statistics*, 2017. https://www.cdc.gov/arthritis/data_statistics/disparities. htm. Accessed May 2018.

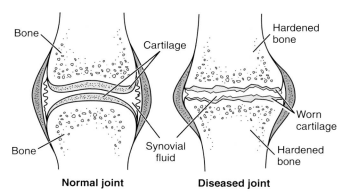

Fig 26.3 Normal Joint and Arthritic (Diseased) Joint.

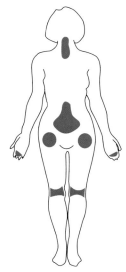

Fig. 26.4 Common Locations for Osteoarthritis.

Many of those with arthritis also have other chronic conditions (comorbidities). Still others are at higher risk for the development of other chronic conditions if they have arthritis. Arthritis is the leading cause of disability for persons in the United States (Table 26.2) (CDC, 2015).

Osteoarthritis

In the United States those with OA and at least 85 years of age are twice as likely to be women and obese. The prevalence of symptomatic knee arthritis increases with each decade with the highest incidence between 55 and 64 years (AF, 2018). A degenerative condition, the normally soft and resilient cartilaginous lining of an affected joint becomes thin and damaged. The joint space narrows, the bones rub together, and the joint itself starts to deteriorate (Fig. 26.3). The joints most commonly affected are the knees, hips, hands, and spine (Fig. 26.4).

OA is the most common cause for arthritis-related hospitalizations (69.9%), many of which are for joint replacements. Those who are non-Hispanic blacks and those with low incomes have lower rates of hip replacements but higher rates of complications and associated mortality. OA is the leading causes of disability among noninstitutionalized adults in the United States and across the globe. Worldwide it is estimated that 9.6% of men and 18% of women have symptomatic OA. More than 30 million adults in the United States have OA, which is the most common form of arthritis (CDC, 2018). In 2015, 23.7 million persons reported an activity limitation of some kind (AF, 2018).

Etiology

The specific causes of OA are unknown; however, it is now believed to be a combination of mechanical forces (e.g., trauma, obesity) and molecular events in the affected joint. Additionally, both modifiable and nonmodifiable factors have been identified (Box 26.3). Classified as idiopathic or secondary, OA

BOX 26.3   Risk Factors for Osteoarthritis

Modifiable
- Obesity (especially for osteoarthritis of the knee and hips)
- Joint injury
- Knee pain
- Occupation requiring excessive or repeated mechanical stress
- Muscle weakness

Nonmodifiable
- Sex (female)
- Age (beginning about age 50 and increases until about 75)
- Race (Asian American/Pacific Islander with lowest risk)
- Familial predisposition

From Centers for Disease Control and Prevention: *Osteoarthritis*, 2018. http://www.cdc.gov/arthritis/basics/osteoarthritis.htm.

is most frequently diagnosed empirically, that is, based on signs and symptoms.

Signs and Symptoms

In classic OA, there is stiffness with inactivity, and pain with activity that is relieved by rest. The stiffness is greatest after extended periods of immobility such as sleep, but usually resolves within 20 to 30 minutes after movement begins. As the joint breakdown advances, so does the pain and duration of stiffness. The stiffness is characterized as difficulty initiating joint movement, immobility, and loss of range of motion (ROM), all quite significant to the older adult and the maintenance of independence. On exam, subluxation, joint instability, swelling, and crepitus are common; all indicators of synovial deterioration. Joint narrowing is evident through x-rays.

As the disease advances, spinal stenosis may develop in the lumbar region and osteophytes in the joints of the fingers. Those in the distal joints are Heberden's nodes and those in the proximal joints are Bouchard's nodes. If present, they appear as deformities in the flexion of these joints. Heberden's nodes are thought to have a hereditary component (Fig. 26.5).

Complications

The complications of OA are all related to the effect of the degenerative changes on function and quality of life, specifically living with pain or the effects of treatment. Fortunately, for advanced disease of the knees and hips, replacements are available and, in many cases, very successful. Persons with advanced OA of the spine often require the support of pain centers (Chapter 27). A serious potential complication with the diagnosis of OA, or presumed diagnosis, is determining if the signs and symptoms are not atypical manifestations of other common late life conditions, for example, the attribution of shoulder pain to OA rather than to an acute myocardial infarction. In 2014 more than one in four persons with arthritis had severe pain (Barbour, 2016). Anxiety is near twice as common as depression among people with arthritis (AF, 2018).

Rheumatoid Arthritis

RA is a systemic inflammatory autoimmune disorder affecting primarily the joints, where it causes pain, swelling, stiffness, and loss of function. Inflammation of the synovium (joint lining) causes destruction of the surrounding cartilage and bone.

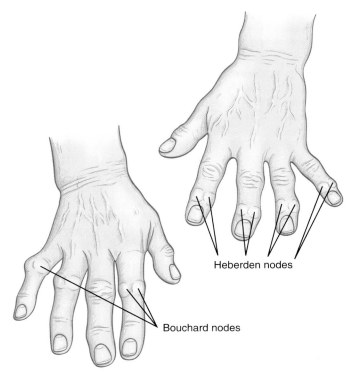

Fig. 26.5 Nodes and Arthritis. (From McCance KL, Huether SE: *Pathophysiology: the biologic basis for disease in adults and children,* ed 7, St Louis, 2014, Elsevier.)

Although the onset of OA is always insidious, the onset of RA may be acute, especially in older adults compared with younger persons (Table 26.3). A diagnosis is made through consideration of the number and types of joints involved (must include one small joint), select serological studies, and the presence of symptoms for at least 6 weeks. However, laboratory findings are less specific in persons with multiple chronic diseases (e.g., most older adults) because there may be multiple other reasons for the same serological abnormalities (Box 26.4). Rapid diagnosis is necessary so treatment can begin as early as possible and therefore provide the greatest chance the joints can be preserved as long as possible.

RA affects about 1.3 million Americans (Genetics Home Reference, 2018). Worldwide the prevalence is about 1%; 1 of 12 women and 1 of 20 men will develop RA in their lifetime (AF, 2018).

	Osteoarthritis	Rheumatoid Arthritis	Gout
Onset	Insidious	More acute in older adults than in younger adults	Sudden/acute
Classic symptoms	Stiffness of joint resolved in <20 minutes after rest	Stiffening lasting more than 20–30 minutes after rest	Acute pain
Classic signs	Affects distal interphalangeal joints, knees, hips, and vertebrae	Affects proximal joints, may be systemic	Inflammation, especially at the base of the great toe
Key management	Initial treatment may be nonpharmacological such as heat and exercise; later acetaminophen and nonsteroidal antiinflammatory drugs (NSAIDs)	Use of disease-modifying antirheumatic drugs (DMARDs) as soon as diagnosis is made	NSAIDs

TABLE 26.3 Comparison of Osteoarthritis, Rheumatoid Arthritis, and Gout.

BOX 26.5 Risk Factors for Rheumatoid Arthritis

- **Age.** Increases with age. The onset of rheumatoid arthritis (RA) is highest among adults in their 60s.
- **Sex.** RA two to three times more common in women.
- **Genetics/inherited traits.** The class II genotypes genes HLA can worsen the illness and the risk of RA may be highest when people with these genes are exposed to environmental factors like smoking or when a person is obese.
- **Smoking.**
- **No live births.**
- **Early life exposures.** Children of lower income parents and those whose mothers smoked have double the risk of developing RA as adults.
- **Obesity.** The more overweight a person is, the higher his or her risk of developing RA.

BOX 26.6 Signs and Symptoms of Rheumatoid Arthritis

- Tender, warm, swollen joints
- Symmetrical pattern of affected joints
- Joint inflammation *often* affecting the wrist and finger joints closest to the hand
- Joint inflammation *sometimes* affecting other joints, including the neck, shoulders, elbows, hips, knees, ankles, and feet
- Fatigue, occasional fevers, loss of energy
- Pain and stiffness lasting for more than 30 minutes in the morning or after a long rest
- Symptoms that last for many years
- Variability of symptoms among people with the disease

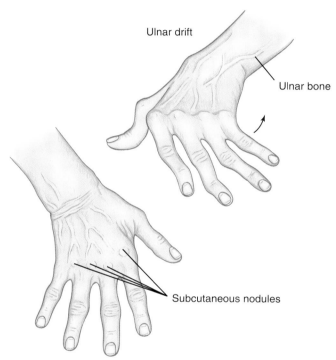

Fig. 26.6 Rheumatoid Arthritis Deformities. (From McCance KL, Huether SE: *Pathophysiology: the biologic basis for disease in adults and children,* ed 7, St Louis, 2014, Elsevier.)

Etiology

A number of risk factors have been associated with the development of RA in older adults (Box 26.5). The exact etiology is unknown but is now believed to be the result of interaction between environmental exposures, genetic factors (HLA-DRB1), and age-related increased autoimmunity (CDC, 2018b; Genetics Home Reference, 2018) (Chapter 3). These and additional studies are under way.

Signs and Symptoms

There are three types of RA: monocyclic, polycyclic, and progressive. In monocyclic RA, the person has one episode lasting 3 to 5 years with no further episodes. In polycyclic RA, the intensity of symptoms varies over time. In progressive RA, symptoms continue to increase in severity and are present at all times. More importantly, RA is now classified as "high risk for" and "definite RA" so that treatment can begin as soon as possible (Aletaha et al, 2010).

Because RA is a systemic disease it affects joints and the body as a whole (CDC, 2018b) (Box 26.6). It can be initially confused with OA or concurrent geriatric syndromes. However, RA is characterized by symmetrical polyarticular limitations affecting five or more joints. The joints are erythematous, painful, and swollen; morning stiffness lasts longer than 30 minutes, compared with the few minutes seen in OA.

RA usually affects the small joints of the wrist, ankle, and hand, although it can also affect the large joints such as the knee. Older adults who have had RA for many years may present with multiple deformities (Fig. 26.6), especially of the hands and feet, and may have to undergo palliative joint replacement or repair surgeries.

Complications

As with OA, the complications of RA include consequences of orthopedic deformities and pain. For those with RA there is also a greater risk of heart disease and obesity (CDC, 2018b). Many are ultimately unable to work. Persons with RA also have a 60% to 70% higher mortality rate overall than those without RA. The majority of deaths are from cardiovascular disease (AF, 2018). The most common orthopedic deformity in RA is the boutonnière deformity or hyperextension of the distal interphalangeal (DIP) joint with flexion of the proximal interphalangeal (PIP) joint, followed by a "swan neck" deformity or flexion of the DIP and extension of the PIP, and a vagus deformity of the knee and volar subluxation of the metatarsophalangeal (MTP) joints.

Gout

Unlike RA, gout is not an autoimmune condition. Instead it is a metabolic disorder and it is related to food, medications, and how each is metabolized in any one person. Gout is characterized by potential deposition of uric acid crystals in the tissues and fluids in the body. It may either be a one-time, very painful acute attack or become chronic, with intermittent, unpredictable flares. Repeated episodes lead to gouty arthritis.

Gout is the most common inflammatory arthritis in the United States affecting about 8.3 million adults (AF, 2018). Men and obese persons suffer from gout most often. Black men in the United States have gout about two times more often than white men (AF, 2018). The risk for gout increases with time, until about 70 years of age when the risk lowers again. (AF, 2018).

Etiology

Gout is a cytokine-mediated inflammatory response to the accumulation of uric acid in the blood and other body fluids, such as the synovial fluid of joints. Gout is the clinical manifestation of either overproduction of uric acid or inadequate excretion. Underexcretion is thought to account for about 80% to 90% of the cases of hyperuricemia (CDC, 2016). Other known factors to influence an acute attack are excessive alcohol consumption, lead toxicity, and a high purine diet (Box 26.7) (Crowther-Radulewicz and McCance, 2014).

BOX 26.7 The Development of Gout

Risk Factors for Gout
Family history of gout
Personal history of an organ transplant
Adult male
Overweight
Drinks alcohol
*Eats foods high in purines*a
Has been exposed to lead

Health Problems That Increase the Risk of Elevated Uric Acid
Renal insufficiency
Hypertension
Hypothyroidism
Kelley-Seegmiller or Lesch-Nyhan Syndromes (rare conditions)

Medications That Increase the Risk of Gout
Diuretics
Salicylates, such as aspirin
Niacin
Cyclosporin
Levodopa

aSee Box 26.10.
From National Institute of Arthritis and Musculoskeletal and Skin Diseases: *Gout*, 2016. https://www.niams.nih.gov/health-topics/gout#tab-risk. Accessed May 2018.

Signs and Symptoms

Gout typically starts with an acute attack. The person complains of exquisite or intense pain in the affected joint or joints, often starting in the middle of the night, awakening one from sleep. They may complain that "even the sheet hurts." The joint is bright red, hot, and too painful to touch. The joint of the great toe is the most typical site; however, it also may occur in the ankle, knee, wrist, or elbow. Fever, malaise, and chills may be present. A laboratory test finding of elevated uric acid is likely, but it also may be within normal limits. The pain of gout may be very responsive to oral anti-inflammatories such as NSAIDs and short courses of steroids or colchicine (CDC, 2018c). Unfortunately, persons who also take anticoagulants cannot take NSAIDs and those with high blood pressure should not. The best approach is to adopt lifestyle changes which decrease risk of reoccurrences.

Complications

An acute attack will resolve in 3 to 10 days even without treatment, however, with prolonged elevations of uric acid, it crystallizes, forming insoluble precipitates that gather in subcutaneous tissue. They are small, white tophi that may be quite painful. If they collect in the kidneys, they can form urate renal stones and cause renal failure. While some have a single episode, 78% have a recurrent flare within 2 years. Gout is associated with an increased risk for death, especially due to cardiovascular disease and kidney disease (AF, 2018).

Osteoporosis

Nurses have an impact on OP in its prevention, treatment to limit the advancement, and the prevention of related complications, specifically bone fractures and pain. Preventive strategies include the promotion of healthy diets and appropriate supplementation, encouragement of physical activity, and protection from injury. The nurse's role includes education about these strategies and the correct use of the medications used for treatment.

Nutrition

While an overall nutritious diet promotes healthy aging, an adequate intake of calcium and vitamin D is especially important in the prevention and treatment of OP.

Calcium. A lifetime of adequate intake of calcium is necessary to achieve and maintain optimal bone health in late life. While one's diet should include calcium-enriched food, supplementation is always recommended. The most common forms of calcium are carbonate and citrate. They are absorbed approximately the same, however, citrate does better on an empty stomach and carbonate with food. Very little calcium is absorbed into the blood stream from the elemental formulation such as "Oyster Shell" and is not recommended. A careful consideration of the timing of when the calcium supplement is taken in relation to other medications and foods is very important (Table 26.4). Many find calcium supplements very constipating and may need to take routine stool softeners. Calcium supplements are necessary even if someone is being treated for OP in some other way.

TABLE 26.4 Examples of Medication-Food-Calcium Interaction.

Product	Interacts With	Solution
H2 Blocker (Zantac, Pepcid, Axid)[a]	Calcium carbonate	Use calcium citrate form
Levothyroxine	Any calcium	At least 1 hour apart
Excess alcohol, protein, salt	Any calcium	Avoid (inhibits calcium absorption)
Caffeine, excess fiber, phosphorus[b]	Any calcium	Avoid (causes excess calcium excretion)
Iron supplements	Calcium supplements or foods (e.g., milk)	At least 2 hours in between
Multivitamin/magnesium	Any calcium supplement or food	At least 30 minutes apart

[a]Not recommended for use in older adults for more than 6 weeks.
[b]Found in processed meats, sodas, preserved foods.

It is important to know that while adequate calcium is necessary to maintain bone health, supplementation has not been found to prevent fractures. The USPSTF currently recommends against supplements under 1000 mg of calcium and 400 IU of vitamin D (see next section) for community dwelling postmenopausal women who do not have OP, previous osteoporotic fracture, or risk factors for falling (USPSTF, 2018).

Vitamin D. To optimize the body's ability to minimize bone loss associated with the development of OP, intake of an adequate amount of vitamin D is necessary. It is essential for calcium uptake into the bones. Sunlight (ultraviolet rays) on the skin stimulates the production of the fat soluble vitamin D. However, older skin is less efficient in producing vitamin D in any circumstances. Supplements are generally recommended for all older women and anyone with a documented deficit. As noted above, the basic dose should exceed 400 IU per day. Adjustments can be made on an individual basis and measurement of 1,25-dihydroxyvitamin D.

Exercise

Regular exercise is recommended at any age, but especially for those at risk for, or with, OP. Weight-bearing activity is that in which bones and muscles work against gravity. This may include walking, jogging, tai chi, stair climbing, dancing, and tennis. There are yoga and Pilates programs that have been designed especially for those who are frailer.

Education

Promoting bone health also includes education about fall prevention (Chapter 19). Risk reduction measures should also be included in all patient or caregiver teaching. Hip protectors can be considered for frail older adults with OP.

Pharmacological Approaches

For those at risk for OP or those with existing OP, pharmacological interventions are often used. While ensuring adequate intake of vitamin D and calcium, the currently available medications include bisphosphonates (e.g., alendronate or Fosamax), selective estrogen reception modifiers (SERMs) (e.g., raloxifene and bazedoxifene, estrogen, parathyroid hormones PTH[1-34], and teriparatide), and the receptor activator of nuclear factor kappa-B ligand (RANKL) inhibitor denosumab. Bisphosphonates are the first line of therapy but are contraindicated in person with renal failure. Each has very specific administration

instructions that must be followed precisely. The nurse needs to be aware of the correct techniques when educating patients or administering the medication at the bedside or clinic. Many of the medications are contraindicated in persons who cannot comply with the procedures needed for safe use. It is no longer the standard of practice to take these indefinitely, and the nurse can work with the patient and provider to determine the appropriate duration of treatment.

⚡ SAFETY ALERT

Oral bisphosphonates must be taken on an empty stomach (when first awake) with a full glass of water, and the person must remain in an upright position for at least 30 minutes and not eat or drink for at least 30 minutes. It must be at least 2 hours before a proton pump inhibitor (PPI) is taken due to the risk for necrosis of the mandible, esophageal erosions, ulceration, or possible rupture, especially when taken incorrectly (Reuben et al, 2017).

PROMOTING HEALTHY AGING: IMPLICATIONS FOR GERONTOLOGICAL NURSING

Gerontological nurses have a direct impact on promoting musculoskeletal health in a number of ways. They are active at all levels of health promotion and disease prevention (*Healthy People 2020* box).

♥ HEALTHY PEOPLE 2020
Goals for Musculoskeletal Wellness

- Reduce the mean level of joint pain among adults with doctor-diagnosed arthritis.
- Reduce the number of adults with diagnosed arthritis who find it "very difficult" to perform joint-related activities.
- Reduce the number of adults with diagnosed arthritis who have difficulty in performing two or more personal care activities, thereby preserving independence.
- Increase the proportion of adults with diagnosed arthritis who receive health care provider counseling.
- Reduce hip fractures among older adults.

Data from U.S. Department of Health and Human Services: *Healthy People 2020,* Office of Disease Prevention and Health Promotion, 2018. http://www.healthypeople.gov/2020.

BOX 26.8 Goals of Nursing Care for the Person With Arthritis

Minimize or prevent pain
Balance rest and activity of joint
Maintain self-esteem
Minimize swelling and inflammation
Maintain function of affected joints

Osteoarthritis and Rheumatoid Arthritis

In caring for those with any form of arthritis, the goals are to minimize disability by preventing further damage and ensuring adequate pain relief (Chapter 27) (Box 26.8). To minimize disability, all affected joints must be used and strengthened, but protected. In the case of RA, protection includes the prompt initiation of appropriate joint-saving medications such as the disease-modifying antirheumatic drugs (DMARDs). Adequate pain relief will allow the person to function at as high a level as possible for as long as possible.

Nonpharmacological Approaches

Nonpharmacological approaches are very important for persons with arthritis. This includes the use of heat and cold, joint support and protection, exercise, and diet. The use of heat and cold is well known for management of arthritic pain. Heat will provide temporary relief in OA, but ice will reduce inflammation. Devices and techniques are available that relieve some of the pressure to the joints and in doing so may decrease pain and improve balance. For example, canes and walkers relieve hip stress. A shoe lift can improve lumbar pain. A brace is useful for knees, especially if there is lateral instability (the knee "gives out"). If the person is no longer able to ambulate, he or she may qualify for mobility assistive devices, including electric wheelchairs and other personal mobility devices (PMDs) (CMS, 2018). Paraffin baths for the hands have been found to be very soothing. These can be purchased or part of the physical therapist's plan of care. When hands are affected, the persons should avoid carrying packages by the fingers, using a cart instead, and use adaptive devices on utensils and household equipment to make a larger grip surface. A variety of adaptive equipment is available to make daily activities less problematic, less traumatic to the joints, and enhance independence.

Exercise is essential for the maintenance of joint function and therefore independence. A skilled physical therapist or rehabilitation nurse specialist can provide an individualized exercise plan to maximize strengths. When performed regularly they will improve flexibility and increase muscle strength, which in turn will better support the affected joints, reduce pain, improve function, and reduce falls. Water exercise is recommended as a gentle way to exercise joints and muscles.

If pain is not adequately controlled (Chapter 27), the person will decrease activity, become deconditioned rapidly, and gain weight. The weight puts more stress on the joints, leading to more pain, less activity, and more debility. A dietitian and nurse work with the person to identify weight and caloric goals and develop meal plans that are culturally acceptable but still balanced and healthy.

The simplest approaches may make big differences in helping persons remain independent. This may include easy-to-use zipper pulls, extension devices to pick up things from a distance (e.g., the floor), or devices to slide on shoes from a sitting position. Velcro closures on clothing are useful for those whose hands are no longer fully functional. Book holders, chairs to sit on while preparing foods, larger light switch changes, and secure stair railings, or even moving heavier objects or those used frequently to lower cabinet shelves, may all be very effective measures.

Surgery

Surgical replacement of the joint (arthroplasty) or joint support through kyphoplasty may be highly successful in reducing intractable pain and restoring all or at least some joint function. Surgical replacements are often recommended for even the very old with a reasonable life expectancy when comorbid conditions are well controlled.

Pharmacological Approaches

If the arthritis pain is mild to moderate, a 3-day course of Tylenol may be effective with minimal side effects. For moderate to severe pain an NSAID may be effective but they may present considerable risk and are contradicted in some cases such as those with hypertension or taking anticoagulants. For intractable joints pain, injections with either steroids or intraarticular hyaluronans (knees only) may be attempted. A number of other products are available (e.g., topicals, Cymbalta, tramadol) as well as nutraceuticals, especially chondroitin. In some cases opioids are necessary to enable the person to fully function with the least amount of pain possible (Reuben et al, 2018).

A third group of medications that are specific for the treatment of RA are the DMARDs. The DMARDs take several weeks to months to provide relief, but they are used specifically to stop the progression of the disease and resultant cartilage damage and bone loss. The DMARD methotrexate is considered first-line treatment, although a number of others are now available (e.g., tumor necrosis factor [TNF]-α inhibitors). All DMARDs are potentially toxic, and the nurse must work closely with the patient and family to be aware of early danger signs (Box 26.9).

For many years, it was thought that people with RA should rest their joints to protect them from damage; however, both rest and exercise are necessary. Therapeutic exercise programs are designed to help maintain or improve the ability to perform

BOX 26.9 Potential Side Effects of Methotrexate Therapy

Hepatic cirrhosis	Mild alopecia and hair thinning
Interstitial pneumonitis	Headache
Severe myelosuppression (rare)	Fatigue
Stomatitis and oral ulcers	Nauseas or diarrhea

From Bingham C, Ruffing V: *Rheumatoid arthritis treatment*, 2013. http://www.hopkinsarthritis.org/arthritis-info/rheumatoid-arthritis/ra-treatment.

ADLs. Even a warm, inflamed joint can be given ROM exercises to maintain movement in the joint. A physical or occupational therapist should be consulted for developing a program of rest and exercise. Splints and assistive devices, such as those discussed earlier, will enhance self-care ability and consequently self-esteem.

Gout

The first goal of treatment during an acute attack of gout is to stop it as promptly as possible and thereby achieve pain relief. This may include NSAIDs, colchicine, and sometimes an injection of long-acting steroids into the joint. If not contraindicated, the nurse ensures that the person drinks an adequate amount of fluids (about 2 L/day) to help flush the uric acid through the kidneys. During drug therapy, the person should not take salicylates, such as aspirin, which may inhibit the effectiveness of other medications being taken.

After the acute attack, the goal is to prevent another attack, systemic spread of the disease, and the development of chronic gout. This may be done by avoiding drugs or foods that are high in purines (Box 26.10) and alcohol, both of which increase uric acid levels, and by taking medications to either decrease uric acid production, such as xanthine oxidase inhibitors (e.g., allopurinol or febuxostat), or increase its excretion (e.g., probenecid) (Reuben et al, 2017). The nurse's role includes teaching the person how to decrease the likelihood of another attack by employing preventive measures.

BOX 26.10 Foods High in Purine

Meat, poultry, and certain fish (maximum 4–6 oz a day)
Organ meats such as mackerel, brains, testicles (severely limit)
Alcohol (limit or avoid)
Peas
Anchovies
Liver
Foods sweetened with high-fructose corn syrup (limit or avoid)

KEY CONCEPTS

- Although several changes occur in the musculoskeletal system, they are not life-threatening but do affect overall mobility and independence and may affect self-esteem.
- OP is diagnosed through the result of a DEXA scan or the person suffering a fragility fracture.
- The most important reason to be concerned about OP and osteopenia is their association with the risk for fractures and subsequent increased mortality and morbidity.
- The majority of persons with OA will have significant limitations at some point, including the inability to care for themselves.
- A major nursing concern in caring for someone with arthritis is helping the person manage pain and thereby preserve function as long as possible.

- One of the differences between OA and RA is the relationship of time to the development of joint stiffening. In OA, stiffening occurs after a period of disuse and resolves 20 to 30 minutes after activity resumes. In RA, the stiffness lasts at least 30 minutes.
- The differentiation between OA and another common and potentially serious condition is often difficult.
- RA affects the joints but can also affect the body in other ways.
- Gout is the result of the deposition of uric acid crystals in a joint or joints. The onset is most often acute.

NURSING STUDY: DOES MRS. SVÖLD NEED A CALCIUM SUPPLEMENT?

Mrs. Svöld is an 80-year-old woman of Scandinavian descent. She is a very petite woman who moved to a nursing home several years ago. She is dependent on others for her mobility. She is only able to get outside at the rare times her sister visits. As you review her medication list you notice that she is not taking any supplements, including calcium and vitamin D. She does, however, take the bisphosphate Fosamax.

- Is your patient at risk for osteoporosis?
- Since she already takes Fosamax, does she need to take supplements?
- What can you do, if anything, to foster bone growth in Mrs. Svöld, and is it necessary since she lives in a nursing home and is immobile?
- Is Mrs. Svöld at any more risk for osteoporosis than some of your other patients? Why or why not?

CRITICAL THINKING QUESTION AND ACTIVITY

1. Analyze your own diet and activities and determine your relative risk for osteoporosis.

RESEARCH QUESTIONS

1. When should women begin to have DEXA scans done?
2. Under what circumstances are DEXA scans appropriate for men?

3. Review the website for Medicare (www.cms.gov) and determine if there is insurance (Medicare) coverage for activities related to bone health.

REFERENCES

Aletaha D, Neogi T, Silman AJ, et al: Rheumatoid arthritis classification criteria, *Arthritis Rheum* 62(9):2569–2581, 2010.

Arthritis Foundation (AF): *Arthritis by the numbers: book of trusted facts & figures* (v. 2), 2018. https://www.arthritis.org/arthritis-cure/scientific-facts/. Accessed March 2019.

Barbour KE, Boring M, Helmick CG, Murphy LB, Qin J: Prevalence of severe joint pain among adults with doctor diagnoses arthritis—United States, 2002-2014, *MMWR Morb Mortal Wkly Rep* 65:1052-1056, 2016.

Centers for Disease Control and Prevention (CDC): *Osteoarthritis (OA)*, 2018a. https://www.cdc.gov/arthritis/basics/osteoarthritis.htm. Accessed May 2018.

Centers for Disease Control and Prevention (CDC): *Rheumatoid arthritis (RA)*, 2018b. https://www.cdc.gov/arthritis/basics/rheumatoid-arthritis.html. Accessed May 2018.

Centers for Disease Control and Prevention (CDC): *Gout*, 2018c. https://www.cdc.gov/arthritis/basics/gout.html.

Centers for Medicare and Medicaid Services (CMS): *PMD documentation requirements* (nationwide), 2017. http://www.cms.gov/Research-Statistics-Data-and-Systems/Monitoring-Programs/Medicare-FFS-Compliance-Programs/Medical-Review/PMDDocumentationRequirementsNationwide.html. Accessed May 2018.

Crowther-Radulewicz CL: Structure and function of the musculoskeletal system. In McCance KL, Huether SE, editors: *Pathophysiology: the biological basis for disease in adults and children*, ed 7, St Louis, 2014, Elsevier, pp 1510–1539.

Crowther-Radulewicz CL, McCance KL: Alterations of musculoskeletal function. In McCance KL, Huether SE, editors: *Pathophysiology: the biological basis for disease in adults and children*, ed 7, St Louis, 2014 Elsevier, pp 1540–1590.

Genetics Home Reference: *Rheumatoid arthritis*, 2018. https://ghr.nlm.nih.gov/condition/rheumatoid-arthritis#sourcesforpage. Accessed June 2018.

Healthy People: *Arthritis, osteoporosis, and chronic back conditions*, 2018. https://www.healthypeople.gov/2020/topics-objectives/topic/Arthritis-Osteoporosis-and-Chronic-Back-Conditions. Accessed June 2018.

McCarthy J, Davis A: Diagnosis and management of compression fractures, *Am Fam Physician* 94(1):44–50, 2016.

Medicare: *Your Medicare coverage: Bone mass measurement (bone density)*. https://www.medicare.gov/coverage/bone-mass-measurements. Accessed March 2019.

Reuben DB, Herr KA, Pacala JT, Pollock BG, Potter JF, Semia TP: *Geriatrics at your fingertips*, ed 19, New York, NY, 2017, American Geriatric Society.

Roberts S, Colombier P, Sowman A, et al: Ageing in the musculoskeletal system: cellular function and dysfunction throughout life, *Acta Orthop* 87(Suppl 363):15–25, 2016.

Sözen T, Özışık L, Basaran NC: An overview and management of osteoporosis, *Eur J Rheumatol* 4(1):46–56, 2017.

U.S. Prevention Services Task Force (USPSTF): *Osteoporosis to prevent fractures: screening*, 2018. https://www.uspreventiveservicestaskforce.org/Page/Document/UpdateSummaryFinal/osteoporosis-screening1?ds=1&s=osteoporosis. Accessed March 2019.

U.S. Prevention Services Task Force (USPSTF): *Final recommendation statement: vitamin D, calcium, or combined supplementation for the primary prevention of fractures in community-dwelling adults: prevention medication*, 2018. https://www.uspreventiveservicestaskforce.org/Page/Document/RecommendationStatementFinal/vitamin-d-calcium-or-combined-supplementation-for-the-primary-prevention-of-fractures-in-adults-preventive-medication. Accessed June 2018.

World Health Organization (WHO): *Musculoskeletal conditions*, 2018. http://www.who.int/news-room/fact-sheets/detail/musculoskeletal-conditions. Accessed June 2018.

27

Pain and Comfort

Kathleen Jett

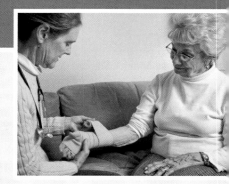

http://evolve.elsevier.com/Touhy/TwdHlthAging

A STUDENT SPEAKS

I know she has pain all of the time, but if I give her too many pills she will get addicted and that would be a bad thing, right?

Ana, age 23

AN OLDER ADULT SPEAKS

It seems to have crept up on me—first one joint, now the other. I wouldn't call it pain really, just an ache that never goes away and keeps me from dancing like I used to.

Gloria, age 78

LEARNING OBJECTIVES

On completion of this chapter, the reader will be able to:

1. Define the concept of pain.
2. Identify factors that affect the pain experience.
3. Identify barriers that interfere with pain assessment and treatment.
4. Describe data to include in a pain assessment.
5. Discuss pharmacological and nonpharmacological pain management therapies.
6. Develop a nursing plan of care for an older adult with pain.

The International Association for the Study of Pain (IASP) defines pain as "an unpleasant sensory and emotional experience associated with actual or potential tissue damage, or described as such" (IASP, 2017). The Society's taxonomy now includes at least 34 different named types, including neuropathic pain (caused by a lesion or disease of the peripheral somatosensory nervous system), often expressed as burning from sources such as postherpetic neuralgia, diabetic neuropathy, and central post-stroke pain (Box 27.1). Nociceptive pain (arising from actual or threatened damage to nonneural tissue) is from somatic sources, such as osteoarthritis (IASP, 2017). All pain is multidimensional with sensory, psychosocial, emotional, personal, and spiritual components. How we respond to it is part of who we are.

Even the words used to describe it are many: an *ache*, a *burn*, a *pester*, or a sense of *despair*—with the language and the willingness to express it a manifestation of the person's cultural heritage and relationship with whom he or she is conversing (Box 27.2). Pain can be a fleeting discomfort or something so pervasive that it wears heavily on one's spirit. Pain is whatever we say it is.

The experience of physical pain is often described as either acute or chronic and persistent. Acute pain is the result of an acute event. The cause is clear (e.g., a fracture or infection), expected, temporary, and usually controllable with adequate analgesic treatment based on the intensity of the pain. It resolves when the underlying cause is resolved. For example, the acute pain of cardiac ischemia is temporarily relieved with nitroglycerin and permanently resolved when oxygen is restored to the myocardium. Acute pain is often associated with autonomic overactivity, such as diaphoresis and tachycardia. Everyone experiences acute physical pain at some point in his or her life. Those at midlife and beyond continue to experience the pain of acute events, but providing comfort becomes more complex due to the frequency of underlying chronic pain and concurrent conditions including those that are psychological in nature such as depression. Acute pain is often superimposed on the persistent pain of preexisting chronic pain.

Chronic pain is pain of some kind that lasts at least 3 to 6 months and is most often associated with progressive disease. It may have periods of exacerbations and remissions. Persistent pain is that which is unremitting and requires constant treatment (Bruckenthal, 2017).

BOX 27.1 Common Conditions That Produce Neuropathic Pain

Stroke
Diabetes
Peripheral vascular disease
Herpes zoster
Degenerative disk disease

BOX 27.2 Possible Effect of Culture on Expressions of Pain

Stoic and non-emotive
  "Grin and bear it" approach—withdrawn, prefers to be alone
  When asked about pain, it is minimized or denied
  Generalized to Northern European and Asian heritage
Emotive
  Wants others around to validate feelings
  Readily cries out in pain
  Generalized to Hispanic, Middle Eastern, Mediterranean

From Carteret M: *Cultural aspects of pain management*, 2010. http://www.dimensionsofculture.com/?s=pain. Accessed July 2018.

BOX 27.4 Barriers to Pain Management in Older Adults

Health Care Professional Barriers
Lack of education regarding pain assessment and management
Concern regarding regulatory scrutiny
Fears of opioid-related side effects/addiction
Belief that pain is a normal part of aging
Belief that cognitively impaired older adults have less pain
Personal beliefs and experiences with pain
Inability to accept self-report without "objective" signs

Patient and Family Barriers
Lack of ability to assess pain in cognitively impaired
Fear of medication side effects
Concerns related to addiction
Belief that pain is a normal part of the aging process
Belief that nothing can be done for pain in "old people"
Fear of being a "bad patient" if complaining/fear of what pain may signal

Health Care System Barriers
Cost
Time
Cultural and political bias concerning opioid use

Modified from Hanks-Bell M, Halvey K, Paice JA: Pain assessment and management in aging. *Online J Issues Nurs* 9:8, 2004.

PAIN IN THE OLDER ADULT

The most common type of pain the gerontological nurse encounters when caring for persons in late life is chronic in nature. It persists most of the time. The perception of pain is altered by many factors, including the person's prior experience and expressions of pain of all types and the person's cultural, cognitive, functional, and psychological status, especially depression and anxiety. Inadequately treated pain of any kind will almost always lead to impaired functional status and in some cases transient cognitive impairment that can become permanent (Bruckenthal, 2017) (Box 27.3).

Pain in older adults is common, more so with the advance of years. More men than women report pain, but the incidence may be anywhere from 12% to 75%, depending on the study, the type of pain, and the confounding variables (Bruckenthal, 2017). The barriers to adequate pain management in older adults are many (Box 27.4), and the impact is significant (Box 27.5).

The gerontological nurse may hear the comment that older adults "feel less pain" than younger adults, especially less than those who are cognitively impaired. The evidence is clear that there are widespread changes that alter the pain experience as we age. However, there is just as much pain but a difference in both pain perception and pain tolerance. With aging there is a decrease in the density of both myelinated and unmyelinated nerve fibers that slightly *delay* the sensation of pain from the periphery. At the same time, there is slower resolution once pain is triggered. Although physical pain may not be felt as quickly, it is less tolerated to some extent (Bruckenthal, 2017).

BOX 27.3 Consequences of Untreated Pain

Falls and other accidents
Functional impairment
Slowed rehabilitation
Mood changes
Increased health care costs
Caregiver strain
Sleep disturbance
Changes in nutritional status
Impaired cognition
Increased dependency and helplessness
Depression, anxiety, fear
Decline in social and recreational activities
Increased health care utilization and costs

From American Geriatrics Society: Pharmacological management of persistent pain in older persons, *J Am Geriatr Soc* 57:1331–1346, 2009.

BOX 27.5 Tips for Best Practice

Potential Impact of Persistent Pain in the Older Adult

Depression
Sleep disturbances
Loss or worsening of physical function and fitness
Loneliness due to loss of social support/withdrawal from social activities
Loss of ability to perform usual role activities
Loss of ability to perform prior leisure activities
Potential for drug/alcohol abuse or misuse

Adapted from Epplin JJ, Higuchi M, Gajendra N, et al: Persistent pain. In Ham RJ, Sloane PD, Warshaw GA, et al, editors: *Primary care geriatrics: a case-based approach*, Philadelphia, 2014, Elsevier, pp 306–314.

In later life, acute pain is often superimposed on chronic pain, and in an effort to treat either, we may add an iatrogenic source of new pain. An example follows:

Ninety-seven-year-old Helen Thomas lives alone, considers herself well, and is almost always bright and cheerful. She has had osteoarthritis for the past 30 years. Her hips ache most of the time and keep her from doing everything she wants to do, but she "does pretty good for an old lady." She takes over-the-counter NSAIDs every day to take away the "sharp" pain. When walking her dog in the snow, she fell and broke a hip. She has considerable postoperative hip pain, but she does not want to "bother the nurses." She becomes less talkative, irritable, and declares that she "just wishes they would give me that pill I take at home." When the nurse conducts a thorough assessment, she finds that Ms. Thomas is slightly confused, is getting very little sleep, and now has a pressure ulcer on her coccyx. She complains that her repaired hip hurts most of the time, as does her "good side" and now her "tail bone." Ms. Thomas has been prescribed Tylenol with codeine as needed but she takes very little of it. She is not given any of the NSAIDs she was taking at home. She is resistive to rehabilitation.

Ms. Thomas had been living with persistent pain when a traumatic event occurred that would ordinarily result in acute pain in anyone. While she was cheerful, there was no reasonable expectation that the persistent pain in the other hip had disappeared. When assessed, she reports ongoing pain but was not being given medications on a regular basis, and therefore both her chronic and acute pain were undertreated or untreated. It is reasonable to believe that the lack of pain management led to her staying in one position for long periods of time, which is now a cause for iatrogenic pain—an immobility-related pressure ulcer. It is most likely that her cognitive status is being compromised by her sleeplessness, undertreated pain, and immobility. Unless there is an interruption in this cycle, Ms. Thomas will likely continue to deteriorate and quickly lose her independence.

Pain in Older Adults With Cognitive Impairments

There is no convincing evidence that peripheral nociceptor responses of pain transmission are impaired in people with dementia, although controversy does exist about central nervous system changes that influence or diminish *interpretation* of pain transmission. Those with dementia may have altered affective responses to pain, probably due to their inability to cognitively process the painful sensation in the context of prior pain experience, attitudes, knowledge, and beliefs (Herr and Decker, 2004, pp. 47–48).

Multiple studies have shown that older adults who are cognitively impaired receive less pain medication, even when they experience the same acutely painful events, such as fractures that would cause pain in others. Many cognitively impaired adults also have persistent nociceptive and neuropathic painful conditions such as arthritis or postherpetic neuralgia. Those with cognitive impairment should be treated for pain whenever a condition exists for which one with cognitive abilities would be treated.

BOX 27.6 Pain Cues in the Person With Communication Difficulties

Changes in Behavior
Restlessness and/or agitation or reduction in movement
Repetitive movements
Physical tension such as clenching teeth or hands
Unusually cautious movements, guarding

Activities of Daily Living
Sudden resistance to help from others
Decreased appetite
Decreased sleep

Vocalizations
Person groans, moans, or cries for unknown reasons
Person increases or decreases usual vocalizations

Physical Changes
Pleading expression
Grimacing
Pallor or flushing
Diaphoresis (sweating)
Increased pulse, respirations, or blood pressure

Providing comfort to those who cannot express themselves requires careful observation of behavior and attention to caregiver reports and knowing when subtle changes have occurred (Box 27.6). In nursing homes and other care settings, certified nursing assistants play an important role.

PROMOTING HEALTHY AGING: IMPLICATIONS FOR GERONTOLOGICAL NURSING

Sudden and acute pain requires a quick assessment and relief, followed by a complex assessment and treatment plan to reach ongoing comfort with and for the older adult. Pain management is that in which both pharmacological and nonpharmacological interventions work in harmony to achieve comfort and maximize function. The basic approach to pain management and control is one suggesting that whatever has worked in the past and been effective without causing harm should be encouraged. This is particularly applicable for older adults with a lifetime of experience at managing pain with both the approaches used in Western medicine and those learned through their personal and cultural heritage.

Assessment

The nurse is often the first one to hear the person's call for comfort of any kind, regardless of the setting, the type of nursing practice, or the means of expression. The assessment provides the information needed to guide the nurse, the older adult, and when present, the caregiver(s) to find a means to address the pain in a culturally acceptable manner. It is of utmost importance that the language and synonyms (e.g., pain, discomfort, ache) used by the nurse are consistent with that of the patient. Specific questions may need to be asked, such as:
- Do you hurt anywhere?
- Do you have pain now?

- Where is your pain?
- Do you have pain every day?
- Does pain keep you from sleeping at night or doing your daily activities?
- What would you be doing if you were not in pain?

Because pain is subjective, only the person experiencing it can describe it or express it and can never be judged by another.

The assessment should be used whenever it is reasonable to presume pain (e.g., after an acute event such as a fracture or at the time of high risk of neuropathic pain such as from an outbreak of shingles, or the pain of acute grief following a loss). In skilled nursing facilities, pain assessments are a required part of the Minimum Data Set (MDS) (Chapter 7) (AAPACN, 2018). All patients in long-term care facilities and nursing homes should be regularly evaluated for their personal experience of pain. It should be repeated at intervals to consistently measure the pain trajectory.

A high-quality comprehensive instrument that incorporates the most important aspects of the assessment is sometimes referred to as a "pain diary." In a pain diary, the person is encouraged to identify (1) location of pain, (2) what was happening/being done at the time of the pain, (3) what medicine was taken, (4) any other treatment/supplement used, (5) intensity of pain, and (6) intensity of pain 1 hour after an intervention designed to relieve it. The assessment includes the person's self-report of both qualitative and quantitative levels of comfort. For the cognitively intact older adult, the assessment begins with identifying the location of the pain. Traditional aspects of the nursing assessment are included in the mnemonic OLD CART: Onset, Location, Duration, Characteristics, Aggravating and Relieving factors, and Treatments used in the past. A comprehensive pain assessment includes the identification of the factors influencing the pain experience, especially depression since it is frequently a comorbid condition. If the cause is something for which there is little control, such as one of the pain syndromes, a "comfort goal" is set (Box 27.7). With this information the nurse can help the patient identify a level of pain that is at least tolerable.

Since it is likely that an older adult has had previous experiences with all types of pain, it is important to discuss these when developing a plan for comfort. The discussion includes what has hurt in the past, what has helped, and how the pain affected function and role (Box 27.8). Awareness of the individual's health and wellness paradigm is especially

---

BOX 27.7　Tips for Best Practice

Setting Pain Goals

Mrs. Smith is a 92-year-old widow who lives alone. Her 74-year-old son lives next door and makes sure she has everything she needs. She has had stomach cancer for the past year. As her tumor enlarged, her pain increased, and eventually around-the-clock morphine was needed for her to continue her usual activities, including baking cakes for the hospice staff! The associated constipation was controlled with a stool softener, but she also had dose-related visual hallucinations. Despite efforts to lower the dose to rid her of these side effects, it was not possible to do so and maintain her pain relief. She finally declared, "I guess I will just have to learn to live with these puppies running around at my feet, better that than hurting. As least I know they are not real!"

BOX 27.8　Tips for Best Practice

Additional Factors to Consider When Assessing Pain

Function: How is the pain affecting the person's ability to participate in usual activities, perform activities of daily living, and perform instrumental activities of daily living?

Alternative expression of pain: Have there been recent changes in cognitive ability or behavior, such as increased pacing, grimacing, or irritability? Is there an increase in the number of complaints? Are they vague and difficult to respond to? Has there been a change in sleep-wake patterns? Is the person resisting certain activities, movements, or positions?

Social support: What are the resources available to the person in pain? What is the person's role in his or her social system, and how is pain affecting this role? How is pain affecting the person's relationship with others?

Pain history: How has the person managed previous experiences with pain? What is the perceived meaning of the past and present pain? What are the cultural factors that affect the person's ability to express pain and receive relief?

---

important in pain assessment (Chapter 4). What does the pain mean? Is the pain believed to be the result of imbalance, a form of punishment, or an infection? A good pain assessment includes a determination of the cause for this pain based on the nurse's knowledge of the person's health status, what has already been attempted to relieve the pain, and what additional strategies are available to provide comfort. Detailed pain assessment and management protocols and videos are available through the University of Iowa at https://geriatricpain.org/pain-management/pain-management-interventions.

Travis and colleagues (2003) use the term iatrogenic disturbance pain (IDP) to describe a type of pain that can be caused by the care provider, such as turning the bedbound patient or even providing personal care to those who are very frail. The authors suggest that, in some circumstances, tasks such as application of a blood pressure cuff, transfers out of bed, bathing, and moving and repositioning patients in the bed may cause an unacceptable level of discomfort. Patients with severe physical limitations (e.g., contractures) and significant cognitive impairment and those persons at the end of life may be particularly likely to experience IDP. In these circumstances, pain diaries are especially important. It is necessary to make special attempts at gentle handling, appropriate lifting devices and techniques, education of staff on proper lifting and moving techniques, and assessment of discomfort during the provision of routine care. Analgesic administration before care or treatments that may cause discomfort may be helpful.

Rating the Intensity of Pain

A key element in the assessment of pain is determining the *intensity of pain as perceived by the person; it is always what the person says it is.* The use of rating scales has become the standard of care. They have been found to be useful for persons who are cognitively intact and in those with mild to moderate cognitive impairment. The same scale must be used each time the pain is reassessed (Box 27.9).

Multiple scales exist, but the most commonly used is for the nurse to ask the person to verbally rank the intensity of pain on a scale of 0 to 10, with 0 being no pain and 10 being the worst pain imaginable. The numbers can also be placed on a drawn and numbered line, a ruler, or a ladder. These are referred to a Numerical Rating Scale (NRS) (Fig. 27.1). The use of an NRS requires that the person has numerical fluency, which can never be assumed.

For those without numerical skills or who express reticence, Verbal Descriptor Scales (VDS) are more appropriate. Descriptors (e.g., sharp, dull, aching) may accompany the placement of the number. The Pain Thermometer is a diagram of a thermometer with word descriptions that show increasing pain intensities that can be read aloud. The Faces Pain Scale Revised (FPS-R) shows a series of faces, with each depicting a different facial expression may also be a useful alternative (Fig. 27.2) (IASP, 2018). Although it was developed for use with children, it has also been found useful for adults; in some situations the FPS-R may be effective with person with cognitive limitations. However, it can also be perceived by the person as an affective scale (e.g., emotional distress as in depression or anxiety) and must be used with caution. A scale of any kind is not useful when working with someone whose culture prohibits both the acknowledgment and expression of pain.

Assessment of Pain in Cognitively Impaired, Nonverbal Older Adults

Scales that are currently available and tested may not be reliable for persons with delirium or more severe impairments (Reuben et al, 2017). The comprehensive pain assessment described previously is only possible when caring for one who is cognitively intact or only minimally impaired so that the conversation can be understood. For all others, an alternate approach is needed (Box 27.10). Instead, nurses, aides, and other caregivers rely on the sometimes subtle and always contradictory cues regarding the person's needs and pain. This has been a system fraught with potential errors as the assessment varies from nurse to nurse and from shift to shift.

A consensus statement on the assessment of pain in older adults is maintained by a group of international pain experts (https://geriatricpain.org/). They recommend that standard assessment instruments specific to those with cognitive impairments be used when the person has advanced dementia. These should always be completed by someone who is not only familiar with the tool but also familiar with the person.

The Pain Assessment in Advanced Dementia Scale (PAINAD Scale) was developed for use with those who either cannot express or cannot reliably express their pain (Warden et al, 2003). It can be administered by all members of the care team. It is a simple, short, focused tool that can be used on a frequent basis; it has demonstrated sensitivity to change with intervention (Table 27.1).

Either the Pain Assessment Checklist for Seniors with Limited Ability to Communicate (PACSLAC) (Fuchs-Lacelle and Hadjistavropoulos, 2004) or the revised PACSLAC-2 is also recommended (Chan et al, 2014). The PACSLAC-2 is a comprehensive behavioral assessment tool that may be very useful as both an initial pain screening and an interval measure.

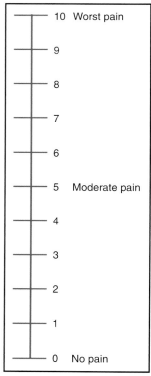

Fig. 27.1 Numerical Rating Scale (NRS). (From Pasero C, McCaffery M: *Pain assessment and pharmacologic management*, St Louis, 2011, Mosby.)

Fig. 27.2 Faces Pain Scale—Revised (FPS-R). Instructions: "The faces show how much pain or discomfort someone is feeling. The face on the left shows no pain. Each face shows more and more pain, and the last face shows the worst pain possible. Point to the face that shows how bad your pain is right NOW." Scoring: Score the chosen face as 0, 2, 4, 6, 8, or 10, counting left to right so 0 = no pain and 10 = worst pain possible. (From Swartz MH: *Textbook of physical diagnosis*, ed 7, St Louis, 2014, Saunders.)

BOX 27.10   Tips for Best Practice

Assessment of Pain in Persons With Impaired Communication Skills and in Noncommunicative Patients

- Attempt to obtain a self-report of pain from the patient; a yes/no response is acceptable.
- If unable to obtain a self-report, document why it cannot be used and report that further observation and investigation are indicated.
- Look for possible causes of pain or discomfort, such as common conditions and procedures that cause pain (e.g., arthritis, surgery, wound care, history of persistent pain, constipation, lifting/moving).
- Medicate before performing any procedure that can cause discomfort.
- Observe and document patient behaviors that may indicate pain or distress or that are unusual from the person's normal patterns and responses. Behavioral observation scales may be used but should be used consistently and with proper training.

- Use surrogate reports (family members, caregivers) of pain and behavior changes, and patient's usual patterns and responses to pain and discomfort. This must be from a person who knows the patient well and should be combined with the other assessment techniques.
- If comfort measures and attention to basic needs (e.g., warmth, hunger, toileting) are not effective, attempt an analgesic trial based on the intensity of the pain and analgesic history. For mild to moderate pain, consider acetaminophen every 6 hours for 24 hours if not contraindicated (maximum 3–4 g). If behaviors improve, continue and add appropriate nonpharmacological interventions. If inappropriate behaviors continue, consider a single low-dose, short-acting opioid and observe effect. May titrate dose upward 25% to 50% if no change in behavior from initial dose. Continue to explore possible causes of behavior; observe for side effects and response.

From Herr K et al: Pain assessment in the nonverbal patient: position statement with clinical practice recommendations, *Pain Manag Nurs* 7:44–52, 2006.

TABLE 27.1   Pain Assessment IN Advanced Dementia—PAINAD.

Items	0	1	2	Score
Breathing independent of vocalization	Normal	Occasional labored breathing Short period of hyperventilation	Noisy labored breathing Long period of hyperventilation Cheyne-Stokes respirations	
Negative vocalization	None	Occasional moan or groan Low level of speech with a negative or disapproving quality	Repeated trouble calling out Loud moaning or groaning Crying	
Facial expression	Smiling or inexpressive	Sad Frightened Frowning	Facial grimacing	
Body language	Relaxed	Tense Distressed pacing Fidgeting	Rigid Fists clenched Knees pulled up Pulling or pushing away Striking out	
Consolability	No need to console	Distracted or reassured by voice or touch	Unable to console, distract, or reassure	
			TOTAL[a]	

[a]Total scores range from 0 to 10 (based on a scale of 0 to 2 for five items), with a higher score indicating more severe pain (0 = no pain to 10 = severe pain).
From Warden V, Hurley AC, Volicer V: Development and psychometric evaluation of the Pain Assessment IN Advanced Dementia (PAINAD) Scale, *J Am Med Dir Assoc* 4:9–15, 2003.

There are six domains of observation: facial expression, verbalizations and vocalizations, body movement, changes in interpersonal interactions, changes in activity patterns or routines, and mental status changes (Chan et al, 2014). The PACSLAC-2 can serve as a guide for care regardless of who is providing it. The observed assessment should occur only when the person is engaged (e.g., walking, eating, transferring). They are complementary to the detailed assessment that is already required for use in skilled nursing facilities (MDS) (Chapter 7). Due to the complexity of assessing pain in a nonverbal adult, the experts recommended that both tools be used to determine the presence or absence of pain. Although the presence of pain may be inferred, the evaluation of the intensity of the pain for these persons is not always possible.

Detailed instructions and downloads of the PACSLAC-2 are available at https://geriatricpain.org/assessment/pain-assessment-cognitively-impaired-older-adults.

Interventions: Providing Comfort

Working with older adults in pain and helping them achieve optimal comfort are especially challenging. Clinical manifestations are complex with multiple potential sources and sites for the pain and confounding variables such as chronic diseases, frailty, and depression. Pain always interferes with health-related quality of life.

Relief of both acute and persistent pain takes commitment and determination of all involved. Nonpharmacological approaches can be time-consuming. Pharmacological approaches are unusually quick and used frequently with high risk. At the same time, the frequency of polypharmacy and the chance of interactions cause some to hesitate, and concerns relating to the use of opioids increase the potential for undertreated or untreated pain. Persons with persistent pain are often afraid of becoming addicted to a pain medication, when they may need pharmacological intervention for the rest of their lives to maintain some level of comfort, function, and independence. Finally, there is often a societal expectation that pain is a natural part of aging or that full relief is not possible, even when quality of life is compromised.

Nonpharmacological Strategies to Promote Comfort

Although pharmacological interventions have been the main-stay of the Western model of pain management, it is now well recognized that nonpharmacological measures alone, or combined with pharmacological approaches, are the most effective and appropriate way to control pain, both persistent and acute pain common in later life. Most approaches have been used for dozens or even thousands of years, with nonpharmacological measures gaining acceptance by both patients and insurers such as Medicare. Several are described here, acknowledging that whole chapters could be devoted to any one approach. The data to support the efficacy of any one approach vary (see www.nih.nccam.gov).

Heat and cold. Many use heat and cold to relieve pain. Cold is ideal for the treatment of acute muscle pain. The purpose is to reduce muscle and nerve irritation. People purchase a product such as Icy Hot, but they more often use something from their freezer. Heat is very comforting to areas affected by arthritis, and a warm cloth or a paraffin bath is ideal as the heat moves into the tissue. Neither should have direct exposure to skin to avoid burns, and cold cannot be used on areas of the body where peripheral vascular disease is present.

Exercise. Both passive and active range of motion and stretching are often used with hot and cold. When pain is from tightened muscles (e.g., a fall), the area of pain can be warmed, stretched, and then cooled. Exercises can be guided by an informed nurse, or when more complex movement and stretching are needed, the person can be referred to a physical therapist.

Transcutaneous electrical nerve stimulation. Transcutaneous electrical nerve stimulation (TENS) and transcutaneous vagal nerve stimulation have been studied for many years. Although there have been promising results in the treatment of acute pain, especially as an adjuvant to pharmacological approaches, there is limited conclusive evidence of its efficacy (Cherian et al, 2015; Vance et al, 2014). Patients often anecdotally report that at least they were doing "something" for their chronic pain. TENS units are now available commercially without a prescription.

Acupuncture and acupressure. Acupuncture uses tiny needles inserted along specific meridians or pathways in the body consistent with the locations used in traditional Chinese medicine. Acupressure is pressure applied with the thumbs or tips of the index finger at the same locations as those used in acupuncture. Acupuncture and acupressure have been used for thousands of years. Evidence supports the benefit of acupuncture for low back pain, neck pain, knee pain/arthritis, and headaches (NCCIH, 2016).

Assistive devices. These are used to "offload" to reduce stress and weight on painful joints.

Energy/touch therapies. Some say the use of touch therapy is a legacy in nursing. Over the years, different kinds of touch have been formalized to include those referred to as the contact

BOX 27.11 Research Notes

In a review of the effectiveness of massage as a form of therapeutic touch, many positive effects have been found. These include reduced pain of rheumatoid arthritis, increased immune response, and reduced depression and anxiety. Resultant changes have been evidenced in the parts of the brain controlling stress and emotional regulation.

therapy of massage (Box 27.11) and noncontact therapies such as healing touch (HT), therapeutic touch (TT), yoga, tai chi, mindfulness meditation, and Reiki. Evidence thus far has been promising but not conclusive (NCCIH, 2017). The acceptability of touch by individual and culture varies considerably. Some physical contact may never be acceptable, such as cross-gender touch in strict Muslim or Orthodox Jewish traditions. The culturally sensitive nurse makes no assumptions and always requests permission before touching a patient.

Relaxation, meditation, and guided imagery. Pain is often accompanied by a strong affective component. Pain is not experienced alone, but with the emotions of anger or frustration or despair (anxiety and depression). We now know that all of these emotional stressors stimulate the sympathetic nervous system, releasing norepinephrine: the strength of the mind-body connection. The norepinephrine in turn increases the sensation of pain. Hence, reducing emotional stressors lessens muscle tension and other physiological manifestations of pain. Distraction, relaxation, and meditation all enable the quieting of the mind and muscles, providing the release of tension and anxiety. Relaxation should be adjunctive to all pharmacological interventions. Meditation, mindfulness meditation, and guided imagery are methods of promoting relaxation. Imagery uses the person's imagination to focus on settings full of happiness and relaxation rather than on the current stressors.

Music. In a review of studies of the effect of music on pain, the results were very slight but differed greatly in part due to the heterogeneity of the studies. All showed a decrease in the intensity of pain and/or opioid requirements for those with pain who listened to music (Vitelli, 2018). Park (2010) found some relief for persons with dementia who listened to their preferred music.

Activity. Activity can be helpful in several ways. It is thought that the less active an individual is, the less tolerable activity becomes. Anyone who becomes inactive may feel more general discomfort than the active person. However, some activities can stimulate pain. Use of analgesics in conjunction with activity may be necessary. The administration of an analgesic medication 20 to 30 minutes before a specific activity may lessen or eliminate discomfort and fear of discomfort during and after the activity and greatly enhance the individual's capacity for that activity. The nurse should learn the patient's body tolerance for activity and work within those parameters.

Cognitive-behavioral therapy and education. Through cognitive-behavioral therapy (CBT), the person learns that self-efficacy and self-care skills are both powerful mediators of pain (Linden et al, 2014). CBT is central to all other approaches to pain management—this means finding ways of best coping with one's circumstances. Through the setting of self-identified

BOX 27.12 Tips for Best Practice

Principles of Pain Management

Every older adult deserves adequate pain management.
The treatment plan must be based on the person's goals.
Follow the basic guide to all pain: *"It is what the person says it is."*
Drug doses may be able to be minimized through the simultaneous use of nondrug therapies.
Prevent/manage side effects promptly.
Perform ongoing evaluation of effectiveness of therapies to know when they need to be adjusted; when goals are no longer reached.
Incorporate all affected members of caregivers, professional and informal, in teaching.
Always use a multimodality, interdisciplinary approach.

Adapted from Ersek M, Polomano RA: Nursing management of pain. In Lewis SL, Dirksen SR, Heitkemper MM, et al, editors: *Medical-surgical nursing: assessment and management of clinical problems*, Philadelphia, 2011, Elsevier, pp 127–152.

goals and treatment contracts with the nurse, the helplessness, hopelessness, and anxiety that often accompany persistent pain can be replaced with determination to expertly manage one's pain, and a small amount of benefit among older adults has been found (Niknejad et al, 2018).

Pharmacological Interventions to Promote Comfort

The pharmacological management of pain in older adults is very difficult. It requires knowledge of both the changes in the pharmacokinetics and pharmacodynamics that accompany aging and the potential food, disease, and medication interactions (Chapter 9). Pharmacological intervention ranges from acetaminophen (Tylenol) to nerve blocks. While treatment regimens vary, all are guided by the same underlying principles (Box 27.12). A balance between potential benefits and harm must always be at the forefront of care.

To achieve the highest level of pain control, it is necessary to ease the "memory of pain," especially for those with persistent pain. This means that it is necessary to prevent the pain, not simply relieve it. The most effective way to do this is to provide around-the-clock (ATC) dosing, at the appropriate dosage; it provides a more stable therapeutic plasma level of the analgesics and eliminates the extremes of overmedication and undermedication. Additional analgesia is prescribed on an as-needed basis (PRN) and should be used freely for pain that "breaks through" the ATC management. Opioid treatment should begin with as-needed doses of short-acting medications and should be titrated based on the amount needed, response obtained, and side effects over at least a 24-hour period and then changed to a long-acting, ATC formulation (e.g., MS Contin). Current recommendations are to start with the lowest anticipated effective dose, monitor the response frequently, and increase the dose slowly to desired effect: "Start low, go slow, but go!"

If a change is needed from one drug to another and the dose of active ingredient is known, then conversion resources are available so that the patient can remain pain free. A conversion table is available at http://clincalc.com/Opioids/.

Nonopioid analgesics. Acetaminophen (APAP, paracetamol) 500 to 1000 mg TID to QID is considered the initial treatment for persistent mild to moderate pain (Bruckenthal, 2017; Reuben et al, 2017). It can only be used with caution in this population, especially when there is any hepatic compromise such as that which comes with alcoholism, malnutrition, and dehydration. It has been found to be effective for the most common causes of pain such as osteoarthritis and back pain. With few side effects or drug interactions, it can be used for ATC dosing if this provides relief. Unfortunately, if used regularly it will increase the risk of bleeding if the person is taking the anticoagulant warfarin. While a maximum of 4 grams (g) in a 24-hour period is appropriate for younger adults, a maximum of only 3 g a day (all sources) should be considered for those who are frail or with renal or hepatic compromise.

A current problem with acetaminophen is that the marketed dosing is 500 mg "extra strength" (interpreted as extra relief) tablets, caplets, gel caps, or topical preparations. Extended-release 650 mg tablets are also available. Many older adults are accustomed to taking two tablets (two 325 mg tablets) every 4 hours. When two 500 mg tablets are taken instead, the maximum dose may be quickly and inadvertently reached.

Nonsteroidal antiinflammatory drugs (NSAIDs) block the pain message from the site to the sensation point in the brain and reduce inflammation. They have been highly useful when persistent pain is of an inflammatory nature (e.g., rheumatoid arthritis) or during a short acute inflammatory event such as following a muscle strain. NSAIDs have a higher side effect profile and drug and disease interactions; unlike acetaminophen, the NSAIDs are particularly dangerous to older adults. They should not be taken by those with hypertension, impaired renal function, or heart failure. NSAIDs cannot be taken concurrently with diuretics, angiotensin-converting enzyme (ACE) inhibitors, or warfarin. The severity of gastrointestinal (GI) toxicity increases with age, especially after 75 years (Bruckenthal, 2017). In some cases, nonacetylated NSAIDs (e.g., trisalicylate) may be alternatives but are associated with more GI toxicity.

The two formulations of NSAIDs most commonly used are ibuprofen (Advil) and naproxen (Aleve, Naprosyn). Many people have ibuprofen available to them at home or it is easily accessible to them. The severity of the GI toxicity increases with age and it is important that the nurse shares this information with each encounter with the person. Naproxen (Naprosyn) appears to be safer than ibuprofen because it has fewer detrimental GI side effects but cannot be used by persons with heart disease.

Two approaches that have been used to address the potentially life-threatening consequences of NSAID use are the introduction of COX-2 inhibitors or the addition of gastroprotective agents to the drug regimen. COX-2 selective inhibitors (e.g., Celebrex) appear to be as effective and have fewer GI side effects. Coadministration of misoprostol or a proton pump inhibitor may be helpful and reasonable, especially for persons at a higher risk for GI bleeding. Celecoxib inhibits cytochrome P450 and enzyme CYP2C9 and in doing so may elevate to plasma concentrations several other drugs, such as beta-blockers (Bruckenthal, 2017).

Finally, pain relieving topical patches, gels, and creams are available. All have fewer systemic side effects but can produce rashes and other skin irritation (Reuben et al, 2017).

Opioid analgesics. For severe pain that has not been relieved with non-opioids, an opioid may be needed. They have more predictable adverse reactions in comparison with the NSAIDs. When moderate to severe acute pain or persistent pain is assessed, a short trial with clear goals is recommended along with careful clinical observation of effect. Sedation, respiratory depression, nausea, constipation, and impaired cognition are common side effects when opioid analgesics are started, or doses increased. All side effects except constipation are likely to resolve with time. Safety measures, such as fall precautions, are needed until the person is stabilized.

> ⚡ **SAFETY ALERT**
>
> Meperidine (Demerol), which is used in younger adults in acute pain, is always contraindicated in the older adult.

If an ATC is being used, the medication used for breakthrough pain should be short acting and comparable to the routine medication so the dose of the latter can be changed appropriately. Unfortunately, too often the titration is not done (i.e., dosages are not adjusted after the original prescription) and pain relief is inadequate, especially in the long-term care setting.

Due to age-related physiological changes, older adults are often more sensitive to opioids, with a resultant higher peak and a longer duration of action. Some side effects may be prevented when the prescribing provider works closely with the patient and the nurse to start with very low doses and then slowly increase the dose of the drug to a point where the best relief can be obtained with the fewest side effects. Because constipation is almost universal when opioids are used, the nurse should ensure that an appropriate bowel regimen is begun at the same time as the opioids. A daily dose of a combination stool softener and mild laxative and an adequate fluid intake are necessary. Prophylactic use of an antiemetic may be helpful for associated nausea until adjustment develops (Bruckenthal, 2017).

Opioids range from the very weak (tramadol, tapentadol, and buprenorphine) to the strongest (morphine and fentanyl patches). Each has its own primary indications, side effects, and precautions.

Older adults without a history of substance abuse are at low risk for abuse when treated for pain. However, opioid misuse is a current public health concern, and nurses at all level of practice can play a part in reducing misuse through the prevention of diversion. This may be helping persons living at home finding ways to keep their medications safe or making sure that the narcotic count at the end of each shift is done consistently and carefully.

Adjuvant pain medications. Adjuvant medications are those intended for another purpose but found to be effective to treat pain, especially neuropathic pain syndromes. They include herbal preparations, antidepressants, and anticonvulsants (e.g., gabapentin) (Wiffen et al, 2017). The early antidepressants such as amitriptyline and doxepin can be effective, but the strong anticholinergic effects prohibit their use with older adults. Most antidepressants (e.g., Prozac) have not been found to be effective, but the selective serotonin epinephrine reuptake inhibitors (SNRIs) (e.g., Cymbalta, Effexor) have been found to be useful, especially in the management of nociceptive pain (Reuben et al, 2017). Finally, cannabis is increasing used, with a growing body of literature to support its effect (Aviram and Samuelly-Leichtag, 2017; Mücke et al, 2018).

Pain Clinics

Pain clinics provide a specialized, often comprehensive and multidisciplinary approach to the management of pain that has not responded to the usual, more standard approaches as described herein. Their use should be encouraged when appropriate. The number and types of pain clinics and programs have increased in response to continued poor pain management in general health care practice. Pain center programs may be inpatient, outpatient, or both. They are generally one of three types: syndrome-oriented, modality-oriented, or comprehensive. Syndrome-oriented centers focus on a specific chronic pain problem, such as headache or arthritis pain. Modality-oriented centers focus on a specific treatment technique, such as relaxation or acupuncture/acupressure. The comprehensive centers tend to be larger and associated with medical centers. These centers include many services and provide a thorough initial assessment (physical, mental, psychosocial) of the person in pain. A comprehensive treatment plan is developed utilizing multiple modalities and a multidisciplinary team of interventionists. The nurse should be familiar with the types of pain management clinics available in their communities to provide the patient and family with necessary information to make a knowledgeable decision in selecting a reputable center.

Evaluation of Effectiveness

The effectiveness of any intervention designed to relieve pain is quantitatively measured with the repeated use of the intensity scale, supplemented by qualitative observations by the nurse. Qualitative indicators of better management or relief include physical changes such as relaxation of muscles that were tense and rigid or a relaxed position rather than one that was constricted. There is an increase in activity and expressions of self-worth. The person is better able to concentrate and focus and has an increased attention span, regardless of cognitive status. The individual is better able to rest, relax, and sleep. It may seem like the person whose pain is finally relieved sleeps for an excessively long period, but this is in response to the exhaustion that the previous pain imposed on the body, mind, and spirit.

The nurse works to advocate for the person so that adjustments of treatment regimens and interventions are based on reassessment findings. Pharmacological treatment must always begin with low doses and increased until relief is obtained. In no other circumstances is it more important than to adequately relieve pain and discomfort than it is in frail older adults who cannot communicate their needs.

KEY CONCEPTS

- The gerontological nurse can advocate for and work with the older adult and significant others to prevent needless suffering and achieve a high level of pain relief and health-related quality of life.
- Multiple modalities are available today to promote comfort, and when used together, in most cases pain can be relieved.
- The experience of pain is multifactorial with physical, psychological, and spiritual components.
- Pain is a subjective experience that is unique to each individual.
- The pain most common in later life is that which is persistent.
- The undertreatment of pain in older adults, especially those in long-term care facilities, is well documented.
- A careful assessment of the presence or absence of pain is possible regardless of the cognitive status of the person.
- If it is reasonable to expect that any person in a particular circumstance would experience pain, it is reasonable to expect that pain is being felt by the person who lacks the ability to express themselves verbally.
- It is never acceptable to fail to treat pain (or the expectation of pain) to the extent possible.
- In many cases, acetaminophen is recommended as the first-line approach for the pharmacological management of mild to moderate pain.
- ATC dosing of the appropriate dose of the appropriate medication will most likely optimize pain relief.
- The use of NSAIDs for pain relief in the older adult must be done with caution, with knowledge of the contraindications and the awareness of the increased risk for associated cardiac events.
- In some cases the use of opioids has been found to be very effective and has the potential to significantly restore function to persons with persistent pain.
- Optimal pain management incorporates both pharmacological and nonpharmacological approaches.

NURSING STUDY: PAIN AND AGING

Ms. P. is a 66-year-old woman with diabetes who, after a stroke, had to relocate to a nursing facility. In a short time, her diabetes began to have uncontrollable fluctuations with blood glucose ranging from 20 to 800 mEq/mL. Some of this was caused by erratic eating habits, almost no exercise, frequent urinary tract infections, and considerable stress related to her condition and her future. She bumped her toe while being assisted into her wheelchair after occupational therapy. In a few days, the bruise had sloughed skin, and an open sore was evident. Despite appropriate treatment, the sore became necrotic and was debrided. Ms. P., who rarely complained, began to moan while she was sleeping and cry a lot during the day. She complained of a continuous burning sensation and said that it felt as if her toe was "on fire." One day she threw her coffee cup across the room complaining that it was not hot enough. Various pain medications were given by mouth on an inconsistent basis, but the relief she experienced was minimal. She began to beg to die. The nurses thought perhaps she was right—after all, her general condition was poor, and life held little satisfaction for her.

- What is the objective and subjective information in the above nursing study?
- Discuss Ms. P.'s situation and her probable prognosis.
- What could be done, on the information you have, to improve Ms. P.'s condition?
- Do you think nurses are concerned about addiction in cases like that of Ms. P.?

CRITICAL THINKING QUESTIONS AND ACTIVITIES

1. Discuss the reasons for sporadic pain medication and inattention to the patient's signals and requests.
2. In what situations do you believe addiction to pain medications is a priority concern?
3. Discuss issues of power and control related to pain management.

RESEARCH QUESTIONS

1. Do pain perceptions generally diminish as one ages?
2. What type of persistent pain do people find most intolerable?
3. How is the pain of arthritis described?
4. What nonpharmacological means of pain control are used most frequently?
5. What nonpharmacological means of pain control are effective, and in what circumstances do they provide pain relief?
6. How effective is patient-controlled analgesia (PCA) when used by older adults?
7. For whom and under what circumstances should the various modalities of pain management be used?
8. How does culture influence pain expression and treatment?
9. What culturally based remedies for pain are used and what is their efficacy?

REFERENCES

American Association of Post-Acute Care Nursing (AAPACN): *Pain interview vs. staff assessment: Are you interviewing everyone possible?* 2018. https://www.aanac.org/Today-in-Long-Term-Care/post/pain-interview-vs-staff-assessment-are-you-interviewing-everyone-possible/2015-01-21.

Aviram J, Samuelly-Leichtag G: Efficacy of cannabis-based medicines for pain management: a systematic review and meta-analysis of randomized controlled trials, *Pain Physician* 20(6):E755–E796, 2017.

Bruckenthal P: Pain in the older adult. In Fillit HM, Rockwood K, Young J, editors: *Brocklehurst's textbook of geriatric medicine and gerontology*, ed 8, Philadelphia, PA, 2017, Elsevier, pp 932–938.

Chan S, Hadjistavropoulos T, Williams J, Lints-Martindale A: Evidence-based development and initial validation of the pain assessment checklist for seniors with limited ability to communicate-II (PACSLAC-II), *Clin J Pain* 30(9):816–824, 2014.

Cherian JJ, Kapadia BH, Bhave A, et al. Use of transcutaneous electrical nerve stimulation device in early osteoarthritis of the knee, *J Knee Surg* 28(4):321–327, 2015.

Epplin JJ, Higuchi M, Gajendra N, et al. Persistent pain. In Ham RJ, Sloane PD, Warshaw GA, et al, editors: *Primary care geriatrics: a case-based approach*, ed 6, Philadelphia, PA, 2014, Elsevier.

Fuchs-Lacelle S, Hadjistavropoulos T: Development and preliminary validation of the pain assessment checklist for seniors with limited ability to communicate (PACSLAC), *Pain Manag Nurs* 51(1):37–49, 2004.

Herr K, Decker S: Assessment of pain in older adults with severe cognitive impairment, *Ann Longterm Care* 12:46–52, 2004.

International Association for the study of pain (IASP): *IASP terminology*, 2017. https://www.iasp-pain.org/terminology?navItemNumber=576.

International Association for the study of pain (IASP): *Faces Pain Scale-Revised home*, 2018. http://www.iasp-pain.org/Education/Content.aspx?ItemNumber=1519.

Linden M, Scherbe S, Cicholas B: Randomized controlled trial on the effectiveness of cognitive behavior group therapy in chronic back pain patients, *J Back Musculoskelet Rehabil* 27(4):563–568, 2014.

Mücke M, Phillips T, Radbruch L, Petzke F, Häuser W: Cannabis-based medicines for chronic neuropathic pain in adults, *Cochrane Database Syst Rev* (3):CD012182, 2018.

National Center for Complementary and Integrative Health (NCCIH): *Relaxation techniques for health*, 2016. https://nccih.nih.gov/health/stress/relaxation.htm.

National Center for Complementary and Integrative Health (NCCIH): *Acupuncture: in depth*, 2017. https://nccih.nih.gov/health/acupuncture/introduction.

Niknejad B, Bolier R, Henderson CR Jr, et al: Association between psychological interventions and chronic pain outcomes in older adults: a systematic review and meta-analysis, *JAMA Intern Med* 178(6):830–839, 2018.

Park H: Effect of music on pain for home-dwelling persons with dementia, *Pain Manag Nurs* 11:141–147, 2010.

Reuben DB, Herr KA, Pacala JT, et al: *Geriatrics at your fingertips*, ed 19, New York, NY, 2017, American Geriatric Society.

Travis SS, Menscer D, Dixon SO, Turner MJ, Thornton M: Assessing and managing iatrogenic disturbance pain for frail, dependent older adults in long-term care situations, *Ann Longterm Care* 11:33, 2003.

Vance CG, Dailey DL, Rakel BA, Sluka KA: Using TENS for pain control: the state of the evidence, *Pain Manag* 4(3):197–209, 2014.

Vitelli R: *Can listening to music help control pain? A new study explores how listening to music can help control pain*, 2018. https://www.psychologytoday.com/us/blog/media-spotlight/201603/can-listening-music-help-control-pain.

Warden V, Hurley AC, Volicer L: Development and psychometric evaluation of the pain assessment in advanced dementia (PAINAD) scale, *J Am Med Dir Assoc* 4:9–15, 2003.

Wiffen PJ, Derry S, Bell RF, et al: Gabapentin for chronic neuropathic pain in adults, *Cochrane Database Syst Rev* (6):CD007938, 2017.

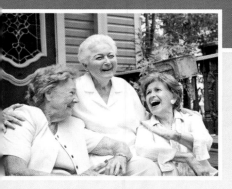

28

Mental Health

Beth M. King, Theris A. Touhy, and Tim Wilson

http://evolve.elsevier.com/Touhy/TwdHlthAging

A STUDENT SPEAKS

I find it a bit depressing to think about getting old. This is such a fun time in my life. But, when you think about it, older adults don't have to worry about school or a job. Some of the older adults I met at the retirement community are busier than I am and don't seem depressed. But, then there are those who are in nursing homes and I am sure they are depressed and lonely. I think it's important to enjoy each day now because you just don't know what life will bring when you're old.

Roseanna, age 23

AN OLDER ADULT SPEAKS

An older adult wrote his philosophy succinctly:
I have no idea about what would constitute happiness for anyone else, considering the differences in taste and preferences, and no spate of ideas about improving the lot of the aged. But I am sure that among other things, a calm acceptance of the facts of life is a great help. I consider serenity and peace of mind two of the greatest gifts I have, although I cannot tell you where they came from or how to get them.

(Burnside, 1975)

LEARNING OBJECTIVES

On completion of this chapter, the reader will be able to:

1. Discuss factors contributing to mental health and wellness in later life.
2. Discuss the effect of common mental health disorders on individuals as they age.
3. List symptoms of anxiety and depression in older adults, and discuss assessment, treatment, and nursing interventions.
4. Recognize older adults who are at risk for suicide, and utilize evidence-based techniques for suicide assessment and interventions.
5. Specify several indications of substance abuse in older adults, and discuss appropriate evidence-based nursing responses.
6. Evaluate interventions aimed at promoting mental health and wellness in older adults.
7. Develop an individualized nursing plan of care for an older adult with depression and bipolar disorder.

Mental health is not different in later life, but the level of challenge may be greater. Developmental transitions, life events, physical illness, cognitive impairment, and situations calling for psychic energy may interfere with mental health in older adults. These factors, though not unique to older adults, often influence coping skills and adaptation. However, anyone who has survived 80 or so years has been exposed to many stressors and crises and has developed tremendous resilience. The majority of older adults face life's challenges with equanimity, good humor, and courage. It is our task to discover the strengths and adaptive mechanisms that will assist them to cope with the challenges.

Well-being in later life can be predicted by cognitive and affective functioning earlier in life. Thus, it is very important to know the older adult's past patterns and life history (Chapter 6). A mentally healthy person is "one who accepts the aging self as an active being, engaging available strengths to compensate for weaknesses in order to create personal meaning, maintain maximum autonomy by mastering the environment, and sustain positive relationships with others" (Qualls, 2001). Defining mental health as an individual ages is complex and there are several factors to consider, "statistical normality, the link between individual functioning and group norms, the extent to which specific disorders can be effectively treated or controlled, and ideas of positive functioning" (Segal et al, 2018, p. 7).

Mental, neurological, and substance (MNS) use disorders are prevalent in all regions of the world and are major contributors to morbidity and premature mortality. Globally, 5% to 7% of older adults experience depression, 3.8% experience anxiety, and approximately 1% have substance use issues (World Health Organization, 2017a). The prevalence of mental health disorders may be even higher than reported statistics because these disorders are both not always reported and not well researched. Predictions are that the number of older adults with mental illness will soon overwhelm the mental health system. The World Health Organization is actively addressing mental health needs globally and supports the United Nations Sustainable Development Goals, specifically goal 3 which promotes mental health and well-being and need for the prevention and treatment of narcotic drug and alcohol abuse (World Health Organization, 2018a).

In both the developed and developing world, mental health care for older adults lags behind that for other age groups and mental disorders have not received adequate attention in global health (Roser and Ritchie, 2018). In response, the World Health Organization created the *Mental Health Action Plan 2013-2020* and the *Mental Health Gap Action Programme and Intervention Guide (mhGAP)* to increase activities and programs and create training manuals for mental, neurological, and substance abuse disorders, particularly in low- and lower-middle income countries (World Health Organization, 2018b) (Box 28.1).

Many individuals in the baby boomer generation have experienced mental health consequences from military conflict, and

BOX 28.1   Resources for Best Practice

- **American Academy of Nursing:** Geropsychiatric Nursing Collaborative
- **American Society of Consultant Pharmacists STAMP Out Prescription Drug Misuse and Abuse Toolkit:** Resource for health professionals to educate older adults and senior services providers about prescription drug misuse and abuse
- **Evidence-Based Practice Guideline: Secondary Prevention of Late-Life Suicide:** https://www.ncbi.nlm.nih.gov/pubmed/30208188.
- **Friendship Line (managed by the Institute on Aging), National Suicide Prevention Lifeline:** Available 24 hours per day, 7 days a week. Friendship Line: 1-800-971-0016; National Suicide Prevention Lifeline: 1-800-273-8255
- **Hartford Institute for Geriatric Nursing:** Geriatric nursing protocol: Depression in Older Adults; Impact of Event Scale-Revised (IES-R); Nursing standard of practice protocol: Substance misuse and alcohol use disorders
- **National Alliance on Mental Illness**
- **National Center for PTSD**
- **National Institute of Mental Health:** Older Adults and Mental Health
- **Online treatment navigator for alcohol use disorder:** Step by step guide for finding professionally led treatment: https://alcoholtreatment.niaaa.nih.gov/
- **Substance Abuse and Mental Health Services Administration:** Promoting Mental Health and Preventing Suicide: A Toolkit for Senior Living Communities (SPARK Kit), screening tools, apps, and research studies; SAFE-T: guide to aid in identification of risk and protective factors, suicide inquiry, risk determination and documentation.
- **World Health Organization:** Mental Health Gap Action and Intervention Guide (mhGAP).

❤ HEALTHY PEOPLE 2020 A

Mental Health and Mental Disorder (Older Adults)

- Reduce the suicide rate.
- Reduce the proportion of persons who experience major depressive episodes.
- Increase the proportion of primary care facilities that provide mental health treatment on-site or by paid referral.
- Increase the proportion of adults with mental disorders who receive treatment.
- Increase the proportion of persons with co-occurring substance abuse and mental disorders who receive treatment for both disorders.
- Increase depression screening by primary care providers.
- Increase the proportion of homeless adults with mental health problems who receive mental health services.

From U.S. Department of Health and Human Services, Office of Disease Prevention and Health Promotion: *Healthy People 2020,* 2014. https://www.healthypeople.gov/.

the 20th century drug culture will also add to the burden of psychiatric illnesses in the future. The baby boomer generation is also more aware of mental health concerns and more comfortable seeking treatment, which will add to the challenges facing the mental health care system. The most prevalent mental health problems in late life are anxiety, severe cognitive impairment, and mood disorders. Alcohol abuse and dependence are also growing concerns among older adults and the incidence of opioid use and misuse is also increasing. Mental health disorders are associated with increased use of health care resources and overall costs of care. *Healthy People 2020* (Office of Disease Prevention and Health Promotion, 2018) includes mental health and mental health disorders as a topic area (Healthy People 2020 A box).

The focus of this chapter is on the differing presentation of mental health disturbances that may occur in older adults and the nursing interventions important in maintaining the mental health and well-being of older adults at the optimum of their capacity. Readers should refer to a comprehensive psychiatric–mental health text for more in-depth discussion of mental health disorders. A discussion of neurocognitive disorders and the behavioral symptoms that may accompany these disorders is found in Chapter 29.

STRESS AND COPING IN LATE LIFE

Stress and Stressors

To understand mental health and mental health disorders in aging, it is important to be aware of stressors and their effect on the functioning of older adults. The experience of stress is an internal state accompanying threats to self. Healthy stress levels motivate one toward growth, whereas stress overload diminishes one's ability to cope effectively. As a person ages, many situations and conditions occur that may create disruptions in daily life and drain one's inner resources or create the need for new and unfamiliar coping strategies resulting in stress overload.

Effects of Stress

There is ongoing research about the connection between emotions and health and illness, but it is known that the mind and body are integrated and cannot be approached as separate entities. Stress may reduce one's coping ability and negatively impact neuroendocrine responses that ultimately impair immune function, and older adults show greater immunological impairments associated with distress or depression. Research on psychoneuroimmunology has explored the relationship between psychological stress and various health conditions such as cardiovascular disease, type 2 diabetes, certain cancers, Alzheimer's disease, frailty, and functional decline. The production of proinflammatory cytokines influencing these and other conditions can be directly stimulated by negative emotions and stressful experiences.

Older adults often experience multiple, simultaneous stressors (Box 28.2). Some older adults are in a chronic state of grief because new losses occur before prior ones are fully resolved; stress then becomes a constant state of being. The ability to tolerate stress varies between individuals and is influenced by current and ongoing stressors, by health, and also by coping ability. For example, if an individual has lost a significant person in the previous year, the grief may be manageable. If he or she has lost a significant person and developed painful, chronic health problems, the consequences may be quite different and can cause stress overload. In the older adult, stress may appear as a cognitive impairment or behavior change that will be alleviated as the stress is reduced to the parameters of the individual's adaptability. Regardless of whether stress is physical or emotional, older adults will require more time to recover or return to prestress levels than younger people.

Any stressors that occur in the lives of older adults may actually be experienced as a crisis if the event occurs abruptly, is unanticipated, or requires skills or resources the individual does not possess. Through a lifetime of coping with stress, some individuals have developed a tremendous stress tolerance, whereas others will be thrown into crisis by changes in their lives with which they feel unable to cope. Important to remember is that there is great individual variability in the definition of a stressor. For some, the loss of a pet canary is a major stressor; others accept the loss of a good friend with grief but without personal disorganization.

Factors Affecting Stress

Researchers concerned with the effects of stress in the lives of older adults have examined many moderating variables and have concluded that cognitive style, coping strategies, social resources (social support, economic resources), personal efficacy, and personality characteristics are all significant to stress management. Social relationships and social support are particularly salient to stress management and coping. Social relationships may reduce stress and boost the immune system by providing resources (information, emotional, or tangible) that promote adaptive behavioral or neuroendocrine responses to acute and chronic stressors. Robins and colleagues (2018) identified the increasing social isolation of community dwelling older adults as a significant factor on the older adult's health and well-being, and weaker social relationships may be associated with higher hospital readmission rates and longer hospital lengths of stay (Valtorta et al, 2018). Some factors that influence one's ability to manage stress are presented in Box 28.3.

Coping

Coping is a complex developmental and multifaceted process that develops over the life span. Some experts suggest that

---

BOX 28.2 Potential Stressors in Late Life

Abrupt internal and external body changes and illnesses
Other-oriented concerns: children, grandchildren, spouse, or partner
Loss of significant people
Functional impairment
Sensory impairments
Memory impairment (or fear of)
Loss of ability to drive (particularly men)
Acute discomfort and pain
Breach in significant relationships
Retirement (lost social roles, income)
Ageist attitudes
Fires, thefts
Injuries, falls
Major unexpected drain on economic resources (house repair, illness)
Abrupt changes in living arrangements to a new location (home, apartment, room, or institution)
Identity theft and fear of scams

BOX 28.3 Factors Influencing Ability to Manage Stress

- Health and fitness
- A sense of control over events
- Awareness of self and others
- Patience and tolerance
- Coping skills
- Resilience
- Hardiness
- Resourcefulness
- Social support
- A strong sense of self

coping may be less effective in older adults because of increased vulnerability to health problems and other stressors. Others postulate that older adults may use more constructive coping strategies in response to stress than younger adults due to life experiences. Coping may also contribute more to the health of older than younger individuals because older adults utilize it to optimize their resources. Further research with older adults is needed, but coping may be a significant component of optimal aging.

Coping Strategies

Coping strategies are the stabilizing factors that help individuals maintain psychosocial balance during stressful periods. Coping strategies involve the identification, coordination, and appropriate use of personal and environmental resources to deal with stressors. Coping is a process that begins with appraisal of the stressor's potential impact and the tools available for dealing with it. The appraisal of the stressor as benign, a threat (potential for harm or loss), or a challenge guides the choice of coping strategies. Individuals use a mixture of coping strategies depending on the situation and their skills and experience. Individuals with more personal (cognition) and environmental resources (social network) use more varied coping strategies, and this may be related to longer life expectancy.

PROMOTING HEALTHY AGING: IMPLICATIONS FOR GERONTOLOGICAL NURSING

Assessment

General issues in the psychosocial assessment of older adults involve distinguishing among normal, idiosyncratic, and diverse characteristics of aging and pathological conditions. Baseline data are often lacking from an individual's earlier years. Using standardized tools and functional assessment is valuable, but the data will be meaningless unless placed in the context of the individual's early life and hopes and expectations for the future. An understanding of past and present history, the person's coping ability, the degree of social support, and the effect of life events are all part of a holistic assessment. Careful listening to the person's life story, an appreciation of the person's strengths, and coming to know each person in his or her own uniqueness are the cornerstones of assessment (Chapter 6).

Assessment of mental health includes examination for cognitive function and conditions of anxiety and adjustment reactions, paranoia, substance use, depression, and suicidal risk. Assessment of mental health must also focus on social intactness and affective responses appropriate to the situation. Attention span, concentration, intelligence, judgment, learning ability, memory, orientation, perception, problem solving, psychomotor ability, and reaction time are assessed in relation to cognitive intactness and must be considered when making a psychological assessment. Assessment includes specific processes that are intact, as well as those that are diminished or compromised. Assessment for specific mental health concerns is discussed throughout this chapter and in Chapter 7. Assessment of cognitive function is discussed in Chapters 7, 23, and 29.

Obtaining assessment data from older adults is best done during short sessions after some rapport has been established. Performing repeated assessments at various times of the day and in different situations will give a more complete psychological profile. It is important to be sensitive to a patient's anxiety, special needs, and disabilities and vigilant in protecting the person's privacy. The interview should be focused so that attention is given to strengths and skills and life challenges.

Interventions

Enhancing functional status and independence, promoting a sense of control, fostering social supports and relationships, and connecting to resources are all important nursing interventions to enhance coping ability. Practices such as meditation, yoga, HeartMath, mindfulness, exercise, and spirituality and religiosity can enhance coping ability. Mind-body therapies that integrate cognitive, sensory, expressive, and physical aspects are most helpful. Reminiscence is useful in understanding the coping style of an older adult, helping the individual to remember how he or she coped successfully, suggesting how these strategies might be applied to the current situation, and enhancing self-esteem and feelings of self-worth (Chapter 6).

FACTORS INFLUENCING MENTAL HEALTH CARE

Attitudes and Beliefs

Older adults with evidence of mental health disorders, regardless of race or ethnicity, are less likely than younger people to receive needed mental health care from mental health specialists. The World Health Organization (2017b) reports that 15% of adults age 60 and older experience a mental disorder, which frequently is not diagnosed or treated. Some of the reasons for this include reluctance on the part of older adults to seek help because of pride of independence, stoic acceptance of difficulty, unawareness of resources, lack of geriatric mental health professionals and services, and lack of adequate insurance coverage for mental health problems. Stigma about having a mental health disorder, particularly for older adults, discourages many from seeking treatment. Ageism also affects identification and treatment of mental health disorders in older adults.

Symptoms of mental health problems may be looked at as a normal consequence of aging or blamed on dementia by both older adults and health care professionals. In older adults, the presence of comorbid medical conditions complicates the recognition and diagnosis of mental health disorders. Also, the myth that older adults do not respond well to treatment is still prevalent.

Other factors—including the lack of knowledge on the part of health care professionals about mental health in late life; inadequate numbers of geropsychiatrists, geropsychologists, and geropsychiatric nurses; and limited availability of psychiatric care, specifically geropsychiatric services—present barriers to appropriate diagnosis and treatment. Increased attention to the preparation of mental health professionals specializing in geriatric care is important to improve mental health care delivery to older adults.

Geropsychiatric Nursing

Geropsychiatric nursing (GPN) is the master's level subspecialty within the adult-psychiatric mental health nursing field. Advanced practice registered nurses (APRNs) must be prepared to care for the growing number of older adults with mental health needs and yet, in a survey of 363 graduate nursing programs, inclusion of GPN continues to remain limited and there were few schools providing GPN programs, tracks, or minors (Stephens et al, 2015). The Geropsychiatric Nursing Initiative (GPNI) is a partnership between the National Hartford Center of Gerontological Nursing Excellence, the American Association of Colleges of Nursing, and the Hartford Institute for Geriatric Nursing (Box 28.1). GPN competency enhancements for entry and advanced practice level education and learning materials to improve the current knowledge and skills of nurses in mental health care for older adults are available (Melillo, 2017). It is essential that both graduate and undergraduate nursing students receive adequate preparation to competently care for the growing numbers of older adults with mental health challenges.

Culture and Mental Health

Mental illness is found in all societies, but the frequencies of different types of mental illness vary, as do the social connotations. The standards that define "normal" behavior for any culture are determined by that culture itself. What may be defined as mental illness in one culture may be viewed as normal behavior in another. Different cultures and communities also exhibit and explain symptoms of mental distress in various ways (Box 28.4). Cultural beliefs also influence who makes health care decisions, help-seeking behavior, preferences for type of treatment, and provider characteristics.

In the United States, disparities in mental health service use by racial and ethnic minority groups are well documented. The report *Racial/Ethnic Differences in Mental Health Service Use Among Adult* (Substance Abuse and Mental Health Services, 2015) offers a review of mental health services' utilization among adults. The findings indicate that persons who identify with two or more races had the highest mental health services utilization (17.1%), followed by whites (16.6%), American Indian or Alaska Native (15.6%), blacks (8.6%), Hispanics (7.3%), and Asians (4.9%). All ethnic/race groups reported that cost of services or lack of health insurance were the main reasons for not seeking mental health care, and the belief that mental health services would not help was the least cited. Furthermore, few racial/ethnic differences were found among all groups related to reasons for not seeking mental health care (p. 1). Differences may result from cultural variation in beliefs about the causes of mental illness and the effects of treatment, past discrimination, and the lack of mental health treatments that are congruent with preferences, values, and beliefs.

Disparities are found in many groups. While not well researched, sexual minority individuals, particularly older gay men, demonstrate higher rates of mental disorders, substance abuse, suicidal ideation, and deliberate self-harm than heterosexual

---

BOX 28.4 Cultural Variations in Expressing Mental Distress

- ***Ataque de nervios (attack of nerves):*** A syndrome among individuals of Latin descent, characterized by symptoms of intense emotional upset, including acute anxiety, anger, grief; screaming and shouting uncontrollably; attacks of crying, trembling, heat in the chest rising into the head; verbal and physical aggression. May include seizure-like or fainting episodes, suicidal gestures. Attacks frequently occur as a result of a stressful event relating to the family (such as death of a relative, conflict with spouse/children, witnessing an accident involving a family member). Symptoms are similar to acute anxiety or panic disorder. Related conditions are "blacking out" in southern United States and "falling out" in West Indies.

- ***Susto (fright):*** A cultural expression for distress and misfortune prevalent among some Latinos in the United States and among people in Mexico, Central America, and South America. Illness is attributed to a frightening event that causes the soul to leave the body and results in unhappiness, sickness, and difficulty functioning in social roles. Symptoms include appetite and sleep disturbances, feelings of sadness, low self-worth, and lack of motivation. Symptoms are similar to posttraumatic stress disorder (PTSD), depression, and anxiety.

- ***Khyâl cap (wind attacks):*** A syndrome found among Cambodians in the United States and Cambodia. Symptoms include dizziness, palpitations, shortness of breath, and cold extremities. Concern that khyâl (a wind-like substance) may rise in the body, along with blood, and cause serious effects such as entering the lungs to cause shortness of breath/asphyxia or entering the brain to cause dizziness, tinnitus, and a fatal syncope. Attacks are frequently brought about by worrisome thoughts. Symptoms include those of panic attacks, generalized anxiety disorder, and PTSD.

---

populations (Hoy-Ellis et al, 2016). Sexual minority stress (gay-related stigma, discrimination or prejudice, concealment of sexual preferences, excessive human immunodeficiency virus [HIV] bereavements) and aging-related stress are thought to contribute to the unique mental health challenges of these individuals (Chapter 33). The effect of minority stress on health disparities in sexual minority individuals, and individuals of different races, ethnicities, and cultures, is an important area of research. Research is also needed on the effect of other stressors such as war, terrorism, displacement, and immigration on mental health.

The newest version of the *Diagnostic and Statistical Manual of Mental Disorders (DSM-5)* (American Psychiatric Association, 2013) has an increased emphasis on culture and mental health, including the range of psychopathology across the globe, not just illnesses common in the United States, Western Europe, and Canada. Another significant change in the *DSM-5* is the developmental approach and examination of disorders across the life span. This is particularly relevant for older individuals because symptoms of mental distress may present differently from the presentation in younger individuals.

Some of the cultural components in the *DSM-5* are presented in Box 28.5. A Cultural Formulation Interview (CFI) (American Psychiatric Association, 2013), including Kleinman's (1980) explanatory model, Leininger's Sunrise Enable Model (Wehbe-Alamah, 2015), and Ray's (2016) Transcultural Caring Dynamics in Nursing and Health Care, guides health care providers in culturally relevant assessment (Box 28.6). An increased understanding of the importance of cultural perspectives for individuals across the life span will facilitate more accurate assessment of mental health disorders, wellness, and illness and lead to less misdiagnosis. Enhancing the cultural proficiency of health care professionals will assist in structuring more culturally appropriate services, thus improving treatment outcomes and decreasing disparities. Box 28.7 presents best practice tips for culture assessment. Research on all aspects of culture and mental health is critical. Chapter 4 discusses culture in more depth.

Availability of Mental Health Care

Dedicated financing for older adult mental health is limited even though about 20% of all Medicare beneficiaries experience some mental disorder each year. Medicare spends five times more on beneficiaries with severe mental illness and substance abuse disorders than on similar beneficiaries without these diagnoses. More than half of dual-eligible persons (those with both Medicare and Medicaid) have mental or cognitive impairments. The 2008 mental health parity legislations ended Medicare's discriminatory practice of imposing a 50% coinsurance requirement for outpatient mental health services. In 2014, coinsurance was reduced to 20%, bringing payments for mental health care in line with those required for all other Medicare Part B services (Center for Medicare Advocacy, 2018).

The Centers for Medicare and Medicaid Services (CMS) health risk assessment and annual wellness visit for Medicare beneficiaries includes screening for depression, questions on alcohol consumption, and detection of cognitive impairment. Medicare also covers a yearly depression screening at no cost to beneficiaries. However, coverage for follow-up care for such problems remains limited (Jeste et al, 2018). Concerns remain about the 190-day lifetime limit for care in inpatient psychiatric facilities and the high out-of-pocket costs of prescription drugs. More comprehensive and integrated mental health care is needed, especially in light of the aging of the baby boomer generation. *Medicare & Your Mental Health Benefits* (Centers for Medicare and Medicaid Services, 2017) will be useful to nurses as they assist older adults to access appropriate mental health services and understand reimbursement issues.

Settings of Care

Older adults receive psychiatric services across a wide range of settings, including acute and long-term inpatient psychiatric units, primary care, and community and institutional settings. The majority of older adults treated for mental health services receive care from primary care providers. Less than 3% receive treatment from mental health professionals (American Psychological Association, 2018). It is critical to integrate mental health and substance abuse with other health services including primary care, specialty care, home health care, and residential community–based care. Primary care providers must routinely screen for mental health problems in older adults and develop working relationships with mental health practitioners in their area to improve access and communication. Successful models include mental health professionals in primary care offices; care managers; community-based, multidisciplinary geriatric mental health treatment teams; and use of advance practice nurses (SAMHSA-HRSA Center for Integrated Health Solutions, 2018).

In acute care settings, nurses will encounter older adults with mental health disorders in emergency departments or in general medical-surgical units. Admissions for medical problems are often exacerbated by depression, anxiety, cognitive impairment, substance abuse, or chronic mental illness and these conditions are often unrecognized by primary care providers. Nurses who can identify mental health problems early and seek consultation and treatment will enhance timely recovery. Advanced practice psychiatric nursing consultation is an important and effective service in acute care settings.

Nursing Homes and Assisted Living Facilities

Nursing homes and, increasingly, residential care/assisted living facilities (RC/ALFs), although not licensed as psychiatric facilities, are providing the majority of care given to older adults with psychiatric conditions. Excluding dementia, individuals with behavioral illness account for close to 50% of all nursing home residents. It is often difficult to find placement for an older adult with a mental health problem in these types of facilities, and few are structured to provide best practice care to individuals with mental illness. Additionally, patients with mental health diagnoses had lower access to high-quality facilities as measured by the overall quality of care and by facility staffing (Temkin-Greener et al, 2018).

The following are some of the obstacles to mental health care in nursing homes and RC/ALFs: (1) shortage of trained personnel; (2) limited availability and access for psychiatric services; (3) lack of staff training related to mental health and mental illness; and (4) inadequate Medicaid and Medicare reimbursement for mental health services. An insufficient number of trained personnel affects the quality of mental health care in nursing homes and often causes great stress for staff.

New models of mental health care and services are needed for nursing homes and RC/ALFs to address the growing needs of older adults in these settings. Psychiatric services in nursing homes, when they are available, are commonly provided by psychiatric consultants who are not full-time staff members and their services are inadequate to meet the needs of residents and staff. Training and education of frontline staff who provide basic care to residents is essential. There is an urgent need for well-designed controlled studies to examine mental health concerns in both nursing homes and RC/ALFs and the effectiveness of mental health services in improving clinical outcomes. Chapter 32 discusses long-term care in more depth.

MENTAL HEALTH DISORDERS

Anxiety Disorders

A general definition of anxiety is unpleasant and unwarranted feelings of apprehension, which may be accompanied by physical symptoms. Anxiety itself is a normal human reaction and part of a fear response; it is rational, within reason. Anxiety becomes problematic when it is prolonged, is exaggerated, and interferes with function.

Prevalence and Characteristics

Epidemiological studies indicate that anxiety disorders are common in the overall population. A large European study of older adults age 65 to 84 found anxiety rates to be 17.2% with agoraphobia being most frequent, followed by panic disorder (PD) and generalized anxiety disorder (GAD); with women having a significantly higher rate of anxiety than men. Interestingly, anxiety rates significantly dropped after the age of 75 (Canuto et al, 2018).

Anxiety disorders are not considered part of the normal aging process, but the changes and challenges that older adults often face may contribute to the development of anxiety symptoms and disorders or reactivate prior anxiety disorders. Increasing frailty, medical illness, losses, pain, lack of social support, traumatic events, medications, poor self-rated health, the presence of another psychiatric illness, and an early-onset anxiety disorder are all risk factors for late-life anxiety disorders.

Late-life anxiety is often comorbid with major depressive disorder, cognitive decline and dementia, and substance abuse. Almost half of older adults diagnosed with major depression also meet the criteria for anxiety. Current evidence suggests that anxiety is even more common than depression in community-dwelling older adults and may precede depressive disorders. There is some evidence to suggest anxiety may be predictive of cognitive decline, but anxiety also develops in response to cognitive decline (Fung et al, 2018). Symptoms of anxiety may occur in 75% of individuals diagnosed with dementia (Clifford et al, 2015). Further investigation is needed on all aspects of anxiety in older adults.

Consequences of Anxiety

Older adults who experience anxiety have more visits to primary care providers with an increased average length of visit. Anxiety symptoms and disorders are associated with many negative consequences including increased hospitalizations, decreased physical activity and functional status, sleep disturbances, increased health service use, substance abuse, decreased life satisfaction, and increased mortality (Brenes et al, 2014).

PROMOTING HEALTHY AGING: IMPLICATIONS FOR GERONTOLOGICAL NURSING

Assessment

Data suggest that approximately 70% of all primary care visits are driven by psychological factors (e.g., panic, generalized anxiety, stress, somatization) (American Psychological Association, 2018). This means that nurses often encounter anxious older adults and can identify anxiety-related symptoms and initiate assessments that will lead to appropriate treatment and management. Whether symptoms represent a diagnosable anxiety disorder is perhaps less important than the fact that the individual will suffer needlessly if assessment and treatment are not addressed. Assessment of anxiety in older adults focuses on physical, social, and environmental factors, past life history, long-standing personality, coping skills, and recent events.

The general and pervasive nature of anxiety may make diagnosis difficult in older adults. In addition, older adults tend to deny the psychological symptoms, attribute anxiety-related symptoms to physical illness, and have coexistent medical

BOX 28.8 Medications That May Cause Anxiety Symptoms

- Anticholinergics
- Digitalis
- Theophylline
- Antihypertensives
- Beta-blockers
- Beta-adrenergic stimulators
- Corticosteroids
- Over-the-counter medications such as appetite suppressants and cough and cold preparations
- Caffeine
- Nicotine
- Withdrawal from alcohol, sedatives, and hypnotics

conditions that mimic symptoms of anxiety. In addition, stigma associated with mental disorders is a factor for older adults. Avoiding previously enjoyed activities and increasing social isolation are major signs of both anxiety and depression. Often, health care providers may attribute these symptoms to "getting older," as a result of age-related stereotypes.

Some of the medical disorders that cause anxiety include cardiac arrhythmias, mitral valve prolapse, delirium, dementia, chronic obstructive pulmonary disease (COPD), heart failure, hyperthyroidism, hypoglycemia, postural hypotension, pulmonary edema, and pulmonary embolism. The presence of cognitive impairment may also make diagnosis complicated. Anxiety is also a common side effect of many drugs (Box 28.8). A review of medications, including over-the-counter (OTC) and herbal or home remedies, is essential with elimination of those that cause anxiety if possible.

It is important to investigate all possible causes of anxiety, such as medical conditions and depression. Diagnostic and laboratory tests may be ordered as indicated to rule out medical problems. Cognitive assessment is included if cognitive impairment is suspected. When comorbid conditions are present, they must be treated. Several assessment/screening tools have been developed specifically for use with older adults: Geriatric Anxiety Inventory (GAI), Adult Manifest Anxiety Scale-Elder (AMAS-E), Geriatric Anxiety Scale (GAS), and Worry Scale (WS) (Balsamo, 2018). If such instruments are used, they should be weighed carefully with other data—complaints, physical exam, history, and collateral interview data.

When assessing anxiety reactions in individuals residing in nursing homes, look for daily disturbances, such as with staff or caregiver changes, room changes, or events over which the individual feels a lack of control or influence. By themselves, these circumstances seldom provoke an anxiety reaction, but they may be "the straw that breaks the camel's back," particularly in frail older adults. Nurses must be alert to the signs of anxiety in frail older adults or those with dementia because symptoms are subtle and the individual may be unable to tell us how they are feeling. Carefully observing behavior and searching for possible reasons for changes in behavior or patterns are important (Chapter 29).

Interventions

Although further research is needed to provide evidence to guide treatment, existing studies suggest that anxiety disorders in older adults can be treated effectively. Treatment choices depend on the symptoms, the specific anxiety diagnosis, comorbid medical conditions, and any current medication regimen. Creighton and colleagues (2018) found that pharmacotherapy was typically the first line of treatment, even though there is growing evidence that nonpharmacological interventions such as cognitive-behavioral therapy (CBT) and alternative medications are the recommended treatments. If the individual has more than one anxiety disorder or suffers from comorbid depression, substance abuse, or medical problems, treatment may be complicated.

Pharmacological Interventions

Pharmacotherapy is a treatment option for many patients with anxiety disorders, either in combination with CBT or as stand-alone treatment. However, research on the effectiveness of medication in treating anxiety in older adults is limited. Age-related changes in pharmacodynamics and issues of polypharmacy make prescribing and monitoring in older adults a complex undertaking. Antidepressants in the form of selective serotonin reuptake inhibitors (SSRIs) are usually the first-line treatment. Within this class of drugs, those with sedating rather than stimulating properties are preferred. Careful monitoring of response and side effects is important.

Second-line treatment may include short-acting benzodiazepines (alprazolam, lorazepam, mirtazapine). Treatment with benzodiazepines should be used for short-term therapy only (less than 3 months) and relief of immediate symptoms, but they must be used carefully in older adults. The American Geriatrics Society Beers' Criteria (2015) includes a strong recommendation to avoid any type of benzodiazepine for the treatment of insomnia or agitation. Use of these medications may be appropriate for only a few select indications, including severe GAD unresponsive to other therapies. However, benzodiazepine use continues to increase with age, growing to nearly one-third of use among those 65 to 80 years. Additionally, only a small proportion of patients who received prescriptions for benzodiazepines were referred to or received psychotherapy or antidepressant therapy. Older adults are not receiving treatments that are both more appropriate and safer (Maust et al, 2016).

Benzodiazepines in older adults can cause cognitive impairment, falls, and other serious side effects. Fall risk is significantly increased with use of benzodiazepines, particularly among older adults with osteoporosis, sensory loss, Parkinson's disease, arthritis, polypharmacy, orthostasis, those who use the restroom frequently at night, and those with a history of falls (Markota et al, 2016). Use of older drugs, such as diazepam or chlordiazepoxide, should be avoided because of their long half-lives and the increased risk of accumulation and toxicity in older people. Nonbenzodiazepine anxiolytic agents (buspirone) may also be used, but are not on an as needed basis (prn). Buspirone has fewer side effects, but it requires a longer period of administration (up to 4 weeks) for effectiveness. See Chapters 9, 17, 29, and 32 for discussions of the use of benzodiazepines in older adults.

Nonpharmacological Interventions

Psychotherapeutic approaches include CBT, exposure therapy mindfulness-based stress reduction (MBSR), and interpersonal therapy. Increasing evidence supports the effectiveness of psychotherapy in treating anxiety in older adults, often in combination with pharmacotherapy. CBT is designed to modify thought patterns, improve skills, and alter the environmental states that contribute to anxiety. CBT may involve relaxation training and cognitive restructuring (replacing anxiety-producing thoughts with more realistic, less catastrophic ones) and education about signs and symptoms of anxiety (Chellingsworth et al, 2016). Telephone-delivered and Internet-based CBT are increasingly available, and preliminary evaluation has shown improved patient outcomes, increased access to care, low cost, and ease of use (Kruse et al, 2017).

MBSR is a new technique that introduces the concept of mindfulness through the practice of techniques such as yoga, mindful breathing, and other forms of meditation (Clifford et al, 2015). Exposure therapy, also used in treatment of posttraumatic stress disorder (PTSD), involves controlled exposure to events/situations that cause anxiety until anxiety lessens and the body and mind are trained to view the situation with less distress.

Complementary and alternative therapies include biofeedback, progressive relaxation, acupuncture, yoga, massage therapy, art therapy, music therapy, dance therapy, meditation, prayer, and spiritual counseling. Music and singing have been found effective in reducing anxiety levels in older adults in a variety of settings and can be a valuable therapeutic nursing intervention (Eells, 2013). A systematic review of relaxation interventions for anxiety and depression with older adults found that yoga, music, and combined relaxation training was most effective for symptoms of anxiety (Klainin-Yobas et al, 2015). The therapeutic relationship between the patient and the health care provider is the foundation for any intervention. Support from family, referral to community resources and support groups, and provision of educational materials are other important interventions. Suggested interventions for anxiety in older adults are presented in Box 28.9.

Posttraumatic Stress Disorder

Although originally considered an anxiety disorder, the *DSM-5* removed PTSD from the classification of anxiety disorders and included it in a new chapter, "Trauma- and Stressor-Related Disorders." In addition to PTSD, this *DSM-5* chapter covers acute stress disorder, adjustment disorders, and reactive attachment disorder. PTSD was once considered a psychological condition of combat veterans who were "shocked" by and unable to face their experience on the battlefield. Individuals with PTSD were labeled as weak, faced rejection from their military peers and society in general, and were removed from combat zones or discharged from the military. Today we know that PTSD is a

BOX 28.9 Tips for Best Practice
Interventions for Anxiety in Older Adults

- Establish a therapeutic relationship and come to know the person.
- Listen attentively to what is said and unsaid; pay attention to nonverbal behavior; use a nonjudgmental approach.
- Support the person's strengths and have faith in his/her ability to cope, drawing on past successes.
- Encourage expression of needs, concerns, and questions.
- Screen for depression.
- Evaluate medications for anxiety side effects; adjust as needed.
- Manage physical conditions.
- Accept the person's defenses; do not confront, argue, or debate.
- Help the person identify precipitants of anxiety and their reactions.
- Teach the person about anxiety, symptoms, and their effects on the body.
- If irrational thoughts are present, offer accurate information while encouraging the expression of the meaning of events contributing to anxiety; reassure of safety and your presence in supporting them.
- Intervene when possible to remove the source of anxiety.
- Encourage positive self-talk, such as "I can do this one step at a time" and "Right now I need to breathe deeply."
- Teach distraction or diversion tactics; progressive relaxation exercises; deep breathing.
- Encourage participation in physical activity, adapted to the person's capabilities.
- Encourage the use of community resources such as friends, family, churches, socialization groups, self-help and support groups, and mental health counseling.

psychobiological mental disorder associated with changes in brain function and structure and can affect survivors of combat experience but also terrorist attacks, natural disasters, mass trauma events, serious accidents, assault or abuse, and even sudden and major emotional losses (National Institute of Mental Health, 2016).

Prevalence

Most of the research on PTSD has been conducted with male veterans of military combat. The lifetime prevalence rate for PTSD for Vietnam veterans is estimated to be 30.9% of men and 26.9% of women; Gulf War veterans: 12.1%, and veterans in Operation Enduring Freedom/Operation Iraqi Freedom: 13.8% (Gradus, 2017). Prevalence rates of PTSD among older adults needs further study, but a recent study by Reynolds and colleagues (2016) reported PTSD rates for older adults (65 and older) to be 2.6%, which is a lower prevalence rates than other age categories.

In addition to military combat, older adults in our care now have also experienced the Great Depression, the Holocaust, Financial Crisis of 2008, and racism—events that also may precipitate PTSD. Although they may have managed to keep symptoms under control, an individual who becomes cognitively impaired may no longer be able to control thoughts, flashbacks, or images. This can be the cause of great distress that may be exhibited by aggressive or hostile behavior. Older adults who are survivors of the Holocaust may experience PTSD symptoms when they are placed in group settings in institutions. Older

BOX 28.10   Clinical Examples of PTSD in Older Adults

Ernie's Story

Ernie may have had PTSD, although it was only speculative after his suicide. On his 18th birthday, Ernie joined the U.S. Army Air Corps (precedent to our present U.S. Air Force) in 1941. He was quickly trained and sent to Burma, China, and India. During his 3-year stint, Ernie survived two airplane crashes, saw several of his companions mutilated in crashes, watched the torture of captured Japanese soldiers, and witnessed the capture of some of his friends. When Ernie returned to the United States, his hair had turned from deep auburn to pure white. He retired from the service after 20 years but was never really able to work after his retirement.

Ernie's life was filled with episodes of alcoholic binges, outbursts of anger, and episodes of abusing others, all seemingly quite out of his control. One friend remained from his service days and visited him periodically until his death in 1996. Other relationships seemed to have been superficial and to have had little meaning for Ernie. On his 78th birthday, which he spent alone, Ernie shot himself. One must wonder how many of the veterans of World War II (WWII), a group at high risk for suicide, are suffering from PTSD.

Jack's Story

An 80-year-old WWII veteran resident with dementia was admitted to a large Veterans Administration (VA) nursing home. Jack's wife told the staff that he had been a high school principal who was very successful in his position. He had recurring frightening dreams throughout his life related to his war experiences and he would always turn off the radio or TV when there were programs about WWII. Now, due to his dementia, he was unable to control his thoughts and feelings. While in the nursing home, he would become very agitated and attempt to hit other residents around him when placed in the large day room. The staff recognized this as a PTSD reaction from his years as a prisoner of war. They always placed him in a smaller day room near the nursing station away from other residents, where he remained calm and pleasant. The aggression stopped without the need for medication.

PTSD, Posttraumatic stress disorder.

women with a history of rape or abuse as a child may also experience symptoms of PTSD when institutionalized, particularly during the provision of intimate bodily care activities, such as bathing. Box 28.10 provides some clinical examples of PTSD.

Symptoms

The *DSM-5* includes four major symptom clusters for diagnosis of PTSD: (1) reexperiencing; (2) avoidance; (3) persistent negative alterations in cognition and mood; and (4) alterations in arousal and receptivity (including irritable or aggressive behavior and reckless or self-destructive behavior) (American Psychiatric Association, 2013). Individuals often reexperience and relive the traumatic event in episodes of fear and experience symptoms such as helplessness, flashbacks, intrusive thoughts, dreams, images, avoidance of thoughts or situations that remind them of the traumatic event, poor concentration, irritability, increased startle reactions, and numbing of emotional responsiveness (detachment, flattened or absent affect). Symptoms may be present within a short time period following the trauma, but a person may have a delayed response from a year to several years.

Consequences

PTSD often co-occurs with physical illness, substance use disorders, depression, and chronic pain. Depression is present in half of individuals with PTSD, making it very important to routinely assess for depression. Co-occurring PTSD and depression is associated with greater symptoms, reduced quality of life, and increased health care utilization than PTSD alone (Rytwinski et al, 2013). In addition, there may be some association between PTSD and a greater incidence and prevalence of dementia, but there is a need for further longitudinal data to fully understand the data (Yoder et al, 2016). More rigorous research is needed in the area of treatment of PTSD, specifically for older adults (Cook and Simiola, 2017).

PROMOTING HEALTHY AGING: IMPLICATIONS FOR GERONTOLOGICAL NURSING

Assessment

PTSD prevention and treatment are only now getting the research attention that other illnesses have received over the years. The care of the individual with PTSD involves awareness that certain events may trigger inappropriate reactions, and the pattern of these reactions should be identified when possible. Knowing the person's history and life experiences is essential in understanding behavior and implementing appropriate interventions. The Hartford Institute for Geriatric Nursing recommends the Impact of Event Scale–Revised (IES-R) (Christianson and Marren, 2013) (Box 28.1).

Assessment of trauma and related symptoms should be routine in older adults because they may not report traumatic experiences or may minimize their importance. Similar to other mental health concerns, older adults may be more likely to report physical concerns, pain, sleep difficulties, or cognitive problems rather than emotional problems. Asking about issues or concerns may prompt a description of emotional reactions. Reports of physical issues should be followed with questions about changes in mood and activities. Cognitive screening for delirium/dementia is important, as is assessment for depression and suicide ideation.

Interventions

Effective coping with traumatic events seems to be associated with secure and supportive relationships; the ability to freely express or fully suppress the experience; favorable circumstances immediately following the trauma; productive and active lifestyles; strong faith, religion, and hope; a sense of humor; biological integrity; and resilience. Research on resiliency may lead to ways to predict who is most likely to develop PTSD following highly stressful events (National Institute of Mental Health, 2016).

The understanding of how to treat PTSD among older adults is still developing. Current treatment recommendations for older adults include CBT and prolonged exposure therapy (PE). A new study, the Warrior Wellness Study (Hall et al, 2018), is examining the effects of exercise with older veterans with PTSD. Other therapies shown to improve PTSD symptoms include cognitive processing therapy, eye movement desensitization and reprocessing, and narrative exposure therapy. Cognitive therapy aims to isolate dysfunctional thoughts and assumptions about the trauma that seem to cause distress. Individuals are encouraged to challenge the truth of the beliefs and to substitute them with more balanced thoughts. Exposure therapy involves recalling distressing memories of the trauma/event via controlled exposure to reminders of the event. Exposure can be done by imagining the trauma, reading descriptions of the event, or visiting the site of the trauma until distress associated with the memory lessens and the body and mind are retrained to view the situation as less dangerous than it was perceived to be.

Evidence-based psychospiritual interventions may also be effective in the treatment of veterans with PTSD and may be more acceptable among those who have a fear of mental illness–related stigma. Individuals able to find meaning and purpose in their traumatic experiences are less likely to develop chronic PTSD. Providers should inquire about the spiritual component of PTSD and help the individual to find meaning in his or her life (Chapter 36). Pharmacological therapy is also used, and sertraline and paroxetine have received approval by the U.S. Food and Drug Administration (FDA) to treat PTSD. Careful monitoring of these medications is necessary in older adults (Chapter 9).

Therapies should be individualized to meet the specific concerns and needs of each unique patient and may include individual, group, and family therapy. Internet-based therapy, self-help therapy, and telephone-assisted therapy are other creative formats to make interventions more widely available, particularly for improving response to mass trauma events. Further research is necessary to understand the various presentations of PTSD in late life and validate and improve the effectiveness of available treatment approaches (Department of Veterans Affairs, 2019). Current practice guidelines for management of PTSD and a treatment protocol for trauma informed care can be found in Box 28.1.

SCHIZOPHRENIA

Prevalence

Older adults are the fastest growing segment of the total population of individuals living with schizophrenia, and the numbers are expected to grow in the coming decades with the increased longevity of the population. The lifetime prevalence for persons living with schizophrenia ranges from 0.3% to 1% with the onset of schizophrenia for men between the ages of 10 to 25 years, for women between the ages of 25 to 35 years, with approximately 3% to 10% diagnosed after the age of 40. Onset of schizophrenia after the age of 45 is identified as late-onset; and after the age of 60 years, the onset of schizophrenia is considered to be rare (American Psychiatric Association, 2013; Sadock et al, 2015).

Symptoms

The main symptoms associated with schizophrenia can be categorized into positive symptoms of delusions, hallucinations,

disorganized speech, disorganized behavior; negative symptoms of flat or blunted affect, anhedonia, avolition; and cognitive symptoms of poor executive functioning, and limited attention span (American Psychiatric Association, 2013). But by age 65, persons living with schizophrenia experience less delusions and hallucinations, with approximately 20% having no active symptoms, while 80% live with some degree of impairment (Sadock et al, 2015). Symptoms of cognitive impairment usually do not improve as the person ages. Mushkin and colleagues (2018) interviewed 20 aging adults living with schizophrenia to develop an understanding of living with schizophrenia and the person's well-being. Interestingly, the findings revealed that the participants viewed old age as "a window of opportunity" and "a chance to live a normal life" (p. 980). Four themes expressed the feeling of well-being: a balanced course of illness in old age, self-fulfillment as promoting well-being, experiencing a sense of belonging, and aging as an opportunity for normalization.

Consequences

Individuals with severe persistent mental illnesses (SPMI) such as schizophrenia form a disenfranchised group whose access to medical care has been limited, leading to greater functional declines, morbidity, and mortality. Persons with schizophrenia have a potential life loss of 14.5 years less than the general population (Hjorthøj et al, 2017). This reduction in years has been attributed to cardiovascular disease related to antipsychotics, poor diet, limited exercise, and smoking (Gates et al, 2015). Continued research is needed specifically to examine the effects of living with schizophrenia as an older adult across the globe.

Schizophrenia is a costly disease both in terms of personal challenges and with regard to medical care costs. The living situations for older adults who have schizophrenia can be challenging, with the majority living in nursing homes, assisted living, boarding houses, or on the streets. Interventions to improve independent functioning, irrespective of age and in conjunction with community services, would decrease the expenses associated with institutionalization. The management of older adults with schizophrenia is expected to become a serious burden for our health care system, requiring the development of integrated models of care across the continuum.

PROMOTING HEALTHY AGING: IMPLICATIONS FOR GERONTOLOGICAL NURSING

Interventions

Treatment for schizophrenia includes both pharmacological and nonpharmacological interventions. First-generation antipsychotics (e.g., haloperidol) have been effective in managing the positive symptoms of schizophrenia but are problematic in older adults and carry a high risk of disabling and persistent side effects, such as tardive dyskinesia (TD). The abnormal involuntary movement scale (AIMS) is useful for evaluating early symptoms of TD (Chapter 9). The second-generation, atypical antipsychotic medications (e.g., risperidone, olanzapine, quetiapine), given in low doses, are associated with a lower risk of extrapyramidal symptoms (EPS) and TD. Another adverse effect of antipsychotics is the potential for weight gain and diabetes. The use of weight-neutral medications is recommended and dietary education, waist circumference, and weight should be routinely included in assessment of individuals with schizophrenia (Hjorthoj et al, 2017). Federal guidelines for the use of antipsychotic medications in nursing homes provide the indications for use of these medications in schizophrenia.

Other important interventions include a combination of support, education, physical activity, and CBT. A positive approach on the part of health care professionals, patients, and their families, combined with interventions to enhance quality of life is important. Families of older adults with schizophrenia experience the burden of caring for a family member with a chronic disability and dealing with their own personal aging. Community-based support services that include assistance with housing, medical care, recreation services, and services that help the family plan for the future of their relative are necessary. There are relatively few services in the community for older adults with schizophrenia. The National Alliance on Mental Illness (NAMI) (Box 28.1) is an important resource for clients and their families.

PSYCHOTIC SYMPTOMS IN OLDER ADULTS

The onset of true psychiatric disorders is low among older adults, but psychotic manifestations may occur as a secondary syndrome in a variety of disorders, the most common being neurocognitive disorders and Parkinson's disease (Chapters 23 and 29).

Paranoid Symptoms

New-onset paranoid symptoms are common among older adults and can present in a number of conditions in late life. Paranoid symptoms can signify an acute change in mental status as a result of a medical illness or delirium, or they can be caused by an underlying affective or primary psychotic mental disorder. Paranoia is also an early symptom of Alzheimer's disease, appearing approximately 20 months before diagnosis. About 30% to 40% of persons with neurocognitive disorders experience paranoid or persecutory delusions (Sadock et al, 2015). Medications, vision and hearing loss, social isolation, alcoholism, depression, the presence of negative life events, financial strain, and PTSD can also be precipitating factors of paranoid symptoms.

Delusions

Delusions are fixed beliefs that guide one's interpretation of events and help make sense out of disorder, even though they are inconsistent with reality. The delusions may be comforting or threatening, but they always form a structure for understanding situations that otherwise might seem unmanageable. A delusional disorder is one in which conceivable ideas, without foundation in fact, persist for more than 1 month.

Common delusions of older adults are of being poisoned, personal objects being stolen, of children taking their assets, of being held prisoner, or of being deceived by a spouse, partner,

---

> **BOX 28.11   Clinical Examples of Delusions**
>
> **Maggie's Story**
> Maggie persistently held on to the delusion that her son was a very important attorney and was coming to force the administration to discharge her from the nursing home. Her son, a factory worker, had been dead for 10 years. The events of her day, her hopes, and her status were all organized around this belief. It is clear that without her delusion she would have felt forlorn, lost, and abandoned.
>
> **Herman's Story**
> Herman was an 88-year-old man in a nursing home who insisted that he must go and visit his mother. His thoughts seemed clear in other respects (often the case with people who are delusional), and one of the authors (P. Ebersole) suspected that he had some unresolved conflicts about his dead mother or felt the need for comforting and caring. P.E. did not argue with him about his dead mother because arguing is never a useful approach to persons with delusions. Rather, she used the best techniques she could think of to assure him that she was interested in him as a person and recognized that he must feel very lonely sometimes. He continued to say that he must go and visit his mother. When P.E. could delay his leaving no longer, she walked with him to the nurses' station and found that his 104-year-old mother did indeed live in another wing of the institution and that he visited her every day.

---

or lover. In older adults, delusions often incorporate significant persons rather than the global grandiose or persecutory delusions. Fear and a lack of trust originating from a basis in reality may become magnified, especially when one is isolated from others and does not receive reality feedback. It is always important to determine if what "appears" to be delusional ideation is, in fact, based in reality. Box 28.11 presents some clinical examples.

Hallucinations

Hallucinations are best described as sensory perceptions that occur in the absence of external stimuli and may be spurred by the internal stimulation of any of the five senses. Although not attributable to environmental stimuli, hallucinations may occur as a combined result of environmental factors. Hallucinations arising from psychotic disorders are less common among older adults, and those that are generated are thought to begin in situations in which one is feeling alone, abandoned, isolated, or alienated. To compensate for insecurity, a hallucinatory experience is stimulated, often an imaginary companion. Imagined companions may fill the immense void and provide some security, but they may also become accusatory and disturbing.

The character and stages of hallucinatory experiences in later life have not been adequately defined. Many hallucinations are in response to physical disorders, such as dementia, Parkinson's disease, sensory disorders, and medications. Older adults with hearing and vision deficits may also hear voices or see people and objects that are not actually present (illusions). Some have explained this as the brain's attempt to create stimulation in the absence of adequate sensory input. If the hallucinations are not disturbing to the person, they do not necessitate treatment (Box 28.11).

PROMOTING HEALTHY AGING: IMPLICATIONS FOR GERONTOLOGICAL NURSING

Assessment

The assessment dilemma is often one of determining if paranoia, delusions, and hallucinations are the result of medical illnesses, medications, dementia, psychoses, sensory deprivation, or overload. Depending on the precipitating factors, treatment will vary. Treatment must be based on a comprehensive assessment and on a determination of the nature of the psychotic behavior (primary or secondary psychosis) and the time of onset of first symptoms (early or late). Treating the underlying cause of a secondary psychosis caused by medical illnesses, dementia, substance abuse, or delirium is a priority.

Assessment of vision and hearing is also important because these impairments may predispose the older adult to paranoia or suspiciousness. Psychotic symptoms and/or paranoid ideation also present with depression, so depression screening should also be conducted. Assessment of suicide potential is also indicated because individuals experiencing paranoid symptoms are at significant risk for harm to self. It is never safe to conclude that someone is delusional or paranoid or experiencing hallucinations unless you have thoroughly investigated his or her claims, evaluated physical and cognitive status, and assessed the environment for contributing factors to the behaviors.

Interventions

Frightening hallucinations or delusions, such as feeling that one is being poisoned, usually arise in response to anxiety-provoking situations and are best managed by reducing situational stress; being available to the person; providing a safe, nonjudgmental environment; and attending to the fears more than the content of the delusion or hallucination. Direct confrontation is likely to increase anxiety and agitation and the sense of vulnerability; it also may disrupt the relationship. A more useful approach is to establish a trusting relationship that is nondemanding and not too intense (Box 28.12).

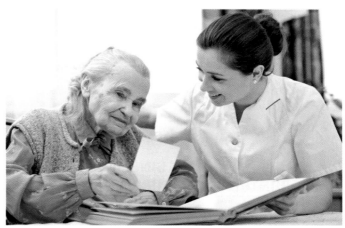

Demonstrating respect and a willingness to listen is the foundation for a caring nurse-patient relationship. (©iStock.com/AlexRaths.)

It is important to identify the individual's strengths and build on them. Demonstrating respect and a willingness to listen to concerns and fears are important. It is important that the nurse be trustworthy, give clear information, and present clear choices. Do not pretend to agree with paranoid beliefs or delusions, but rather ask what is troubling to the person and provide reassurance of safety. It is important to try to understand the person's level of distress, and how he or she is experiencing what is troubling. Other suggestions are to avoid television, which can be confusing, especially if the person awakens and finds it on or has a hearing or vision impairment. In addition, reduce clutter in the person's room and eliminate shadows that can appear threatening. Provide glasses and hearing aids to maximize sensory input and decrease misinterpretations.

If symptoms are interfering with function and interpersonal and environmental strategies are not effective, antipsychotic drugs may be used. The newer atypical antipsychotics (risperidone, olanzapine) are preferred but must be used judiciously, with careful attention to side effects and monitoring of response. None of the antipsychotic medications are approved for use in treatment of behavioral responses in individuals with neurocognitive disorders. Atypical antipsychotic medications include a black box warning related to an increased risk of death when prescribed for older adults with dementia-related psychosis (Centers for Medicare & Medicaid Services Medicaid Program Integrity Education, 2015). See Chapter 29 for further discussion of behavior and psychological symptoms in dementia and nonpharmacological interventions.

BIPOLAR DISORDER

The *DSM-5* defines bipolar disorder (BD) as a recurrent mood disorder that includes periods of mania and/or hypomania and major depression (bipolar I) or major depression and hypomanic episodes (bipolar II) (American Psychiatric Association, 2013). The length of the phases of depression and mania varies, lasting from days to weeks. BD is a lifelong disease that usually begins in adolescence, but 20% of older adults with BD experience their first episode after 50 years of age. With the aging of

---

BOX 28.12   Clinical Example: Is It Hallucinations?

One older woman in a nursing home who had Alzheimer's disease and was experiencing agnosia would look in the mirror and talk to "the nice lady I see in there." "Do you want to eat or go out for a walk with me?" she would ask. It was comforting to her, and therefore she did not need medication for her "hallucination," as some would have labeled her behavior. As is the case with many disease symptoms, frail older adults do not typically manifest the cardinal signs we have been taught to associate with certain physical and mental disorders. Diagnostic criteria, and often evidence-based practice guidelines, have been developed out of observation and research with younger people and may not always fit the older adult. Until knowledge and research on the unique aspects of aging increase, nurses and other health care professionals are urged to individualize their assessment and treatment of older people using available guidelines specific to older people.

the population, predictions are that there will be a drastic increase of older adults with BD in the coming decades. BDs often stabilize in late life, and individuals tend to have longer periods of depression. Mania is a more frequent cause of hospitalization than depression, but depression may account for more disability. Similar to other psychiatric disorders in older adults, comorbidities often mask the presence of the disorder and it is frequently misdiagnosed, underdiagnosed, and undertreated.

PROMOTING HEALTHY AGING: IMPLICATIONS FOR GERONTOLOGICAL NURSING

Assessment

Assessment includes a thorough physical examination and laboratory and radiological testing to exclude physical causes of the symptoms and identify comorbidities. A medication review should be conducted because symptoms can be a side effect of medications. Obtaining an accurate history from the individual, and the family, is important and should include assessment of symptoms associated with depression, mania, hypomania, and a family history of BD. Episodes of mania combined with depressed features and a family history of BD are highly indicative of the diagnosis (Box 28.13).

Interventions

Pharmacotherapy

Lithium, the most commonly used substance for individuals with BDs, has neurological effects that make it difficult for older adults to tolerate. Lithium also has a long half-life (more than 36 hours), and dosing needs to be adjusted based on renal function. Medications that can affect urine production (diuretics) can alter lithium levels. Lithium levels, blood urea nitrogen (BUN) levels, and creatinine plasma levels need to be monitored closely (Sadock et al, 2015). Anticonvulsant medications such as valporic acid, divalproex sodium, and lamotrigine are more commonly used in BD treatment, although use of lamotrigine calls for monitoring for Stevens-Johnson syndrome. Medication levels and liver function tests must be monitored. Many of the anticonvulsant medications have an FDA warning that their use may increase suicide risk, so careful monitoring for changes in mood and behavior and signs of suicidal ideation is important.

Antidepressants such as fluoxetine, paroxetine, and venlafaxine can be used to treat depression in BD disorder in combination with other medications. Because these medications can trigger mania, careful assessment is important. Atypical antipsychotic drugs are also sometimes used, but with the same safety warnings discussed earlier, and are not to be used if neurocognitive disorders are suspected. Olanzapine, aripiprazole, and quetiapine are all approved for the treatment of BD and may relieve symptoms of severe mania and psychosis (U.S. Food and Drug Administration, 2017).

Psychosocial Approaches

Patient and family education and support are essential, and the family must understand that the individual is not able to control mania and irritating behaviors because of a chemical imbalance in the brain. Treatment with medication and intensive psychotherapy; CBT; interpersonal and rhythm therapy (improving relationships with others and managing regular daily routines); and family-focused therapy have been reported to be effective in improving recovery rates.

Psychoeducation is an important component of all psychosocial interventions, and nurses can assist patients in learning about BD and its treatment. Psychoeducation should include developing an acceptance of the disorder, becoming aware of factors influencing symptoms and signs of relapse, learning how to communicate with others, and establishing regular sleep and activity habits. Teaching patients to keep a log to monitor mood changes, activity levels, stressors, and amount of sleep is important. Medication regimens can be complicated, and many individuals struggle to remain adherent. An important nursing intervention is educating patients and families about the benefits and risks of prescribed medications, the importance of monitoring therapeutic effects, side effects, and the value of medication management systems.

DEPRESSION

Depression is not a normal part of aging, and studies show that most older adults are satisfied with their lives (National Institute on Aging, 2017). To understand depression, the nurse must understand the influence of late-life stressors and changes and the beliefs older adults, society, and health professionals may have about depression and its treatment.

Prevalence

Depression is a significant public issue and remains underdiagnosed and undertreated in the older adult population. The prevalence of depression among older adults ranges from 1% to 5% but rates are at least two times higher in primary care and medical settings with 6% to 9% meeting the criteria for major depression (Bruce and Sirey, 2018; Centers for Disease Control and Prevention, 2017). Furthermore, depression is the leading cause of disability globally and a major factor in the burden of disease worldwide (World Health Organization, 2018c). The prevalence of depressive disorders in older adults is expected to more than double by 2050 (Jeste et al, 2018).

Estimates are that 17% of older adults have symptoms of depression that do not meet the criteria for MDD; these symptoms are referred to as subsyndromal depression, dysthymic depression, and mild depression (Bruce and Sirey, 2018). The *DSM-5* utilizes the term *persistent* depressive disorder to describe symptoms that are long standing (lasting 2 years or longer) but do not meet the

---

BOX 28.13   Focus on Genetics

Research on the genetic basis for mental health disorders such as depression, schizophrenia, and bipolar disorder is being conducted by the National Institute of Mental Health Center for Collaborative Genetic Studies on Mental Disorders (https://www.nimhgenetics.org/).

The latest genome-wide study identified shared genetic risk factors between schizophrenia and bipolar disorder, bipolar disorder and depression, and schizophrenia and depression, the first evidence of overlap between these disorders. Continuous research on gene discovery for mental health disorders is ongoing.

criteria for MDD. Recognition and treatment are important because persistent depressive disorder has a negative impact on physical and social functioning and quality of life for many older adults and is associated with an increased risk of a subsequent major depression. There is limited research about older adults with mild depressive disorders.

Prevalence rates of depression in older adults likely underestimate the extent of the problem. The stigma associated with depression may be more prevalent in older adults, and they may not acknowledge depressive symptoms or seek treatment. Perceived stigma may be less of a concern for the future older adult population who are more aware of mental health concerns and more likely to seek treatment. Many older adults, particularly those who have survived the Great Depression, both world wars, the Holocaust, and other tragedies, may see depression as shameful, evidence of a flawed character, self-centered, a spiritual weakness, and sin or retribution. Freeman and colleagues (2016) found that a negative view of aging impacted the persistence of depression and anxiety.

Health professionals often expect older adults to be depressed and may not take appropriate action to assess for and treat depression. The differing presentation of depression in older adults and the increased prevalence of medical problems that may cause depressive symptoms also contribute to inadequate recognition and treatment. Even if depression is identified, most older adults with significant depression do not receive guideline-consistent, if any, depression treatment (Bruce and Sirey, 2018). All health care professionals must receive adequate education about depression in older adults in order to provide safe, effective care.

Consequences

Depression is a common and serious medical condition second only to heart disease in causing disability and harm to an individual's health and quality of life. Depression and depressive symptomatology are associated with negative consequences, such as delayed recovery from illness and surgery, excess use of health services, cognitive impairment, exacerbation of coexisting medical illnesses, malnutrition, decreased quality of life, and increased suicide and non–suicide-related deaths. It is highly likely that nurses will encounter a large number of older adults with depressive symptoms in all settings. Recognizing depression and enhancing access to appropriate mental health care are important nursing roles to improve outcomes for older adults.

Etiology

The causes of depression in older adults are complex and must be examined in a bio-psychosocial framework. Factors of health, gender, developmental needs, socioeconomics, environment, personality, losses, and functional decline are all significant to the development of depression in later life. Biological causes, such as neurotransmitter imbalances, have a strong association with many depressive disorders in late life. This may be a factor in the high incidence of depression in individuals with neurological conditions such as stroke, Parkinson's disease, and neurocognitive disorders.

Serious symptoms of depression occur in 30% to 50% of individuals with Alzheimer's disease and depression is also a risk factor for dementia, particularly early-onset, recurrent,

severe depression (Cipriani et al, 2015; Ryu, 2017). Among individuals with Alzheimer's disease, depression is the earliest observable symptom in at least one-third of cases (Jeste et al, 2018). Depression in individuals with Alzheimer's disease may be due to an awareness of progressive decline, but research suggests that there may also be a biological connection between depression and Alzheimer's disease.

Medical disorders and medications can also result in depressive symptoms (Boxes 28.14 and 28.15). Other important factors influencing the development of depression are alcohol abuse, loss of a spouse or partner, loss of social supports, lower income level, caregiver stress (particularly caring for a person with dementia), and gender. Some common risk factors for depression are presented in Box 28.16.

BOX 28.14   Medical Conditions and Depression

Cancers
Cardiovascular disorders
Endocrine disorders, such as thyroid problems and diabetes
Neurological disorders, such as Alzheimer's disease, stroke, and Parkinson's disease
Metabolic and nutritional disorders, such as vitamin B_{12} deficiency, malnutrition, diabetes
Viral infections, such as herpes zoster and hepatitis
Vision and hearing impairment

BOX 28.15   Medications and Depression

Antihypertensives
Angiotensin-converting enzyme (ACE) inhibitors
Methyldopa
Reserpine
Guanethidine
Antiarrhythmics
Anticholesteremics
Antibiotics
Analgesics
Corticosteroids
Digoxin
L-Dopa

BOX 28.16   Risk Factors for Depression in Older Adults

- Chronic medical illnesses, disability, functional decline
- Alzheimer's disease and other dementias
- Bereavement
- Caregiving
- Female (2:1 risk)
- Socioeconomic deprivation
- Family history of depression
- Previous episode of depression
- Admission to long-term care or other change in environment
- Medications
- Alcohol or substance abuse
- Living alone
- Widowhood

PROMOTING HEALTHY AGING: IMPLICATIONS FOR GERONTOLOGICAL NURSING

Assessment

Making the diagnosis of depression in older adults can be challenging, and symptoms of depression present differently in older adults. Older adults who are depressed report more somatic complaints such as insomnia, loss of appetite, weight loss, memory loss, and chronic pain. It is often difficult to distinguish somatic complaints from the physical symptoms associated with chronic illness. Both symptoms must be evaluated.

Decreased energy and motivation, lack of ability to experience pleasure, increased dependency, poor grooming and difficulty completing activities of daily living (ADLs), withdrawal from people or activities enjoyed in the past, decreased sexual interest, and a preoccupation with death or "giving up" are also signs of depression in older adults. Feelings of guilt and worthlessness, seen in younger depressed individuals, are less frequently seen in older adults.

Individuals often present with complaints of memory problems and a cognitive impairment of recent onset that mimics dementia but subsides upon remission of depression (previously called pseudodementia). It is important to note that a large percentage of these patients progress into irreversible dementia within 2 to 3 years, so recognition and treatment of depression are important. It is essential to differentiate between dementia and depression, and older adults with memory impairment should be evaluated for depression. Symptoms such as agitation, physically aggressive behavior, and repetitive verbalizations in persons with dementia may be indicators of depression (Cipriani et al, 2015) (Chapter 29).

Comprehensive assessment involves a systematic and thorough evaluation using a depression screening instrument, interview, psychiatric and medical history, physical (with focused neurological exam), functional assessment, cognitive assessment, laboratory tests, medication review, determination of iatrogenic or medical causes, and family interview as indicated. Assessment for depressogenic medications, for alcohol and substance abuse, and for related comorbid physical conditions that may contribute to or complicate treatment of depression must also be included (Box 28.17).

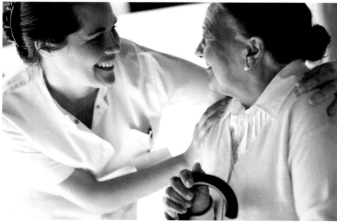

Creating hopeful environments in which meaningful activities and supportive relationships can be enjoyed is an important nursing role in the treatment of depression. (©iStock.com/Yuri.)

BOX 28.17 Tips for Best Practice

Assessment of Depression

- Utilize a depression screening tool (GDS or Cornell if cognitive impairment).
- Assess for suicide—ask direct question, "Have you thought of killing or harming yourself?"
- Investigate somatic complaints and look for underlying acute or chronic stressful events.
- Investigate sleep patterns, changes in appetite or weight, socialization pattern, level of physical activity, and substance abuse (past and present).
- Ask direct questions about psychosocial factors that may influence depression: elder abuse, poor environmental conditions, and changes in the patient role after death or disability of a spouse/partner.
- Obtain psychiatric and medical histories.
- Perform a physical exam including a focused neurological exam.
- Evaluate and treat chronic illnesses to improve outcomes and prevent exacerbations.
- Complete a functional assessment (pay close attention to changes in activities of daily living (ADL) function).
- Perform a cognitive assessment; depressed patients may show little effort during examination, answer "I don't know," and have inconsistent memory loss and performance during exam.
- Conduct a medication review (assessment for medications that may cause depressive symptoms).
- Assess for psychotic symptoms (delusions, hallucinations) and symptoms of bipolar disorder.
- Perform laboratory tests as appropriate to rule out other causes of symptoms (e.g., thyroid-stimulating hormone (TSH), T_4, serum B_{12}, vitamin D, folate, complete blood count, urinalysis).
- Utilize family/significant others in obtaining key information to correlate patient's symptoms with others' observations; always assess and interview patient first.

Screening of all older adults for depression should be incorporated into routine health assessments across the continuum of care—in hospitals, primary care, long-term care, home care, and community-based settings. The Geriatric Depression Scale (GDS) was developed specifically for screening older adults and has been tested extensively in a number of settings. The Cornell Scale for Depression in Dementia (CSDD) is recommended for the assessment of depression in older adults with dementia (Chapter 7).

Interventions

The goals of depression treatment in older adults are to decrease symptoms, reduce relapse and recurrence, enhance function and quality of life, and reduce mortality and health care costs. Interventions are individualized and are based on history, severity of symptoms, concomitant illnesses, and level of disability. There are a wide range of treatments for depression, and outcomes for older adults are generally similar to those observed for younger populations. However, this may not be true for frail, very old patients with multiple medical comorbidities (Kok and Reynolds, 2017). Guidelines suggest that effective treatment for major depression is a combination of pharmacological therapy and psychotherapy or counseling with psychotherapy alone recommended as a first-line treatment in mild major depression. Psychotherapy is comparable with the effectiveness of antidepressants (Kok and Reynolds, 2017).

Nonpharmacological Approaches

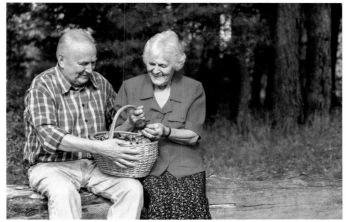

Older adults enjoying an activity together. (©iStock.com/FredFroese.)

Evidence-based nonpharmacological treatment options are needed for the treatment of depression, especially in primary care. CBT meets the highest level of evidence with a small but beneficial effect after metaanalysis. However, there are other promising options for treatment, particularly in community settings, that could be delivered by nurses. Types of nonpharmacological treatment that have been found to be helpful in depression include family and social support, education, grief management, exercise, humor, spirituality, CBT, brief psychodynamic therapy, interpersonal therapy, reminiscence and life review therapy (Chapter 6), problem-solving therapy, and complementary therapy (e.g., tai chi) (Holvast et al, 2017). Exercise has been associated with a significant reduction in depressive symptoms (Seo and Chao, 2018) (Chapter 18) (Research Highlights box). The development of effective, simplified, and accessible psychotherapeutic approaches, including Internet-based programs, geared toward older adults is important.

There are few systematic studies testing the efficacy of behavioral interventions for mild depression in individuals with neurocognitive disorders but several interventions hold promise. Problem-adaptive therapy (PATH), a home-delivered intervention that also involves caregivers, has been found to reduce depressive symptoms. Reminiscence therapy has been reported to improve depressive symptoms in individuals with mild to moderate dementia. Another intervention, behavior therapy-positive events (BT-PE), teaches caregivers to increase the patient's engagement in pleasant activities and positive interactions. Exercise therapy and caregiver problem-solving skills have been shown to be superior to placebo (Bohlken et al, 2017; Cipriani et al, 2015).

Despite evidence-based guidelines calling for combined pharmacological and psychotherapeutic treatment, and the fact that older adults often prefer psychotherapy to psychiatric medications, psychological interventions are often not offered as an alternative. Reasons for this include time, reimbursement constraints, and a limited well-trained geriatric mental health workforce.

Integrated care. The majority of older adults prefer to be treated for depression by primary care providers rather than mental health specialists. New models of care providing both primary and behavioral care in the same setting are designed to promote collaboration between primary care providers and mental health specialists in planning and treating older adults. There is evidence that integrated care improves access, quality, and outcomes of depression treatment for older adults. The most effective models involve systematic depression screening, a depression care manager to work directly with the patients over time (often nurses), and the use of evidence-based depression treatment (Bruce and Sirey, 2018; Gilbody et al, 2017). Several collaborative interventions delivered in the home have also shown effectiveness in reducing depression symptoms, depression remission, and improved quality of life (Bruce and Sirey, 2018) (Box 28.18).

🔲 RESEARCH HIGHLIGHTS

The purpose of this systematic review was to determine the impact of exercise on depressive symptomology experienced by older adults living in a community setting in the United States. Based on the inclusion criteria of the study, 10 studies were reviewed; seven randomly controlled studies and three quasi-experimental. The exercise interventions varied by study; from walking, yoga, tai chi, aerobic exercises, and weight lifting. In addition, the exercise intensity and duration varied by study. The majority of the studies reviewed reported a reduction of depressive symptomatology when measured immediately after exercise, but only three studies measured the effect on depressive symptoms over a period of time. Several limitations were identified in the studies: small sample size, various exercise modalities, and varied measurements of outcomes. More rigorous study designs and methodology are recommended to assess the long-term effect of exercise on depressive symptoms in a population of older adults.

From Seo JY, Chao Y: Effects of exercise interventions on depressive symptoms among community-dwelling older adults in the United States, *J Gerontol Nurs* 44(3):31–38, 2018.

BOX 28.18 Exemplar Program

PEARLS (Problem-Solving to Overcome Depression)

- Targets homebound older adults with chronic conditions to provide "housecalls" for depression, particularly in underserved communities.
- Incorporates program into existing community-based programs that deliver care and resources to clients.
- Designed to treat minor depression and persistent depressive disorder by teaching behavioral and problem-solving techniques and pleasant activities scheduling.
- Utilizes the Chronic Care and Collaborative Care Models.
- Uses a psychiatrist-led team with trained counselors to work one-on-one with participants in eight in-home sessions followed by a series of maintenance telephone session contacts.
- A supervising psychiatrist reviews cases regularly, addresses other causes of depression, and works with the individual's primary care provider to assess treatment effectiveness and need for more formal depression treatment including medications.
- Results show reduction in depression symptoms, lower rates of hospitalization, and improved function, emotional well-being, and quality of life.
- Program included in SAMSHA's National Registry of Evidence-Based Programs and Practices and Agency for Healthcare Research and Quality Innovation Exchange.

From Health Promotion Research Center: *PEARLS*. www.pearlsprogram. org. Accessed March 2019.

Pharmacological Approaches

Antidepressants may effectively treat depression in older adults but have a high risk for adverse effects because of multiple medical comorbidities and drug-drug interactions from polypharmacy. Two-thirds of older adults who use antidepressants receive drugs that are either contraindicated or have the potential for moderate to major interactions (Holvast et al, 2017; Kok and Reynolds, 2017). Choice of medication depends on comorbidities, drug side effects, and the type of effect desired. People with agitated depression and sleep disturbances may benefit from medications with a more sedating effect, whereas those who are not eating may do better taking medications that have an appetite-stimulating effect.

The most commonly prescribed antidepressants are the SSRIs. These agents work selectively on neurotransmitters in the brain to alleviate depression. The SSRIs are generally well tolerated in older adults but anticholinergic and sedative effects may be associated with physical and cognitive impairment. For those who do not respond to an adequate trial of SSRIs, there is another group of antidepressants that combines the inhibition of both serotonin and norepinephrine reuptake inhibitors (SNRIs) (e.g., venlafaxine [Effexor]). These also may be preferred by those who are engaged in or who anticipate sexual activity because they are less likely to have sexual side effects. One of the atypical antidepressants, such as bupropion [Wellbutrin] or trazodone, may be used. In the context of reducing polypharmacy, Wellbutrin also reduces nicotine dependency, and trazodone is sedating—for the person who has difficulty getting to or staying asleep. Since the development of the SSRIs and SNRIs, the older monoamine oxidase (MAO) inhibitors and tricyclic antidepressants are no longer indicated due to their high side effect profile, including risk for falls.

All antidepressant medications must be closely monitored for side effects and therapeutic response. There are more than 20 antidepressants approved by the FDA for the treatment of depression in older adults, and several may have to be evaluated to determine the medication most effective for the individual. Similar to other medications for older adults, doses should be lower at first (50% of the target dose) and titrated as indicated until adequate treatment effect is ensured. If the patient has responded to treatment, it is not clear how long the medication should be continued, but if there is a lifetime history of depression, recommendations are that pharmacotherapy should be maintained for at least 2 years to prevent recurrence (Kok and Reynolds, 2017) (Chapter 9).

Other Treatments

Electroconvulsive therapy (ECT) is the most effective treatment for older adults with major depression with efficacy ranging from 60% to 80%. ECT is also indicated for patients at risk for severe harm because of psychotic depression, suicidal ideation, severe malnutrition, or a medical condition that worsens because they refuse medication (Kok and Reynolds, 2017). ECT results in a more immediate response in symptoms and is also a useful alternative for frail older adults with multiple comorbid

BOX 28.19   **Tips for Best Practice**
Family and Professional Support for Depression
• Provide relief from discomfort of physical illness. • Enhance physical function (i.e., regular exercise and/or activity; physical, occupational, recreational therapies). • Develop a daily activity schedule that includes pleasant activities. • Increase opportunities for socialization and enhance social support. • Provide opportunities for decision-making and the exercise of control. • Focus on spiritual renewal and rediscovery of meanings. • Reactivate latent interests, or develop new ones. • Validate depressed feelings as aiding recovery; do not try to bolster the person's mood or deny his or her despair. • Help the person become aware of the presence of depression, the nature of the symptoms, and the time limitation of depression. • Emphasize depression as a medical, not mental, illness that must be treated like any other disorder. • Provide easy-to-use educational materials to older adults and family members, such as those available through the National Institute of Mental Health (NIMH). • Involve family in patient teaching, particularly younger family members who may have different life experiences related to depression and its treatment. • Provide an accepting atmosphere and an empathic response. • Demonstrate faith in the person's strengths. • Praise any and all efforts at recovery, no matter how small. • Assist in expressing and dealing with anger. • Do not stifle the grief process; grief cannot be hurried. • Create a hopeful environment in which self-esteem is fostered and life is meaningful.

conditions who are unable to tolerate antidepressant treatment. ECT is much improved, but older adults will need a careful explanation of the treatment because they may have many misconceptions.

Rapid transcranial magnetic stimulation (rTMS) is a treatment approved in 2008 by the FDA to treat MDD in adults for whom medication was not effective or tolerated. The treatment consists of administering brief magnetic pulses to the brain by passing high currents through an electromagnetic coil adjacent to the patient's scalp. The targeted magnetic pulses stimulate the circuits in the brain that are underactive in patients with depression with the goal of restoring normal function and mood. For most patients, treatment is administered in 30- to 40-minute sessions over a period of 4 to 6 weeks. The effectiveness of the treatment is still being evaluated in older adults. TMS is contraindicated for persons who have seizures, stroke, brain injury/trauma/surgery, pacemakers, or intracranial magnetic devices. Box 28.19 presents suggestions for families and professionals caring for older adults with depression.

SUICIDE

Some of the highest suicide rates in the United States and globally are among older adults. Suicide attempts are more frequent among adolescents and young adults, but older men and women have the highest suicide rate in the United States, with rates reaching as high as 48.7/100,000 among white older men (Butcher and Ingram, 2018). Older widowers are thought to be the most vulnerable because they have often depended on their wives to maintain the comforts of home and the social network of family and friends. Among racial/ethnic populations, in 2016, whites had the highest suicide rate, followed by American Indian/Alaska Natives (American Foundation for Suicide Prevention, 2016). Women in all countries have much lower suicide rates, possibly because of greater flexibility in coping skills based on multiple roles that women fill throughout their lives. Despite these alarming statistics, there is little research on suicide ideation and behavior among older adults.

Possible contributing factors to rising suicide rates include the economic downturn, intentional overdoses associated with the increase in use of prescription opioids, other substance use, and a cohort effect based on the high suicide rates of this age group in their adolescent years. Butcher and Ingram (2018) raise the question of the effect of ageism and suicide. Older adults may internalize the negative stereotypes of aging, and health care professionals can also reflect ageism in practice (Chapter 2). "It is common for health care providers to view suicidal thinking as a normal reaction in older adults" (2018, p. 21). These statistics contribute to the concern about the increasing mental health problems in future generations of older adults and call for increased prevention efforts in this age group.

In most cases, depression and other mental health problems, including anxiety, contribute significantly to suicide risk. Common precipitants of suicide include physical or mental illness, death of a spouse or partner, substance abuse, chronic pain, limited social support, living alone, financial strain, and a history of suicide attempts (Choi et al, 2015). One of the major differences in suicidal behavior in the old and the young is the lethality of method. Eight out of 10 suicides for men older than 65 were with firearms, and firearms account for 51% of all suicides (American Foundation for Suicide Prevention, 2016).

Many older adults who die by suicide reached out for help before they took their own life. Three-fourths of older adults who commit suicide had seen their physician within 1 month before death; 40% had visited within 1 week of the suicide, and 20% had visited the physician on the day of the suicide (American Psychological Association, 2018). Depression is frequently missed, and older adults with suicide ideation or with other mental health concerns often present with somatic complaints. The statistics suggest that opportunities for assessment of suicidal risk are present, but the need for intervention is not seen as urgent or even recognized. Consequently, it is very important for providers in all settings to inquire about recent life events, implement depression screening for all older adults, evaluate for anxiety disorders, assess for suicidal thoughts and ideas based on depression assessment, and recognize warning signs and risk factors for suicide. Behavioral clues and risk and protective factors are presented in Box 28.20

BOX 28.20 Warning Signs and Suicide Risk and Recovery Factors

Risk Factors and Signs

Male gender
Psychiatric diagnosis
Physical illness
Functional impairment
Depression
Loss of social support
Social isolation
Alcohol and substance misuse and abuse
Major loss, such as the death of a spouse or partner
History of major losses
Financial insecurity
Recent suicide attempt
History of suicide attempts
Major crises or transitions, such as retirement or relocation to an assisted living or nursing facility
Major crises in the lives of family members
Loss of mobility
Time of care transitions, especially following hospitalizations
Preoccupation with death
Poorly controlled pain
Expression of the belief that one is in the way, a burden
Giving away favorite possessions, money
Cognitive loss

Recovery Factors

A capacity for the following:
 Understanding
 Relating
 Benefiting from experience
 Benefiting from knowledge
 Accepting help
 Being loving
 Expressing wisdom
 Displaying a sense of humor
 Having a social interest
 Accepting a caring and available family
 Accepting a caring and available social network
 Accepting a caring, available, and knowledgeable professional and health network

From Westefeld JS, Casper D, Galligan P, et al: Suicide and older adults: risk factors and recommendations. *Loss Trauma* 20:491–508, 2015.

PROMOTING HEALTHY AGING: IMPLICATIONS FOR GERONTOLOGICAL NURSING

Assessment

Older adults with suicidal intent are encountered in many settings. It is our professional obligation to prevent, whenever possible, an impulsive destruction of life that may be a response to a crisis or a disintegrative reaction. The lethality potential of an older adult must always be assessed when elements of depression, disease, and spousal loss are evident. Any direct, indirect, or enigmatic references to the ending of life must be taken seriously and discussed. In the nursing home setting, the

Minimum Data Set (MDS) (Chapter 7) includes screening for suicide risk and mandates that long-term care facilities have effective protocols for managing suicide risk.

The Joint Commission released an alert that recommends suicide risk screening in all settings (Jahn, 2017). "Suicide prevention cannot be limited to hospital, primary care, and clinic settings, but rather must reach into communities and culture" (Butcher and Ingram, 2018, p. 29). However, every older adult should be screened for suicidal ideation at each primary care visit. Early detection is the first level of suicide prevention, and crisis intervention follows as a second level of prevention support for older adults at risk. If the older adult has personal, medical, or situational risk factors, screening should take place every 6 months or more frequently if indicated.

Assessment should include (1) identification of risk factors, medical problems, medications, functional status, nutritional status, personal and family psychiatric history, alcohol or substance drug use, and complete physical and neurological exam, (2) evaluation of cognitive function, (3) psychological strengths, coping skills, spirituality, sexuality, suicidal ideation, past attempts at suicide, and (4) quantity and quality of social support, financial status, legal history, and potential for elder abuse (Butcher and Ingram, 2018, p. 22). The Columbia-Suicide Severity Rating Scale (C-SSRS) is an evidence-based suicide assessment tool used by many hospitals and organizations. The American Psychiatric Nurses Association and American Association of Suicidology utilize the acronym, IS PATH WARM, as a component of suicide warning signs (Box 28.21). Other resources can be found in Box 28.1.

The most important consideration for the nurse is to establish a trusting and respectful relationship with the person. Because many older adults have grown up in an era when suicide bore stigma and even criminal implications, they may not discuss their feelings in this area. It is also important to remember that in older adults, typical behavioral clues such as putting personal affairs in order, giving away possessions, and making wills and funeral plans are indications of maturity and good judgment in late life and cannot be construed as indicative of suicidal intent. Even statements such as "I won't be around

long" or "I'm ready to die" may be only a realistic appraisal of the situation in old age.

If there is suspicion that the older adult is suicidal, use direct and straightforward questions such as the following:
- Have you ever thought about killing yourself?
- How often have you had these thoughts?
- How would you kill yourself if you decided to do it?

> **⚡ SAFETY ALERT**
> Always ask direct questions of the patient and family about suicide risks and suicide ideation.

Interventions

It is important to have a suicide protocol in place that clearly defines how the nurse will intervene if a positive response is obtained from any of the questions. The person should never be left alone for any period of time until help arrives to assist and care for him or her. Patients at high risk should be hospitalized, especially if they have current psychological stressors and/or access to lethal means. Patients at lower risk may be treated as outpatients provided they have adequate social support and no access to lethal means. Other crisis interventions include partial hospitalization, day treatment, antidepressant medications, communicating risk to family, care management, counseling, support groups, assistance with financial stress, increased social involvement, and increased activity with faith community (Butcher and Ingram, 2018).

Suicide is a taboo topic for most of us, and there is a lingering fear that the introduction of the topic will be suggestive to the patient and may incite suicidal action. Precisely the opposite is true. By introducing the topic, we demonstrate interest in the individual and open the door to honest human interaction and connection on the deep levels of psychological need. It is the nature of our concern and our ability to connect with the alienation and desperation of the individual that will make a difference. Working with isolated, depressed, and suicidal older adults challenges the depths of nurses' ingenuity, patience, and self-knowledge.

SUBSTANCE USE DISORDERS

Substance abuse among older adults is one of the fastest growing health problems in the United States (Chhatre et al, 2017). With the aging of the baby boomer generation, the number of adults older than age 50 with substance use disorders is projected to reach 5.7 million by 2020 (Mattson et al, 2017). The baby boomer generation has had more exposure to alcohol and illegal drugs in their youth and has a more lenient attitude about substance abuse. Additionally, psychoactive drugs became more readily available for dealing with anxiety, pain, and stress. While alcohol remains the most frequent reason for admission to substance abuse treatment, this proportion is declining. Cocaine- and heroin-related admissions are on the rise in the older adults and the incidence of opioid abuse and misuse is also increasing (Chhatre et al, 2017; Jeste et al, 2018). Despite these increases, substance abuse in older adults

---

BOX 28.21   Warning Signs/Behaviors Related to Suicide Risk: IS PATH WARM Mnemonic

I	Ideation
S	Substance abuse
P	Purposelessness
A	Anxiety
T	Trapped
H	Hopelessness
W	Withdrawal
A	Anger
R	Recklessness
M	Mood changes

From American Association of Suicidology: *Know the warning signs of suicide.* http://www.suicidology.org/resources/warning-signs. Accessed March 2019.

remains an underrecognized and undertreated public health concern (Jeste et al, 2018). The Healthy People 2020 B box presents objectives for substance abuse in adults.

 HEALTHY PEOPLE 2020 B

Substance Abuse Objectives for Adults

- Increase the proportion of persons who need alcohol and/or illicit drug treatment and received specialty treatment for abuse or dependence in the past year.
- Increase the proportion of persons who are referred for follow-up care for alcohol problems, drug problems after diagnosis, or treatment for one of these conditions in a hospital emergency department.
- Increase the number of Level I and Level II trauma centers and primary care settings that implement evidence-based alcohol Screening and Brief Intervention (SBI).
- Reduce the proportion of adults who drank excessively in the previous 30 days.
- Reduce average alcohol consumption.
- Reduce the past-year nonmedical use of prescription drugs (pain relievers, tranquilizers, stimulants, sedatives, any psychotherapeutic drug).
- Decrease the number of deaths attributable to alcohol.

From U.S. Department of Health and Human Services, Office of Disease Prevention and Health Promotion: *Healthy People 2020,* 2014. https://www.healthypeople.gov/.

Alcohol Use Disorder
Prevalence and Characteristics

In the United States, alcohol use disorders are reported in 11% of adults aged 54 to 64 years and about 6.7% of those older than 65 years. Alcoholism is the third most prevalent psychiatric disorder (after dementia and anxiety) among older men. Most severe alcohol abuse is seen in people ages 60 to 80 years, not in those older than 80 years. Two-thirds of older adults with alcohol abuse are early-onset drinkers (alcohol use began at age 30 or 40), and one-third are late-onset drinkers (use began after age 60). Late-onset drinking may be related to situational events such as illness, retirement, or death of a spouse and includes a higher number of women (Campbell et al, 2014). Alcohol-related problems in older adults often go unrecognized, although the residual effects of alcohol abuse complicate the presentation and treatment of many chronic disorders.

Gender Issues

While men (particularly older widowers) are four times more likely to abuse alcohol than women, the prevalence in women may be underestimated. The number and impact of older female drinkers are expected to increase over the next 20 years as the disparity between men's and women's drinking decreases. Women of all ages are significantly more vulnerable to the effects of alcohol misuse including faster progression to dependence and earlier onset of adverse consequences. Even low-risk drinking levels (no more than one standard drink per day) can be hazardous for older women. Older women also experience unique barriers to detection of and treatment for alcohol problems. Health care providers often assume alcohol use symptoms are related to other conditions in aging (Goldstein et al, 2015).

Physiology

Older adults, especially females, develop higher blood alcohol levels because of age-related changes (increased body fat, decreased lean body mass, and total body water content) that alter absorption and distribution of alcohol. Decreases in hepatic metabolism and kidney function also slow alcohol metabolism and elimination. A decrease in the gastric enzyme alcohol dehydrogenase results in slower metabolism of alcohol and higher blood levels for a longer time. Risks of gastrointestinal ulceration and bleeding related to alcohol use may be higher in older adults because of the decrease in gastric acidity that occurs in aging (Goldstein et al, 2015).

Consequences

The health consequences of long-term alcohol use disorder include cirrhosis of the liver, cancer, immune system disorders, cardiomyopathy, cerebral atrophy, dementia, and suicide (Goldstein et al, 2015). Other effects of alcohol in older adults include urinary incontinence, which results from rapid bladder filling and diminished neuromuscular control of the bladder; gait disturbances from alcohol-induced cerebellar degeneration and peripheral neuropathy; depression; functional decline, increased risk for injury; and sleep disturbances and insomnia. Alcohol misuse has also been implicated as a major factor in morbidity and mortality as a result of trauma, including falls, drownings, fires, motor vehicle crashes, homicide, and suicide.

Alcohol use also exacerbates conditions such as osteoporosis, diabetes, hypertension, and ulcers. Many drugs that older adults use for chronic illnesses cause adverse effects when combined with alcohol (Box 28.22). All older adults should be given precise instructions regarding the interaction of alcohol with their medications.

Alcohol Guidelines for Older Adults

The possible health benefits of alcohol in moderation have been reported in the literature (reduced risk of coronary artery disease, ischemic stroke, Alzheimer's disease, and vascular dementia). As a result, older adults may not perceive alcohol use as potentially harmful, but clinically significant adverse effects can occur in some individuals consuming as little as two to three drinks per day over an extended period. A drink is defined as

---

BOX 28.22   Medications Interacting With Alcohol

Analgesics
Antibiotics
Antidepressants
Antipsychotics
Benzodiazepines
H_2-receptor antagonists
Nonsteroidal antiinflammatory drugs (NSAIDs)
Herbal medications (echinacea, valerian)
Acetaminophen taken on a regular basis, when combined with alcohol, may lead to liver failure
Alcohol diminishes the effects of oral hypoglycemics, anticoagulants, and anticonvulsants

From National Institute on Alcohol Abuse and Alcoholism: *Mixing alcohol with medicines.* https://pubs.niaaa.nih.gov/publications/Medicine/medicine.htm. Accessed June 2018.

5 ounces of wine, 12 ounces of beer, or 1.5 ounces of 80-proof distilled spirits or liquor.

Because of the increased risk of adverse effects from alcohol use, the National Institute of Alcohol Abuse and Alcoholism defines "at-risk drinking" for men and women aged 65 years and older as more than one drink per day. Binge drinking is a pattern of drinking by men consuming more than five drinks and women more than four drinks within 2 hours (Centers for Disease Control and Prevention, 2018). Health professionals must share information with older adults about safe drinking limits and the deleterious effects of alcohol intake.

PROMOTING HEALTHY AGING: IMPLICATIONS FOR GERONTOLOGICAL NURSING

Assessment

Alcohol- and substance use-related problems among older adults are too frequently undetected by health care professionals. Assessment challenges include poor symptom recognition, lack of provider training, inadequate knowledge of screening instruments, lack of time, skepticism about benefits, fear of patient reactions, and the belief that patients will not be candid about alcohol use (DiBartolo et al, 2017). Alcohol-related problems may be overlooked in older adults because they do not drastically disrupt their lives or are not clearly linked to physical disorders. Health care providers may also be pessimistic about the ability of older adults to change long-standing problems.

The U.S. Preventive Services Task Force (2018) recommends that clinicians screen adults 18 years and older in primary care for alcohol misuse. Screening should be a part of health visits for people older than the age of 60 years in primary, acute, and long-term care settings (Sorrell, 2017). Although alcohol is the drug most often used among older adults, assessment should include all substances used (recreational drugs, prescription, nicotine, and OTC medications) (Han et al, 2018). The Hartford Institute of Geriatric Nursing recommends that the Short Michigan Alcoholism Screening Test–Geriatric Version be used with older adults because it is more age appropriate than other instruments (Table 28.1). A single question can also be used for alcohol screening: "How many times in the past year have you had 5 or more drinks in a day (if a man), or 4 or more drinks (if you are a woman older than 65 years of age)?" If the individual acknowledges drinking that much, follow-up assessment is indicated.

Assessment of depression is also important because depression is often comorbid with alcohol abuse. Alcohol and depression screenings should be offered routinely at health fairs and other sites where older adults may seek health information. A medication review should be conducted, and screening should be done both before prescribing any new medications that may interact with alcohol and as needed after life-changing events. Alcohol abuse should be suspected in an older adult who presents with a history of falling, unexplained bruises, or medical problems associated with alcohol abuse problems.

Alcoholism is a disease of denial and not easy to diagnose, particularly in older adults with psychosocial and functional decline from other conditions that may mask decline caused by alcohol. Early signs such as weight loss, irritability, insomnia, and falls may not be recognized as indicators of possible alcohol problems and may be attributed to "just getting older." Box 28.23 presents signs and symptoms that may indicate the presence of alcohol problems in older adults.

Alcohol users often reject or deny the diagnosis, or they may take offense at the suggestion of it. Feelings of shame or disgrace may make older adults reluctant to disclose a drinking problem. Families of older adults with substance use disorders, particularly their adult children, may be ashamed of the problem and choose not to address it. Health care providers may feel helpless over alcoholism or uncomfortable with direct questioning or may approach the person in a judgmental manner. A caring and supportive approach that provides a safe and open atmosphere is the foundation for the therapeutic relationship. It is always important to search for the pain beneath the behavior.

Interventions

Alcohol problems affect physical, mental, spiritual, and emotional health. Interventions must address quality of life in all of these spheres and be adapted to meet the unique needs of the older adult. Abstinence from alcohol is seen as the desired goal, but a focus on education, alcohol reduction, and reducing harm is also appropriate. Increasing the awareness of older adults

TABLE 28.1 Short Michigan Alcoholism Screening Test—Geriatric Version (S-MAST-G).	Yes (1)	No (0)
1. When talking with others, do you ever underestimate how much you drink?		
2. After a few drinks, have you sometimes not eaten, or been able to skip a meal, because you didn't feel hungry?		
3. Does having a few drinks help decrease your shakiness or tremors?		
4. Does alcohol sometimes make it hard for you to remember parts of the day or night?		
5. Do you usually take a drink to relax or calm your nerves?		
6. Do you drink to take your mind off your problems?		
7. Have you ever increased your drinking after experiencing a loss in your life?		
8. Has a doctor or nurse ever said they were worried or concerned about your drinking?		
9. Have you ever made rules to manage your drinking?		
10. When you feel lonely, does having a drink help?		
TOTAL S-MAST-G SCORE (1–10)		

Scoring: 2 or more "Yes" responses indicate an alcohol problem.
From the Regents of the University of Michigan: *Short Michigan alcohol screening test—geriatric version (S-MAST-G)*. Ann Arbor, MI, 1991, University of Michigan Alcohol Research Center.

BOX 28.23 Signs and Symptoms of Potential Alcohol Problems in Older Adults

Anxiety
Irritability (feeling worried or "crabby")
Blackouts
Dizziness
Indigestion
Heartburn
Sadness or depression
Chronic pain
Excessive mood swings
New problems making decisions
Lack of interest in usual activities
Falls
Bruises, burns, or other injuries
Family conflict, abuse
Headaches
Incontinence
Memory loss
Poor hygiene
Poor nutrition
Insomnia
Sleep apnea
Social isolation
Out of touch with family or friends
Unusual response to medications
Frequent physical complaints and physician visits
Financial problems

about the risks and benefits of alcohol consumption in the context of their own situation is an important goal. Treatment and intervention strategies include cognitive-behavioral approaches, individual and group counseling, medical and psychiatric approaches, referral to Alcoholics Anonymous, family therapy, case management and community and home care services, and formalized substance abuse treatment. Treatment outcomes for older adults have been shown to be equal to or better than those for younger people (Campbell et al, 2014). Providing education about alcohol use to older adults and their families and referring to community resources are important nursing roles and essential to best practices.

Unless the person is in immediate danger, a stepped-care intervention approach beginning with brief interventions followed by more intensive therapies, if necessary, should be used. The U.S. Preventive Services Task Force (2018) recommends brief counseling interventions to reduce alcohol use for adults. Brief intervention is a time-limited, patient-centered strategy focused on changing behavior and assessing patient readiness to change. Sessions can range from one meeting of 10 to 30 minutes to four or five short sessions. The goals of brief intervention are to (1) reduce or stop alcohol consumption and (2) facilitate entry into formalized treatment if needed. Research results indicate that this type of intervention, with counseling by nurses in primary care settings, is effective for reducing alcohol consumption, and older adults may be more likely to accept treatment given by their primary care provider.

Long-term self-help treatment programs for older adults show high rates of success, especially when social outlets are emphasized and cohort supports are available. A significant concern is the lack of programs designed specifically for older adults, particularly older women, whose concerns are very different from those of a younger population who abuse drugs or alcohol. Health status, availability of transportation, and mobility impairments may further limit access to treatment. Development of treatment sites in senior centers and ALFs and telemedicine programs would increase accessibility. Pharmacological treatment has not played a major role in the long-term treatment of alcohol-dependent older adults, but two medications, naltrexone (Revia) and acamprosate (Campral), are approved for treatment and have been used effectively with older adults. Disulfiram (Antabuse) is seldom used in older adults due to concerns about cardiovascular adverse effects (Campbell et al, 2014). Additional resources are presented in Box 28.1.

Acute Alcohol Withdrawal

When there is significant physical dependence, withdrawal from alcohol can become a life-threatening emergency. Detoxification should be done in an inpatient setting because of the potential medical complications and because withdrawal symptoms in older adults can be prolonged. Older adults who drink are at risk of experiencing acute alcohol withdrawal if admitted to the hospital for treatment of acute illnesses or emergencies. All patients admitted to acute care settings should be screened for alcohol use and assessed for signs and symptoms of alcohol-related problems. Older adults with a long history of consuming excess alcohol, previous episodes of acute withdrawal, and/or a history of prior detoxification are at increased risk of acute alcohol withdrawal.

Symptoms of acute alcohol withdrawal vary but may be more severe and last longer in older adults. Minor withdrawal (withdrawal tremulousness) begins 6 to 12 hours after a patient has consumed the last drink. Symptoms include tremor, anxiety, nausea, insomnia, tachycardia, and increased blood pressure and frequently may be mistaken for common problems in older adults. Major withdrawal is seen 10 to 72 hours after cessation of alcohol intake, and symptoms include vomiting, diaphoresis, hallucinations, tremors, and seizures.

Delirium tremens (DTs) is the term used to describe alcohol withdrawal delirium; it usually occurs 24 to 72 hours after the last drink but may occur up to 10 days later. DTs occur in 5% of patients with acute alcohol withdrawal and are considered a medical emergency. Other signs and symptoms include confusion, disorientation, hallucinations, hyperthermia, and hypertension. The Clinical Institute Withdrawal Assessment (CIWA) scale is recommended as a valid and reliable screening instrument (MSD Manual, 2018).

Recommended treatment is the use of short-acting benzodiazepines at one-half to one-third the normal dose around-the-clock or as needed during withdrawal. The use of oral or intravenous alcohol to prevent or treat withdrawal is not established. The CIWA aids in medication adjustments. Other interventions include assessing mental status, monitoring vital signs, and maintaining fluid balance without overhydrating. Calm and quiet surroundings, no unnecessary stimuli, consistent caregivers, frequent reorientation, prevention of injury, and support and caring are additional suggested interventions.

Other Substance Abuse Concerns

A more common concern seen among older adults is the misuse and abuse of prescription psychoactive medications. Dependence on sedative, hypnotic, or anxiolytic drugs, often prescribed for anxiety or insomnia and taken for many years with resulting dependence, is especially problematic for older women, who are more likely than men to receive prescriptions for these drugs (Markota et al, 2016).

Some of the reasons for the abuse of psychoactive prescription medications may be inappropriate prescribing and ineffective monitoring of response and follow-up. In many instances, older adults are given prescriptions for benzodiazepines or sedatives because of complaints of insomnia or nervousness, without adequate assessment for depression, anxiety, or other conditions that may be causing the symptoms. Older adults may not be informed of the side effects of these medications, including interactions with alcohol, dependence, and withdrawal symptoms. More importantly, conditions such as anxiety and depression may not be recognized and treated appropriately. STAMP Out Prescription Drug Misuse and Abuse Toolkit is an excellent resource for health care professionals to use in education about prescription drug misuse and abuse in older adults (Box 28.1).

■ KEY CONCEPTS

- Mental health is a fluctuating situation for most individuals, with peaks and valleys of happiness and pain.
- The prevalence of mental health disorders is expected to increase significantly with the aging of the baby boomers.
- Mental health disorders are underreported and underdiagnosed among older adults. Somatic complaints are often the presenting symptoms of mental health disorders, making diagnosis difficult.
- The incidence of psychotic disorders with late-life onset is low among older adults, but psychotic manifestations can occur as secondary symptoms in a variety of disorders, the most common being Alzheimer's disease. Psychotic symptoms in Alzheimer's disease necessitate different assessment and treatment than do long-standing psychotic disorders.
- Anxiety disorders are common in later life, and reestablishing feelings of adequacy and control is the heart of crisis resolution and stress management.

- Depression remains underdiagnosed and undertreated in the older adult population and is considered a significant public health issue. Depression in older adults can be effectively treated. Unfortunately, it is often neglected or assumed to be a condition of aging that one must "learn to live with." An important nursing intervention is assessment of depression.
- Suicide is a significant problem among older men, particularly widowers. Many are seen by a health care professional with physical complaints shortly before they commit suicide, and assessment of depression and suicidal intent is important.
- Substance abuse, particularly alcohol, and misuse of psychoactive prescription drugs are often under recognized and undertreated problems of older adults, particularly older women. Screening and appropriate assessment and intervention are important in all settings.
- Treatment outcomes for substance abuse for older adults are equal to or better than those for younger people.

NURSING STUDY: BIPOLAR DISORDER

Myra is a 71-year-old white woman who was admitted to the geropsychiatry inpatient unit for alcohol abuse and noncompliance with her lithium, which had been prescribed for a diagnosed bipolar disorder. Myra's primary mode of coping with her depression and mood swings has been to drink alcohol, meet abusive men, and play bingo. However, when she stops taking her dose of lithium, she begins to have flight of ideas, argues with her daughters, and tries to pick up men in her apartment complex. After seeing her at home, you discover that she has a long history of being physically abused by her husband, now deceased for 8 years, and has been living with one daughter who also has emotionally and physically abused her, causing Myra to be hospitalized. Myra's ability to test reality is compromised because of years of denial and low self-esteem. She says, "I used to have lots of times when I felt really good in between the depressions. Now I feel depressed most of the time." She tells you that her daughters harass her and interfere in her life. Your goals as a community-based nurse are to facilitate her independence (being able to live in her own apartment), to assist her with medication compliance, and to intervene with Myra to improve relationships with her daughters. Home visits are approved through Medicare for 1 month after hospital discharge.

Based on the case study, develop a nursing care plan using the following procedure[a]:

- List Myra's comments that provide subjective data.
- List information that provides objective data.
- From these data, identify and state, using an accepted format, two nursing diagnoses you determine are most significant to Myra at this time. List two of Myra's strengths that you have identified from the data.
- Determine and state outcome criteria for each diagnosis. These criteria must reflect some alleviation of the problem identified in the nursing diagnosis and must be stated in concrete and measurable terms.
- Plan and state one or more interventions for each diagnosed problem. Provide specific documentation of the sources used to determine the appropriate intervention. Plan at least one intervention that incorporates Myra's existing strengths.
- Evaluate the success of the intervention. Interventions must correlate directly with the stated outcome criteria to measure the outcome success.

[a]Students are advised to refer to their nursing diagnosis text and identify possible or potential problems.

CRITICAL THINKING QUESTIONS AND ACTIVITIES

1. How will you evaluate Myra's ability to live independently?
2. What particular strategies are necessary to meet the goals of the nursing care plan?
3. Given that Myra's primary coping strategy is drinking alcohol, how will you facilitate her sobriety and help her deal with stress?
4. How much involvement with Myra's daughters do you believe is necessary to assist with her transition back into her own apartment?

5. Given the limited number of visits covered by Medicare, what information does Myra need to provide self-care? In other words, the nurse must be teaching Myra how to live independently after discharge from home health care. What does Myra need to know?
6. Discuss the meanings and thoughts triggered by the student's and the elder's viewpoints expressed at the beginning of the chapter. How do these vary from your own experience?

NURSING STUDY: DEPRESSIVE DISORDER WITH SUICIDAL THOUGHTS

Jake had cared for his wife, Emma, during a long and painful illness until she died 4 years ago. He found that alcohol provided a way to cope with the stress. Within a year after her death, Jake met a lady to whom he was very attracted, and a few months later she moved in with him. Jake managed to move his things around until some space was made for her personal items, but neither of them was very comfortable with this. He really did not like to move his things from their usual place and, because her allotted space was so small, she felt like an intruder. He collected guns, and she shuddered when she saw them. He was an avid fan of John Wayne movies, and she preferred going to the symphony. He liked meat and potatoes, and she was a vegetarian. She also disapproved of his increasing reliance on alcohol. The blending of two such different lifestyles proved difficult. In a few months she moved out, and Jake blamed himself. He said over and over, "I should have done more for her. I'm not good for anything anymore." His friends began to pull away from him, just when he needed them most, because he seemed to talk of nothing but his various aches, pains, and pills and his general discouragement with life. Jake's consumption of alcohol increased markedly.

He had some health problems: a mild heart failure, a lack of exercise, dairy products gave him diarrhea, he was somewhat obese, and his knees were painful most of the time. He routinely visited his allergist, his internist, his orthopedist, and his cardiologist. However, it seemed the more he went to these specialists, the worse he felt. He was taking several medications, and each time he saw one of his clinicians, he came away with another prescription. No one asked about his drinking, and he never mentioned it. He awoke one morning feeling very dizzy, so he went to his internist later in the day. He began to share the litany of his discomforts, and the physician reminded him that at 76 years of age he could not expect to always feel in top shape.

When he returned from seeing the physician, Jake called his daughter and surprised her by saying he had just decided he would take a week off and go to Hawaii to see if the sun and sand would revive him. Jake was not usually impulsive. His daughter, fortunately, was a psychiatric nurse and was concerned about the change in his behavior.

Based on the case study, develop a nursing care plan using the following procedure[a]:

- List Jake's comments that provide subjective data.
- List information that provides objective data.
- From these data, identify and state, using an accepted format, two nursing diagnoses you determine are most significant to Jake at this time. List two of Jake's strengths that you have identified from the data.
- Determine and state outcome criteria for each diagnosis. These criteria must reflect some alleviation of the problem identified in the nursing diagnosis and must be stated in concrete and measurable terms.
- Plan and state one or more interventions for each diagnosed problem. Provide specific documentation of the source used to determine the appropriate intervention. Plan at least one intervention that incorporates Jake's existing strengths.
- Evaluate the success of the intervention. Interventions must correlate directly with the stated outcome criteria to measure the outcome success.

[a]Students are advised to refer to their nursing diagnosis text and identify possible or potential problems.

CRITICAL THINKING QUESTIONS AND ACTIVITIES

1. Discuss the variations in symptoms of depression in older adults and younger adults.
2. Describe some of the reasons that may make older adults vulnerable to depression.
3. Describe a time when you were depressed and the feelings you had. What did you do about it?
4. Given the situation in this case, discuss what your thoughts would be if you were Jake's daughter.
5. Given his daughter's background, what are her responsibilities in this case?
6. What is the responsibility of a student nurse in the case of suspected suicidal thoughts?

7. Would you address the possibility of suicidal thoughts if you were the nurse in a primary care setting? When and how would you take on this task?
8. What action should be taken for Jake's protection?
9. Would you expect that Jake is still grieving over the death of his wife? What are your thoughts about this situation?
10. What are the clues or indications that an older adults is thinking of committing suicide?
11. What are some of signs of suicidal intent in young adults? How are these signs different from those of older adults?
12. Under what conditions do you think a person has a right to take his or her life?

13. What are your thoughts about Jake's use of alcohol?
14. Do you think suicide is a sign of weakness or strength?
15. Do you agree or disagree with the following statements on the basis of the evidence about depression and suicide in older adults?
    - Normally older adults feel depressed much of the time.
    - Older adults are more likely than young people to admit to depression.
    - Most older adults talk about suicide but rarely try to kill themselves.
    - Depression of the older adult is helped by medications.
    - Depression may be the cause of forgetfulness.
    - Depression in the older adult is often linked with illness and alcoholism.

RESEARCH QUESTIONS

1. What is the prevalence of mental health disorders in community-dwelling older adults? What mental health care is nursing able to provide in the home?
2. How common is alcohol abuse a strategy of self-care used by the older adult with emotional concerns?
3. What types of interventions are most appropriate for older adults with alcohol or drug abuse problems?
4. Is psychiatric home care a more cost-effective alternative than institutional care?
5. What are the cardinal symptoms of depression in the oldest-old?
6. How many primary care providers consider or evaluate for the presence of depression in older adults who see them for physical complaints?
7. What are the most reliable tools for identifying depression in cognitively intact and cognitively impaired older adults?
8. What is the meaning of depression in older adults of different races, cultures, and ethnicities?
9. What modifications need to be made in assessment and treatment of mental health disorders to enhance cultural appropriateness?

REFERENCES

American Foundation for Suicide Prevention: *Suicide statistics,* 2016. https://afsp.org/about-suicide/suicide-statistics/. Accessed June 2018.

American Geriatrics Society 2015 Beers Criteria Update Expert Panel: American Geriatrics Society 2015 updated Beers Criteria for potentially inappropriate medication use in older adults, *J Am Geriatr Soc* 63(11):2227–2246, 2015.

American Psychiatric Association: *Diagnostic and statistical manual of mental disorders,* ed 5, Arlington, VA, 2013, American Psychiatric Publishing.

American Psychological Association: *Growing mental and behavioral concerns facing older adults,* 2018. http://www.apa.org/advocacy/health/older-americans.aspx. Accessed June 2018.

Balsamo M, Cataldi F, Carlucci L, Fairfield B: Assessment of anxiety in older adults: a review of self-report measures, *Clin Interv Aging* 13:573–593, 2018.

Bohlken J, Weber SA, Siebert A, Forstmeier S, Kohlmann T: Reminiscence therapy for depression in dementia, *GeroPsych* 30(4):145–151, 2017.

Butcher H, Ingram T: Evidence-based practice guideline. Secondary prevention of late-life suicide, *J Gerontol Nurs* 44(11):20–32, 2018.

Brenes GA, Danhauer SC, Lyles MF, Miller ME: Telephone-delivered psychotherapy for rural-dwelling older adults with generalized anxiety disorder: study protocol of a randomized controlled trial, *BMC Psychiatry* 14:34, 2014.

Bruce ML, Sirey JA: Integrated care for depression in older primary care patients, *Can J Psychiatry* 63(7):439–446, 2018.

Burnside IM: Listen to the aged, *Am J Nurs* 75(10):1800–1803, 1822, 1975.

Campbell J, Resnick B, Warshaw G: Alcoholism. In Ham R, Sloane P, Warshaw G, editors: *Primary care geriatrics,* ed 6, Philadelphia, PA, 2014, Elsevier, pp 365–371.

Canuto A, Weber K, Baertschi M, et al: Anxiety in old age: psychiatric comorbidities, quality of life, and prevalence according to age, gender, and country, *Am J Geriatr Psychiatry* 26(2):174–185, 2018.

Center for Medicare Advocacy: *Part B,* 2018. http://www.medicareadvocacy.org/medicare-info/medicare-part-b/. Accessed June 2014.

Centers for Disease Control and Prevention: *Self-directed violence surveillance: uniform definitions and recommended data elements,* 2011. https://www.cdc.gov/violenceprevention/pdf/Self-Directed-Violence-a.pdf. Accessed June 2018.

Centers for Disease Control and Prevention: *Depression is not a normal part of growing older,* 2017. https://www.cdc.gov/aging/mentalhealth/depression.htm. Accessed June 2018.

Centers for Disease Control and Prevention: *Fact sheets-binge drinking,* 2018. https://www.cdc.gov/alcohol/fact-sheets/binge-drinking.htm. Accessed June 2018.

Centers for Medicare & Medicaid Services Medicaid Program Integrity Education: *Atypical antipsychotic medications: use in adults,* 2015. https://www.cms.gov/Medicare-Medicaid-Coordination/Fraud-Prevention/Medicaid-Integrity-Education/Pharmacy-Education-Materials/Downloads/atyp-antipsych-adult-factsheet11-14.pdf. Accessed June 2018.

Centers for Medicare and Medicaid Services: *Medicare & your mental health benefits,* 2017. https://www.medicare.gov/Pubs/pdf/10184-Medicare-Mental-Health-Bene.pdf. Accessed June 2018.

Chellingsworth M, Kishita N, Laidlaw K: *A clinician's guide to CBT with older adults,* 2016, p 20. https://www.uea.ac.uk/documents/246046/8314842/LICBT_BOOKLET_FINAL_JAN16.pdf/48f28e80-dc02-45b6-91cd-c628d36e8bca. Accessed June 2018.

Chhatre S, Cook R, Mallik E, Jayadevappa R: Trends in substance use admissions among older adults, *BMC Health Serv Res* 17:584, 2017.

Choi NG, DiNitto DM, Marti CN: Middle-aged and older adults who had serious suicidal thoughts: who made suicide plans and nonfatal suicide attempts? *Int Psychogeriatr* 27(3):491–500, 2015.

Christianson S, Marren J: *Impact of Event Scale-Revised (IES-R),* New York, NY, 2013, Hartford Institute for Geriatric Nursing.

Cipriani G, Lucetti C, Carlesi C, Danti S, Nuti A: Depression and dementia: a review, *Eur Geriatr Med* 6(5):479–486, 2015.

Clifford KM, Duncan NA, Heinrich K, Shaw J: Update on managing generalized anxiety disorder in older adults, *J Gerontol Nurs* 41(4):10–20, 2015.

Cook JM, Simiola V: Trauma and PTSD in older adults: prevalence, course, concomitants and clinical considerations, *Curr Opin Psychol* 14:1–4, 2017.

Creighton AS, Davison TE, Kissane DW: The prevalence, reporting, and treatment of anxiety among older adults in nursing homes and other residential aged care facilities, *J Affect Disord* 227: 416–423, 2018.

DiBartolo MC, Jarosinski JM: Alcohol use disorder in older adults: challenges in assessment and treatment, *Issues Ment Health Nurs* 38(1):25–32, 2017.

Department of Veterans Affairs: *PTSD treatment basics,* 2019. https://www.ptsd.va.gov/understand_tx/tx_basics.asp. Accessed March 2019.

Freeman AT, Santini ZI, Tyrovolas S, Rummel-Kluge C, Haro JM, Koyanagi A: Negative perceptions of aging predict the onset and persistence of depression and anxiety: findings from a prospective analysis of The Irish Longitudinal Study on Aging (TILDA), *J Affect Disord* 199:132–138, 2016.

Fung AWT, Lee JSW, Lee ATC, Lam LCW: Anxiety symptoms predicted decline in episodic memory in cognitively health older adults: a 3-year prospective study, *Int J Geriatr Psychiatry* 33(5):748–754, 2018.

Gates J, Killackey E, Phillips L, Álvarez-Jiménez M: Mental health starts with physical health: current status and future directions of non-pharmacological interventions to improve physical health in first-episode psychosis, *Lancet Psychiatry* 2:726–742, 2015.

Gilbody S, Lewis H, Adamson J, et al: Effect of collaborative care vs. usual care on depressive symptoms in older adults with sub-threshold depression: the CASPER randomized clinical trial, *JAMA* 317(7):728–737, 2017.

Goldstein NS, Hodgson N, Savage CL, Walton-Moss B: Alcohol use and the older adult woman, *J Nurse Pract* 11(4):436–442, 2015.

Gradus JL: *Epidemiology of PTSD. U.S. Department of Veterans Affairs,* 2017. https://www.ptsd.va.gov/professional/treat/essentials/epidemiology.asp. Accessed March 2019.

Hall KS, Morey MC, Beckham JC, et al: The Warrior Wellness study: a randomized controlled exercise trial for older veterans with PTSD, *Transl J Am Coll Sports Med* 3(6):43–51, 2018.

Han BH, Moore AA: Prevention and screening of unhealthy substance use by older adults, *Clin Geriatr Med* 34(1):117–129, 2018.

Hjorthøj C, Stürup AE, McGrath JJ, Nordentoft M: Life expectancy and years of potential life lost in schizophrenia: a systematic review and meta-analysis, *Lancet Psychiatry* 4(4):295–301, 2017.

Holvast F, Massoudi B, Oude Voshaar RC, Verhaak PFM: Non-pharmacological treatment for depressed older patients in primary care: a systematic review and meta-analysis, *PLOS One* 12(9):e0184666, 2017.

Hoy-Ellis CP, Ator M, Kerr C, Milford J: Innovative approaches address aging and mental health needs in LGBTQ communities, *J Am Soc Aging* 40(2):56–62, 2016.

Jahn DR: Suicide risk in older adults: the role and responsibility of primary care, *J Clin Outcomes Manag* 24(4):181–190, 2017.

Jeste DV, Peschin S, Buckwalter K, et al: Promoting wellness in older adults with mental illnesses and substance use disorders: call to action to all stakeholders, *Am J Geriatr Psychiatry* 26(6):617–630, 2018.

Klainin-Yobas P, Oo WN, Suzanne Yew PY, Lau Y: Effects of relaxation interventions on depression and anxiety among older adults: a systematic review, *Aging Ment Health* 19(12):1043–1055, 2015.

Kleinman A: *Patient and healers in the context of culture: an exploration of the borderland between anthropology, medicine, and psychiatry.* Berkeley, 1980, University of California Press.

Kok RM, Reynolds CF III: Management of depression in older adults a review, *JAMA* 317(20):2114–2122, 2017.

Kruse CS, Krowski N, Rodriguez B, Tran L, Vela J, Brooks M: Telehealth and patient satisfaction: systematic review and narrative analysis, *BMJ Open* 7(8):e016242, 2017.

Markota M, Rummans TA, Bostwick JM, Lapid MI: Benzodiazepine use in older adults: dangers, management, and alternative therapies, *Mayo Clin Proc* 91(11):1632–1639, 2016.

Mattson M, Lipari RN, Hays C, Van Horn SL: A day in the life of older adults: substance use facts. *The CBSSQ Report.* Rockville, MD, 2017, Substance Abuse and Mental Health Services Administration. https://www.ncbi.nlm.nih.gov/books/NBK436750/pdf/Bookshelf_NBK436750.pdf. Accessed June 2018.

Maust DT, Kales HC, Wiechers IR, Blow FC, Olfson M: No end in sight: benzodiazepine use among older adults in the United States, *J Am Geriatr Soc* 64(12):2546–2553, 2016.

Melillo KD: Geropsychiatric nursing: what's in your toolkit? *J Gerontol Nurs* 43(1):3–6, 2017.

MSD Manual Professional Version: *CIWA-AR Clinical Institute Withdrawal Assessment for Alcohol scale,* 2018. https://www.msdmanuals.com/professional/multimedia/clinical-calculator/ciwa%20ar%20clinical%20institute%20withdrawal%20assessment%20for%20alcohol%20scale. Accessed June 2018.

Multicultural Mental Health Resource Centre: *Cultural formulation,* 2018. http://www.multiculturalmentalhealth.ca/clinical-tools/cultural-formulation/. Accessed June 2018.

Mushkin P, Band-Winterstein T, Avieli H: "Like every normal person?!" The paradoxical effect of aging with schizophrenia, *Qual Health Res* 28(6):977–986, 2018.

National Institute of Mental Health: *Post-traumatic stress disorder,* 2016. https://www.nimh.nih.gov/health/topics/post-traumatic-stress-disorder-ptsd/index.shtml. Accessed June 2018.

National Institute of Mental Health: *Suicide,* 2018. https://www.nimh.nih.gov/health/statistics/suicide.shtml. Accessed June 2018.

National Institute of Mental Health: *Older adults and mental health.* https://www.nimh.nih.gov/health/topics/older-adults-and-mental-health/index.shtml. Accessed June 2018.

National Institute on Aging: *Depression and older adults,* 2017. https://www.nia.nih.gov/health/depression-and-older-adults. Accessed June 2018.

Office of Disease Prevention and Health Promotion: *About the data,* 2018. www.healthypeople.gov/2020/data-search/About-the-Data. Accessed June 2018.

Ray M: *Transcultural caring dynamics in nursing and health care,* Philadelphia, PA, 2016, FA Davis.

Reynolds K, Pietrzak RH, Mackenzie CS, Chou KL, Sareen J: Post-traumatic stress disorder across the adult life span: findings from a nationally representative survey, *Am J Geriatr Psychiatry* 24(1):81–93, 2016.

Robins LM, Hill KD, Finch CF, Clemson L, Haines T: The association between physical activity and social isolation in community dwelling older adults, *Aging Ment Health* 22(2): 175–182, 2018.

Roser M, Ritchie H: *Mental health,* 2018. https://ourworldindata.org/mental-health. Accessed June 2018.

Rytwinski NK, Scur MD, Feeny NC, Youngstrom EA: The co-occurrence of major depressive disorder among individuals with posttraumatic stress disorder: a meta-analysis, *J Trauma Stress* 26:299–309, 2013.

Ryu SH, Jung HY, Lee KJ, et al: Incidence and course of description in patients with Alzheimer's disease, *Psychiatry Investig* 14(3): 271–280, 2017.

Segal DL, Qualls SH, Smyer MA: *Aging and mental health,* ed 3, Hoboken, NJ, 2018, John Wiley & Sons.

Seo JY, Chao YY: Effects of exercise intervention on depressive symptoms among community-dwelling older adults in the United States: a systematic review, *J Gerontol Nurs* 44(3):31–38, 2018.

SAMHSA-HRSA Center for Integrated Health Solutions: *Behavioral health in primary care,* 2018. https://www.integration.samhsa.gov/integrated-care-models/behavioral-health-in-primary-care. Accessed June 2018.

Sorrell JM: Substance use disorders in long-term care settings: a crisis of care for older adults, *J Psychosoc Nurs Ment Health Serv* 55(1):24–27, 2017.

Stephens CE, Harris M, Buron B: The current state of U. S. Geropsychiatric graduate nursing education: results of the National Geropsychiatric Graduate Nursing Education Survey, *J Am Psychiatr Nurses Assoc* 21(6):385–394, 2015.

Substance Abuse and Mental Health Services Administration: *Racial/ethnic differences in mental health service use among adults,* HHS Publication No. SMA-15-4906, Rockville, MD, 2015, Substance Abuse and Mental Health Services. https://www.integration.samhsa.gov/MHServicesUseAmongAdults.pdf. Accessed June 2018.

Temkin-Greener H, Campbell L, Cai X, Hasselberg MJ, Li Y: Are post-acute patients with behavioral health disorders admitted to lower-quality nursing homes? *Am J Geriatr Psychiatry* 26(6):643–654, 2018.

U.S. Department of Health and Human Services (USDHHS), Office of Disease Prevention and Health Promotion: *Healthy People 2020,* 2014. https://www.healthypeople.gov/. Accessed March 2019.

U. S. Food and Drug Administration: *The facts on bipolar disorder and FDA-approved treatments,* 2017. https://www.fda.gov/ForConsumers/ConsumerUpdates/ucm530107.htm. Accessed June 2018.

U.S. Preventive Services Task Force: *Unhealthy alcohol use in adolescents and adults: screening and behavioral counseling interventions,* 2018. https://www.uspreventiveservicestaskforce.org/Page/Document/UpdateSummaryDraft/unhealthy-alcohol-use-in-adolescents-and-adults-screening-and-behavioral-counseling-interventions. Accessed June 2018.

Valtorta NK, Moore DC, Barron L, Stow D, Hanratty B: Older adults' social relationships and health care utilization: a systematic review, *Am J Public Health* 108(4):e1–e10, 2018.

Wehbe-Alamah H: Madeleine Leininger's theory of culture care diversity and universality. In Smith MC, Parker ME, editors: *Nursing theories and nursing practice,* ed 4, Philadelphia, PA, 2015, FA Davis, pp 303–319.

Westefeld JS, Casper D, Galligan P, et al: Suicide and older adults: risk factors and recommendations, *J Loss Trauma* 20:491–508, 2015.

World Health Organization: *Mental health of older adults,* 2017a. http://www.who.int/news-room/fact-sheets/detail/mental-health-of-older-adults. Accessed June 2018.

World Health Organization: *mhGAP training manuals for the mhGAP Intervention Guide for mental, neurological, and substance use disorders in non-specialized health settings –version 2.0,* 2017b. http://www.who.int/mental_health/mhgap/training_manuals/en/. Accessed June 2018.

World Health Organization: *Sustainable development knowledge platform,* 2018a. https://sustainabledevelopment.un.org/post2015/transformingourworld. Accessed June 2018.

World Health Organization: *Mental health. Key publications,* 2018b. http://www.who.int/mental_health/publications/en/. Accessed June 2018.

World Health Organization: *Depression,* 2018c. http://www.who.int/news-room/fact-sheets/detail/depression. Accessed June 2018.

Yoder M, Norman S: *Co-occurring PTSD and neurocognitive disorder (NCD),* 2016, US Department of Veterans Affairs. https://www.ptsd.va.gov/professional/treat/cooccurring/ncd_assess_cooccur.asp. Accessed March 2019.

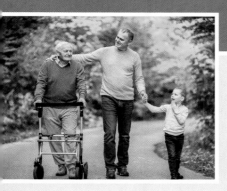

29

Care of Individuals With Neurocognitive Disorders

Debra Hain, María Ordóñez, and Theris A. Touhy

http://evolve.elsevier.com/Touhy/TwdHlthAging

A STUDENT SPEAKS

It is one thing to learn about neurocognitive disorders from a textbook or a lecture; it is something entirely different to care for and interact with individuals who are living with one of these disorders. My first contact as a nursing student with a person living with dementia was during a clinical experience at a skilled nursing facility (SNF) in a unit that had people with moderate to severe stage dementia. As students, we fed and bathed them, held their hands, and talked to them without any knowledge of whether they understood or even consciously registered any of what was said, or whether their responses were purely instinctual. Nonetheless, we had a caring approach to meeting their physical needs while preserving their dignity. Somehow, I lacked insight into their lives before the SNF and didn't even realize that I had not considered what happens in the community.

Later, as an RN-to-BSN student, I had a completely different engagement when I began my community nursing immersion experience at the Louis and Anne Green Memory and Wellness Center at Florida Atlantic University. There, older adults with concerns about their memory would come to the clinic to undergo a comprehensive geriatric evaluation of their cognitive status, be diagnosed, and obtain recommendations on how to potentially slow the progression of a neurocognitive disorder. Similarly, patients with a diagnosis of dementia would come to the day center as participants to attend cognitive stimulating and socially activating classes aimed at slowing the progression of their dementia and supporting their care partners. The caring wholeness of the center truly inspired me. I learned that there is much more to dementia than what you learn from books or hear from the news. I learned that older adults come with a history that is important to understand and respect. I embraced the concept of coming to know the person while discovering what matters most to the individual and their family. Having this inspiring experience as a student has led to my current position at the Center and my love for older adults living with neurocognitive disorders and their families.

Ismo Hujanen, BSN, RN, age 34

A NURSE SPEAKS
KNOW ME

Know who I am before you tell me what to do
I have history that makes me who I am
I am a daughter
I am a wife, mother, and grandmother, but remember,
I am not a child no matter what I do,
I have a lifetime of memories that may take time to retrieve
So just, take a few minutes to come to know me as the person I have been and will be
Take time to authentically listen and discover what matters most to me
My speech may be jumbled, so I may communicate through my behavior
So look at me; see me for who I am before you silence me with drugs
Know who I am before you care for me

Debra Hain, PhD, written with love of those with dementia whom I have cared for over many years

LEARNING OBJECTIVES

On completion of this chapter, the reader will be able to:

1. Identify the characteristics of delirium and differentiate between delirium, mild and major neurocognitive disorders (NCDs), dementia, and depressive disorders.
2. Discuss prevention, treatment, and nursing interventions for individuals with delirium.
3. Describe nursing models of care for individuals with mild and major NCDs.

4. Discuss common concerns in care of individuals with mild and major NCDs (communication, behavior, personal care, safety, nutrition) and nursing interventions.
5. Discuss strategies to enhance well-being and quality of life for both individuals with mild and major NCDs and their caregivers.

CARING FOR INDIVIDUALS WITH NEUROCOGNITIVE DISORDERS

This chapter focuses on care of older adults living with mild and major neurocognitive disorders (NCDs) and delirium with an emphasis on nursing interventions. The term dementia has been replaced with mild and major NCDs in the *Diagnostic and Statistical Manual of Mental Disorders*, ed 5, *DSM-5* (American Psychiatric Association, 2013), but the terms *dementia* and *cognitive impairment* will also be used in this chapter. Chapter 23 presents further information about NCDs including classification, etiology, disease-specific information, and pharmacological treatment. Cognitive functioning and aging is discussed in Chapter 5 and cognitive assessment in Chapter 7.

Person and Family-Centered Care

It has been said that prevention is the best and most important treatment for dementia; however, current research does not provide us with the answers or means to prevent all the cases. Therefore, the most important aspect of care for an individual after being diagnosed with dementia is to take a person- and family-centered care approach (this approach is incorporated into all care activities and will be integrated throughout the chapter). Person-centered and person/family-centered care are used interchangeably; however, they always refer to the same concept: caring for the person and family as a whole. Regardless of the circumstances, a diagnosis of dementia affects not only the person with the diagnosis but also his or her whole support system. Person-centered care is "essential to good dementia care and the underlying philosophy of the 2018 Alzheimer's Association Dementia Care Practice Recommendations" (Fazio et al, 2018a, p. S10). It is imperative that the philosophy of person-centered care for individuals with mild and major NCDs guide health promotion strategies in this population, regardless of the stage of dementia.

Person-centered care looks beyond the disease and the tasks we must perform to the person within and our relationship with them. The focus is not on what we need to do to the person but on the person himself or herself and how to enhance their well-being and quality of life. The principles of autonomy, independence, and self-determination are core to person-centered care (Lepore et al, 2017). "The person with dementia is not an object, not a vegetable, not an empty body, not a child,

but an adult, who, given support, might exercise choices and respond to a respectful approach" (Woods, 1999, p. 35). Person-centered care fosters abilities, supports limitations, ensures safety, enhances quality of life, prevents excess disability, and offers hope.

The Centers for Medicare and Medicaid Services (CMS) includes person-centered care as one of the six essential themes for nursing home care, regulation, and enforcement. Person-centered care is the foundation for identifying and meeting the needs of individuals through interpersonal relationships that maintain selfhood of the person with dementia. In many instances, there is a need for organizational culture change from the traditional medical model to person-centered care by making the community more homelike and less like an institution (Evans, 2017; Fazio et al, 2018b). Gerontological nurses play a key role as patient advocates in the culture-change movement, which is discussed in more depth in Chapter 32.

All older adults with NCDs are deserving of nursing interventions aimed toward maintaining or achieving the highest level of physical and cognitive function possible while promoting health and well-being. To promote well-being that can lead to positive health outcomes of older adults with NCDs, it is essential that gerontological nurses embrace evidence-based practice in development and implementation of person-centered interventions. Evidence-based practice takes the best available evidence (i.e., research, clinical practice guidelines, quality improvement), clinician expertise, person/family wishes, and preferences for care as they engage in shared decision making.

Strong interprofessional collaboration is important to high-quality care of individuals with dementia. Establishing a person/family and care provider partnership allows for shared power and shared decision making between older adults with NCDs, family, and the interprofessional team. In this model of care, individuals and their families are recognized as experts on their lives, wishes and preferences for care are honored, and providers are seen as experts in dementia care. Together they establish realistic and attainable goals and a plan of care that respects all parties involved (Gilster et al, 2018; Hain et al, 2011). Box 29.1 presents research on an innovative nurse practitioner–led, dementia-specific, community-based model of care being developed by two of the chapter's authors, Drs. Hain and Ordonez.

BOX 29.1   Translational Research in Gerontological Nursing: Bridging the Gap: Providing Specialized Dementia Care and Supportive Services Through Community Partnerships (BGDCS-CP)

This quality improvement project was supported with grant funding from the Alzheimer's Disease Initiative: Specialized Supportive Services Project.

An innovative nurse practitioner (NP)–led model of care incorporated a patient/family-provider-community partnership paradigm that aims to develop a person-centered relationship where trust between the provider and person receiving care is an essential aspect of shared decision making. The uniqueness of this approach was the establishment of this partnership with older adults with, or/at risk of, Alzheimer's disease and related dementias (ADRD), their caregivers, health care professionals with expertise in dementia care (i.e., nurse practitioner, neurologist, neuropsychologist, social worker), and community partners (i.e., senior centers, faith-based community, independent living facility). The goal of the project was to identify those with or/at risk of ADRD and address unmet needs by implementing person-centered, evidence-based interventions. The project investigators expanded the dementia specialized and supportive services offered at the Memory and Wellness Center (MWC) to the community. Through this project, we have been able to identify and intervene in communities of racial and ethnic diverse populations, who often don't have access to specialized care and supportive services offered at the MWC. We are currently, analyzing the data but preliminary findings are promising indicating that an NP-led, dementia-specific, community-based model of care is an effective way to improve health outcomes of those with or/at risk of ADRD and their caregivers.

Ordóñez M, Hain D: *Bridging the Gap: Providing Specialized Dementia Care and Supportive Services through Community Partnerships (BGDCS-CP,* 2015-8*).* Funded by Administration on Aging—Alzheimer's Disease Initiative: Specialized Supportive Services Project.

NEUROCOGNITIVE DISORDER: DELIRIUM

Although delirium is common in older adults, it often goes unrecognized, which increases the risk of functional decline, mortality, and health care costs (Inouye et al, 2014). Nurses play a key role in early identification and implementation of interventions aimed at reducing delirium and associated risks. Depression, delirium, and the mild and major NCDs (dementia) are called the *three D's* of cognitive impairment because they occur frequently in older adults. These important geriatric syndromes are not a normal consequence of aging, even though the incidence and prevalence are highest in older adults.

Because cognitive and behavioral changes characterize all three D's, it can be difficult to diagnose delirium, delirium superimposed on mild or major NCDs (dementia) (DSD), or depression (Chapter 28). In the presence of depression, it is difficult to determine the true contribution of cognitive impairment; thus, depression should be treated and the individual should undergo reevaluation of cognitive status once stable. It is also important to note that an individual should not be newly diagnosed with dementia while in the hospital because it is very likely that the person has delirium superimposed on a cognitive disorder (DSD) that may be mild but interpreted as more advanced.

Differences Among Delirium, Dementia (Mild and Major NCD), and Depression

Delirium is characterized by an acute or subacute onset, with symptoms developing over a short period of time (usually hours to days). Symptoms tend to fluctuate over the course of the day, often worsening at night. People often experience reduced ability to focus, sustain, or shift attention, which leads to cognitive or perceptual disturbances. Perceptual disturbances are often accompanied by delusional (paranoid) thoughts and behavior and hallucinations. Often the hallucinations are related to seeing deceased family members, for example the person may report talking with his or her mother.

In contrast, major and mild NCDs typically have a gradual onset and a slow, steady pattern of decline without alterations in consciousness. These disorders represent serious pathological alterations and require assessment and interventions. However, a change in cognitive function in older adults is often seen as normal and therefore is not investigated. Any change in mental status in an older adult requires a comprehensive geriatric assessment with a strong focus on cognitive function (Chapters 5, 7, and 23). Knowledge about cognitive function in aging and appropriate assessment and evaluation are keys to differentiating these three syndromes. Table 29.1 presents the clinical features and the differences in cognitive and behavioral characteristics in delirium, mild and major NCDs, and depression. The accepted criteria for a diagnosis of delirium are presented in the *DSM-5* (American Psychiatric Association, 2013).

Etiology

Regardless of the etiology, the goal of delirium care is prevention and early identification. It is important to note that the development of delirium is a result of complex interactions among multiple causes. Delirium results from the interaction of predisposing factors (e.g., vulnerability on the part of the individual due to predisposing conditions, such as underlying cognitive impairment, functional impairment, depression, acute illness, sensory impairment) and precipitating factors/insults (e.g., medications, procedures, restraints, iatrogenic events, sleep deprivation, bladder catheterization, pain, and environmental factors). For example, an older adult with preexisting dementia may experience delirium after receiving just a single dose of sleep medication. Although a single factor, such as an infection, can trigger an episode of delirium, several coexisting factors are also likely to be present. A highly vulnerable older individual requires a lesser amount of precipitating factors to develop delirium (Inouye, 2018).

The exact pathophysiological mechanisms involved in the development and progression of delirium remain uncertain. One single cause or mechanism is not likely, but rather emerging evidence supports the theory of complex interaction of biological factors leading to the disruption of neuronal networks (Inouye et al, 2014). Inouye (2018) proposes that "baseline and precipitating factors contribute to delirium in independent and substantive ways" (p. 448). This means that the relationship between these two models is not independent but rather

TABLE 29.1	Differentiating Delirium, Depression, and Dementia (Mild or Moderate NCD).		
Characteristic	**Delirium**	**Depression**	**Dementia**
Onset	Sudden, abrupt	Recent, may relate to life change; can be chronic	Insidious, slow, over years and often unrecognized until deficits obvious In vascular dementia will see stair step pattern so may see sudden change in cognitive function but should always be evaluated
Course over 24 hours	Fluctuating, often worse at night	Fairly stable, may be worse in the morning	Fairly stable, may see changes with stress some individuals have more symptoms toward nighttime (sundowning); may see sudden change when microvascular infarct occurs in vascular dementia
Consciousness	Reduced	Clear	Clear
Alertness	Increased, decreased, or variable	Normal	Generally normal
Psychomotor activity	Increased, decreased, or mixed Sometimes increased, other times decreased	Variable, agitation or retardation	Normal, may have apraxia or agnosia
Duration	Hours to weeks	Variable and may be chronic	Years
Attention	Disordered, fluctuates	Most often no impairment; however, can see difficulty concentrating	Generally normal but may have trouble focusing
Orientation	Usually impaired, fluctuates	Usually normal; may answer "I don't know" to questions or may not try to answer	Often impaired; may make up answers or answer close to the right thing or may confabulate but try to answer
Speech	Often incoherent, slow, or rapid; may call out repeatedly or repeat the same phrase	May be slow	Difficulty finding word, perseveration
Affect	Variable but may look disturbed, frightened	Flat	Slowed response, may be labile

NCD, Neurocognitive disorder.
Modified from Sendelbach S, Guthrie PF, Schoenfelder DP: Acute confusion/delirium, *J Gerontol Nurs* 35(11):11–18, 2009.

multiplicative. The causes of delirium are potentially reversible; therefore, accurate assessment and diagnosis are critical. Delirium is given many labels: acute confusional state, acute brain syndrome, confusion, reversible dementia, metabolic encephalopathy, and toxic psychosis.

Incidence and Prevalence

Delirium is a prevalent and serious neuropsychiatric syndrome that commonly occurs in older adults across the continuum of care. It is associated with short- and long-term consequences that can negatively influence health outcomes. Among medical inpatients, delirium is present on admission to the hospital in 10% to 31% of older patients. During hospitalization, 11% to 42% of older adults develop delirium. Up to 80% of patients in the intensive care unit (ICU) develop delirium. In subacute settings, a delirium is highly prevalent and persistent, still present on discharge and up to 3 months after discharge (Forsberg, 2017; Miu et al, 2016). A recent study in a Korean nursing home (Moon and Park, 2018) found the incidence of delirium was twice as high as that of patients in ICUs and hospitals.

Delirium Superimposed on Dementia (DSD)

Older adults with mild and major NCDs are three to five times more likely to develop delirium; however, delirium is less likely to be recognized and treated as compared to delirium that occurs in those without mild and major NCD. The prevalence of DSD in community and hospital populations ranges from 22% to 89%. An incidence of 40% in the community was reported in a recent study (Moon and Park, 2018). The presence of delirium can accelerate the trajectory of cognitive decline in older adults with preexisting NCD. DSD is associated with high mortality and morbidity among hospitalized older adults. Changes in the mental status of older adults with dementia are often attributed to underlying dementia, or "sundowning," and therefore is not identified or even considered as a possible reason for changes in cognitive function. Despite its prevalence, DSD has not been well investigated and there is a need for more research on this topic as well as development of protocols for assessment and treatment (Morandi et al, 2017).

Recognition of Delirium

Delirium, one of the most significant geriatric syndromes, is considered a medical emergency. Interestingly, as previously stated, despite a high incidence and prevalence of delirium, it is underrecognized. A comprehensive review of the literature suggests "nurses are missing key symptoms of delirium and appear to be doing superficial mental status assessments" (Steis and Fick, 2008, p. 47). Delirium in the ICU may be difficult to identify because of sedation and hypoactive disorders (Birge and Aydin, 2017). Other factors contributing to the lack of recognition of delirium among health care professionals include inadequate education about delirium, limited use of formal assessment methods, a view that delirium is not as essential to the patient's well-being in light of more serious medical problems, and ageist attitudes. Failure to recognize delirium, identify the underlying causes, and implement timely interventions contributes to the negative sequelae associated with the condition.

In a study of interventions nurses use to assess, prevent, and treat delirium in the acute care setting, cognitive changes in older adults are often labeled as confusion, frequently accepted as part of normal aging, and rarely questioned. Confusion in a child or younger adult would be recognized as a medical emergency, but confusion in older adults may be accepted as a natural occurrence. Nurses reported that caring for patients with delirium was seen as "annoying, frustrating, and not interesting" and interfered with the "real work" of caring for a medical-surgical patient (Dahlke and Phinney, 2008, p. 45). The authors conclude that nurses are faced with the predicament of fitting care for older adults into a system that does not recognize the unique needs of this population.

Clearly, attitudes about care of older adults and education about delirium assessment, prevention, and treatment are essential to improve care outcomes. Several recent studies investigating the effect of educational interventions on nurses' knowledge and practice of delirium care reported positive findings. A quasiexperimental study conducted in ICU investigated the effect of nonpharmacological interventional training on delirium recognition and intervention strategies.

The findings support that educating nurses can help reduce the incidence of delirium through early recognition of delirium (Birge and Aydin, 2017). Research conducted by D'Avolio (Research Highlights A box) showed that a blended educational intervention on nurses' delirium knowledge and skills was effective in increasing screening of older adults with risk for delirium. Once delirium was identified, the nurses implemented nonpharmacological interventions. Dr. D'Avolio's current research focuses on engaging caregivers through a remote monitoring and technology-assisted nurse coaching intervention that offers both access and support for delirium prevention. Delirium prevention among family caregivers of older adults with dementia remains unexplored. Addressing this gap is important because family caregivers have valuable insight about subtle changes in cognition.

Precipitating Factors for Delirium

There are many predisposing and precipitating factors for delirium (Box 29.2). The risk of delirium increases with the number of risk factors present. The more vulnerable the individual, the greater the risk. Identification of high-risk patients, risk factors, early and appropriate assessment, and continued surveillance is the cornerstone of delirium prevention. Among the most predictive risk factors are immobility, functional deficits, use of restraints or indwelling catheters, medications, acute illness, infections, alcohol or drug abuse, sensory impairments, malnutrition, dehydration, respiratory insufficiency, surgery, and cognitive impairment. Unrelieved or

---

🎓 RESEARCH HIGHLIGHTS A

A Blended Educational Intervention for Delirium

Purpose: The purpose of this study was to determine the feasibility of a blended educational intervention on nurses' delirium knowledge and skills. The Delirium Education Intervention (DEI) integrated didactic education along with bedside teaching to demonstrate application of the intervention to clinical practice with a variety of adult patients. The nurse participants reported that the clinical demonstrations and an opportunity to perform delirium assessment with supervision were the highlights of the DEI.

Method: We used a quasiexperimental, one-group pretest-posttest design ($O_1 \times O_2$) design to collect data from participant nurses who evaluated patients for delirium. All of the nurses ($n = 52$) reported (1) lack of delirium education in their core curriculum and (2) lack of knowledge related to the utilization of a standardized delirium assessment tool. The study participants received a delirium packet for review before receiving an on-unit educational intervention. After the educational intervention, nurses participated in bedside teaching demonstrating delirium assessment and interventions. Nursing assessments and interventions included (1) review of medications, (2) diagnostic tests, (3) orientation, (4) sensory, (5) nutrition, (6) toileting, (7) sleep, (8) pain, (9) mobility, (10) social needs, (11) safety, and (12) nurse specialist consultation.

Results: After the study implementation, the data demonstrated that 80% of 643 patients were assessed using the Confusion Assessment Method and provided nonpharmacological interventions. Nurses screened 643 patients, 12% of patients were positive for delirium.

Conclusion: The findings highlight gaps in clinical practice, which were filled by a cost-effective, blended educational intervention. The DEI did improve the ability of nurses to provide delirium assessment and nonpharmacological interventions. The nurse participants reported that the clinical demonstrations and an opportunity to perform delirium assessment with supervision were the highlights of the DEI. This study is significant because it examined an intervention consisting of didactic, bedside teaching and a toolkit. These findings contribute to the development of a feasible, cost-effective approach to delirium detection. Future studies in implementation science are needed to determine the most effective educational interventions and the sustainability of these interventions.

Current Study: Dr. Deborah D'Avolio became interested in delirium among older adults through her experiences as a researcher, nurse practitioner, and, more importantly, as a family caregiver of loved ones with dementia. Older adults with dementia who develop delirium have a greater risk of adverse outcomes. Delirium is preventable, treatable, frequently misdiagnosed, and often not recognized by health care providers and family caregivers. In her current study, funded by the Network for the Investigation of Delirium: Unifying Scientists, Dr. D'Avolio is working toward a possible solution—engaging caregivers through a remote monitoring and technology-assisted nurse coaching intervention. Delirium prevention among family caregivers of older adults with dementia remains unexplored. Addressing this gap is important because family caregivers have valuable insight about subtle changes in cognition. This project addresses the needs of family caregivers, and offers both access and support to delirium prevention.

D'Avolio D: *Evaluation of an Educational Intervention for Increasing Delirium Recognition and Intervention Among Hospitalized Older Adults: A Feasibility Study,* 2012. Faculty Grant, Northeastern University.

BOX 29.2 Precipitating Factors for Delirium

- Age greater than 65 years
- Cognitive impairment
- Severe illness or comorbidity burden
- Hearing or vision impairment
- Current hip fracture
- Presence of infection
- Inadequately controlled pain
- Polypharmacy and use of psychotropic medications (benzodiazepines, anticholinergics, antihistamines, antipsychotics)
- Depression
- Alcohol use
- Sleep deprivation or disturbance
- Renal insufficiency
- Aortic procedures
- Anemia
- Hypoxia or hypercarbia
- Poor nutrition
- Dehydration
- Electrolyte abnormalities
- Poor functional status
- Immobilization or limited mobility
- Risk of urinary retention or constipation
- Use of invasive equipment, restraints

From American Geriatrics Society: *Clinical practice guidelines for postoperative delirium in older adults*, 2014. https://geriatricscareonline.org/ProductAbstract/american-geriatrics-society-clinical-practice-guideline-for-postoperative-delirium-in-older-adults/CL018. Accessed April 2019.

BOX 29.3 What Causes Delirium?

D	Dementia
E	Electrolytes
L	Lungs, liver, heart, kidney, brain
I	Infection
Rx	Polypharmacy, psychotropics
I	Injury, pain, stress
U	Unfamiliar environment
M	Metabolic

There is usually more than one cause.

BOX 29.4 Clinical Subtypes of Delirium

Hypoactive Delirium
- "Quiet or pleasantly confused"
- Reduced activity
- Lack of facial expression
- Passive demeanor
- Lethargy
- Inactivity
- Withdrawn and sluggish state
- Limited, slow, and wavering vocalizations

Hyperactive Delirium
- Excessive alertness
- Easy distractibility
- Increased psychomotor activity
- Hallucinations, delusions
- Agitation and aggressive actions
- Fast or loud speech
- Wandering, nonpurposeful repetitive movement
- Verbal behaviors (yelling, calling out)
- Removing tubes
- Attempting to get out of bed
- Unpredictable fluctuations between hypoactivity and hyperactivity

inadequately treated pain significantly increases the risk of delirium. Invasive equipment, such as nasogastric tubes, intravenous (IV) lines, catheters, and restraints, also contributes to delirium by interfering with normal feedback mechanisms of the body.

Medications can contribute to delirium, and all medications, particularly those with anticholinergic effects and any new medications, should be considered suspect. The Beers' Criteria for potentially inappropriate medication use in older adults is a resource for potential problem medications (American Geriatrics Society, 2015). The Beers' Criteria lists select medications that should be avoided or have the dose adjusted based on an individual's kidney function; this is critical in older adults. Baseline kidney function needs to be evaluated and monitored throughout the hospital stay. This can be done using an estimated glomerular filtration rate (eGFR). Determining the necessary dose reduction of medication by using the creatinine clearance is also important (Chapter 9). Certain high-risk medications should be avoided, if possible; however, it is equally important to start medications when needed. For example, uncontrolled pain can lead to delirium, so starting an analgesic may be the best treatment. A mnemonic representing causes of delirium can be found in Box 29.3.

Clinical Subtypes of Delirium

Delirium is categorized according to the level of alertness and psychomotor activity. The clinical subtypes are hyperactive, hypoactive, and mixed. Box 29.4 presents the characteristics of

each of hyperactive and hypoactive delirium. Because of the increased severity of illness and the use of psychoactive medications, hypoactive delirium may be more prevalent in the ICU. Although the negative consequences of hyperactive delirium are serious, the hypoactive subtype may be more often missed and is associated with a worse prognosis because of the development of complications such as aspiration, pulmonary embolism, pressure ulcers, and pneumonia.

Consequences of Delirium

Delirium is a terrifying experience for the individual and his or her family and significant others, and people often think the individual is "going crazy." Delirium is associated with increased length of hospital stay and hospital readmissions, increased services after discharge, and increased morbidity, mortality, and institutionalization, independent of age, coexisting illnesses, or illness severity (Flaherty et al, 2017; Salluh et al, 2015).

Posttraumatic stress disorder (PTSD) symptoms (nightmares, flashbacks, memories, and dreams individuals were unable to comprehend), although often not recognized, may occur in adults with delirium (Battle et al, 2017) (Chapter 28)

(Box 29.5). Resources on delirium including video descriptions of delirium by patients can be found in Box 29.6.

Although the majority of hospital inpatients recover fully from delirium, a substantial minority will never recover or recover only partially. Each episode of delirium increases the vulnerability of the brain, which further enhances the risk of dementia (Inouye, 2018; Inouye et al, 2014). The persistence of delirium after discharge may interfere with the ability to manage chronic conditions and contribute to poor outcomes (Hain et al, 2012). Further research is needed to determine the reasons for the long-term poor outcomes, whether characteristics of the delirium itself (subtype or duration) influence prognosis, and how the long-term effects might be decreased.

BOX 29.5 Patient Descriptions of Delirium Experiences

Being handcuffed to a railing among criminals in the city jail, fighting to get free and guards standing by to shoot him if he escaped

Children running around without heads; kids with animal heads

Seeing helicopters evacuating patients from an impending tornado, leaving her behind

Blood seeping through holes and cracks in my skin, forming a puddle of red around me

A horror show of people trying to kill her, ants crawling on faces, finding herself on a raft, in a space pod, in the Arctic, in the desert—each with its own terrible narrative

From Amoss M: Treating the trauma of intensive care, *Johns Hopkins Magazine*, 2013, http://hub.jhu.edu/magazine/2013/summer/ptsd-intensive-care. Accessed June 2018; Edmunds L: Delirium, *Johns Hopkins Medicine*, 2014, http://www.hopkinsmedicine.org/news/publications/hopkins_medicine_magazine/features/delirium. Accessed June 2018; Hoffman J: Nightmares after the ICU, *The New York Times*, July 22, 2013, http://well.blogs.nytimes.com/2013/07/22/nightmares-after-the-i-c-u. Accessed June 2018.

BOX 29.6 Resources for Best Practice

Delirium and Dementia

Advance Directive for Dementia: www.dementia-directive.org

Hartford Institute for Geriatric Nursing: Delirium: Nursing Standard of Practice Protocol: Prevention, early recognition, and treatment; Assessment and management of delirium in older adults with dementia; Confusion Assessment Method (CAM), CAM ICU

Hartford Institute for Geriatric Nursing: Dementia Series

Hospital Elder Life Program (HELP): Program materials, Family-HELP program, The Family Confusion Assessment Method (FAM-CAM)

ICU Delirium and Cognitive Impairment Study Group: Patient and Family Report: Memories from the ICU

ICU-DIARY.org: Informal network for all health care workers interested in the ICU diary

Nursing Home Toolkit: Promoting Positive Behavioral Health: http://www.nursinghometoolkit.com/

Society of Critical Care Medicine: Clinical practice guidelines for the management of pain, agitation, and delirium in adult patients in the ICU

WeCare Advisor: http://www.programforpositiveaging.org/wecareadvisor/

ICU, Intensive care unit.

⚡ SAFETY ALERT

Older adults with risk factors for delirium should be screened for delirium upon admission to the hospital, when transitioning from one area of care to another, and before discharge to other care settings or home. Individuals who experience delirium are at risk for no recovery or partial recovery postdischarge from acute care facility (Cole et al, 2017). The highest risk for adverse events (i.e., death, hospitalization, emergency department [ED] visits) is within the first 3 months of discharge, especially for those with preexisting ADRD (Alzheimer's disease and related disorders). Older adults who don't recover may have an underlying health condition (i.e., persistent physical illness, medication toxicity, frailty) that may impact their cognitive status (Cole et al, 2017). Therefore, it is imperative that older adults experiencing delirium undergo a comprehensive geriatric assessment with a particular focus on cognitive status and potential reversible causes of delirium.

PROMOTING HEALTHY AGING: IMPLICATIONS FOR GERONTOLOGICAL NURSING

Assessment

Assessment of Delirium

Prevention of delirium is the first step in caring for vulnerable older adults who are at risk of delirium. An awareness and identification of the risk factors for delirium and a formal assessment for delirium are the first-line interventions for prevention. Delirium has been called a critical vital sign of cognitive health, and assessment should be given the same attention as other vital signs (Fick, 2018). Nurses play a pivotal role in the identification of delirium and the earlier we intervene the greater the chance for positive health outcomes.

Assessment begins with a thorough history and identification of key diagnostic features. Several instruments can be used to assess the presence and severity of delirium. To detect changes, it is very important to determine the person's baseline cognitive status. If the person cannot tell you this, family members or other caregivers who are with the older adult can be asked to provide this information. Family members and other caregivers know the person well and will notice subtle changes in behavior. They can give information about whether or not these behaviors are normal for this person and, if not, when they first appeared.

If the patient is alone, the responsible party or the institution transferring the patient can provide this information by phone. Determining baseline cognitive function is essential. Do not assume the person's current mental status represents his or her usual state, and do not attribute altered mental status to age alone or assume that dementia is present. All older adults, regardless of their current cognitive function, should have a formal assessment with valid and reliable instruments to identify possible delirium when admitted to the hospital.

The Montreal Cognitive Assessment (MoCA) is a brief screening instrument to detect cognitive impairment. It is a paper-and-pencil tool that takes about 10 minutes to administer and is scored out of 30 points. The test and instructions are freely available on the MoCA website (www.mocatest.org). No permission is required for clinical or educational use. Chapter 7 provides more information regarding assessment of cognitive status. Several delirium-specific assessment instruments are available, such as the Confusion Assessment Method (CAM) (Inouye et al, 1990) and the NEECHAM (Neelon and Champagne) Confusion Scale (Neelon et al, 1996).

The CAM-ICU is another instrument specifically designed to assess delirium in an intensive care population and has been validated for use in critically ill, nonverbal patients who are on mechanical ventilation (Ely et al, 2001; Rigney, 2006). Many acute care settings have made the CAM a part of the electronic medical record. The Confusion Assessment Method-Family Assessment Method (CAM-FAM) (Steis et al, 2012) can be used to identify symptoms based on reports from family members and highly correlates with the CAM in identification of delirium (Flanagan and Spencer, 2015) (Box 29.6).

Once an individual is identified as having delirium, reassessment should be conducted every shift. Documenting specific objective indicators of alterations in mental status rather than using the global, nonspecific term confusion will lead to more appropriate prevention, detection, and management of delirium and its negative consequences. Findings from assessment using a validated instrument are combined with nursing observation and assessment, chart review, and physiological findings such as laboratory studies. Delirium often has a fluctuating course and can be difficult to recognize, so assessment must be ongoing and include multiple data sources.

Interventions

Nonpharmacological Approaches

Because the etiology of delirium is multifactorial, interventions that are multicomponent and address more than one risk factor are more likely to be effective. There is strong evidence that multicomponent interventions can prevent delirium in both medical and surgical settings and less robust evidence that they reduce the severity of delirium. Early engagement of the interdisciplinary team in assessment of risk factors as soon as the patient is admitted is key to a successful delirium prevention program (Oberai et al, 2018). Continued research is needed to evaluate what type of approach has the most beneficial effect in different clinical settings. A person-centered approach to care, rather than a disease-focused approach, can yield the best outcomes (Box 29.7).

A well-researched program of delirium prevention in the acute care setting, the Hospital Elder Life Program (HELP) (Hshieh et al, 2015; Inouye et al, 1999), focuses on managing six risk factors for delirium: cognitive impairment, sleep deprivation, immobility, visual impairments, hearing impairments, and dehydration. An interprofessional team of geriatric specialists, including nurses, takes a multifaceted approach to maintain cognitive and physical function for high-risk older adults, maximize independence at discharge, assist with transitions, and prevent unnecessary readmissions. Trained volunteers are also utilized in the HELP program. The program is used in more than 200 hospitals in the United States and internationally. The Family-HELP program (Box 29.6), an adaptation and extension of the original HELP program, trains family caregivers in selected protocols (e.g., orientation, therapeutic activities, vision, and hearing). Initial research demonstrates

> ### BOX 29.7 Clinical Exemplar: Delirium
>
> Mrs. J is an 88-year-old female who has end-stage kidney disease (ESKD) who experienced sudden onset of confusion resulting in admission to an acute care facility. Her husband reports she was talking to her deceased mother at night when she would go to bed and had a sudden onset of urinary incontinence. The internal medicine resident notified the adult/gerontological nurse practitioner (AGNP) that Mrs. J has dementia, and that we should consider discontinuing dialysis and consider hospice care. The AGNP had known Mrs. J for many years and was surprised by this new diagnosis of dementia. The important first step of providing the best care for Mrs. J was performing a comprehensive geriatric assessment of that included evaluating her cognitive status and possible reversible cause of acute confusion. The laboratory studies indicated that Mrs. J was not uremic (buildup of waste products normally excreted by the kidneys). The computed tomography (CT) scan of her brain revealed no evidence of stroke, acute changes, or other brain injury. White blood cell count was elevated, there were positive findings on urinalysis and this, along with the clinical picture of a sudden onset of urinary incontinence and hallucinations, indicated that she had a urinary tract infection. Her confusion abated after a course of antibiotics.
>
> Lessons learned from this encounter are not to assume an older adult with acute confusion has dementia and that a comprehensive geriatric assessment must be conducted to determine the reason for delirium. Most importantly, nurses must advocate for older adults with possible delirium as the AGNP did for this patient. The AGNP educated the internal medicine resident about delirium in older adults with ESKD so he will not make another premature diagnosis that could result in an inappropriate discontinuation of a lifesaving intervention. After discharge from the hospital, Mrs. J returned to dialysis until her death 2 years later. Mrs. J and her husband were so grateful that the AGNP took the time to come to know her and cared enough to be her advocate.

From Debra Hain, PhD, ARNP, AGPCNP-BC, Nephrology Nurse Practitioner.

that active engagement of family caregivers in preventive interventions for delirium is feasible and supports a culture of family-oriented care.

Most of the interventions in the HELP program can be considered quite simple and part of good nursing care. Interventions include the following: offering herbal tea or warm milk instead of sleeping medications, keeping the ward quiet at night by using vibrating beepers instead of paging systems, removing catheters and other devices that hamper movement as soon as possible, encouraging mobilization, assessing and managing pain, and correcting hearing and vision deficits. Fall risk–reduction interventions—such as bed and chair alarms, low beds, reclining chairs, volunteers to sit with restless patients, and keeping routines as normal as possible with consistent caregivers—are other examples of interventions. Box 29.8 presents suggested interventions for delirium.

The use of an intensive care diary has been shown to assist patients to make sense of their experience of delirium and improve communication with their families about their experiences. The practice of writing a diary has been widely used in European countries, especially those in Scandinavia, since the 1970s as a low-cost technology to improve the quality of life after critical illness. ICU diaries are being implemented and evaluated in the United States, and the use of diaries may be a simple and practical nursing intervention that may reduce the level of PTSD-related symptoms for patients and relatives after critical illness (Blair et al, 2017). Entries into the diary are made

BOX 29.8   Tips for Best Practice

Prevention of Delirium

- Sensory enhancement (ensuring glasses, hearing aids, listening amplifiers)
- Mobility enhancement (ambulating at least twice a day if possible)
- Bedside presence of a family member whenever possible
- Cognitive orientation and therapeutic activities (tailored to the individual)
- Pain management
- Cognitive stimulation (if possible, tailored to individual's interests and mental status)
- Simple communication standards and approaches to prevent escalation of behaviors
- Nutritional and fluid repletion enhancement
- Sleep enhancement (sleep hygiene, nonpharmacological sleep protocol)
- Medication review and appropriate medication management
- Adequate oxygenation
- Prevention of constipation
- Minimize the use of invasive medical devices, restraints, or immobilizing devices
- Pay attention to environmental noise, light, temperature
- Normalize the environment (provide familiar items, routines, clocks, calendars)
- Minimize the number of room changes and interfacility transfers

Adapted from American College of Surgeons NSQIP and American Geriatrics Society: *Optimal perioperative management of the geriatric patient.* https://www.facs.org/,/media/fi les/quality%20programs/geriatric/acs%20nsqip%20geriatric%202016%20guidelines.ashx; and American Geriatrics Society: *Clinical practice guidelines for postoperative delirium in older adults,* 2014. http://www.sciencedirect.com/science/article/pii/S1072751514017931. Accessed February 2016.

by nurses and also by relatives during the patient's stay. The diary is written directly to the patient in everyday language using an empathetic and reflective style and therapeutic communication. It contains daily entries on the current status of the patient and descriptions of situations and surroundings in which the patient might find recognition. The text is often supported by photos (Box 29.6).

Pharmacological Approaches

Pharmacological interventions to treat the symptoms of delirium may be necessary for patients who are in danger of harming themselves or others, or if nonpharmacological interventions are not effective. However, pharmacological interventions should be viewed as one approach in a multicomponent program of prevention and treatment but should not replace thoughtful and careful evaluation and management of the underlying causes of delirium. Research on the pharmacological management of delirium is limited, but with increased understanding of the neuropathogenesis of delirium, drug therapy may become more important.

Antipsychotic drugs are routinely used to treat delirium even though the U.S. Food and Drug Administration has not approved their use for treating the condition. A systematic review and meta-analysis evaluating the effectiveness of antipsychotics for the prevention or treatment of delirium concluded that current evidence does not support the use of these medications (Neufield et al, 2016). A recent experimental study reported that the use of haloperidol (Haldol) or ziprasidone

(Geodon), as compared with placebos, in patients with acute respiratory failure or shock and hypoactive or hyperactive delirium in the ICU did not significantly alter the duration of delirium (Girard et al, 2018). Limited use of antipsychotics may be considered if the patient's life or safety is at risk because of severe agitation. If these drugs are used, it is important to reduce the duration and discontinue as soon as possible based on the older adult's clinical presentation.

The Society of Critical Care Medicine (2018) created guidelines on clinical practice for adult patients in the ICU regarding pain, agitation, and delirium (Box 29.6). These guidelines place great emphasis on the use of valid and reliable tools for assessment of (1) pain, agitation/sedation, and delirium in patients in the ICU; (2) the use of an interprofessional team approach; (3) avoidance of oversedation; (4) encouragement of more active participation in spontaneous awakening and breathing trials; (5) early mobilization programs; (6) pain management; and (7) environmental strategies to preserve sleep-wake cycles.

Caring for patients with delirium can be a challenging experience since the individual has difficulty communicating and may demonstrate disturbing behaviors, such as pulling out IV lines or attempting to get out of bed, disrupt medical treatment, and compromise their own safety or that of others. It is essential that nurses realize any behavior is an attempt to communicate something and express needs so it is important to implement strategies to address these unmet needs. Older adults experiencing delirium feel frightened and may have a sense of lost control of their lives. The calmer and more reassuring the nurse is, the safer the patient will feel. Box 29.9 presents some communication strategies that are helpful in caring for individuals experiencing delirium.

BOX 29.9   Tips for Best Practice

Communicating With a Person Experiencing Delirium

- Know the person's past patterns.
- Look at nonverbal signs, such as tone of voice, facial expressions, and gestures.
- Speak slowly.
- Be calm and patient.
- Face the person and keep eye contact; get to the level of the person rather than standing over him or her.
- Explain all actions.
- Smile.
- Use simple, familiar words.
- Allow adequate time for response.
- Repeat if needed.
- Tell the person what you want him or her to do rather than what you do not want him or her to do.
- Give one-step directions; use gestures and demonstration to augment words.
- Reassure person's safety.
- Keep caregivers consistent.
- Assume that communication and behavior are meaningful and an attempt to tell us something or express needs.
- Do not assume that the person is unable to understand or experiencing cognitive impairment.

CARE OF INDIVIDUALS WITH NEUROCOGNITIVE DISORDERS (NCDs)

Nurses provide direct care for people with NCDs in the community, hospitals, and long-term care facilities. They also work with families and staff, teaching best practice approaches to care and providing education and support. With the rising incidence of NCDs, nurses will play an even larger role in the design and implementation of evidence-based practice and provision of education, counseling, and supportive services to individuals with NCDs and their caregivers. A model caring-based nurse-managed memory center with experts in NCDs that provides comprehensive care for individuals with NCDs and their caregivers is described in Box 29.10.

The overriding goals in caring for older adults with NCDs are to maintain function and prevent excess disability, structure the environment and relationships to maintain stability, compensate for the losses associated with the disease, and create a therapeutic milieu that nurtures the personhood of the individual and maintains well-being and quality of life. Box 29.11 presents an overview of person-centered nursing interventions in the care of individuals with NCDs.

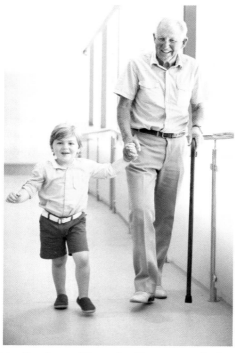

Maintaining Function and Preventing Unnecessary Decline Are Important. (©iStock.com/Squaredpixels.)

Nutrition, activities of daily living (ADLs), maintenance of health and function, safety, communication, behavioral changes, caregiver needs and support, and quality of life are the major care concerns for patients, families, and staff caring for individuals with dementia. Five common care concerns for individuals with a diagnosis of a major NCD and nursing interventions are discussed in the remainder of this chapter: communication, behavior concerns, ADL care, wandering, and nutrition. Caregiving for persons with NCDs is discussed in

BOX 29.10   An Exemplar Program for Comprehensive Dementia Care

About the Center

The Louis and Anne Green Memory and Wellness Center (MWC) is a unique Center of the Christine E. Lynn College of Nursing at Florida Atlantic University in Boca Raton, Florida. Grounded in the philosophy of caring espoused by the College, the MWC provides compassionate and innovative programs of care that reflect best practice, research, and education. The MWC is a state-designated Memory Disorder Clinic and the first adult day center in Florida to receive the designation of "Specialized Alzheimer's Services Center."

Model of Care

Clinical practice at the MWC is illuminated philosophically and operationally by caring science and utilizes a nurse practitioner (NP)-led model designed to provide comprehensive, coordinated care. NPs function as the dementia-specific care providers and care managers within a core physician-NP-psychologist-neuropsychologist-social worker team.

Services

Comprehensive memory and wellness evaluations are conducted by a trilingual interprofessional team within a patient/family-provider partnering framework. Driving assessment, physical, occupational, and speech therapy evaluations and treatment, and a cognitive rehabilitation program are also available. Hearing and honoring the story of the patient and family guide assessment, diagnosis, and ongoing care. Educational programs for caregivers, self-preservation activities such as yoga, caregiver consultations with a certified care manager, psychotherapy, a caregiver library, and caregiver support groups are offered. Support groups are offered for adult children as well as younger individuals with neurocognitive disorders. A variety of educational programs and classes are also offered for the formal and informal care providers in the community.

Adult Day Center

Provides a wide array of evidence-based therapeutic programs designed to maintain and enhance cognitive and physical function and quality of life. Activities include chair yoga, reminiscence, cognitive stimulation activities, health education (nutrition, exercise, spirituality, mental health/well-being), and creative arts such as painting and drawing, music, cards, puzzles, and board games.

Student Education and Research

Clinical practice experiences for students of the Colleges of Nursing, Medicine, Social Work, and other professions are supervised by MWC staff. Continuous engagement in research within the College of Nursing creates the possibility to advance knowledge related to care of individuals living with dementia.

From María de los Ángeles Ordóñez, DNP, CNS, APRN, GNP-BC, PMHNP-BC, Director, Louis and Anne Green Memory and Wellness Center From Memory Disorder Clinic Coordinator; Tappen R, Ordóñez M, Curtis B: Designing a nurse-managed center grounded in caring: the aesthetics of place and space, *J Art Aesthet Nurs Health Sci* 2(1): 22, 2014.

Chapter 34, and other care concerns such as falls and incontinence are discussed in earlier chapters of this book.

Differing Needs in Younger-Onset Dementia and Mild NCD

While the focus of this chapter is on care concerns of individuals with major NCDs, it is important to note that the concerns of individuals and their caregivers living with younger-onset dementia (onset before 65 years), mild NCD, and early stages

BOX 29.11 Person-Centered Nursing Interventions in Care of Individuals With NCD

- Come to know the person
- Build and nurture authentic caring relationships
- Recognize and accept the person's reality
- Obtain input from the individual, engage in shared decision making to the extent possible
- Maximize abilities to make choices
- Structure daily living to maximize remaining abilities and support limitations
- Identify characteristics of the social and physical environment that may cause distress for the person or exacerbate behavior and psychological symptoms
- Provide meaningful activities and relationships to enhance quality of life
- Ensure safety
- Monitor general health and impact of the NCD on management of other medical conditions.
- Collaborate with caregivers in the areas of problem-solving, resource access; long-range planning, emotional support, and respite
- Support advance care planning and advance directives.

NCD, Neurocognitive disorder.
Adapted from Fazio S, Pace D, Maslow K, et al: Alzheimer's Association dementia care practice recommendations, *Gerontologist* 58(S1–S9), 2018.

of major NCD are quite different. To date, the preponderance of research and intervention programs has been directed toward persons and their families living with major NCD and has focused on preparing caregivers to cope with issues such as behavior problems, incontinence, ADL care, and nursing home placement. Many of these issues are not relevant to those with younger-onset dementia and mild NCD, therefore they will not be of interest to them, and can even be frightening and misleading.

A significant number of individuals are diagnosed with dementia earlier in their lives, even as young as in their 30s and 40s. According to the Alzheimer's Association (2018), up to 5% of Americans living with Alzheimer's disease belong to that group. Therefore, the current language guidelines suggest using the term *younger-onset dementia* instead of the previously used *early-onset dementia*, since it could be confused with early stages of symptoms of dementia at any age. Individuals with younger-onset dementia report difficulties both in the process of receiving a diagnosis and afterward. Diagnosis felt "unexpected, out of time (too young to have dementia), and led to changes in self-identity, powerlessness and changes in relationships. Social exclusion was common and loss of meaningful activity exacerbated a difficult situation" (Greenwood and Smith, 2016). The individual may have dependent children at home and still be employed. They may be forced to retire and experience a loss of income, work roles, and related benefits during prime working years. Most dementia services are designed for older adults and do not meet the specific needs of younger individuals. Because the individual is younger, he or she is likely to be in better health than older adults and meeting the safety needs of someone who is still physically able can be challenging (Greenwood and Smith, 2016; Sakamoto et al, 2017).

Areas of concern for caregivers of persons with mild NCD and early-stage NCD center less on personal care needs and more on communication, behavior, and relationships. Interventions that help both the person and his or her caregiver to deal with changing roles, stress, frustration, loss, communication difficulties, and the couple relationship are particularly needed (Research Highlights B box). Continued research and development of programs of support and services for individuals with mild NCD, younger-onset stage dementia, and early stage major NCD and their caregivers are a priority, as is continued evaluation of the effectiveness of interventions in practice. Research must include the voices of those experiencing the health challenge of living with an NCD. Chapter 34 discusses caregiving for individuals with NCDs.

RESEARCH HIGHLIGHTS B

Using Narratives of Individuals and Couples Living With Mild to Moderate NCDs to Guide Practice

A descriptive phenomenological approach was used to understand the experience of living with a mild to moderate NCD from the person, the spouse, and the dyad of the person and spouse. Six couples were interviewed individually and as a couple and asked to tell the story of their experience living with dementia. The themes that emerged from the caregiver narratives indicated that they were trying to do the best they could to ensure that their loved ones receive optimal health care and that life can be as pleasurable as possible. Persons living with an NCD were also trying to do their best from the perspective of slowing the disease and not being a burden to their spouse.

Communication difficulties with a loved one can be a major source of stress for caregivers. Persons living with mild-moderate NCDs experienced frustration in trying to communicate effectively and, most importantly, they were quite aware of their own difficulties. Opportunities for both the person living with the disease and the caregiver to express frustration and anger over communication difficulties and receive validation of their feelings are important aspects of clinical practice. Effective strategies to maintain and enhance communication and deal effectively with stress can be taught and role-modeled. Participation in programs that enhance cognitive and physical functioning and slow the progression of the disease process were of great importance to the individual. Feeling competent and capable in learning new things, participating in stimulating activities, socializing with people who have similar interests, and feeling respected rather than patronized were noted as valuable components of the day program they attended. This finding reinforces the importance of person-centered respectful communication.

The findings support the importance of living one day at a time by doing the best one can do to promote health and not becoming overwhelmed by what the future may bring. This study provides evidence of how important it is to take a person-centered approach to care and to develop programs that consider the needs of persons living with NCDs, their spouse, and the couple dyad throughout the trajectory of the disease process. Interventions to enhance couples' relationships are important and promote more positive outcomes for the person living with dementia and for the caregiver. Programs and activities aimed at helping the person maintain maximum cognitive, physical, and social function for as long as possible are important and are beneficial for both the person and the caregiver.

NCDs, Neurocognitive disorders.
From Hain D, Touhy TA, Sparks-Compton D, et al: Using narratives of individuals and couples living with early stage dementia to guide practice, *J Nurs Appl Rev Res* 4:82–93, 2014.

Need for Ongoing Assessment

Assessment of individuals and their caregivers is an especially important nursing role and the quality of dementia care is contingent upon quality, person-centered assessment and care planning. Person-centered assessment is an opportunity to come to know the person and the caregiver and develop caring relationships. Beginning at the time of diagnosis and continuing through the course of the disease, individuals and their caregivers require ongoing assessment and monitoring of disease progression and response to therapy. Needs change as the disease progresses and "what matters most at any particular time in the course of the patient's experience will change as the disease progresses, the person's perspective changes, and challenges occur that may threaten equilibrium and/or provide opportunities for growth" (Molony et al, 2018, p. S37). Assessment should occur at least every 6 to 12 months or any time there is a change in behavior or increase in the rate of decline. In long-term care facilities, frequency of assessment is guided by regulations. Medicare now provides reimbursement for a clinical visit that includes a multidimensional assessment and comprehensive care plan for persons with a documented cognitive impairment.

The focus of assessment is to support strengths and abilities while supporting losses and limitations to enhance the ability of the individual and the caregiver to "live fully with dementia" (Molony et al, 2018, p. S36). The perspective of the individual living with dementia should be a priority and the individual should be involved in all discussions to the extent possible. Ongoing assessment of the ability to comprehend benefits and harm of treatment options is essential when making decisions related to health care or obtaining informed consent. Molony and colleagues (2018) provide detailed guides for comprehensive person-centered assessment. Caregiver assessment is discussed in Chapter 34.

End-of-Life Discussions

Meaningful advance care planning is usually not addressed until far too late in the course of the illness. It is not common for health care providers to inform individuals and families about end-stage dementia and the need to make wishes and preferences for care early in the disease trajectory while the individual can express their desires. Health care professionals need to provide education, explore values and preferences, and facilitate end-of-life planning. The individual and the family will need information, honest communication, and ongoing support as they think about these important decisions. Although in the early stages, the palliative care movement has gained momentum as health care professionals recognize the value of palliative care in this population. Palliative care should be considered when a person is diagnosed so there is a skilled and competent team of experts supporting the individual with NCD and their family along the disease trajectory.

Palliative care occurs on a spectrum from the beginning of a life-limiting illness where care needs may not be substantial to later in the disease trajectory where care needs are the greatest and the person meets eligibility for hospice care. Palliative care is focused on symptom management, comfort care, and psychological, social, and spiritual support. In addition, bereavement support is available for the caregivers when the individual with dementia dies (Chapter 35). There is ample evidence that individuals with end-stage dementia receive suboptimal end-of-life care and often experience unrelieved suffering that not only deprives the patient and family of compassionate end-of-life care but can also result in overly aggressive treatments (Lee et al, 2017; Sekerak and Stewart, 2014). "Health care surrogates and clinicians struggle with decision making and are often unsure whether the care they provide is what the individual would want" (Gaster, 2017, p. 2175).

Standard advance directives may not be helpful for individuals with dementia since they typically address what the individual would want if death were imminent or there is a permanent coma state. "Dementia is a chronic, life-limiting disease with a variable trajectory. Dementia progresses slowly over many years and leaves people with a long time-frame of diminishing cognitive function and loss of ability to guide their own care" (Gaster, 2017). Gaster (2017) has developed an advanced directive for dementia that addresses the differing needs at varying stages of dementia and suggests that this may be a document that individuals could complete before they develop signs of dementia and could be used as a supplement to a standard advance directive form (Box 29.6).

COMMUNICATION

The experience of losing cognitive and expressive abilities is both frightening and frustrating. Early in the disease, word finding is difficult (anomia), and remembering the exact facts of a conversation is challenging (Box 29.12). As the disease progresses, memory, speech, and communication also decline. NCD affects both receptive and expressive communication components and alters the way people speak. Automatic language skills (e.g., hello) are retained for the longest time. The person may wander from the topic of conversation and bring up seemingly unrelated topics. The person may fail to pick up on humor or sarcasm or abstract ideas in conversation. Nonverbal and behavioral responses become especially important as a way of communication as verbal skills become more limited. As the disease progresses, verbal output may become less frequent although the grammar and sounds of the language being spoken remain relatively intact. Even in the later stages of NCD, the individual may understand more than you realize and still

---

BOX 29.12 Patient's Descriptions of Communication Difficulties

"I forget words. Sometimes it doesn't mean much and other times it means a great deal. I have learned ways to avoid making mistakes like shaking hands when I don't remember the person's name, joking, looking at their faces for a reaction."

(Hain et al, 2014, p. 85)

"There are a range of things you want to say over and over because I think it was a word that was important to say and I'll forget . . . I hope that what I am saying makes sense."

(Hain et al, 2010)

needs opportunities for interaction and caring communication, both verbal and nonverbal.

Communication is essential to person-centered care. No group of patients is more in need of supportive relationships with skilled, caring healthcare providers. People with cognitive and communication impairments "depend on their relationship with and trust of others to provide emotional support, solve problems, and coordinate complex activities" (Buckwalter et al, 1995, p. 15). Communication with individuals experiencing NCDs requires special skills and patience. Caregivers experience frustration and anxiety when their attempts to communicate with the person who has cognitive limitations are unsuccessful, often resulting in short interactions which are mostly task-oriented. Communication may be seen as a low priority because of heavy workloads and lack of awareness of the importance of communication. When individuals cannot communicate their needs, behavioral problems may occur (Machiels et al, 2017).

To effectively communicate with a person experiencing an NCD, it is essential to believe that the person is trying to communicate something that is important. It is critical that nurses recognize various ways a person with dementia may communicate by knowing the person. The best thing we can do is discover what the person is trying to communicate and intervene according to needs. However jumbled it may seem, the person is attempting to tell us something. It is our responsibility as professionals to understand and know how to respond. The person with NCD cannot change his or her communication; we must change ours (Box 29.13).

Nurses can overcome barriers to communication by taking a person-centered approach. Such framework encourages coming to know the person by taking time to find out the individual's story: "Who am I?" In some cases, people are unable to disclose a lifetime of memories but taking the time to find out what their background is and making time to be present can contribute to effective communication. A recent communication intervention in long-term care demonstrated the value of tailored communication plans based on the abilities of the residents with dementia. The plans included how to communicate with the individual, how the resident communicates with others, and an "about me" section which gives information about

the person (where he or she was born, work, family, interests). The results suggest that the communication intervention had positive effects on residents' quality of living (QOL) and care providers' mood and burden (McGilton et al, 2017).

Evidence-Based Communication Strategies

Classic research conducted by Ruth Tappen of Florida Atlantic University (Boca Raton, FL) and colleagues (Tappen et al, 1997, 1999) provided insight into communication strategies that were helpful in creating and maintaining a therapeutic relationship with people with moderate to major NCDs. In these studies, conversations between 23 participants in the middle and late stages of AD and a clinical nurse specialist were analyzed to clarify what type of communication techniques were helpful in creating and maintaining a therapeutic relationship. Interviewers were told to "avoid frequent correction of the individual, encourage the individual to engage in conversation, attempt to make the conversation as meaningful as possible, and to assume that any attempt at communication had some meaning to it, however difficult it was to ascertain that meaning" (Tappen et al, 1997, p. 250).

Findings of this study were compared with recommendations in the literature, and specific communication strategies were developed. More than 80% of the participants' responses were relevant in the context of the conversation. The research challenged some of the commonly held beliefs about communication with persons with NCDs, for example, avoiding the use of open-ended questions and keeping communication focused only on simple topics, task-oriented topics, and questions that can be answered with yes or no responses.

Findings of this study provided suggestions for specific communication strategies effective in various nursing situations and hope for nurses to establish meaningful relationships that nurture the personhood of people with NCDs (Box 29.14). Communication strategies differ depending on the purpose of communication (e.g., performing ADLs, encouraging expression of feelings). Approaches to communication must be adapted not only to the person's ability to understand but also to the purpose of the interaction. What is appropriate for assessment may be a barrier to conversation that is designed to facilitate expression of concerns and feelings.

In the past, structured programs of reality orientation (RO) (orienting the person to the day, date, time, year, weather, upcoming holidays) were often used in long-term care facilities and chronic psychiatric units as a way to stimulate interaction and enhance memory. This intervention is still often noted as being of benefit to persons with NCDs. However, structured RO may place unrealistic expectations on persons with major NCDs and may be distressing if the individual cannot remember these things. Families and professional caregivers can often be heard asking people with NCDs to name relatives, state their birth year, and remember other current facts. One can imagine how upsetting and demoralizing this might be to a person unable to remember.

This does not imply that we should not orient the person to daily activities, time of day, and other important events, but it should be offered without the expectation that the person will

---

BOX 29.13 Tips for Best Practice

Communicating Effectively With Individuals With Dementia

Envision a tennis game: The caregiver is like the tennis coach, and whenever the coach plays the ball, he or she seems to be able to put the ball where the person on the other side of the net can return it. The coach also returns the ball in such a way as to keep the rally going; he or she does not return it to score a point or win the match, but rather returns the ball so that the other player is able to reach it and, with encouragement, hit it back over the net again. Similarly, in our communication with people with dementia, our conversation and words must be put into play in such a way such that the person can respond effectively and share thoughts and feelings.

From Kitwood T: *Dementia reconsidered: the person comes first,* Bristol, 1999, Open University Press.

BOX 29.14 Four Useful Strategies for Communicating With Individuals Experiencing Cognitive Impairment

Simplification Strategies

Simplification strategies are useful with ADLs:

- Give one-step directions.
- Speak slowly and clearly.
- Allow time for response.
- Reduce distractions.
- One-to-one conversations; avoid multiple caregivers interacting at the same time.
- Give clues and cues as to what you want the person to do. Use gestures or pantomime to demonstrate what it is you want the person to do—e.g., put the chair in front of the person, point to it, pat the seat, and say, "Sit here."

Facilitation Strategies

Facilitation strategies are useful in encouraging expression of thoughts and feelings:

- Establish commonalities.
- Share self.
- Allow the person to choose subjects to discuss.
- Speak as if to an equal.
- Use broad openings, such as "How are you today?"
- Employ appropriate use of humor.
- Follow the person's lead.

Comprehension Strategies

Comprehension strategies are useful in assisting with understanding of communication:

- Identify time confusion (in what time frame is the person operating at the moment?).
- Find the theme (what connection is there between apparently disparate topics?). Recognize an important theme, such as fear, loss, or happiness.
- Recognize the hidden meanings (what did the person mean to say?).

Supportive Strategies

Supportive strategies are useful in encouraging continued communication and supporting personhood:

- Introduce yourself, and explain why you are there. Reach out to shake hands, and note the response to touch.
- If the person does not want to talk, go away and return later. Do not push or force.
- Sit closely, and face the person at eye level.
- Limit corrections.
- Use multiple ways of communicating (gestures, touch).
- Search for meaning in all communication.
- Know the person's past life history, and daily life experiences and events.
- Recognize feelings, and respond.
- Treat the person with respect and dignity.
- Show interest through body posture, facial expression, nodding, and eye contact. Assume a pleasant, relaxed attitude.
- Attend to vision and hearing losses.
- Do not try to bring the person to the present or use reality orientation. Go to where the person is, and enjoy the conversation.
- When leaving, thank the person for his or her time and attention, and information.
- Remember that the quality, not the content or quantity, of the interaction is basic to therapeutic communication.

ADLs, Activities of daily living.

remember. Caregivers can provide orienting information as part of general conversation (e.g., "It's quite warm for December 10, but it will be a beautiful day for our lunch date"). Rather than structured RO, a better approach is to go where the person is in his or her own world rather than trying to bring the person's world into yours. For example, if the individual insists that he or she needs to leave the house to meet the school bus, it is more helpful to ask the individual to talk about the times he or she did this activity rather than informing the person that his or her children are grown and do not ride the school bus.

Validation therapy, developed by Naomi Feil in the 1980s, involves following the person's lead and responding to feelings expressed rather than interrupting to supply factual data. Communication techniques include using nonthreatening words to establish understanding; rephrasing the person's words; maintaining eye contact and a gentle tone of voice; responding in general terms when meaning are unclear; and using touch if appropriate (Scales et al, 2018). "Although the evidence base for validation therapy is underdeveloped, the concept of honoring the feelings of the person living with dementia has face validity as part of person-centered dementia care" (Scales et al, 2018, p. S95). Helping families and caregivers understand validation therapy can assist in enhancing quality time with their loved ones.

PROMOTING HEALTHY AGING: IMPLICATIONS FOR GERONTOLOGICAL NURSING

Care and communication that respect and value the dignity and the worth of every person and use of research-based communication techniques will enhance communication and personhood. Gerontological nurses who are sensitive to communication and interaction patterns can assist both formal and informal caregivers in using more personal verbal and nonverbal communication strategies that are humanizing and show respect for the person.

BEHAVIOR CONCERNS AND NURSING MODELS OF CARE

Behavioral and psychological symptoms of dementia (BPSD) occur in 97% (at least one symptom) of individuals with NCD and can become more common as the disease progresses. Symptoms often co-occur, increasing their impact even more. BPSDs occur in clusters or syndromes identified as psychosis (delusions and hallucinations), agitation, aggression, depression, anxiety, apathy, disinhibition (socially and sexually inappropriate behaviors), motor disturbances, nighttime behaviors, and appetite and eating problems. The most common symptoms are apathy, depression, and anxiety. Symptoms often co-occur, increasing their impact even more. Lifelong psychiatric disorders (Chapter 28) and their management may also affect the development of these symptoms (Kales et al, 2015).

BPSDs appear to be a consequence of multiple, but sometimes modifiable, interacting factors. These factors are both external and internal and result in part from heightened vulnerability to the environment as cognitive function declines. Neurodegeneration associated with dementia also plays a role in BPSDs (Molony et al, 2018; Scales et al, 2018). The quality of the interaction between the caregiver and the person living with dementia also influences behavioral symptoms (Kales et al, 2015). A recent scoping review of the evidence on determinants of BPSDs reported the following causes as common across several behavioral symptoms: neurodegeneration, type of dementia, severity of cognitive impairments, declining functional abilities, caregiver burden, poor communication, and boredom (Kolanowski et al, 2017).

BPSD should be viewed as a form of communication that is meaningful (rather than a problem), an expression of unmet needs, and/or a reflection of lower tolerance for stressors in the physical and psychosocial environment. They are the individual's best attempt to communicate a variety of unmet needs. BPSDs symptoms cause a great deal of distress to the person and the caregivers, contribute to increased financial cost, caregiver burden, and nursing stress, poor quality of life for the person with dementia and their caregiver, significant declines in function, risk for physical abuse, and often precipitate institutionalization (Austrom et al, 2018; Kolanowski et al, 2017). Clinically significant BPSDs, if untreated, are associated with faster disease progression than in the absence of such symptoms.

Several nursing models of care are helpful in recognizing and understanding the behavior of individuals with NCDs and can be used to guide practice and assist families and staff in providing care from a more person-centered framework. The *Progressively Lowered Stress Threshold (PLST)* model and the *Need-Driven Dementia-Compromised Behavior (NDDB)* model focus on the close interplay between person, context, and environment. These models propose that behavior is used to communicate or express, in the best way the person has available, unmet needs (physiological, psychosocial, disturbing environment, uncomfortable social surroundings) and/or difficulty managing stress as the disease progresses.

The Progressively Lowered Stress Threshold Model

The PLST model (Hall, 1994; Hall and Buckwalter, 1987) was one of the first models used to plan and evaluate care for people with NCDs in every setting. The model suggests that environmental antecedents produce stress, which is met by a coping response that is compromised by the impact of dementia (Scales et al, 2018). Symptoms such as agitation are a result of a progressive loss of the person's ability to cope with demands and stimuli when the person's stress threshold is exceeded. An example is the person who becomes agitated in response to excess noise in the environment (loudspeaker, loud talk). Some stressors that may trigger these symptoms are presented in Box 29.15.

Using this model, care is structured to decrease the stressors and provide a safe and predictable environment. Positive outcomes from use of the model include improved sleep; decreased sedative and tranquilizer use; increased food intake and weight; increased socialization; decreased episodes of aggressive, agitated, and disruptive behaviors; increased caregiver satisfaction with care; and increased functional level. Box 29.16 presents the principles of care derived from the PLST model.

BOX 29.15 Stressors Triggering BPSDs (PLST Model)

Fatigue
Change of environment, routine, or caregiver
Misleading stimuli or inappropriate stimulus levels
Internal or external demands to perform beyond abilities
Physical stressors such as pain, discomfort, acute illness, and depression

BPSDs, Behavioral and psychological symptoms of dementia; *PLST*, Progressively Lowered Stress Threshold.

BOX 29.16 Principles of Care Derived From PLST Model

1. Maximize functional abilities by supporting all losses in a prosthetic manner.
2. Establish a caring relationship and provide the person with unconditional positive regard.
3. Use patient behaviors indicating anxiety and avoidance to determine appropriate limits of activity and stimuli.
4. Teach caregivers to try to find causes of behavior and to observe and evaluate verbal and nonverbal responses.
5. Identify triggers related to discomfort or stress reactions (factors in the environment, caregiver communication).
6. Modify the environment to support losses and promote safe function.
7. Evaluate care routines and responses on a 24-hour basis and adjust plan of care accordingly.
8. Provide as much control as possible; encourage self-care, offer choices, explain all actions, do not push or force the person to do something.
9. Keep the environment stable and predictable.
10. Provide ongoing education, support, care, and problem solving for caregivers.

PLST, Progressively Lowered Stress Threshold.
Adapted from Hall GR, Buckwalter KC: Progressively Lowered Stress Threshold: a conceptual model for care of adults with Alzheimer's disease, *Arch Psychiatr Nurs* 1:399–406, 1987.

Need-Driven Dementia-Compromised Behavior Model

The NDDB model (Algase et al, 2003; Kolanowski, 1999; Richards et al, 2000) is a framework for the study and understanding of behavioral symptoms. All behaviors have meaning and are a form of communication, particularly as verbal communication becomes more limited. The NDDB model proposes that the behavior of persons with NCDs carries a message of need that can be addressed appropriately if the person's history and habits, physiological status, and physical and social environment are carefully evaluated. Rather than behavior being viewed as disruptive, it is viewed as having meaning and expressing needs. Behavior reflects the interaction of background factors (cognitive changes as a result of dementia, gender, ethnicity, culture, education, personality, responses to stress) and proximal factors (physiological needs such as hunger or pain, mood, physical environment [e.g., light, noise, temperature]) with social environment (e.g., staff stability and mix, presence of others).

Optimal care is provided by manipulating the proximal factors that precipitate behavior and by maximizing strengths and minimizing the limitations of the background factors. For instance, sleep disruptions are common in people with dementia. If the person is not getting adequate sleep at night, agitated or aggressive behavior during the day may signal the need for more rest. Interventions to modify proximal factors interfering with sleep, such as noise, frequent awakenings during the night, and daytime boredom, can help meet the need for rest and sleep and decrease agitation or aggression.

PROMOTING HEALTHY AGING: IMPLICATIONS FOR GERONTOLOGICAL NURSING

Assessment

The focus must be on understanding that behavioral expressions communicate distress, and the response is to investigate the possible sources of distress and intervene appropriately. There are many possible reasons for BPSDs. After ruling out medical problems (e.g., pneumonia, dehydration, impaction, infection/sepsis, fractures, pain, or depression) as a cause of the behavior, continued assessment to identify why distressing symptoms are occurring is important. Conditions such as constipation or urinary tract infections can cause great distress for individuals with cognitive impairment and may lead to marked changes in behavior. In a study of community-dwelling older adults with dementia, 36% had undetected illness associated with BPSDs, making adequate assessment and treatment essential. Side effects of drugs or drug-drug interactions can also contribute to the development of symptoms (Kales et al, 2015).

Pain and discomfort are associated with aggressive behaviors in individuals with dementia. After careful assessment of other possible causes of pain or discomfort, treatment with a trial of analgesics should be considered. Treatment of pain is challenging, especially in today's opioid epidemic where providers often are afraid to prescribe these medications. In some circumstances the person is not receiving enough medicine to control the pain so may act out due to an inability to verbally express symptoms. It is essential for nurses to discover nonpharmacological approaches to pain and to advocate for appropriate pharmacological interventions.

Understanding what triggers behavior is essential for development of interventions that address the individual's unmet need. Fear, discomfort, unfamiliar surroundings and people, illness, fatigue, depression, need for autonomy and control, caregiver approaches, communication strategies, and environmental stressors are frequent precipitants of behavioral symptoms. "For the individual with late-stage dementia, a good deal of their discomfort comes from nonphysiological sources, for example, from difficulty sorting out and negotiating everyday life activities" (Kovach et al, 1999, p. 412). The need for socialization and support and stimulation to address boredom can also contribute to changes in behavior. "Lack of meaningful activity is cited by people living with dementia and family members as one of the most persistent and critical unmet needs. The provision of individualized meaningful activities may help prevent or alleviate BPSDs by enhancing quality of life through engagement, enhanced social interaction, and opportunities for self-expression and self-determination" (Scales et al, 2018, p. S96). Box 29.17 presents precipitating factors for BPSDs.

BOX 29.17 Conditions Precipitating Behavioral Symptoms in Individuals With Dementia

- Communication deficits
- Pain or discomfort
- Acute medical problems
- Sleep disturbances
- Perceptual deficits
- Depression
- Need for social contact
- Hunger, thirst, need to toilet
- Loss of control
- Misinterpretation of the situation or environment
- Crowded conditions
- Changes in environment or people
- Noise, disruption
- Being forced to do something
- Fear
- Loneliness
- Psychotic symptoms
- Fatigue
- Environmental overstimulation or understimulation
- Depersonalized, rushed care
- Restraints
- Psychoactive drugs

BOX 29.18 Framework for Asking Questions About the Meaning of Behavior

What?
What is being sought? What is happening? Does the behavior have a physical or emotional component or both? What are the person's responses? What would be done if the person was 20 years old instead of 80? What is the behavior saying? What is the emotion being expressed?

Where?
Where is the behavior occurring? What are the environmental triggers?

When?
When does the behavior most frequently occur: after activities of daily living (ADLs), family visits, mealtimes?

Who?
Who is involved? Other residents, caregivers, family?

Why?
What happened before? Poor communication? Tasks too complicated? Physical or medical problem? Person being rushed or forced to do something? Has this happened before and why?

What Now?
Approaches and interventions (physical, psychosocial)
Changes needed and by whom?
Who else might know something about the person or the behavior or approaches? Communicate to all and include in plan of care.

Putting yourself in the place of the person with an NCD and trying to see the world from his or her eyes will help you understand his or her behavior. Questions of what, where, why, when, who, and what now are important components of the assessment of behavior. Box 29.18 presents a framework for asking

BOX 29.19   Examples of Behavior and Environmental Modification Strategies for Managing BPSD

Behavior	Strategy
Hearing voices	Evaluate hearing or adjust amplification of hearing aids.
	Assess quality and severity of symptoms.
	Determine whether they present an actual threat to safety or function.
	Assess noise around patient's room (e.g., staff talking in hallway).
Aggression	Determine and modify underlying causes of aggression (e.g., pain, caregiver interaction, being forced to do something).
	Teach caregiver not to confront individual, use distraction, observe facial expression and body posture, leave individual alone if safe, return later for the task (e.g., bathing).
	Create a calmer, more soothing environment.
Repetitive questioning	Respond with a calm, reassuring voice.
	Use calm touch for reassurance.
	Place warm water bottle covered with soft fleece cover on the lap or abdomen.
	Inform individual of events only as they occur.
	Structure daily routines.
	Involve person in meaningful activities.

BPSDs, Behavioral and psychological symptoms of dementia.
Adapted from Kales H, Gitlin L, Lyketsos C, et al: Management of neuropsychiatric symptoms of dementia in clinical settings: recommendations from a multidisciplinary expert panel, *J Am Geriatr Soc* 62:762–769, 2014.

questions about the possible meanings and messages behind observed behavior. Asking caregivers to play back the situation "as if in a movie" is often helpful in eliciting details and understanding the circumstances associated with the problematic behavior. Except in late-stage NCD, when verbal communication may be problematic, the perspective of the individual should be elicited to determine what he or she can describe about the situation. It is also important to understand what aspect of the behavior is most problematic or distressing for the individuals and the caregiver and design individually tailored interventions (Molony et al, 2018).

Use of a behavioral log or diary over a 2- to 3-day period to track when the behavior occurs, the circumstances, and the response to interventions is recommended and required in SNFs. The Behave-AD, the Cohen-Mansfield Agitation Inventory, and the Neuropsychiatric Inventory for Nursing Homes are examples of reliable instruments that can be used in assessment. The WeCare Advisor (Box 29.6) is a web-based application designed to enable family caregivers to assess, manage, and track BPSDs using nonpharmacological approaches. Further testing of the tool is ongoing (Kes et al, 2017) (Box 29.6). Box 29.19 presents examples of some common behaviors and possible strategies.

Interventions
Pharmacological Approaches

All evidence-based guidelines endorse an approach that begins with comprehensive assessment of the behavior and possible causes followed by the use of nonpharmacological interventions as a first line of treatment except in emergency situations when BPSDs could lead to imminent danger or compromise safety (American Geriatrics Society, 2014). However, it is also recognized that medications, including antipsychotics, may be necessary and appropriate for the palliation of patient distress when nonpharmacological interventions fail (Kerns et al, 2018). The atypical psychotics may be more effective for symptoms

such as anger, aggression, and paranoid ideas (Kales et al, 2015). Strict federal regulations monitor the use of psychotropic medications in SNFs. Antipsychotic medication use in nursing homes may be considered after all possible causes of behavior have been investigated and, if used, should be given at the lowest possible dosage for the shortest period of time, monitored closely for side effects, and subject to gradual dose reduction and rview (CMS, 2013). Pharmacological approaches may be considered, in addition to nonpharmacological approaches, if there has been a comprehensive assessment of reversible causes of behavior; the person presents a danger to self or others; nonpharmacological interventions have not been effective; and the risk/benefit profiles of the medications have been considered. There must be documentation of all care planning related to the individual's behaviors and use and effectiveness of nonpharmacological interventions.

Nonpharmacological Approaches

Nonpharmacological approaches are person-centered approaches that are informed by careful assessment of the cause and meaning of the individual's behavioral and psychological symptoms. Nonpharmacological approaches can be grouped into three categories: (1) those targeting the individual, (2) those targeting the caregiver, and (3) those targeting the environment (Kales et al, 2015). Approaches include the following: sensory practices (aromatherapy, massage, multisensory stimulation, bright-light therapy), psychosocial practices (validation therapy, reminiscence therapy, music therapy, animal-assisted therapy, meaningful activities), environmental design (e.g., special care units, homelike environment, gardens, safe walking areas), changes in mealtime and bathing environments, consistent staffing assignments and structured care protocols (bathing, mouth care), and support for caregivers (Scales et al, 2018). There is a large amount of literature on nonpharmacological interventions, and these approaches are recommended in the culture change movement (Chapter 32). In general, these interventions, despite a lack of rigorous testing, have shown promise for improving quality of life for persons with dementia at home and in residential care, have no harmful side effects, and require minimal to moderate investment (Scales et al, 2018). Nonpharmacological approaches with the strongest evidence-base are those based on family caregiver interventions, which have been shown to have greater effect than antipsychotics (Kales et al, 2015).

Use of iPads to both prevent and address agitation in individuals with dementia holds interesting possibilities. While further research is needed related to what types of applications and programs are effective, preliminary findings suggest that even individuals with major NCDs were able to interact with the device and episodes of agitation and restlessness were reduced (Ross et al, 2015). Box 29.20 presents an exemplar on use of the iPad to calm agitation behavior. Music therapy, personalized for the individual, has been shown to be an enjoyable and effective approach to alleviate BPSDs and enhance well-being (Scales et al, 2017).

Continued attention to translating these interventions into real-world practice across settings in feasible and cost-effective ways is needed. Resnick and colleagues (2016) note that "despite regulatory requirements and availability of educational materials focused on nonpharmacological management of BPSDs, less than 2% of nursing homes consistently implement behavioral approaches" (p. 571). Identified barriers include lack of knowledge, skills, and hands-on experience with the many different approaches, belief that medication use is more effective, lack of belief in the effectiveness of nonpharmacological approaches, inadequate staffing, and lack of administrative support.

A toolkit approach that provides a variety of interventions may be useful in improving the use of nonpharmacological interventions in long-term care facilities. An online toolkit, *Promoting Positive Behavioral Health: A Nonpharmacological Toolkit for Senior Living Communities* (Kolonowski and Van Haitsma, 2013), provides many resources for nurses, other caregivers, and families including behavior assessment tools, clinical decision-making algorithms, and evidence-based approaches to ameliorate or prevent BPSDs (Box 29.6). Practical suggestions about using nonpharmacological approaches that emerged from focus groups with direct care providers are presented in Box 29.21.

Despite recommendations for treatment of BPSD, antipsychotic medications are often given as the first-line response across settings without appropriate assessment of factors contributing to the behaviors (Kolanowski et al, 2017). Prevalence rates of antipsychotic use declined in nursing homes as a result of several proactive measures (Chapter 32). However, rates of antipsychotic use among individuals with dementia living in the community are rising. Recommendations are to expand the efforts to curb the use of these drugs beyond nursing homes (Marselas, 2018).

A study of providers and families investigating factors influencing the use of medications for BPSDs despite recommendations reported the following: (1) medications were seen as safer and more effective than nonpharmacological interventions;

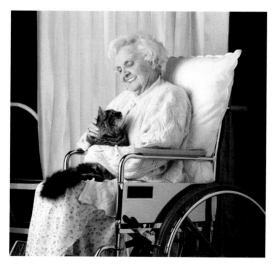

A nursing home resident enjoying pet therapy. (Courtesy Corbis.)

(2) medications are frequently prescribed by physicians who are not familiar with nonpharmacological approaches; and (3) resources that facilitate and encourage alternate therapies are inadequate and underutilized. Families and experienced nurses in the study recognized there were times when even "optimally applied . . . nonmedication approaches did not work to relieve patients' distressing symptoms . . . caregivers expressed a strong need to alleviate patient distress and were uncomfortable about not intervening when symptoms affected quality of life. If medications were effective, almost all caregivers supported their use as worth the potential side effects" (Kerns et al, 2017, p. e41).

Clearly, the role of medications and nonpharmacological interventions to treat BPSDs needs further study. Health care providers and family caregivers can benefit from training, better access, and practical assistance in implementing approaches for behavioral concerns. Behavioral health programs must be better integrated with medical care for individuals with dementia. Collaborative care management programs for the treatment of AD, often led by advanced practice nurses, have been shown to improve quality of care, decrease the incidence of BPSDs, and decrease caregiver stress (Callahan et al, 2006; Fortinsky et al, 2014; Reuben et al, 2014).

PROVIDING CARE FOR ACTIVITIES OF DAILY LIVING

The losses associated with dementia interfere with the person's communication patterns and ability to understand and express thoughts and feelings. Perceptual disturbances and misinterpretations of reality contribute to fear and misunderstanding. Often, bathing and the provision of other ADL care, such as dressing, grooming, and toileting, are the cause of much distress for both the person with dementia and the caregiver.

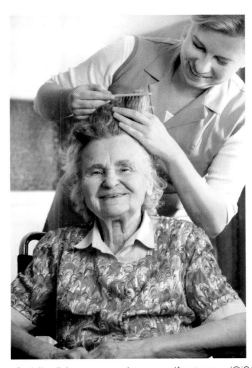

Activities of daily living care enhance self-esteem. (©iStock.com/AlexRaths.)

BOX 29.22 Understanding Behavior: Seeing Through the Eyes of the Person
You are asleep in the chair at home when suddenly you are awakened by a person you have never seen before trying to undress you. Then he or she puts you naked into a hard, cold chair and wheels you down a hallway. Suddenly cold water hits you in the face and the person is touching your private areas. You don't understand why the person is trying to do this to you. You are embarrassed, frightened, cold, and angry. You hit and scream at this person and try to get away.

Bathing

Bathing is the ADL associated with the highest frequency of BPSDs expressions of distress (Scales et al, 2018). Bathing is an essential aspect of everyday life that most people enjoy. However, bathing can be perceived as a personal attack by persons with dementia who may respond by screaming or striking out. In institutional settings, a rigid focus on tasks or institutional care routines, such as a shower three mornings each week, can contribute to the distress and precipitate distressing behaviors. Being touched or bathed against one's will violates the trust in caregiver relationships and can be considered a major affront (Rader and Barrick, 2000). The behaviors that may be exhibited are not deliberate attacks on caregivers by a violent person, but rather a way to express self in an uncertain situation. The message is, in the words of Rader and Barrick: "Please find another way to keep me clean, because the way you are doing it now is intolerable" (2000, p. 49) (Box 29.22).

PROMOTING HEALTHY AGING: IMPLICATIONS FOR GERONTOLOGICAL NURSING

Assessment and Interventions

In research conducted in nursing homes, Rader and Barrick (2000) have provided comprehensive guidelines for bathing people with NCDs in ways that are pleasurable and decrease distress. Asking the question "What is the easiest, most comfortable, least frightening way for me to clean the person right now?" guides the choice of interventions. *Bathing Without a Battle* is an approach that can be used to create a better bathing experience for people with dementia. These techniques show positive results in reducing BPSD (Box 29.23). Another innovative approach being investigated in Sweden is caregiver singing and the use of background music during ADL care in nursing homes. Caregivers play and sing familiar songs during care routines. When compared to usual care practices, this approach enhanced the expression of positive moods and emotions, increased the mutuality of communication, and reduced aggression and resistive care behaviors (Hammar et al, 2011). The provision of oral care is another ADL that often precipitates anxiety and agitation for individuals with NCDs. Person-centered oral care protocols are discussed in Chapter 15.

BOX 29.23   Tips for Best Practice

Techniques for Bathing Without a Battle

1. Rethink the bathing experience.
   - Make the experience comfortable and pleasurable.
   - Consider what makes the individual feel good.
   - Do not be in a hurry.
2. Approach techniques such as "let's go get freshened up for the day" and avoiding bathing terminology (e.g., "it's time for your bath") can create a more positive environment. Tell person it is time to get freshened up and try not to ask, "do you want a bath?" because the answer may be no.
3. Have the room ready.
   - Keep the room warm and low-lit.
   - Hand-held showerhead wets one area at a time.
   - Have a large towel or blanket to preserve dignity and keep person warm.
4. Begin bathing least sensitive area first.
   - Wash legs and feet first, followed by arms, trunk, perineum area, and face last.
5. Save washing hair until last or do separately.
6. Use distraction techniques.
   - Consider using music, calming sounds, or singing songs that the person likes.
   - Consider having the person hold a towel or something to provide distraction.
7. Consider a towel bath, under clothes bath, or sponge bath

From University of North Carolina Cecil G. Sheps Center for Health Services Research: *Bathing without a battle.* http://bathingwithoutabattle.unc.edu/. Accessed July 2018.

WANDERING

Wandering associated with NCDs is one of the most difficult management problems encountered in home and institutional settings. Wandering is a complex behavior and is not well understood. Wandering is defined as "a syndrome of dementia-related locomotion behavior having a frequent, repetitive, temporally disordered and/or spatially disoriented nature that is manifested in lapping, random and/or pacing patterns, some of which is associated with eloping, eloping attempts or getting lost unless accompanied" (Algase et al, 2007, p. 696). Risk factors for wandering include visuospatial impairments, anxiety and depression, poor sleep patterns, unmet needs, and a more socially active and outgoing premorbid lifestyle. One in five persons with dementia wander and wandering frequency tends to increase as cognitive function decreases (Futrell et al, 2014). There is a need for more research and interventions for this behavior.

Wandering presents safety concerns in all settings. Wandering behavior affects sleeping, eating, safety, and the caregiver's ability to provide care, and it also interferes with the privacy of others. The behavior can lead to falls, elopement (leaving the home or facility), injury, and death. The stimulus for wandering arises from many internal and external sources. Wandering can be considered a rhythm, intrinsically and extrinsically driven. Box 29.24 presents insight into the behavior of wandering from the perspective of individuals with an NCD.

BOX 29.24   Patient Perspectives on Wandering Behavior

"Wandering and restlessness is one of the by-products of Alzheimer's disease. . . . When the darkness and emptiness fill my mind, it is totally terrifying. . . . Thoughts increasingly haunt me. The only way I can break the cycle is to move."

(Davis, 1989, p. 96)

"Very often, I wander around looking for something which I know is very pertinent, but then after a while I forget all about what it was I was looking for. When I'm wandering around, I'm trying to touch base with—anything, actually. If anything appeared, I'd probably enjoy it, or look at it or examine it and wonder how it got there. I feel very foolish when I'm wandering around not knowing what I'm doing and I'm not always quite sure how to do any better. It's not easy to figure out what the heck I'm looking for."

(Henderson, 1998)

PROMOTING HEALTHY AGING: IMPLICATIONS FOR GERONTOLOGICAL NURSING

Assessment and Interventions

Careful assessment of physical problems that may trigger wandering, such as acute illness, exacerbations of chronic illness, fatigue, medication effects, and constipation, is important. Unmet needs or pain can increase wandering (Futrell et al, 2014). Wandering behaviors can be predicted through careful observation and awareness of the person's patterns. For example, if the person with dementia starts wandering or trying to leave the home in the afternoon every day, meaningful activities such as music, exercise, and refreshments can be provided at this time. Research suggests that wandering may be less likely to occur when the person is involved in social interaction. There are also several instruments to assess risk for wandering, and nurse researcher May Futrell and her colleagues (2010, 2014) developed an evidence-based protocol for wandering. Box 29.25 presents other suggested interventions.

Wandering behavior may also result in people with NCD going outside and getting lost. All people with dementia are considered capable of getting lost. Caregivers must prevent people with NCDs from leaving homes or care facilities unaccompanied, register the person in the Alzheimer's Association Safe Return program and Silver Alert if available, and have a plan of action in case the person does become lost. Protocols must be in place in care facilities that include identification of individuals who may wander; a wandering prevention program to ensure safety; and an elopement response plan (Futrell et al, 2014). There are a number of assistive technology devices and programs that can enhance the safety of persons who wander (Chapter 20).

NUTRITION

Older adults with NCDs are particularly at risk for weight loss and inadequate nutrition. Weight loss often becomes a considerable concern in later stages and 76% of institutionalized older adults with NCDs need to be fed, refuse food, or choke

BOX 29.25   Tips for Best Practice

Interventions for Wandering or Exiting Behaviors

- Face the person and make direct eye contact (unless this is interpreted as threatening).
- Gently touch the person's arm, shoulders, back, or waist if he or she does not move away from a door or other exit.
- Call the person by his or her formal name (e.g., Mr. Jones).
- Listen to what the person is communicating verbally and nonverbally; listen to the feelings expressed.
- Repeat specific words or phrases, or state the need or emotion (e.g., "You need to go home." You're worried about your husband.").
- If such repetition fails to distract the person, accompany him or her, talking calmly, repeating phrases and the emotion you identify.
- Provide orienting information only if it calms the person. If it increases distress, stop talking about the present situations. Do not "correct" the person or belittle his or her agenda.
- At intervals, redirect the person toward the facility or his or her home by suggesting: "Let's walk this way now" or "I'm so tired, let's turn around."
- If orientation and redirection fail, continue to walk, allowing the person control but ensuring safety.
- Make sure you have a backup person, but he or she should stay out of eyesight of the person.
- Have someone call for help if you are unable to redirect. Usually the behavior is time limited because of the person's attention span and the security and trust between you and the person.

Adapted from Rader J, et al: How to decrease wandering, a form of agenda behavior, *Geriatr Nurs* 6(4):196–199, 1985.

BOX 29.26   Myths and Facts About PEG Tubes in Advanced Dementia and End-of-Life Care

Myths

- PEGs prevent death from inadequate intake.
- PEGs reduce aspiration pneumonia.
- PEGs improve albumin levels and nutritional status.
- PEGs assist in healing pressure injuries.
- PEGs provide enhanced comfort for people at the end of life.
- Not feeding people is a form of euthanasia, and we cannot let people starve to death.

Facts

- PEGs do not improve quality of life.
- PEGs do not reduce risk of aspiration and increase the rate of pneumonia development. In one study, the use of feeding tubes was associated with an increased risk of pressure injuries among nursing home residents with advanced cognitive impairment (Teno et al, 2012).
- PEGs do not prolong survival in dementia.
- Nearly 50% of patients die within 6 months following PEG tube insertion.
- PEGs cause increased discomfort from both the tube presence and the use of restraints.
- PEGs are associated with infections, gastrointestinal symptoms, and abscesses.
- PEG tube feeding deprives people of the taste of food and contact with caregivers during feeding.
- PEGs are popular because they are convenient and labor beneficial.

PEG, Percutaneous endoscopic gastrostomy.
Data from Aparanji K, Dharmarajan T: Pause before a PEG: a feeding tube may not be necessary in every candidate, *J Am Med Dir Assoc* 11:453–456, 2010; Teno J, Gozalo P, Mitchell S, et al: Feeding tubes and the prevention or healing of pressure ulcers, *Arch Intern Med* 172(9):697–701, 2012; Vitale C, Monteleoni C, Burke L, et al: Strategies for improving care for patients with advanced dementia and eating problems: optimizing care through physician and speech pathologist collaboration, *Ann Longterm Care* 17:32–39, 2009.

on liquid or solid foods. Nutritional concerns are a major source of distress for people living with NCDs and their caregivers and are identified as a top-10 research priority (Abelhamid et al, 2016). Some of the predisposing factors to nutritional inadequacy include lack of awareness of the need to eat, depression, loss of independence in self-feeding, agnosia, apraxia, vision impairments (deficient contrast sensitivity), wandering, pacing, and behavior disturbances. Weight loss increases the risk for infection, pressure injury development, poor wound healing, and hospitalization and is associated with higher mortality and morbidity rates. Nurses, as members of interprofessional teams, play a significant role in assessing nutrition in older adults with NCDs. Chapter 14 discusses nutritional needs and interventions in depth.

Tube Feeding in End-Stage Dementia

Increasing evidence indicates that tube feeding in the end-stage of dementia does not prolong survival or improve quality of life. In fact, enteral feeding increases the risk of several complications, including aspiration and pressure injuries (Box 29.26). The proportion of nursing home residents with advanced dementia receiving feeding tubes has decreased by 50% between 2000 and 2014. However, even though feeding tube use decreased across racial groups, it has remained relatively higher among black residents (Mitchell et al, 2016). The American Geriatrics Society (AGS) (2014) does not recommend feeding tubes for older adults with advanced dementia and suggests that careful hand feeding is at least as good as tube feeding for the outcomes of death, aspiration pneumonia, functional status, and patient comfort.

As discussed in Chapter 14, food and eating are closely tied to socialization, comfort, pleasure, love, and the meeting of basic biological needs. Feeding is often equated with caring, and not providing adequate nutrition may be viewed as cruel and inhumane. Decisions about feeding tube placement are challenging and require thoughtful discussion with patients and caregivers, who should be free to make decisions without duress and with careful consideration of the patient's advance directives, if available. Many considerations factor into decisions families and providers make about enteral feeding, including the individual's wishes in an advanced directive, cultural, religious and ethical beliefs, legal and financial concerns, and emotions.

Most feeding tube insertions occur during acute hospitalization and decisions to place a feeding tube are often taken without completely exhausting every means to maintain a normal oral intake. Research has shown that discussions surrounding the decision are often inadequate (Teno et al, 2015). Discussion about advance directives and feeding support should begin early in the course of NCDs rather than waiting until a crisis develops. The best advice for individuals is to state preferences for the use of a feeding tube in a written advance directive. Individuals should be given information about the risks and benefits of enteral feeding in the end stages of NCDs (see Box 29.6 for reference to an advanced directive in dementia). The decision should never be understood as a question of tube feeding versus no feeding. No family member should be made to feel that he or she is starving his or her loved one to death if a decision is made not to institute enteral feeding. Efforts to provide nutrition should continue, and patients should be able to take any type of nutrition they desire any time they desire (Ying, 2015). Regardless of the decision, an important nursing role is to journey with the patient's loved ones, providing support and encouraging expression of feelings. Making these decisions is very difficult and loved ones "have to make peace with their decisions" (Teno et al, 2015).

PROMOTING HEALTHY AGING: IMPLICATIONS FOR HEALTHY AGING

Assessment and Interventions

There has been little research on specific interventions to support food and fluid intake in individuals with NCDs and results of a systematic review found no definitive evidence on effectiveness, or lack of effectiveness, of specific interventions. Further research is needed and should include individuals with different NCDs, at different stages, and in different settings. However, Abdelhamid and colleagues (2016) suggest that individuals and their caregivers have to deal with eating problems despite a lack of evidence. Some promising interventions reported include: (1) establishing a routine so that the individual does not have to remember time and places for eating; (2) continue to serve foods and fluids that the person likes and has always eaten; (3) provide nutrient-dense foods (e.g., peanut butter, protein bars, yogurt); (4) pay attention to mealtime ambience; (5) allow as much time as needed to eat the foods that are preferred; (6) make food available 24 hours a day; and (7) allow the person to follow his or her accustomed eating schedule (e.g., late breakfast, early dinner). Other suggestions to enhance food intake are presented in Box 29.27. Comprehensive nutritional assessment and nursing interventions for nutritional concerns are discussed in Chapter 14.

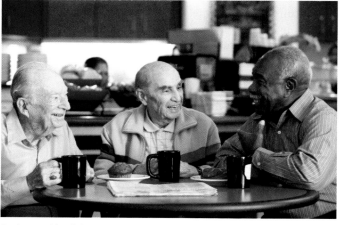

A pleasurable dining experience. (©iStock.com/monkeybusinessimages.)

BOX 29.27 Tips for Best Practice

Improving Intake for Individuals With Neurocognitive Disorders

- Serve only one dish at a time.
- Provide only one utensil at a time.
- Consider using a "spork" (combination spoon-fork).
- Serve finger foods such as fried chicken, chicken strips, pizza in bite-size pieces, fish sticks, sandwiches.
- Serve soup in a mug.
- Remove any hot items or items that should not be eaten.
- Cut up foods before serving.
- Sit next to the person at his or her level.
- Demonstrate eating motions that the person can imitate.
- Use hand-over-hand feeding technique to guide self-feeding.
- Use verbal cueing and prompting (e.g., take a bite, chew, swallow).
- Use gentle tone of voice, and avoid scolding or demeaning remarks.
- Provide verbal encouragement to participate in eating by talking about food taste and smell.
- Offer small amounts of fluid between bites.
- Help person focus on the meal at hand; turn off background noise, remove clutter from the table.
- Avoid patterned dishes or table coverings.
- Use red plates/glasses/cups; food intake may increase when food is served with high-contrast tableware.
- Use unbreakable dishes that will not slide around.
- Serve smaller, more frequent meals rather than expecting the person to complete a big meal.
- Family style meals.
- Eat with carers.
- Involve in preparation of food, smelling the food cook.

Data from Dunne T, Neargarder S, Cipolloni P, et al: Visual contrast enhances food and liquid intake in advanced Alzheimer's disease, *Clin Nutr* 23(4):533–538, 2004; Spencer P: *How to solve eating problems common to people with Alzheimer's and other dementias.* https://www.caring.com/articles/alzheimers-eating-problems. Accessed June 2015; and How to solve eating problems common to people with Alzheimer's and other dementias. https://www.caring.com/articles/alzheimers-eating-problems. Accessed June 2018; Abdelhamid et al: Effectiveness of interventions to directly support food and drink intake in people with dementia: a systematic review and meta-analysis, *BMC Geriatrics* 16:26, 2016.

NURSING ROLES IN THE CARE OF PERSONS WITH DEMENTIA

Caregiving for someone with an NCD by family members, or formal caregivers, requires special skills, knowledge of evidence-based practice, and a deep understanding of the person. Caring is paramount and it is not an area of nursing that "just anyone can do" (Splete, 2008, p. 11). A major focus of nursing education and continued education of practicing nurses should be on providing in-depth information on best practice care of individuals with NCDs. Current practice often does not reflect person-centered care and can cause great distress and poor outcomes for the individual and their caregivers.

Rader and Tornquist (1995) reflect on the knowledge required and provide a view of caregiving roles that is quite useful and understandable for all caregivers. The authors have found that nurses and family caregivers can truly relate to the practical wisdom in these words.

Magician role: To understand what the person is trying to communicate both verbally and nonverbally, we must be a magician who can use our magical abilities to see the world through the eyes, the ears, and the feelings of the person. We know how to use tricks to turn an individual's behavior around or prevent it from occurring and causing distress.

Detective role: The detective looks for clues and cues about what might be causing distress and how it might be changed. We have to investigate and know as much about the person as possible to be a good detective.

Carpenter role: By having a wide variety of tools and selecting the right tools for the job, we build individualized plans of care for each person.

Jester role: Many people with NCDs retain their sense of humor and respond well to the appropriate use of humor. This does not mean making fun of but rather sharing laughter and fun. "Those who love their work and do it well employ good doses of humor as part of the care of others, and for self-care" (Rader and Barrick, 2000, p. 42). The jester spreads joy, is creative, energizes, and lightens the burdens (Laurenhue, 2001; Rader and Barrick, 2000).

Fig. 29.1 presents a nursing situation that one nurse experienced in caring for individuals with NCDs who was

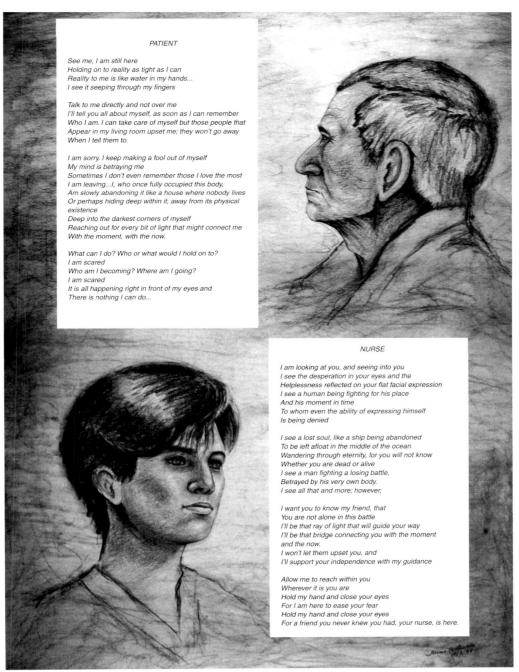

Fig. 29.1 Nurse and Patient. (Copyright ©1998 by Jaime Castaneda, Lake Worth, FL.)

being admitted to a nursing home. Written from the perspective of the nurse and his knowledge of the patient, the story provides insight into important nursing responses, such as providing person-centered care, implementing therapeutic communication, and establishing meaningful relationships. It is a lovely example of expert gerontological nursing for individuals and a fitting way to end this chapter.

KEY CONCEPTS

- Nurses must advocate for thorough assessment of any older adult who appears to be experiencing cognitive decline and inability to function in important aspects of life. Evidence supports that the pathology of Alzheimer's-type dementia is present years before the person may have symptoms so it is important to consider self-reported changes in cognitive function, that may warrant further evaluation. Caregiver reports of changes in a loved one's cognitive function is also an important indicator for evaluation of cognitive status.

- Delirium results from the interaction of predisposing factors (e.g., vulnerability on the part of the individual due to predisposing conditions such as cognitive impairment, severe illness, and sensory impairment) and precipitating factors/insults (e.g., medications, procedures, restraints, iatrogenic events). Delirium is characterized by an acute onset, fluctuating levels of consciousness, and frequent misperceptions and illusions. It often goes unrecognized and is attributed to age or dementia. Individuals with NCDs are more susceptible to delirium. Knowledge of risk factors, preventive measures, and treatment of underlying medical problems are essential to prevent serious consequences.

- Acute illness (e.g., urinary tract infections, respiratory tract infections), medications, and pain are frequently the causes of delirious states in older adults. In individuals with NCDs, a change in environment can precipitate delirium. Always make sure you consider medications as a cause.

- In older adults experiencing delirium, a new diagnosis of a NCD cannot be made until the delirium is resolved.

- It is essential to view all behavior as meaningful and an expression of needs. The focus must be on understanding that behavioral expressions communicate distress, and the response is to investigate the possible sources of distress and intervene appropriately.

- All evidence-based guidelines endorse an approach that begins with comprehensive assessment of the BPSDs and possible causes followed by the use of nonpharmacological interventions as a first line of treatment except in emergency situations when BPSDs could lead to imminent danger or compromise safety, or as palliative care approach when the individual is distressed and nonpharmacological interventions have not lead to alleviation of symptoms.

- Fear, discomfort, unfamiliar surroundings and people, illness, fatigue, depression, need for autonomy and control, caregiver approaches, communication strategies, and environmental stressors are frequent precipitants of behavioral symptoms.

- Individuals with NCDs respond best to calmness and patience, adaptations of communication techniques, and environments and relationships that enhance function, support limitations, ensure safety, and provide opportunities for a meaningful quality of life. Because individuals may be unable to express their feelings and needs in ways that are easily understood, the gerontological nurse must always try to understand the world from their perspective.

NURSING STUDY: MAJOR NCD: BEHAVIOR

Pat is an 83-year-old retired nurse who was diagnosed with major neurocognitive disorder (NCD) 3 years ago. Her other diagnoses include hypertension and osteoarthritis. She had a hip replacement 6 years ago and also has pain in her shoulders and knees from the osteoarthritis and some limitation of movement that affects her mobility. She lives with her daughter, who has brought her to the clinic for a medication check.

Her daughter tells you, the nurse, that things have not been going well. The daughter states that Pat has been verbally and physically abusive to her when she tries to bathe and dress her. She hits her and screams "You're hurting me!" The daughter says that her mother was a very fastidious person and always wanted to look nice, so she cannot understand why she resists bathing and dressing. The daughter tries to give her mother a shower at least every other day, but the battles have gotten so bad that she has not been able to keep this schedule. The daughter tells you that her mother never took showers, preferring either a tub bath or sponge bathing at the sink. However, the shower is more convenient for the daughter and her mother cannot get in the whirlpool tub at her house. She is concerned over her mother's appearance and also deeply hurt that her mother has been so mean to her. Her mother has been a lovely woman

and never acted like this before. She asks you what she can do and if her mother needs some kind of tranquilizer.

Based on the nursing study, develop a nursing care plan using the following procedure[a]:

- List Pat's comments that provide subjective data.
- List information that provides objective data.
- From these data, identify and state, using an accepted format, two nursing diagnoses you determine are most significant to Pat at this time. List two of Pat's strengths that you have identified from the data.
- Determine and state outcome criteria for each diagnosis. These must reflect some alleviation of the problem identified in the nursing diagnosis and must be stated in concrete and measurable terms.
- Plan and state one or more interventions for each diagnosed concern. Provide specific documentation of the source used to determine the appropriate intervention. Plan at least one intervention that incorporates Pat's existing strengths.
- Evaluate the success of the intervention. Interventions must correlate directly with the stated outcome criteria to measure the outcome success.

[a]Students are advised to refer to their nursing diagnosis text and identify possible or potential problems.

CRITICAL THINKING QUESTIONS AND ACTIVITIES

1. What internal and external factors could be influencing Pat's behavior?
2. What nursing framework for understanding behavior would be helpful in this situation?
3. Discuss some specific interventions that might be helpful in promoting comfort during bathing for persons with dementia.
4. What type of communication techniques would be helpful in assisting with ADLs for a person with dementia?
5. How might you help the daughter in understanding and reacting to her mother's behavior?

RESEARCH QUESTIONS

1. What barriers do nurses encounter in recognizing delirium in hospitalized older adults?
2. How does delirium influence the ability of older adults discharged from the hospital to manage their care (i.e., medications)?
3. What is the relationship between hospitalized older adults with delirium and 30-day rehospitalization?
4. What are student nurses' feelings about caring for individuals with NCDs?
5. What types of programs affect the health and well-being of older adults with NCDs?
6. What nonpharmacological interventions are most effective in the home setting for individuals with NCDs who wander?
7. What are the effects of an interprofessional team approach to for individuals with BSPDs who reside in nursing homes?
8. What type of dining options encourage intake in long-term care facilities?
9. Do educational programs for informal and formal caregivers of older persons with NCDs improve understanding and management of behavioral problems?

REFERENCES

Algase DL, Beel-Bates C, Beattie ERA: Wandering in long-term care, *Ann Longterm Care* 11:33–39, 2003.

Algase DL, Moore DH, Vandeweerd C, Gavin-Dreschnack DJ: Mapping the maze of terms and definitions in dementia-related wandering, *Aging Ment Health* 11:686–698, 2007.

Abdelhamid A, Bunn D, Copley M, et al: Effectiveness of interventions to directly support food and drink intake in people with dementia: systematic review and meta-analysis, *BMC Geriatr* 16:26, 2016.

American Geriatrics Society 2015 Beers Criteria Update Expert Panel: American Geriatrics Society 2015 updated Beers Criteria for potentially inappropriate medication use in older adults, *J Am Geriatr Soc* 63(11):2227–2246, 2015.

American Geriatrics Society: *Choosing wisely: ten things physicians and patients should question*, 2015. https://www.choosingwisely.org/societies/american-geriatrics-society/. Accessed April 2019.

American Psychiatric Association: *Diagnostic and statistical manual of mental disorders*, ed 5, Washington, DC, 2013, American Psychiatric Association.

Alzheimer's Association: *Younger/early onset Alzheimer's & Dementia*, 2018. https://www.alz.org/alzheimers_disease_early_onset.asp.

Austrom MG, Boustani M, LaMantia MA: Ongoing medical management to maximize health and well-being for persons living with dementia, *Gerontologist* 58(Suppl 1):S48–S57, 2018.

Battle CE, James K, Bromfield T, Temblett P: Predictors of post-traumatic stress disorder following critical illness: a mixed methods study, *J Intensive Care Soc* 18(4):289–293, 2017.

Blair KTA, Eccleston SD, Binder HM, McCarthy MS: Improving the patient experience by implementing an ICU diary for those at risk of post-intensive care syndrome, *J Patient Exp* 4(1):4–9, 2017.

Callahan CM, Boustani MA, Unverzagt FW, et al: Effectiveness of collaborative care for older adults with Alzheimer disease in primary care: a randomized controlled trial, *JAMA* 295: 2148–2157, 2006.

Centers for Medicare and Medicaid Services (CMS): *Center for clinical standards and quality/survey and certification group* (Memo), May 14, 2013. http://www.cms.gov/Medicare/Provider-Enrollment-and-Certification/SurveyCertificationGenInfo/Downloads/Survey-and-Cert-Letter-13-35.pdf. Accessed June 2018.

Cole MG, McCusker J, Bailey R, et al: Partial and no recovery from delirium after hospital discharge predict increased adverse events, *Age Ageing* 46:90–95, 2017.

Dahlke S, Phinney A: Caring for hospitalized older adults at risk for delirium: the silent, unspoken piece of nursing practice, *J Gerontol Nurs* 34:41–47, 2008.

Ely EW, Margolin R, Francis J, et al: Evaluation of delirium in critically ill patients: validation of the Confusion Assessment Method for the intensive care unit (CAM-ICU), *Crit Care Med* 29:1370–1379, 2001.

Evans J: Person-centered care and culture change, *Caring Ages* 18(8):6, 2017.

Fazio S, Pace D, Maslow K, Zimmerman S, Kallmyer B: Alzheimer's Association dementia care practice recommendations, *Gerontologist* 58(Suppl 1):S1–S9, 2018a.

Fazio S, Pace D, Flinner J, Kallmyer B: The fundamentals of person-centered care for individuals with dementia, *Gerontologist* 58(Suppl 1):S10–S19, 2018b.

Fick DM: The critical vital sign of cognitive health and delirium: whose responsibility is it? *J Gerontol Nurs* 44(8):3–5, 2018.

Flanagan NM, Spencer G: Informal caregivers and detection of delirium in postacute care: a correlational study of the confusion assessment method (CAM), confusion assessment method-family assessment method (CAM-FAM) and DSM-IV criteria, *Int J Older People Nurs* 11(3):176–183, 2015.

Fortinsky RH, Delaney C, Harel O, et al: Results and lessons learned from a nurse practitioner-guided dementia care intervention for primary care patients and their family caregivers, *Res Gerontol Nurs* 7(3):126–137, 2014.

Forsberg MM: Delirium update for postacute care and long-term care settings: a narrative review, *J Am Osteopath Assoc* 117:32-38, 2017.

Futrell M, Melillo KD, Remington R, Schoenfelder DP: Evidence-based practice guideline: wandering, *J Gerontol Nurs* 36:6–16, 2010.

Futrell M, Melillo KD, Remington R, Butcher HK: Evidence-based practice guideline: wandering, *J Gerontol Nurs* 40(11): 16–23, 2014.

Gaster B, Larson EB, Curtis JR: Advance directives for dementia: meeting a unique challenge, *JAMA* 318(22):2175–2176, 2017.

Gilster SD, Boltz M, Dalessandro JL: Long-term care workforce issues: practice principles for quality dementia care, *Gerontologist* 58(Suppl 1):S103–S113, 2018.

Girard TD, Exline MC, Carson SS, et al: Haloperidol and ziprasidone for treatment of delirium in critical illness, *N Engl J Med* 379:2506–2516, 2018.

Greenwood N, Smith R: The experiences of people with young-onset dementia: a meta-ethnographic review of the qualitative literature. *Maturitas* 92:102-109, 2016.

Hain D, Dunn DJ, Tappen RM: Patient-provider partnership in a memory disorder center, *J Am Acad Nurse Pract* 23(7):351–356, 2011.

Hain DJ, Tappen R, Diaz S, Ouslander JG: Cognitive impairment and medication self-management errors in older adults discharged home from a community hospital, *Home Healthc Nurse* 30(4):246–254, 2012.

Hain DJ, Touhy TA, Compton Sparks D, et al: Using narratives of individuals and couples living with early stage dementia to guide practice, *J Nurs Pract Appl Rev Res* 4:82–93, 2014.

Hain D, Touhy T, Engstrom G: What matters most to carers of people with mild to moderate dementia as evidence for transforming care, *Alzheimers Care Today* 11:162–171, 2010.

Hall GR: Caring for people with Alzheimer's disease using the conceptual model of progressively lowered stress threshold in the clinical setting, *Nurs Clin North Am* 29:129–141, 1994.

Hall GR, Buckwalter KC: Progressively lowered stress threshold: a conceptual model for care of adults with Alzheimer's disease, *Arch Psychiatr Nurs* 1:399–406, 1987.

Hammar LM, Emami A, Engström G, Götell E: Communicating through caregiver singing during morning care situations in dementia care, *Scand J Caring Sci* 25(1):160–168, 2011.

Hshieh TT, Yue J, Oh E, et al: Effectiveness of multicomponent nonpharmacological delirium interventions: a meta-analysis, *JAMA Intern Med* 175(4):512–520, 2015.

Inouye SK, Bogardus ST Jr, Charpentier PA, et al: A multicomponent intervention to prevent delirium in hospitalized older patients, *N Engl J Med* 340:669–676, 1999.

Inouye SK, van Dyck CH, Alessi CA, Balkin S, Siegal AP, Horwitz RI: Clarifying confusion: the confusion assessment method: a new method for detection of delirium, *Ann Intern Med* 113:941–948, 1990.

Inouye SK, Westendorp RG, Saczynski JS: Delirium in elderly people, *Lancet* 383:911–922, 2014.

Inouye SK: Delirium-a framework to improve acute care for older persons, *J Am Geriatr Soc* 66(3):446–451, 2018.

Kales HC, Gitlin LN, Lyketsos CG: Assessment and management of behavioral and psychological symptoms of dementia, *BMJ* 350:h369, 2015.

Kales HC, Gitlin LN, Stanislawski B, et al: We Care Advisor™: the development of a caregiver-focused, web-based program to assess and manage behavioral and psychological symptoms of dementia, *Alzheimer Dis Assoc Disord* 31(3):263–270, 2017.

Kerns JW, Winter JD, Winter KM, Kerns CC, Etz RS: Caregiver perspectives about using antipsychotics and other medications for symptoms of dementia, *Gerontologist* 58(2):e35–e45, 2018.

Kolanowski AM: An overview of the need-driven dementia-compromised behavior model, *J Gerontol Nurs* 25:7–9, 1999.

Kolanowski A, Boltz M, Galik E, et al: Determinants of behavioral and psychological symptoms of dementia: a scoping review of the evidence, *Nurs Outlook* 65:515–529, 2017.

Kolanowski A, Van Haitsma K: *Promoting positive behavioral health: a non-pharmacologic toolkit for senior living communities*, 2013. https://www.nursinghometoolkit.com/toolkitoverview.html. Accessed June 2018.

Laurenhue K: Each person's journey is unique, *Alzheimers Care Q* 2:79–83, 2001.

Lee RP, Bamford C, Poole M, McLellan E, Exley C, Robinson L: End of life care for people with dementia: the views of health professionals, social care service managers and frontline staff on key requirements for good practice, *PLoS One* 12(6):e0179355, 2017.

Lepore M, Lines LM, Wiener JM, Gould E: Person-centered and person-directed dementia care, *Generations ACL Suppl* 79-81, 2017.

Machiels M, Metzelthin SF, Hamers JP, Zwakhalen SM: Interventions to improve communication between people with dementia and nursing staff during daily nursing care: a systematic review, *Int J Nurs Stud* 66:37–46, 2017.

Marselas K: Not just a nursing home problem: antipsychotic use increasing in elderly, community-dwelling dementia patients, *McKnight's Long-Term Care News*, April 24, 2018. https://www.mcknights.com/news/aarps-elizabeth-carter-efforts-to-reduce-off-label-use-need-to-be-expanded/article/760609/. Accessed July 2018.

McGilton KS, Rochon E, Sidani S, et al: Can we help care providers communicate more effectively with persons having dementia living in long-term care homes? *Am J Alzheimers Dis Other Demen* 32(1):41–50, 2017.

Mitchell SL, Mor V, Gozalo PL, Servadio JL, Teno JM: Tube feeding in US nursing home residents with advanced dementia, 2000-2014, *JAMA* 316(7):769–770, 2016.

Miu DK, Chan CW, Kok C: Delirium among elderly patients admitted to a post-acute care facility and 3-months outcome, *Geriatr Gerontol Int* 16(5):586–592, 2016.

Molony SL, Kolanowski A, Van Haitsma K, Rooney KE: Person-centered assessment and care planning, *Gerontologist* 58(Suppl 1): S32–S47, 2018.

Morandi A, Davis D, Bellelli G, et al: The diagnosis of delirium superimposed on dementia: an emerging challenge, *J Am Med Dir Assoc* 18(1):12–18, 2017.

Neelon VJ, Champagne MT, Carlson JR, Funk SG: The NEECHAM confusion scale: construction, validation, and clinical testing, *Nurs Res* 45:324–330, 1996.

Neufeld KJ, Yue J, Robinson TN, Inouye SK, Needham DM: Antipsychotic medication for prevention and treatment of delirium in hospitalized adults: a systematic review and meta-analysis, *J Am Geriatr Soc* 64(4):705–714, 2016.

Oberai T, Laver K, Crotty M, Killington M, Jaarsma R: Effectiveness of multicomponent interventions on incidence of delirium in hospitalized older patients with hip fracture: a systematic review, *Int Psychogeriatr* 30(4):481–492, 2018.

Öztürk Birge A, Tel Aydin H: The effect of nonpharmacological training on delirium identification and intervention strategies of intensive care nurses, *Intensive Crit Care Nurs* 41:33–42, 2017.

Moon KJ, Park H: Outcomes of patients with delirium in long-term care facilities: a prospective cohort study, *J Gerontol Nurs* 44(9):41–50, 2018.

Rader J, Barrick A: Ways that work: bathing without a battle, *Alzheimers Care Q* 1(4):35–49, 2000.

Rader J, Tornquist E: *Individualized dementia care*, New York, NY, 1995, Springer.

Resnick B, Kolanowski A, Van Haitsma K, et al: Pilot testing of the EIT-4-BPSD intervention, *Am J Alzheimers Dis Other Demen* 31(7):570–579, 2016.

Reuben DB, Ganz DA, Roth CP, McCreath HE, Ramirez KD, Wenger NS: Effect of nurse practitioner comanagement on the care of geriatric conditions, *J Am Geriatr Soc* 61(8):857–867, 2014.

Richards K, Lambert C, Beck C: Deriving interventions for challenging behaviors from the need-driven dementia-compromised behavior model, *Alzheimers Care Q* 1:62–72, 2000.

Rigney TS: Delirium in the hospitalized elder and recommendations for practice, *Geriatr Nurs* 27(3):151–157, 2006.

Ross L, Ramirez S. Bhatt A, et al: *Tables devices (iPad) for control of behavioral symptoms in older adults with dementia*. Presented at the American Association for Geriatric Psychiatry (AAGP) 2015 Annual Meeting, March 31, 2015.

Sakamoto ML, Moore SL, Johnson ST: "I'm still here": personhood and the early-onset dementia experience, *J Gerontol Nurs* 43(5):12–17, 2017.

Salluh JI, Wang H, Schneider EB, et al: Outcome of delirium in critically ill patients: systematic review and meta-analysis, *BMJ* 350:h2538, 2015.

Scales K, Zimmerman S, Miller SJ: Evidence-based nonpharmacological practices to address behavioral and psychological symptoms of dementia, *Gerontologist* 58:S88–S102, 2018.

Sekerak R, Stewart J: Caring for the patient with end-stage dementia, *Ann Longterm Care* 22(12): 36–43, 2014.

Society of Critical Care Medicine: Guidelines for the prevention and management of pain, agitation/sedation, delirium, immobility, and sleep disruption in adult patients in the ICU. *Crit Care Med*, 46(9):e825–e873, 2018.

Splete H: Nurses have special strategies for dementia, *Caring Ages* 9:11, 2008.

Steis MR, Fick DM: Are nurses recognizing delirium? A systematic review, *J Gerontol Nurs* 34:40–48, 2008.

Steis MR, Evans L, Hirschman KB, et al: Screening for delirium using family caregivers: convergent validity of the Family Confusion Assessment Method and interviewer-rated Confusion Assessment Method, *J Am Geriatr Soc* 60(11):2121–2126, 2012.

Tappen RM, Williams C, Fishman S, Touhy T: Persistence of self in advanced Alzheimer's disease, *Image J Nurs Sch* 31:121–125, 1999.

Tappen RM, Williams-Burgess C, Edelstein J, Touhy T, Fishman S: Communicating with individuals with Alzheimer's disease: examination of recommended strategies, *Arch Psychiatr Nurs* 11:249–256, 1997.

Teno JM, Freedman VA, Kasper JD, Gozalo P, Mor V: Is care for the dying improving in the United States? *J Palliat Med* 18(8):662–666, 2015.

Woods B: Dementia challenges and assumptions about what it means to be a person, *Generations* 13:39, 1999.

Ying I: Artificial nutrition and hydration in advanced dementia, *Can Fam Physician* 61(3):245–248, 2015.

30

Economics and Health Care in Later Life

Kathleen Jett

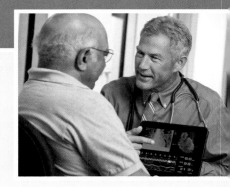

http://evolve.elsevier.com/Touhy/TwdHlthAging

A STUDENT SPEAKS

We went on a home visit with our preceptors today. I could hardly stand it.
The house was almost bare. The only food was left over from the "home-delivered meals"
he gets from the local service organization. The preceptor said that he was doing
the best he could with what he had.

Evelyn, age 21

AN OLDER ADULT SPEAKS

When I was growing up, life was hard. We were so poor we couldn't do much but to hold on
tight. When I was lucky, I could get work plowing a field for $1 an acre. You work hard, and
you make do. There were not such things as going to a doctor or hospital; you just pray you
don't get sick. . . . Then when I turned 65 I got a little check from the government and a red,
white, and blue insurance card [Medicare card]. The check [SSI] isn't much, about $521 a
month but I consider myself blessed and much better off than ever before. And now I don't
worry about my health; I will be taken care of, praise the Lord.

Aida, age 74 in 1994

LEARNING OBJECTIVES

On completion of this chapter, the reader will be able to:

1. Briefly explain the history of Social Security and Supplementary Security Income.
2. Explain how health care is financed in the United States.
3. Compare the types of health care services available under Medicare.
4. Describe the role of the nurse-advocate in relation to health and economic issues of concern to the older adult.

ECONOMICS IN LATE LIFE

Social Security

Considered by many to be one of the most successful federal programs in the United States, Social Security was established in 1935 by President Franklin Delano Roosevelt during the depths of the Great Depression (Chapter 1). The primary function was to provide monetary benefits to older retired workers to prevent or minimize the financial burden on younger members of society (National Archives, 2016). It was based on the societal belief that older adults were uniformly poor in relation to younger adults.

Social Security and several programs that followed were established as "age-entitlement" programs. This means that eligible individuals (beneficiaries) could receive monthly monetary benefits simply because of their age, regardless of their actual financial need (Box 30.1). However, the benefits were and are limited to those who have paid taxes on a requisite amount of income (Box 30.2). In 2018 more than 63 million Americans received almost $1 trillion in benefits. Nine out of 10 persons at least 65 years of age receive Social Security benefits. Among these, many depend on Social Security for at least 50% of their income; 50% of married couples and 71% of those unmarried (SSA, 2018) (Fig. 30.1). For 23% of those who are married and 43% of those who are unmarried, Social Security makes up 90% of their income. In 2018 the average monthly income from Social Security was $1404 with a maximum of $2687 for those who had reached the "age of full retirement." The monthly payment increases every year one *delays* receiving the benefit between their "full retirement age" and the age of 70. Depending on the state of the economy of the country, beneficiaries may receive an annual cost-of-living increase. The program is managed on what is called a pay-as-you-go system. In most cases

BOX 30.1 Criteria for Eligibility for Social Security

American citizens or legal residents, at least 62 years of age, who are totally and permanently disabled (including blind) or who are married to or an eligible partner of or dependent of someone who is eligible to receive Social Security benefits.

BOX 30.2 Amount of Annual Wages Needed to Receive Social Security Income

To receive even the minimal monthly income from Social Security, a person must have worked enough to have earned 40 "credits." In 2017, one credit was equal to an income of $1300 with a maximum of four credits possible in any one year. Only income from which Social Security taxes are withheld can be used toward a credit. For the current cohort of older adults, this calculation has been most beneficial to white men, who are more likely to have worked the most consistently and at higher salaries than all other groups of workers. It is least beneficial to those who were low wage-earners, who never worked out of the home (e.g., housewives and homemakers), or who took time out of the job market for caregiving and child-rearing activities.

Social Security taxes are collected from a percentage of one's income matched by employers. The funds, although individually deposited, are not reserved for any one person (i.e., no one has an account set aside in his or her name). A portion of the funds not immediately paid out to beneficiaries are "borrowed" by the federal government for regular operating expenses. The government converts the remainder into bonds and places these in a "trust fund" overseen by trustees. Details of the changing status of this fund are provided to the public annually and may be accessed at http://www.ssa.gov/oact/progdata/funds.html.

If the amount of contributions from workers exceeds that paid to beneficiaries, the program, as designed, can remain solvent. However, the combination of the increasing number of beneficiaries, the decreasing number of workers (in proportion to the beneficiaries), and the intangible nature of the "trust fund" has resulted in concern that the program will cease to exist in the near future. This is potentially a serious threat to the millions who depend on Social Security as their sole source of income. The extent of this threat continues to be hotly debated. While the depth of the concern varies from year to year, a solution has not been found. To delay the problem, legislation was passed in 1983 to gradually increase the age when one could reach "full retirement," and therefore eligible to receive Social Security (Table 30.1).

Supplemental Security Income

Not all older people living in the United States have income from any source that is adequate to provide even the most basic necessities of life. This is especially true for persons who have spent their lives employed in the agriculture industry, in the food industry, or as domestic workers and were paid very low wages, or on a cash basis. Supplemental Security Income (SSI) was established in 1965 to provide a minimal level of economic support to persons age 65 and older such as Aida (see earlier), those who are blind, or disabled. SSI either provides "total support" or supplements a low Social Security benefit (Box 30.3).

Other Late Life Income

Finally, late life income may come from private retirement investments and/or employer pensions. These monies are held for the beneficiary until such a time when they must begin to "withdraw" some portion of this, at the age determined by the fund but no later than 70 ½ years of age. Some

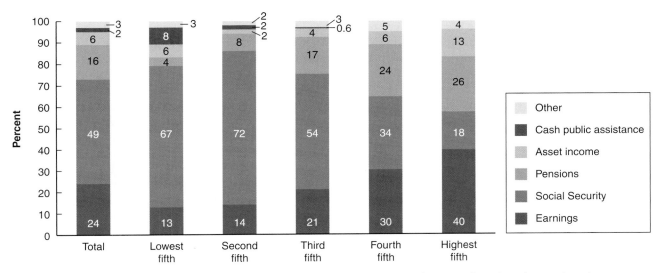

NOTE: The definition of "other" includes, but is not limited to, unemployment compensation, workers' compensation, veterans' payments, and personal contributions. Quintile limits are $12,492, $19,245, $19,027, and $47,129. Estimates may not sum to the totals because of rounding. Reference populations: These data refer to the civlian noninstitutionalized population.
SOURCE: U.S. Census Bureau, Current Population Survey, Annual Social and Economic Supplement.

Fig. 30.1 Percentage Distribution of Sources of Family Income for Persons Age 65 and Older, 2014. (From Federal Interagency Forum on Aging-Related Statistics: *Older Americans 2016: key indicators of well-being,* Washington, 2016, U.S. Government Printing Office.)

TABLE 30.1	Full Retirement Age.
Year of Birth[a]	Full (Normal) Retirement Age
1937 or earlier	65
1938	65 and 2 months
1939	65 and 4 months
1940	65 and 6 months
1941	65 and 8 months
1942	65 and 10 months
1943–1954	66
1955	66 and 2 months
1956	66 and 4 months
1957	66 and 6 months
1958	66 and 8 months
1959	66 and 10 months
1960 and later	67

[a]If you were born on January 1, you should refer to the previous year. From Social Security: *Benefits planner: retirement.* n.d. http://www. socialsecurity.gov/retire2/agereduction.htm. Accessed July 2018.

BOX 30.3   A Monthly Stipend for the Lowest Income: The SSI Program

In 2018, the Supplementary Security Income (SSI) program provided for a maximum benefit of $750 a month for an eligible individual ($1125 per couple) to provide for basic needs. The determination of the total income the person has already includes the value of "gifts" such as housing (e.g., living with a child). Most of the recipients are those older than age 65.

private retirement plans offer several choices for receipt of funds. The retiree could elect to take his or her pension in one lump sum, a monthly amount based on his or her own life expectancy alone, or based on the life expectancy of the retiree and spouse or partner. In other words, a person may establish a plan so that he or she receives all or most of the benefit during his or her *expected* lifetime rather than providing for any survivor benefit. Notification of the potential survivor is now required but was not always so in the past. This may still affect some of the oldest survivors (Box 30.4).

BOX 30.4   A Surprising Change of Income

Mrs. Jones lived in a small rural community. Her husband had worked for the same company from the time he was 18 until he died. He had a limited but adequate pension to meet their day-to-day needs, but nothing extra. His Social Security benefit was small due to his lifelong low wages. When Mr. Jones died suddenly, Mrs. Jones was informed that she would no longer receive support from his pension. He had opted for the "no survivor benefit" when he enrolled, meaning that all benefits would cease upon his death.[a] Because she had never worked outside of the home, Mrs. Jones was dependent solely on her husband's survivor Social Security benefit. She was in danger of losing her home because she could not afford her taxes.

[a]Note: This is no longer legal without the express permission of the potentially surviving spouse.

ECONOMICS AND HEALTH CARE

Before the industrial revolution of the late 1800s people in most countries and cultures worked until they were no longer physically able to do so. In many cases the type of work changed as they aged, but the expectation was that the person would continue to contribute to the family or the community until shortly before death. In turn, family members and the community provided care to those who were no longer able to care for themselves. While this is still the case in some countries and cultures, as countries industrialized, care of members of the family with diminished capacity became problematic in both social and economic terms. As younger members of the family joined the urban workforce, many older adults stayed behind in agricultural areas of the country with less social and caregiving support (Achenbaum and Carr, 2014).

In the early 1900s, almshouses and poor houses emerged to provide care for the frail and ill indigent who did not have family available or were unable to care for themselves. Most of these facilities were initially supported by charitable groups, especially religious organizations. Governments eventually became involved when the primary population of the home was frail older adults and the disabled; they became essentially public nursing institutions. In some communities, public monies replaced or supplemented charitable offerings. Local governments were authorized to purchase land and erect facilities through taxes to others. The care of indigent elderly was considered a public responsibility; however, because of the long-held social belief in personal responsibility, those residing in such care facilities were required to contribute any property they owned and most or all of their income to help cover the expenses related to their care (Achenbaum and Carr, 2014).

Economic factors are always driving forces in the delivery of health care, regardless of who pays for it and where it is provided. While some higher-income countries are struggling to keep up with the escalating costs of technology, persons in low-income countries may not receive even the most rudimentary care. In countries with universal health care, it is supported to a large extent by significant payroll taxes. The insurance risk is shared among all residents of the country. That is, some level of health care is available to all those living in the country. The expectation is that all people can use services while being protected from associated financial hardship. However, at this time there is a very wide variation in who is actually eligible for the "universal health care" and if it even exists within any one country (World Health Organization [WHO], 2017).

With few exceptions health care has always been a purchased service in the United States. In most cases it is not considered a right. However, the federal government is the major purchaser of health care through its insurance plans (Medicare, Railroad Medicare, Medicaid, and TRICARE) or provided directly through Veterans Services. The major insurance plan available to and used by eligible adults at least 65 years of age living in the United States is Medicare. For those with very low incomes, they may also be eligible for Medicaid, an insurance plan that is jointly funded by state and federal resources.

Changes in Health Care for Older Adults

When Social Security was put into place in 1934, President Roosevelt also proposed a universal health insurance plan but because of the opposition to it, Roosevelt removed it to avoid losing Social Security (Corning, 1969). The American Medical Association opposed any national program of health insurance, believing it to be "socialized medicine," and successfully prevented its implementation (Goodman, 1980). *Fortune* magazine polled the American public in 1942 and found that 76% of those questioned opposed government-financed medical care (Cantril, 1951).

In the early 1960s President Lyndon Johnson recognized that the numbers of poor children, those with serious disabilities, and older persons, were increasing significantly and that these vulnerable groups were most often without access to health services of any kind. Although opposition continued, Johnson proposed amendments to the Social Security program to address this widespread public health problem. In Senate and House hearings, some legislators described the amendments as steps that would continue to destroy independence and self-reliance and would tax the poor and middle classes to subsidize the health care of the wealthy (Social Security, n.d.). Nonetheless, legislation was passed in 1965 and 1966 to expand the Social Security system by establishing Medicare and Medicaid, and Medicare for retired railroad workers.

A short time after implementation of these plans, millions more people could receive health care and the associated costs escalated rapidly. Prescription drug coverage (Medicare Part D) was added in 2006 by President George W. Bush's administration. The Affordable Care Act of the Obama administration (2010) contained several provisions with the potential to further impact health care services for older adults, especially coverage for preventive services (Table 30.2).

Medicare

Medicare is the insurance plan specifically designed to provide almost universal health care for those eligible for Social Security.

It is administered by a special entity, the Centers for Medicare and Medicaid Services (CMS). Medicare is made up of three components: the age-entitlement Medicare A, the purchased Medicare B or the alternative Advantage Plans (Medicare C), and the purchased Prescription Drug Plan (PDP) (Medicare D).

As soon as a person is 65 (or meets special disability requirements), he or she is automatically enrolled in Medicare A and receives a "red, white, and blue" card indicating coverage in most cases. The choices associated with Medicare Parts B/C, and D are selected based on personal preference and availability. In most cases selection and enrollment must take place during a 6-month period beginning 3 months before and ending 3 months after a person's 65th birthday to avoid late enrollment penalties and higher premiums (CMS, 2018a). In 2018 more than 59 million persons received Medicare benefits, almost all of them age 65 or older (CMS, 2018b).

At the time of this writing, two comprehensive no-cost health promoting services are available to older adults. A one-time "Welcome to Medicare" visit (Box 30.5) and Annual "Wellness Visits" beginning 12 months after the initial exam (Box 30.6). These are both specifically designed to promote healthy aging

---

TABLE 30.2 Major Components of the Affordable Care Act That Affect Older Adults.

Component	Description
Primary care	Incentives to providers based on quality and not just quantity of care ("evaluation of quality-based indicators")
Bundled payments	Payment to hospital for the entire "bundle of care," which includes both the hospital stay and the medical needs for a period of time after discharge
Five-star programs	Yearly evaluation and ranking of Medicare Parts C and D
Decreasing out-of-pocket costs for prescription medications	Reduce current size of the donut hole and decrease the copay in the donut hole from 100% to 25%; donut hole set to be closed by 2020
No copays for those preventive services with most evidence of usefulness	Increased access to preventive services

---

BOX 30.5 The "Welcome to Medicare" Exam

Must be obtained within 12 months of enrolling in Medicare Part B and must include the following:
- Review of medical record including family history, current health conditions, prescriptions
- Review of social history related to your health
- Education and counseling about preventive services
- Health screenings, immunizations, or referrals for other care as needed
- Height, weight, and blood pressure measurements
- Calculation of body mass index
- Simple vision test
- Review of risk for depression and level of safety
- An offer to discuss advance directives
- Written preventive health plan
- Make sure person is up to date on recommended cancer screens and immunizations

---

BOX 30.6 Yearly "Wellness" Visit[a]

Completion of a "Health Risk Assessment"
- A review of medical and family history, including medications, herbs, and dietary supplements taken
- Developing or updating a list of current providers
- Height, weight, blood pressure, and other routine measurements
- Screening for any cognitive impairment or indications of depression
- Screening for potential functional impairments or safety risks
- Personalized health advice related to assessment, including health risks identified, and treatment options
- A screening schedule for appropriate preventive services

[a]First one at least 12 months after "Welcome" visit. Cannot include a physical exam of any kind.
See http://www.medicare.gov/coverage/your-medicare-coverage.html to determine coverage, copay, and eligibility for screenings.

through prevention and early detection (primary and secondary prevention).

Like Social Security, Medicare was designed as a pay-as-you-go system; that is, Medicare taxes collected from employers and employees are used for the payment of specific health-related expenses of current beneficiaries. The funds are not earmarked for any particular taxpayers' future medical expenses. While the federal government pays most of the health-related costs covered by Medicare, the beneficiaries contribute in the form of premiums and copays.

Medicare Part A

Medicare Part A is a hospital insurance plan covering acute care, short-term rehabilitation in a skilled nursing facility or at home and most of the costs associated with hospice care (Box 30.7). There is no premium. Those who have not paid an adequate amount into the U.S. Social Security system (Social Security taxes) may be eligible to purchase Part A coverage for a monthly fee.

BOX 30.7 Health Services Provided Through Medicare Part A

Designed to partially cover the costs of acute hospitalization semiprivate rooms and any necessary medical services and supplies; care as listed below:
1. There is a deductible for days 1 to 60 (each stay)
2. Days 60 to 120 copay amounts increase over time
3. There is no coverage after 150 days
4. Deductibles and copays increase every year
5. The deductibles and copays are either paid out-of-pocket or reimbursed by Medicaid or Medigap policies

Skilled rehabilitative nursing care in a health care facility (only when care by a licensed nurse or physical or occupational therapist is needed):
1. Only after a minimum of 72-hour acute care hospital admission *(not observation)*
2. The first 20 days are covered at 100% if skilled care is needed the entire time
3. Days 21 to 100 with a daily copay of more than $100
4. No coverage after 100 days
5. Coverage ceases the day skilled care is no longer needed

Home health services requiring skilled care (only when care by a licensed nurse or physical or occupational therapist is needed):
1. Intermittent skilled care for the purpose of rehabilitation provided in the home
2. The person must be ill enough to be considered homebound
3. Medicare may pay 80% of the approved amount for durable medical equipment and supplies (e.g., hospital bed)

Hospice care is provided for terminally ill persons expected to live less than 6 months who elect to forgo traditional medical treatment for the terminal illness:
1. Copay of $5 for Medicare
2. Copay of 5% for limited respite or pain management stays
3. Replaces Medicare Parts A and B for all costs associated with the terminal condition

Inpatient psychiatric care:
1. Limited to 190 days in a lifetime
2. Partial payment
3. Other significant restrictions apply

BOX 30.8 Health Services Provided Through Medicare Part B

Designed to cover some of the costs associated with outpatient or ambulatory services. Deductibles and copays are required in most cases:
1. Physician, nurse practitioner, or physician assistant medically necessary services
2. Limited prescribed supplies
3. Medically necessary diagnostic tests
4. Physical, occupational, and speech therapy for the purpose of rehabilitation
5. Limited durable medical equipment if prescribed by a *physician* and for documented medical necessity
6. Outpatient hospital treatment, blood, and ambulatory surgical services
7. Some preventive services (many with no copay or deductible)
8. Diabetic supplies (excluding insulin and other medications) (Chapter 24)

Medicare Part B

Medicare B (referred to as *Original Medicare*) provides insurance coverage for many of the services provided on an outpatient basis, such as visits to providers' offices (Box 30.8). After January 1, 2007, the premium for Medicare B was based in part on one's income as reported to the Internal Revenue Service. Advantages of *Original* Part B are choice of the primary care provider and referrals are not usually necessary. Providers who "accept assignment" have agreed to charge only an "allowable fee" that Medicare determines annually. The provider receives 80% of this amount from Medicare and the patient is responsible for the remaining 20% and any deductible. If the service is provided independently by a nurse practitioner, the reimbursement rate is 85% of the 80% (AANP, 2013).

A provider who does not accept assignment may charge the patient up to 15% more than the total allowable charge. A combination of an increasing number of wealthy older adults and fewer primary care providers has spawned an industry of "boutique" services, including physician practices. For an additional "membership," "convenience," or "surcharge," patients are eligible for a wide range of special services from immediate access to an emergency room to unlimited access to the provider (e.g., via private cell phone).

Medicare Part C

When enrolling or changing Medicare plans one might select *Original* Medicare B or Medicare Part C. Otherwise referred to as a Medicare Advantage Plans (MAP), Medicare Part C uses a prospective payment system and includes traditional health maintenance organizations (HMOs) and other similar programs. All traditional services covered by *Original* Medicare Part A and Part B must be provided, and additional services, copays, and deductibles are predetermined. MAPs may or may not provide prescription drug benefits; if so, they are referred to as MAP-PDs. Not all MAPs are offered at all locations in the United States; premiums vary depending on location and range of services. In some cases no premium is charged to the member and is paid directly by the federal government.

MAPs may provide a cost savings to the member, and extra benefits in comparison to the Original Medicare Plan. However, special rules must be followed, including the requirement that no care is obtained without a referral from the assigned primary care provider. This person serves as a "gate-keeper" in an effort to ensure that only the highest quality medically necessary care is received. Should a member obtain services without a referral, there is no coverage and all costs are "out-of-pocket."

Medicare C plans are now rated once a year in a 5-star program, on a scale of 0 to 5 with the results available to the public. This information can be used if one wants to change from one program to another (at designated times of the year). This is an attempt to hold the Medicare C (Advantage) Plans more accountable for the quality of care they provide (Medicare, n.d.a.).

Alternatives to Medicare C. Several programs have emerged as health care finance is changing in the United States. One of these is the *Medicare Cost Plan* available in certain areas of the country. Another is the Medicare Medical Savings Account (MSA) plan. The federal government makes monthly payments directly into the person's saving account. When health services are needed, the person pays for them directly. There are also demonstration plans and a Medication Therapy Management program available to accompany Medicare D Medication plan (Medicare, n.d.b.).

Medicare Part D PDP

The Medicare Modernization Act of 2003 established Medicare Part D, a prescription drug plan (PDP) for eligible recipients of Medicare (Box 30.9). It is an *elective* PDP with associated out-of-pocket premiums and copayments. All persons with Medicare, except those in MAP-PD programs, are eligible to voluntarily purchase a PDP. However, if one chooses to do so, the same rules and timing related to enrollment and incurring of penalties seen in Medicare B apply. People can change their plans during the "open enrollment" periods each year without penalty or when they have a change of circumstances, such as entering a long-term care facility. Help with the associated costs is available for persons with low incomes. For persons with both Medicare and Medicaid the plan is mandatory, and in most cases the person is arbitrarily assigned to a particular PDP.

BOX 30.9 Medicare Prescription Drug Plans

Most prescription drug plans (PDPs) are set up in a similar way with deductibles and copays; however, to be a provider in Medicare Part D, the insurance plan must meet the following specific guidelines. Premiums based on the plan (usually dependent on the range of medications covered) plus a payment based on your income (reported to the Internal Revenue Service: e.g., family income $17,000 or less, pay nothing above your premium; family income more than $428,000, pay $69.30 above your premium).

1. Annual deductible as low as zero
2. Copay of medications dependent on plan until the "donut hole" is reached[a]
3. Donut hole: out-of-pocket cost is 47.5% of the 50% required manufacturer discount (down from 100% when it was established with no manufacturer discount)
4. After having spent a set amount in any one year, you receive what is called "catastrophic coverage" and all medications are at a minimum amount or percentage

[a]Note: Under the current plan, the size of the donut hole gets smaller every year. It is scheduled to close in 2020.

As with Medicare C Advantage Plans, a 5-star rating plan is used. Each year the commercial companies that provide Medicare D plans are evaluated and the results are posted on the CMS website. Established by the Affordable Care Act, this is an attempt to hold these plans more accountable for the quality of the product they provide, including pricing and patient safety.

Supplemental Insurance/Medigap Policies

Because of potentially high deductibles and copayments, people who have the financial resources often purchase Medicare supplement insurance plans, often referred to as Medigap. Most older adults who don't have a Medigap from their former employer, purchase one from a commercial carrier or through Medicare. While Medicare (A, B/C) remains the "primary" insurance, and therefore billed first, the Medigap plans serve as a "secondary insurance." A monthly premium is paid and, in exchange, many or all of the copays and deductibles not covered by the "primary insurance" (i.e., Medicare) are paid. Persons searching for an appropriate plan can be referred to the Medicare website for their state or can request a printed copy of the standard plans (available at www.cms.gov).

Medicaid

Medicaid was established in 1965 as part of the revisions to the Social Security Act at the same time as Medicare. It is a health insurance program jointly funded by federal and state governments using tax dollars. CMS administers the program at the federal level, and a state agency administers it at each state level.

Medicaid covers the costs of health services for low-income children, pregnant women, those who are permanently disabled, and persons age 65 and older. Eligibility is determined by the state and is based on income and assets, categorical need, and lack of ability to afford any insurance premiums, including those associated with Medicare. Only a limited number of people can receive Medicaid regardless of their situation due to their state's fiscal health and political priorities.

Medicaid covers all Medicare premiums, copays, and deductibles and may provide additional health benefits. Persons who are dually eligible for both Medicare and Medicaid are frequently required to be enrolled in MAP-PD plans. Federal law requires states to provide a certain minimal level of service, and states may add other coverage such as vision care, dentures, prostheses, case management, and other medical or rehabilitative care provided by a licensed health care practitioner. Medicaid pays for the majority of the care provided in nursing homes in the United States.

Consistent with the early expectations in the almshouses, if institutional long-term care is needed, the person is expected to be fiscally responsible for his or her own care to the extent possible before depending on the tax support of the community. That is, the person is required to use his or her own assets (e.g., Social Security) first to pay for care. When assets are no longer (or ever) available, then Medicaid (funded through taxes) provides a "safety net" to ensure that the poorest, most disabled, and frailest persons receive care.

For a person who requires the financial support of Medicaid for a nursing home stay and has a spouse who is able to remain in the community, Congress enacted provisions in 1988 to protect him or her from "spousal impoverishment." Burial funds and only one-half of the combined value of the household goods, including the automobile (up to a limit), are counted as belonging to the patient, are used to determine eligibility, and are not expected to be used to pay for care. On the death of both spouses, it is expected that the amount that Medicaid has spent on the care (and only up to that point) be reimbursed with any remaining funds in the couple's estate (Medicaid, n.d.).

In the past, some people who believed they would soon need nursing home care transferred funds (sometimes large amounts) to others to be eligible for Medicaid to avoid using their own funds to pay for their care. While some transfers are permitted, such as to a spouse or a disabled, dependent child, any other transfer (i.e., to another person or to a trust) is considered Medicaid fraud. When a person applies for Medicaid, a "look-back period" is done to determine if funds have been transferred that would normally be available to the applicant. If transfers were made, Medicaid support will not begin until the costs incurred equal the amount of the transfer. For example, an income-eligible person (monthly income less than the state's determination of institutional Medicaid) who transfers $100,000 and is in a nursing home where the monthly rate is $10,000 would not be eligible for Medicaid for 10 months. This is known as "spend-down." These regulations attempt to ensure that individuals pay what they can for the care they need but still provide a safety net when funds are exhausted.

The majority of the Medicaid funds are used to provide extended long-term nursing home care for older and disabled adults but persons who are near-poor and without assets and with monthly incomes greater than the "low income" limit set by the state are not eligible for assistance with health care expenses under Medicaid. In the absence of the availability of informal caregivers, providing for those who need assistance continues to be a major social and public health problem in the United States (Chapter 32).

Other Means to Finance Health Care

In some parts of the country (and for some persons), alternative plans have been developed to both finance and provide for health needs while aging.

Indian Health Services

The Indian Health Service (IHS) is a federal health program for and with American Indians and Alaskan Natives (http://www.ihs.gov). Services are provided both at the tribal level and through Urban Indian Health Programs. The provision of health services is complex among this population. Persons who are American Indians and military veterans are eligible for care through Veterans' Services but not through the IHS. Retired workers are most likely eligible for Medicare and if low income, they may also qualify for Medicaid. Traditional IHS care ensures that all documented members of one of the many Indian Nations have care. However, it is limited to those who have no other source of care. There are a number of programs in development and implementation is intended to promote health among American Indians at all ages, ranging from those who

are aging healthfully to those caring for aging and debilitated older adults (http://www.ihs.gov/ElderCare).

Program of All-Inclusive Care for the Elderly

The Program of All-inclusive Care for the Elderly (PACE) is a program for Medicaid-eligible seniors providing comprehensive care in community settings. Services vary by site. There is no cost to the participants. For a detailed description, see Chapter 32.

Care for Veterans

The Veterans Health Administration (VA) system has long held a leadership position in gerontological care. A great deal of the research and innovations in care that guided gerontologists in earlier years was generated through the VA system. In addition, many geriatric fellowships to train geriatricians have been provided through VA hospitals. The system has been a forerunner of the various continua of care providers now in place. Since early on, this system provided VA-administered nursing homes, home care and community-based programs, respite care, blindness rehabilitation, mental health, and numerous other services.

In the past, veterans' hospitals and services were available on an as-needed basis for anyone who had served in the uniformed services at any time and for any length of time. It was not necessary for individuals to use their Medicare benefits. However, this system has undergone significant change as the number of veterans has increased. One of the first changes noted included restrictions placed on the use of veterans' hospitals and services. Instead of coverage of any health problem, priorities were set for those health problems that are deemed "service connected" in some way; in other words, the health care problem began when the person was on active duty.

The older veteran is now expected to obtain and use Medicare for non–service-connected health problems. They are responsible for copays and deductibles the same as those for other Medicare beneficiaries. An outcry among veterans and veteran groups resulted in the development of a free Medigap policy known as TRICARE for Life (TFL).

TRICARE for Life. TRICARE is a free Medigap policy provided by the Department of Defense for Medicare-eligible beneficiaries ages 65 and older and their dependents or widows or widowers older than age 65. This plan requires that the person enroll in both Medicare Part A and Part B and pay the premiums for Part B. TFL covers those expenses not covered by Medicare, such as copays and costs for prescription medicines obtained through the VHA. Dependent parents or parents-in-law may be eligible for pharmacy benefits if they turned age 65 on or after April 1, 2001, and are also enrolled in Medicare Part B. For more information about this, see http://www.military.com/benefits/tricare.

Veteran Aid. For those veterans or surviving spouses at least 65 or officially disabled, who served at least 1 day during war time and receive a military pension, there is monetary support (up to $2230 in 2019) available if assistance with is needed. These funds can be used for home care, nursing home, and assisted living facilities. The program is referred to Aid and Attendance and Household Pension (Senior Veterans, 2018).

The range of program services and eligibility criteria is complex. The reader is referred to https://www.payingforseniorcare.com/longtermcare/resources/veterans_pension.html.

Long-Term Care Insurance

Some are electing to purchase additional insurance for their potential future long-term care needs. Ideally, these policies would cover the expenses related to copays for long-term care and coverage for what is called custodial care, that is, help with day-to-day needs (as opposed to skilled care). Traditionally, these policies were limited to care in long-term care facilities and provided a flat-rate reimbursement to residents for their costs. However, these policies are becoming more creative and innovative and may, under some circumstances, cover home care costs instead of or in addition to care in long-term care facilities. Many plans are being marketed. To offer assistance to older adults, nurses can refer the person to the websites provided by the Administration on Aging (https://longtermcare.acl.gov/costs-how-to-pay/what-is-long-term-care-insurance/) or the American Association for Long-Term Care Insurance (www.aaltci.org).

The purchaser of a long-term care policy is cautioned to read the policy carefully and understand all the details, limitations, and exclusions, such as if the plan covers the amount and type of service that the person would desire if it were needed. They may have a benefit period or a lifetime value. The benefit period may be in days or in dollars spent. Particular concerns are related to dementia because many of the early policies excluded these individuals from home benefits and included very limited institutional benefits. It is advisable to suggest that the persons speak to an independent financial advisor and refer to consumer reports of the chosen insurance company and its reliability before applying for a policy.

KEY CONCEPTS

- The Social Security system in the United States provides a guaranteed income for persons who have paid a requisite amount into the system earlier in their lives.
- Both the Social Security and the Medicare insurance programs are based on a "pay-as-you-go" arrangement with funds from current workers used to support current retirees.
- Social Security provides an income to the majority of retired persons in the United States.
- Medicare is a near-universal health insurance plan for persons who are age 65, blind, permanently disabled, or with end-stage renal disease.

- Medicare is composed of Parts A, B, C, and D. There is no premium for Medicare Part A, hospitalization. There are considerable differences between Parts B and C, which must be selected at the age of eligibility.
- Medigap policies can be purchased to cover the out-of-pocket costs associated with Medicare.
- Medicaid provides coverage for the out-of-pocket medical expenses for poor Medicare beneficiaries.

CRITICAL THINKING QUESTIONS AND ACTIVITIES

1. Ask a person who is insured under Medicare what is the most helpful. What is least helpful?
2. How would older adults like to see Medicare changed?
3. What are the prevalent attitudes of a person at least 65 years of age with whom you are acquainted regarding their economic future?

RESEARCH QUESTIONS

1. Whom do older adults most frequently contact when they need legal and economic advice?
2. How many older adults feel secure about their economic future?
3. What are the current average out-of-pocket costs for health care combining Medicare and Medigap policies?
4. How do people feel about the rationing of health care based on age or survivability?

REFERENCES

American Association of Nurse Practitioners (AANP): *Fact sheet: Medicare reimbursement,* 2013. https://www.aanp.org/legislation-regulation/federal-legislation/medicare/68-articles/325-medicare-reimbursement. Accessed July 2018.

Achenbaum WA, Carr LC: A brief history of aging services in the United States, *Generations: American Society on Aging,* 2014. http://www.asaging.org/blog/brief-history-aging-services-united-states. Accessed July 2018.

Cantril H: *Public opinion 1935-1946,* Princeton, NJ, 1951, Princeton University Press.

Centers for Medicare and Medicaid Services (CMS): *Enrolling in Medicare part A & part B,* 2018a. https://www.medicare.gov/pubs/pdf/11036-Enrolling-Medicare-Part-A-Part-B.pdf. Accessed July 2018.

Centers for Medicare and Medicaid Services (CMS): *Medicare enrollment dashboard,* 2018b. https://www.cms.gov/Research-Statistics-Data-and-Systems/Statistics-Trends-and-Reports/Dashboard/Medicare-Enrollment/Enrollment%20Dashboard.html. Accessed July 2018.

Corning P: *The evolution of Medicare: from idea to law* (Research report no. 29), Washington, DC, 1969, U.S. Department of Health, Education and Welfare, Social Security Administration, Office of Research and Statistics, U.S. Government Printing Office.

Goodman JC: *The regulation of medical care: is the price too high?* (Cato public policy research monograph no. 3). San Francisco, 1980, Cato Institute.

Medicaid.gov: *Spousal impoverishment.* https://www.medicaid.gov/medicaid/eligibility/spousal-impoverishment/index.html. Accessed July 2018.

Medicare.gov: *5-star special enrollment period.* https://www.medicare.gov/sign-up-change-plans/when-can-i-join-a-health-or-drug-plan/five-star-enrollment/5-star-enrollment-period.html. Accessed July 2018.

Medicare.gov: *Other Medicare plans.* https://www.medicare.gov/sign-up-change-plans/medicare-health-plans/other-health-plans/other-medicare-health-plans.html. Accessed July 2018.

National Archives: *Social Security marks 75th anniversary,* August 14, 2016. http://www.archives.gov/press/press-releases/2010/nr10-128.html. Accessed July 2018.

Senior Veterans: *Who is eligible for the pension benefit with Aid and Attendance?* 2018. https://www.veteransaidbenefit.org/eligibility_aid_attendance_pension_benefit.htm. Accessed July 2018.

Social Security: *Historical background and development of Social Security.* https://www.ssa.gov/history/briefhistory3.html. Accessed July 2018.

Social Security: *Fact sheet: Social Security,* 2018. https://www.ssa.gov/news/press/factsheets/basicfact-alt.pdf. Accessed July 2019.

World Health Organization (WHO): *Tracking universal health coverage: 2017 global monitoring report,* 2017. http://www.who.int/health-info/universal_health_coverage/report/2017/en/. Accessed July 2018.

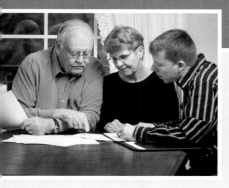

31

Common Legal and Ethical Issues

Kathleen Jett

http://evolve.elsevier.com/Touhy/TwdHlthAging

A STUDENT SPEAKS

When I was asked to go on a home visit to Mr. Jones it was obvious that he did not take care of himself. His clothes were dirty, and he smelled like urine. But he had no significant health problems and seemed undisturbed by the situation. I really didn't know what to think or do.

Steffen, age 19

AN OLDER ADULT SPEAKS

I have had a feeding tube in my stomach for a long time due to cancer. I had been in the hospital recently and even though I disagreed, the social worker was concerned that I could not take care of myself at home. They sent a nurse out to check on me and sure enough, just as she drove up I was pouring my daily beer into my tube. I was so glad she didn't say anything about that, just asked how I was doing!

Henry, age 68

LEARNING OBJECTIVES

On completion of this chapter, the reader will be able to:

1. Describe the nurse's responsibility to respect decision making for those with limited capacity.
2. Differentiate the mechanisms for the protection of those who have limited decision-making capacity and discuss the advantages and disadvantages of each, from least restrictive to most restrictive.
3. Identify the nurse's responsibility for the protection of those with limited capacity.
4. Differentiate between abuse and neglect.
5. Understand the meaning of undue influence and describe how it might be identified.
6. Describe cultural differences in the perception and response to abuse.
7. Identify the ethical conflicts between beneficence and autonomy in self-neglect.
8. Define the nurse's role in the prevention of mistreatment of older adults.

In the day-to-day practice of caring for older adults, gerontological nurses face questions that are ethical in nature, often with legal implications. In the first section of this chapter, decision-making from a process perspective is considered, specifically when the individual is suspected to have limited decision-making capacity. In the second section, the ethical and legal ramifications of "elder" mistreatment are examined relative to the nurse's role. Although gerontological nurses (unless also attorneys) cannot provide any legal advice, it is imperative that they are able to discuss several key ethical and legal issues frequently encountered in their work.

DECISION MAKING

Consent is a concept that arises from the ethical principle of *self-determination* or *autonomy*. In the health care setting, self-determination is documented or expressed through what we refer to as *informed consent*. In most circumstances the consent is implied, such as when the person accepts a medication that is offered or cooperates with a dressing change.

More complex consent is needed under certain circumstances (Box 31.1). Except for an emergency, a person must be free from the effect of sedating medications before formal informed consent can be obtained (Zorowitz, 2014). In older adults, it is also important that the nurse ensures that any special needs are addressed (e.g., functional hearing aids, reading glasses) (Box 31.2). Most courts have upheld the requirements of providing information in such a way that an average person could understand it before being asked to decide. Consent to participate in research is a more detailed and extensive process because treatments received in such circumstances may not necessarily provide benefit to the participant and the risks may not be known. Research with the very frail and those with changing levels of capacity (for any reason) has been difficult and has limited the advancement of science in some areas due to the overriding need to protect the participant.

Informed consent in health care is only possible with the assumption that adults have decision-making *capacity* or in its absence, that someone else has decision-making authority for them. Decisional capacity means that a person can understand a problem, the risks and benefits of a decision, the alternative options, and the consequences of the decision. Capacity is presumed when the legal age of "adult" is reached, unless adjudicated (decided by a court) to lack such capacity. However, even in the absence of an adjudication of incapacity, it is sometimes necessary to make professional judgments that influence accepting consent from a person, such as someone who has been given sedatives or pain medicine, is clearly in emotional distress, or is cognitively impaired.

Until the 1980s to 1990s, medical decision making in Western medicine was based on the ethical principle of paternalism. That is, patients were expected to put blind trust in the physician to make decisions that "he" thought was best for them. Autonomous decision making is now expected and the provider has a legal responsibility to inform the individual of the health problem at hand and the possible risks, benefits, and alternatives of treatment proposed (The Joint Commission, 2016). The individual has the right and responsibility to make his or her decisions whenever possible (Chapter 4). When dealing with older adults, the provider must take note that they may have been brought up under the paternalistic model and may now need to come to grips with the necessity of making the type of decision autonomously that they never had to deal with. It is now expected that decisions are made within the context of the individual's health values and needs (Box 31.3). In many other belief systems and cultures, decisions, including those related to health care, are either shared or delegated responsibilities (Chapter 4).

In day-to-day gerontological practice with frail older adults, it is important to differentiate between legally determined incapacity and day-to-day decision making. While the person may still be legally competent, does he or she have the capacity to understand at the level needed for the decision at hand? Deciding which foods to accept is very different from deciding to undergo a surgical procedure or begin a regimen of chemotherapy or dialysis. He or she may have no or limited capacity for one type of decision but full capacity for another. A guiding principle is to provide protection to those with questionable capacity and ensure that the person's needs are met and personal rights are protected.

There are a range of modes of protection that can be provided, with the expectation that the least restrictive one is used whenever possible. These options include powers of attorney, conservatorship, and guardianship. It is important that nurses understand the differences and meaning of each and that there are differences from state to state.

Advance Care Planning

Gerontological nurses have the responsibility to encourage their patients, neighbors, and family members to discuss their wishes regarding potential incapacity and end-of-life care, otherwise referred to as "advance care planning." It is acceptable to encourage older adults to legally appoint a surrogate (see following sections) or otherwise formally document one's wishes. The use of living wills and do not resuscitate (DNR) orders are addressed in Chapter 35.

Power of Attorney

A power of attorney (POA) is a person (agent) who has been legally appointed to act on behalf of another in ways that are specifically indicated in a legal document. This may include appointing the person to complete a transaction or asking the person to assume full responsibility for the assets of another. In some jurisdictions there are two types—a general POA and a durable POA for health care. In both cases the appointment of the POA has been made in advance as a part of advance care planning in anticipation of future needs. The person named as a general POA most often represents the person in matters of business but not those of health care. In many cases, the authority of the general POA is no longer in effect if the person is determined to be incapacitated. A *durable* POA continues after persons can no longer speak for themselves.

The person appointed as a *durable power of attorney for health care*, referred to as a *health care surrogate*, or *proxy* in some states, is responsible for making medical decisions for persons specifically when they are unable to do so for themselves. Whether the surrogate can make end-of-life decisions is determined by state statutes. As soon as the person regains abilities or chooses to end the authority of the POA, it is no longer in force. The nurse should encourage the person appointing an agent to do so with utmost care and to do so only after in-depth discussions of wishes and values. It will need to be someone who can and will follow the person's wishes. It is possible that a spouse may not be the best person for this task.

Designation of an agent is the least restrictive form of decision-making assistance. All rights and responsibilities afforded by law are retained. An important aspect of this approach is that the person given decision-making rights is someone who has been chosen by the individual rather than appointed by a court.

Health Care Proxy

Most state statutes and cultures provide a "hierarchy" of those who have the authority to act on a person's behalf or when the person has lost (either temporarily or permanently) the capacity to make decisions and has not documented his or her preferences. For example, in the state of Florida it is written into Statute 765.401 that all health care facilities have the legal responsibility to follow this "order of decision-maker" (Box 31.4). The decision-making responsibilities proceed down the list until a willing proxy is obtained (Florida, 2018).

Both surrogates and proxies are expected to use *"substituted judgment"* in making decisions, that is, based on what they believe the person would decide if able to do so and not necessarily the surrogate's choice in a similar situation (Zorowitz, 2014) (Box 31.5). As the gerontological nurse works with people who are making decisions about the selection of a surrogate, like a POA, the nurse can encourage persons to carefully consider someone who is willing to uphold their wishes or holds similar values.

BOX 31.4   Hierarchy of Appointments of Health Care Proxy by Florida State Statute, From First to Last

Guardian
Spouse
Majority of adult children
Parents
Majority of adult siblings reasonably available for consultation
Adult relative who has exhibited special care and has regular contact and familiar with the person's beliefs
Close friend
Licensed clinical social worker selected by bioethics committee

From State of Florida: *The 2017 Florida Statutes*, 2017. http://www.leg.state.fl.us/statutes/index.cfm?App_mode=Display_Statute&URL=0700-0799/0765/Sections/0765.401.html. Accessed February 2018.

BOX 31.5   "I Know That Is What She Would Want but That Is Not What I Want"

Mr. and Mrs. Jones had been married for 60 years. She had developed Alzheimer's disease a number of years earlier and reached a point where she did not always know what to do with food in her mouth. She no longer recognized her husband and did not respond in any verbal way. In almost daily distress, her husband intermittently pleaded that a "feeding tube" be placed into her so she could "eat." However, Mrs. Jones had made it very clear to her husband and to all who knew her that she "never wanted artificial nutrition" or anything done to stop a natural death when she worsened. When Mr. Jones asked for a feeding tube, the only thing we could say was that we were very sorry, but her wishes had been made very clearly and that is what we were bound to follow. He agreed that those indeed were her wishes and started to cry.

Guardians and Conservators

Guardians and conservators are individuals, agencies, or corporations that have been appointed to take care, custody, and control of an incapacitated person and ensure that his or her needs are met and handled responsibly (Box 31.6). Such appointments can only be made at court hearings in which someone demonstrates the older adult is incapacitated in some way.

BOX 31.6   Conservators and Guardians

Conservators
Appointed to manage the finances of the ward and continue in that role until the court appointment is rescinded. Each state is slightly different in how this is handled and defined.

Guardians of the Person
Appointed by the court to help the incapacitated person make informed decisions (or makes decisions for the person) about personal and health matters. The guardian is expected to ensure that the ward remains safe and receives adequate and appropriate food, shelter, and personal hygiene. The guardian provides appropriate consent for medical or other professional care as needed and, in some cases, is reflective of the previously expressed wishes of the person. *In some cases, the Guardian is also "of the Property."*

In some states it is not required that the older adult be present. If the judge agrees that this level of protection is needed, the person is declared incapacitated. Like surrogates and proxies, conservators and guardians are expected to use substituted judgment in all decision making.

In some states limits are set in the appointment of guardianship according to the degree of protection needed. Total dependency means that the person lacks all decision-making capacity and cannot meet even basic needs in any self-sustaining way. Partial dependency means the person may be able to manage certain challenges of life, but health or cognitive abilities interfere with more complex decision making. In the latter situation, a guardian is appointed to protect the person in very specific ways.

Conservatorships and guardianships are expensive and may deplete the patient's assets, leaving little to care for the patient. There have also been reports of exploitation. The use of these mechanisms of care is the most restrictive, and in most cases the person loses all rights to self-determination and should only be considered in cases of severe impairment, such as for persons with advanced dementia. Nurses working with older adults and their families can encourage the use of advance care planning as alternatives that are less restrictive, noting that the definitions and rules vary from state to state. If someone is seeking to establish a guardianship over the opposition of the patient, the patient may need to hire an attorney skilled in this type of litigation. The National Academy of Elder Law Attorneys and the State Bar Elder Law Section are good resources.

MISTREATMENT OF OLDER ADULTS

Mistreatment of older adults is a complex phenomenon that includes "elder" abuse and neglect. It is the infliction of actual harm, or a risk for harm, to vulnerable older persons through the action or behavior of others (American Psychological Association [APA], 2017). It is a universal problem and occurs in all educational, racial, cultural, religious, and socioeconomic groups, in any family configuration, and in every setting. It is one of our most unrecognized and underreported social problems today. While there are no reliable statistics available related to the prevalence on a worldwide basis, the World Health Organization (WHO) estimates that up to 15.7% of those older than age 60 have been or will be mistreated. However, this number is strongly suspected to be an underestimate (WHO, 2018). In a survey of nursing homes in the United States, 36% of staff reported having witnessed at least one incident of physical abuse in the previous year, 10% admitted committing at least one act of physical abuse, and 40% admitted to perpetrating physiological abuse (WHO, 2018). As the population of older adults grows (Chapter 1), so does the expectation that the prevalence of mistreatment will increase as well. The risk is further exacerbated as family caregivers have increasing responsibilities outside of the home (Chapter 34).

For mistreatment to occur, the perpetrator and a vulnerable older adult must have a trusting relationship of some kind. This may be as simple as a salesperson (financial exploitation) or as complex as a long-time caregiver such as a spouse or a child.

BOX 31.7   A Lifelong History of Abuse

A young adult woman was the 24-hour caregiver to her dying grandfather. While he was weak, he could still move about his hospital bed and even get out of it alone from time to time. We noticed that he appeared to regularly make suggestive remarks to his granddaughter and reach toward her. She seemed frightened and always tried to back away. When we were finally able to talk to her alone she quietly said that she was afraid of him; he had sexually assaulted her all her life. She was assigned by the family to be his caregiver because she was disabled and could not work outside of the home.

BOX 31.8   More Likely to Mistreat and Be Mistreated

More Likely to Abuse or Neglect
- Family member
- One with emotional or mental illnesses
- One who is abusing alcohol or other substances
- History of family violence
- Cultural acceptance of interpersonal violence
- Caregiver frustration
- Social isolation
- Impaired impulse control of caregiver

More Likely to Be Abused or Neglected
- Cognitively impaired, especially with aggressive features
- Dependent on abuser
- Physically or mentally frail
- Having abused the caregiver earlier in life
- Women either living alone or in a household with family members
- Having been abused in the past
- Behavior that is considered aggressive, demanding, or unappreciative
- Living in an institutional setting
- Feeling deserving of abuse due to personal inadequacies

From National Council on Aging: *Elder abuse facts*, 2018. https://www.ncoa.org/public-policy-action/elder-justice/elder-abuse-facts/. Accessed February 2018.

Most often "elder mistreatment" occurs in the context of family caregiving. This may be a lifelong pattern that intensifies in the current situation (Box 31.7). The risk factors for one to become an abuser or be abused are often interconnected (Box 31.8).

Mistreatment at the hands of formal (hired) caregivers also occurs. When several different persons are giving care, monitoring becomes especially difficult. Situations of increased potential for formal caregiver abuse include those in which there is inadequate supervision of patient care, poor coordination of services, inadequate staff training, theft or fraud, drug and alcohol abuse by staff, tardiness and absenteeism, unprofessional and criminal conduct, and inadequate record keeping. The nurse should pay attention to the person who is alone with a formal caregiver for extended periods of time, with no support from others and no opportunities for respite for the caregiver.

In recognition of this escalating social and personal problem, countries have been working hard to understand the issue in their own countries and many have developed proactive programs and policies to identify and provide services to persons at risk (Box 31.9). With the support of the United Nations,

BOX 31.9 Tips for Best Practice

Making a Difference: Opportunities to Reduce Mistreatment of Older Adults

The World Health Organization and the United Nations have exerted a considerable amount of effort to help countries better understand elder mistreatment and develop programs and policies to address this growing problem. To hear concerns from the elder's viewpoint, see the free download *Missing voices: views of older persons on elder abuse* at http://www.who.int/ageing/projects/elder_abuse/missing_voices/en/.

BOX 31.11 Factors Increasing the Risk of Elder Abuse

Cultural or societal tolerance of violence, especially against women
Shame and embarrassment
Fear of retaliation
Fear of institutionalization
Social isolation
Unacceptability of emotional expression, especially that of fear or distress

From World Health Organization: *Elder abuse*, 2018. http://www.who.int/mediacentre/factsheets/fs357/en/. Accessed February 2018.

creative programs have been implemented in countries across Europe (Brunne, 2013). In the United States there has been an increase in the number of training programs for persons at the "front line," such as health professionals and police officers, and passage of more stringent laws against mistreatment. Mistreatment of older adults is categorized as either abuse or neglect. However, unlike the case with children, if the older adult maintains capacity, nothing can be done without the person's permission.

Abuse

Abuse is intentional and may be physical, psychological, medical, financial, confinement, or sexual (Box 31.10) (APA, 2017;

BOX 31.10 Types of Abuse of Older Adults

Physical abuse: The use of physical force that results in the threat of or the infliction of bodily injury, physical pain, or impairment. It includes, but is not limited to, acts of violence such as striking (with or without an object), pushing, shaking, pinching, and burning. It includes the use of physical restraints, force-feeding, and physical punishment.

Sexual abuse: Nonconsensual sexual contact of any kind, including with those persons unable to give consent. It includes unwanted touching of any kind and sexual assault or battery—such as rape, sodomy, coerced nudity, and forced sexually explicit photographing.

Psychological abuse: The infliction of anguish, pain, or distress through verbal or nonverbal acts, including intimidation or enforced social isolation. This includes verbal assaults, insults, threats, intimidation, humiliation, and harassment. It can include belittling the person in front of others and forced social isolation from family, friends, or usual activities.

Medical abuse: Subjecting a person to unwanted medical treatments or procedures. Examples of this include venipuncture or the insertion of a urinary catheter (also sexual abuse) in those with dementia who refuse the procedure. The use of chemical restraints (e.g., sedatives) for the convenience of care rather than for the protection of the person (**medical neglect:** failure to provide needed medical care).

Financial abuse or material exploitation: The illegal or improper use of another's funds, property, or assets. Exploitation may be accomplished through coercion (undue influence), such as demanding that the person sign checks or other documents, including deeds to property, with the threat of withholding care.

Discrimination: The illegal cultural or social behavior such as that which is demeaning, belittling, or the withholding of full rights to persons, especially those who are at risk of physical, emotional, or sexual abuse or of financial exploitation as a result of the discrimination.

Abandonment: The desertion of a person by an individual who had assumed the responsibility of providing care or assistance.

Hall et al, 2016; NCOA, 2018). It occurs in relationships where there is or has been an expectation of trust; it is a violation of human rights (WHO, 2018). Should harm occur, the abuser can be sued for the older adult's injuries. If the abuse escalates to a criminal act or if the abuse includes theft of property or money, the perpetrator is subject to criminal prosecution. Many states require certain persons, including nurses, who become aware of abuse, neglect, or exploitation to report it to the appropriate authorities immediately. The designated authority can be found in each state's laws (Stetson, 2016).

Most abuse occurs in the home setting; almost 60% of abuse is perpetrated by a family member (NCOA, 2018). Unfortunately, many factors interfere with the identification of those who are mistreated (Box 31.11). It is further complicated by varying cultural perspectives on abuse. The practitioner should be sensitive to the cultural background of the patient and family as there may be differences in how people view the same situation and how they elect to care for older adults in their community. However, whatever the cultural beliefs, the practitioner must focus on ensuring the safety of the person while respecting his or her articulated wishes (Box 31.12).

Whereas physical abuse often has external signs, it is more difficult to detect financial exploitation. Care is costly, and the person's assets may be gone before it is noticed that charges have been excessive or misappropriated. Changes in banking practices, access to a bank account by an unauthorized person, failure to pay medical or other bills, unexpected changes in a will, or the disappearance of personal items are all suggestions of possible financial exploitation and undue influence. However, in some cultures this may not be considered abuse due to the common belief it is appropriate to share funds within families, even at the expense of one's own needs (WHO, 2018). Also "invisible," the most common form of abuse is verbal/emotional/psychological (NCEA, 2016).

Undue Influence

Undue influence is the substitution of one person's will for the true desires of another. . . . Undue influence takes place when one person uses his or her role and power to exploit the trust, dependency or fear of another to gain psychological control over the weaker person's decision making, usually for financial gain.

(Quinn 2002, p. 11)

BOX 31.12 Potential Cultural Variations Regarding Abuse and Neglect and Risk for Exploitation[a]

Latino
- *Machismo:* Expectation of men to neglect self on behalf of others if necessary
- *Marianismo:* Role expectation of women to tolerate abuse and focus on service of others
- *Vergüenza:* Need to protect the family from shame (above all things)
- *La familia:* Emphasis on the family instead of outsiders
- Extreme level of guilt not to provide care to older members of the family at home regardless of the difficulty to do so

Asian/Pacific Islander
- Ability to endure violence as a symbol of strength and honor
- Not familiar with the terms of abuse; instead use terms "sacrifice" and "suffering"
- Psychological abuse considered the worst possible type of abuse and the most commonly experienced
- Strong belief in filial duty to care for parents may result in excessive burden on single caregivers due to other obligations such as to financially support oneself
- Defined only within a family setting
- Unacceptability to express emotions

Chinese
- Must be kept in family
- Disrespect most important form of mistreatment
- Cultural disparities in expectations between younger adults and older adults

Asian Indian
- Children leaving the family home may be considered a form of elder abandonment
- Oldest son handles all finances, without question
- As age is venerated, physical abuse very uncommon

Japanese
- 80% report psychological abuse is the worst type of abuse to endure
- Emotional abuse, neglect, physical abuse reported to be perpetrated by daughters-in-law
- Lack of caring for elder is a sign of disrespect and socially unacceptable
- Suffering is expected to be done in a stoic manner
- Fatalism to suffering, should it occur
- Self-blame
- Those who expose a family "shame" may be considered a traitor and be sanctioned

Korean
- Financial exploitation as defined in the United States not considered a form of abuse
- High tolerance for neglect
- Placing in nursing home shameful and a form of abuse

Vietnamese
- Family problems to be kept at home; cannot be disclosed to outsiders
- Neglect brings shame to family
- Psychological "silent treatment" most serious

[a]May or may not be applicable to any one subcultural group. It is always recommended for the nurse to find the correct language used and not make assumptions; these are gross generalizations. Note that the groups identified as Latino is very broad. The subgroups of Korean and others are more specific. Please further note that the information in this box is drawn from multiple sources.

Undue influence is a means of financial or material exploitation. Undue influence may occur in an insidious way if the perpetrator isolates the victim from friends and family in some way, such as with the suggestion that he or she is the only one who cares. In other situations, the older adult meets a "new friend," who offers to provide "lifelong" care in exchange for the title to property such as one's home. A salesman may make an "offer you just can't refuse" or claims an unneeded repair or replacement.

Undue influence can also occur outside of the caregiving situation; for example, a person provides false affection and even marriage to a lonely person *for the purpose of defrauding the person of assets.* In these cases, intervention is difficult because the victim has developed trust and reliance on the abuser and has entered the relationship voluntarily. Affection and kindness to the older adult in and of itself is not considered undue influence. It only reaches that point when the relationship leads to persuasion or coercion that limits the person's ability to make independent or informed choices. Quinn (2002) has developed guidelines for nurses attempting to identify signs of undue influence (Box 31.13).

Impact of Abuse

The abuse of older adults has effects that are far more reaching than is usually discussed. Posttraumatic stress syndrome and lowered self-efficacy even after the termination of the abusive

situation may never be resolved. Those subjected to even minimal abuse have been found to have a 300% higher risk for death than those who have never been abused (NCOA, 2017). In addition, older adults who have been victims of violence have more health problems than other older adults, including increased bone or joint problems, digestive problems, depression or anxiety, chronic pain, hypertension, and cardiovascular disease.

Neglect

Abuse is an act of commission—that is, doing something to another—while neglect is a type of mistreatment that is an omission, or the *failure* of action by a caregiver through one's own behavior or choices. Neglect of self and neglect by caretakers are often difficult to define because they are intertwined with energy, lifestyle, and resources.

Nurses are particularly challenged by issues of self-neglect when the ethical principle of beneficence (do good) counters that of autonomy (self-determination). In either case, the needs of the individual may not become known until there is a medical crisis when the person's unmet needs become visible to others.

Neglect by a Caregiver

Neglect by a caregiver requires a socially (formally or informally) recognized role and responsibility of a person to provide care to a vulnerable other. Neglect is most often passive mistreatment, such as an act of omission. Passive neglect is the

BOX 31.13 Signs of Undue Influence

- Actions inconsistent with his or her life history. Actions run counter to the person's previous lifelong values and beliefs.
- Makes sudden changes with regard to financial management. Examples include cashing in insurance policies or changing titles on bank accounts or real estate property.
- Elder changes his or her will and previous disposition of assets.
- Elder is taken to practitioners different from those he or she has always trusted. Examples include bankers, stockbrokers, attorneys, physicians, and realtors.
- Elder is systematically isolated from or is continually monitored when with others who care about him or her.
- Someone unexpectedly moves into the person's home, or the person is moved into someone's home under the guise of providing better care.
- Someone attempts to get income checks directed differently from the usual arrangement.
- Documents are suddenly signed frequently as the elder nears death.
- A history of mistrust exists in the elder's family, especially with financial affairs, and the elder places unusual trust in newfound acquaintances.
- Statements of the elder and the alleged abuser vary concerning the elder's affairs or disposition of assets.
- A power imbalance exists between the parties in matters of finances or health.
- The stronger person unduly benefits by the transaction.
- The elder is never left alone with anyone. No one is allowed to speak to the elder without the alleged abuser having a way of finding out about it.
- Unusual patterns arise in the elder's finances. For instance, numerous checks are written out to "cash," always in round numbers, and often in large amounts.
- The elder reports meeting a "wonderful new friend who makes me feel young again." The elder then becomes suspicious of family and begins to avoid family gatherings.
- The elder is pressed into a transaction without being given time to reflect or contact trusted advisors.

Adapted from Quinn M: Undue influence and elder abuse: recognition and intervention strategies. *Geriatr Nurs*, 23, 11–16, 2002.

failure to provide the goods and services, such as food, medication, medical treatment, and personal care necessary for the well-being of the care recipient, but also the failure or inability to recognize one's responsibility to provide care. Active neglect or willful deprivation occurs in the situation when care is withheld deliberately and for malicious reasons (NCOA, 2018). In some cases, this level of neglect would also be considered abuse. Neglect by caregivers occurs for many reasons (Box 31.14).

BOX 31.14 Examples of Causes of Neglect by Caregivers

Caregiver personal stress and exhaustion
Multiple role demands
Caregiver incompetence
Unawareness of importance of the neglected care
Financial burden of caregiving limiting resources available
Caregivers' own frailty and advanced age
Unawareness of community resources available for support and respite

Self-Neglect

Self-neglect is a behavior in which people fail to meet their own basic needs in the way the average person would in similar circumstances. It generally manifests itself as a refusal to, or failure to, provide themselves with adequate safety, food, water, clothing, shelter, personal hygiene, or health care. It may be due to diminished capacity, but it also may be the result of a long-standing lifestyle, homelessness, alcoholism, or other substance abuse. It is important for the nurse to remember that there are many mentally competent people who understand the consequences of their decisions and make conscious and voluntary decisions to engage in acts that threaten their health or safety as a matter of personal choice. There are both ethical and legal questions as to how much health care professionals can and should intervene in these situations.

PROMOTING HEALTHY AGING: IMPLICATIONS FOR GERONTOLOGICAL NURSING

Nurses are expected to provide safety and security to the persons under their care to the extent possible. When caring for vulnerable older adults, it also may mean wrestling with difficult and problematic legal and ethical issues. This may include questioning the person's decision-making capacity related to informed consent (Box 31.2). It may involve contacting the designated protective services when there is evidence of potential abuse or even working for an abuse hotline or international program for the protection of older adults.

Clues to Potential Incapacity

As noted, unless adjudicated (declared by the courts) otherwise, all adults have a presumed capacity to control their lives, including what happens to their bodies; that is, they have the autonomous legal and ethical right to make health-related decisions. It is always necessary to determine whether the appearance of incapacity is truly one of impairment or whether it is simply the manifestation of choices that are inconsistent with the preferences, expectations, or values of the health care system or the nurse, caregiver, surrogate, or proxy.

Lack of capacity is *not* a question of preference or a question of the person's values or choices, but the ability to understand the problem at hand, the choice made, and its consequences. The nurse is expected to work toward preserving the individual's integrity, independence, dignity, and assets to the extent possible. Lack of capacity also does *not* necessarily mean the patient has refused care (UChicago Medicine, 2012) but has the right to refuse treatment and to leave a hospital or nursing home without "signing out AMA". One cannot hold a patient against her or his will unless he or she is in immediate danger to self or others.

What Is the Nurse's Responsibility Regarding Issues of Capacity?

In many settings where gerontological nurses provide care to older adults, ethical and legal questions of capacity and decision-making authority can occur quickly. While working in a nursing facility, the author regularly heard from previously distant or uninvolved relatives of older adults who were still able to make all but the most complex decisions. The presumed relative would insist that he or she was the person's POA and therefore had the right to override an individual's decisions or would insist on access to the person's medical and health information. In such a situation, several nursing actions are expected, including asking the person's opinion on the situation and requiring that the presumed relative produce the documents granting authority (Box 31.15).

If the older adult lacks capacity and the facility is provided with authentic documentation that a person is the resident's guardian, then all requests and instructions must be followed. The patient cannot revoke the guardianship; this can only be done by the court that awarded it. Those who appointed health care surrogates or health care proxies can revoke this designation at any time.

As an advocate, the nurse has a responsibility to protect the patient from neglect or exploitation from all sources, including guardians, surrogates, or proxies. Nurses who are consulted about legal issues should not attempt to provide legal advice but, instead, should refer the person to a law attorney, preferably one who is certified by the National Academy of Elder Law Attorneys, the State Bar Elder Law Section, or National Elder Law Foundation (www.nelf.org). The nurse who is interested can also access this site for more detailed information related to elder law. Additionally the American Bar Association Commission on Law and Aging has a wealth of information online which will be helpful to nurses working with seniors.

Mistreatment of Older Adults

When working with frail and vulnerable older adults, nurses must always be vigilant and sensitive to the signs and symptoms of mistreatment. In addition to the obvious indicators of physical abuse (e.g., unexplained bruises or weight loss), the nurse looks for more subtle signs (Box 31.16). For the person who is clearly competent and refuses assessment, it cannot be done. For a person with questionable capacity and unmet needs or other signs of abuse or neglect, intervention is required. It is important to remember that what some might consider "poor judgement" is not the same as incapacity.

A full and specialized assessment includes the immediate determination of the person's safety. Further assessment of mistreatment involves several very sensitive components and tools developed by experts in the field that may be very useful

(Box 31.17). Assessment of mistreatment in the cross-cultural setting is especially difficult; however, helpful guidelines can be found at the National Center on Elder Abuse. Because of the sensitive nature of such an assessment, specialized training is recommended for all gerontological nurses (https://ncea.acl.gov/).

Mandatory Reporting

In most states in the United States, in the Virgin Islands, and in Guam, licensed nurses are included in those known as "mandatory reporters." This means that persons who know or have reasonable cause to believe that vulnerable persons are being abused, neglected, or exploited are required to report this promptly to authorities identified by the jurisdiction where the person lives. Usually these reports are anonymous (Brent, 2019).

If abuse occurs in an institutional setting, it would be very unusual for the nurse not to inform one's employer of the situation.

In many states, nursing homes or licensed assisted living facilities, the nurse has the additional resource of calling the state long-term care ombudsman for help when the situation is less conclusive.

Ombudsmen are either volunteers or paid staff members who are responsible for acting as advocates for vulnerable residents in institutions (www.ltcombudsman.org) (Consumer Voice, 2016). All reports, either to the state ombudsman or the state's protective services will be investigated. A unique aspect of elder abuse compared with child abuse is that the physically frail (and even abused or neglected) but mentally competent adult can, and often does, refuse intervention due to several factors including fear of retaliation or lack of alternative caregiver. These adults cannot be removed from harmful situations without their permission, much to the frustration of the nurse and other health care providers.

Prevention of Abuse

In the ideal situation, gerontological nurses are alert to potential mistreatment of vulnerable older adults and take steps to prevent the occurrence of abuse or neglect. In some situations, the abuse may have been prevented. If the mistreatment is the result of psychopathological conditions, especially if the situation is long-standing, the nurse probably cannot prevent the abuse. However, nurses can make sure that the potential victims know how to get help if it is needed and are aware of the resources that are available to them. The nurse can also work with the older adult, caregiver, and community support groups to increase the social network and help to create shelters for this group of at-risk persons (e.g., promote more community activities and involve older adults in the lives of their neighbors).

If the abusive behavior is learned or a response to stress, the situation may be subject to change. Learned abuse, theoretically, can be unlearned and may respond to a close working relationship with a mentoring professional who can demonstrate positive problem solving and new ways of managing difficult situations.

If the abuse is triggered by the stress of caregiving, nurses can be very proactive and help all involved find ways to lessen the stress. This may include finding respite services, changing the situation entirely (giving permission to the caregiver to relinquish the role), referring to support groups for expression of frustrations and peer support, teaching people how to use crisis hotlines, and providing access to professional consultation,

---

BOX 31.18 Tips for Best Practice

Prevention of Elder Mistreatment

- Determine (if possible) if what appears as mistreatment is lack of caregiver skills.
- Make professionals aware of potentially abusive situations.
- Help families develop and nurture informal support systems.
- Link families with support groups.
- Teach families stress management techniques.
- Arrange comprehensive care resources.
- Provide counseling for troubled families.
- Encourage the use of respite care and day care.
- Obtain necessary home health care services.
- Inform families of resources for meals and transportation.
- Encourage caregivers to pursue their individual interests.

---

victim support groups, or victim volunteer companions. Most importantly, thoughtful and compassionate care is imperative for both the victim and the perpetrator. See Box 31.18 for tips on the prevention of mistreatment of older adults.

Finally, for older adults who become incapacitated, legal protection at some level may be necessary. Gerontological nurses can become familiar with the laws that specifically affect older adults in their state. This can be accomplished by attending continuing education programs to update their knowledge in the field of elder law and protection. Nurses are able to assist older adults and family members seek legal representation when necessary and to help them find solutions that may solve potential caregiving problems in as least restrictive a manner as possible. Although initiating these interventions is usually the responsibility of the social worker and enacted by lawyers and judges, the nurse should understand the basic concepts and the types of legal protection for elders and other incapacitated persons.

Advocacy

An advocate is one who maintains or promotes a cause; defends, pleads, or acts on behalf of another; and fights for someone who cannot fight for themselves.

Topics for advocacy can include protection of specific rights (e.g., promoting the least restrictive residential alternative), finding the best nursing home, or testifying at the judicial appointment of a conservator. Other areas of advocacy include the rights of medical patients, the right to have the in-home supportive services needed to assist with care, and the right to access government programs that support caregiving and help prevent abuse (e.g., Area Agencies on Aging, veterans' programs). Nurse-advocates function in various arenas: with their own and other disciplines within their own agencies, with other agencies, with physicians, with families, with neighbors and community representatives, with professional organizations, with legislators, and with courts.

Nurses act as advocates when they support people as autonomous free agents who have the right to make decisions and to be involved in all conversations about their health care needs. In a health care setting, advocacy is acting for or on behalf of another in terms of supporting the best interests of that other person with respect to choose the receipt of, as appropriate, and refusal of health care. However, situations occur in the care of older adults when the person is either not strong enough or does not have the capacity to exert measures to protect his or

her own interests. When this occurs, the nurse's role is to ensure not only that the person is protected but also that his or her voice is not lost even when he or she cannot express himself or herself.

KEY CONCEPTS

- Informed consent is based on the ethical principle of autonomy, which requires the capacity to understand a situation, the choices that are available, and the consequences of a decision.
- In the health care setting, an individual may have legal capacity but have diminished or varying levels of capacity to make health-related decisions.
- Varying levels of protection are available to protect a person with diminished capacity and to ensure that his or her voice is still heard.

- Elder mistreatment is an umbrella term that covers abuse, neglect, exploitation, and abandonment.
- The nurse has a legal responsibility to report mistreatment of frail or disabled older adults that is known or responsibly believed to have occurred/is occurring.

NURSING STUDY: WHEN CAN YOU INTERVENE?

Mrs. Henry, 87 years old, is admitted to the medical/surgical floor of a community hospital with a fractured right orbit and ruptured eye globe. Her husband attends to her with care and concern, trying to anticipate her needs. He is active and appears much younger than his stated age of 85. The emergency department report states the cause of the injury as "fall at home." Although Mrs. Henry is alert and oriented, she appears very thin, frail, and withdrawn. Her husband also voices concern that she seems confused at times. When the gerontological clinical nurse specialist arrives to do a basic assessment, she reports to the nurses that she is concerned that Mrs. Henry has been abused. Her husband answers all the questions posed to his wife, and, as he does so, Mrs. Henry seems to withdraw even further from both him and the staff. Mr. Henry does not leave his wife's side for hours. Finally, he leaves for a quick cup of coffee, and

the nurse who had been providing care quickly goes into the room and asks Mrs. Henry what happened. She begins to cry and says that her husband hit her. She is immediately offered shelter and protection. She declines, saying that she has nowhere else to go but back home and that she will be okay. The husband returns to find the nurse talking to his wife privately and immediately gathers up her things, and they leave the hospital against medical advice.
- Identify the risk factors for abuse in this situation.
- Provide the subjective data suggesting abuse.
- Provide the objective data suggesting abuse in this situation.
- Describe the nurse's legal responsibility to Mrs. Henry at this time.
- Describe the next step the nurse can take on the departure of a patient who reports abuse but declines intervention.

CRITICAL THINKING QUESTIONS AND ACTIVITIES

1. After reading this chapter, discuss with a classmate why you believe some older adults feel that they have no options but to endure abuse of any kind.

2. If you were the nurse making home visits to the man and his granddaughter described in Box 17.7, what would you do? What if this were your neighbor?
3. Why might Mrs. Henry believe she has no options?

RESEARCH QUESTIONS

1. What are your responsibilities for reporting elder abuse in your state?

2. What resources are available to frail older adults in your community who are attempting to escape from abuse?

REFERENCES

American Psychological Association (APA): *Elder abuse and neglect: in search of solutions,* 2017. http://www.apa.org/pi/aging/resources/guides/elder-abuse.aspx?item=1. Accessed February 2018.
Brent N: *Nurses and mandatory reporting laws,* 2019, CPH and Associates. https://www.cphins.com/nurses-and-mandatory-reporting-laws/. Accessed March 2019.
Brunne V: *6th meeting of the working group on ageing: policy brief on abuse of older persons,* 2013. https://www.unece.org/fileadmin/DAM/pau/age/wg6/Presentations/UNECE_PolicyBrief.pdf. Accessed February 2018.

Hall J, Karch DL, Crosby A: *Elder abuse surveillance: uniform definitions and recommended core data elements,* 2016. https://www.cdc.gov/violenceprevention/pdf/EA_Book_Revised_2016.pdf. Accessed February 2018.
National Center on Elder Abuse (NCEA): *Research: statistic/data,* 2016. https://ncea.acl.gov/whatwedo/research/statistics.html#prevalence. Accessed February 2018.
Nursing Home Abuse Center: *Elder abuse statistics: statistics over time,* 2019. https://www.nursinghomeabusecenter.com/elder-abuse/statistics/. Accessed March 2019.
Quinn M: Undue influence and elder abuse: recognition and intervention strategies, *Geriatr Nurs* 23:11–16, 2002.

The Joint Commission: *Informed consent: more than getting a signature,* 2016. https://www.jointcommission.org/assets/1/23/Quick_Safety_Issue_Twenty-One_February_2016.pdf. Accessed February 2018.

UChicago Medicine: *Do patients pay when they leave against medical advice?* 2012. http://www.uchospitals.edu/news/2012/20120203-billing.html. Accessed February 2018.

World Health Organization (WHO): *Elder abuse,* 2018. http://www.who.int/mediacentre/factsheets/fs357/en/. Accessed February 2018.

Zorowitz RA: Ethics. In Ham RJ, Sloane D, Warshaw GA, et al, editors: *Primary care geriatrics: a case-based approach,* ed 6, Philadelphia, 2014, Elsevier, pp 77–91.

32

Long-Term Care

Theris A. Touhy

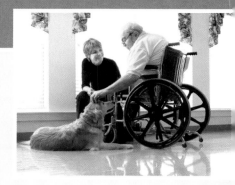

http://evolve.elsevier.com/Touhy/TwdHlthAging

A STUDENT SPEAKS

I feel so depressed when I see all the older people in nursing homes. I don't know how families can put loved ones into a nursing home and I have promised my parents that I will never do that to them.

John, age 25

AN OLDER ADULT SPEAKS

This nursing home is my home now. We are all like a family, and I will die here. The girls that help me during the day, we treat one another like family members. We have some days when we are grumpy, some days we are happy, and we don't hold our feelings back, just like you would do with your own family at home.

Helen, age 88

LEARNING OBJECTIVES

On completion of this chapter, the reader will be able to:

1. Define long-term care and describe the long-term care system.
2. Describe factors influencing the provision of long-term care.
3. Identify differences between the focus of acute and long-term care.
4. Discuss long-term care as a component of the health care system in the United States.
5. Describe several long-term care options for older adults including continuing care retirement communities, residential care facilities, skilled nursing facilities, and community-based programs such as Program of All-Inclusive Care for the Elderly (PACE) and adult day health.
6. Discuss interventions to improve care for older adults in skilled nursing facilities including quality improvement, culture change, and transitional care.

The term long-term care (LTC) is often only associated with nursing homes and with care of older adults but LTC describes a variety of services, including medical and nonmedical care, provided on an ongoing basis to people of all ages who have a chronic illness or physical, cognitive, or developmental disabilities. LTC can be provided informally or formally in a range of environments, from an individual's home to the home of a friend or relative, an adult day health center, independent and assisted living facilities (ALFs), continuing care retirement communities (CCRCs), skilled nursing facilities, and hospice.

Long-term services and supports (LTSS) consist predominantly of assistance or supervision with activities of daily living (ADLs), such as bathing, dressing, toileting, or eating, or with instrumental activities of daily living (IADLs), such as shopping or cleaning. Older adults receive the majority of LTSS (80%) on a yearly basis but children and younger adults also receive this type of care. Children younger than age 18 are a small percentage of the total population requiring LTSS but can have substantial needs that will last a lifetime. Most people with LTSS needs live in their own home with family, friends, and volunteers (as well as hired personnel) providing most of the care. However, the bulk of LTC throughout the developed world is informal unpaid care provided by friends and relatives. The nature of family caregiving is changing as more individuals are discharged early from acute settings with increasingly complex medical care needs to be met in the home. Without family caregivers, the present level of LTC could not be sustained (Chapter 34).

FUTURE PROJECTIONS

The number of older adults needing LTSS is dramatically increasing year after year, and the challenge of ensuring the quality and financial stability of care provision is one faced by governments in both developed and developing countries. On average, 52% of people who turned 65 years of age in 2017 will develop a severe disability that will require long-term services and supports at some point. The average duration of need, over a lifetime, is about 2 years; only 14% are expected to need LTC for 5 years or more (Nguyen, 2017). In the coming years, most families will have a member with a need for LTC services and supports. However, with shrinking family sizes, there will be fewer potential caregivers and reliance on formal care services can be expected to expand (Chapter 34). Estimates are that spending on LTC will increase fivefold by 2045 in the United States.

COSTS OF LONG-TERM CARE

The total U.S. LTC spending is currently financed through a mixture of Medicaid, Medicare, out-of-pocket spending, private LTC insurance, and appropriations from the Older Americans Act (Chapter 30). LTC is expensive and becoming more expensive; costs have outpaced inflation since 2003 (Table 32.1). The cost of LTSS continues to be much higher than what most people can afford and only people in the wealthiest 10% to 20% of older adult households have savings that could absorb the risks of high LTSS spending (Reinhard et al, 2017). Finding a way to pay for LTC is a growing concern for people of all ages, especially older adults, individuals with disabilities, and their families. Most people have not planned for their LTC needs and are not knowledgeable about existing resources.

Medicaid

Medicaid is the primary payer for LTSS for people who have low incomes and who deplete their personal savings to pay for medical and LTC. Medicaid accounts for more than 62% of national LTC spending in the United States. Of this amount, about 47% is for institutional care and 53% is for home and community-based services (HCBS) (Nguyen, 2017). Without affordable private-insurance options or public insurance alternatives, such as a national LTC insurance system or expanded coverage for Medicare beneficiaries, there will be continued reliance on the Medicaid program.

TABLE 32.1	Costs of U.S. Long-Term Care Services and Support Programs.
Service	**Cost**
Homemaker services	National median hourly rate: $21
Home health aide	National median hourly rate: $21.50
Adult day health	National median daily rate: $70
Assisted living facility	National median monthly rate: $3750 Annual cost: $45,000
Nursing home care	National median daily rate (semiprivate room): $235 National median monthly rate $7148 Annual cost: $85,783

Data from Genworth 2017 Cost of Care Survey: http://newsroom.genworth.com/2017-09-26-Genworth-2017-Annual-Cost-of-Care-Survey-Costs-Continue-to-Rise-Across-All-Care-Settings. Accessed March 2018.

The Medicaid program is administered by the states and there is wide variation in support of LTSS funding. Where you live really matters because there are huge differences across the states in how well they are doing in expanding and funding LTSS. While there are some states developing innovative, coordinated, and accessible LTSS systems, a recent report found that most states aren't doing a great job of helping people needing such care (Fig. 32.1). Proposals to reduce Medicaid spending further jeopardize the availability and affordability of long-term care supports and services. National and state initiatives are being directed toward changing the bias from institutional care to more HCBS that can be less expensive and reflective of the desires of people to "age in place." While progress has been made, it is not adequate to meet the needs of aging baby boomers and beyond. Recommendations from experts suggest that the pace of change needs to triple or quadruple to meet the needs of an aging population (Reinhard et al, 2017).

Medicare

Medicare is not designed to provide coverage for LTC services and only covers acute and postacute medical care for people 65 years of age and older and for younger populations who qualify for Social Security because of disability. Many people think that Medicare covers LTC; however, in reality, it provides limited coverage for short-term skilled nursing facility stays and home health services for postacute rehabilitation care (Chapter 30). Fifty-seven percent of care in nursing facilities is paid for by Medicaid; 14% by Medicare; and 29% by private insurance plans and private individuals (out-of-pocket) (American Healthcare Association, 2018). Medicare does not cover the costs of care in chronic, custodial, and LTC units. If the older adult was admitted to the nursing home because of a dementia diagnosis and the need for assistance with ADLs and maintenance of safety, Medicare would not cover the cost of care unless there was some skilled need.

Private Long-Term Care Insurance

LTC insurance covers many types of LTC and benefits, including palliative and hospice care. The exact coverage depends on the type of policy purchased and what services are covered. Policies cover nursing home care only or can be more comprehensive and cover both facility and home care. Relatively few people have purchased this type of insurance. Barriers to the purchase of LTC insurance include the inability of many people to afford coverage, the belief that LTC is covered by their general policies or by Medicare, and the reluctance of private insurers to write policies for those in poor health (the individuals most likely to require LTC services). Some new and more cost-effective options for LTC insurance are emerging, as are proposed reforms to encourage more individuals to obtain coverage, such as the Partnership for Long-Term Care program.

Out-of-Pocket Spending

For those who do not qualify for Medicare or Medicaid benefits, the costs of LTC are paid out-of-pocket. Out-of-pocket spending accounts for about 17% of national spending for LTC

State Ranking on Overall LTSS System Performance

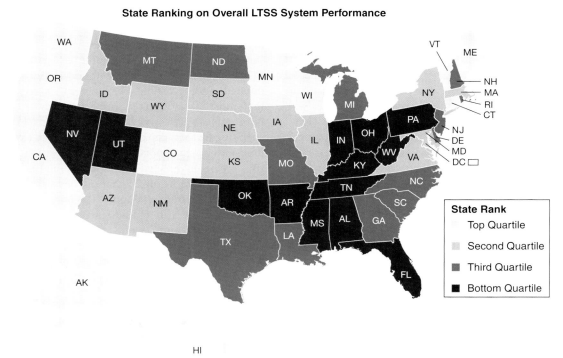

Fig. 32.1 State Ranking on Overall Long-Term Services and Supports *(LTSS)* System Performance, **2017.** (From http://www.longtermscorecard.org/. Accessed March 2018.)

(Nguyen, 2017). LTC is the largest expenditure for older adults in the United States.

LTC AND THE US HEALTH CARE SYSTEM

The U.S. health care system has been focused on delivering acute care needs and addressing time-limited and specific illnesses or injuries as they occur in episodes, driven by restrictions of Medicare, Medicaid, and private insurance. Such a system does not address the increasingly complex and long-term needs of people with chronic conditions who need acute and long-term services and support systems. Traditionally, health care has been made up of two sectors: acute care and ambulatory care. Each setting has been viewed as an independent entity with little coordination or recognition of LTC as an integral part of the continuum of care.

Today, the total spectrum of care has been expanded to include long-term and postacute care (LTPAC) services, which includes nursing homes, ALFs, home care, and hospice (Fig. 32.2). However, in the United States today, the LTPAC system is complex and fragmented, isolated from other service providers, and poorly funded; it also is confusing and difficult for the individual and the caregiver to access and negotiate. Access to services is dependent on funding governed by a mix of federal, state, and local rules and procedures. Separate agencies have unique eligibility rules, intake, and assessment processes. When individuals need LTC, they and their families must find and arrange for services on their own, sometimes on short notice when the need arises from a medical event or with a change in the individual's functional capacity.

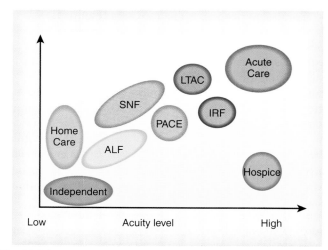

Fig. 32.2 Long-Term and Postacute Care Spectrum of Care. *ALF,* Assisted living facility; *IRF,* inpatient rehabilitation facility; *LTAC,* long-term acute care facility; *PACE,* Programs of All-Inclusive Care for the Elderly; *SNF,* skilled nursing facility. (From John F. Derr, RPh; JD and Associates Enterprises, Inc.)

There is no comprehensive approach to care coordination in the LTC system. As a result, services and supports may not be provided in the most appropriate setting by the most appropriate provider, the individual's needs and preferences may not be met, and caregivers may experience substantial stress trying to arrange for or provide care. This fragmented, provider- and setting-centered approach (as opposed to a person-centered approach) results in unmet needs, risk for injuries, and adverse outcomes (Box 32.1). There is also a critical shortage of

BOX 32.1 One Woman's Story

Myra is an 86-year-old woman who lives in her own condominium apartment in Florida. Her diagnoses include osteoarthritis and hypertension. She is a widow with no children or close relatives. She has about $80,000 in savings and is very careful living on a limited income monthly budget. Her hands are so deformed by arthritis that she cannot dress herself or turn the knob on her kitchen stove. She is very alert but is having increasing difficulty living alone. Friends and neighbors have been helping as much as they can. She has been on a waiting list for home and community-based services for a month. Due to her savings, she is not eligible for assistance with in-home care under Medicaid and the cost of a homemaker or aide is more than she can afford. Her savings do not make her eligible for Medicaid and she would have to spend down to $2000 to qualify.

She visits her primary care provider for her annual exam and asks about how she can get care services so that she can stay in her own home. Her primary care provider tells her she is not safe to live alone and she is given a list of nursing homes. She is shocked to discover that the nursing home can cost up to $90,000 yearly and is not covered by Medicare unless she has a skilled need. If she became ill and was discharged to a nursing home, Medicare would pay for a short-term nursing home stay (full coverage for 20 days and partial coverage for up to 80 days if she had a prior 3-day hospital admission) and skilled care needs. Upon discharge from the nursing home, if she still required skilled care, she could receive part-time home health care (registered nurse [RN] supervision, therapy, home health aide a couple of hours per day for personal care).

BOX 32.3 Goals of Long-Term Care

1. Provide a safe and supportive environment for chronically ill and functionally dependent people.
2. Restore and maintain highest practicable level of functional independence.
3. Preserve individual autonomy.
4. Maximize quality of life, well-being, and satisfaction with care.
5. Provide comfort and dignity at the end of life for residents and their families.
6. Provide coordinated interdisciplinary care to subacutely ill residents who plan to return to home or a less restrictive level of care.
7. Stabilize and delay progression, when possible, of chronic medical conditions.
8. Prevent acute medical and iatrogenic illnesses, and identify and treat them rapidly when they do occur.
9. Create a homelike environment that respects the dignity of each resident.

well-prepared health care professionals and direct care staff to provide LTC, putting the individual who needs LTC at further risk of poor outcomes (Chapter 2).

Health care professionals who have not had experience in the LTC system are often unaware of the many differences between acute care and LTC. Unless they have experienced the need for LTC in their own families, they may be unaware of the challenges associated with obtaining quality care for individuals with long-term needs. It is important for health care professionals, especially nurses, to understand the total spectrum of care and the differences between acute and LTC (Boxes 32.2 and 32.3). "Without addressing the obstacles discussed above, we will continue to move forward with a partial view of older adults—one seen through an acute and medical lens, rather than seeing a person with a story, a family system, and a community" (Golden and Shier, 2012–2013, p. 11).

BOX 32.2 Focus of Acute and Long-Term Care

Acute Care Orientation	Long-Term Care Orientation
• Illness	• Function
• High technology	• High touch
• Short term	• Extended
• Episodic	• Interdisciplinary model
• One-dimensional	• Ongoing
• Professional	• Multidimensional
• Medical model	• Paraprofessional and family
• Cure	• Care

GLOBAL APPROACHES TO LTC

Most countries are facing increasing challenges surrounding LTC for the growing numbers of older adults. Many of the developed countries have been preparing for big increases in their older populations and the associated growth in the need for LTC services for many years. Every developed country in the world, except for the United States and the United Kingdom, has some system for universal LTC. The United States and the United Kingdom (excluding Scotland) are the only developed countries that still operate a means-tested system (Medicaid in the United States). Most governments have established collectively financed systems for personal and nursing home care cost. It may be social insurance (e.g., Germany, Japan, Korea), a personal care benefit (e.g., paying informal caregivers in cash or in-kind for services) (e.g., France, Italy, Australia), or fully integrated social care (e.g., Sweden, Norway) (Box 32.4).

All nations need to take steps to prepare for the growing numbers of older adults by creating sustainable financing systems, developing better ways to support informal caregivers, and focusing efforts on prevention and chronic care management. By sharing best practices, nations can learn from one another in designing systems of care that support the health and well-being of their citizens. As the United States looks to improving the LTC system, there is a slow shift away from a solely acute medical model and more emphasis on managing chronic disease and LTC and prevention while lowering costs and preserving quality. The US Senate Commission on Long-Term Care's *Report to the Congress* (2013) provides a comprehensive look at the existing system and offers many excellent best practice recommendations for improvement. A few are presented in Box 32.5.

PROMOTING HEALTHY AGING: IMPLICATIONS FOR GERONTOLOGICAL NURSING

We know we can do better providing care to those with long-term needs even in times of fiscal restraint through creative planning and utilization of best practices. Gerontological nurse

---

BOX 32.4 A Swedish Example of Long-Term Care

Roger is an 87-year-old widowed man who lives alone in the home he has owned for more than 40 years. He fell and broke his hip and received care in the hospital in his local municipality. All of his care in the hospital, including rehabilitation, was covered by the government. When he was ready for discharge, a care plan meeting with Roger, his family/significant others, the district nurse in his municipality, social worker, and therapists was held to evaluate how much care he will need following discharge. He will not be discharged until the plan is decided. If Roger is able to return home safely, he will receive personal care up to several times a day (getting up, dressing, grooming, toileting, meals, going to bed) at no charge to him. Services are supported through taxes and administered through the local municipalities.

If his family wants to provide some of this care, they can receive a stipend equivalent to the salary of the paid caregivers. Care plan meetings are held with the team to determine the type of services he needs, and the frequency; however, he can receive home assistance until his function improves and he is able to live safely at home. If he continues to need extensive care at home (24 hours/day) that is more expensive than nursing home care, he will be evaluated for nursing home care. If he needs to go to a nursing home, he must go to a home in his area. Individuals with the greatest need have priority and sometimes there is a waiting period before admission. He may pay a small fee for the nursing home depending on his income level but probably not more than $150 to $200 per month. The remaining costs are covered through the government benefits. The district nurse will continue to coordinate his care and evaluate his status while he is in the nursing home.

In person communication, February 2016, Gabriella Engstrom RN, PhD.

BOX 32.5 U.S. Senate Commission on LTC: Selected Recommendations

- Strengthen long-term services and supports (LTSS) financing through private options for financial protection (long-term care [LTC] insurance, tax preference for LTC policies, protection for catastrophic LTC costs).
- Strengthen LTSS financing through social insurance (comprehensive Medicare benefit for LTSS through increase in Medicare payroll tax and creation of Part A premium).
- Eliminate the 3-day hospital stay requirement for skilled nursing facility (SNF) coverage.
- Reconsider the requirement for home health services under Medicare that the individual be "homebound."
- Create a more responsive, integrated, person-centered and fiscally responsible LTSS delivery system that ensures people can access quality services in settings they choose.
- Promote active involvement of individuals and family caregivers in making care decisions and ensuring delivery of care in the least restrictive setting consistent with their preferences.
- Establish a single point of contact for LTSS on the care team (personal navigator, care coordinator).
- Develop a standardized assessment tool that can produce a single care plan across care settings.
- Enhance options and improve focus on quality across settings, with particular attention to home and community-based care.
- Create livable communities and more opportunities to "age-in-place" (Chapter 20).
- Develop a national strategy to support family caregivers.
- Create meaningful career ladders for direct care workers to improve access to career advancement opportunities and improved compensation.

From United States Senate, Commission on Long-Term Care: *Report to the Congress,* September 13, 2013. https://www.gpo.gov/fdsys/pkg/GPO-LTCCOMMISSION/content-detail.html. Accessed March 2018.

---

educators, researchers, and providers must be knowledgeable about the full spectrum of LTPAC so that they can assist individuals and their caregivers to obtain the most appropriate care to enhance health and well-being. Nurses also must advocate for improved financing and delivery of LTSS services so that quality, equitable, seamless, and affordable person-centered care is available for all in need of such services.

FORMAL LONG-TERM CARE SERVICE PROVIDERS

The following section describes some of the types of facilities and programs providing LTC services in the United States. Services available and characteristics of the individuals served are discussed. It is important for nurses in all practice settings to be knowledgeable about the range of services so that they can assist older adults and their families in making decisions when the need for LTC arises. Nurses who practice in acute care need to know the characteristics of the setting from which the patient is admitted, and to which they will be discharged, to create appropriate discharge plans and effective transitions of care. Most nurses work in one setting and are not familiar with the requirements of other settings or the needs of individuals in these settings. As a result, there are often significant misunderstandings and criticisms of care in different settings across the continuum. We can no longer work in our individual "silos" and not be concerned with what happens after the patient is out of our particular institution.

Community Care
Program for All-Inclusive Care for the Elderly

This program is a Medicaid and Medicare program that provides community services to individuals who would otherwise need a nursing home level of care. Participants must meet the criteria for nursing home admission, prefer to remain in the community, and be eligible for Medicare/Medicaid. It is a full service model that covers the cost of primary care, hospitalization, emergency department visits, approved specialty services, rehabilitation, home care, medication and treatment, and social and recreational services in a community center environment. The All-Inclusive Care for the Elderly (PACE) program has been the only Medicare program that has required and paid for interdisciplinary team care using a capitated payment. Nursing has been central to the PACE care model since its inception. Outcomes of PACE include increased use of ambulatory services, lower rates of nursing home use and in-patient hospitalization, lower rates of functional decline, and better reported health status than among a comparison population (Cortes and Sullivan-Marx, 2016).

PACE is recognized as a permanent provider under Medicare and a state option under Medicaid. Currently, there are 123 PACE programs operating 250 PACE centers in 31 states serving over 45,000 participants. PACE has been approved by the U.S. Department of Health and Human Services (USDHHS) Substance Abuse and Mental Health Services Administration (SAMHSA) as an evidence-based model of care. Models such as PACE are innovative care delivery models, and continued development of such models is important as the population ages (National PACE Association, 2019) (Box 32.6).

Adult Day Services

Adult day services (ADSs) are community-based group programs designed to provide social and some health services to adults who need supervised care in a safe setting during the day. They also offer caregivers respite from the responsibilities of caregiving, and most provide educational programs, support groups, and individual counseling for caregivers. Adult day centers are serving populations with higher levels of physical disability and chronic disease.

Increasingly, ADSs are being utilized to provide community-based care for conditions like Alzheimer's disease and for transitional care and short-term rehabilitation following hospitalization. Nearly half of all ADS participants have some level of dementia. Staff ratios in ADS are one direct care worker to six clients. Almost 80% of centers have professional nursing staff, 50% have a social worker, and 60% offer case management services. Most also offer transportation services.

Some ADSs are private pay, and others are funded through Medicaid home and community-based waiver programs, state and local funding, and the Veterans Administration (Table 32.1). ADSs hold the potential to meet the need for cost-efficient and high-quality LTC services, and continued expansion and funding are expected. ADSs are an important part of the LTPAC continuum and a cost-effective alternative or supplement to home care or institutional care. Although further research is needed on patient and caregiver outcomes of ADS, findings suggest that they improve health-related quality of life for participants and improve caregiver well-being. Local area agencies on aging are good sources of information about ADSs and other community-based options.

Continuing Care Retirement Communities (CCRCs)

Life care communities, also known as CCRCs, provide the full range of residential options, from single-family homes to skilled nursing facilities all in one location. Most of these communities provide access to these levels of care for a community member's entire remaining lifetime, and for the right price, the range of services may be guaranteed. Having all levels of care in one location allows community members to make the transition between levels without life-disrupting moves. For married couples in which one spouse needs more care than the other, life care communities allow them to live nearby in a different part of the same community. Most CCRCs are managed by not-for-profit organizations. Entrance fees can range from as low as $20,000 for a non-purchase (rental) agreement to buy-in fees among the most expensive CCRCs of up to $500,000 or more depending on the size and location of the unit and the community. Monthly costs can be as low as $500 at some communities and as high as $3000 or more depending on type of contract and service plan. Costs of CCRCs are paid out-of-pocket and not covered by Medicare or Medicaid.

Residential Care/Assisted Living

Residential care/assisted living (RC/AL) facilities are non-medical facilities that provide room, meals, housekeeping, supervision and distribution of medication, and personal care assistance with basic activities like hygiene, dressing, eating, bathing, and transferring. This level of care is for individuals who are unable to live by themselves but who do not need 24-hour nursing care. RC/AL are known by more than 30 different names across the country, including adult congregate facilities, foster care homes, personal care homes, homes for the elderly, domiciliary care homes, board and care homes, rest homes, family care homes, retirement homes, and assisted living facilities (ALFs).

BOX 32.6   Resources for Best Practice

Alzheimer's Association: Dementia Care Practice Recommendations for assisted living facilities (ALFs) and Nursing Homes

American Assisted Living Nurses Association: Certification, Scope and Standards of Practice

American Healthcare Association/National Center for Assisted Living: Information, educational resources, guide to choosing an assisted living facility and skilled nursing facility

Argentum (formerly the Assisted Living Federation of America): Information, educational resources, guide to choosing an ALF

Centers for Medicare and Medicaid Services: Guide to choosing a nursing home; Nursing Home Compare; Nursing Home Quality Care Collaborative (NHQCC) Learning; Partnership to Improve Dementia Care in Nursing Homes; Quality Assurance and Performance Improvement (QAPI)

Eden Alternative

National Adult Day Services Association

National Programs of All-Inclusive Care for the Elderly (PACE) Association

Pathway Health, Interact Program: Quality improvement for nursing homes. http://www.pathway-interact.com/interact-tools/interact-tools-library/interact-version-4-0-tools-for-nursing-homes/

The Green House Project

The National Nursing Home Quality Improvement Campaign: Evidence-based and model-practice resources to support quality improvement

National Consumer Voice for Long-Term Care: National voice representing consumers in issues related to long-term care; information and resources to help insure quality care; Guide to Choosing a Nursing Home

Pioneer Network: Culture change information and toolkit

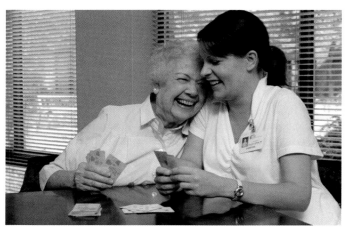

Providing nursing services in assisted living facilities promotes physical and psychosocial health. (From Potter PA: *Basic nursing: essentials for practice,* ed 7, St Louis, 2010, Mosby.)

RC/AL are viewed as more cost-effective than nursing homes while providing more privacy and a homelike environment. Medicare does not cover the cost of care in these types of facilities. The majority of individuals in RC/AL pay for their care from their personal resources and 47% of facilities accept Medicaid. Private and LTC insurance may also cover some costs. The rates charged and the services those rates include vary considerably, as do regulations and licensing. States are responsible for regulating RC/AL and there are no federal quality standards or mandatory reporting on quality similar to Nursing Home Compare.

Assisted living. A popular type of RC/AL is ALFs, also called *board and care homes* or *adult congregate living facilities.* Box 32.7 presents information about the typical ALF resident. ALF settings may be a shared room or a single-occupancy unit with a private bath, kitchenette, and communal meals. They all provide some support services but if care needs increase, there is usually a charge for services. If the individual has a skilled need, Medicare will cover a portion of the care in the setting similar to coverage in the home.

Assisted living is more expensive than independent living and less costly than skilled nursing home care, but it is not inexpensive (Table 32.1). Costs vary by geographical region, size of the unit, and relative luxury. Forty-two percent of ALFs are small with four to ten beds and 33% have between 26 and 100 beds. Most ALFs offer two or three meals per day, light weekly housekeeping, and laundry services, and optional social activities. Each added service increases the cost of the setting but also allows for individuals with resources to remain in the setting longer, as functional abilities decline. Consumers are advised to inquire as to exactly what services will be provided and by whom if an ALF resident becomes more frail and needs more intensive care.

Many older adults and their families prefer ALFs to nursing homes because they cost less, are more homelike, and offer more opportunities for control, independence, and privacy. However, many residents of ALFs have chronic care needs and over time may require more care than the facility is able to provide. Services (e.g., home health, hospice, homemakers) can be brought into the facility, but some question whether this adequately substitutes for 24-hour supervision by registered nurses (RNs). Only 17% of residential care facilities (RCFs) reported having registered, licensed practical, or vocational nurses on staff. RCFs are not required to provide licensed nursing on a 24-hour basis, even though there is evidence that many residents in some facilities are frail, with many chronic illnesses, impaired self-care needs and cognition, and unmet care needs (Harrington et al, 2017).

With the growing numbers of older adults with dementia residing in ALFs, many are establishing dementia-specific units. It is important to investigate services available, and staff training, when making decisions about the most appropriate placement for older adults with dementia. Continued research is needed on best care practices and outcomes of care for people with dementia in both ALFs and nursing homes. The Alzheimer's Association has issued a set of dementia care practices for ALFs and nursing homes (Alzheimer's Association, 2009).

The nonmedical nature of ALFs is a primary factor in keeping costs more reasonable than those in nursing facilities, but costs are still high for those without adequate funds. Appropriate standards of care must be developed, and care outcomes monitored to ensure that residents are receiving quality care in this setting, which is almost devoid of professional nursing. Available data about facility to resident ratios raise questions about care quality (Harrington et al, 2017). "The absence of oversight and regulations requires families to do extra due diligence before choosing a facility" (Gleckman, 2018). Further research is needed on care outcomes of residents in ALFs and the role of unlicensed assistive personnel, and RNs, in these facilities.

Advanced practice gerontological nurses are well suited to the role of primary care provider in ALFs, and many have assumed this role. The American Assisted Living Nurses Association has established a certification mechanism for nurses working in these facilities and has also developed a *Scope and Standards of Assisted Living Nursing Practice for Registered Nurses.* The Assisted Living Federation of America and the National Center for Assisted Living provide a consumer guide for choosing an AL residence (Box 32.6).

BOX 32.7   Profile of a Resident in an Assisted Living Facility

- 32% 75 years to 84 years; 51% over 85 years
- Female (72%)
- 38% need help with 3–5 activities of daily living; 61% need help with bathing; 45% need help dressing; 37% need help with toileting; 18% need help with eating; 25% need help with bed transfer
- About 52% are cognitively impaired
- The median length of stay is about 22 months
- 59% move to a nursing facility
- 33% die while a resident of an assisted living facility

From National Center for Assisted Living: https://www.ahcancal.org/ncal/Pages/index.aspx. Accessed March 2018.

Skilled Nursing Facilities (Nursing Homes)

Nursing homes are the settings for the delivery of around-the-clock care for those needing specialized care that cannot be provided elsewhere. Nursing homes are a complex health care setting that is a mix of hospital, rehabilitation facility, hospice, and dementia-specific units, and they are a final home for many older adults. When used appropriately, nursing homes fill an important need for families and older adults.

Characteristics of Nursing Homes

The settings called *nursing homes* or *nursing facilities* most often include up to two levels of care: a *skilled nursing care* (also called *subacute care*) facility is required to have licensed professionals with a focus on the management of complex medical needs; and a *chronic care* (also called *long-term* or *custodial*) facility is required to have 24-hour personal assistance that is supervised and augmented by professional and licensed nurses. Often, both kinds of services are provided in one facility.

There are approximately 15,655 certified nursing homes in the United States with 1.7 million beds. The majority of nursing homes (70%) are for-profit organizations (American Healthcare Association/National Center Assisted Living [HCA/NCAL], 2018). The number of nursing home beds is decreasing in the United States as a result of the increased use of RCFs and more reimbursement by Medicaid programs for community-based care alternatives. However, in most areas of the country, the supply and use of nursing homes is still greater than those of other LTC service options. Of the 3.9 million individuals needing care, 22% have stays of less than 100 days and 78% have stays of 100 days or more (CDC, 2017). Long-term chronic care nursing home residents represent the most frail of all older adults. Their needs for 24-hour care could not be met in the home or RC setting or may have exceeded what the family was able to provide.

Subacute Care (Short Term)

Subacute care is more intensive than traditional nursing home care and several times more costly, but far less costly than care in a hospital. Skilled nursing facilities are the most frequent site of postacute care in the United States. The expectation is that the patient will be discharged home or to a less intensive setting. Length of stay is usually no more than 1 to 3 months. In addition to skilled nursing care, rehabilitation services are an essential component of subacute units. Length of stay is usually less than 1 month and is largely reimbursed by Medicare. Patients in subacute units are usually younger and less likely to be cognitively impaired than those in traditional nursing home care. Generally, higher levels of professional staffing are found in the subacute setting than those in the traditional nursing home setting because of the acuity of the patient's condition (Chapter 2).

Chronic Care (Long Term)

Nursing homes also care for patients who may not need the intense care provided in subacute units but still need ongoing 24-hour care. This may include individuals with severe strokes, dementia, or Parkinson disease, and those receiving hospice

care. Residents of long-term chronic care facilities are predominantly women, 80 years or older, widowed, and dependent in ADLs and IADLs. About 50% of these residents are cognitively impaired, and these types of facilities are increasingly caring for people at the end of life. Twenty-three percent of Americans die in nursing homes, and this figure is expected to increase to 40% by 2040 (Stanford School of Medicine, 2019; Teno et al, 2013). While the percentage of older adults living in nursing homes at any given time is low (4% to 5%), those who live to age 85 will have a one in two chance of spending some time in a nursing home. This could be for subacute care, ongoing LTC, or end-of-life care.

Interprofessional Team Model in Subacute and Long-Term Care

An interprofessional team, working with the resident and family, assesses, plans, and implements care in nursing homes and all facilities that provide rehabilitation and restorative programs (Box 32.8). Rehabilitation and restorative care is increasingly important in light of shortened hospital stays that may occur before conditions are stabilized and the older adult is not ready to function independently. The opportunity to work collaboratively with a team is one of the most exciting aspects of practice in LTC facilities.

Professional Nursing in Long-Term Care

There are a wide range of opportunities for professional nursing in skilled nursing facilities and projections of an increase in the need in the coming years (Chapter 2). The setting provides opportunities for learning and practice in areas that are core to 21st century nursing: managing chronic illness and palliative care in ways that are patient-centered and evidence-based, working with interdisciplinary teams, supervising unlicensed caregivers, and developing systems for quality improvement. Professional nursing practice in this setting is different from acute care in terms of competencies, focus, and goals of care. LTC should be marketed as a bright future career for young nurses that requires excellent technical and critical thinking skills and is more autonomous than other areas of nursing (Sherman and Touhy, 2017). Nursing education programs and

---

BOX 32.8 Interprofessional Teams in Nursing Homes

Patient
Family/significant others
Nurse
Primary care provider: physician, nurse practitioner
Physical, occupational, speech therapists
Social worker
Dietitian
Discharge planner/case manager
Psychologist
Prosthetist and orthotist
Audiologist

facility orientation and training programs must prepare nurses to practice competently in this important and growing care setting (Research Highlights box).

⚡ RESEARCH HIGHLIGHTS

This qualitative focused ethnography explored the complexities of care; working environments; and knowledge, skills, and efforts of care aides who work in nursing homes. Twenty female and two male care aides from one privately funded and four publicly funded nursing homes in a western Canadian province were interviewed. Swanson's Middle Range Theory of Caring was used as a framework for the study. Interview data were analyzed in a two-stage process. Descriptive analysis was used to identify their perceptions and experiences and then the fit between their perceptions and experiences, context of care, and Swanson's Middle Range Theory of Caring was explored.

The following four themes were identified: (1) desiring the ideal relationship; (2) establishing relationships with residents and their families; (3) maintaining relationships with residents and their families; and (4) the reality of care aide work. Forming and maintaining relationships was viewed as a foundational and significant component of care aide work. The work occurs within a helping and caring framework and is not "just completing tasks." Care aides are the central and most accessible service providers in nursing homes and the caring between the care aides and the residents/families is to be valued and nurtured. The authors state: "The complexities of care and working environments are not well understood, and the knowledge, skills, and efforts of those who have chosen careers in residential care remain obscure and undervalued" (p. 24). Further research is needed to more fully explore the nature and expression of caring in nursing homes and its potential to improve both outcomes and quality of life.

From Andersen E, Spiers J: Care aides' relational practices and caring contributions, *J Gerontol Nurs* 42(11):24–30, 2016.

Nursing homes are often blamed for all of the societal problems associated with the aging of our population. Daily, millions of dedicated caregivers in nursing homes are providing competent and compassionate care to very sick older adults against great odds, such as a lack of support, inadequate salaries and staff, inadequate funding, and a lack of respect. It is time for their stories to be told, and it is time to recognize their needs for adequate and well-trained staff to do this very important work. Although there are continued challenges and opportunities to improve care in nursing homes (and care in all settings for older adults) and in the fabric of the LTC system, many nursing homes provide an environment that truly represents the best of caring and quality of life. "The many positive aspects of nursing in LTC facilities are often overshadowed by an uncomplimentary image of care in this setting, influenced by a history laden with scandals and the media's readiness to highlight the abuses and substandard conditions demonstrated by a small minority. This negative image is compounded by reimbursement policies that significantly limit the ability to provide high-quality care" (Eliopoulos, 2010, p. 365).

Since the 1990s, more than 150 research studies have examined the effect of nurse staffing levels and improved quality outcomes in states with higher minimum staffing levels, particularly registered nurse staffing, on care outcomes, with most finding positive effects with higher staffing levels and improved quality outcomes. Benefits of higher staffing levels, especially RNs, include lower mortality rates; improved physical functioning; less antibiotic use; fewer pressure ulcers, catheterized residents, and urinary tract infections; lower hospitalization rates; and less weight loss and dehydration. In addition to staffing levels, nursing staff training and competency have been identified as critical factors in ensuring high quality care (Harrington et al, 2017). The use of nurse practitioners in nursing homes is also associated with improved patient outcomes and satisfaction (Chapter 2).

Despite the evidence of improved outcomes associated with professional nurse presence in nursing homes, federal rules require only one RN in the nursing facility for 8 hours a day, a figure quite shocking considering the ratio of RNs to patients in acute care, even in the face of shortages in this setting. Federal regulations require adequate staffing to meet the needs of the residents, and most nursing homes go beyond this minimal RN staffing, particularly in subacute units. However, the federal government has not acted to mandate increases in minimum RN staffing requirements. Many groups dealing with issues of the aging, as well as the American Nurses Association (ANA), have supported the critical need for adequate staffing in nursing homes. An expert panel on nursing homes provided comprehensive recommendations for improved RN staffing and increased gerontological nursing education requirements for all staff (Box 32.9). Continued research on new models of care delivery and the appropriate mix of all levels of nursing staff in subacute and long-term units is needed to improve outcomes.

Nursing Assistants

Although it is important to promote professional nursing care for all older adults, nursing assistants provide the majority of direct care in nursing homes and significantly contribute to the quality of life for residents. Research results support the deep commitment and passion that nursing assistants bring to their jobs (Box 32.10). The significance and importance of close personal relationships between nursing assistants and residents, often described as "like family," is emerging as a central dimension of quality of care and positive outcomes. The commitment and dedication of nursing home staff must be honored and supported. They have much to teach us about aging, nursing, and caring. Box 32.11 presents a description of caring themes expressed by nursing home caregivers.

BOX 32.9   Expert Panel Recommendations: Professional Nursing in Nursing Homes

Bachelor of science in nursing (BSN) degree for directors of nursing
Increased staffing ratios for registered nurses (RNs), licensed practical nurses (LPNs), and nursing assistants
Most nursing homes should have a full-time clinical nurse specialist (CNS) or gerontological nurse practitioner (GNP) on staff

From Harrington C, Kovner C, Mezey M, et al: Experts recommend minimum staffing standards for nursing facilities in the United States. *Gerontologist* 40(1):5–16, 2000.

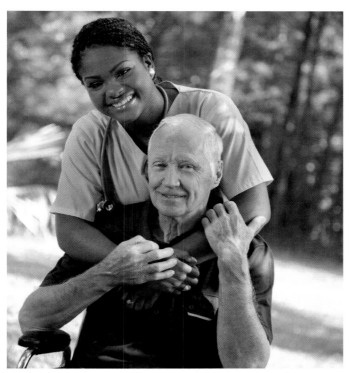

Caring relationships between staff and residents in long-term care enhance quality of care. (©iStock.com/Pamela Moore.)

BOX 32.11 Bill of Rights for Long-Term Care Residents

- The right to voice grievances and have them remedied
- The right to information about health conditions and treatments and to participate in one's own care to the greatest extent possible
- The right to choose one's own health care providers and to speak privately with one's health care providers
- The right to consent to or refuse all aspects of care and treatments
- The right to manage one's own finances, if capable, or to choose one's own financial advisor
- The right to be transferred or discharged only for appropriate reasons
- The right to be free from all forms of abuse
- The right to be free from all forms of restraint to the extent compatible with safety
- The right to privacy and confidentiality concerning one's person, personal information, and medical information
- The right to be treated with dignity, consideration, and respect in keeping with one's individuality
- The right to immediate visitation and access at any time for family, health care providers, and legal advisors; the right to reasonable visitation and access for others

Note: This list of rights is a sampling of federal and several states' lists of rights of residents or participants in long-term care. Nurses should check the rules of their own state for specific rights in law for that state.

BOX 32.10 How We Care: Voices of Nursing Home Staff

Responding to What Matters
Taking time to do the little things, competence, cleanliness, meeting basic needs, safe administration of medications, kindness and consideration

Caring as a Way of Expressing Spiritual Commitment
Spiritual beliefs lead staff to long-term care and continue to motivate and guide the special care they give to residents; they reflect a spiritual commitment to caring for residents as expressed in the golden rule: "Do unto others as you would like done to you."

Devotion Inspired by Love for Others
Deep connection between staff and residents described as being like family, caring for residents as you would for your own mother or father, sharing of good and bad times, going out on a limb to be an advocate, listening, and staying with residents when others had given up

Commitment to Creating a Home Environment
Nursing home is the resident's home, staff are guests in the home; the importance of cleanliness, privacy, good food, and feeling part of a family

Coming to Know and Respect Person as Person
Treating residents, families, and one another with respect and dignity, being recognized for the person you are, intimate knowing of likes and dislikes, individualized care

Adapted from Touhy T, Strews W, Brown C: Expressions of caring as lived by nursing home staff, residents, and families, *Int J Human Caring* 9:31, 2005.

Critical shortages of nursing assistants exist now in RCFs, skilled care, and home care, and these shortages will worsen in the future. Recruitment, retention, and high turnover rates are a problem in nursing homes. Several recent studies have investigated the relationship of factors such as turnover, work satisfaction, staffing, and power relations to quality of care and positive outcomes in nursing homes. Results support the importance of developing a culture of respect in which the work of nursing assistants is understood and valued at all levels of the organization. An important nursing role in LTC is the supervision and education of nursing assistants to enable them to competently perform in their role as an essential member of the care team.

Currently, federal standards for education and training for certified nursing assistants require a minimum of 75 training hours. As a result of the increasing complexity of the clinical setting, regulatory changes in requirements may be indicated. A recent study reported that 151.6 total training hours and a ratio of twice as many clinical hours to didactic hours are needed to promote quality of care in nursing homes (Trinkoff et al, 2017).

One of the most important components of the culture change movement (discussed later) is the creation of models of care that value and honor the important work of nursing assistants. Culture change must be equally concerned about the needs of residents and the well-being of staff (Thomas and Johansson, 2003). "An organization that learns to give love, respect, dignity, tenderness, and tolerance to all members of the staff will soon find these same virtues being practiced by the staff" (Thomas and Johansson, 2003, p. 3).

Until health care professionals and our society make a real commitment to providing adequate wages, individual supports (e.g., health insurance, education, career ladders), and an appreciation of their significant contribution to quality of nursing home care, these neglected workers cannot be expected to have the energy or incentive to extend themselves to the older adults in their care. Care of the frail older adult and seriously ill persons is labor intensive and costly and requires specialized knowledge. Reasonable workloads, enhanced education and training, and adequate reimbursement are essential. The meaning and value of the work of nursing assistants must be supported by professional nurses and communicated to nursing home owners, managers, legislators, and other health care professionals (Andersen and Spiers, 2016).

Resident Bill of Rights

Regulations have also been created to protect the rights of the residents of nursing homes. Residents in LTC facilities have rights under both federal and state laws. The staff of the facility must inform residents of these rights and protect and promote their rights. The rights to which the residents are entitled should be conspicuously posted in the facility (Box 32.12). Also, the Long-Term Care Ombudsman Program is a nationwide effort to support the rights of both the residents and

---

BOX 32.12 Quality Measures for Nursing Homes

Percentage of Short-Stay Residents With:
- Moderate to severe pain
- Pressure ulcers that are new or worsened
- Seasonal influenza vaccine
- Pneumococcal vaccine
- Antipsychotic medication
- Improvements in function
- Any cause hospital readmission
- Community discharge for 100 days without readmission
- Outpatient emergency department visit

Percentage of Long-Term Residents With:
- One or more falls with a major injury
- Urinary tract infections
- Moderate to severe pain
- Pressure ulcers that are new or worsened
- Loss of bowel and bladder control
- Use of a bladder catheter
- Physical restraints
- A need for increased help with daily activities
- Weight loss
- Depressive symptoms
- Antipsychotic medication
- Seasonal influenza vaccine
- Pneumococcal vaccine
- Ability to move independently worsened
- Antianxiety or hypnotic medication

From Harrington C, Wiener J, Musumeci M: Key issues in long-term care services and supports quality, *The Henry J Kaiser Family Foundation Issue Brief*, October 2017. https://www.kff.org/report-section/key-issues-in-long-term-services-and-supports-quality-appendix/. Accessed March 2018.

---

the facilities. In most states, the program provides trained volunteers to investigate rights and quality complaints or conflicts. All reporting is anonymous. Each facility is required to post the name and contact information of the ombudsman assigned to the facility.

QUALITY OF CARE IN SKILLED NURSING FACILITIES

Nursing homes are one of the most highly regulated industries in the United States. The Omnibus Budget Reconciliation Act (OBRA) of 1987 and the frequent revisions and updates are designed to improve the quality of resident care and have had a positive impact. Some of the requirements of OBRA and subsequent legislation include the following: comprehensive resident assessments (Minimum Data Set [MDS]) (Chapter 7), increased training requirements for nursing assistants, elimination of the use of medications and restraints for the purpose of discipline or convenience, higher staffing requirements for nursing and social work staff, standards for nursing home administrators, and quality assurance activities. The Quality Assurance Performance Improvement (QAPI) requires all nursing homes participating in Medicare or Medicaid programs to implement a QAPI program to assess quality of care provided to residents and to improve outcomes. The National Nursing Home Quality Improvement Campaign provides free, easy access to evidence-based and model-practice resources to support continuous quality improvement (Box 32.6). The Skilled Nursing Facility Value-Based Purchasing Program (SNF VBF), beginning in 2019, rewards skilled nursing facilities with incentive payments for the quality of care they give to individuals with Medicare (CMS, 2018).

Nursing homes undergo regular unannounced surveys every 9 to 15 months and surveys are also conducted in response to complaints. Detailed inspection data and penalties for violations for individual nursing homes are reported on CMS's Nursing Home Compare website (www.medicare.gov/NHCompare). Nursing homes were the first to publish online quality information, which is now available for hospitals and other health care organizations. Nursing home also receive an overall quality rating using CMS's Five-Star Rating System based on annual inspection and complaint investigation data provided by state agencies; facility-reported nurse staffing hours/resident day; and quality measures based on MDS resident data.

Most nursing home quality measures have improved over time. Between 2011 and 2016, the use of physical restraints and antipsychotic medications, pressure ulcers among high risk residents, the percentage of residents experiencing pain and urinary tract infections, and the proportion of residents with ADL impairments that got worse declined. In 2014, 23.9% of long-stay nursing home residents were receiving an antipsychotic medication; since then there has been a decrease of 35.4% to a national prevalence of 15.4% (CMS, 2019). The prevalence rate of antipsychotic use declined in nursing homes as a result of several proactive measures but rates of antipsychotic use among individuals with dementia living in the community are rising. Recommendations are to expand the efforts to curb the use of these drugs beyond nursing homes (Carter, 2018).

Disparities in care quality are associated with resident race/ethnicity; for profit/nonprofit status (higher quality is associated with the non-profit status); and staffing levels. In spite of the benefits of using report cards, a recent study found that most hospital patients do not receive data about nursing home quality and receive only lists of nursing homes. Nurses involved in discharge planning are encouraged to use the CMS report cards so patient's choices are based on quality data (Harrington et al, 2017). Box 32.12 presents quality measures.

Improving Quality of Transitional Care in Nursing Homes

Transitional care is discussed in depth in Chapter 2, but some further information related to improving the quality of transitional care in nursing homes is presented in this section. Most current models of transitional care focus on care transitions from hospital to home, but increasing attention is being directed to other types of transitions such as hospital to nursing home, nursing home to hospital, and nursing home to home. Providing a seamless continuum of care through improved coordination of acute care, postacute care, and LTC services and better management of transitions between care settings are essential in health care today to address both cost and quality issues.

Medicare patients admitted to a postacute care facility following hospital discharge have an increased risk of readmission, with more than a quarter readmitted to the hospital in the first week and one-fifth readmitted within 30 days. Up to two-thirds of these hospital transfers are rated as potentially avoidable by expert LTC health professionals (http://www.pathway-interact.com/). However, the rate of potentially avoidable hospitalizations among SNF residents has fallen by nearly a third in recent years as a result of many quality improvement initiatives (Mongan, 2016). Hospitalization of nursing home residents potentially causes harm, both mentally and physically, to the resident and increases stress for the family/significant others.

The QAPI program requirements discussed above include attention to improving transitional care processes and effectively managing acute changes in an individual's condition while in the nursing home. Components of transitional care models and best practices in transitional care are presented in Chapter 2.

Interventions to Reduce Acute Care Transfers (INTERACT) is an exemplary program for reducing the frequency of transfers to the acute hospital from nursing homes. INTERACT is a quality improvement program with communication tools, care paths or clinical tools, and advance care planning tools to assist nursing homes in identifying and managing acute changes in condition without hospital transfer when safe and feasible (interact2.net). Other successful interventions include the use of nurse practitioners working in collaborative teams with physicians, standardized admission assessments, palliative care consultations for residents with recurrent hospitalizations, and interprofessional case conferences.

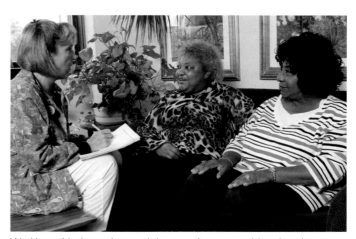

Working with the patient and the caregiver to provide education to enhance self-care abilities and to facilitate linkages to resources is important for the consideration of promoting safe discharges and transitions to home and other care settings. (From Potter, P.A. (2010). *Basic nursing: essentials for practice* (7th ed.). St Louis: Mosby.)

Choosing a Quality Nursing Home

While the national rating system for nursing homes is helpful for evaluating quality, Centers for Medicare and Medicaid Services (CMS) advises consumers to use additional sources of information because the rating system provides only a "snap shot" of the care in individual nursing homes following one inspection and should not substitute for visiting nursing homes. The most appropriate method of choosing a nursing home is to personally visit the facility, meet with the director of nursing, observe care routines, discuss the potential resident's needs, and use a format such as the one presented in Box 32.13 to ask questions. CMS provides a nursing home checklist on its website, and the National Consumer Voice for Quality Long-Term Care also provides resources for choosing a nursing home and understanding quality measures (Box 32.6).

Nurses play an important role in helping individuals and their family/significant others understand the discharge process and their posthospital needs, particularly if discharge to a skilled nursing facility is planned. CMS recommends that an evaluation of discharge be performed at least 48 hours before discharge, but ideally, discharge planning should begin on admission. Patient and family education should include the role of skilled nursing facilities in rehabilitation, role of members of the interprofessional team, interpretation of five-star ratings, and other information on how to choose a facility.

The Culture Change Movement

Across the United States, and internationally, the movement to transform nursing homes from the typical medical model into "homes" that nurture quality of life for older adults and support and empower frontline caregivers is changing the face of LTC. Begun by the Pioneer Network, a national not-for-profit organization that serves the culture change movement, many facilities are changing from a rigid institutional approach to one that is person centered. CMS has endorsed culture change in the federal nursing home regulations and has also released a

---

BOX 32.13 Selecting a Nursing Home

Central Focus
- Residents and families are the central focus of the facility.

Interaction
- Staff members are attentive and caring.
- Staff members listen to what residents say.
- Staff members and residents smile at one another.
- There is a prompt response to resident and family needs.
- Meaningful activities are provided on all shifts to meet individual preferences.
- Residents engage in activities with enjoyment.
- Staff members talk to cognitively impaired residents; cognitively impaired residents are involved in activities designed to meet their needs.
- Staff members do not talk down to residents, talk as if they are not present, ignore yelling or calling out.
- Families are involved in care decisions and daily life in facility.

Milieu
- Calm, active, friendly
- Presence of community, volunteers, children, plants, animals

Environment
- No odor, clean, and well maintained
- Rooms personalized
- Private areas
- Protected outside areas
- Equipment in good repair

Individualized Care
- Restorative programs for ambulation, ADLs
- Residents well dressed and groomed
- Resident and family councils
- Pleasant mealtimes, good food, residents have choices
- Adequate staff to serve meals and assist residents
- Flexible meal schedules, food available 24 hours per day
- Ethnic food preferences available

Staff
- Well trained, high level of professional skill
- Professional in appearance and demeanor
- RNs involved in care decisions and care delivery
- Active staff development programs
- Physicians and advanced practice nurses involved in care planning and staff training
- Adequate staff (more than the minimum required) on each shift
- Low staff turnover

Safety
- Safe walking areas indoors and outdoors
- Monitoring of residents at risk for injury
- Restraint-appropriate care, adequate safety equipment and training on its use

ADLs, Activities of daily living; *RNs,* registered nurses.
Adapted from Rantz MJ, Mehr DR, Popejoy L, et al: Nursing home care quality: a multidimensional theoretical model, *J Nurs Care Qual* 12:30–46, 1998.

---

self-study tool for nursing homes to assess their own progress toward culture change.

Culture change is the "process of moving from a traditional nursing home model—characterized as a system unintentionally designed to foster dependence by keeping residents, as one observer put it, 'well cared for, safe, and powerless'—to a regenerative model that increases residents' autonomy and sense of control" (Brawley, 2007, p. 9). The ultimate vision of culture change is to improve the lives of residents and staff by centering facility's philosophies, organizational structures, environmental designs, and care around practices that support residents' needs and preferences. Older adults in need of LTC want to live in a homelike setting that does not look and function like a hospital. They want a setting that allows them to make decisions they are used to making for themselves, such as when to get up, take a bath, eat, or go to bed. They want caregivers who know them and understand and respect their individuality and their preferences. Box 32.14 presents some

---

BOX 32.14 Institution-Centered Versus Person-Centered Culture

Institution-Centered Culture
- Schedules and routines are designed by the institution and staff, and residents must comply.
- Focus is on tasks that need to be accomplished.
- Rotation of staff among units occurs.
- Decision making is centralized with little involvement of staff or residents and families.
- There is a hospital environment.
- Structured activities are provided to all residents.
- There is little opportunity for socialization.
- Organization exists for employees rather than residents.
- There is little respect for privacy or individual routines.

Person-Centered Culture
- Emphasis is on relationships between staff and residents.
- Individualized plans of care are based on residents' needs, usual patterns, and desires.
- Staff members have consistent assignments and know the residents' preferences and uniqueness.
- Decision making is as close to that of the resident as possible.
- Staff members are involved in decisions and plans of care.
- Environment is homelike.
- Meaningful activities and opportunities for socialization are available around the clock.
- There is a sense of community and belonging—"like family."
- There is involvement of the community—children, pets, plants, outings.

Adapted from The Pioneer Network. www.pioneernetwork.net. Accessed March 2018.

BOX 32.15 Principles of Culture Change

- Care and activities are directed by the residents.
- The environment and care practices support a homelike atmosphere.
- Relationships among staff and residents are supported and fostered.
- Increased attention to respect of staff and the value of caring are promoted.
- Staff is empowered to respond to the residents' needs and desires.
- The organizational hierarchy is flattened to support collaborative decision making for staff.
- Comprehensive and continuous quality improvement underscores all activities and decisions to sustain a person-directed organizational culture.

Adapted from Mueller C, Burger S, Rader J, et al: Nurse competencies for person-directed care in nursing homes, *Geriatr Nurs* 34:101–104, 2013.

BOX 32.16 Nursing Home Culture Change Competencies for Nurses

Models, teaches, and utilizes effective communication skills such as active listening, giving meaningful feedback, communicating ideas clearly, addressing emotional behaviors, resolving conflict, and understanding the role of diversity in communication.

Creates systems and adapts daily routines and "person-directed" care practices to accommodate resident preferences.

Views self as part of team, not always the leader.

Evaluates the degree to which person-directed care practices exist in the care team and identifies and addresses barriers to person-directed care.

Views the care setting as the residents' home and works to create attributes of home.

Creates a system to maintain consistency of caregivers for residents.

Exhibits leadership characteristics/abilities to promote resident-directed care.

Role models person-directed care.

Problem solves complex medical/psychosocial situations related to resident choice and risk.

Facilitates team members, including residents and families, in shared problem solving, decision making, and planning.

From Mueller C, Burger S, Rader J, et al: Nurse competencies for person-directed care in nursing homes, *Geriatr Nurs* 34:101–104, 2013.

of the differences between an institution-centered culture and a person-centered culture.

While further research is needed, some results suggest that person-centered care is associated with improved organizational performance, including higher resident and staff satisfaction, better workforce performance, and higher occupancy rates. Examples of philosophies and programs of culture change are the Eden Alternative (companion animals, indoor plants, frequent visits by children, involvement with the community), the Green House Project (small homes designed for 10 to 12 residents), and the Wellspring Model. The Eden Alternative is best known for the addition of animals, plants, and visits from children to nursing homes. However, cats and dogs are not the heart of culture change. Truly transforming a nursing home starts at the top and requires involvement of all levels of staff and changes in values, attitudes, structures, and management practices. The principles central to culture change are presented in Box 32.15.

Nurses should take a leadership role in the culture change movement. Box 32.16 presents nursing home cultural change competencies for nurses. Strategic and cost-efficient methods of assisting nursing homes to implement culture change are needed and will require strong nursing leadership.

PROMOTING HEALTHY AGING: IMPLICATIONS FOR GERONTOLOGICAL NURSING

Nurses play a key role in improving quality of care in nursing homes through evidence-based practice and leadership in quality improvement initiatives. Nursing research has contributed significantly to the evidence-based interventions to improve quality of care in the nursing home. Further research needs to be directed to other LTPAC settings. For many, nursing in LTC offers the opportunity to practice the full scope of nursing, establish long-term relationships with patients and families, and make a significant difference in patient outcomes. While medical management is important, the need for expert nursing is the most essential service provided. More and more nursing graduates will practice in LTPAC settings, and education must prepare them for these roles. Nurses are increasingly recognized as important to improved health outcomes for the individual with LTC needs.

▌ KEY CONCEPTS

- LTC describes a variety of services, including medical and nonmedical care (assistance with ADLs and IADLs), provided on an ongoing basis to people of all ages who have a chronic illness or physical, cognitive, or developmental disabilities.
- LTC can be provided informally or formally in a range of environments, from an individual's home to the home of a friend or relative, an adult day health center, independent and ALFs, CCRCs, skilled nursing facilities, long-term chronic care facilities, and hospice.
- The total spectrum of health care in the United States has been expanded to include LTPAC services, which include nursing homes, ALFs, home care, and hospice.

- The bulk of long-term care throughout the developed world is informal unpaid care provided by family members. Without family caregivers, the present level of LTC could not be sustained.
- The number of older adults needing LTSS is dramatically increasing year after year, and the challenge of ensuring the quality and financial stability of care provision is one faced by governments in both the developed and the developing world.
- LTC coverage in the United States is expensive, fragmented, overly reliant on institutional care, and primarily financed by individuals themselves or their caregivers or by Medicaid.

- Nursing homes are the settings for the delivery of around-the-clock care for those needing specialized care that cannot be provided elsewhere. Nursing homes are a complex health care setting that is a mix of hospital, rehabilitation facility, hospice, and dementia-specific units, and they are a final home for many older adults.

- Quality of care in nursing homes is improving. In skilled nursing facilities nationwide, the average performance has improved. Professional nurse staffing results in improved outcomes.
- Culture change in nursing homes is a growing movement to develop models of person-centered care and improve outcomes and quality of life.

NURSING STUDY: TRANSITIONS ACROSS THE CONTINUUM

Ray is 85 years old and was recently admitted to the hospital from his own home following a fall with resultant fracture of the right hip. He was brought to the hospital by paramedics after a neighbor checked on him because they had not heard any sounds from his apartment. He had been lying on the floor for 8 hours unable to call for help. He lives alone in a one-bedroom condominium. His wife of 50 years died 4 years ago. His three adult children and their families live out of state but keep in close contact with their father and visit several times a year. The last time they saw their father was 4 months before his hospitalization.

Before the hip fracture, Ray was fairly capable of taking care of himself but since the death of his wife, his memory and mood have declined. He is hard of hearing in both ears but often refuses to wear his hearing aids, claiming that they distort all sounds and are a bother. He only occasionally left his apartment and had lost a great deal of weight. His neighbors reported that he was falling frequently and there were repeated calls to 911 for assistance. He had several "fender-benders" and had limited his driving to shopping and church. His children were becoming increasingly worried about him living alone. He refused to consider moving to live nearer or with his children or to an assisted living facility. He did not want to be a bother to his children. His home is full of family pictures, pictures from his worldwide travels with his wife, memorabilia from his days as a police officer, and antique furniture. He has a little dog who gives him great enjoyment.

Following a surgical repair of his fractured hip, he experienced delirium and his mental status declined. He received physical therapy but had difficulty following the orders for partial weight bearing on the affected leg. He became incontinent and required an adult brief. He also developed a necrotic pressure ulcer on his right heel. The hospital case manager recommended to the family that he be transferred to a skilled nursing facility for further rehabilitation, treatment of the pressure ulcer, and possible long-term care placement. It was felt that he could

not return safely to his home because of his mental status and functional decline. His finances were limited, so a home that accepted both Medicare and Medicaid was recommended.

Even though the family had promised their father that they would never put him in a nursing home and felt terrible, they agreed with the decision and felt relieved that he would not be living alone. Worried that he would be upset, they decided not to tell him that he would not be going home. They decided to sell his apartment to provide some money for his nursing home care. The children divided the furniture and memorabilia between them and sold the remaining household items. They chose not to tell him that they had done this and when he asked, they said: "When you get better, then you can go home." Ray's mental status continued to decline. He was unable to walk independently, experienced weight loss and sleep problems, and became more withdrawn.

Based on the case study, develop a nursing care plan using the following procedure[a]:

- List Ray's and the family comments that provide subjective data.
- List information that provides objective data.
- From these data, identify and state, using an accepted format, two nursing diagnoses you determine are most significant to Ray at this time. List two of Ray's strengths that you have identified from the data.
- Determine and state outcome criteria for each diagnosis. These must reflect some alleviation of the problem identified in the nursing diagnosis and must be stated in concrete and measurable terms.
- Plan and state one or more interventions for each diagnosed problem. Provide specific documentation of the source used to determine the appropriate intervention. Plan at least one intervention that incorporates Ray's strengths.
- Evaluate the success of the interventions. Interventions must correlate directly with the stated outcome criteria to measure the outcome success.

[a]Students are advised to refer to their nursing diagnosis text and identify possible or potential problems.

CRITICAL THINKING QUESTIONS AND ACTIVITIES

1. If you were in the role of a hospital case manager, how might you have helped this family with the discharge decision?
2. Would Ray be appropriate for an ALF upon discharge from the hospital? Why or why not? What services would need to be in place for him to be discharged to an ALF? How would he pay for these services?
3. Would Ray be appropriate for discharge home following hospitalization? What would home health provide under Medicare? What other services might he need? How would he pay for these services?
4. What are some of the obstacles that families of older adults face when their loved one needs a great deal of care? Do you

think that families should provide the care rather than placing loved ones with 24-hour care needs in nursing homes? If this was your family, what challenges might present in providing 24-hour care for a loved one?
5. Would you be willing to pay more taxes or be required to purchase LTC insurance to pay for LTC? Do you think individuals should be responsible for paying for their own LTC needs?
6. Would you consider nursing practice in LTC? Why or why not? What can education programs do to more adequately prepare students for practice in LTC and encourage them to consider working in these settings?

RESEARCH QUESTIONS

1. What are the experiences of older adults seeking care assistance to remain in their own homes?
2. What are the differences in the characteristics of residents of ALFs and nursing homes?
3. How do outcomes of care differ for older adults living in ALFs and nursing homes?
4. What are the best practice approaches to the provision of long-term care for older adults?

5. How do younger adults and older adults in different countries feel about increased taxes for government support of long-term care?
6. Are younger people preparing for their future LTC needs?
7. What is the relationship between a culture change model and care outcomes in nursing homes?
8. How does the role of the professional nurse differ between acute and long-term care?

REFERENCES

Alzheimer's Association: *Dementia care practice: recommendations for assisted living residences and nursing homes,* 2009. https://www.alz.org/national/documents/brochure_DCPRphases1n2.pdf. Accessed March 2018.

Andersen EA, Spiers J: Care aides' relational practices and caring contributions, *J Gerontol Nurs* 42(11):24–30, 2016.

Brawley E: What culture change is and why an aging nation cares, *Aging Today* 28:9–10, 2007.

Centers for Disease Control and Prevention (CDC): *Fast facts: nursing home care,* 2017. https://www.cdc.gov/nchs/fastats/nursing-home-care.htm. Accessed March 2018.

Centers for Medicare and Medicaid Services (CMS): *National Partnership to Improve Dementia Care in Nursing Homes: Antipsychotic medication use data report,* 2019. https://www.nhqualitycampaign.org/files/AP_package_20180131.pdf. Accessed March 2018.

Centers for Medicare and Medicaid Services (CMS): *The skilled nursing facility value-based purchasing program (SNF VBP),* 2018. https://www.cms.gov/Medicare/Quality-Initiatives-Patient-Assessment-Instruments/Value-Based-Programs/Other-VBPs/SNF-VBP.html. Accessed March 2018.

Carter SE: *Off-label antipsychotic use in older adults with dementia: not just a nursing home problem,* 2018. https://www.healio.com/psychiatry/alzheimers-disease-dementia/news/online/%7Bfd3bb4c1-2b69-472c-895f-d7a303636f3f%7D/off-label-antipsychotic-use-rising-among-community-dwelling-dementia-patients. Accessed April 2018.

Cortes TA, Sullivan-Marx EM: A case exemplar for national policy leadership, *J Gerontol Nurs* 42(3):9–14, 2016.

Eliopoulos C: *Gerontological nursing,* Philadelphia, PA, 2010, Wolters Kluwer/Lippincott Williams & Wilkins.

Gleckman H: What we don't know—but should—about assisted living facilities, *Forbes,* 2018. https://www.forbes.com/forbes/welcome/?toURL=https://www.forbes.com/sites/howardgleckman/2018/02/05/what-we-dont-know-but-should-about-assisted-living-facilities/&refURL=https://www.google.com/&referrer=https://www.google.com/. Accessed March 2018.

Genworth: *Genworth 2017 annual cost of care survey: costs continue to rise across all settings,* 2017. http://newsroom.genworth.com/2017-09-26-Genworth-2017-Annual-Cost-of-Care-Survey-Costs-Continue-to-Rise-Across-All-Care-Settings. Accessed March 2018.

Golden R, Shier G: What does "care transitions" really mean? *Generations* 36(4):6–12, 2012-2013.

Harrington C, Kovner C, Mezey M, et al: Experts recommend minimum staffing standards for nursing facilities in the United States, *Gerontologist* 40(1):5–16, 2000.

Harrington C, Wiener JM, Ross L, Musumeci M: Key issues in long-term services and supports quality. *The Henry J Kaiser Family Foundation Issue Brief,* 2017. https://www.kff.org/report-section/key-issues-in-long-term-services-and-supports-quality-appendix/. Accessed March 2018.

Mongan E: 6 new quality measures coming to nursing home compare, five-star rating system, *McKnights Long-Term Care News,* 2016. https://www.mcknights.com/news/6-new-quality-measures-coming-to-nursing-home-compare-five-star-rating-system/article/481007/. Accessed March 2018.

Mueller C, Burger S, Rader J, Carter D: Nurse competencies for person-directed care in nursing homes, *Geriatr Nurs* 34:101–104, 2013.

National PACE Association: *What is PACE?* 2019. https://www.npaonline.org/. Accessed March 2019.

Nguyen V: Fact sheet long-term support and services, *AARP Public Policy Institute,* 2017. https://www.aarp.org/content/dam/aarp/ppi/2017-01/Fact%20Sheet%20Long-Term%20Support%20and%20Services.pdf. Accessed March 2018.

Reinhard S, Accius J, Houser A, Ujvari K, Alexis J, Fox-Grage W: *Picking up the pace of change, 2017: a state scorecard on long-term services and supports for older adults, people with physical disabilities, and family caregivers,* 2017, AARP, Commonwealth Fund, SCAN Foundation. http://www.longtermscorecard.org. Accessed March 2018.

Sherman R, Touhy T: An exploratory descriptive study to evaluate Florida nurse leader challenges and opportunities in nursing home setting, *SAGE Open Nurs* 3:1–7, 2017.

Stanford School of Medicine: *Palliative care,* 2019. https://palliative.stanford.edu/home-hospice-home-care-of-the-dying-patient/where-do-americans-die/. Accessed March 2019.

Teno JM, Gozalo PL, Bynum JP, et al: Change in end-of-life care Medicare beneficiaries, *JAMA* 309(5):470–477, 2013.

Thomas WH, Johansson C: Elderhood in Eden, *Top Geriatr Rehabil* 19:282–290, 2003.

Touhy T, Strews W, Brown C: Expressions of caring as lived by nursing home staff residents, and families, *Int J Hum Caring* 9:31–37, 2005.

Trinkoff AM, Yang BK, Storr CL, Zhu S, Lerner NB, Han K: Determining the CNA training-hour requirement for quality care in U.S. nursing homes, *J Nurs Regul* 8(1):4–10, 2017.

United States Senate, Commission on Long-Term Care: *Report to the Congress,* 2013. http://www.gpo.gov/fdsys/pkg/GPO-LTCCOMMISSION/content-detail.html. Accessed March 2018.

33

Intimacy and Sexuality

Theris A. Touhy

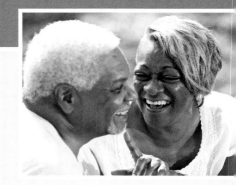

http://evolve.elsevier.com/Touhy/TwdHlthAging

A STUDENT SPEAKS

I'm sorry but I cannot imagine my grandparents having sexual intercourse or being interested in information about sexual health. I never thought much about sexuality and older adults but, I must say, I do hope that I will have a fulfilling sexual life when I am old.

Jennifer, age 21

AN OLDER ADULT SPEAKS

These early morning hours are terribly lonely ... that's when I have such a longing for someone who loves me to be there just to touch and hold me ... and to talk to.

Sister Marilyn Schwab
From Schwab, M. (1986). A gift freely given: the personal journal of Sister Marilyn Schwab, Mt Angel: Benedictine Sisters.

LEARNING OBJECTIVES

On completion of this chapter, the reader will be able to:

1. Discuss touch and intimacy as integral components of sexuality.
2. Discuss the physiological, social, and psychological factors that affect sexual function as people age.
3. Identify the effects of illness on sexual function and adaptations to enhance sexual health.
4. Describe the various approaches to sexuality assessment that may reduce nurse-client anxiety in discussing a sensitive area.
5. Discuss challenges related to intimacy and sexuality for individuals with dementia and those residing in long-term care facilities.
6. Discuss the rising incidence of HIV/AIDS and sexually transmitted diseases among older adults and interventions to promote safe practices.
7. Develop a plan of care for an older adult to promote sexual health.

TOUCH

Touch is the first of our senses to develop and provides us with our most fundamental means of contact with the external world. It is the oldest, most important, and most neglected of our senses, stronger than verbal or emotional contact. All other senses have an organ on which to focus, but touch is everywhere. Touch is unique because it frequently combines with other senses. An individual can survive without one or more of the other senses, but no one can survive and live in any degree of comfort without touch.

In the absence of touching or being touched, people of all ages can become sick and become touch starved. Touch is experienced physically as a sensation, and affectively as emotion and behavior. The interaction of touch affects the autonomic,

reticular, and limbic systems, and thus profoundly affects the emotional drives. The human yearning for physical contact is embedded in our language in such figurative terms as "keep in touch," "handle with care," and "rubbed the wrong way." We will focus on touch as an overt expression of closeness, intimacy, and sexuality. We believe an individual must recognize the power of touch and its intimacy to fully comprehend sexuality. Touch and intimacy are integral parts of sexuality, just as sexuality is expressed through intimacy and touch. Together, touch and intimacy can offer the older adult a sense of well-being. Throughout life, touch provides emotional and sensual knowledge about other individuals—an unending source of information, pleasure, and pain.

Response to Touch

The Touch Model proposed by Hollinger and Buschmann (1993) suggests that attitudes toward touch and acceptance of touch affect the behaviors of both caregivers and patients. Two types of touch occur during the nurse-patient relationship: procedural and nonprocedural. Procedural touch (task-oriented or instrumental touch) is physical contact that occurs when a particular task is being performed. Nonprocedural touch (expressive physical touch) does not require a task and is affective and supportive in nature, such as holding a patient's hand.

Everyone has definite feelings, opinions, and comfort with touch based on his or her own life experience. The boundaries of tactual communication are learned culturally. Cultural and religious norms determine the appropriateness and acceptability of touch. For example, touch of any kind between members of the opposite sex outside of the family is strictly forbidden in traditional Muslim religion. The nurse should ask the person's permission before touching and not assume that a person likes or wants to be touched (Chapter 4).

Of all health care professionals, nurses have the most frequent opportunities to provide gentle, reassuring, renewing touch. Therapeutic, caring touch by the nurse is a potent healing intervention. It is important that touching be done with respect regarding the person's comfort and with the nurse's intention of providing a comforting and healing modality within the nurse-patient relationship.

Touch Zones

Hall (1969) identifies different categories of touching—expanding or contracting zones around which every individual extends the sensory experience of touching, smelling, hearing, and seeing. The categories of touching include the intimate, vulnerable, consent, and social zones (Fig. 33.1). Providing care in the zone of intimacy, which is identified as generally the area within an arm's length of the individual's body and is the space used for comforting, protecting, and lovemaking, is part of the

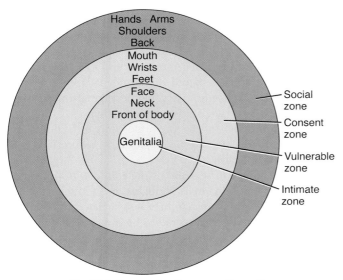

Fig. 33.1 Zones of Intimacy or Sexuality.

nurse's function. The vulnerable zone is highly sexually charged and will be protected. The most intimate area, the genitalia, is the most personally protected area of the body and causes the most stress and anxiety when approached, touched, or viewed by the caregiver. The consent zone requires the nurse to seek out or ask permission to touch or initiate procedures to these areas. The social zone includes the areas of the body that are the least sensitive or embarrassing to be touched and that do not necessarily require permission to be handled.

Illness, confinement, and dependency seen in hospitalization and institutionalization are stresses on the intimate zone of touch. Just as caregivers enter a room without knocking, so they often intrude into the intimate circle of touch without asking. A person's need for privacy and personal space is strongly related to acceptance and response to touch. If the need for privacy and distance is great, touch should be used judiciously.

Therapeutic Touch

Touch is a powerful healer and a therapeutic tool that nurses can use to satisfy "touch hunger" of older adults. Nursing has recognized the importance of touch and has the social sanctions to touch the body in the intimate and personal care of a person, an opportunity too often not fully used for the betterment of the older adult's adaptation to environment and location in time and space. Touch can serve as a means of providing sensory stimulation, reducing anxiety, relieving physical and psychological pain, comforting the dying, and sexual expression.

Krieger's experiments with therapeutic touch (1975) demonstrate physiological and psychological improvement in patients who are exposed to consistent "doses" of touch. Hands-on healing and energy-based interventions have been found in cultures throughout history, dating back at least 5000 years. "Laying on of the hands" and the power of touch to heal had largely disappeared with the scientific revolution. The phenomenon has reemerged as healing touch and therapeutic touch movements. A growing body of research supports the healing power of touch, and *Energy Field, Disturbed* is an approved nursing diagnosis.

Many nurses have learned how to perform therapeutic and healing touch and use these modalities in their practice with people of all ages. Positive outcomes of interventions utilizing touch in nursing homes, particularly with people with dementia and agitated behaviors, have been reported (Wang et al, 2017). Further research on the use of touch with older adults is needed. Touch is a powerful tool to promote comfort and well-being when working with older adults.

INTIMACY

Intimacy is the degree to which we express and have a need for closeness with another person. Although intimacy is often thought of in the context of sexual performance, it encompasses more than sexuality and includes five major relational components: commitment, affective intimacy, cognitive intimacy, physical intimacy, and interdependence (Youngkin, 2004). It is a warm, meaningful feeling of joy. Intimacy includes the need for close friendships; relationships with family, friends, and formal caregivers; spiritual connections; knowing that one matters in someone else's life; and the ability to form satisfying social relationships with others (Syme, 2015). "Closeness, intimacy, and touch are lifelong needs that do not get old, even when we do" (Clark, 2015).

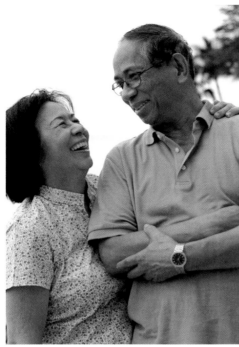

Older couples enjoy love and companionship. (©iStock.com/DanielBendjy.)

Older adults may be concerned about changes in sexual intimacy, but "social relationships with people important in their lives, the ability to interact intellectually with people who share similar interests, the supportive love that grows between human beings (whether romantic or platonic), and physical nonsexual intimacy are equally—and in many instances more—important than the physical intimacy of direct sexual relations. All of these facets of intimate life are integrally woven into the fabric of aging, along with other influences that can make life rewarding" (Youngkin, 2004, p. 46). Intimacy needs change over time, but the need for intimacy and satisfying social relationships remains an important component of healthy aging.

SEXUALITY

Sexuality is a central aspect of being human throughout life and encompasses sex, gender identities and roles, sexual orientation, eroticism, pleasure, intimacy, and reproduction. Sexuality is experienced and expressed in thoughts, fantasies, desires, beliefs, attitudes, values, behaviors, practices, roles, and relationships. While sexuality can include all of these dimensions, not all of them are always experienced or expressed. Sexuality is influenced by the interaction of biological, psychological, social, economic, political, cultural, legal, historical, religious, and spiritual factors (World Health Organization, 2018). "Sexuality begins *in utero* as we are developing as human beings and ends

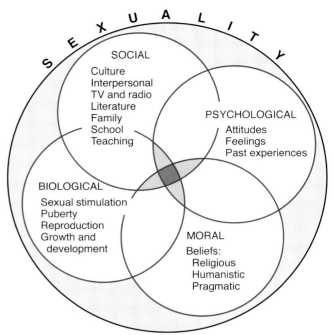

Fig. 33.2 Interrelationship of Dimensions of Sexuality.

with our death. Sexuality is the total expression of who we are as human beings. It is the most complex human attribute and encompasses our whole psychosocial development—our values, attitudes, physical appearance, beliefs, emotions, attractions, our likes/dislikes, our spiritual selves" (Clark, 2017). As a major aspect of intimacy, sexuality includes the physical act of intercourse, and many other types of intimate activity. Enjoying and expressing one's sexuality leads to feelings of pleasure and well-being that are essential at any age to meet human needs for intimacy and belonging. Sexuality also allows a general affirmation of life (especially joy) and a continuing opportunity to search for new growth and experience.

Sexuality, similar to food and water, is a basic human need, yet it goes beyond the biological realm to include psychological, social, and moral dimensions (Fig. 33.2). The constant interaction among these spheres of sexuality works to produce harmony. The linkage of the four dimensions composes the holistic quality of an individual's sexuality. "Historically, sexuality has been perceived more narrowly in a biomedical context, with emphasis placed on the sexual response cycle, heteronormative behaviors (e.g., penile-vaginal intercourse), and heterosexist and ageist assumptions" (Syme, 2015, p. 36). A holistic view better reflects the philosophy of healthy aging for all individuals. The *Healthy People 2020* box presents goals related to sexual health.

The social sphere of sexuality is the sum of cultural factors that influence the individual's thoughts and actions related to interpersonal relationships, and sexuality related to ideas and learned behavior. Television, radio, literature, and the more traditional sources of family, school, and religious teachings combine to influence social sexuality. The belief of that which constitutes masculine and feminine is deeply rooted in the individual's exposure to cultural factors (Chapter 4).

The psychological domain of sexuality reflects a person's attitudes, feelings toward self and others, and learning from experiences. Beginning with birth, the individual is bombarded with cues and signals of how a person should act and think about the use of "dirty words" or body parts. Conversation is self-censored in the presence of or in discussion with certain people. The moral aspect of sexuality, the "I should" or "I shouldn't," makes a difference that is based in religious and cultural beliefs or in a pragmatic or humanistic outlook.

The final dimension, biological sexuality, is reflected in physiological responses to sexual stimulation, reproduction, puberty, and growth and development. Because of the interrelatedness, these dimensions affect each other directly or indirectly whenever an aspect of sexuality is out of harmony.

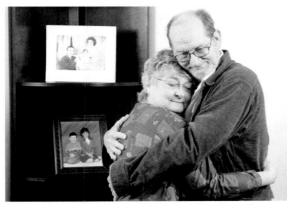

Love and affection are important to older adults. (From Sorrentino SA, Gorek B: *Mosby's textbook for long-term care assistants* ed 5, St Louis: Mosby.)

Acceptance and Companionship

Sexuality validates the lifelong need to share intimacy and have that offering appreciated. Sexuality is love, warmth, sharing, and touching between people, not just the physical act of coitus. Margot Benary-Isbert, in her book *The Vintage Years* (1968), expresses the essence of sexuality most eloquently (p. 200):

> Let us not forget old married couples who once shared healthy and happy days as they now share the unavoidable limitations of old age and grow even closer together in love and patience. When they exchange a smile, a glance, one can guess that they still think each other beautiful and loveable.

SEXUAL HEALTH

The World Health Organization defines sexual health as a state of physical, emotional, mental, and social well-being in relation to sexuality; it is not merely the absence of disease, dysfunction or infirmity. Sexual health requires a positive and respectful approach to sexuality and sexual relationships, and the possibility of having pleasurable and safe sexual experiences, free of coercion, discrimination, and violence. For sexual health to be attained and maintained, the sexual rights of all persons must be respected, protected, and fulfilled (World Health Organization, 2018).

Sexual health is a realistic phenomenon that includes four components: personal and social behaviors in agreement with individual gender identity; comfort with a range of sexual role behaviors and engagement in effective interpersonal relations with both sexes in a loving relationship or long-term commitment; response to erotic stimulation that produces positive and pleasurable sexual activity; and the ability to make mature judgments about sexual behavior that is culturally and socially acceptable. These interpretations address the multifaceted nature of the biological, psychosocial, cultural, and spiritual components of sexuality and imply that sexual behavior is the capacity to enhance self and others. Sexual health is individually defined and wholesome if it leads to intimacy (not necessarily coitus) and enriches the involved parties.

Factors Influencing Sexual Health

Older adults are becoming increasingly open in their attitudes and beliefs about sexuality. However, a large number of cultural, biological, psychosocial, and environmental factors can influence the sexual behavior of older adults. The older adult may be confronted with barriers to the expression of his or her sexuality by reflected attitudes, health, culture, economics, opportunity, and historic trends. Factors affecting a person's attitudes on intimacy and sexuality include family dynamics and upbringing and cultural and religious beliefs (Chapter 4).

Older adults often internalize the broad cultural proscriptions of sexual behavior in late life that hinder the continuance of sexual expression. There remains a prevailing assumption that as we age, we become sexually undesirable, incapable of sex, or asexual. "It is erroneously believed that older adults (especially older women) are unattractive, that older sex is disgusting, risky, or 'wrong,' aging entails sexual dysfunction and sex, as a rule, should be discouraged in old age homes and other facilities" (Dhingra et al, 2016). Health care professionals are not immune to these stereotypes and may assume sexual issues are of lesser concern to older adults and neglect to address this important aspect of healthy aging. It is refreshing to see more movies with older actors that incorporate more positive views of older adults enjoying intimate and satisfying, sexual relationships (e.g., *Best Exotic Marigold Hotel* and *Our Souls at Night*).

Much sexual behavior stems from incorporating other people's reactions. Older adults do not feel old until they are faced with the fact that others around them consider them old. Similarly, older adults do not feel asexual until they are continually

BOX 33.1 Sexuality and Aging Women: Common Myths

- Masturbation is an immature activity of youngsters and adolescents, not older women.
- Sexual prowess and desire wane during the climacteric, and menopause is the death of a woman's sexuality.
- Hysterectomy creates a physical disability that results in the inability to function sexually.
- Sex has no role in the lives of older adults, except as perversion or remembrance of times past.
- Sexual expression in old age is taboo.
- Older adults are too old and frail to engage in sex.
- The young are considered lusty and virile; older adults are considered lecherous.
- Sex is unimportant or over in the lives of the older adults.
- Older women do not wish to discuss their sexuality with professionals.

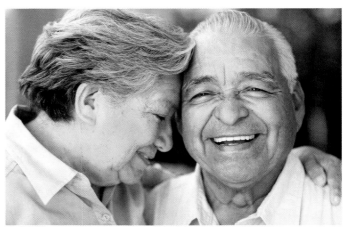

Sexuality is an important need in late life and affects pleasure, adaptation, and a general feeling of well-being. (©iStock.com/Aldo Murillo.)

treated as such. An often quoted statement by Alex Comfort (1974) sums it up nicely: "In our experiences, old folks stop having sex for the same reasons they stop riding a bicycle—general infirmity, thinking it looks ridiculous, no bicycle." Box 33.1 presents some of the myths about sexuality in older women that may be held by older adults themselves and by society in general.

Activity Levels

For both heterosexual and lesbian, gay, bisexual, transgender (LGBT) individuals, research supports that liberal and positive attitudes toward sexuality, greater sexual knowledge, satisfaction with a long-term relationship or a current intimate relationship, good social networks, psychological well-being, and a sense of self-worth are associated with greater sexual interest, activity, and satisfaction. Both early studies of sexual behavior in older adults and more recent ones indicate that older adults are continuing to enjoy active sex lives well into their 70s and 80s. More than half of men and almost a third of women over the age of 70 years reported that they were still sexually active, with a third of these men and women having sex at least twice a month, although sexual problems are relatively prevalent (Heidari, 2016).

Determinants of sexual activity and functioning include the interaction of each partner's sexual capacity, physical health, motivation, conduct, and attitudes, and the quality of the dyadic relationship. Having a sexual partner, frequent intercourse, good health, low level of stress, and an absence of financial worries enhanced a happy sexual relationship. Sexual activity is closely tied to overall health, and individuals with better health are more likely to be sexually active. The most common reason for sexual inactivity among heterosexual couples is the male partner's health. Patterns of sexual activity in earlier years are a major predictor of sexual activity in later life, and individuals with higher levels of sexual activity in middle age show less decline as they age. Regular sexual expression enhances psychological and physical well-being in older adulthood and may improve cognitive functioning (Schafer, 2018; Wright et al, 2017).

Cohort and Cultural Influences

The era in which a person was born influences attitudes about sexuality. Women in their 80s today may have been strongly influenced by the prudish Victorian atmosphere of their youth and may have experienced difficult marital adjustments and serious sexual problems early in their marriages. Sexuality was not openly expressed or discussed, and this was a time when pleasurable sex was for men only; women engaged in sexual activity to satisfy their husbands and to make babies. These kinds of experiences shape beliefs and knowledge about sexual expression and comfort with sexuality, particularly for older women. It is important to come to know and understand the older adult within his or her social and cultural background and not make judgments based on one's own belief system.

The next generation of older adults (baby boomers) has experienced other influences, including more liberal attitudes toward sexuality, the women's movement, a higher number of divorced adults, the human immunodeficiency virus (HIV) epidemic, and increased numbers of LGBT individuals, that will affect their views and attitudes as they age. The baby boomers and beyond, as they find themselves experiencing sexuality beyond the age they had assigned to their elders, may alter current perceptions. Most of what is known about sexuality in aging has been gained through research with well-educated, healthy, white older adults. Further research is needed among culturally, socially, and ethnically diverse older adults; those with chronic illness; and LGBT older adults.

Biological Changes

Acknowledgment and understanding of the age changes that influence sexual physiology, anatomy, and the stages of sexual response may partially explain alteration in sexual behavior to accommodate these changes and facilitate continued pleasurable sex. Characteristic physiological changes during the sexual response cycle do occur with aging, but these vary among individuals

TABLE 33.1   Physical Changes in Sexual Responses in Old Age.

Female	Male
Excitation Phase	
Diminished or delayed lubrication (1 to 3 minutes may be required for adequate amounts to appear)	Less intense and slower erection (but can be maintained longer without ejaculation)
Diminished flattening and separation of labia majora	Increased difficulty regaining an erection if lost
Disappearance of elevation of labia majora	Less vasocongestion of scrotal sac
Decreased vasocongestion of labia minora	Less pronounced elevation and congestion of testicles
Decreased elastic expansion of vagina (depth and breadth)	
Breasts not as engorged	
Sex flush absent	
Plateau Phase	
Slower and less prominent uterine elevation or tenting	Decreased muscle tension
Nipple erection and sexual flush less often	No color change at coronal edge of penis
Decreased capacity for vasocongestion	Slower penile erection pattern
Decreased areolar engorgement	Delayed or diminished erectile and testicular elevation
Labial color change less evident	
Less intense swelling or orgasmic platform	
Less sexual flush	
Decreased secretions of Bartholin's glands	
Orgasmic Phase	
Fewer number and less intense orgasmic contractions	Decreased or absent secretory activity (lubrication) by Cowper's gland before ejaculation
Rectal sphincter contraction with severe tension only	Fewer penile contractions
	Fewer rectal sphincter contractions
	Decreased force of ejaculation (approximately 50%) with decreased amount of semen (if ejaculation is long, seepage of semen occurs)
Resolution Phase	
Observably slower loss of nipple erection	Vasocongestion of nipples and scrotum slowly subsides
Vasocongestion of clitoris and orgasmic platform	Very rapid loss of erection and descent of testicles shortly after ejaculation
	Refractory time extended (time required before another erection ranges from several to 24 hours, occasionally longer)

depending on general health factors. The changes occur abruptly in women starting with menopause but more gradually in men, a phenomenon called andropause. The "use it or lose it" phenomenon applies here: the more sexually active the person is, the fewer changes he or she is likely to experience in the pattern of sexual response. Changes in the appearance of the body (wrinkles, sagging skin) may also affect the older person's security about his or her sexual attractiveness. Table 33.1 summarizes physical changes in the sexual response cycle. A major nursing role is to provide information about these changes and appropriate assessment and counseling within the context of the individual's needs.

SEXUAL RESPONSE

The most prevalent sexual problem in men is erectile dysfunction (ED). ED is defined as the inability to achieve a full erection or the inability to maintain an erection adequate for sexual intimacy. Although most men will experience periodic episodes of ED, these episodes tend to become more frequent with advancing age. Approximately 60% of men at 60 years old and 70% of men at 70 years old have ED (Mobley et al, 2017). When discussing ED with older men, it is important to also provide education about

normal age-related changes. Older men require more physical penile stimulation and a longer time to achieve erection, and the duration of orgasm may be shorter and less intense.

An erection is governed by the interaction among the hormonal, vascular, and nervous systems. A problem in any of these systems can cause ED. Multiple causes can contribute to this problem in older men. Nearly one-third of ED is a complication of diabetes. Cardiovascular disease (CVD) and hypertension cause a narrowing and hardening of the arteries, leading to reduced blood flow to the corporal bodies, which is essential for achieving an erection. Recent studies have confirmed that ED also serves as a predictor of future CVD and individuals who present with ED and CVD risk factors should be evaluated for silent CVD (Mobley et al, 2017; Patel and Bennett, 2016). Alcohol abuse, smoking, medications, prostate cancer and treatment, obesity, anxiety, depression, and relationship discord are also causes of ED in older men (Marchese, 2017). The new nerve-saving microsurgical techniques used for prostatectomies often spare erectile function.

The use of phosphodiesterase inhibitors such as sildenafil (Viagra), vardenafil (Levitra), and tadalafil (Cialis) has revolutionized treatment for ED regardless of cause. Some have commented that this can be called "the Viagratization of the older population." Contraindications to the use of these medications include use of nitrate therapy, heart failure with low blood pressure, certain antihypertensive regimens, and other medications and cardiovascular conditions (Chapter 9).

Before the availability of these medications, intracavernosal injections with the drugs papaverine and phentolamine, vasoactive agents that reduce resistance of arteriolar and cavernosal smooth muscle tissue of the penis, were used. Penile implants of the semirigid, adjustable-malleable, or hinged and inflatable types are available when impotence does not respond to other treatments or is irreversible. The hinged and inflatable types, which are inserted in the testicular area, are the most popular. Another alternative is the vacuum pump device, which works by creating a vacuum that draws blood into the penis, causing an erection. Vacuum pumps are available in manual and battery-operated versions and may be covered by Medicare if deemed medically necessary.

Our understanding of the female response is still not well understood and the definition and diagnostic criteria of sexual dysfunction are controversial and still under development (Chen et al, 2013). Difficulties reported by sexually active women related to becoming sexually aroused and achieving orgasm (Lee et al, 2016). Female sexual function can be influenced by factors such as culture, ethnicity, emotional state, age, and previous sexual experiences, and age-related changes in sexual response. Frequency of intimacy depends more on the age, health, and sexual function of the partner or the availability of a partner, rather than on their own sexual capacity. Postmenopausal changes in the urinary or genital tract as a result of lower estrogen levels can make sexual activity less pleasurable. Dyspareunia, resulting from vaginal dryness and thinning of the vaginal tissue, occurs in one-third of women older than age 65. In many instances, using water-soluble lubricants such as K-Y Jelly, Astroglide, Slip, and HR lubricating jelly during foreplay or intercourse can resolve the difficulty. Topical low-dose estrogen creams, rings, or pills that are introduced into the vagina may also help to plump tissues and restore lubrication, with less absorption than oral hormones.

Women can experience arousal disorders resulting from drugs such as anticholinergics, antidepressants, and chemotherapeutic agents and from lack of lubrication from radiation, surgery, and stress. Orgasmic disorders also may result from drugs used to treat depression. Unlike ED, studies of vascular insufficiency are less clear in women. Prolapse of the uterus, rectoceles, and cystoceles can be surgically repaired to facilitate continued sexual activity. Urinary incontinence (UI) is another condition that may affect sexual activity for both men and women. Appropriate assessment and treatment are important because many causes of UI are treatable (Chapter 16).

LESBIAN, GAY, BISEXUAL, AND TRANSGENDER SEXUALITY

Estimates are that 2.4% of adults (2.7 million) 50 years of age and older in the United States self-identify as LGBT, and this population will increase dramatically over the next few decades given the significant aging of the population. The total number of older adults who self-identify as LGBT, have engaged in same-sexual behavior or romantic relationships, and/or are attracted to members of the same sex is estimated to increase to more than 20 million by 2060 (Fredriksen-Goldsen and Kim, 2017). Chapter 34 discusses LGBT relationships in more detail.

Discrimination in health and social systems affects gay, lesbian, bisexual, and transgender individuals of all ages. Discrimination ranges from refusal of care, biases or incorrect assumptions, to overt derogatory statements (American Geriatrics Society, 2015). Older adults may be even more at risk for discrimination as a result of lifelong experiences with marginalization and oppression. They may have been shunned by family or friends, religious organizations, and the medical community; ridiculed or physically attacked; or labeled as sinners, perverts, or criminals. In the 1950s same-sex behaviors were typically characterized as sodomy, were criminal, and the American Psychiatric Association classified homosexuality as a psychiatric disorder (Fredriksen-Goldsen, 2016). It was not until 1973 that homosexuality was removed from the *Diagnostic and Statistical Manual of Mental Disorders.* LGBT individuals may face dual discrimination due to their age and their sexual orientation or gender identity and older women in lesbian relationships face the triple threat of being women, being old, and having a different sexual orientation (American Psychological Association, 2018).

As a result of lifelong discrimination and negative experiences with health care agencies and personnel, LGBT older adults are much less likely than their heterosexual peers to access needed health and social services or identify themselves as gay or lesbian to health care providers. As a result, they are at greater risk for poorer health than their heterosexual counterparts. While many LGBT adults manifest resilience and good health despite marginalization, compared to heterosexuals of similar age, gay and bisexual adults 50 years of age and older are more likely to report higher prevalence of poor general health, disabling chronic conditions, high rates of substance abuse, and suicide (Franc et al, 2018). An increased rate of stroke or heart attack has also been reported in this population (Fredriksen-Goldsen and Kim, 2017). Transgender and bisexual older adults and individuals living with HIV are at greater risk for disparities and poorer health outcomes (Emlet, 2016).

Sexual orientation and gender identity have been identified as key gaps in health disparities research, with LGBT older adults an especially understudied population (Fredriksen-Goldsen and Kim, 2017). The landmark Aging with Pride: National Health, Aging, and Sexuality/Gender Study is the first federally funded longitudinal national project designed to better understand the aging, health, and well-being of LGBT midlife and older adults and their families. With over 2400 LGBTQ adults ranging in age from 50 to over 100, this project will deepen our understanding of how various life experiences are related to changes in aging, health, and well-being over time. Most health surveys do not include sexual identity questions, so there are limited data on this population. Some population-based surveys, such as the National Health Interview Survey, have added sexual identity questions, as have some state-level efforts made through the Behavioral Risk Factor Surveillance System surveys. *Healthy People 2020* highlighted LGBT people for the first time as a health disparate population and outlined goals to improve their health, safety, and well-being.

There is a dearth of research addressing LGBT health. Research has been conducted primarily with middle-class white gay men and lesbians in urban areas. Even less is known about bisexual and transgender older adults. Nursing as a whole, particularly gerontological nursing, continues to remain relatively silent on LGBT in health and aging. Nurse researchers are encouraged to consider study designs, methods, and procedures that support inclusion and visibility of LGBT older adults (Cloyes, 2016).

PROMOTING HEALTHY AGING: IMPLICATIONS FOR GERONTOLOGICAL NURSING

Assessment

Health care providers may assume that their LGBT patients are heterosexual and neglect to obtain a sexual history, discuss sexuality, or be aware of their particular medical needs. Providers receive little education and training in the needs of this population and may lack sensitivity when caring for older LGBT individuals (American Geriatrics Society, 2015). Health history forms need to be inclusive and not heterosexist. Use gender neutral questions for identification of a same-sex partner by using terms like partner or significant other is much better than asking, "Are you married?" (Franc et al, 2018). This form of the question allows the nurse to look beyond the rigid category of family. You can ask individuals if they consider themselves as primarily heterosexual, homosexual, or bisexual. This question conveys recognition of sexual variety. Euphemisms are frequently used for a life partner (e.g., roommate, close friend). An older lesbian woman in a health care situation may refer to herself indirectly by saying "people like us." Nurses need to become more aware of these nuances and try to understand the fear of discovery that is apparent in the older gay man and lesbian woman. These older adults are of a generation in which they were, and may still be, closeted because of the homophobic experiences they had throughout their younger years.

To treat a transgender individual with respect, you treat them according to their gender identity, not their sex at birth. Someone who lives as a woman today is called a transgender woman and should be referred to as "she" and "her." A transgender man who lives as a man should be referred to as "he" and "him." Some transgender individuals identify as neither a man or a woman, or as a combination of male and female and may use terms like nonbinary or genderqueer to describe their gender identity. Those who are nonbinary often prefer to be referred to as "they" and "them." If the patient identifies as transgender, it is important to ask how the patient wishes to be addressed. Use the name the person has asked you to call them and the pronouns they want you to use (National Center for Transgender Equality, 2016).

Better support and care services for LGBT individuals by care providers should include working through homophobic attitudes and discomfort discussing sexuality, learning about special issues facing LGBT individuals, and becoming aware of resources in the community specific to this population. Appropriate health teaching materials, including those that depict same-sex couples, are important, as is not making assumptions about a person's sex based on his or her appearance. LGBT individuals look for indications of an inclusive and welcoming environment, which may include the display of nondiscrimination policies or a rainbow flag (Franc et al, 2018). When caring for transgender older adults, it is important to use discretion and sensitivity when obtaining medical and surgical histories and performing physical examinations (Jablonski et al, 2013). Facilities or agencies in the community need to be assessed from the perspective of the client, patient, or resident who may be gay, lesbian, bisexual, or transgender. It is important that service providers create programs that are inclusive and culturally appropriate for all individuals (Chapter 4). Programs to increase awareness of the needs of LGBT older adults and reduce discrimination are necessary especially in light of the anticipated increase in older LGBT individuals (Fredriksen-Goldsen, 2016).

INTIMACY AND CHRONIC ILLNESS

Chronic illnesses and their related treatments may bring many challenges to intimacy and sexual activity. Physical capacity for sexual activity may be affected by illness, and psychological factors (anxiety, depression). Patients and their partners are given little or no information about the effect of illnesses, on sexual activity or strategies to continue sexual activity within functional limitations. Individuals want and need information on sexual functioning, and health care professionals need to become more knowledgeable and more actively involved in sexual counseling (Byrne et al, 2017). Table 33.2 presents suggestions for individuals with chronic illness. Timing of intercourse (mornings or when energy level is highest), oral or anal sex, masturbation, appropriate pain relief, and different sexual positions are all strategies that may assist in continued sexual activity. There is no consensus on what kind of position the individual should assume for sexual activity, but a lesser amount of energy is expended with the person on the bottom during use of the missionary position. Alternative positions may require less energy and may be more comfortable depending on the situation (Fig. 33.3) (Steinke, 2013; Steinke et al, 2013).

For individuals with cardiac conditions, manual stimulation (masturbation) may be an alternative that can be used to maintain sexual function if the practice is not objectionable to the patient. Studies show that masturbation is less taxing on the heart and makes less oxygen demand. Although self-stimulation is steeped in myth and fear, masturbation is a common and healthy practice in late life. Individuals without partners or those whose spouses are ill or incapacitated find that masturbation is helpful. As children, today's older population was discouraged from practicing this pleasurable activity with stories of the evils of fondling a person's own genitals.

Attitudes have changed over the years and the National Social Life, Health, and Aging Project (NSHAP) study reported that more than 50% of male participants and 25% of female

TABLE 33.2   Chronic Illness and Sexual Function: Effects and Interventions.

Condition	Effects/Problems	Interventions
Arthritis	Pain, fatigue, limited motion Steroid therapy may decrease sexual interest or desire	Advise patient to perform sexual activity at time of day when less fatigued and most relaxed Suggest use of analgesics and other pain-relief methods before sexual activity Encourage use of relaxation techniques before sexual activity, such as a warm bath or shower, application of hot packs to affected joints Advise patient to maintain optimal health through a balance of good nutrition, proper rest, and activity Suggest that he or she experiment with different positions, use pillows for comfort and support Recommend use of a vibrator if massage ability is limited Suggest use of water-soluble jelly for vaginal lubrication
Cardiovascular disease	Most men have no change in physical effects on sexual function; one-fourth may not return to pre–heart attack function; one-fourth may not resume sexual activity Women do not experience sexual dysfunction after heart attack Fear of another heart attack or death during sex Shortness of breath	Encourage counseling on realistic restrictions that may be necessary **Post–myocardial infarction (MI):** Those able to engage in mild to moderate physical activity without symptoms can generally resume sexual activity; those with a complicated MI may need to resume sexual activity gradually over a longer period of time Avoid large meals several hours before sex Avoid anal sex Instruct patient and spouse on alternative positions to avoid strain and allow for unrestricted breathing Stop and rest if chest pain is experienced, take nitroglycerin if prescribed, and seek emergency treatment for sustained chest pain **Post-CABG or pacemaker or ICD insertion:** Avoid strain or direct pressure on device/incision Individuals with poorly controlled arrhythmias should not engage in sexual activity until the condition is well managed Instruct individual that ICD could fire with sex, although uncommon; a change in device setting may be needed
Cerebrovascular accident (stroke)	Depression May or may not have sexual activity changes Often erectile disorders occur Change in role and function of partners Decreased physical endurance, fatigue Mobility and sensory deficits Perceptual and visual deficits Communication deficits Cognitive and behavioral deficits Fear of relapse or sudden death	Encourage counseling Instruct patient to use alternative positions Suggest use of a vibrator if massage ability is limited Suggest use of pillows for positioning and support Suggest use of water-soluble jelly for lubrication Suggest alternate forms of sexual expression acceptable to the individuals
Chronic obstructive pulmonary disease (COPD)	No direct impairment of sexual activity, although affected by coughing, exertional dyspnea, positions, and activity intolerance Medications may lead to erectile difficulties	Encourage patient to plan sexual activity when energy is highest Instruct patient to use alternative positions; use ample pillows for support and elevate the upper body, or use a sitting upright position; avoid any pressure on the chest Advise patient to plan sexual activity at time medications are most effective Suggest use of oxygen before, during, or after sex, depending on when it provides the most benefit Teach partner to observe for breathing difficulty and allow time for change of positions and time to catch breath when needed
Diabetes	Sexual desire and interest unaffected Neuropathy and/or vascular damage may interfere with erectile ability; about 50% to 75% of men have erectile disorders; a small portion have retrograde ejaculation Some men regain function if diagnosis of diabetes is well accepted, if diabetes is well controlled, or both Women have less sexual desire and vaginal lubrication Decrease in orgasms/absence of orgasm can occur; less frequent sexual activity; local genital infections	Recommend possible candidates for penile prosthesis Suggest use of alternative forms of sexual expression Recommend immediate treatment of genital infections

TABLE 33.2 Chronic Illness and Sexual Function: Effects and Interventions.—cont'd

Condition	Effects/Problems	Interventions
Cancers		
Breast	No direct physical affect; there is a strong psychological effect: loss of sexual desire, body-image change, depression/reaction of partner	Refer to support groups, sex therapists, counselors Encourage open expression of sexual concerns
Prostate	Incontinence can occur following surgery Erectile dysfunction Psychological effects Use of nerve-sparing surgery causes less dysfunction	Kegel exercises and routine toileting Use of phosphodiesterase inhibitors Provide information related to sexual functioning/continence
Most other cancers	Men and women may lose sexual desire temporarily Men may have erectile dysfunction; dry ejaculation; retrograde ejaculation Women may have vaginal dryness, dyspareunia Both men and women may experience anxiety, depression, pain, nausea from chemotherapy, radiation, hormone therapy, and nerve damage from pelvic surgery	New sexual positions may be helpful; explore alternative sexual activities

CABG, Coronary artery bypass graft; *ICD,* implantable cardioverter-defibrillator.
Data from Steinke EE: Sexuality and chronic illness, *J Gerontol Nurs* 39(11):18–27, 2013.

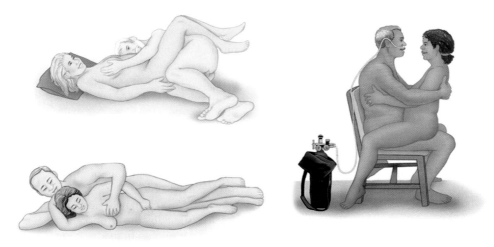

Fig. 33.3 Adaptations of Sexual Positions for Individuals With Chronic Illness.

participants acknowledged masturbating, regardless of whether or not they had a sexual partner (Lindau et al, 2010). Masturbation provides an avenue for resolution of sexual tensions, keeps sexual desire alive, maintains lubrication and muscle tone of the vagina, provides mild physical exercise, and preserves sexual function in individuals who have no other outlet for sexual activity and gratification of their sexual need.

One couple, who had long sustained a satisfactory sexual relationship, was unable to imagine engaging in alternative modes of sexual expression (cunnilingus, mutual masturbation, and repositioning) that were suggested when the wife developed severe osteoarthritis. The old gentleman brought the worn and dog-eared illustrative pamphlet back to the nurse in the health clinic. "She just won't go for it, nurse!" In such cases, the most well-meant advice may not be useful. To resolve such incompatible needs, the nurse may best counsel the most sexually active and liberal partner in ways to achieve orgasm while still remaining sexually comforting for the other partner.

INTIMACY AND SEXUALITY IN LONG-TERM CARE FACILITIES

Research is needed on sexuality in residential care facilities, but surveys suggest that a significant number of older adults living in these settings might choose to be sexually active if they had privacy and a sexual partner (Syme et al, 2017). Intimacy and sexuality among residents includes the opportunity to have not only intercourse but also other forms of intimate expressions, such as touching, hugging, kissing, hand holding, and masturbation. The sexual needs of older adults in long-term care facilities should receive the same attention as nutrition, hydration, and other well-accepted needs. The institutionalized older adult has the same rights as the noninstitutionalized older adult to engage in or refrain from sexual activity

Attitudes about intimacy and sexuality among long-term care staff and, often, family members may reflect general societal attitudes that older adults do not have sexual needs or that sexual activity is inappropriate. Families may have difficulty understanding that their older relative may want to have a new relationship. Nursing home staff generally have limited knowledge of late-life sexuality and may view residents' sexual acts as problems rather than as expressions of the need for love and intimacy. Reactions may include disapproval, discomfort, and embarrassment, and caregivers may explicitly or implicitly discourage or deny intimacy needs. LGBT older adults are particularly at risk for being discriminated against by both staff and other residents and may not receive care that is culturally safe and appropriate (Neville et al, 2014). Fears of being outed, disrespected, mistreated, and harmed are common and they often choose to stay in the closet (Steelman, 2018).

The majority of nursing facilities do not have policies addressing any aspect of resident sexuality and provide little training for staff. The evidence is clear that communication between older adults and health care professionals about sexual issues is currently poor (Syme et al, 2016). Privacy is a major issue in care facilities that can prevent fulfillment of intimacy and sexual needs. Suggestions for providing privacy and an atmosphere accepting of sexual activity include the availability of a private room, not interrupting when doors are closed and sexual activity is taking place, allowing residents to have sexually explicit materials in their rooms, and providing adaptive equipment, such as side rails or trapezes and double beds. In one facility where the author worked, the staff would assist one of the female residents to be freshly showered, perfumed, and in a lovely nightgown when she and her partner wanted to have sexual relations.

Interventions

Staff, family, and resident education programs to promote awareness, provide education on sexuality and intimacy in later life, involve residents in discussions of sexuality, and discuss interventions to respond to residents' needs are important in long-term care settings. Staff education should include the opportunity to discuss personal feelings about sexuality, changes associated with aging, the impact of diseases and medications on sexual function, sexual expression among same-sex residents, and role-playing and skill training in sexual assessment and intervention. The facility should clearly demonstrate its acceptance of sexuality and the rights and needs of residents of all sexual orientations to have their sexual needs accepted. Information about sexuality and sexual health in informational booklets, promotional flyers, and other documents produced for current and future residents would assist in normalizing the expression of sexuality in care environments.

Sexual expression policies need to be developed with input from staff, residents, and families, displayed prominently, and reviewed with staff members (Palacios-Ceña et al, 2016). Special attention is needed to ensure that LGBT identity is respected in long-term care facilities. Issues related to sexuality and sexual

health should be discussed without anxiety or discomfort so that older adults receive optimal care and treatment (Bauer et al, 2016). The care facility should be a place where all older adults can be comfortable living (Neville et al, 2014).

INTIMACY, SEXUALITY, AND DEMENTIA

Intimacy and sexuality remain important in the lives of persons with dementia and their partners throughout the illness. Intimacy and sexuality may serve as a nonverbal form of communication and intimacy when other cognitive skills and functions have declined. A recent study reported that the majority of partnered older men and women who experience mild to moderate changes in cognition are sexually active, including 40% of partnered people age 80 to 91 years. One-quarter of men and 1 in 10 women in the dementia group reported masturbating. Most people, including men and women with lower cognition, regarded sexuality as an important part of life and reported having sex less often than they would like. Yet sexual behavior between life partners when one has dementia is not often addressed, and individuals with dementia may be viewed as asexual. Individuals with lower cognitive scores infrequently discuss sex with a physician, and physicians rarely counsel individuals with dementia, especially women, about sexual changes that may result from dementia or other medical conditions (Lindau et al, 2018). Nurses need to have an awareness of the sexual needs of the individual with dementia and their partner and be comfortable discussing this area with both. Communication can be encouraged by asking the question, How has dementia affected your sexual relationship?

As dementia progresses, particularly in individuals living in care facilities, intimacy and sexuality issues may present challenges, especially regarding the cognitively impaired individuals who may lack sexual consent capacity, or the ability to make one's own sexual decisions (Jones and Moyle, 2018; Syme et al, 2016). Inappropriate sexual behavior (exposing oneself, masturbating in public, or making inappropriate sexual advances or sexual comments) may also occur in long-term care settings. These behaviors are most distressing to families, staff, and other residents. Sexual inappropriateness (sexual disinhibition) is one of the least understood aspects of dementia. Individuals with subtypes of dementia that include frontal lobe impairment (Pick's disease and alcoholic dementia) may exhibit more sexually inappropriate behavior.

These kinds of behaviors may be triggered by unmet intimacy needs or may be symptoms of an underlying physical problem, such as a urinary tract or vaginal infection. The lack of privacy in care facilities may lead to sexually inappropriate behavior in public areas. Social cues such as explicit television shows may also precipitate behaviors. Bodily contact, such as in bathing residents, may be misinterpreted as a sexual act or romantic advance.

A resident with dementia might be mistaking another person for his or her spouse and begin exhibiting unwelcome intimate behavior toward that person. On the other hand, sexual expression between residents could indicate development of a new relationship, as beautifully depicted in the 2007 movie with Julie Christie, Away from Her. *Former Supreme Court*

Justice Sandra Day O'Connor poignantly described the relationship between her husband, who had Alzheimer's disease, and another resident in a residential care setting. (www.usatoday.com/news/nation/2007-11-12-court_N.htm) (Rheaume and Mitty, 2008, p. 348)

An interprofessional sexual assessment is helpful in determining the underlying need that the individual is expressing and how it might be addressed. Encouraging family and friends to touch, hug, kiss, and hold hands when visiting may help to meet touch and intimacy needs and decrease inappropriate sexual behavior. Also, allowing the person to stroke a pet or hold a stuffed animal may be helpful. Behavioral and nonpharmacological interventions are first-line treatment. Aggressive or violent behavior may require limit setting, working with the resident and family, providing for sexual expression in a nonharmful manner, and pharmacological treatment if indicated. Staff will need opportunities for discussion and assistance with interventions.

Sexuality among nursing home residents with dementia is a sensitive topic, and there are no national guidelines for determining sexual consent capacity among individuals with severe dementia. This topic is poorly understood and inadequately researched and consensus about standard of care on this issue is limited (American Medical Directors Association, 2016). Determination of ability to consent for sexual activity for an individual with cognitive impairment involves concepts of voluntary participation, mental competence, and an understanding of the risks and benefits. The Hebrew Home in Riverdale, New York, initiated model sexual policies in 1995 with the most recent update in 2014. The National Institute on Aging and the Alzheimer's Association provide helpful resources on sexuality and dementia (Box 33.2).

HIV/AIDS AND OLDER ADULTS

An increasingly significant trend in the global HIV epidemic is the growing number of people aged 50 years and older who are living with HIV. This trend is occurring in both developed and developing countries. While rates of HIV/AIDS have remained relatively stable and even declined a little in younger age groups, the number of older adults infected with the virus is growing. In 2015, it was estimated that 50% of all individuals living with HIV in the United States were ages 50 and older, a proportion predicted to rise to 70% by 2020. Gay and bisexual men remain disproportionally affected by HIV and 59% of infections among men in this older age group are attributed to male-to-male sexual contact. Women older than age 60 make up one of the fastest-growing risk groups and most contracted the virus from sex with infected partners. Transgender women are also at disproportionate risk for HIV, but prevalence data on older transgender individuals are not available (Karpiak and Brennan-Ing, 2016). The incidence among older adults is expected to continue to increase as more individuals become infected later in life, and those who were infected in early adulthood live longer as a result of advances in disease treatment.

The compromised immune system of an older adult makes him or her even more susceptible to HIV or AIDS than a younger adult. Older women who are sexually active are at high risk for HIV/AIDS (and other sexually transmitted infections) from an infected partner, resulting, in part, from normal age changes of the vaginal tissue—a thinner, drier, friable vaginal lining that makes viral entry more efficient. Studies show that sexually active older men and women do not routinely use condoms, thus increasing their risk of sexually transmitted diseases (STDs). Recently widowed or divorced individuals may not understand the need for practicing safe sex because they do not worry about an unwanted pregnancy and may not understand the risk of STDs. Older women are more likely than their younger counterparts to be in noncommitted relationships and difficulty negotiating safe sexual relationships can contribute to increased HIV risk (Coleman, 2017). Box 33.3 presents some other risk factors.

Assessment

Physicians, nurse practitioners, and other health professionals need to increase their knowledge of HIV in older adults and become comfortable taking a complete sexual history and talking about sex with all older adults. Sexual health issues such as sexually transmitted infections, sexual functioning, and the sexual history of adult patients should be

---

BOX 33.2   Resources for Best Practice

- **Administration on Aging:** Older Adults and HIV Toolkit
- **Centers for Disease Control and Prevention (CDC):** Guide to Taking a Sexual History
- **Hartford Institute for Geriatric Nursing:** Wallace, M: Issues regarding sexuality, Protocol: Sexuality in the Older Adult: See Assessment Series for video illustrating use of PLISSIT model
- **Hebrew Home for the Aged at Riverdale:** The Center for Older Adult Sexuality: Policy and guidelines for sexual expression among individuals with dementia in long-term care
- **HIVAge.org:** Resources, research
- **National Center for Transgender Equality**
- **National Institute on Aging:** Sexuality in later life, changes in intimacy and sexuality in Alzheimer's disease, HIV, AIDS and older people.
- **National Resource Center for LGBT Aging (SAGE):** Resources aimed at improving the quality of services and supports offered to lesbian, gay, bisexual and transgender (LGBT) older adults.
- **The Fenway Guide to LGBT Health**

BOX 33.3   Risk Factors for HIV

- You are sexually active and do not use a latex or polyurethane condom.
- You do not know your partner's drug and sexual history. Questions you should ask: "Has your partner been tested for HIV/AIDS?" "Has he or she had a number of different sexual partners?" "Has your partner ever had unprotected sex with someone or shared needles?" "Has he or she injected drugs or shared needles with someone else?" Drug users are not the only people who might share needles. People with diabetes who inject insulin or draw blood to test glucose level might share needles.
- You have had a blood transfusion or operation in a developing country at any time or a blood transfusion in the United States between 1978 and 1985.

incorporated as a routine part of the medical history throughout life (Ports et al, 2014). The idea that older adults are not sexually active limits health care providers' objectivity to recognize HIV/AIDS as a possible diagnosis. AIDS in older adults has been called the "Great Imitator" because many of the symptoms, such as fatigue, weakness, weight loss, and anorexia, are common to other disease conditions and may be attributed to normal aging. Additionally, older adults may blame possible symptoms on aging or be reluctant to seek testing or share symptoms due to the stigma they associate with the disease.

Most U.S. guidelines recommend HIV testing among high-risk groups regardless of age, but routine screening recommendations differ and some have a cut-off age of 65 years. The Joint Academy of HIV Medicine, the American Geriatrics Society, and the AIDS Community Research Initiative of America recommend routine opt-out screening, regardless of age (HIVAge. org, 2017). Late diagnosis of HIV can occur because health care providers may not always test older adults for HIV infection (CDC, 2017a). Medicare covers annual screenings for HIV for those who are at increased risk and those who ask for the test. Also covered is annual screening for those who are at increased risk for STDs. An HIV test system is made by the Home Access Health Corporation and is the only home system approved by the US Food and Drug Administration (FDA). It is available at retail pharmacies.

Interventions

Lack of awareness about HIV in older adults results in diagnosis late in the course of the disease, late start to treatment, possibly more damage to their immune system, and poorer prognoses than younger individuals (CDC, 2018). Women tend to be diagnosed with HIV later in their disease than men and fewer women are getting HIV treatment (The Well Project, 2018). HIV-infected older adults may also be at increased risk of geriatric syndromes that complicate their treatment and face higher rates of CVD, diabetes, hypertension, and cancer. HIV and its treatment can also have profound effects on the brain. Although AIDS-related dementia, once relatively common among people with HIV, is now rare, researchers estimate that more than 50% of people with HIV have HIV-associated neurocognitive disorder (HAND), which may include deficits in attention, language, motor skills, memory, and other aspects of cognitive function that may significantly affect a person's quality of life. People who have HAND may also experience depression or psychological distress. Researchers are studying how HIV and its treatment affect the brain, including the effects on older adults living with HIV (National Institute of Neurological Disorders and Stroke, 2018).

Highly active antiretroviral therapy (HAART) can be more complicated if there are chronic illnesses, comorbidities, and polypharmacy. Long-term effects of HAART are also not well studied. However, there is no evidence that response to therapy is different in older adults than in younger individuals and some data suggest that older individuals may be more adherent to HAART. Presently, guidelines for care of adults 60 to 80 years of age with HIV are somewhat limited because this population

---

BOX 33.4 Disease-Stage Summary of Care (HIV/AIDS) in Older Adults

Early-Stage Care
- Discuss sexual history.
- Perform routine screening for HIV.
- HIV symptoms are often atypical in older adults.
- If HIV positive, antiretroviral therapy should be started in all older patients regardless of CD4 T-lymphocyte count.
- No specific guidelines exist for choosing antiretroviral drugs in HIV-positive older adults.
- Choice of highly active retroviral therapy (HAART) depends on factors such as pill burden, dosing frequency, comorbid disease, drug interactions, and local drug availability.
- Provide education on HIV transmission reduction strategies and adherence to drug therapy.

Chronic-Stage Care
- HIV-associated non–AIDS conditions are more likely to impact mortality than HIV.
- Management of comorbidities should be prioritized (cardiovascular, hepatic, renal, bone, central nervous system).
- Modifiable lifestyle risk factors, focusing on health maintenance and prevention, should be addressed.
- Risk for polypharmacy and drug interactions should be considered.
- Risk for social isolation should be considered since social support can influence health outcomes.

Advanced-Stage Care
- Provide ongoing discussions of end-of-life preferences, choice of living environment, and safety.
- Prognosis is an increasingly important component of decision making related to screening, adding medications, and considering invasive treatments.
- Palliative care is an important consideration in older HIV-positive patients.
- Best models of care are not well defined but will require integration of HIV, primary care, and geriatric expertise.

Adapted from Greene M, Justice AC, Lampiris HW, et al: Management of human immunodeficiency virus infection in advanced age, *JAMA* 309(13): 1397–1405, 2013.

---

has not been studied in clinical trials or pharmacokinetic trials. Box 33.4 presents a disease-stage summary of care.

Misinformation about HIV is more common in older adults and they may know less about the disease than younger individuals. Educational materials and programs aimed at older adults need to be developed, particularly for older women. Educational materials should include information about what HIV/AIDS is and how it is (and is not) transmitted, risk-reduction counseling, symptoms of which to be aware, and the treatments that are available. For older women, including opportunities to practice communication skills with sexual partners, may be helpful in sexual discussions with partners later. Small, peer-aged groups may be more successful for providing education than larger groups (Coleman, 2017). Brochures and prevention posters need to depict older adults and be designed for older learners. Jane Fowler of the National HIV Wisdom for Older Women's Program asks the question: "How often does a wrinkled face appear on a prevention poster?" Box 33.2 provides additional resources.

There have been significant increases in the rate of other STDs in older adults. Older adults who are sexually active may be at risk for diseases such as syphilis, chlamydia infection, gonorrhea, genital herpes, hepatitis B, genital warts, and trichomoniasis. Risk factors are similar to those for AIDS and include the increasing number of divorced older adults, unsafe sexual practices (seniors have the lowest rate of condom use compared to other age groups), access to medications to aid in sexual function, and inadequate assessment and testing for STDs in this population. Older adults are more likely to receive a diagnosis of an STD when it is too late and then are unable to benefit from the available medications in the early stages. Many older adults are embarrassed to ask to be tested for STDs. Assessment of older adults needs to include screening for STDs and sex education for prevention (Benjamin Rose Institute on Aging, 2018; CDC, 2017b).

PROMOTING HEALTHY AGING: IMPLICATIONS FOR GERONTOLOGICAL NURSING

Nurses have multiple roles in the area of sexuality and older adults. The nurse is a facilitator of a milieu that is conducive to the person asking questions and expressing his or her sexuality. The nurse is also an educator and provides information and guidance to those who need it. Some older adults remain or want to remain sexually active, whereas others do not see this as an important part of their lives. Nurses should open the door to discussions of sexual concerns in a nonjudgmental manner, helping those who want to continue to be sexually active, and making it clear that stopping sex is an acceptable option for others.

Assessment

Sexuality and intimacy are crucial to healthy aging, and the way these are expressed among older adults is changing, particularly with the aging of the baby boomers and upcoming generations. When promoting healthy aging, nurses must consider increasingly open attitudes toward sexuality, dating and developing new relationships, the challenges of facilitating intimacy in residential settings, and the importance of promoting sexual health and safe sex practices. Being aware of one's own feelings about sexuality and attitudes toward intimacy and sexuality in older adults of all sexual preferences is important. Only after confronting one's own attitudes, values, and beliefs can the nurse provide support without being judgmental. Discussion and assessment of sexual health of healthy older adults and those with dementia need to be included in nursing education programs (Jones and Moyle, 2018).

Validation of the normalcy of sexual activity and a discussion of the physiological changes that occur either with age or as a result of illness are important. Anticipation of problems in older individuals' sexual experiences can ward off anxiety, misconceptions, and an arbitrary cessation of sexual pleasure. Adaptations that will promote sexual function for individuals with chronic illness should be provided. Screening for HIV/AIDS and other STDs and education about safe sexual practices are also important (Box 33.5).

In addition, the myth that adults do not engage in sexual activity must be put to rest. When questions about sexual issues are asked or when the older adult is examined, the nurse needs to be particularly cognizant of the era and culture in which the individual has lived to understand the factors affecting conduct. Box 33.6 provides other suggestions for assessment, from the perspective of the older adult. Currently, there are no instruments that could be used in clinical practice or research to assess the sexual health of the older population. Nurse researcher Meredith Kazer and colleagues (2013) report on the preliminary development of the Geriatric Sexuality Inventory and note that having a self-report instrument to replace open-ended questions may be an effective strategy to decrease the discomfort of health care providers and older adults in discussing sexuality. The Centers for Disease Control and Prevention (CDC) provides a guide to taking a sexual history (Box 33.2).

- A medication review is essential because many medications affect sexual functioning. Often, medications are prescribed to both older men and women without attention to the sexual side effects. If medications that affect sexual function are necessary, adjustment of doses, use of alternative agents, and prescription of antidotes to reverse the sexual side effects are important (Box 33.7) (Chapter 9).

The PLISSIT Model (Annon, 1976) is a helpful guide for discussion of sexuality (Box 33.8).

- **Permission:** Obtain permission from the client to initiate sexual discussion. Allow the person to discuss concerns related to sexual issues, and gather information about what might have changed in the person's life to affect sexual needs and response. Questions such as the following can be used: "What concerns or questions do you have about fulfilling your sexual needs?" or "In this era of HIV and other sexually transmitted infections, I ask all my patients about sexual practices and concerns. Are there any questions I can answer for you?"
- **Limited Information:** Provide the limited information to function sexually. Offer teaching about the normal age-associated

BOX 33.6 Tips for Best Practice

Guidelines for Health Care Providers in Talking to Older Adults About Sexual Health

Health Care Providers Should Spend Time With Older Adults
- Be available to discuss the subject.
- Give us your full attention.
- Allow time to ask questions.
- Take time to answer questions.
- Health care providers should use clear and easy-to-understand words and everyday language.

Health Care Providers Should Help Older Adults Feel Comfortable Talking About Sex
- Help us to break the ice.
- Make us feel comfortable in asking questions.
- Offer permission to express feelings and needs.
- Do not be afraid or embarrassed to discuss sexuality problems.

Health Care Providers Should Be Open-Minded and Talk Openly
- Do not assume there are no concerns.
- Be open.
- Ask direct questions about sexual activity and attitudes.
- Discuss sexual concerns freely.
- Answer questions honestly.
- Just talk about it.
- Do not evade sexual concerns.
- Be willing to discuss sexual problems.
- Probe sexual concerns if older adult wishes.

Health Care Providers Should Listen
- Listen so that we feel you are interested in our problems.
- Let us talk.

Health Care Providers Should Treat Older Adults With a Respectful and Nonjudgmental Attitude
- See us as individuals with sexual needs.
- Accept us for what we are: gay, straight, bisexual, transgender.
- Be nonjudgmental.
- Show genuine concern and respect.

Health Care Providers Should Encourage Discussion
- Make opportunities for one-to-one discussion.
- Provide privacy.
- Promote candid discussion.
- Provide discussion groups to ask questions.
- Develop support groups.

Health Care Providers Can Give Advice or Suggestions
- Provide information.
- Offer to find solutions and alternatives to given situations.
- Provide explicit pamphlets; explain sexual positions, lubrication.
- Discuss old taboos.
- Give suggestions of ways to help solve sexual problems.

Health Care Providers Need to Understand That Sex Is Not Just for the Young
- Try to eliminate the idea that sex and love are just for younger people.
- Acknowledge that sexual impulses are healthy and do not disappear as individuals age.
- Treat older adults as normal sexual beings and not as asexual people.
- Recognize that sex can improve—can become even better—when one is older.

BOX 33.7 Medications That May Affect Sexual Health

Antihypertensive agents
Medications for prostate diseases
Cholesterol medications
Antidepressant agents
Other medications that affect mood
Anticholinergic agents
Pain medications (narcotics)
Osteoporosis medications
Oral hypoglycemic agents
Insulin
Chemotherapy for cancer

BOX 33.8 PLISSIT Model

P   **Permission** from the client to initiate sexual discussion
LI   Providing the **Limited Information** needed to function sexually

SS   Giving **Specific Suggestions** for the individual to proceed with sexual relations
IT   Providing **Intensive Therapy** surrounding the issues of sexuality for the clients (may mean referral to specialist)

Compiled from Annon J: The PLISSIT model: a proposed conceptual scheme for behavioral treatment of sexual problems, *J Sex Educ Ther* 2:1–15, 1976.

changes that affect sexual performance or how illness may affect sexuality. Encourage the person to learn more about the concern from books and other sources.
- **Specific Suggestions:** Offer suggestions for dealing with problems such as lubricants for atrophic vaginitis; use of condoms to prevent sexually transmitted infections; proper use of ED medications; how to communicate sexual and other needs; ways to increase comfort with coitus or ways to be intimate without coital relations.
- **Intensive Therapy:** Refer as appropriate for complex problems that require specialist intervention.

Interventions

Interventions will vary depending on the needs identified from the assessment data. Following a comprehensive assessment, interventions may center on the following categories: (1) education regarding age-associated change in sexual function; (2) compensation for age-associated changes and effects of chronic illness; (3) effective management of acute and chronic illness affecting sexual function; (4) provision of education on HIV and STDs and reduction of risk factors; (5) removal of barriers associated with fulfilling sexual needs; and (6) special interventions to promote sexual health in older adults with cognitive impairment (Box 33.2).

KEY CONCEPTS

- Touch provides sensory stimulation, reduces anxiety, and provides pain relief, comfort, and sexual expression.
- The absence of touch, a powerful sense, threatens survival.
- Sexuality is love, sharing, trust, warmth, and physical acts. Sexuality provides an individual with self-identity and affirmation of life.
- Sexual activity continues in aging, though adaptations are needed for the age-related changes of the male and female genital systems.
- Generally speaking, medications, ill health, and lack of a partner affect sexual activity.
- Further research is needed to promote knowledge and understanding of the sexual health of LGBT older adults.

- AIDS awareness and the practice of safe sex among older adults are still lacking. Health professionals, too, do not consider older adults at risk for AIDS and STDs, even though the incidence of both in older adults is rapidly increasing.
- The major role of the nurse in enhancing the sexual health of older adults in the community or in long-term care settings is education and counseling about sexual function; adaptations for age-related changes and chronic conditions; prevention of HIV/AIDS and STDs in sexually active older adults; and the maintenance of sexuality for the older adult's health, well-being, and pleasure.

NURSING STUDY: SEXUALITY IN LATE LIFE

George was a 70-year-old man who had been widowed for 6 years. He lived alone in a lovely home in the hills of San Francisco. His many friends tried to introduce him to a lady who would be attractive to him, but they were unaware of his real concerns. Although George was attracted to young, energetic women, often barely older than his daughters, he was justifiably cautious regarding their sincere attraction to him because he had a considerable estate. In addition, his sexual desire was waning and his capacity for sexual performance was unpredictable. One thing George expressed fairly frequently was, "I don't like demands made on me." To further complicate the picture, George had begun to take medication to reduce his benign prostatic hypertrophy (BPH) that had become increasingly troublesome. The medication further reduced his sexual desire. In addition, George's sleep pattern was disturbed by the need to arise three or four times each night to void. George came to the clinic for follow-up evaluation of his BPH, and, while talking with the nurse, he began crying uncontrollably, much to his embarrassment and the nurse's surprise because George had always seemed to be a rather solid and stoic fellow who was reluctant to discuss feelings.

Based on the case study, develop a nursing care plan using the following procedure[a]:

- List George's comments that provide subjective data.
- List information that provides objective data.
- From these data, identify and state, using an accepted format, two nursing diagnoses you determine are most significant to George at this time. List two of George's strengths that you have identified from the data.
- Determine and state outcome criteria for each diagnosis. These criteria must reflect some alleviation of the problem identified in the nursing diagnosis and must be stated in concrete and measurable terms.
- Plan and state one or more interventions for each diagnosed problem. Provide specific documentation of the sources used to determine the appropriate intervention. Plan at least one intervention that incorporates George's existing strengths.
- Evaluate the success of the intervention. Interventions must correlate directly with the stated outcome criteria to measure the outcome success.

[a]Students are advised to refer to their nursing diagnosis text and identify possible or potential problems.

CRITICAL THINKING QUESTIONS AND ACTIVITIES

1. How would you begin discussing sexuality with George?
2. What are the factors that may be underlying George's sexual distress?
3. With a partner, role-play and demonstrate your interpersonal interaction with George in this situation.
4. What resources or recommendations would you suggest for George?

RESEARCH QUESTIONS

1. What do women find are the most troubling changes in their sexuality as they grow older?
2. What do men find are the most troubling changes in their sexuality as they grow older?
3. What are the differences in sexual feelings and expression in the 60-year-old, the 70-year-old, the 80-year-old, and the 90-year-old individual?
4. What are the chronic disorders that most affect sexual performance of men and women, and how are individuals affected?
5. How many individuals older than age 60 have ever been given the opportunity to provide a thorough sexual history?
6. What community and health resources are available to meet the needs of LGBT older adults?
7. What is the knowledge level about HIV/AIDS for people older than age 65?

REFERENCES

American Geriatrics Society: American Geriatrics Society Care of Lesbian, Gay, Bisexual, and Transgender Older Adults Position Statement, *J Am Geriatr Soc* 63:423–426, 2015.

American Medical Directors Association: *Capacity for sexual consent in dementia in long-term care,* 2016. https://paltc.org/amda-white-papers-and-resolution-position-statements/capacity-sexual-consent-dementia-long-term-care. Accessed April 2018.

American Psychological Association: *Lesbian, gay, bisexual and transgender aging,* 2018. http://www.apa.org/pi/lgbt/resources/aging.aspx. Accessed April 2018.

Annon JS: The PLISSIT model: a proposed conceptual scheme for behavioral treatment of sexual problems, *J Sex Educ Ther* 2:1–15, 1976.

Bauer M, Haesler E, Fetherstonhaugh D: Let's talk about sex: older people's views on the recognition of sexuality and sexual health in the health-care setting, *Health Expect* 19(6):1237–1250, 2016.

Benary-Isbert M: *The vintage years,* New York, NY, 1968, Abingdon Press.

Benjamin Rose Institute on Aging: *Sexually transmitted diseases in older adults,* 2018. http://www.benrose.org/resources/article-stds-older-adults.cfm. Accessed April 2018.

Byrne M, Murphy P, D'Eath M, Doherty S, Jaarsma T: Association between sexual problems and relationship satisfaction among people with cardiovascular disease, *J Sex Med* 14(5):666–674, 2017.

Centers for Disease Control and Prevention (CDC): *STD and HIV screening recommendations,* 2017a. https://www.cdc.gov/std/prevention/screeningreccs.htm. Accessed April 2018.

Centers for Disease Control and Prevention (CDC): *Sexually transmitted disease surveillance,* 2017b. https://www.cdc.gov/std/stats/default.htm. Accessed April 2018.

Centers for Disease Control and Prevention: *HIV among people aged 50 and older,* 2018. https://www.cdc.gov/hiv/group/age/olderamericans/index.html. Accessed April 2018.

Chen CH, Lin YC, Chiu LH, et al: Female sexual dysfunction: definition, classification, and debates, *Taiwan J Obstet Gynecol* 52(1):3–7, 2013.

Clark T: *The circles of sexuality and aging,* 2015, American Society on Aging. https://www.asaging.org/blog/circles-sexuality-and-aging. Accessed March 2019.

Cloyes KG: The silence of our science: nursing research on LGBT older adult health, *Res Gerontol Nurs* 9(2):92–104, 2016.

Coleman CL: Women 50 and older and HIV. Prevention and implications for health care providers, *J Gerontol Nurs* 43(12):29–34, 2017.

Comfort A: Sexuality in old age, *J Am Geriatr Soc* 22:440–442, 1974.

Dhingra I, De Sousa A, Sonavane S: Sexuality in older adults: clinical and psychosocial dilemmas, *J Geriatr Ment Health* 3(2):131–139, 2016.

Emlet CA: Social, economic, and health disparities among LGBT older adults, *Gen J West Gerontol Soc* 40(2):16–21, 2016.

Franc L, Moukoulou L, Scott L, Zerwic J: LGBT inclusivity in health assessment textbooks. *J Prof Nurs* 34(6):483–487, 2018.

Fredriksen-Goldsen KI: The future of LGBT + aging: a blueprint for action in services, policies, and research, *Gen J West Gerontol Soc* 40(2):6–15, 2016.

Fredriksen-Goldsen KI, Kim HJ: The science of conducting research with LGBT older adults—an introduction to aging with pride: National Health, Aging, and Sexuality/gender study (NHAS), *Gerontologist* 57(Suppl 1):S1–S14, 2017.

Hall ET: *The hidden dimensions,* Garden City, NY, 1969, Doubleday.

Heidari S: Sexuality and older people: a neglected issue, *Reprod Health Matters* 24(48):1–5, 2016.

HIVAge.org: *Detection and screening for HIV in older adults clinical recommendations,* 2017. http://hiv-age.org/2017/08/22/detection-screening-hiv-older-adults/. Accessed April 2018.

Jones C, Moyle W: Are gerontological nurses ready for the expression of sexuality by individuals with dementia? *J Gerontol Nurs* 44(5):2–4, 2018.

Karpiak S, Brennan-Ing M: Aging with HIV: the challenges of providing care and social supports, *Gen J Am Soc Aging* 40(2):23–25, 2016.

Kazer MW, Grossman S, Kerins G, Kris A, Tocchi C: Validity and reliability of the Geriatric Sexual Inventory, *J Gerontol Nurs* 39(11):38–45, 2013.

Krieger D: Therapeutic touch: the imprimatur of nursing, *Am J Nurs* 75:784–787, 1975.

Lee DM, Nazroo J, O'Connor DB, Blake M, Pendleton N: Sexual health and well-being among older men and women in England: findings from the English Longitudinal Study of Ageing, *Arch Sex Behav* 45(1):133–144, 2016.

Lindau ST, Gavrilova N: Sex, health, and years of sexually active life gained due to good health: evidence from two US populations based cross sectional surveys of ageing, *BMJ* 340:c810, 2010.

Lindau ST, Dale W, Feldmeth G, et al: Sexuality and cognitive status: a U.S. nationally representative study of home-dwelling older adults, *J Am Geriatr Soc* 66:1902-1910, 2018.

Marchese K: An overview of erectile dysfunction in the elderly population, *Urol Nurs* 37(3):157-170, 2017.

Mobley DF, Khera M, Baum N: Recent advances in the treatment of erectile dysfunction, *Postgrad Med J* 93:679–685, 2017.

National Center for Transgender Equality: *Understanding transgender people: The basics,* 2016. https://transequality.org/issues/resources/understanding-transgender-people-the-basics. Accessed April 2018.

National Institute of Neurological Disorders and Stroke: *Clinical trials,* 2019. https://www.ninds.nih.gov/Disorders/Clinical-Trials/Anakinra-Recombinant-Human-IL-1-Receptor-Antagonist-Neuroinflammation-HIV. Accessed March 2019.

Neville SJ, Adams J, Bellamy G, Boyd M, George N: Perceptions towards lesbian, gay and bisexual people in residential care facilities: a qualitative study, *Int J Older People Nurs* 10(1):73–80, 2014.

Palacios-Ceña D, Martínez-Piedrola RM, Pérez-de-Heredia M, Huertas-Hoyas E, Carrasco-Garrido P, Fernández-de-Las-Peñas C: Expressing sexuality in nursing homes: the experience of older women: a qualitative study, *Geriatr Nurs* 37(6):470–477, 2016.

Patel CK, Bennett N: Advances in the treatment of erectile dysfunction: what's new and upcoming? *F1000Res 5,* 2016.

Ports KA, Barnack-Tavlaris JL, Syme ML, Perera RA, Lafata JE: Sexual health discussions with older patients during periodic health exams, *J Sex Med* 11(4):901–908, 2014.

Rheaume C, Mitty E: Sexuality and intimacy in older adults, *Geriatr Nurs* 29:342–349, 2008.

Schafer MH, Upenieks L, Iveniuk J: Putting sex into context in later life: environmental disorder and sexual interest among partnered seniors, *Gerontologist* 58(1):181–190, 2018.

Steelman RE: Person-centered care for LGBT older adults, *J Gerontol Nurs* 44(2):3–5, 2018.

Steinke EE: Sexuality and chronic illness, *J Gerontol Nurs* 39(11):18–29, 2013.

Steinke EE, Jaarsma T, Barnason SA, et al: Sexual counseling for individuals with CVD and their partners: a consensus statement from the American Heart Association and the ESC Council on Cardiovascular Nursing and Allied Professions (CCNAP), *Circulation* 128:2075–2096, 2013.

Syme ML: *Sexual health in older adulthood: defining the goals,* 2015. http://asaging.org/blog/sexual-health-older-adulthood-defining-goals. Accessed April 2018.

Syme ML, Yelland E, Cornelison L, Poey JL, Krajicek R, Doll G: Content analysis of public opinion on sexual expression and dementia: implications for nursing home policy development, *Health Expect* 20:705–713, 2017.

TheWell Project: *Women and HIV,* 2018. http://www. thewellproject.org/hiv-information/women-and-hiv. Accessed April 2018.

Wang Y, Wu J, Wang Z: The effectiveness of massage and touch on behavioural and psychological symptoms of dementia: a quantitative systematic review and meta-analysis, *J Adv Nurs* 73(10):2283–2295, 2017.

Wright H, Jenks RA, Demeyere N: Frequent sexual activity predicts specific cognitive abilities in older adults, *J Gerontol B Psychol Sci Soc Sci,* 74(1):47–51, 2019.

World Health Organization: *Defining sexual health,* 2018. http://www. who.int/reproductivehealth/topics/sexual_health/sh_definitions/ en/. Accessed April 2018.

Youngkin EQ: The myths and truths of mature intimacy: mature guidance for nurse practitioners, *Adv Nurse Pract* 12:45–48, 2004.

Relationships, Roles, and Transitions

Theris A. Touhy

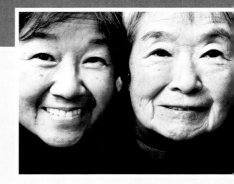

http://evolve.elsevier.com/Touhy/TwdHlthAging

A STUDENT SPEAKS

I'm really worried about retirement! That is ridiculous at my age, but I keep reading and hearing about Social Security and Medicare running out of money for the baby boom generation. Those are my parents! What about me?

Joseph, age 30

AN OLDER ADULT SPEAKS

I thought when my children left home that my most important job was done. But they came home again and again, and then my mother-in-law came to live with us. Finally, the kids were really on their own and married, so now I take care of the grandchildren while they both work to make ends meet. I just pray daily that my husband will remain healthy. I don't think I could deal with one more thing.

Esther, age 64

LEARNING OBJECTIVES

On completion of this chapter, the reader will be able to:

1. Explain the issues involved in adapting to transitions and role changes in later life.
2. Discuss changes in family structure and functions in society today.
3. Examine family relationships in later life.
4. Identify the range of caregiving situations and the potential challenges and opportunities of each.
5. Discuss nursing responses with older adults experiencing caregiver roles or other transitions.

This chapter examines the various relationships, roles, and transitions that characteristically play a part in later life. Important roles include those of spouse, partner, parent, grandparent, great-grandparent, sibling, friend, and caregiver. The role functions of these relationships shift as societal norms and economics change. Even more changes are expected as the first wave of baby boomers enters young-old age. The major concerns of this group are maintaining health and independence, having adequate health care coverage, ensuring the preservation of Social Security, and meeting caregiving demands. This major change in the aging landscape is only one of the massive social changes that have altered the patterns of work, family, and kinship structure in recent decades.

Concepts of family structure and function—the transitions of retirement, widowhood, widowerhood, and caregiving—are examined. Nursing interventions to support older adults in maintaining fulfilling roles and relationships and adapting to transitions are discussed.

LATER LIFE TRANSITIONS

Role transitions that occur in later life include retirement, grandparenthood, widowhood, and becoming a caregiver or recipient of care. These transitions may occur predictably or may be imposed by unanticipated events. Retirement is an example of a predictable event that can and should be planned long in advance, although for some, it can occur unexpectedly as a result of illness, disability, or being terminated from a job. To the degree that an event is perceived as expected and occurring at the right time, a role transition may be comfortable and even welcomed. Those persons who must retire "too early" or are widowed "too soon" will have more difficulty adapting than those who are at an age when these events are expected.

The speed and intensity of a major change may make the difference between a transitional crisis and a gradual and comfortable adaptation. Most difficult are the transitions that incorporate losses rather than gains in status, influence, and opportunity. The move from independence to dependence and becoming a care recipient is particularly difficult. Conditions that influence the outcome of transitions include personal meanings, expectations, level of knowledge, preplanning, and emotional and physical reserves. Cohort, cultural, and gender differences are inherent in all of life's major transitions. Those transitions that make use of past skills and adaptations may be less stressful. The ideal outcome is when gains in satisfaction and new roles offset losses.

Retirement

Issues of work and retirement for older adults are a cultural universal topic because every culture has mechanisms for retiring their older citizens. While retirement patterns differ across the world, in industrialized nations, and in many developing nations, the expectation is that older workers will cease full-time career job employment and be entitled to economic support. However, whether that support will be adequate, or even available, is a growing concern worldwide. In the United States and many European countries and in Australia, the problems are emerging as the generation born after World War II moves into retirement. Developing countries face similar issues with the growth of the older population combined with decreasing birth rates. Governments may not be able to afford retirement systems to replace the tradition of children caring for aging parents. Most countries are not ready to meet what is projected to be one of the defining challenges of the twenty-first century.

Retirement, as we formerly knew it, has changed. The transitions are blurring, and the numerous patterns and styles of retiring have produced more varied experiences in retirement. Retirement is no longer just a few years of rest from the rigors of work before death. It is a developmental stage that may occupy 30 or more years of one's life and involve many stages. Some individuals will be retired longer than they worked. Retirees are living longer, and declining birth rates mean there will be fewer workers to support them. Countries are scaling down retirement benefits and raising the age when individuals can collect them.

Individuals can expect to work longer before retirement and many plan to continue to work after they retire. Some do so because of economic need, whereas others have a desire to remain involved and productive. At this time, 30% of individuals 65 to 69 years old, 30% of those 70 to 74 years old, and 8.4% of those aged 75 years and older are still working. Almost all of those who worked for pay in retirement enjoy working and staying active and involved. However, financial reasons also had an influence on working: 67% worked to buy extras, 42% needed money to make ends meet, 23% worked because of a decrease in the value of their savings, and 13% worked to keep health insurance or other benefits (Employee Benefit Research Institute, 2017; Morley, 2017).

People are starting to retire later as they realize the obstacles financial challenges or obligations present to successful retirement and future independence (Plawecki and Plawecki, 2016). Since 2017, retirees are less likely to feel confident that they will be able to afford medical care and long-term care and that Medicare will continue as is (Employee Benefit Research

Institute, 2018). More than one in five older Americans receive 90% or more of their total retirement income from Social Security, and another quarter receive between 50% and 90% of their income from that source (Applebaum and Cummins, 2017). More than half of the world's working population claims they are not preparing adequately for a comfortable retirement, with a sizable percentage of workers reporting they have no or very little money in savings and investments (Employee Benefit Research Institute, 2017). Single senior households, mostly women, are at even greater financial vulnerability.

Special Considerations in Retirement

The three-legged stool for retirement (Social Security, savings, and private pensions) has become one-legged for a sizable proportion of Americans because of limited personal retirement savings and decline in pension plans (Morley, 2017). Older adults with disabilities, those who had less access to education or held low-paying jobs with no benefits, and those not eligible for Social Security are at increased economic risk during retirement years. Older minority women, never-married women, and divorced women are more likely to be in poverty and are less likely to receive Social Security (Shelton, 2016). Prior to the legalization of same-sex marriage in the United States, individuals were denied access to Social Security survivor benefits. After legalization of same-sex marriage, married same-sex couples now have access to Social Security survivor benefits, Medicaid spend-downs, bereavement leave, and tax exemptions upon inheritance of jointly owned real estate and personal property.

Inadequate coverage for women in retirement is common because their work histories have been sporadic and diverse. Women often retire earlier than anticipated because of family needs. Whereas most men have always worked outside the home, it is only within the past 30 years that this has been the expectation of women. Therefore large cohort differences exist. Traditionally, the variability of women's work histories, interrupted careers, the residuals of sexist pension policies, Social Security inequities, and low-paying jobs created hazards for adequacy of income in retirement. The scene is gradually changing in many respects, but the gender bias remains (Chapter 30).

Retirement Planning

Current research suggests that retirement has positive effects on life satisfaction and health, although this may vary depending on the individual's circumstances. Decisions to retire are often based on financial resources; attitudes toward work, family roles, and responsibilities; the nature of the job; access to health insurance; chronological age; health; and self-perceptions of ability to adjust to retirement. Retirement planning is advisable during early adulthood and essential in middle age. However, people differ in their focus on the past, present, and future and their realistic ability to "put away something" for future needs.

Retirement preparation programs are usually aimed at employees with high levels of education and occupational status, those with private pension coverage, and government employees. Thus, the people most in need of planning assistance may be those least likely to have any available, let alone the resources for an adequate retirement. Individuals who are retiring in poor health, minorities, women, those in lower socioeconomic levels, and those with the least education may experience greater concerns in retirement and may need specialized counseling and targeted education efforts.

PROMOTING HEALTHY AGING: IMPLICATIONS FOR GERONTOLOGICAL NURSING

Successful retirement adjustment depends on socialization needs, energy levels, health, adequate income, variety of interests, amount of self-esteem derived from work, presence of intimate relationships, social support, and general adaptability (Box 34.1). Nurses may have the opportunity to work with people in different phases of retirement or participate in retirement education and counseling programs.

Talking with clients older than age 50 about retirement plans, providing anticipatory guidance about the transition to retirement, identifying those who may be at risk for lowered income and health concerns, and referring to appropriate resources for retirement planning and support are important nursing interventions. Additionally, the period of preretirement and retirement may be an opportune time to enhance the focus on health promotion and illness and injury prevention (Chapter 1). It is important to build on the strengths of the individual's life experiences and coping skills and to provide appropriate counseling and support to assist individuals to continue to grow and develop in meaningful ways during the transition from the work role. In ideal situations, retirement offers the opportunity to pursue interests that may have been neglected while fulfilling other obligations. However, for too many individuals, retirement presents challenges that affect both health and well-being, and nurses must be advocates for policies and conditions that allow all older adults to maintain quality of life in retirement.

Death of a Spouse or Life Partner

Losing a spouse or other life partner after a long, close, and satisfying relationship is the most difficult adjustment one can face, aside from the loss of a child. This loss is a stage in the life

---

BOX 34.1   Predictors of Retirement Satisfaction

- Good health
- Functional abilities
- Adequate income
- Suitable living environment
- Strong social support system characterized by reciprocal relationships
- Decision to retire involved choice, autonomy, adequate preparation, higher-status job before retirement
- Retirement activities that offer an opportunity to feel useful, learn, grow, and enjoy oneself
- Positive outlook, sense of mastery, resilience, resourcefulness
- Good marital or partner relationship
- Sharing similar interests to spouse/significant other

BOX 34.2   Common Widower Bereavement Reactions

- Search for the lost mate
- Neglect of self
- Inability to share grief
- Loss of social contacts
- Struggle to view women as other than wife
- Erosion of self-confidence and sexuality
- Protracted grief period

---

course that can be anticipated but seldom is considered. Spousal bereavement in later life is a high probability for women and, while less common among men, still a significant event. Older women are substantially more likely to be widowed (and not remarried) than older men (37% vs. 13%) and the majority of these older widowed women live alone. Men are about half as likely as women to live alone today and men are more likely than women to remarry after divorce or widowhood (Stepler, 2016). The number of widows has declined, especially for women whose spouses are now living longer. The decline in widowhood in recent decades also results from a rising share of divorced older Americans who have not remarried, particularly among those aged 65 to 74 years (Stepler, 2016).

Although change in marital status is accepted as a normal life experience, the death of a spouse is a significant life event for older adults. With the loss of the intimate partner, several changes occur simultaneously in almost every domain of life and have a significant impact on well-being: physical, psychological, social, practical, and economic. Individuals who have been self-confident and resilient seem to fare best. Having frequent contact with family and friends is key to resilience in handling the loss. The transitional phase of grief, if handled appropriately, leads to the confirmation of a new identity, the end of one stage of life, and the beginning of another.

Gender differences on widowhood are found in the literature. Bereaved husbands may be more socially and emotionally vulnerable. Suicide risk is highest among men older than 80 years of age who have experienced the death of a spouse (Chapter 28). Widowers adapt more slowly than widows to the loss of a spouse and often remarry quickly. Loneliness and the need to be cared for are factors influencing widowers to pursue new partners. Having associations with family and friends, being members of a church community, and continuing to work or engage in activities can all be helpful in the adjustment period following the death of a wife. Common bereavement reactions of widowers are listed in Box 34.2 and should be discussed with male clients.

PROMOTING HEALTHY AGING: IMPLICATIONS FOR GERONTOLOGICAL NURSING

Assessment

Nurses working with bereaved individuals will need to review Lindemann's classic grief studies to understand the initial somatic responses of the bereaved (Lindemann, 1944) (Chapter 35). There is an elevated risk of morbidity and mortality, particularly in the early bereavement period. The likelihood of a heart attack or stroke doubles in the critical 30-day period after a partner's death. The risk seems likely to be the result of adverse physiological responses associated with acute grief. The bereavement period is also associated with an elevated risk of multiple psychiatric disorders, particularly if the death was unexpected. This is an important time for nurses to assess the health status of the individual and provide interventions to assist in coping. However, the risks of effects of spousal bereavement and increasing age on health, particularly chronic issues, remain elevated even among those long past the event (10+ years), so ongoing surveillance and assessment are indicated.

Interventions

Nurses will interact with bereaved older adults in many settings. Knowing the stages of transition to a new role as a widow or widower will be useful in determining interventions, although each individual is unique in this respect. Individuals respond to losses in ways that reflect the nature and meaning of the relationships and the unique characteristics of the bereaved. Patterns of adjustment are presented in Box 34.3. With adequate support, reintegration can be expected in 2 to 4 years. People with few familial or social supports may need professional help to get

through the early months of grief in a way that will facilitate recovery. Additional information about dying, death, and grief can be found in Chapter 35.

RELATIONSHIPS IN LATER LIFE

The classic study of Lowenthal and Haven (1968) has been reviewed in detail and elaborated many times since its inception. The importance of caring relationships and the presence of a confidante as a buffer against "age-linked social losses" are demonstrated in the study. Maintaining a stable intimate relationship was more closely associated with good mental health and high morale than was a high level of activity or elevated role status. Individuals seem able to manage stresses if some relationships are close and sustaining.

Increasingly evident is that a caring person may be a significant survival resource. Frequently nurses become the caring other in an older adult's life, especially among those living in nursing homes (Touhy, 2001) (Chapter 32). Social bonding increases health status through as yet undetermined physiological pathways, though studies in psychoneuroimmunology are giving us clues. Social support is related to psychological and physical well-being, and participation in meaningful social activities is also a modifying factor that may offset the risk of dementia.

Friendships

Friends are often a significant source of support in late life. The number of friends may decline, but the majority of older adults have at least one close friend with whom they maintain close contact, share confidences, and can turn to in an emergency. The social network may narrow as one ages with intimate personal relationships being maintained and the more instrumental relationships discontinued. Research across the globe supports the value of friendship for older adults in promoting health and well-being.

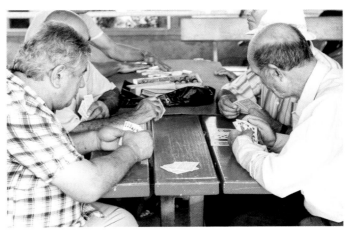

Friends play an important role in the lives of older adults. (By Michal Osmenda, Brussels, Belgium [CC BY 2.0 (http://creativecommons.org/licenses/by/2.0)], via Wikimedia Commons.)

BOX 34.3 Patterns of Adjustment to Widowhood

Stage 1: Reactionary (First Few Weeks)
Early responses of disbelief, anger, indecision, detachment, and inability to communicate in a logical, sustained manner are common. Searching for the mate, visions, hallucinations, and depersonalization may be experienced.
Intervention: Support, validate, be available, listen to individual talk about mate, reduce expectations.

Stage 2: Withdrawal (First Few Months)
Depression, apathy, physiological vulnerability; movement and cognition are slowed; insomnia, unpredictable waves of grief, sighing, and anorexia occur.
Intervention: Protect individual against suicide, monitor health status, and involve in support groups.

Stage 3: Recuperation (Second 6 Months)
Periods of depression are interspersed with characteristic capability. Feelings of personal control begin to return.
Intervention: Support accustomed lifestyle patterns that sustain and assist individual to explore new possibilities.

Stage 4: Exploration (Second Year)
Individual begins new ventures, testing suitability of new roles; anniversaries, holidays, birthdays, and date of death may be especially difficult.
Intervention: Prepare individual for unexpected reactions during anniversaries. Encourage and support new trial roles.

Stage 5: Integration (Fifth Year)
Individual will feel fully integrated into new and satisfying roles if grief has been resolved in a healthy manner.
Intervention: Assist individual to recognize and share own pattern of growth through the trauma of loss.

Friendships are often sustaining in the face of overwhelming circumstances. Friends provide the critical elements of satisfactory living that families may not, providing commitment and affection without judgment. Personality characteristics between friends are compatible because the relationships are chosen and caring is shared without obligation. Trust, demonstrations of caring, and mutual problem solving are important aspects of the friendships. Friends may share a lifelong perspective or may bring a totally new intergenerational viewpoint into one's life. Late-life friendships often develop out of changing situations, such as relocation to retirement or assisted living communities, widowhood, and involvement in volunteer pursuits. As desires and pursuits change, some friendships evolve that the person never would have considered in his or her youth.

Considering the obvious importance of friendship, it seems to be a neglected area of exploration and a seldom considered resource for professionals working with older adults. Because close friendships have such influence on the sense of well-being of older adults, anything done to sustain them or assist in building new friendships and social networks will be helpful. Internet access and social media offer new opportunities to interact with friends or even to form new friendships. Generally, women tend to have more sustaining friendships than do men, and this factor contributes to resilience, a characteristic linked to successful aging (Chapter 28).

Nurses may include questions about the individual's friendships and their importance and availability in their assessment of older adults. While friendships do provide much support, they are also a further source of grief in old age. The loss of friends through death occurs often and nurses must appreciate the nature of this loss. Encouraging intergenerational friendships and linking older adults to resources for social participation and meaningful activities are important interventions.

FAMILIES

Changing Family Structure

The idea of family evokes strong impressions of whatever an individual believes the typical family should be. Because everyone comes from a family, these impressions have powerful symbolic meanings. However, in today's world, the definition of family is in a state of flux. As recently as 100 years ago, the norm was the extended family made up of parents, their grown children, and the children's children, often living together and sharing resources, strengths, and challenges. As cities grew and adult children moved in pursuit of work, parents did not always come along, and the nuclear family evolved. The norm in the United States became two parents and their two children (nuclear family), or at least that was the norm in what has been considered mainstream America. This pattern was not as common among ethnically diverse families where the extended family is often the norm. However, families are changing, and today the nuclear family is much less common.

Changing family patterns pose significant challenges for the future of long-term care because 80% to 90% of all long-term care services and supports are provided by spouses, adult children, and other informal caregivers. Baby boomers are more likely to live alone than previous generations, and single-person households are increasing (Vespa and Schondelmyer, 2015). Other countries are also experiencing changes in family composition, and even values, as the numbers of older adults increase and the younger members of society become more mobile and move away from their home. In China, the extended family is disappearing and in 2013 the country enacted a new law mandating that family members must attend to the spiritual needs of older family members and visit them frequently if they live apart. Nearly half of the country's seniors live apart from their children (United Nations Economic and Social Commission for Asia and the Pacific, 2018).

A decrease in fertility rates has reduced family size, and American families are smaller today than ever before. The high divorce and remarriage rate results in households of blended families of children from previous marriages and the new marriage. The new modern family includes single-parent families, blended families, gay and lesbian families, domestic partnerships, and childless families. Older adults without families, either by choice or by circumstance, may create their own "families" through communal living with siblings, friends, or others. Indeed, it is not unusual for childless older adults residing in long-term care facilities to refer to the staff as their new "family."

Multigenerational Families

The U.S. Census Bureau defines multigenerational families as those consisting of more than two generations living under the same roof. One in five Americans lives in a multigenerational household, about 19% of the population. In the United States, multigenerational families have grown by approximately 60% since 1990 (Cohn and Passel, 2016). Multigenerational families are more common among other cultures but it is growing among nearly all U.S. racial groups and Hispanics, among all age groups, and among both men and women. In recent years, young adults have been the age group most likely to live in multigenerational households (previously, it had been older adults). Among 25- to 29-year-olds, 31% live in multigenerational households (Cohn, 2016). The growth of multigenerational households in the United States accelerated during the economic downturn, and this growing trend is expected to continue. "Multigen" remodeling or new home building to accommodate intergenerational families is an increasing trend. Box 34.4 presents tips when planning to add an older adult to the household.

Family Relationships

Family members, however they are defined, form the nucleus of relationships for the majority of older adults and their support system if they become dependent. A long-standing myth in society is that families are alienated from their older family members and abandon their care to institutions. Nothing could be further from the truth. Family relationships remain

BOX 34.4 Tips for Best Practice
Adding an Older Adult to the Household

Questions to Ask
- What are the needs of the new member and of the family?
- Where will space be allotted for the new member?
- How will the new member be included in existing family patterns?
- How will responsibilities be shared?
- What resources in the community will assist in the adjustment phase?
- Is the environment safe for the new member?
- How will family life change with the added member, and how does the family feel about it?
- What are the differences in socialization and sleeping patterns?
- What are the older adult's needs and expectations?
- What are the older adult's skills and talents?

Modifications That May Need to Be Made
- Arrange semiprivate living quarters if possible.
- Regularly schedule visits to other relatives to give each family time for respite and privacy.
- Arrange adult day health programs and senior activities for the older adult to help keep contact with members of his or her own generation. Consider how the older adult will feel about giving up familiar surroundings and friends.

Potential Areas of Conflict
- Space: especially if someone has given up his or her space to the older relative.
- Possessions: older adults may want to move possessions into the house; others may not find them attractive or may insist on replacing them with new things.
- Entertaining: times when old and young feel the need or desire to exclude the other from social events.
- Responsibilities and chores: the older adult may feel useless if he or she does nothing and may feel in the way if he or she does something.
- Expenses: increased cost of home maintenance, food, clothing, and recreation may not be shared appropriately.
- Vacations: whether to go together or alone; young persons may feel uneasy not taking the older adult out and may feel resentful if they must.
- Childrearing: disagreement over childrearing policies.
- Childcare: finding a balance between the amount of responsibility grandparents will assume for childcare if desired and family needs/desires.

Ways to Decrease Areas of Conflict
- Respect privacy.
- Discuss space allocations.
- Discuss the older adult's furnishings before the move.
- Make it clear in advance when social events include everyone or exclude someone.
- Make clear decisions about household tasks; all should have responsibility geared to ability.
- Have the older adult pay a share of expenses if able.

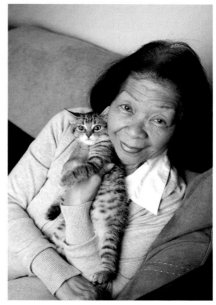

Pets are a part of the family and are particularly beneficial to older adults. They provide companionship, comfort, and caring. (©iStock.com/michellegibson.)

As families change, the roles of the members or expectations of one another may also change. Grandparents may assume parental roles for their grandchildren if their children are unable to care for them; or grandparents and older aunts and uncles may assume temporary caregiving roles while the children, nieces, and nephews work. Adult children of any age may provide limited or extensive caregiving to their own parents or aging relatives who may become ill or impaired. A spouse, sibling, or grandchild may also become a caregiver.

Close-knit families are more aware of the needs of their members and work to resolve problems and find ways to meet the needs of members, even if they are not always successful. Emotionally distant families are less available in times of need and have greater potential for conflict. If the family has never been close and supportive, it will not magically become so when members grow older. Resentments long buried may crop up and produce friction or psychological pain. Long-submerged conflicts and feelings may return if the needs of one family member exceed those of the others.

In coming to know the older adult, the gerontological nurse also comes to know the family, learning of their special gifts and their life challenges. The nurse works with the older adult within the unique culture of his or her family of origin, present family, and support networks, including friends.

Types of Families
Traditional Couples
The marital or partnered relationship in the United States is a critical source of support for older adults, and over half of older noninstitutionalized older adults live with their spouse (including partner). The proportion living with their spouse decreases with age, especially for women. Women older than age 65 are three times as likely as men of the same age to be widowed.

strong in old age, and most older adults have frequent contact with their families. Most older adults possess a large intergenerational web of significant people, including sons, daughters, stepchildren, in-laws, nieces, nephews, grandchildren, and great-grandchildren, and partners and former partners of their offspring. Families provide the majority of care for older adults. Changes in family structure will have a significant impact on the availability of family members to provide care for older adults in the future.

Almost half of women 75 years and older live alone (Administration on Aging, Administration for Community Living, U.S. Department of Health and Human Services, 2017). Men who survive their spouse into old age ordinarily have multiple opportunities to remarry if they wish. Even among the oldest-old, the majority of men are married. A woman is less likely to have an opportunity for remarriage in late life.

Often, older couples live together but do not marry because of economic and inheritance reasons. An increasing number of adults ages 50 years and older are in cohabiting relationships and the rate of cohabitation has risen 75% since 2007. The rising number of cohabiters often coincides with rising divorce rates among this group. Most cohabiters ages 50 and older have previously been married, including a majority who are divorced. The percentage of cohabiters who are widowed rises among older adults 65 years and older (Stepler, 2016).

The needs, tasks, and expectations of couples in late life differ from those in earlier years. Some couples have been married more than 60 or 70 years. These years together may have been filled with love and companionship or abuse and resentment, or anything in between. However, in general, marital status (or the presence of a long-time partner) is positively related to health, life satisfaction, and well-being. For all couples, the normal physical and sociological circumstances in late life present challenges. Some of the issues that strain many of these relationships include (1) the deteriorating health of one or both partners; (2) limitations in income; (3) conflicts with children or other relatives; (4) incompatible sexual needs; and (5) mismatched needs for activity and socialization.

Divorce. In the past, divorce was considered a stigmatizing event. Today, however, it is so common that a person is inclined to forget the ostracizing effects of divorce from years ago. Older couples are becoming less likely to stay in an unsatisfactory marriage, and with the aging of the baby boomers, divorce rates will continue to rise. The divorce rate among people 50 years of age and older has doubled in the past 25 years. Among adults 50 years and older who divorced in the past year, about a third had been in their prior marriage for at least 30 years and 12% had been married for 40 years or more. Research indicates that many late-life (gray) divorcees have grown unsatisfied with their marriages over the years and are seeking opportunities to pursue their own interests and independence for the remaining years of their lives. Health care professionals must avoid making assumptions and be alert to the possibility of marital dissatisfaction among older adults. Nurses should ask, "How would you describe your marriage?"

Long-term relationships are varied and complex, with many factors forming the glue that holds them together. Marital breakdown may be more devastating in older adults because it is often unanticipated and may occur concurrently with other significant losses. Nurses and other health care professionals must be concerned with supporting a client's decision to seek a divorce and with assisting him or her in seeking counseling in the transition. Divorce will initiate a grieving process similar to the death of a spouse, and a severe disruption in coping capacity may occur until the individual adjusts to a new life. The grief may be more difficult to cope with because no socially sanctioned patterns have been established. In addition, tax and fiscal policies favor married couples, and many divorced older women are at a serious economic disadvantage in retirement.

LGBT Couples

As the variations in families grow, so do the types of coupled relationships. Among the types of couples we see today are lesbian, gay, bisexual, and transgender (LGBT) couples. Although the number of LGBT people of any age has remained elusive given the reluctance many have about disclosing their status, an estimated 2.7 million Americans more than 60 years of age are LGBT with projections that this figure is likely to double by 2030 (Chapter 33).

Most LGBT adults older than age 60 are single because the ability to legally marry is a recent occurrence. Many have been part of a live-in couple at some time during their life, but as they age, they are more likely to live alone. Gay and bisexual men older than age 50 are twice as likely as heterosexual men of the same age to live alone, while older lesbian and bisexual women are about one-third more likely to live alone. Approximately one-third of the lesbian women "come out" after age 50. Many lesbians married, raised children, divorced, and led double lives.

In the case of transgender individuals, medical providers for many years required candidates for sex reassignment surgery to divorce their spouses, move to a new place, and construct a false personal history consistent with their new gender expression. These practices resulted in transgender people losing even more of their social and personal support systems than might otherwise have been the case.

It is important to recognize that there are considerable differences in the experiences of younger LGBT individuals when compared with those who are older. Older LGBT individuals did not have the benefit of antidiscrimination laws and support for same-sex partners and are more likely to have kept their relationships hidden than those who grew up in the modern-day gay liberation movement. Those LGBT older adults who came out to family members and faced the negative consequences of becoming estranged from their families of origin often created "families of choice," or chosen families. Chosen families are individuals that are chosen to play a significant role in the life of the individual even though they are not biologically or legally related. Families of choice usually include partners, friends, coworkers, neighbors, and ex-partners—individuals who provide the same supportive functions as would be expected from one's family of origin (Orel and Coon, 2016).

Transgender and bisexual individuals are less likely to "be out." Some LGBT individuals may have developed social networks of friends, members of their family of origin, and the larger community, but many lack support. Because many LGBT couples may have no or fewer children, they will have fewer caregivers as they age. Organizations that serve LGBT older adults in the community need to enhance outreach and support mechanisms to enable them to maintain independence and age safely and in good health. Box 34.5 presents resources for LGBT older adults.

Increasing numbers of same-sex couples are choosing to have families, and this will necessitate greater understanding of

BOX 34.5 Resources for Best Practice

Administration on Aging: National Resource Center on Lesbian, Gay, Bisexual, and Transgender (LGBT) Aging

Agency for Healthcare Research and Quality: Care for the Caregiver Program Implementation Guide

Alzheimer's Association: EssentiALZ—Care training resources, e-learning workshops, DVDs, online care training for dementia care and certification for professionals

American Grandparents Association: grandparents.com

Caregiver Action Network: Resources, education

Association of American Retired Persons (AARP): Caregiver resource

Administration for Community Living: National family caregiver support program

Family Caregiver Alliance

Facebook online support group for grandparents and relatives raising children

Grandparents raising grandchildren: http://www.grandparentingblog.com/

Home Alone Alliance: Short videos in English and Spanish on caregiving techniques (wound care, mobility, managing medications)

Lavender Health: Site maintained by a team of nurses; educational resources and PowerPoint presentations on LGBT health issues and best practices for LGBT communities

Lesbian and Gay Aging Issues Network (LGAIN): A constituent group of the American Society on Aging that works to raise awareness about the concerns of LGBT older adults and the unique barriers they encounter in gaining access to housing, health care, long-term care, and other needed services

National Alliance for Caregiving: International resources and best practices in caregiving

National Resource Center on LGBT Aging: Technical assistance resource center aimed at improving the quality of services and supports offered to LGBT older adults

Preparedness for Caregiving Scale: https://consultgeri.org/try-this/general-assessment/issue-28.pdf

Services and Advocacy for Gay, Lesbian, Bisexual, and Transgender Elders (SAGE)

U.S. Administration on Aging: National Family Caregiver Support Program

these "new" types of families, young and old. The majority of research has involved gay and lesbian couples, and much less is known about bisexual and transgender relationships. Much more knowledge of cohort, cultural, and generational differences among age groups is needed to understand the dramatic changes in the lives of LGBT individuals in family lifestyles.

Older Adults and Their Adult Children

In adulthood, relationships between the generations become increasingly important for most people. Older parents enjoy being told about the various activities and successes of their offspring, and these adult children begin to see aspects of themselves that have developed from their parents. At times, the relationships may become strained because the younger adults are more concerned with their own spouses, partners, and children. The parents are no longer central to their lives, though offspring may be central to the lives of their parents. The most difficult situations occur when the parents are openly critical or judgmental about the lives of their offspring. In the best of situations, adult

children shift to the role of friend, companion, and confidant to the older adult, a concept known as filial maturity.

By and large, older adults and their children have relationships that are reciprocal in nature and characterized by affection and mutual support. These relationships are both the most important and potentially the most conflicted. Family resources are shared from birth and usually in some way until and after death. These resources may be tangible, such as money, belongings, and housing. Intangible resources may include advice, support, guidance, and day-to-day assistance with life. Older adults provide a family history perspective, models for growing old, assistance with grandchildren, a sense of continuity, and a philosophy of aging.

Most older adults see their children on a regular basis, and even children who do not live close to their older parents maintain close connections, so *"intimacy at a distance"* can occur. Nine in ten older adults living with others say they are in contact with their children at least weekly and about four in ten say they communicate with their children on a daily basis (Stepler, 2016).

Never-Married Older Adults

The number of adults who have never married is increasing in the United States. Older adults who have lived alone most of their lives often develop supportive networks with siblings, friends, and neighbors. Never-married older adults may demonstrate resilience to the challenges of aging as a result of their independence and may not feel lonely or isolated. Furthermore, they may have had longer lifetime employment and may enjoy greater financial security as they age. Single older adults will increase in the future because being single is increasingly more common in younger years.

Grandparents

The role of grandparenting, and increasingly great-grandparenthood, is experienced by most older adults. The numbers of grandparents are at record highs and still growing at more than twice the overall population growth rate. Most Americans (83%) 65 years and older have grandchildren. Of these grandparents, two-thirds have at least four grandchildren. Seventy-two percent think being a grandparent is the single most important and satisfying thing in their life (American Grandparents Association, 2017–2018). Great-grandparenthood will become more common in the future in light of projections of healthier aging (Krogstad, 2015).

As the term implies, the "grands" are a step beyond parents in their concerns, exposure, and responsibility. The majority of grandparents derive great emotional satisfaction from their grandchildren. Historically, the emphasis has been on the progressive aging of the grandparent as it affects the relationship with the grandchild, but little has been said about the effects of the growth and maturation of the grandchild on the relationship. Many young adults who have had close contact with their grandparents report that this relationship was very meaningful in their lives. Growing numbers of adult grandchildren are assisting in caregiving for their grandparents.

The age, vitality, and proximity of both grandchild and grandparent produce a kaleidoscope of possible activities and

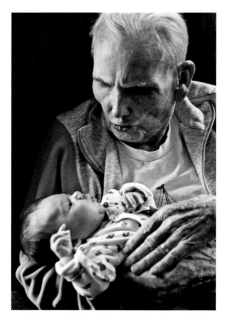

The author's grandson and his maternal great-grandfather. (Photo courtesy Ben Aronoff, Fogline Studios.)

interactions as both progress through their aging processes. Grandparents are in frequent contact with their grandchildren, with 60% in contact on at least a weekly basis (Stepler, 2016). Geographic distance does not significantly affect the quality of the relationship between grandparents and their grandchildren. The Internet is increasingly being used by distant grandparents as a way of staying involved in their grandchildren's lives and forging close bonds (Chapter 5).

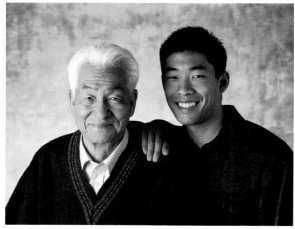

Grandparenting is an important role for older adults. (Copyright ©Getty Images.)

Younger grandparents typically live closer to their grandchildren and are more involved in childcare and recreational activities (Box 34.6). Older grandparents with sufficient incomes may provide more financial assistance and other types of instrumental help. Grandparent-headed households are one of the fastest growing U.S. family groups, and this phenomenon is also taking place in other countries. Approximately 27 million

BOX 34.6   A Grandmother as Seen by an 8-Year-Old Child

"A grandmother is a woman who has no children of her own. That is why she loves other people's children."

"Grandmothers have nothing to do. They are just there: when they take us for a walk they go slowly, like caterpillars along beautiful leaves. They never say, 'Come on, faster, hurry up!'"

"Everyone should try to have a grandmother, especially those who don't have a TV."

grandparents are responsible for raising their grandchildren in the United States (Taylor et al, 2017). This phenomenon is discussed later in the chapter.

Siblings

Late-life sibling relationships are poorly understood and have been neglected by researchers. As individuals age, they often have more contact with siblings than they did in the years when family and work demands were more pressing. About 80% of older adults have at least one sibling, and they are often strong sources of support in the lives of never-married older adults, widowed persons, and those without children. For many older adults, these relationships become increasingly important because they have a long history of memories and are of the same generation and similar backgrounds.

Sibling relationships become particularly important when they are part of the support system, especially among single or widowed older adults living alone. The strongest of sibling bonds is thought to be the relationship between sisters. When blessed with survival, these relationships remain important into late old age. Service providers should inquire about sibling relationships of past and present significance.

The loss of siblings has a profound effect in terms of awareness of one's own mortality, particularly when those of the same gender die. When an older adult reaches the age of the sibling who died, the reaction can be quite disruptive. Not only is grieving activated, but also rehearsal for one's own death may occur. In some cases in which an older sibling survives younger ones, there may be not only a deep grief but also pangs of guilt: "Why them and not me?" (Chapter 35).

Fictive Kin

Fictive kin are nonblood kin who serve as "genuine fake families," as expressed by Virginia Satir. These nonrelatives become surrogate family and take on some of the instrumental and affectional attributes of family. Fictive kin are important in the lives of many older adults, especially those with no close or satisfying family relationships and those living alone or in institutions. Fictive kin includes both friends and, often, paid caregivers. Primary care providers, such as nursing assistants, nurses, or case managers, often become fictive kin. Professionals who work with older adults need to recognize the instrumental and emotional support, and the mutually satisfying relationships, that occur between friends, neighbors, and other fictive kin who assist older adults who are dependent.

CAREGIVING

There are four kinds of people in the world: those who have been caregivers, those who are currently caregivers, those who will be caregivers, and those who will need caregivers.

(Rosalyn Carter, Alzheimer's Reading Room, 2013)

Family caregiving has become a normative experience (similar to marriage, working, or retirement) for many of America's families and cuts across racial, ethnic, and social class distinctions. Gerontological nurses are most likely to encounter older adults with their family and friends in situations relating to caregiving of some kind. Informal caregivers (family members and other unpaid caregivers) provide the majority of care for older adults in the United States. Thirty-two percent of informal caregivers are caring for their parent and 36% are caring for their spouse. At any given point, about 6% of adult children are providing care for a parent but about 17% will provide care at some point in their lives. Many of these caregivers are also employed outside the home and often face great stressors in trying to manage jobs and families while parent caring (Oldenkamp et al, 2016; Wettstein and Zulkarnain, 2017).

Caregivers are evenly split between men and women, although we know very little about the male caregiver experience (Accius, 2017). Family structures have changed, as have family caregiving networks. It is important for nurses to understand the complexity of caregiving and the many forms it may take. Defining caregiving as a dyad of a caregiver and care recipient does not reflect today's patterns of caregiving (Epps et al, 2019). Informal care provided by caregivers is universally recognized as the foundation of the long-term care system. Informal caregivers basically provide free services to care recipients. It would cost an estimated $470 billion to replace the care that family caregivers provide, more than the amount of total Medicaid spending (Feinberg and Levine, 2015–2016). Without family caregivers, the present level of long-term care could not be sustained. Box 34.7 presents some statistics on caregiving.

Caregiving in the LGBT community follows a different pattern. Nine percent of caregivers self-identify as LGBT and LGBT older adults largely care for each other. However, LGBT baby boomers and millennials also take care of their aging parents at a disproportionate rate (National Resource Center on LGBT Aging, 2016). Spouses, partners, and friends provide almost 90% of the care received by LGBT older adults. The pattern reflects the importance of a "chosen family" in the lives of LGBT older adults. "These chosen families provide care to the LGBT older adult, but they often go unrecognized and are not provided with adequate information to care for patients or not acknowledged as caregivers in medical settings. Nurses need to give them the support, assistance, and information they need to provide proper care to their loved one" (Wardecker and Johnston, 2018, pp. 2–3). These patterns may change for future generations of LGBT older adults who have had the benefits of marriage equality, greater social acceptance, and having children.

The concern over encountering anti-LGBT bias increases the demand for informal caregiving because LGBT older adults will go to great lengths to avoid entering senior housing and are often determined to age-in-place at all costs. They are also less likely to access supportive in-home services because of fear of discrimination and bias. In a number of areas across the country, LGBT community members have launched efforts to create senior housing and retirement communities specifically designed with their needs in mind. Many of these projects are still in development stages and are primarily designed for affluent individuals. Hopefully, as the community continues to advocate on behalf of LGBT seniors, a greater variety of housing options will ultimately be available. Local and national LGBT organizations can be another vital resource in locating community agencies that are sensitive and supportive (Family Caregiver Alliance, 2015; Knauer, 2016) (Chapter 32).

Caregiving is considered a major public health issue across the globe, and attention to the physical and mental health of caregivers is receiving increased attention. Due to demographic changes, the demand for family caregivers of adults over the age of 65 years is increasing significantly but we do not have an eldercare system properly equipped to support them (Eldercare Workforce Alliance, 2018). Current trends suggest that the use of paid, formal care by older adults in the community has been decreasing, while their sole reliance on family caregivers has been increasing. The need for family caregivers will increase substantially, but the number of family caregivers who are available to provide care is also decreasing substantially. The

---

BOX 34.7   Facts About Caregiving

- Approximately 34.2 million caregivers have provided care to an adult aged 50 or older in the past 12 months in the United States.
- Family caregivers are children (41.3%), spouses (38.4%), and other family and friends (20.4%).
- The average duration of a caregiver's role is 4.6 years.
- Sixty-six percent of caregivers are female and their average age is 48. Older caregivers are more likely to care for a spouse or partner; their average age is 63 years and one-third of them are in poor health.
- The number of male caregivers is smaller but increasing, and continued research is needed to address their unique needs. Among spousal caregivers 75 years and older, both sexes provide equal amounts of care.
- Between 12% and 18% of the total adult caregivers in the United States are estimated to be between the ages of 18 and 24, a group known as emerging adults, and they have many of the same caregiving responsibilities as older adults.
- About 43.5 million adult family caregivers care for someone who has Alzheimer's disease or other dementia. They provide care an average of 1 to 4 years more than caregivers of individuals with other illnesses.
- Almost half of lesbian, gay, bisexual, and transgender (LGBT) older adults provide caregiving assistance to families or origin or families of choice.
- More than 2.7 million grandparents are providing primary care (custodial grandparents) for grandchildren in the United States and grandparent-headed households are one of the fastest-growing U.S. family groups.
- Caregiving can have serious negative effects on mental and physical health. Approximately 40% to 70% of caregivers have clinically significant symptoms of depression.
- Caregiving can also present financial burdens, and women who are family caregivers are 2.5 times more likely than noncaregivers to live in poverty.

Data from National Alliance for Caregiving Family Caregiver Alliance: *Caregiving in the U.S. 2015.* http://www.caregiving.org/caregiving2015/. Accessed May 2018.

"caregiver support ratio" will start to drop when the first baby boomers begin to turn 80 in just 10 years (by 2026) and by 2050, the ratio will fall to less than three potential caregivers for every person 80 years and older (Feinberg and Levine, 2015–2016). Additionally, there is a growing shortage of formal caregivers (nursing assistants, licensed practical nurses [LPNs] and registered nurses [RNs]) for long-term care services across the continuum (Chapter 2).

Some suggest that the conception of caregiving is different among the baby boomer generation. While they recognize their responsibility to care for ill family members, they view themselves as partners in the organization of care and want to negotiate and set limits to the amount and kind of care they wish to undertake. This will require the existence of alternative resources to family care and policy and practice that no longer takes family caregiving for granted. Baby boomer caregivers and upcoming generations will expect more support and formal assistance from national and local agencies in a coordinated long-term care network (Chapter 32).

Impact of Caregiving

Although caregiving is a means to "give back" to a loved one and can be a source of joy in the giving, it is also stressful. "Caregiving is a very complex issue, and assuming a caregiving role is a time of transition that requires a restructuring of one's goals, behaviors, and responsibilities. It requires taking on something new, but it is also about loss—of what was and what could have been" (Lund, 2005, p. 152). Caregivers are considered to be *the hidden patient* (Schulz and Beach, 1999, p. 2216).

Family caregiving has been associated with increased levels of depression and anxiety, poorer self-reported physical health, compromised immune function, higher rates of insomnia, increased alcohol use, and increased mortality (Tang et al, 2018). Caregiver burden encompasses physical, psychological, emotional, relational, social, and financial problems due to caregiving (Pristavec, 2018). Unrelieved caregiver stress increases the potential for abuse and neglect (Chapter 31). There are certain circumstances that are more likely to cause challenges with caregiving (Box 34.8).

Caregiving can be both rewarding and distressing, generating both feelings of benefit and burden for some caregivers and even with high burden, caregivers may experience high benefits. Caregivers experiencing benefits have better mental health and

BOX 34.8   Circumstances Associated With Caregiver Stress

- Competing role responsibilities (e.g., work, home)
- Advanced age of the caregiver
- High-intensity caregiving need
- Insufficient resources
- Financial difficulty
- Poor self-reported health
- Living in the same household with the care recipient
- Dementia of the care recipient
- Length of time caregiving
- Prior relational conflicts between the caregiver and care recipient

continue in the caregiving role longer than those experiencing burden (Pristavec, 2018). Positive benefits of caregiving may include enhanced self-esteem and well-being, personal growth and satisfaction, and finding or making meaning through caregiving. Caregiving is more likely to be perceived as rewarding if the caregiver feels needed and useful, has a close and reciprocal relationship with the care recipient, believes their help is appreciated by the care recipient, and has an adequate support network (Monin et al, 2017). The positive benefits of caregiving have been given more attention in recent years, but further research is needed to help understand what factors influence how caregivers perceive the experience and how assistance programs can focus on increasing the perception of benefits (Pristavec, 2018). Boxes 34.9 and 34.10 present further information on caregiver needs and tips for reducing stress.

Patricia Archbold and colleagues (1990) studied caregiving as a role and examined how the relationships between the caregiver and care recipient (mutuality) and the preparation of the caregiver for the tasks and stresses of caregiving (preparedness) influence reactions to caregiving. Most caregivers are not prepared for the many responsibilities they face and receive no formal instruction in caregiving activities. Lack of preparedness can greatly increase the caregiver's stress. Caregivers who report a high level of preparedness for the caregiving experience lower levels of caregiver strain after hospitalization of older adults and during cancer care and treatment (Zwicker, 2018). Several validated caregiver assessment instruments are available including the Preparedness for Caregiving Scale (Fig. 34.1) and the Modified Caregiver Strain Index (Fig. 34.2). Further research is needed to understand the complexities of the caregiving and care-receiving role and provide a theory base for nursing interventions.

Caregiving of Individuals With Dementia

Caregivers of individuals with dementia provide more intensive help than nondementia caregivers and experience greater financial, emotional, and physical challenges (Gaugler et al, 2017). Services for individuals with dementia used to be primarily institutional, such as in nursing homes, but now more than two-thirds to three-quarters of individuals with dementia live in the community (Lepore and Wiener, 2017). Factors that increase the stress of caregiving for an individual with dementia include grief over the multiple losses that occur, the physical demands and duration of caregiving (up to 20 years), communication difficulties, and a lack of resource availability. Demands are intensified if the care recipient demonstrates behavioral disturbances and impairments in activities of daily living (ADLs) and instrumental activities of daily living (IADLs) (Gaugler et al, 2017) (Chapter 29).

A recent study of African American and white caregivers of individuals with Alzheimer's disease (Wilks et al, 2018) reported that spirituality was an important factor in overcoming stressful situations for both ethnic groups, but spiritual support's impact was stronger among the African American caregivers. The authors suggest further research is needed to understand the role of spirituality in the caregiving process (Chapter 36).

RESEARCH HIGHLIGHTS

My interest in dementia developed with participation in a project to improve content on the care of older adults in nursing curricula. Later, I witnessed a family member with Alzheimer's disease struggling to maintain a close marital relationship and was moved to investigate approaches to support couples. The effects of Alzheimer's disease and related dementias (AD) on marital relationships can be devastating for both partners. In individuals with dementia, communication abilities decline as the AD progresses. Without communication, marital intimacy is replaced by loneliness, frustration, and estrangement. The purpose of the study was to evaluate the effects of the CARE intervention (Communicating About Relationships and Emotions) on the quality of communication between spouse caregivers and their partners with AD. The sample included 15 couples living at home in South Florida. One partner had moderate stage AD and the other self-identified as the caregiver. The researchers met with couples weekly at their homes for 10 weeks. The CARE intervention followed a manual for couples covering common AD communication challenges and coaching in applying effective communication strategies. Caregiver spouses learned to focus on valuing partners' contributions to conversation. They practiced responding to their partners' communication difficulties with empathy and facilitating participation

in conversation. Spouses with AD practiced social behaviors such as making eye contact and expressing relationship-focused thoughts and feelings. At the end of each session, couples were asked to converse about a topic of their choosing and the conversations were video recorded.

Recordings were later analyzed for changes in communication behavior over time. The analysis showed that caregivers' spouses learned to avoid communication that blocked further conversation. For example, they learned that questions such as "Don't you remember?" seemed like criticism and discouraged conversation whereas questions such as "What do you think?" demonstrated caregivers' willingness to engage. Both spouses improved their communication. Nurses encounter couples like the study participants in many health care situations and can use these opportunities to assess communication quality and promote spouses' engagement with one another.

Williams CL, Newman D, Hammer LM: Preliminary study of a communication intervention for family caregivers and spouses with dementia. *Int J Geriatr Psychiatry* 33(2):e343–349, 2018.

Williams CL: Maintaining caring relationships in spouses affected by Alzheimer's disease, *Int J Human Caring* 19(3):12–18, 2015.

BOX 34.9 Caregiver Needs

- Finding time for myself
- Keeping the person I care for safe
- Balancing work and family responsibilities
- Managing emotional and physical stress
- Finding easy and satisfying activities to do with the care recipient
- Learning how to talk to physicians
- Making end-of-life decisions
- Moving or lifting the care recipient; bathing and dressing
- Managing incontinence or toileting problems
- Managing the challenging behaviors of the care recipient
- Negotiating health care and home- and community-based services
- Managing complex medication schedules or high-tech medical equipment
- Choosing a home health agency, assisted living, or skilled nursing facility
- Finding non-English educational material

BOX 34.10 Tips for Best Practice

Reducing Caregiver Stress

- Educate yourself about the disease or medical condition.
- Contact the appropriate disease-related organization to learn about resources and education and support groups to help you adapt to the challenges you encounter.
- Find a health care professional who understands the disease.
- Consult with other experts to help plan for the future (legal, financial).
- Tap your social resources for assistance.
- Take time for relaxation and exercise.
- Use community resources.
- Maintain your sense of humor.
- Explore religious beliefs and spiritual values.
- Participate in pleasant, nurturing activities such as reading a good book, taking a warm bath.
- Seek supportive counseling when you need it.
- Identify and acknowledge your feelings; you have a right to ALL of them.
- Set realistic goals.
- Attend to your own health care needs.

Adapted from Mayo Clinic: *Caregiver stress: tips for taking care of yourself,* January 19, 2018. https://www.mayoclinic.org/healthy-lifestyle/stress-management/in-depth/caregiver-stress/art-20044784. Accessed May 2018.

Nurse researcher Dr. Christine Williams discusses her innovative research on enhancing communication between spousal caregivers and their loved one with dementia (Research Highlights box). The Alzheimer's Reading Room presents a summary of some of the communication strategies from Dr. William's research that were found helpful in sustaining spouse caregiver relationships (https://www.alzheimersreadingroom.com/2017/10/alzheimers-study-reveals-communication-patterns-that-sustain-spouse-caregiver-relationships.html).

Spousal Caregiving

Eighty percent of older adults who live with spouses with disabilities provide care for them. More wives than husbands provide care, but this is changing as the life expectancy for men increases. Caregiving spouses experience more mental and physical health problems from their caregiving, provide more intensive, time-consuming care than other family caregivers, and are less likely to receive assistance from other family members (Oldenkamp et al, 2016; Polenick and DePasquale, 2018). Older spouses often take on greater burden than they can

reasonably handle and get by with significantly less help in the home than other types of caregivers, yet their responsibilities increase over time (Park, 2017). Spousal caregivers who perceive a great deal of strain are almost two times more likely to die than caregivers reporting some strain (Perkins et al, 2013).

Older spouses caring for partners who are ill also face many role changes. Older women may need to learn to drive, manage money, or make decisions by themselves. Male caregivers may need to learn how to cook, shop, do laundry, and provide personal care to their wives. Spousal caregivers also deal with the added responsibilities of caregiving while at the same time dealing with the anticipated loss of their spouse. Nurses should be alert to situations in which health care personnel may be able to

YOUR PREPARATION FOR CAREGIVING

We know that people may feel well prepared for some aspects of giving care to another person, and not as well prepared for other aspects. We would like to know how well prepared you think you are to do each of the following, even if you are not doing that type of care now.

	Not at all prepared	Not too well prepared	Somewhat well prepared	Pretty well prepared	Very well prepared
1. How well prepared do you think you are to take care of your family member's physical needs?	0	1	2	3	4
2. How well prepared do you think you are to take care of his or her emotional needs?	0	1	2	3	4
3. How well prepared do you think you are to find out about and set up services for him or her?	0	1	2	3	4
4. How well prepared do you think you are for the stress of caregiving?	0	1	2	3	4
5. How well prepared do you think you are to make caregiving activities pleasant for both you and your family member?	0	1	2	3	4
6. How well prepared do you think you are to respond to and handle emergencies that involve him or her?	0	1	2	3	4
7. How well prepared do you think you are to get the help and information you need from the health care system?	0	1	2	3	4
8. Overall, how well prepared do you think you are to care for your family member?	0	1	2	3	4

9. Is there anything specific you would like to be better prepared for? _____

_____

_____

_____

_____

MEAN SCORE of the number of items answered: _____

Fig. 34.1 Caregiver Preparedness Scale. (From Archbold PG, Stewart BJ, Greenlick MR, et al: Mutuality and preparedness as predictors of caregiver role strain, *Res Nurs Health* 13:375–385, 1990. Reprinted with permission from John Wiley & Sons.)

provide supports and resources that make it possible for an individual to assume new responsibilities without being totally overwhelmed. Adult day programs, respite care services, or periodic assistance from a home health aide or homemaker may make it possible for the couple to continue to live together and ease the strain of caregiving. It is important to pay attention to the physical and mental health needs of the caregiver and those of the care recipient.

Aging Parents Caring for Adult Children With Intellectual and Developmental Disabilities

Although we tend to think of caregivers as middle-aged adults caring for older adults, an unknown number of older adults are caring for their middle-aged children with intellectual and developmental disabilities (I/DD). In the past century, children with I/DD were typically in institutions and usually died before reaching adulthood. Today, about 75% of adults with I/DD now live with their parents or other family members and more than 25% live with parents aged 60 years and older (Baumbusch et al, 2017). For the first time in history, individuals with I/DD are outliving their parents, and planning for their future is an area posing challenges for older adults and for service providers internationally.

With increased survival, adults with I/DD are also at risk for developing chronic illness and will need more care and services. For example, individuals with Down syndrome are more likely to develop dementia. Often, the burden of caring for a child with I/DD has been carried by parents for their entire adult

Directions: Here is a list of things that other caregivers have found to be difficult. Please put a checkmark in the columns that apply to you. We have included some examples that are common caregiver experiences to help you think about each item. Your situation may be slightly different, but the item could still apply.

	Yes, On a Regular Basis = 2	Yes, Sometimes = 1	No = 0
My sleep is disturbed (For example: the person I care for is in and out of bed or wanders around at night)	_____	_____	_____
Caregiving is inconvenient (For example: helping takes so much time or it's a long drive over to help)	_____	_____	_____
Caregiving is a physical strain (For example: lifting in or out of a chair; effort or concentration is required)	_____	_____	_____
Caregiving is confining (For example: helping restricts free time or I cannot go visiting)	_____	_____	_____
There have been family adjustments (For example: helping has disrupted my routine; there is no privacy)	_____	_____	_____
There have been changes in personal plans (For example: I had to turn down a job; I could not go on vacation)	_____	_____	_____
There have been other demands on my time (For example: other family members need me)	_____	_____	_____
There have been emotional adjustments (For example: severe arguments about caregiving)	_____	_____	_____
Some behavior is upsetting (For example: incontinence; the person cared for has trouble remembering things; or the person I care for accuses people of taking things)	_____	_____	_____
It is upsetting to find the person I care for has changed so much from his/her former self (For example: he/she is a different person than he/she used to be)	_____	_____	_____
There have been work adjustments (For example: I have to take time off for caregiving duties)	_____	_____	_____
Caregiving is a financial strain	_____	_____	_____
I feel completely overwhelmed (For example: I worry about the person I care for; I have concerns about how I will manage)	_____	_____	_____

[Sum responses for "Yes, on a regular basis" (2 pts each) and "yes, sometimes" (1 pt each)]

Total Score =

Fig. 34.2 Modified Caregiver Strain Index. (From Thornton M, Travis SS: Analysis of the reliability of the Modified Caregiver Strain Index, *J Gerontol B Psychol Sci Soc Sci* 58(2):S129, 2003. Copyright ©The Gerontological Society of America. Reproduced by permission of the publisher.)

life and will end only with the death of the parent or the adult child. Parental caregivers who are aging face changes in their financial resources and health that affect their continued caregiving ability.

A majority of these caregivers worry how their child will receive care if they develop a debilitating illness or die. A recent study reported that aging parents were increasingly aware of their own aging process and the implications for their ability to continue providing care. They were fostering connections with both informal and formal sources of care that could supplement or replace their care activities. It was important to shift their care activities from providing physical support to a focus on social-economic support and communicating their intimate knowledge of their relative with I/DD to others who could provide care in the future. Engaging in conversations and planning for end-of-life care was a major challenge and depended to a certain extent on their relative's understanding of death and dying and their emotional readiness to live without their main care provider (Baumbusch et al, 2017).

In the United States, the Planned Lifetime Assistance Network (PLAN), available in some states through the National Alliance for the Mentally Ill, provides lifetime assistance to individuals with disabilities whose parents or other family members are deceased or can no longer provide for their care. The Alzheimer's Association and other aging organizations offer education and support programs for both parents and their developmentally disabled adult children in some communities. There is a continued need for the development of both in-home and community options for developmentally disabled adults who are aging. Additionally, there is a need for research exploring the experience of aging families caring for adult children with I/DD.

Grandparents Raising Grandchildren

Over the past decade grandparents have assumed the primary caregiving responsibility for their grandchildren at an unprecedented rate. Global figures indicate that grandparents represent the majority of all kinship carers and are the largest providers of formal childcare between birth and 12 years of age (McLaughlin et al, 2017). More than 2.7 million grandparents are providing primary care (custodial grandparents) for grandchildren in the United States and grandparent-headed households are one of the fastest-growing U.S. family groups. About 39% of grandparent caregivers are over the age of 60.

The reasons grandparents take a child into the home without his or her parents vary among countries, groups, and individuals. Many grandparents have become, by default, the primary caregivers of grandchildren because the parents are unable to provide the care needed as a result of child abuse, teen pregnancy, imprisonment, joblessness, military deployment, drug and alcohol addictions, illness, death, and other social problems. Drug addiction, especially to opioids, is behind much of the rise in the number of grandparents raising their grandchildren (Generations United, 2016a).

Research related to the effect of grandparent caregiving on health status is lacking, but existing literature suggests that there are economic, health, and social challenges inherent in this role. As with other types of caregiving, there are both blessings and burdens and caregivers' experiences will be unique. For many grandparents, the challenges may include limited income and financial support through the welfare system, lack of informal support systems, loss of leisure activities in retirement, and shame or guilt related to their children's inability to parent (McLaughlin et al, 2017). Physical and mental stressors appear to be greater when grandparents are raising a chronically ill or

special-needs child or a child with behavioral problems, or experiencing chronic illness themselves.

Often, crisis situations precipitate the decision of a grandparent to assume caring for a grandchild, and time for preparation is not available. In many cases, grandparents assume care so that their grandchildren's care is not taken over by the public care system. However, many custodial grandparents are not licensed in the foster care system and are not eligible for the same services and financial support as licensed foster parents (Wiltz, 2016). About 25% of grandparent-headed households are in poverty, and over half of grandmothers raising grandchildren live in poverty. Housing, food, and child care assistance are minimal for grandfamilies outside the system and only a small percentage get the help they need (Generations United, 2017).

The benefits for the children cared for by grandparents are better than for children in nonrelative care and include increased stability, greater safety, better behavioral and mental health outcomes, more positive feelings about placements, more likely to report they "always felt loved," more likely to live with or stay connected to siblings, and greater preservation of cultural identity and community connections (Generations United, 2016b).

Interventions

Routine screening and monitoring of the psychological distress of primary care grandparents and offering support, advice, and referral to reduce stressors are important. Currently, evidence suggests that cognitive-behavioral interventions have the most empirical support for improving grandparent caregiver's psychological well-being. Promising approaches that require further research to support their effectiveness include support groups, interdisciplinary case management, and psychoeducational interventions (McLaughlin et al, 2017). Another successful service is kinship navigator programs, which provide a single point of entry for connecting to housing, household resources, physical and mental health services, and financial and legal assistance (Generations United, 2017). Some grandparent caregivers may be reluctant to seek assistance and often neglect their own health concerns. Delivering health promotional and financial assistance information within the nonjudgemental environment of grandparent support groups may be effective (Taylor et al, 2017). Resources to support grandparent caregivers should be available in communities and could be offered through health care institutions, schools, and churches. Web-based interventions can also be evaluated. Nurses can be instrumental in developing and conducting these types of interventions.

Recommendations from major reports on grandparent caregiving include the following: (1) reforms of the federal welfare financing system to encourage a continuum of tailored services and supports for grandparents; (2) ensuring access to financial assistance needed to meet children's needs through the Temporary Assistance for Needy Families; (3) addressing barriers to licensing relatives as foster parents so they can receive necessary financial support and services; and (4) establishing a national federal task force and technical assistance center on grandfamilies (Generations United, 2017). As of the time of writing, the Supporting Grandparents Raising Grandchildren Act, coauthored by Senator

Interventions With Grandparent Caregivers

- Early identification of at-risk grandparents
- Comprehensive assessment of physical, psychosocial, and environmental factors affecting those in the caregiving role for grandchildren
- Anticipatory guidance and counseling about child growth and development and other child-raising issues
- Referral to resources for support, counseling, and financial assistance
- Advocacy for policies supportive of grandparents who have assumed a caregiving role

Susan Collins and Senator Bob Casey, which would create a federal task force charged with supporting grandparents raising grandchildren, is moving through Congress (Collins, 2018).

The National Family Caregiver Support Program (NFCSP), under the Older Americans Act program, provides support services, education and training, counseling, and respite care and should be encouraged in all states. Nurses can refer the grandparents to their local area agency on aging to inquire about available resources. Box 34.5 presents resources for grandparents, and suggestions for nursing interventions with older adults providing primary care to their grandchildren are presented in Box 34.11.

Long-Distance Caregiving

Because of the increasing mobility of today's global society, more children move away for education or employment and do not return home. When the parent needs help, it must be provided "long distance." This is perhaps one of the most difficult situations, and it presents unique challenges. The usual impulse is to want to move the older adult into the family's home or to a more accessible location for the family, but this may not be best for the older adult or for the family (Box 34.4). Issues that need to be considered in long-distance caregiving include identifying a local person who will be available quickly in emergency situations; identifying reliable individuals or services that will provide daily monitoring if necessary; identifying acceptable facilities for assisted living or nursing home care if that becomes necessary; determining which family member is most likely to be free to travel to the older adult if needed; and being sure that legalities regarding advance directives, a will, and power of attorney (for health care and financial) have been established.

A profession and industry has emerged to assist the geographically distant family member to ensure that an older relative will receive care. This profession is made up of geriatric care managers, some of whom are nurses or social workers. A care manager can be hired to do everything a family member would do if able, from being available in an emergency, to helping with estate planning, to making arrangements for a move to a nursing home. These services are available primarily to those who are able to pay for them because they are not covered by private insurance, Medicare, or any public agencies. Although these services are expensive, they may be far less expensive than alternative living arrangements or institutional placement.

Similar services may be available for persons with very low incomes through the local Area Agency on Aging "Community Care for the Elderly" programs. When incomes are too high to qualify for Medicaid and too low to pay for private care managers, the individual and their families must do the best they can. Long-distance care then depends on the goodness of neighbors, local friends, and apartment managers and frequent trips by the long-distance caregiver to the older adult.

PROMOTING HEALTHY AGING: IMPLICATIONS FOR GERONTOLOGICAL NURSING

Assessment
Family Assessment
A comprehensive assessment of the older adult includes assessment of the family. Often, nurses see families in times of crisis when an older family member needs care. When working with families, it is important for the nurse to be aware of his or her vision of what a "family" should be and what a "family" should do. Our values should not enter into assessment and intervention with clients and families should not be judged or labeled as dysfunctional (Feinberg and Levine, 2015–2016). It is necessary to identify the strengths within each family and to build on those strengths while recognizing the family's limitations in providing support and caregiving. Thus, the nurse's role is to teach, monitor, and strengthen the family system so as to maintain health and wellness of the entire family structure.

Family Caregiver Assessment
Family caregiver assessment is a systematic process of gathering information about a caregiving situation to identify the specific problems, needs, strengths, and resources of the family caregiver, and the caregiver's ability to contribute to the needs of the care recipient (Feinberg and Levine, 2015–2016). Assessment also includes how the health care team can help the person providing care. Assessment data are used to develop a personalized plan of care for the family. Although vitally important, family caregiver assessment is weak in long-term care support and service programs and rare in health care settings (Feinberg and Levine, 2015–2016).

Family caregivers are often performing tasks that nurses typically perform including injections, tube feedings, operating special equipment, managing multiple medications, catheter and colostomy care, and other complex care responsibilities— "the same tasks that make nursing students tremble the first time they have to perform them" (Kennedy, 2017). And, almost half of these family caregivers are doing these medical/nursing tasks without any preparation and few visits from home care providers (Reinhard et al, 2017). Only about a third of family caregivers reported that a doctor, nurse, or social worker asked them what was needed to care for their loved one, and even less said a health or social provider had asked what they needed to care for themselves (Feinberg and Levine, 2015–2016).

In response to these concerns, new laws in support of family caregivers have been enacted at both the state and federal levels. The Caregiver Advise, Record, and Enable or CARE Act is in effect in nearly three-quarters of the United States Provisions of the laws vary from state to state but the CARE Act generally institutes three basic reforms that require hospitals to (1) let patients identify a family caregiver when they're admitted; (2) notify the family caregiver in advance when the patient will be discharged; and

BOX 34.12 Goals of a National Family Caregiving Strategy

- Identify actions that the government, communities, health providers, employers, and others can take to support family caregivers
- Promote greater adoption of person-centered care and family-centered care in health settings and long-term care settings
- Training for family caregivers
- Respite options for family caregivers
- Ways to increase financial security for family caregivers
- Workplace policies to help family caregivers keep working
- Collect and share information about innovative family caregiving models
- Assess federal programs around family caregiving
- Address disparities and meet the needs of the diverse caregiving population

From Eisenberg R: What the new RAISE Family Caregivers Act will do, *Forbes Personal Finance* Jan. 10, 2018. https://www.forbes.com/sites/nextavenue/2018/01/10/what-the-new-raise-family-caregivers-act-will-do/#9711f9870b9d. Accessed April 2018.

BOX 34.13 Tips for Best Practice

Nursing Actions to Create and Sustain a Partnership With Caregivers

- Surveillance and ongoing monitoring
- Coaching: helping caregivers apply knowledge and develop skills
- Teaching: providing information and instruction
- Providing accurate and complete information about services; determine with the family referrals for services based on needs and preferences of caregiver and care recipient; mutually determine with the family services that are affordable, acceptable, and logistically feasible
- Fostering partnerships: fostering communication and collaboration between the caregiver and the care recipient and between them and the nurse
- Providing psychosocial support: attending to psychosocial well-being; help the caregiver and family identify effective coping strategies
- Coordinating: orchestrating the work of other health care team members and the activities of the caregiver

(3) provide a simple instruction of the medical tasks they will be performing when their loved one returns home (Kennedy, 2017). In 2018, the Recognize, Assist, Include, Support, and Engage (RAISE) Family Caregivers Act was signed into law (Govtrack, 2018). The law directs the U.S. Secretary of Health and Human Services (HHS) to develop, maintain, and update an integrated national strategy to support family caregivers (Box 34.12).

Interventions

In designing interventions to support caregiving, a partnership model, combining the nurse's professional expertise with the caregiver's knowledge of the family member, is recommended. Given the range of caregiving situations and the uniqueness of each, interventions must be tailored to individual needs and build on the caregiver's existing strengths and resources. Interventions include risk assessment, education about caregiving and stress, needed care skills, caregiver health and home safety, support groups, linkages to ongoing support, counseling, resource identification, relief/respite from daily care demands, and stress management.

Education provided by nurses to help prepare the caregiver for the caregiving role, particularly at the time of discharge from the hospital or nursing home, can help to prevent role strain and lessen burden. Questions to be addressed with the caregiver include the following (Reinhard et al, 2017):

- What questions do you have regarding care today?
- What questions do you have about care at home?
- How are you doing and what are your needs?

With many caregivers trying to balance caregiving responsibilities while working, educational programs offered in the workplace can be beneficial for both the caregiver and the employer. When the nurse works with a family from a different culture that may have rituals and routines unfamiliar to him or her, the nurse needs to be particularly careful to respect these differences. Service providers need to enhance cultural competence and design programs that are culturally acceptable (Chapter 4).

Linking caregivers to community resources, such as respite care, adult day programs, and financial support resources, is important. Respite care allows the caregiver to take a break

from caregiving for various periods of time. Respite care may be provided in institutions, in the home, or in other community settings. Nurses should be aware of respite care resources in their communities, and the local Area Agency on Aging can provide information on respite care and other caregiver services. These interventions, when available, can alleviate much of the stress of caregiving but are utilized infrequently or very late in the course of caregiving in the United States. Many countries in Europe offer generous respite care services as part of the long-term care system. The *Healthy People 2020* box presents objectives for long-term services and supports. Box 34.13 presents nursing interventions for caregivers.

♥ HEALTHY PEOPLE 2020

Long-Term Services and Supports

- Reduce the proportion of unpaid caregivers of older adults who report an unmet need for caregiver support services.
- Reduce the proportion of noninstitutionalized older adults with disabilities who have an unmet need for long-term services and supports.

Data from U.S. Department of Health and Human Services, Office of Disease Prevention and Health Promotion: *Healthy People 2020*, 2012. http://www.healthypeople.gov/2020.

Tailored multicomponent interventions designed to match a specific target population seem to have the most positive outcomes on caregiver burden and stress—for example, groups designed to assist caregivers caring for individuals with early-stage dementia or those with Parkinson's disease. Programs that work collaboratively with care recipients and their families and are more intensive and modified to the caregiver's needs are also more successful. There are wide variations in caregiving experiences and the needs of an adult child caring for a parent with dementia may be quite different from those of a gay man or woman caring for a friend with cancer. Online training and support programs and telehealth tools seem to have great potential and need further research (Chi and Demiris, 2017; Egan et al, 2018).

Interventions with caregivers must always consider the great variability in family structures, resources, traditions, and history. The range of adaptations is enormous, and the goal is always to restore the balance of the system to the greatest extent possible and support caregivers in their caring. Research suggests that differences exist in caregiving quality of life among individuals of different ages, male and female caregivers, and different racial and minority groups. Greater caregiving responsibilities are reported among females, racial and ethnic minorities, and low-income caregivers (Cook and Cohen, 2018). Further research is needed to provide the foundation of nursing interventions with diverse caregivers (Bonds and Lyons, 2018). Resources for caregiving are presented in Box 34.5.

KEY CONCEPTS

- Roles define individual and societal expectations of function.
- The ability to successfully negotiate transitions and develop new and gratifying roles depends on personal and environmental supports, timing, clarity of expectations, personality, and degree of change required.
- Numerous patterns of retirement exist, and therefore retirement per se cannot be viewed categorically.
- Preretirement planning and postretirement follow-up significantly affect positive adaptation to the transition.
- Older adults and their family members carry a long history. Current family dynamics must be understood within the context of family history.
- Loss of a spouse/life partner is the role change that has the greatest potential for life disruption, and nursing support can make a significant positive difference in the transition.

- Widowers are a neglected group in the literature and in the service arena. These men are particularly vulnerable to physical and mental stress.
- Family members and other unpaid caregivers provide 80% of care for older adults in the United States.
- Grandparents are increasingly assuming primary caregiving roles with grandchildren.
- Caregiving activities are one of the most major social issues of our time and a significant global public health problem.
- Nursing interventions with caregivers include risk assessment, education about caregiving and stress, needed care skills, caregiver health and home safety, support groups, linkages to ongoing support, counseling, resource identification, relief/respite from daily care demands, and stress management.

NURSING STUDY: RETIREMENT

Sandy was a professor at a small, private college in a metropolitan area. Although she had taught nursing for 25 years and loved her work, it had been a demanding year, and she was very tired. A rumor had recently circulated that the college was in trouble financially. Some of the most affluent alumni could no longer be counted on for gifts and endowments because the football coach had not produced a winning team for several years. Because the tuition was becoming exorbitant, the college had recently lost some students to one of the three state college campuses within driving distance of the city. The trustees of the college, in a move to cut expenses, offered an incentive to professors who were willing to retire early; an extra year of service credit was presented for every 6 years worked. Sandy was only 55 years old but thought that the 4 years of extra credit would bring her near the minimum retirement age for Social Security (an error, of course, because her age did not change with her service credit). Rather impulsively, Sandy decided to accept the offer after telling colleagues, "Well, you know how I love to travel. Why wait until I'm too old to enjoy retirement? Why don't you think about the offer, too? This is a once-in-a-lifetime opportunity." Near the end of the academic year, the celebrations began: recognition, plaques, expressions of gratitude from students, and envy from her associates. The send-off was wonderful. In the summer, Sandy withdrew her savings and booked a cruise to the Greek islands. The journey was lovely, and she enjoyed every moment. Sandy began to feel depressed when she got off the ship but knew it was only because the elegant cruise was over. However, as fall came around, Sandy began to feel more depressed. Most of her friends were teachers, and they were all back at work. Sandy briefly thought of going to Pittsburgh to visit her sister but decided against the idea because she and her sister had really never been very compatible. Then Sandy was hit with some of the realities of early retirement: she was unable to withdraw any of her considerable tax-deferred savings before she was 59 ½ years of age without significant penalty, her health insurance coverage was considerably less comprehensive after retirement, her colleagues were all busy, and she was very bored. Then the real blow fell. The college, in desperation, had dipped into the retirement funds to remain solvent, and the retirees' pensions were now at risk. Sandy's sister, who was a nurse, called to announce that she wanted to come and stay a few days while she attended a conference in the city. When she arrived, Sandy overwhelmed her with the litany of woes. If you were Sandy's sister, what would you do?

Based on the nursing study, develop a nursing care plan using the following procedure[a]:

- List Sandy's comments that provide subjective data.
- List information that provides objective data.
- From these data, identify and state, using an accepted format, two nursing diagnoses you determine are most significant to Sandy at this time. List two of Sandy's strengths that you have identified from the data.
- Determine and state outcome criteria for each diagnosis. These criteria must reflect some alleviation of the problem identified in the nursing diagnosis and must be stated in concrete and measurable terms.
- Plan and state one or more interventions for each diagnosed problem. Provide specific documentation of the source used to determine the appropriate intervention. Plan at least one intervention that incorporates Sandy's existing strengths.
- Evaluate the success of the intervention. Interventions must correlate directly with the stated outcome criteria to measure the outcome success.

[a]Students are advised to refer to their nursing diagnosis text and identify possible or potential problems.

CRITICAL THINKING QUESTIONS AND ACTIVITIES

1. Identify several important family and social roles that older members of your family fulfill.
2. What are the factors to consider in role transitions, and how can transitions be made smoother?
3. What factors must be considered in the decision to retire?
4. Discuss the differences you would expect in adaptation to retirement between an individual who retired because of ill health and one who retired because he or she desired to do so.
5. How do you think retirement differs for men and women?
6. Describe what you think would be an ideal retirement.
7. Discuss how you think an individual can prepare for widowhood.
8. Discuss the meanings and the thoughts triggered by the young person's and older adult's viewpoints expressed at the beginning of the chapter. How do these vary from your own experience?
9. In your own family, who will provide care to an aging family member if needed? Does the family/older adult worry about being able to pay for long-term care? What provisions have been made for this possibility?

RESEARCH QUESTIONS

1. What are the challenges associated with older adults working longer?
2. What are the patterns of adaptation of widowers? How do the patterns differ for young-old and old-old?
3. Who divorces in later life and for what reasons?
4. What are the differences between grandparenting and great-grandparenting?
5. Are there differences in the experience of primary grandparent caregivers based on ethnicity, race, and culture?
6. How do adults who were raised by grandparents view this experience?
7. Do interventions to improve the physical health of caregivers relate to less reported stress and improved health outcomes?
8. What are the reactions of older adults to the care given by their offspring?
9. How do upcoming generations view caregiving responsibilities?

REFERENCES

Accius J: *Breaking stereotypes: spotlight on male family caregivers,* 2017. AARP Public Policy Institute. https://www.aarp.org/ppi/info-2017/breaking-stereotypes-spotlight-on-male-family-caregivers.html. Accessed March 2019.

Administration on Aging, Administration on Community Living, US Department of Health and Human Services: *Profile of older Americans,* 2017. https://acl.gov/aging-and-disability-in-america/data-and-research/profile-older-americans. Accessed March 2019.

Alzheimer's Reading Room: *Caregiver quote of the day,* 2013. http://www.alzheimersreadingroom.com/2009/11/quote-of-day-caregivers.html. Accessed May 2018.

Applebaum R, Cummins P: From rock 'n' roll to rock "n" chair: are baby boomers financially ready for retirement? *Generations* 41(2):88–94, 2017.

Archbold PG, Stewart BJ, Greenlick MR, Harvath T: Mutuality and preparedness as predictors of caregiver role strain, *Res Nurs Health* 13:375–384, 1990.

Baumbusch J, Mayer S, Phinney A, Baumbusch S: Aging together: caring relations in families of adults with intellectual disabilities, *Gerontologist* 57(2):341–347, 2017.

Bonds K, Lyons KS: Formal service use by African American individuals with dementia and their caregivers: an integrative review, *J Gerontol Nurs* 44(6):33–39, 2018.

Chi NC, Demiris D: The roles of telehealth tools in supporting family caregivers: current evidence, opportunities, and limitations, *J Gerontol Nurs* 43(2):3–4, 2017.

Cohn D, Passel JF: *A record 64.6 million Americans live in multigenerational households,* 2016. Washington, DC: Pew Research Center. http://www.pewresearch.org/fact-tank/2018/04/05/a-record-64-million-americans-live-in-multigenerational-households/. Accessed March 2019.

Collins S: *Casey bill to support grandparents caring for their grandchildren, as the opiod crisis increases their numbers,* 2018. https://www.collins.senate.gov/newsroom/bill-help-grandparents-raising-grandchildren-due-opioid-crisis-passes-senate. Accessed April 2018.

Cook S, Cohen S: Sociodemographic disparities in adult child informal caregiving intensity in the United States, *J Gerontol Nurs* 44(9):15-20, 2018.

Egan KJ, Pinto-Bruno ÁC, Bighelli I, et al: Online training and support programs designed to improve mental health and reduce burden among caregivers of people with dementia: a systematic review, *J Am Med Dir Assoc* 19:200–206.e1, 2018.

Eldercare Workforce Alliance: *Advancing a well-trained workforce to care for us as we age,* 2018. http://eldercareworkforce.org/. Accessed May 2018.

Employee Benefit Research Institute: *Retirement Confidence Survey – 2017 results,* 2017. https://www.ebri.org/retirement/retirement-confidence-survey. Accessed March 2019.

Employee Benefit Research Institute: *28th Annual Retirement Confidence Survey,* 2018. https://www.ebri.org/retirement/retirement-confidence-survey. Retrieved March 2019.

Epps F, Rose K, Lopez R: Who's your family? African American caregivers of older adults with dementia, *Res Gerontol Nurs* 12(1):20–26, 2018.

Family Caregiver Alliance, National Center on Caregiving: *LGBT caregiving: frequently asked questions,* 2015. https://www.caregiver.org/print/32. Accessed April 2018.

Feinberg LF, Levine C: Family caregiving: looking to the future, *Generations* 39(4):1119, 2015–2016.

Gaugler J, Jutkowitz E, Peterson CM: An overview of dementia caregiving in the United States, *Generations Fall* (ACL Suppl): 37–42, 2017.

Generations United: *State of grandfamilies: In loving arms: the protective role of grandparents and other relatives in raising children exposed to trauma,* 2017. http://gu.org/OURWORK/Grandfamilies/TheStateofGrandfamiliesinAmerica/TheStateofGrandfamiliesinAmerica2017.aspx. Accessed April 2018.

Generations United: *Raising the children of the opiod epidemic: solutions and supports for grandfamilies,* 2016a. https://www.gu.org/resources/the-state-of-grandfamilies-in-america-2016/. Accessed March 2019.

Generations United: *Children thrive in grandfamilies,* 2016b. http://grandfamilies.org/Portals/0/16-Children-Thrive-in-Grandfamilies.pdf. Accessed May 2018.

GovTrack: *HR 3759 (115th) RAISE Family Caregivers Act,* 2018. https://www.govtrack.us/congress/bills/115/hr3759. Accessed April 2018.

Kennedy MS: Family caregivers need our help–and now it's the law, *Am J Nurs* 117(12):7, 2017.

Knauer NJ: LGBT older adults, chosen family and caregiving, *J Law Relig* 31(2):150–168, 2016.

Krogstad JM: *5 facts about American grandparents,* 2015. Washington, DC: Pew Research Center. http://www.pewresearch.org/fact-tank/2015/09/13/5-facts-about-american-grandparents/. Accessed March 2019.

LePore M, Wiener J: Improving services for people with Alzheimer's disease and related dementias and their caregivers, *Generations Fall* (Suppl):3–6, 2017.

Lindemann E: Symptomatology and management of acute grief, *Am J Psychiatr* 151:155–160, 1944.

Lowenthal MF, Haven C: Interaction and adaptation: intimacy as a critical variable, *Am Sociol Rev* 33:20–30, 1968.

McLaughlin B, Ryder D, Taylor MF: Effectiveness of interventions for grandparent caregivers: a systematic review, *Marriage Fam Rev* 53(6):509–531, 2017.

Monin JK, Brown SL, Poulin MJ, Langa KM: Spouses' daily feelings of appreciation and self-reported well-being, *Health Psychol* 36(12):1135–1139, 2017.

Morley J: Vicissitudes: retirement with a long post-retirement future, *Gener J Am Soc Aging* 41(2):101–107, 2017.

National Resource Center on LGBT Aging: *Fact sheet: LGBT caregiving.* New York, 2016, Sage (Services & Advocacy for Gay, Lesbian, Bisexual, and Transgender Elders).

Oldenkamp M, Hagedoorn M, Slaets J, Stolk R, Wittek R, Smidt N: Subjective burden among spousal and adult-child informal caregivers of older adults: results from a longitudinal cohort study, *BMC Geriatr* 16:208, 2016.

Orel NA, Coon D: The challenges of change: how can we meet the care needs of the ever-evolving LGBT family? *Gener J Am Soc Aging* 40(2):41–45, 2016.

Park M: In sickness and in health: spousal caregivers and the correlates of caregiver outcomes, *Am J Geriatr Psychiatry* 25(10):1094–1096, 2017.

Perkins M, Howard VJ, Wadley VG, et al: Caregiving strain and all-cause mortality: evidence from the REGARDS study, *J Gerontol B Psychol Sci Soc Sci* 68(4):504–512, 2013.

Plawecki HM, Plawecki LH: Challenges of retirement, *J Gerontol Nurs* 42(11):3–5, 2016.

Polenick CA, DePasquale N: Predictors of secondary role strains among spousal caregivers of older adults with functional disability, *Gerontologist* 59(3):486–495, 2019.

Pristavec T: The burden and benefits of caregiving: a latent class analysis, *Gerontologist,* 2018. doi:10.1093/geront/gny022.

Reinhard SC, Capezuti E, Bricoli B, Choula RB: Feasibility of a family-centered hospital intervention, *J Gerontol Nurs* 43(6):9–16, 2017.

Schulz R, Beach SR: Caregiving as a risk factor for mortality: the caregiver health effects study, *J Am Med Assoc* 282(23):2215–2219, 1999.

Shelton A: *Social Security: a key retirement resource for woman,* 2016. AARP Public Policy Institute. https://www.aarp.org/work/social-security/info-2014/social-security-a-key-retirement-income-source-for-older-minorities-ppi.html. Accessed March 2019.

Stepler R: *Smaller share of women ages 65 and older are living alone,* Washington DC, 2016. Pew Research Center. http://www.pewsocialtrends.org/2016/02/18/smaller-share-of-women-ages-65-and-older-are-living-alone/. Accessed March 2019.

Tang SH, Chio O, Chang LH, et al: Caregiver active participation in psychoeducational intervention improved caregiving skills and competency, *Geriatr Gerontol Int* 18(5):750–757, 2018.

Taylor MF, Marquis R, Coall DA, Batten R, Werner J: The physical health dilemmas facing custodial grandparent caregivers: policy considerations, *Cogent Med* 4(1), 2017.

Touhy TA: Nurturing hope and spirituality in the nursing home, *Holist Nurs Pract* 15:45–56, 2001.

United Nations Economic and Social Commission for Asia and the Pacific: *China has a law that mandates children to care for their elderly parents,* 2018. http://www.unescap.org/ageing-asia/did-you-know/364/china-has-law-mandates-children-care-their-elderly-parents. Accessed April 2018.

Vespa J, Schondelmyer E: *A gray revolution in living arrangements,* 2015. United States Census Bureau Census Blogs. https://www.census.gov/newsroom/blogs/random-samplings/2015/07/a-gray-revolution-in-living-arrangements.html. Accessed May 2018.

Wardecker B, Johnston T: Seeing and supporting LGBT older adults' caregivers and families, *J Gerontol Nurs* 44(11):2–4, 2018.

Wettstein G, Zulkarnain A: *How much long-term care do adult children provide?* Chestnut Hill, MA, 2017, Center for Retirement Research at Boston College.

Wilks SE, Spurlock WR, Brown SC, Teegen BC, Geiger JR: Examining spiritual support among African American and Caucasian Alzheimer's caregivers: a risk and resilience study, *Geriatr Nurs* 39(6):663–668, 2018.

Zwicker D: Preparedness for caregiving scale, *Try This* (28), 2018. https://consultgeri.org/try-this/general-assessment/issue-28.pdf. Accessed May 2018.

35

Loss, Death, and Palliative Care

Kathleen Jett

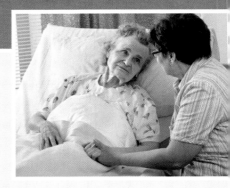

http://evolve.elsevier.com/Touhy/TwdHlthAging

A STUDENT SPEAKS

*When I started nursing school I was so afraid that I would have to take care
of someone who was dying—or maybe even died! Then I found out that to share the
time before death with a person is a special privilege.*

Ana, age 20

AN OLDER ADULT SPEAKS

*When we were in our 60s, my friends and I met over cards, went on trips, and experienced
all of the joys of retirement. We didn't have much time to worry about aches and
pains. In our 70s we had less time to play because we were busy visiting one
another in the hospital or in nursing homes. In our 80s we met frequently
again, but it was usually at our friends' funerals, leaving little time for cards or
travel. Now that I am in my 90s, hardly any of my friends are still alive; you know it gets
kind of lonely, so you just have to make new younger friends!*

Theresa, age 93

LEARNING OBJECTIVES

On completion of this chapter, the reader will be able to:

1. Compare and contrast the needs of older adults in response to varying types of losses.
2. Differentiate the types of grief and the needs of the griever.
3. Discuss the attributes that are needed by the nurse to provide the highest quality of care to those experiencing loss or death.
4. Discuss the benefits and limitations of the available conceptual frameworks for dying and grieving.
5. Identify aspects of palliative care in which there is a special need to work within the cultural boundaries.
6. Develop interventions that will enhance coping and the reestablishment of equilibrium within the family.
7. Differentiate living wills from do-not-resuscitate (DNR) orders and explain the roles and responsibilities of the nurse as they relate to each of them.

LOSS, GRIEF, AND BEREAVEMENT

Loss, dying, and death are universal, incontestable events of the human experience. With age, the number of losses increases. Some of these are associated with normal changes, such as the loss of joint flexibility (Chapter 26). Other losses are related to changes in everyday life and transitions, such as moving and retirement (Chapter 34). Still others include the loss of loved ones through death or the anticipation of one's own approaching death. Some deaths are considered normative and expected, such as that of older parents, while the death of adult children or grandchildren is always nonnormative and unexpected.

Loss of any kind has the potential to trigger grief and mourning. The terms *grief* and *mourning* and a third term, *bereavement*, are often used interchangeably. It has been suggested that bereavement can be used to refer to the fact that a loss has occurred. Grief is the response to a loss, and mourning is the outward expression of grief. Mourning is a socially and culturally prescribed behavior following, and around the time of a loss, especially from death. In many traditions, wearing black is part of mourning behavior. Although there are well-defined rituals in response to loss through death, no guidelines exist for many other losses, such as independent functional ability, the long-time companionship of a pet, or self-concept following a mastectomy.

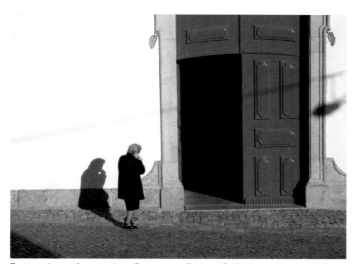

Expressions of mourning. Funeral on Friday. (©JB55, https://www.flickr.com/photos/jb55/.)

In later life one loss and its accompanying grief is often superimposed on others. No sooner has the individual begun to grieve for one when another occurs. When the losses accumulate in quick succession, the griever may become incapacitated and require careful and skilled support and guidance. This phenomenon can lead to a continual state of grieving, known as *bereavement overload.*

This chapter addresses grief as a response to loss, palliative care, and some of the ethical and legal issues surrounding end-of-life decision-making. The purpose of this chapter is to provide gerontological nurses the basic information needed to promote effective grieving and good and appropriate deaths. Loss is considered broadly to include anything that has meaning to the person.

GRIEF WORK

Researchers have tried for years to understand the grieving process *(grief work)*, resulting in a number of models and theories to explain and predict the human response. Pioneer thanatologist (one who studies the dying process) Elisabeth Kübler-Ross is best known for describing what became known as the stages of dying (1969). Grievers are expected to first begin to deny what is happening, then move to anger, bargaining, depression,

and finally acceptance. Each of the early theorists described successful grieving as movement steadily through predictable stages, phases, or tasks until one eventually was able to "let go" of that which was lost (Hall, 2011). These early models have strongly influenced how nurses, physicians, other health care professionals, and society in general have thought about grieving and dying.

Newer approaches have described grief work as more of a flexible process in which a continued attachment to that which has been lost, at some level, is "normal" (Hall, 2011). Although the theories are intended to describe physical death and related grief, we propose that these same models can serve as a framework for understanding other types of meaningful losses in the lives of older adults.

The Loss Response Model

The Loss Response Model (LRM) is influenced by the systems' work of nurse theorist Dr. Betty Newman (Alward, 2010) and the writing of nurse Barbara Giacquinta (1977), psychiatrist Avery Weisman (1979), and thanatological scholars Doka (2002) and Neimeyer and Sands (2011). It can be used to improve the understanding of grieving and to assist nurses in caring and comforting those who have experienced, or are experiencing, a loss. A framework is provided from which nursing interventions can be easily developed.

In the LRM, those who grieve are viewed as part of a system that is striving to maintain equilibrium or stability (Fig. 35.1) (Jett and Jett, 2014). However, the *impact* of the loss (or the anticipation of it) results in *disequilibrium* or instability within the system. The system is in chaos, the grievers are emotionally and functionally compromised *(functional disruption)*, and it is difficult for them to accomplish their usual activities of daily living (Chapter 7). Common, simple activities, such as dressing, that normally take a few minutes may take much longer. Deciding which clothing to wear may seem too complex a task. Even as the tasks are accomplished, the person may complain of feeling distracted, restless, "at loose ends," and numb (Richardson et al, 2015). Men who complained of numbness have been found to have higher cortisol levels (i.e., indicators of physiologically prolonged stress) than comparative women (Richardson et al, 2015).

Nurses can make a significant contribution to the family in fostering even momentary stability by knowing what questions to ask at the time of death, such as: What cultural or familial

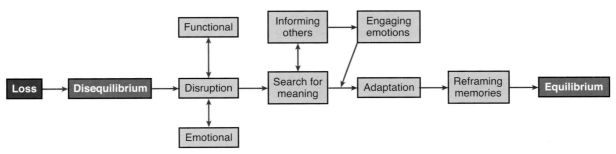

Fig. 35.1 The Loss Response Model.

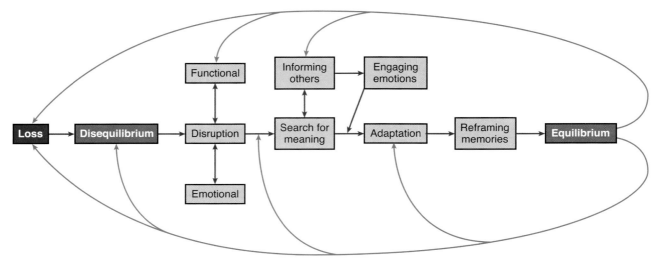

Fig. 35.2 The Loss Response Model and Cyclical Loss.

rituals are important right now? Is there anyone who should be called at this time? Would a spiritual advisor be a support for you right now? Have funeral arrangements already been made? If not, who can help you with this? Parallel questions can be used in the situations of other types of loss such as, what furniture will you be moving from your apartment to the assisted-living facility?

As the system attempts to stabilize and grievers attempt to make sense of the chaos and integrate the loss into their lives, they *search for meaning,* asking such questions as the following: Why did this happen to us (me)? How will we survive the loss? In reacting to the loss of a child or a grandchild, thoughts of "Why wasn't it me?" are common. Searching for meaning is difficult, and as it is done, *others are informed of the loss.* Each time the story is repeated, *emotions are engaged* in ways that are consistent with the griever's culture and personality. While acute grief may be triggered at each telling, the intensity of the sorrow becomes less and the duration shorter. Movement toward a new equilibrium progresses as the person incorporates the loss.

As roles and situations change, *adaptation* is necessary. In the language of the LRM, adaptation is a process in which the system changes to survive. For example, when a person is no longer able to do a task due to loss of ability, someone else must step in to perform it; when the patriarch dies, it may be a cultural expectation that the eldest son assumes his father's roles and responsibilities.

Finally, if the system is to survive, it must redefine itself. This is accomplished not by forgetting or ignoring the loss but by *reframing memories.* In the case of a death, family portraits and reunions will still be possible, just different from how they were before, and new memories can and will be made perhaps starting with a word or so to honor the person who is no longer there. Similarly, if celebrations had always been at the home of the matriarch (eliciting the sights, smells, and memories of childhood), her move to a nursing home will prevent this custom. Adaptation leads to the development of new memories when the celebrations are held at the home of another, such as that of a child. The system can return to a new but different

steady state. The nurse serves as a role model who displays the behavioral qualities of responsiveness, authenticity, commitment, and competence, that is, caring.

However, grieving is not linear, especially in later life (Fig. 35.2). At any point in the movement toward stabilization, new disturbances may lead to renewed instability. The grievers are finding ways to adapt to the functional disruption related to one loss when another occurs. A home has been rearranged to make it safe for the person who has suffered a stroke when she falls and breaks her hip, necessitating a nursing home stay, either short-term or permanent, due to the combined losses. A cyclic LRM is most appropriate, especially for those with multiple underlying chronic conditions.

Types of Grief

Grieving takes enormous amounts of physical and emotional energy. It is the hardest thing anyone can do and may be especially hard for those who are accumulating losses, as one does with aging, or are facing multiple losses at the same time, such as following a catastrophic event. The most common types of grief are anticipatory, acute, shadow (a type of chronic grief), and complicated. Another type, disenfranchised or unspeakable grief, may be occurring and hidden for one reason or another, but nonetheless can be quite significant.

Anticipatory Grief

Anticipatory grief is the response to a real or perceived loss before it occurs—a dress rehearsal, so to speak. One grieves in preparation for a potential loss, such as the loss of belongings (e.g., selling a home), moving (e.g., into a nursing home), knowing that a body part or function is going to change (e.g., amputation), or in anticipation of the death of a loved one. Behaviors that may signal anticipatory grief include preoccupation with the pending loss, unusually detailed planning, or a sudden change in attitude toward the thing or person to be lost. Some feel more in control of the situation because anticipatory grief facilitates planning and preparation for death by saying goodbyes or preparing for burials if that is accepted in the person's culture. In other cases anticipatory grief leads to declines in spousal health even before the death (Toyama and Honda, 2016).

If the loss is certain but the timing is either uncertain or not occurring as expected, anticipatory grieving may be particularly difficult, not because the loss is desired, but in response to the emotional ups and downs of the waiting, with the system staying in a state of disequilibrium. Glaser and Strauss (1968) describe this as an *interruption in sentimental order;* no one knows quite how to behave. Family and friends, and nurses as professional grievers, usually deal much more easily with known losses at a known time or in a set manner (Glaser and Strauss, 1968).

Anticipatory grief can also result in the phenomenon of premature detachment from an individual who is dying or detachment of the dying person from others. Pattison (1977) calls the latter *sociological death* and the former *psychological death.* In either case, the person who is dying, moving to a nursing home, or losing someone is no longer involved in day-to-day activities of living and essentially suffers a premature death.

Acute Grief

Acute grief is a crisis. It has a definite syndrome of somatic, functional, and emotional symptoms of distress that occur in waves of varying lengths of time during the period of impact. Symptoms may occur every time others are informed of the loss or acknowledged by the self or others in the form of condolences. Preoccupation with the loss is a phenomenon similar to daydreaming and is accompanied by a sense of unreality. Depending on the situation, feelings of self-blame or guilt may be present and manifest themselves as hostility or anger toward friends and family. The intense stress of acute grief may lead to significant declines in physical health and the manifestation of depressive symptoms. The older adult who is acutely grieving may say things like "If only I had forced him/her to see the doctor sooner!" or "How could they do this to me?"

Acute grief will be the most intense in the months immediately following the loss and lessen over time. Acute grief is experienced at a national or global level after catastrophic events, such as the hurricanes Katrina in 2005 and Irma in 2017 (Shear et al, 2013) or the eruption of volcano Kilauea in 2018.

Shadow Grief

Grieving takes time, but over the months, the intense pain of the acute period of impact lessens as memories are reframed. But the old memories never go away completely. There are often moments of intermittent sadness referred to as *shadow grief* (Horacek, 1991). It may temporarily inhibit some function but is considered a normal response. While most often discussed in the context of perinatal death, a type of shadow death can occur at any age. It may be triggered by anniversary dates (birthdays, holidays, anniversaries) or by sensory stimuli, such as the smell of perfume, a color, or a sound (Carr et al, 2014) (Box 35.1).

People deal with this in many different ways. Each year, hundreds of people visit the Vietnam Veterans Memorial in Washington, DC, to remember and leave items that connect them to those who have died. Similarly, individuals make

pilgrimages to the Wailing Wall in Jerusalem, praying and placing prayer papers in the crevices of the wall. In Mexico, the annual holiday called "Day of the Dead" is a time when people visit the graves of their family members, leave food, grieve anew, and feel a renewed sense of connection with those who have died before them.

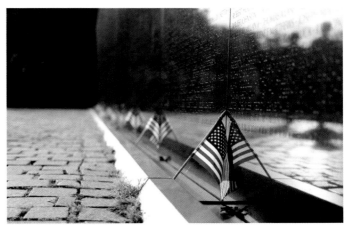

Remembering Those Lost. U.S. flags at the Vietnam Veterans Memorial Wall in Washington, DC. (©Austin Kirk, https://www.flickr.com/photos/aukirk/.)

Complicated Grief

Shadow grief is a type of chronic grief that is considered healthy and restorative. Yet for others, the shadows are debilitating. Those who are survivors of major tragedies, war, rape, abuse, and other horrific events are also grieving; the "shadows" are now recognized as posttraumatic stress. This is a form of complicated grief.

Complicated grief also comes in the form of acute grief that does not significantly lessen over the months and even years after the loss. Obstacles of one form or another interfere with the evolution toward the *reestablishment of equilibrium;* stability is elusive. The memories resist being reframed. Issues of guilt, anger, and ambivalence toward the person who has died are factors that will impede the grieving process until these issues are resolved. Reactions are exaggerated and memories are experienced as if they are fresh, over and over again.

Signs of possible complicated grief, in the form of a prolonged grief disorder, include excessive yearning and longing, decreased interest in everyday activities, and insomnia that lingers for an extended period of time or surfaces months or years later. It may trigger a new major depressive episode or cause one to reappear (Maciejewski et al, 2016). If the depression is manifested in cognitive difficulties, it may be misinterpreted as dementia, especially in the very frail (Chapter 28). Complicated grief requires the professional intervention of a grief counselor, a psychiatric nurse practitioner, or a psychologist who is skilled in helping one cope with complicated grief (Rosner et al, 2018).

Disenfranchised Grief

The person whose loss cannot be openly acknowledged or publicly mourned experiences what is called *disenfranchised* or *unspeakable grief.* The grief is stigmatizing, socially disallowed, or unsupported (Doka, 2002). The death may be one that is not socially condoned, such as that associated with capital punishment, or when a survivor does not have a socially recognized right to be perceived as a person in bereavement. The relationship is not recognized, the loss is not sanctioned, the griever is not recognized, and public mourning is not acceptable. Disenfranchised grief frequently occurs when same-sex partnerships or marriages are not acknowledged by the family of the deceased or in secret relationships (e.g., extramarital), and the griever may not be able tell others of the meaning or depth of the attachment (Bristowe et al, 2016). It may follow the death of an estranged family member, death caused by suicide, death due to AIDS, or by families of death row inmates (Beck and Jones, 2007–2008; Jones and Beck, 2007–2008).

The person in late life can experience disenfranchised grief when family or friends do not understand the full meaning of the loss, for example, of a person's forced retirement, the death of a pet, or gradual losses caused by chronic conditions. Families coping with a member who has Alzheimer's disease may also experience disenfranchised grief when others perceive the death as a "blessing" and fail to support the griever or caregiver who has struggled for years with anticipatory grief and now must cope with the actual death.

Factors Affecting Coping With Loss

To cope effectively with loss is to have the ability to move from a state of chaos (i.e., disequilibrium and instability) to one of stability and equilibrium. It is to find meaning in the loss and be able to find a way to *reframe memories.* Many factors affect the ability to cope with loss and grief (Box 35.2).

Psychiatrist Avery Weisman (1979, pp. 42–43) described those who are more likely to effectively deal with loss as "good copers"—individuals or families who have successfully navigated through crises in the past (Box 35.3). In other words, they can acknowledge the loss and try to make sense of it. They can maintain composure when necessary, can generally use good judgment, and can remain optimistic and appropriately hopeful without denying the loss. Good copers seek guidance when it is needed.

On the contrary, those who cope less effectively have few, if any, of these abilities. They tend to be more rigid, pessimistic, and demanding. They are more likely to be dogmatic and expect perfection in themselves and others. Ineffective copers are more likely to live alone, socialize little, and have few close friends or have an ineffective support network. They may have

---

BOX 35.2 Factors Influencing the Grieving Process

Physical
Number of concurrent medical conditions
Use of sedatives (delays but does not lessen grief)
Nutritional state: if inadequate, reduces the ability to cope or meet demands of daily living; inadequate rest can lead more quickly to mental and physical exhaustion
Exercise: if inadequate, limits emotional outlet; may increase aggressive feelings, tension, and anxiety

Emotional
Unique nature and meaning of loss
Individual coping behavior, personality, and mental health
Individual level of maturity and intelligence
Previous experience with loss or death
Social, cultural, ethnic, religious, or philosophic background
Sex-role conditioning
Immediate circumstances surrounding loss
Timeliness of the loss
Perception of preventability (sudden vs. expected)
Perceived importance of the loss or relationship to that which is lost
Number, type, and quality of secondary losses
Presence of concurrent stresses or crises

Social
Individual support systems and the acceptance of assistance of its members
Individual sociocultural, ethnic, religious, or philosophic background
Educational, economic, and occupational status
Ritual

Modified from Beare PG, Myers JL: *Adult health nursing,* ed 3, St Louis, 1998, Mosby.

BOX 35.3 Identifying Those With Better Coping Skills

- Avoid avoidance
- Confront realities, and take appropriate action
- Focus on solutions
- Redefine problems
- Consider alternatives
- Have good communication with others
- Seek and use constructive help
- Accept support when offered
- Can keep up their morale

From Weisman A: *Coping with cancer,* New York, 1979, McGraw-Hill.

---

a history of mental illness or have guilt, anger, or ambivalence toward the person who has died or that which has been lost. The person is more likely to have unresolved past conflicts or be facing the loss at the same time as secondary life stressors. In some cases they will have fewer opportunities as a result of the loss. They are the persons who are most in need of the expert interventions of grief counselors and skilled, sensitive gerontological nurses.

PROMOTING HEALTHY AGING WHILE GRIEVING: IMPLICATIONS FOR GERONTOLOGICAL NURSING

Loss, grief, and death are parts of the lives of all of us and occur with increasing frequency as we age. The goal of the gerontological nurse is not to prevent grief but to support those who are coping with grief and facilitate the return of equilibrium to the system each time a new loss occurs. Although the acute emotions associated with the impact of the loss will usually abate, any long-term detrimental effects can be ameliorated. While promoting healthy aging, the nurse works with the grieving as part of the normal workday; this is both a privilege and a responsibility. It is one of the few areas in nursing in which small actions can make a large difference in the lives of the persons to whom we provide care.

Assessment

The goal of the grief assessment is to differentiate those who are likely to cope effectively from those who are less likely so that appropriate interventions can be planned (Boxes 35.3 and 35.4). A grief assessment is based on "coming to know" the grievers. Information is obtained through observation in the context of culture (Burke et al, 2017).

A grief assessment is based on listening to the expression of spiritual or existential concerns and needs and the relationship to that which has been or will be lost. How many other stressful or demanding events or circumstances are going on in the griever's life? How meaningful is the loss? Answers to these questions will help determine the potential intensity of support needed and the risk for complicated grieving.

The nurse determines what stress management techniques are normally used and if they have been helpful (e.g., talking it out) or detrimental (e.g., substance abuse) in the past. Are usual support systems available? Was the griever's identity closely tied to that which is lost, such as a lifelong athlete who is faced with never walking again? If the loss is of a partner, how was the relationship? The loss of an abusive or controlling partner may liberate the survivor, who may feel guilty for not feeling the grief that others expect (Box 35.5). For many older women who depended on their spouses financially, death may leave them impoverished, significantly complicating their grief. A survivor may be suddenly homeless after the loss of a domestic partner in jurisdictions in which such relationships are unrecognized. Knowing more about the loss and its effect on the person's life will enable the nurse to construct and implement appropriate and caring interventions.

Interventions

Weisman (1979) described the work of health care professionals as "countercoping." Although he was discussing working with people with cancer, it is equally applicable to working with people who are grieving other losses. "Countercoping is like counterpoint in music, which blends melodies together into a basic harmony. The patient copes; the therapist [nurse] countercopes; together they work out a better fit" (Weisman, 1979, p. 109).

BOX 35.4 Assessment of the Dying Patient and Family

Patient
Age
Gender
Coping styles and abilities
Social, cultural, ethnic background
Previous experience with illness, pain, deterioration, loss, grief
Mental health
Lifestyle
Fulfillment of life goals
Amount of unfinished business
The nature of the illness (death trajectory, problems particular to the illness, treatment, amount of pain)
Time passed since diagnosis
Response to illness
Knowledge about the illness or disease
Acceptance or rejection of the diagnosis
Amount of striving for dependence or independence
Feelings and fears about illness
Location of the patient (home, hospital, nursing home)
Family rules, norms, values, and past experiences that might inhibit grief or interfere with a therapeutic relationship

Family
Developmental stage of the family
Existing subsystems
Geographic proximity of support network
Degree of flexibility or rigidity
Type of communication
Rules, norms, expectations
Values, beliefs
Quality of emotional relationships
Dependence, interdependence, freedom of each member
Closeness or disengaged from the dying member
Established extrafamilial interactions
Strengths and vulnerabilities of the family
Style of leadership and decision-making
Unusual methods of problem solving, crisis resolution
Family resources (personal, financial, community)
Current problems identified by the family
Quality of communication with the caregivers
Immediate and long-range anticipated needs

From Hess PA: Loss, grief, and dying. In Beare P, Myers J, editors: *Adult health nursing*, ed 3, St Louis, 1998, Mosby.

BOX 35.5 "Now I Can Buy That Blouse I Have Been Wanting!"

Sam and Hannah had been married more than 50 years. During that time Hannah's children often encouraged her to leave Sam since he was consistently psychologically abusive and controlling. In the last couple of years of his life, these qualities intensified so that she was forbidden to purchase only the necessities of life, even with her own money. He died after a prolonged illness, but even before the elaborate funeral expected in her culture, she exclaimed (to those closest to her), "Now I can buy that blouse I have been wanting, and maybe a new couch, too!"

Helping Grievers Move Through the Impact of Loss to the Reestablishment of New Memories

Functional Disruption
- Provide functional assistance

Searching for Meaning
- Provide reliable sources of information (e.g., websites)
- Inform appropriate providers of the person's need for information and make sure they receive it
- Active listening

Engaging Emotions
- "Give permission" to express emotions
- Offer physical presence
- Offer to locate usual sources of support during times of crisis (e.g., minister, tribal elder)
- Active listening

Informing Others
- Offer physical presence
- Active listening

Adaptation
- Identify meaningful events influenced by the loss
- Help find new ways of replacing that which has been lost
- Offer discussions of how the loss has affected life
- Active listening

Reframing Memories
- Offer to discuss mechanisms to develop new memories without denying connection with that or with whom has been lost
- Encourage reminiscence
- Facilitate opportunities for culturally based and desired bereavement rituals
- Assure grievers that stability will return
- Active listening

Like good copers, good gerontological nurses must be flexible, practical, resourceful, gently realistic, and abundantly optimistic. Nurses introduce themselves, establish rapport, learn the cultural rules regarding the situation, and explain their roles (e.g., nurse practitioner, charge nurse, staff nurse) and the time they will be available. The nurse fosters the griever's movement from disequilibrium and instability to a new, albeit modified, steady state (Box 35.6).

Impact and Functional Disruption

If it is the time of *impact* (e.g., just after a new serious diagnosis, at the death of a family member, at the time of a move to a care facility), nurses can provide a safe environment ensuring that basic needs, such as meals and rest, are met. At all times, active listening is preferable to giving advice. When listening, the nurse soon discovers that it is not necessarily the actual loss that is of utmost concern but, rather, the fear associated with the loss. If the nurse listens carefully to both the stated and the implied expressions, statements such as the following may be heard: "How will I go on?" "What will I do now?" "What will become of me?" "I don't know what to do." "How could he (she)

do this to me?" Because the nurse knows that there will be some resolution, such comments may seem exaggerated or melodramatic, but to the one who is grieving, there seems to be no end to the pain. The person who is actively grieving cannot yet look ahead or know that the despair and other feelings will resolve. The nurse can soften the despair by fostering *reasonable and appropriate hope*, such as, "You will make it through one moment at a time, and I will be here to help."

Nurses observe for *functional disruption* and offer support and direction. When the death is imminent, the nurse may have to ask difficult questions, such as the following: Does the person have a living will? Who is the proxy? Who needs to be notified; does this include a spiritual advisor? The nurse helps the family establish priorities and determine how to accomplish them, encouraging them to delay what they can. The nurse can either complete the task (e.g., tell them that you are going to wash the dishes; do not ask) or find a friend or other family member who is less affected and able to step in to minimize the functional disruption.

Searching for Meaning, Engaging Emotions, and Informing Others

As grievers search for meaning, the nurse facilitates coping with loss by helping them get the information they feel they need, consider alternatives, and find ways to make their grief manageable. In this way clarification is supported (Weisman, 1979).

Sometimes families are looking for information about a disease or trying to understand how to find the best hospital for a treatment or the best nursing home for a long-term stay (Chapter 32). The nurse assists in obtaining the information whenever possible. With the availability of Internet search engines and devices such as touch screens and tablets, this is often straightforward even as simply as providing key search terms. While paying attention to health literacy, many sources provide reliable information in a range of languages. Active listening often helps grievers make sense of the loss and find meaning in it as they experience a change in their reality. Often this means helping the person contact a health care provider, an elder in their culture, or a spiritual leader.

Expressions of emotion, be they through panic, hysteria, or silence, may make grief less frightening. In some cultures catharsis is expected, and in others it is the nurse who gives the griever the "permission" needed to emote. Sometimes it is a spiritual search and help is in the form of finding a resource or a place of peace, such as the chapel. Often, what is needed most is someone to listen to the existential and unanswerable questions, the "whys" and "hows," without giving answers. At other times it may be appropriate to be directive, such as suggesting that "This is not a good time to make any major decisions" (Weisman, 1979).

Sometimes nurses feel a need to help *inform others* for the grievers, thinking that this is an expression of caring. While it appears to be, it is more therapeutic for grievers or designated cultural spokespersons to talk to others about the losses, and nurses should refrain from intervening in this way. Instead, the nurse can offer to find a phone number or just offer to "be there" when the news is being shared. In this way, the nurse

Helping the Person Reframe Memories of a Former Ritual

The grandmother who had always hosted her eldest daughter's birthday party can still do that even if she is now a resident in a long-term care facility. The nurse can help the resident reserve a private space within the facility, send out invitations, and have the birthday party as always but now reframe it as catered by the facility in the person's new "home."

provides support when the griever's emotions engage and at the same time shows respect for the person's and family's cultural roles.

Adaptation

As the person or family moves toward equilibrium after the impact of a loss, be it a death, a move to a nursing home, or other change, the nurse can help the person reorganize this new life. The nurse talks with the person who is grieving about what was most valued about that which has been lost, determines what habits and rituals were comforting related to this, and finds ways to incorporate these in a new way to the new environment (Box 35.7). For example, if the person always had a cup of tea before bed but now does not have access to a kitchen, "cup of tea at bedtime" can become part of the individualized plan of care.

Memories Reframed and the Return to Equilibrium and a New Steady State

For the system to return to equilibrium and a new steady state, however fleeting, new memories are needed. Reminiscence is often helpful in creating these. The nurse collaborates with grievers by encouraging them to share stories with others and repeat them as often as needed (Weisman, 1979). Listening to the story, endlessly repeated, is difficult to do and it is likely to change with each retelling, but this means that memories are being reframed as a new steady state is approaching. Reminiscence allows the reality of the loss to filter slowly into the unconscious mind. It helps the griever acknowledge that the loss is indeed real and that life can go on, even though the future may be experienced in a different way. At the time when new memories are being developed, drawing out anecdotes and vignettes of his or her life before the loss will allow the person to see a different perspective. The nurse serves as a role model who displays the behavioral qualities of responsiveness, authenticity, commitment, and competence, that is, caring.

DYING AND DEATH

Before the 1900s, most women and men died at home. Women often died during childbirth, and men often died of unknown causes. During times of war, most men died in battle or from battle-associated injuries. The life expectancy at birth in 1900 was 46.3 years for men and 48.3 years for women (United States). Now both men and women live well into their 70s and beyond (Chapter 1). While most people prefer to die at home, they most often die in acute care

hospitals with wide variation in prevalence by country of residence. In an exploratory study, physicians found patient characteristics, physical environment, and support networks were stronger than other factors influencing a patient's ability to die at home (Wales et al, 2018).

Dying is both a challenging life experience and a private one. How people deal with their own dying is often a reflection of the way they responded to earlier losses and stressors. Most people probably die as they have lived, that is, the manner in which one faces dying is an expression of personality, circumstances, illness, and culture.

Although not all older adults have had fulfilling lives or have a sense of completion, transcendence, or self-actualization (Chapter 36), their deaths at the age of or after that of their parents is considered normative. If dying occurs after a particularly prolonged or painful illness, it is sometimes rationalized as a relief, at least in part. The deaths of the older community members at the time of war are never considered an acceptable loss of human potential. A major question arises when considering dying and death in late life. When is a person with multiple chronic or repeated acute or progressive health problems considered to be "dying"? Both manageable chronic conditions and those associated with an irreversible terminal condition often occur at the same time, more so as we age. While the signs and symptoms attributed to terminal conditions may appear obvious, they can easily be confused with frailty and exacerbations of chronic diseases. However, the nurse can look for signs of an approaching death when the person begins using "coded communication," such as saying goodbye instead of the usual goodnight, giving away cherished possessions as gifts, urgently contacting friends and relatives with whom the person has not communicated with for a long time, and having direct or symbolic premonitions that death is near.

Anxiety, depression, restlessness, and agitation are behaviors that are frequently categorized as manifestations of confusion or dementia but may also be responses to the inability to express feelings of foreboding and a sense of life escaping one's grasp. Ensuring that the person remains comfortable, whether the condition is chronic, acute, or terminal, is the work of the nurse and other members of the caring team. Many people have said that death is not the problem; it is the dying that takes the work. This is true for all involved: the person who is dying, the loved ones, the professional caregivers such as the nurses, and the nursing assistants in care facilities, who are too often invisible grievers.

The Family

Today's older adults are usually members of both multigenerational and complex family constellations, consisting of ex-spouses and partners, step-grandchildren, and fictive kin (those considered family as a result of affective bonds). Although members may be geographically distant, in many cases some degree of filial ties exists (Chapter 34). When a person in late life becomes seriously or terminally ill and cannot uphold his or her role or obligation, the family balance or dynamics is significantly altered (*functional disruption*).

For example, new arrangements are needed when the older adults who had been providing childcare or help with meal preparation are no longer able to do so. This change may cause considerable familial distress, as will the need for personal care when day-to-day help seems impossible due to the work demands and schedules of adult children, grandchildren, nieces, and nephews. Even he or she who is single and relies on friends and neighbors finds a change in the relationships. Depending on the role the individual has in the family/friend constellation, while changes may not occur at the time of diagnosis, they will as any associated frailty advances (Chapter 21). Roles and traits of the person who is now considered to be dying may create adjustment difficulties in the soon-to-be survivors, whether they are partners, spouses, adult children, or grandchildren. Adult children often begin to see their own mortality through the death of their parents as the family is reframed.

The idea that family members can remain involved with the dying person may be a source of constant conflict as they anticipate and plan for life without the dying family member. This change requires enormous energy by family members who are already burdened with their own anticipatory grief, daily living, and, in many cases, raising their own children and possibly grandchildren. Family members have to separate their own identities from that of the patient and learn to tolerate the reality that another family member will die while they live on. The ability of the family to support, love, and provide intimacy may lead to exhaustion, impatience, anger, and a sense of futility if the dying is prolonged. Family members may be at different points in grief than the patient or each other, which can hinder communication when it is needed the most. As the illness worsens, physical disability increases, and the patient's needs intensify, so may the family members' feelings of helplessness and frustration.

Responding to the effects of grief requires acknowledging feelings that surface before and after the death. Coming to terms with the reality of the impending loss means that family members often go through a period of self-reflection. Because people are "supposed to" die in old age according to social norms, the grief responses may not be exceptionally intense and this can lead to either guilt or relief for the person who is suffering.

The family may feel extremely pressured to provide very personal care during the final days of a relative's life. They may feel caught between experiencing the present and remembering the person as he or she was, between pushing for more interventions with the potential to extend the dying or letting life take its natural course. Nurses often hear families lament that they "can't give up on them," even if this runs counter to the dying person's wishes (Chapter 31).

Despite the family's grief and pain, they must give the patient permission to die; let the loved one know that it is all right to let go and leave them. This gesture is the last act of love and dignity that the family can offer. Occasionally, no family is available to say, "It's okay to let go." The task then falls to the nurse who has developed a meaningful relationship with the person through care.

PROMOTING A GOOD DEATH: IMPLICATIONS FOR GERONTOLOGICAL NURSING

The needs of the dying are like threads in a piece of cloth. Each thread is individual but necessary to the integrity and completeness of the fabric. If one thread is pulled, it touches the other threads, affecting the fabric's appearance, the thread placement, and the stability of the piece. When one need is unmet, it will affect all others because they are all interwoven. Separating the physical, psychological, and spiritual needs of the dying in late life to identify specific interventions and approaches is difficult because of their interconnection. There are several ways to approach an understanding of the needs of persons who are dying and the responsibilities of the nurse in the promotion of a healthy death (Fig. 35.3).

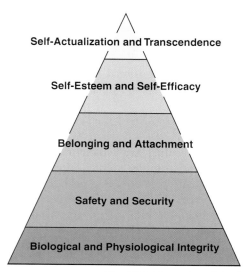

Self-Actualization and Transcendence — To share and come to terms with the unavoidable future / To perceive meaning in death

Self-Esteem and Self-Efficacy — To maintain respect in the face of increasing weakness / To maintain independence to the extent possible / To feel like a normal person, a part of life right to the end / To preserve personal identity

Belonging and Attachment — To talk / To be listened to with understanding / To be loved and to share love / To be with a caring person when dying

Safety and Security — To be given the opportunity to voice hidden fears / To trust those who care for him or her / To feel that he or she is being told the truth / To be secure

Biological and Physiological Integrity — To obtain relief from physical symptoms / To conserve energy / To be free from pain

Fig. 35.3 Hierarchy of the Dying Person's Needs, Based on Maslow.

The 6 C's Approach

Psychiatrist Avery Weisman (1979) identified six needs of the dying: care, control, composure, communication, continuity, and closure (the 6 C's). The importance of each to the person is influenced by his or her personality, culture, experiences, religious and philosophical beliefs, orientation, the prior degree of life involvement, and perhaps gender. Weisman's approach can provide a framework for the nurse in the development of interventions when caring for those who are dying.

Care

The dying person should have the best care possible; this means freedom from pain, conservation of energy, expert management of symptoms, and support at all times. Common symptoms include dyspnea, fatigue, pain, and those that are more specific to the cause of the terminal condition. In aging they accompany the symptoms the person has due to concurrent chronic disease. It is never acceptable for any of the person's *symptoms* to remain either untreated or undertreated.

The chronic pain that often accompanies dying is not going to stop and usually requires a regimen of narcotic and adjuvant drug therapy administered around the clock and on time, not just "as requested" by the patient (Chapter 27). Providing adequate relief must be done without concern of addiction or overall effect on respiratory status; relief of pain is paramount.

Pain goes beyond the physical to that which is spiritual and psychological, induced by depression, anxiety, fear, and other unresolved emotional concerns that are just as strong and just as real. When emotional needs are not met, the total pain experience is exacerbated or intensified. Medication alone cannot relieve this pain. Instead, empathetic listening and allowing those who are dying to verbalize what is on their minds are important interventions that must be based on the energy and stamina that are available at any one time. If tears and sadness are present, silence and touch, if acceptable, are worth more than words can convey. Gentleness, closeness, and sitting near the person may be appropriate. The counsel of the person's spiritual advisor may be needed.

Diversional activity can sometimes ease pain: a backrub to relieve tension, a foot massage, radio or television, or exposure to art and music. If hearing is impaired, headphones are very useful. If vision is impaired, audio books or a volunteer reader can be found. In many instances, psychological pain can be relieved if the person feels safe and has someone close by to converse, to listen, and to be with.

Dying requires much energy to cope with the physical assault of illness on the body and the spiritual and emotional unrest that dying initiates. Care means helping the person conserve energy. How much can the individual do without becoming physically and emotionally taxed? What activities of daily living are most important for the person to do independently? How much energy is needed for the patient to talk with those who are the most important without becoming exhausted? Only the person who is dying can answer these questions, and the nurse can advocate for the person to be given the opportunity to do so. By meeting the needs for freedom from pain and conservation of energy, the nurse has already begun to ensure that the person receives optimal care in order to maximize the quality of life to the extent possible for the time that remains.

Control

As death gets closer, people often feel that they have less and less control over their lives and bodies. The person is in the process of losing everything he or she has ever known or would ever know. The potential loss of identity, independence, and control over bodily functions can lead to threatened self-esteem. The person may begin to feel ashamed, humiliated, and like a "burden." Control is the need to remain in a collaborative role relating to one's own living and dying and as active a participant in the care as desired. The nurse can help the person meet these needs by taking every opportunity to return the control to the person and, in doing so, bolster self-esteem. Essential to the facilitating of self-esteem is the premise that the values of the patient must figure significantly in the decisions that will affect the course of dying. Whenever possible, the nurse can have the person decide when to groom, eat, wake, and sleep, and so on. The nurse never has the right to determine the activities of the individual, especially relating to visitors and how time is spent.

Composure

Dying is an emotional activity—for the dying and for those around them. The need for composure is that which enables the person to modulate emotional extremes within cultural norms as is appropriate. This is not to avoid the sadness; this is to have moments of relief.

Communication

The need for communication is broad, from the need for information to make decisions, to the need to share information. Although the type and content of communication that is acceptable to the person vary, the nurse has a responsibility to ensure that the person has an opportunity for the communication he or she desires.

Communication includes auditory, visual, and tactile stimulation to appropriately nurture and foster quality of life while dying. Verbal and nonverbal communication is necessary to convey positive messages. Hand-holding, placing an arm around the shoulder, or sitting on the edge of the bed as culturally appropriate conveys to the person that the nurse or caregiver is available to listen.

In a classic study of terminal illness in the hospital, Glaser and Strauss (1965) identified four types of communication: *closed awareness*, *suspected awareness*, *mutual pretense*, and *open awareness*. Each of these influenced the work on the hospital unit. Closed awareness is described as "keeping the secret." Hospital staff and the family and friends know that the patient is dying, but the patient does not know it or also keeps the secret. Generally, caregivers invent a fictitious future for the patient to believe in (e.g., next year we are going on the cruise we always wanted), in hopes that it will boost the patient's morale. Although this happens less today with the legislation related to patients' rights, it still occurs. In suspected awareness, the patient suspects that he or she is going to die. Hints are bandied back and forth, and a contest ensues for control of the information. Mutual pretense is a situation of "let's pretend." Everyone knows the death is approaching, but the patient, family, friends, nurses, and physicians do not talk about it—real feelings are kept hidden, and too often, so are questions. Open awareness acknowledges the reality of approaching death. The patient may ask, "Will I die?" and "How and when will I die?" "What is it going to be like?" The patient becomes resigned to dying, and the family grieves with the patient rather than for the patient. The nurse can encourage open awareness whenever possible while respecting the patient's cultural patterns and behaviors. It is essential to note that what is said and to whom is culturally determined. Talking about dying or death may be considered taboo and speaking to the wrong person may be very inappropriate (Brown, 2017; Bryant, 2017; Coolen, 2012).

Continuity

The need for continuity is fulfilled by preserving as normal a life as possible while dying; by transcending the present, continuity helps to maintain self-esteem. Often a dying patient can feel shut off from the rest of the world at a time when he or she is still capable of being involved and active in some way. Providing stimuli such as photographs and mementos, enabling the individual to stay at home, or enabling individuality or other culturally appropriate experiences in the institutional setting engenders continuity and self-esteem. Self-esteem and dignity complement each other. Dignity involves the individual's ability to maintain a consistent self-concept.

Loneliness may be the result of a loss of continuity with one's life and a diminution of one's concept of self and results in spiritual or existential distress. The nurse may ask about the person's life and those things most valued and work with the family and the patient or nursing home resident on a plan to remain engaged in as many of the activities and past roles as long as possible. A father who watches a certain ballgame with his son every Sunday can continue to do this regardless of the need to be in a hospital, a nursing home, or an inpatient hospice unit. If the person is bed-bound at home, it may be more practical to have the bed in a central area rather than in a distant room. Treating the person as an intelligent adult says, "I care" and "You're not alone" and "You are important." Others prefer some time alone and value solitude (Box 35.8). This too can be respected as a way of enhancing the continuity of a long life. The nurse can determine the personal preferences and values of the person and work toward honoring these.

Closure

The need for closure is the need for the opportunity for reconciliation, transcendence, and self-actualization (Chapter 36) (Maslow, 1943). Reminiscence is one way of putting life in order, to evaluate the pluses and minuses of life, and to think about the legacies left behind. It is a means of resolving conflicts, giving up prized possessions, and making final goodbyes. Learning to say "goodbye" today leaves open the possibility of many more "hellos." Pain and other symptoms that are not well cared for interfere with this reconciliation, making appropriate interventions by the nurse especially important.

BOX 35.8 Meditation Coping

Mrs. Herbert was a spry 76-year-old white woman. She was the sole caregiver of her husband with midstage Alzheimer's disease. The hospital had arranged for her husband to share a room with her while her diagnostic tests were completed and her symptoms stabilized before she went home. She had just been diagnosed with metastatic breast cancer, with a terminal diagnosis. The nurses thought that she was becoming increasingly irritable and agitated after her initial calmness. As an advanced practice nurse on an oncology unit, I was called to assess Mrs. Herbert and recommend a treatment plan. We talked for a while—about her life, her plans for the future, and her usual coping mechanisms. She explained that she had everything under control and had already made arrangements for home care in the process of planning for the eventual long-term care needs of her husband. As she started to cry, she said, "It's just so hard with my life disrupted here. Every morning for years I have meditated for 30 minutes. My husband respects my need for quiet, and afterward I think I can do anything! I have not been able to meditate since I have been here; the nurses and staff are always coming in my room or calling on the room's intercom—I can't find any moments of peace!" The nurses and I worked out a plan with Mrs. Herbert. Every morning between 6:00 and 6:30 AM, she would not be disturbed. A "Do Not Disturb" sign would be placed on the intercom at the nurses' station and on her door. A noticeable change was seen in just a few days; Mrs. Herbert was calmer and coping well again. She was most appreciative to "have my life back again."

For some, closure means coming to terms with their spiritual selves, with the Great Spirit, Jesus, God, Allah, or Buddha—of that which has meaning to the person. If the patient has existential or spiritual needs, arranging for pastoral care may be offered but should never be done without the person's permission. The nurse can foster transcendence by providing patients with the time and privacy for self-reflection and an opportunity to talk about whatever they need to talk about, especially about the meanings of their lives and the meanings of their deaths.

Spirituality

In 2002, a group of experts in palliative care gathered to develop and subsequently update consensus documents for the provision of hospice and palliative care. The 2013 guidelines were driven in part by discovery that while addressing the spiritual needs of persons who are dying had long been an expectation of providers of hospice and palliative care, they were not often met. The responsibility of health care professionals to assess spiritual and existential needs during the dying process is stressed. When needs are identified, nurses are expected to ensure that the needs are addressed. A fourth guideline became available in 2019. The *Guideline* emphasize the importance of the interdisciplinary team, including the chaplain or other spiritual advisor. The nurse is reminded of the importance of attending to spiritual and cultural rituals that are important to the patient and family as a means of comfort and support (National Coalition for Hospice and Palliative Care, 2019).

The spiritual dimension of persons who are dying deals with the transcendental or existential relationship between the dying person and another—between the person and his or her god or the person and significant others. Signs of spiritual distress while dying include expressions of hopelessness, meaninglessness, guilt, and despair, all of which can emerge

BOX 35.9 Indicators of an Appropriate and Good Death

- Care needed is received, and it is timely and expert.
- One is able to control one's life and environment to the extent that is desired and possible and in a way that is culturally consistent with one's past life.
- One is able to maintain composure when necessary and to the extent desired.
- One is able to initiate and maintain communication with significant others for as long as possible.
- Life continues as normal as possible while dying with the added tasks that may be needed to deal with and adjust to the inevitable death.
- One can maintain *desirable* hope at all times.
- One is able to reach a sense of closure in a way that is culturally consistent with one's practices and life patterns.

indirectly through anxiety, depression, or anger. At the specific direction of the patient, interventions may involve calling the patient's choice of a religious leader; sharing spiritual readings that are consistent with the patient's beliefs; reciting meditative poems and playing music of the person's choice; obtaining religious articles such as amulets, a Bible, or a rosary; or praying. *The nurse is strongly cautioned that these interventions must be consistent with the culture and express wishes of the patient and may not at any time be suggested based on the nurse's belief system.*

Hope

Hope is a fluid concept that changes as dying comes closer. At the beginning, the person hopes for a cure. When a prognosis is given, the hope may change to have "as much time as possible." As death approaches, the hope may be for a good death, one that is symptom free (Box 35.9).

Hope is expectancy of fulfillment, an anticipation, or relief from something. Hope is based on the belief of the possible, the support of meaningful others, a sense of well-being, overall coping ability, and a purpose in life. Hope empowers, generates courage, motivates action and achievement, and can counter physiological, spiritual, and emotional dysfunction. Hope involves faith and trust.

It can be classified as desirable or expectational (Pattison, 1977). Expectational hope sounds like "I hope to get better" or "I hope my children get here in time." If this hope is a reflection of expectations that are not realistic, they can increase stress for the person and caregiver. However, this hope can be modified without being lost. In desirable hope, the wishes are something that would be appreciated if it were to occur without the fixed expectation that it will, will not, or must occur. The nurse can respond to the comment "I hope I get better" from someone who is rapidly declining with "That would be really great; in the meantime, there is so much we can do."

Nurses seldom recognize the small things they do, routinely and unconsciously, to impart hope. The act of helping with grooming conveys a quiet belief that the person matters. Pain relief and comfort measures show that the individual's needs are important and reinforce the value of the person.

Promoting Equilibrium for the Family

The nurse is often present and supporting the family at the moment of death and in the moments both preceding and following it. Regardless of the age of the survivors, they, too, have needs and nurses have a responsibility to care for them. This may be in the form of the interventions that promote equilibrium to a system now in chaos. Nursing interventions include actions that empower the family to cope with the death in a manner consistent with their traditions. In a small ethnography, Herbert and colleagues (2008) found that family caregivers most needed prognostic information prior to death and were unlikely to ask. Hearing from the provider what the death would "look like" was a key ingredient the families found missing.

PALLIATIVE CARE

According to the World Health Organization, palliative care is "an approach to care that improves the quality of life of patients and their families who are facing problems associated with life-threatening illness" through the prevention, assessment, and treatment of pain and other physical, psychological, and spiritual problems (World Health Organization, 2018). Providing such care is part of day-to-day practice of gerontological nurses who routinely care for older adults having life-limiting conditions, such as Alzheimer's disease or Parkinson's disease (Chapter 23). The primary goal of palliative care is to prevent or minimize suffering. It is often provided through interdisciplinary formal systems to help people understand their options and make health-related decisions that are consistent with their values and to facilitate seamless transitions when movement from one care setting is necessary.

Most importantly, palliative care is offered simultaneously with life-prolonging or stabilizing care for those living with chronic conditions (Fig. 35.4). When working with older adults and their families, the focus is very often on amelioration of cognitive and functional limitations and support to the caregivers who are coping with multiple issues simultaneously.

Purely palliative care may be elected when previously curative treatments are no longer effective, such as with end-stage cancer, AIDS, or end-stage heart disease. It may also be appropriate when

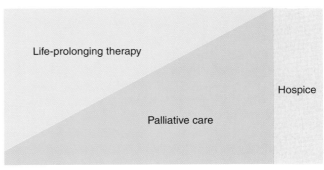

Fig. 35.4 Palliative care is offered simultaneously with life-prolonging and curative therapies for persons living with serious, complex, and advanced illness. (From Ham RJ, Sloane PD, Warshaw GA, et al: *Primary care geriatrics*, ed 6, Philadelphia, 2014, Elsevier.)

an individual with multiple comorbid conditions or a health care proxy makes the decision to forgo any aggressive treatment of chronic or new health problems. It must be noted that the provision of palliative care does not mean that any simple curative treatments to transient new problems are automatically withheld, such as the treatment of a urinary tract infection or other infection when the terminal illness is something else, such as heart disease, cancer, or chronic obstructive pulmonary disease (COPD).

Whereas initially palliative care was provided primarily by specialized organizations, today it is provided regardless of setting and by anyone sharing these goals and skills. This may be in the ambulatory care clinic when the focus of the care of the person with neurodegenerative disorders is comfort (Chapter 23) or in specialized beds in an acute care or long-term care facility.

Providing Palliative Care Through Hospice Services

The model for the modern-day hospice is based on the medieval concept of hospitality in which a community assists the traveler at dangerous points along a journey. The dying are also travelers along the continuum of life and wellness, in a community consisting of friends, family, and health care providers. However, for many years, providing comfort to those approaching death was lacking. In 1952 Englishwoman Dame Cicely Saunders, a nurse, social worker, physician, and writer, began working at St. Joseph's Hospice in London. The goal of her work and study was to reduce pain. In 1967 she established Saint Christopher's Hospice, also in London, based on the principles of teaching, clinical research, and the provision of expert and holistic pain and symptom relief (St. Christopher's, n.d.). Inspired by the work of Dame Saunders, Dr. Florence Wald, the Dean of the College of Nursing at Yale University, and physician Dr. Elisabeth Kübler-Ross championed the hospice concept in the United States. In 1974 Dr. Wald, two pediatricians, and a chaplain founded Connecticut Hospice in Branford, Connecticut.

Hospice programs in the United States started out as small, free-standing organizations supported entirely by charitable contributions and volunteer effort; services were available to all, regardless of ability to pay, and were provided exclusively in the person's home. The number of organizations providing formal hospice care grew rapidly, especially after the services were approved for reimbursement by Medicare, Medicaid, and many private insurers (Chapter 30). While they were initially all non-profit, in 2017 the majority (67%) of hospices were for-profit corporations (National Hospice and Palliative Care Organization [NHPCO], 2018). The variations in origins and styles reflect the style of leadership, funding sources, political forces, and available resources for health and social services in the community in which they were established or continue to exist. While the care provided is palliative, it is within the specific context of a signed agreement between the individual and the organization in which the person has elected to receive only comfort care. Hospice services are limited to those for whom two physicians have agreed that the person has a prognosis of 6 months or less.

At a minimum, services include medical, nursing, nursing assistant, chaplain, social work, and volunteer support. Potential services may also include massage, music, art, pet therapy, and other nonpharmacological interventions to promote comfort

and quality of life. Hospices provide care not only to the dying but also to their families and friends through support groups and other bereavement services before and after the deaths.

The majority of hospice care is provided in people's homes to support an identified informal caregiver. The home becomes the primary center of care, provided by family members or friends, who are taught basic care techniques as needed, including diet, exercise, and medication management with intermittent visits from the hospice staff. Volunteers, as members of the team, are a unique aspect of care; chores are performed, and friendship and companionship are provided to the patient and family.

Many hospices today have free-standing care centers where a patient may go to provide caregivers with short periods of respite or when intense symptom management is more than is possible at home. Those hospices without centers may have agreements with skilled nursing homes or acute care hospitals where the same symptom management can be achieved. When and if stabilized, the person returns home.

The unprecedented contribution of hospice continues to be the provision of comfort for those who are dying and of support for those close to them. Through both pharmacological and non-pharmacological means, control of pain and other symptoms can often be accomplished without denying the patient's full alertness and the ability to communicate with others. The crux of accomplishing this end is the anticipation of symptoms and intervention by the caregiver before problems occur. Both hospice and other palliative care programs support and guide the family in patient care and ensure safe passage (i.e., for the patient, that he or she will not die alone; and that the family will not be abandoned).

Nursing practice in hospice incorporates the expression of the mind-body continuum. Nursing is considered the cornerstone of hospice care. The nurse provides much of the direct care and functions in a variety of roles: as staff nurse giving direct care, as coordinator implementing the plan of the interdisciplinary team, as advocate for the patient and hospice in the clinical and political arena, and sometimes as executive officer responsible for research and educational activities.

DECISION-MAKING AT THE END OF LIFE

Who makes end-of-life decisions has been the subject of research, debate, and federal legislation in the United States. Although people have always had opinions about their wishes, in the past these were made in the context of the prevailing principle of paternalism, that is, reliance on physicians to make the decisions they would make for their own children. This perspective has been replaced by presumed autonomy in the health care setting based on a Euro-American or Western perspective (Chapters 4 and 31). Persons from many other culture groups place less emphasis on the individual and more, if not all, on identified cultural or familial decision-makers (Mazanec and Panke, 2015).

Decision-making about life-prolonging measures when death is inevitable is a legal, ethical, medical, and professional issue faced by gerontological nurses in their daily work. Yet the lines between living and dying are quite blurred, especially for the medically frail, or for an older adult with a multitude of chronic conditions. Considerable ethical conflicts arise from the technological advances available in some parts of the world or when there is ambivalence of whether death is to be fought or allowed to proceed naturally. Nonetheless, the nurse is obligated to know legal restrictions related to decision-making and then work with the individual and family on how these are consistent with their cultural patterns and rituals related to the end of life. For example, Hispanic older adults are more likely to defer decision-making to other members of the family based on the belief that they know and will act on their wishes.

Living Wills

Since the passage of the Patient Self-Determination Act (PSDA) in 1991 in the United States, any agency that is reimbursed by Medicare for services is required to provide all adult patients with information about their rights to make their own health care decisions, accept or refuse treatment, and complete an advance directive (AD) (Chapter 30) of some kind, especially living wills (LWs). In the outpatient setting, providers (e.g., physicians, nurse practitioners, and physician assistants) are encouraged, but not obligated to provide this information.

The PSDA recognized an LW as an AD that is specifically related to a situation in which a person is facing a terminal illness and unable to speak for herself or himself. It is a morally and, in some jurisdictions, legally binding document in which adults could express their wishes regarding end-of-life decisions for some future time when they were unable to do so for themselves. LWs may be as limited as decisions regarding the use of resuscitation or as detailed as decisions about dialysis, antibiotics, tube feedings, and so on (Box 35.10). The LW includes the appointment of a proxy to uphold patients' wishes when they are no longer able to do so. As the proxy is selected by the individual, the legal assumption is that a designated person has more authority than the next-of-kin (if that person is not the proxy).

An LW can be revoked only by the individual, either verbally or in writing. The person may also indicate revocation by tearing, burning, or destroying the document, preferably in front of witnesses. Directives may also be amended; formal language is not necessary, and one can add items in writing or cross out unwanted passages, but only the creator of the document may do so. If the person becomes incompetent, revocation is no longer possible, and the last statement of wishes stands. Nurses should know the details of AD and LW requirements in the state, country, or other jurisdiction in which they practice. The nurse should also be familiar with the LW form or forms available in the organization in which he or she is employed. The exact format and signature requirements (e.g., notary) for ADs including LWs vary from state to state.

Barriers to Completing Advance Directives

In a review of the literature of advanced care plans (ACPs) among persons from ethnic/minorities groups, completion ranged from 40% to 59.1%. Sociodemographic, health status, literacy, and experiences, cultural values, and spirituality factors all served in some way as barriers to completion. Those living in the community completed ACPs less often than their white majority counterparts or their minority counterparts who were seriously ill or hospitalized. Those who were disadvantaged including economically, with low health literacy levels or having reduced knowledge of ACP, had fewer of these completed.

Those coming from a collectivist culture were significantly less likely to have an ACP. Instead, such decisions were left to the decision-makers in the family. Those with strong beliefs in God or a higher power were much more likely to have their religious beliefs guide their end-of-life decisions than have completed an ACP of any kind (Hong et al, 2018) (Box 35.11). Interpreters, used to assist the health care professional with explanations to their non–English-speaking patients, may not facilitate a clear translation of an AD because of cultural beliefs surrounding death or anticipation of poor health, for example many in the Haitian culture believe that speaking of death is taboo and may cause it to occur more quickly (Coolen, 2012).

To ensure that one's end-of-life decisions transfer accurately from one care facility to another, the POLST (*Physicians Orders for Life-Sustaining Treatment*) document was created. The document is signed by the physician (or nurse practitioner, depending on the state) after a discussion with the patient and a review of such documents as their LW. The POLST goes with the patient between settings (National POLST Paradigm, 2019). The POLST is not an AD; it is a health care provider order to emergency personnel and health care facilities. The POLST is not recognized in all states or organizations, yet without this or a similar document, emergency providers are required to do everything necessity to prolong life (National POLST Paradigm, 2019).

BOX 35.11 Cultural Barriers to the Completions of Advance Directives, Including Living Wills

Distrust of the health care system (especially in groups who have experienced violence or discrimination in the United States or their country of origin)

Cultural pattern of collectivism: family or designated others rather than individual are"decision-makers"

Preference for physician, as expert, to make the decision

Taboo to talk about death or dying

Influence of faith and spirituality: illness as a test of faith

Belief that life is a gift from God that must be protected at all costs

Death as a part of the cycle of life and must not be disturbed

Dying away from home may lead to a disturbance of the spirits

Cannot die at home as the spirit will linger

From Coolen PR: Cultural relevance in end-of-life care, *EthnoMed*, May 1, 2012. https://ethnomed.org/clinical/end-of-life/cultural-relevance-in-end-of-life-care. Accessed July 2018.

BOX 35.10 Tips for Best Practice

A living will is not the same as a do-not-resuscitate (DNR) order or a do-not-hospitalize (DNH) order, which are medical directives to health care professionals and are not personal advance directives. Neither the DNR order nor the DNH order should be written without a discussion of the implications with the patient and/or proxy. The nurse is often the one to facilitate this order in either case.

PROMOTING HEALTHY AGING: IMPLICATIONS FOR GERONTOLOGICAL NURSING

Although nurses cannot provide legal information, they do serve as resource persons ready to discuss many of the questions people have about end-of-life decision-making, especially how these affect their care (Box 35.12). The nurse must consider the factors previously discussed and must ensure that patients are informed of their rights related to the PSDA in a culturally sensitive manner. The nurse may be responsible to inquire about the presence of an existing AD, to offer and explain the option, and to ensure that any existing directive still reflects the person's wishes. The nurse is also responsible for ensuring that existing or newly created ADs are available in the appropriate locations in the medical record.

The nurse can help the person understand interventions (e.g., cardiopulmonary resuscitation [CPR], intubations, and artificial nutrition) and their consequences. The nurse can explain that choosing no further intervention is not "giving up" but is an active decision to allow a natural death to occur. Personal bias cannot be injected into the discussion (e.g., religious affiliation or otherwise) under any circumstances. The nurse is an impartial advocate for the patient regardless of decision or setting, but it is particularly important in the long-term care environment. There, the nurse advocates for the self-determination of all patients to the best possible extent, even those with limited cognitive function (ANA, 2016; Ferguson, 2018). The nurse also acts as a patient advocate by bringing together decision makers, older adults, and health care providers to discuss anything from the person's wishes to difficult issues that may arise in executing a directive.

No one can think of all possible contingencies that might require decisions regarding life-limiting conditions. The use of values' assessments may help clarify what the person holds important in his or her life and how this relates to his or her desires for health care, quality, and quantity of life. Does the older adult want measures to be taken to prolong life at all costs, or does he or she wish for a natural death? What are the boundaries in which suffering can be minimized? Are there any persons the person who is dying feels comfortable with, who can act as a proxy and will ensure that the person's wishes will be carried out? Answers to these questions are essential in the promotion of an appropriate and good death. Before a directive is completed, the family and support persons should discuss whether those who are to be involved are comfortable with the decisions and will adhere to the directive. For older adults without family, the nurse may become a sounding board, but he or she must take care to not influence the outcome and may never serve as a proxy in a patient's LW or durable power of attorney.

Approaching Death

As long ago as 1991, the U.S. Supreme Court reviewed the case of *Cruzan v. State of Missouri* and confirmed a person's right to refuse unwanted treatment. No distinction was made between withholding and withdrawing treatment. Later, case law characterized tube feeding and intravenous feeding as medical treatments (also referred to as *artificial sustenance*) and therefore these could also be refused. Nonetheless, questions remained. These rights have not always been granted, and questions have been raised regarding the relationship between patients' wishes and the responsibilities and activities of health care providers. The questions have become more and more complex as states and countries wrestle with questions of physician-assisted suicide, euthanasia, terminal sedation, and double effect.

Physician-Assisted Suicide

The potential for a person's ultimate control of his or her dying has risen to state and Supreme Court levels in the United States and to equivalent levels in other countries. In 1994 and again in 1997, voters in Oregon were the first to pass legislation legalizing a person's right to end his or her life in very specific circumstances. The voters in Washington State passed similar legislation in 2008 with identical restrictions. Vermont, Hawaii, Colorado, the District of Columbia, and New Jersey (2019) followed. Montana courts ruled that there was nothing in the state law prohibiting physician-assisted suicide, but no definitive laws have been passed (Death with Dignity National Center, 2018). In 2015 a law was enacted in California allowing physician-assisted suicide. However, in 2018 the law was overturned in court (PEW Charitable Trust [1996-2019]).

Physician-assisted suicide is legal in Canada, Columbia, part of Australia, Switzerland, Germany, South Korea, Japan, and Finland. In many other countries, persons' involvement is subject to criminal prosecution. The status of any one state or country is subject to change. The numbers of people who have chosen this route to end their suffering have been relatively few. At the same time, the number of referrals to palliative care programs and hospice services has increased.

Palliative Sedation

In 1997, the U.S. Supreme Court declared that while universal physician-assisted suicide was illegal, pharmacological sedation for the relief of refractory symptoms (e.g., pain, nausea and vomiting, dyspnea), by whatever means necessary, was acceptable. This has been referred to as *terminal sedation* but is more accurately *palliative sedation* (Cherny et al, 2018).

The intent of the sedation is to provide comfort but to go no further. This is based on the concept of *double effect*—that is, if the sedation provides comforts even if it is possible that death is hastened, it is considered neither assisted suicide nor euthanasia and is acceptable. While replete with ethical questions, the *intention* must be to relieve the suffering with treatment and to that extent only (Seale et al, 2015). Active euthanasia, wherein the goal is relief through death, remains illegal everywhere in the United States but both euthanasia and physician-assisted suicide are legal in Belgium, the Netherlands, Luxemburg, Austria (2019), and Colombia (MDMD, 2018).

PROMOTING HEALTHY DYING WHILE AGING: IMPLICATIONS FOR GERONTOLOGICAL NURSING

Nurses are professional grievers, in caring for those who are frail and dying in any setting; we are repeatedly exposed to the death of our patients. Some consider the death of a patient a failure—they have "lost" the person they cared for. However, when it is a good death, it can be viewed as a professional success because the nurse provided safe conduct for the dying and gentle care for the survivors (Box 35.13). We can use the reminders of our own mortality as motivation to live the best we can with the time we have. Nurses can seek support and offer support to each other. As grievers, we too may need to tell the story of the dying person to those professionals around us, in either formal or informal support groups; and we need

---

BOX 35.13 Tips for Best Practice

Safe Conduct

The responsibility of the nurse is to provide what is referred to as "safe conduct," helping the dying and their families navigate through unknown waters to a good and appropriate death (i.e., one that a person would choose if choosing were possible). A good and appropriate death is one in which one's needs are met for as long as possible, and life is never without meaning.

---

to listen to our colleagues' stories, over and over again if necessary.

Caring for older adults requires knowledge of the grieving and dying processes and skills in providing relief of symptoms or palliative care (Table 35.1). However, it is also acknowledged that working daily with the grieving or dying is an art. The development of the art necessitates inner strength. The nurse needs to have spiritual strength—strength from within. This does not mean that the nurse must have a specific religious orientation or affiliation but, rather, that he or she has a positive belief in self, a connection to others, and a belief that life has meaning and there is such a thing as a good death. The effective nurse has developed a personal philosophy of life and of death. Although this may change over time and cannot be assumed to

---

TABLE 35.1 Best Nursing Practice: Signs and Symptoms of Approaching Death.

Physical	Rationale	Intervention
Coolness	Diminished peripheral circulation to increase circulation to vital organs	Socks, light cotton blankets or warm blankets if needed; do not use electric blanket
Increased sleeping	Conservation of energy	Respect need for increased rest; inquire as to their wishes regarding timing of companionship
Disorientation	Metabolic changes	Identify self by name before speaking to patient; speak clearly, and truthfully
Fecal and/or urinary incontinence	Increased muscle relaxation	Change bedding as needed; use bed pads; avoid indwelling catheters
Noisy respirations	Poor circulation of body fluids, immobilization, and the inability to expectorate	Elevate the head with pillows, or raise the head of the bed, or both; gently turn the head to the side to drain
Restlessness	Metabolic changes and relative cerebral anoxia	Calm the patient by speech and action; reduce light; gently rub back, stroke arms, or read aloud; play soothing music; do not use restraints
Decreased intake of food and fluids	Body conservation of energy for function	Provide nutrition within limits expressed by patient or in advance directive; semisolid liquids easiest to swallow; protect mouth and lips from discomfort of dryness
Decreased urine output	Decreased fluid intake and decreased circulation to kidney	None
Altered breathing pattern	Metabolic and oxygen changes	Elevate the head of bed; speak gently to patient
Emotional or Spiritual	**Presumed Rationale**	**Intervention**
Withdrawal	Prepares the patient for release and detachment and letting go	Continue communicating in a normal manner using a normal voice tone; identify self by name; give permission to "let go"
Vision-like experiences of dead friends or family; religious vision	Preparation for transition	Accept the reality of the experience for the person; reassure him or her that the experience is normal
Restlessness	Tension, fear, unfinished business	Listen to patient express his or her fears, sadness, and anger; facilitate completion of business if possible
Unusual communication	Signals readiness to let go	Say what needs to be said to the dying patient; kiss, hug, cry with him or her as appropriate

be held by anyone else, one's beliefs about life and death will help the nurse through difficult times. Emotional maturity allows the nurse to deal with disappointment and postponement of immediate wants or desires. Maturity means that the nurse can reach out for help for self when needed. Finally, to provide comfort to grieving persons, nurses must be comfortable with their own lives or at least be able to set aside their own sadness and grief while working with that of others (Box 35.14).

It is always important to remember that some nurses are unable to care for the dying because of their own unresolved conflicts and should not be expected to function in these roles. This may be a temporary situation associated with events in the nurse's life or something deeper, such as a traumatic experience in the death of a loved one. The nurse should recognize his or her limitations and should defer care to another nurse when appropriate. In doing so, the nurse gives the most compassionate care possible.

> ### BOX 35.14 Nursing Skills Needed for the Practice of Palliative/End-of-Life Care
>
> - Have ability to talk to patients and families about dying.
> - Be knowledgeable about symptom control and pain-control techniques.
> - Have ability to provide comfort-oriented nursing interventions.
> - Recognize physical changes that precede imminent death.
> - Deal with own feelings.
> - Deal with angry patients and families.
> - Be knowledgeable and deal with the ethical issues in administering end-of-life palliative therapies.
> - Be knowledgeable and inform patients about advance directives.
> - Be knowledgeable of the legal issues in administering end-of-life palliative care.
> - Be adaptable and sensitive to religious and cultural perspectives.

Modified from White KR, Coyne PJ, Patel UB: Are nurses adequately prepared for end-of-life care? *J Nurs Scholarsh* 33:147–151, 2001. Sigma Theta Tau International.

KEY CONCEPTS

- Grief is a physical, emotional, and spiritual/existential response to loss.
- The Loss Response Model can be used to guide the development of nursing interventions designed to optimize the quality of life for those who are grieving and those who are dying.
- Persons who are at risk for complicated grieving should receive specialized and skilled supportive care.
- The individual's response to loss and grief is similar to how he or she has dealt with other stressors in life.
- An individual is living until he or she has died; the nurse works with the person and significant others to maintain as high a quality of life as possible before, during, and after the loss or death.
- Hope is fluid and empowering; it can be appropriately supported during any aspect of the process of loss, grief, and mourning. Hope generates courage and resilience.

- Palliative care is that which focuses on comfort rather than cure.
- Hospice is a specific interprofessional approach to the provision of palliative care.
- Palliative care can be provided regardless of setting.
- Advance directives and living wills provide persons the opportunity to express their end-of-life wishes and appoint a proxy to act on those wishes, when they are unable to do so for themselves.
- Physician-assisted suicide is now legal or permitted in several states and countries. As a result of the law, the care of the dying has improved.
- Double effect is the accepted practice that permits the provision of as much medication as needed to relieve suffering, even if the amount has the potential to hasten death. It occurs in the context of palliative sedation.

NURSING STUDY: COPING WITH DYING

Jesse was simply unable to believe that his wife was dying. The physician told Jesse that Jeanette was in the early stages of multiple myeloma, and that she might die in less than a year or she might have remissions and live another decade. Jesse and his wife had worked hard all their lives and raised two sons. Now they were both retired and financially secure and thought the best years of their lives were ahead of them. However, both Jesse and Jeanette were the type who approached a problem head-on. They gathered all the relevant material they could find about multiple myeloma and assiduously studied it. Jeanette said that she did not want to mention her problem to others because she thought that she was unable to deal with "their piteous cancer looks." She also stressed that she expected to have long remissions and to live at least 10 more years. So why trouble friends and family? As a result of her decision, Jesse was unable to share his fear and grief because he had promised to respect Jeanette's wishes in that regard. She began a series of chemotherapeutic drugs, and friends began to

notice her lethargy. They began to worry about her, but she insisted, "I'm just fine." Six months passed with a steady downward course in Jeanette's condition. Her sons began to suspect she had a malignancy, and one son, Rob, asked outright, "Are you hiding a serious illness from us?" She denied it, but Rob also noticed that Jesse was withdrawing into himself and that he was drinking more than usual. Rob knew something was wrong but was at a loss. When Rob went to the family physician for his annual checkup, the office nurse said, "Oh, Rob, how is your mother doing?"

- Considering the situation and the current regulations about the protection of patient privacy, how would you respond to the son's next question if you were the nurse?
- As a nurse, how could you promote communication within this family to help them move toward open awareness?
- What is your priority in attending to the needs of Jesse? Of Jeanette? Of their children?

CRITICAL THINKING QUESTIONS AND ACTIVITIES

1. Explore your likely responses to being given a terminal diagnosis. What coping mechanisms work for you?
2. With which level of awareness approach would you be most comfortable? As a nurse? As a patient?
3. If you believe that you are able, discuss your grief process when you dealt with the loss of someone special in your life.
4. Practice with a partner several methods that you will use to introduce the topic of dying with a patient who is critically ill and is not expected to live long.
5. Describe how you would deal with a dying person and his or her family when these family members are especially protective of each other.
6. Discuss and strategize how you would bring up the topic of advance directives.
7. Explore with family and friends their thoughts on completing an advance directive.

RESEARCH QUESTIONS

1. What advance directive is legally recognized in your state?
2. What is the American Nurses Association viewpoint on nurses' involvement in assisted suicide?
3. Select a culture other than your own and explore loss, grief, and morning rituals. How often are they used?

REFERENCES

Alward PD: Betty Newman's system model. In Parker ME, Smith MC, editors: *Nursing theories and nursing practice,* ed 3, Philadelphia, 2010, FA Davis, pp 182–201.

ANA: *Nurses' roles and responsibilities in providing care and support at the end of life,* 2016. ANA Position Statement. https://www.nursingworld.org/~4af078/globalassets/docs/ana/ethics/endoflife-positionstatement.pdf. Accessed March 2019.

Beck E, Jones SJ: Children of the condemned: grieving the loss of a father on death row, *Omega (Westport)* 56(2):191–215, 2007–2008.

Bristowe K, Marshall S, Harding R: The bereavement experiences of lesbian, gay, bisexual and/or trans* people who have lost a partner: a systematic review, thematic synthesis and modeling of the literature, *Palliat Med* 30(8):730–744, 2016.

Brown J: Five death rituals to give you a new view on funerals, *NewScientist,* 2017. https://www.newscientist.com/article/2152283-five-death-rituals-to-give-you-a-new-view-on-funerals/. Accessed July 2018.

Bryant S: *Death and dying: How different cultures view the end,* 2017. https://countrynavigator.com/blog/expert-view/death/. Accessed July 2018.

Burke A, Burgess SL, Cadet T: Utilizing evidence-based assessment instruments to detect well-being and distress in English and Spanish-speaking caregivers of individuals affected by dementia, *Dementia (London)* 2017. doi:10.1177/1471301217739095.

Cherny N, Smith TJ, Savarese DMF: *Palliative sedation,* 2018. https://www.uptodate.com/contents/palliative-sedation. Accessed July 2018.

Coolen PR: *Cultural relevance in end-of-life care,* 2012. https://ethnomed.org/clinical/end-of-life/cultural-relevance-in-end-of-life-care. Accessed July 2018.

Death with Dignity: *Take action in your state: Death with dignity around the U.S.,* 2018. https://www.deathwithdignity.org/take-action/. Accessed July 2018.

Doka KJ: *Disenfranchised grief: new directions, challenges, and strategies for practice,* Champaign, IL, 2002, Research Press.

Ferguson R: Care coordination at end of life: The nurse's role, *Nursing* 48(2):11–13, 2018.

Giacquinta B: Helping families face the crisis of cancer, *Am J Nurs* 77:1585–1588, 1977.

Glaser B, Strauss A: *Awareness of dying,* Chicago, 1965, AVC.

Glaser BG, Strauss AL: *Time for dying,* Chicago, 1968, Aldine.

Hall C: Beyond Kübler-Ross: recent developments in our understanding of grief and bereavement, *InPsych* 33(6), 2011. http://www.psychology.org.au/publications/inpsych/2011. Accessed July 2018.

Herbert RS, Schultz R, Copeland V, Arnold RM: What questions do family caregivers want to discuss with health care providers in order to prepare for the death of a loved one? An ethnographic study of caregivers of patients at end of life, *J Palliat Med* 11:476–483, 2008.

Hong M, Yi EH, Johnson KJ, Adamek ME: Facilitators and barriers for advance care planning among ethnic and racial minorities in the U.S.: a systematic review of the current literature, *J Immigr Minor Health* 20(5):1277–1287, 2018.

Horacek BJ: Toward a more viable model of grieving and consequences for older persons, *Death Stud* 15:459–472, 1991.

Jett KJ, Jett SW: *The loss response model,* 2014, unpublished manuscript.

Jones SJ, Beck E: Disenfranchised grief and nonfinite loss as experienced by the families of death row inmates, *Omega (Westport)* 54(4):281–299, 2007–2008.

Kübler-Ross E: *On death and dying,* New York, 1969, Macmillan.

Maciejewski PK, Maercker A, Boelen PA, Prigerson HG: "Prolonged grief disorder" and "persistent complex bereavement disorder," but not "complicated griefs," are one and the same diagnostic entity: an analysis of data from the Yale bereavement stud, *World Psychiatry* 15(3):266–275, 2016.

Maslow AH: A theory of human motivation, *Psychol Rev* 50:370–396, 1943.

Mazanec P, Panke JT: Cultural considerations in palliative care. In Ferrell BR, Coyle N, editors: *Oxford textbook of palliative nursing,* ed 4, New York, 2015, Oxford University Press, pp 701–713.

My Death My Decision: *Assisted dying in other countries,* 2018. https://www.mydeath-mydecision.org.uk/info/assisted-dying-in-other-countries/.

NHPCO: *NHPCO facts and figures: Hospice care in America,* 2018, National Hospice and Palliative Care Organization. https://www.nhpco.org/. Accessed July 2018.

National Coalition for Hospice and Palliative Care: *Clinical practice guidelines for quality palliative care,* ed 4, 2019. https://www.nationalcoalitionhpc.org/ncp. Accessed March 2019.

National POLST Paradigm: *Guidance for health care professionals to identify appropriate patients for POLST*, 2019. https://polst.org/professionals-page/?pro=1. Accessed March 2019.

Neimeyer RA, Sands DC: Meaning reconstruction in bereavement: from principles to practice. In Neimeyer RA, Harris DL, Winokuer HR, Thornton GF, editors: *Grief and bereavement in contemporary society: bridging research and practice*, New York, 2011, Routledge.

Pattison EM: The experience of dying. In Pattison EM, editor: *The experience of dying*, Englewood Cliffs, NJ, 1977, Prentice-Hall.

PEW Charitable Trust: *Judge overturn's California's physician-assisted suicide law,* 1996-2019. https://www.pewtrusts.org/en/research-and-analysis/blogs/stateline/2018/05/16/judge-overturns-californias-physicianassisted-suicide-law. Accessed March 2019.

Richardson VE, Bennett KM, Carr D, Gallagher S, Kim J, Fields N: How does bereavement get under the skin? The effects of late-life spousal loss on cortisol levels, *J Gerontol B, Psychol Sci Soc Sci* 70(3):341–347, 2015.

Roser R, Rimane E, Vogel A, Rau J, Hagl M: Treating prolonged grief disorder with prolonged grief-specific cognitive behavioral therapy: study protocol for a randomized controlled trial, *Trials* [Published online], 2018. doi:10.1186.s13063-018-2618-3. Accessed March 2019.

Seale C, Raus K, Bruinsma S, et al: The language of sedation in end-of life care: the ethical reasoning of care providers in three countries, *Health (London)* 19(4):339–354, 2015.

Shear MK, Ghesquiere A, Glickman K: Bereavement and complicated grief, *Curr Psychiatry Rep* 15(11):406, 2013.

St. Christopher's: *Dame Cicely Saunders—her life and her work.* http://www.stchristophers.org.uk/about/damecicelysaunders. Accessed July 2018.

Toyama H, Honda A: Using narrative approach for anticipatory grief among family caregivers at home, *Glob Qual Nurs Res* 3, 2016.

Wales J, Kurahashi AM, Husain A: The interaction of socioeconomic status with place of death: a qualitative analysis of physician experiences, *BMC Palliat Care* 17(1):87, 2018.

Weisman A: *Coping with cancer*, New York, 1979, McGraw-Hill.

World Health Organization: *Palliative care,* 2018. http://www.who.int/news-room/facts-in-pictures/detail/palliative-care. Accessed July 2018.

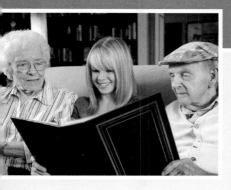

36

Self-Actualization, Spirituality, and Transcendence

Priscilla Ebersole[a] and Theris A. Touhy

http://evolve.elsevier.com/Touhy/TwdHlthAging

A STUDENT SPEAKS

Well, I always went to church with my parents when I was a child, but it was really boring. Now, I sometimes go with my grandmother to make her happy. I see how important it is to her, and I wonder if it will be important to me when I get really old. I'm just too busy right now.

Lori, age 22

AN OLDER ADULT SPEAKS

This is a real problem! I have three children and don't want them to squabble over my things when I'm gone. I would like it if they would each choose something special that would remind them of me, but every time I bring it up they cut me off and won't talk about it. I know there will be a big fight over the piano!

Mabel, age 84

LEARNING OBJECTIVES

On completion of this chapter, the reader will be able to:

1. Provide a comprehensive definition of self-actualization and identify several qualities of self-actualized older adults.
2. Discuss the nursing role in relation to the self-actualization of older adults.
3. Describe several examples of transcendence as experienced by older adults.
4. Specify various types of creative self-expression and describe their positive impact on health, illness, and quality of life among older adults.
5. Understand the meaning of spirituality in the lives of older adults and discuss nursing interventions to facilitate spiritual health.
6. Define the concept of legacy and name several types of legacies and ways that the nurse can facilitate their expression.

Self-actualization, *spirituality*, and *transcendence* are vague, ambiguous terms that mean whatever the theorist thinks. These expressions also serve as umbrella terms for other conditions and situations that are addressed throughout this chapter. These terms overlap a great deal, but we have attempted to tease out the meanings for the reader, knowing that the perception of the reader will cast a particular interpretation that we may not have thought or intended. These conditions are ineffable, within the awareness of the individual but often inexpressible. Why, if these concepts are so obscure, do we include them as the final chapter in a text for nurses working with older adults? Because these concepts are the life tasks of aging, seldom fully

approached earlier. Concerns of the young are to become established as adults; middle-aged persons are overwhelmed with the requirements of success and survival.

Older adults are more in touch with their inner psychological life than at any other point in the life cycle. Ferreting out the reason for being and the meaning of life is the concern of older adults. "As people age, confronting mortality is part of it, but as things change, they begin to recognize who they are and who they aren't, the strengths they have and haven't. They begin to think about the value and meaning of life. Tending to look more inwards rather than outwards often happens when we are 45 to 50, but there's a screaming need for it when we reach

---

[a]Special thanks to Dr. Priscilla Ebersole, the original author of this chapter, for her foundational and very wise contributions.

BOX 36.1 Developmental Phases in the Second Half of Life

Midlife reevaluation: Early 40s to late 50s and characterized by seriously confronting the sense of one's own mortality and thinking about time remaining instead of time gone by. A catalyst for uncovering unrealized creative sides of ourselves.

Liberation: Mid-50s to mid-70s and characterized by a sense of personal freedom to speak one's mind and do what needs to be done. With retirement comes a new experience of personal liberation and having time to experiment with something different.

Summing-up: Late 60s to the 80s and beyond and characterized by the desire to find larger meaning in the story of one's life and to deal with unresolved conflicts and unfinished business. Motivation to give the wisdom accrued throughout life, share lessons and fortunes through autobiography and personal storytelling, philanthropy, community activism, and volunteerism.

Encore: Any time from the late 70s to the end of life and characterized by the desire to restate and reaffirm major themes in one's life and explore new variations on those themes or further attend to unfinished business or unresolved conflicts and a desire to live well until the end.

From Cohen G: Research on creativity and aging: the positive impact of the arts on health and illness, *Generations* 30(1):7–15, 2006.

---

85 or 90" (Bernstein, 2009). An understanding of the developmental phases in the second half of life assists in understanding the journey toward self-actualization (Box 36.1).

Nurses will likely see numerous older adults who are apparently not seeking any of these esoteric states of existence and have never tried to cultivate their deepest inner nature. We live in a mechanistic, scientifically based culture in which cultivation of immeasurable states of being has not been necessarily regarded or regarded at all. The dramatic increase in the population of older adults has been considered a problem to be solved in an era of dwindling resources rather than a resource to enrich society.

Despite all the human efforts for the past millennia, we have not been able to completely grasp or dissect the human soul. I have many times approached this subject incorrectly by asking individuals what it is like to be old. Now that I am old, what it is like seems too concrete. What is the meaning of this stage of life? Every nurse must ask this question of his or her older clients, friends, and parents. Do not ask on your way out the door. For many people, this notion will take some pondering. For some, it will open the door of their later lives just a crack. Others will be enlightened and will teach you a great deal.

SELF-ACTUALIZATION

Self-actualization is the highest expression of one's individual potential and implies inner motivation that has been freed to express the most unique self or the "authentic person" (Maslow, 1959, p. 3). The crux of self-actualization is defining life in such a way as to allow room for continual discovery of self. A critical consideration in developing self-actualization is an underlying sense of mastery and a sense of coherence in the life situation. This effort depends to a large extent on individual attributes and self-esteem. In this chapter, we hope to expose the nurse to the myriad evidences of self-actualization

in old age and suggest ways in which the nurse can assist older adults in seeking their own unique way of living, growing, and making meaning. The focus is on nursing actions that may encourage older adults to seek new possibilities within themselves.

Characteristics of the Self-Actualized

As we age, threats to self-esteem are strong if value is measured only by attainment, containment, power, and influence. Ethics, values, humor, courage, altruism, and integrity flourish in people who continue to grow toward self-actualization. Numerous other attributes can be mentioned. We focus only on those qualities that seem most pertinent to the older adult whom health care professionals are serving (Box 36.2).

Courage

Courage is the quality of mind or spirit that enables a person to conquer fear and despair in the face of difficulty, danger, pain, or uncertainty. An older adult with diabetes, amputations, and failing vision sits in his room at the retirement home, looking out the window for hours each day, for weeks, months, and years. Yet he retains his positive spirit and love of life. This is courage. An older lady crippled with arthritis attends her ailing spouse, who no longer recognizes her. This is courage. When asking older adults how they keep going day by day, various answers are given. No one has ever said to me, "It is because I am courageous." Older adults need to be told. A gold star can be given to people who have lived and survived the long battle of living many years filled with both joy and pain. Memorials are made for people who die in battle, but few monuments are raised to those who courageously wake every morning with no great purpose or challenge to push them out of bed.

Tara Cortes, executive director of the Hartford Institute for Geriatric Nursing, shares the following quote from a 91-year-old gentleman: "It's a decision I make every morning when I

BOX 36.2 Traits of Self-Actualized People

- Time competent: The person uses past and future to live more fully in the present.
- Inner directed: The person's source of direction depends on internal forces more than on others.
- Flexible: The person can react situationally, without unreasonable restrictions.
- Sensitive to self: The person is responsive to his or her own feelings.
- Spontaneous: The person is able and willing to be himself or herself.
- Values self: The person accepts and demonstrates strengths as a person.
- Accepts self: The person approves of self, in spite of weaknesses or deficiencies.
- Positively views others: The person sees both the bad and the good in others as essentially good and constructive.
- Positively views life: The person sees the opposites of life as meaningfully related.
- Acceptance of aggressiveness: The person is able to accept own feelings of anger and aggressiveness.
- Capable of intimate contact: The person is able to develop warm interpersonal relationships with others.

wake up. I have a choice; I can spend the day in bed recounting the difficulty I have with parts of my body that no longer work, or get out of bed and be thankful for the ones that do. Each day is a gift, and as long as my eyes open, I'll focus on the new day and all the happy memories I've stored away just for this time in my life" (Cortes, 2013). The capacity of the spirit to find meaning in existence is often remarkable. Nurses may ask, "What sustains you in your present situation?"

Altruism

A high degree of helping behaviors is present in many older adults. The very old will remember the Great Depression and the altruism that kept people physically and spiritually alive. Neighbor helped neighbor long before the government came to the rescue. Apparently, a sense of meaning in life is strongly tied to survival and is derived from the conviction of, in some way, being needed by others. Many nurses are in the field because of altruistic motives and can understand the importance of assisting others. This idea might be discussed with the older adult.

Volunteering often involves new role development and endeavors that expand one's awareness. When volunteer services are considered as a means of personal enrichment and an expression of altruism, it is important for the older adult to augment some latent interest areas and launch into pursuits perhaps unavailable earlier because of time constraints or other commitments. Nurses may question older adults about latent interests and talents that they may want to cultivate.

Humor

Metcalf (1993) explains humor: it originates in the Latin root *humour,* meaning fluid and flexible, able to flow around and wear away obstacles. In the same way that water sustains our life and well-being, humor sustains our mental well-being. Cousins (1979) and many other researchers have recognized the importance of humor in recovery from illness. The physiological effects of humor stimulate production of catecholamines and hormones and increase pain tolerance by releasing endorphins.

Older adults often initiate humor, and, in our seriousness, we may overlook the dry wit or, worse, perceive it as confusion. Older adults are not a humorless group and frequently laugh at themselves. Objections to jokes about old age seem to emanate from the young far more than the old. Perhaps the old, from the vantage point of a lifetime, can more clearly see human predicaments. Ego transcendence (Peck, 1955) allows one to step back and view the self and situation without the intensity and despair of the egocentric individual.

Continuous Moral Development

The moral development of mankind, on an individual and collective basis, has been of interest to philosophers and religious leaders throughout history. The driving forces of morality are love (Plato) and intellect (Aristotle).

Kohlberg's refinements of his original theories have focused on the evidence, derived from autobiographies, that in maturity, transformations of moral outlook take place. Kohlberg posited old age as a seventh stage of moral development that goes beyond reasoning and reaches awareness of one's relative participation in universal morality. This stage of moral development involves identification with a more enduring moral perspective than that of one's own life span (Kohlberg and Power, 1981). This effort involves moral expansion and the exemplary impact of the fully developing older adult on the following generations, born and unborn. We have come to believe that these exemplary lives may be the most important function of older adults as we decry the honor and recognition given to individuals who seem to have little integrity or reliability. Youngsters must have models of honorable, truthful, and honest older adults if we hope to cultivate these qualities in society and human experience.

Self-Renewal

Self-renewal is an ongoing process that ideally continues through adult life as one becomes self-actualized (Hudson, 1999). According to Hudson, self-renewal involves the following:

- Commitment to beliefs
- Connecting to the world
- Times of solitude
- Episodic breaks from responsibility
- Contact with the natural world
- Creative self-expression
- Adaptation to changes
- Learning from down times

Collective Self-Actualization

The collective power of self-actualized older adults has already brought about many changes in society. Power is a term describing the capacity of an individual or group to accomplish something, to take command, to exert authority, and to influence. The self-actualized older adult is powerful and confident. Power is the gateway to resources and recognition.

The age-equality movement, older citizens returning to school, and the revolution of older adults in movements such as the Gray Panthers have produced major changes in the status and recognition of older adults. Gray Panthers recognize that issues of aging are not narrow or exclusive but, rather, are representative of human rights for people of all ages. Maggie Kuhn (1979), founder of the Gray Panthers, died in 1995 at the age of 89, but her beliefs and followers survive. Kuhn perceived that the issues confronting older adult are not those of self-interest. As "elders of the tribe," the old should seek "survival of the tribe" (Kuhn, 1979, p. 3).

WISDOM

Wisdom is an ancient concept that has historically been associated with the older adults of a society. Wisdom represents the pinnacle of human development and can be compared to Maslow's self-actualization or Erickson's ego integrity. In many cultures, older adults are respected for their years of experience and are awarded the role of wise older adult in political, judicial, cultural, and religious systems.

In recent years, there has been renewed interest in the concept of wisdom and the capacity of the aging brain to develop unique capacities. Many skills improve with age but are not identified on standard cognitive screens, and certain testing conditions have exaggerated age-related declines in cognitive performance (Chapter 5). The bulk of research has focused on cognitive declines and strategies to help older adults find ways to overcome cognitive failings. Because of this emphasis, research on cognitive capacities in aging and possible ways to stimulate wisdom has been limited.

Moving beyond Piaget's formal operational stage of cognitive development, adult development theories propose a more advanced cognitive stage, the postformal operational stage. In this stage, individuals develop the skills to view problems from multiple perspectives, utilize reflection, and communicate thoughtfully in complex and emotionally challenging situations (Parisi et al, 2009). Recent neuroimaging research has suggested that changes in the brain, once seen only as compensation for declining skills, are now thought to indicate development of new capacities (Chapter 5).

Characteristics of Wisdom

One does not become wise simply because one grows old. Nor is wisdom achieved simply because of an accumulation of life experiences. Most agree that the achievement of wisdom is a developmental process that requires the ability to "integrate experiences across time and utilize these experiences in a reflective manner" (Parisi et al, 2009, p. 867). Maturity, integrity, generativity, the ability to overcome negative personality characteristics such as neuroticism or self-centeredness, superior judgment skills in difficult life situations, the ability to cope with difficult challenges in life, and a strong sense of the ultimate meaning and purpose of life are also associated with wisdom (Ardelt, 2004) (Box 36.3). Wisdom is a major contributor to successful aging (Reichstadt et al, 2010). The renewed emphasis on wisdom and other cognitive capabilities that can develop with age provides a view of aging that reflects the history of many cultures and provides a much more hopeful view of both aging and human development.

Paths to growing older and wiser can be fostered throughout life. Viewing older adults as resources for younger people, our society places the reason for and the immense value of aging at the center of focus. This is in contrast to the view of aging as inevitable decline, personal diminishment, disengagement from life, and a drain on society. Nursing too must turn to the wise leaders who came before us as we chart our course for the future (Chapter 2). Priscilla Ebersole, one of the geriatric nursing pioneers, and coauthor of this chapter, shares her reflections on wisdom from the perspective of her 90 years (Box 36.4).

With the prospect of longer and healthier lives, older adults are looking for more meaningful and challenging ways to foster continued growth and contribute to society. Programs such as Foster Grandparents, the Experience Corps, and the Sage-ing Guild are examples of this new view.

BOX 36.3   Dimensions of Wisdom

- Cognitive: Knowledge and acceptance of the positive and negative aspects of human nature, the limits of knowledge, and of life's unpredictability and uncertainties; a desire to know the truth and comprehend the significance and deeper meaning of experiences, phenomena, and events
- Reflective: Being able to perceive phenomena and events from multiple perspectives; self-awareness, self-examination, self-insight; absence of subjectivity and projections (e.g., the tendency to blame other people or circumstances for one's own situation, decisions, or feelings)
- Affective: Sympathetic and compassionate love for others; positive emotions and behaviors toward others

From Ardelt M: Wisdom as expert knowledge system: a critical review of a contemporary operationalization of an ancient concept, *Hum Dev* 47:257–285, 2004.

BOX 36.4   Reflections on Wisdom: Priscilla Ebersole, Geriatric Nursing Pioneer

In thinking about wisdom, I wonder what it is and if we ever achieve anything near that in one lifetime. I now have more questions about life than I have answers.

- Where are we in the process of human evolution? We seem to be consumed with speed and technical wonders. What about the extrasensory perceptions and amazing coincidences that seemingly arise randomly? Are we still primitives?
- Dying: Doesn't it present more questions? I have become immunized as so many I love have preceded me, but it would be wonderful to know how much time I have—or would it?
- How can one develop true compassion? I have flashes of it, but find I still have many judgmental feelings about many persons and events. Is this not practical?
- How can I learn more from others? I am rather trapped in my own skin and imperfections.
- Is it true that our hormones really affect us so much? Yes, undoubtedly I have become much more aggressive with the almost total loss of estrogen. Do I care?
- Is the search for prolongevity a worthy goal? Only when one is healthy and has something to offer the world. But, really, what is healthy? Only function? Mind health?
- Does history really teach us anything? Though we seem to repeat so much of it yet pondering it and our roots remains significant for me. And what about the universe, both macro and micro of which we really still know so little? Pondering and wondering, I will never know even a bit of all I wish.

Yet becoming old is *becoming* as life seems to hold many lifetimes in one. There are so many challenges and circumstances that change one's perspective and beliefs. One begins to feel a part of and connected to every living thing. The youth and elders in one's lifetime are so significant in one's philosophy. Grandchildren and great grandchildren open new vistas of thought and opportunities to redo some of the faltering actions of parenthood.

It seems one important goal is to learn to enjoy life in spite of all the bumps one experiences along the way. Maybe learning to be content with whatever one is and whatever one can do and one's tribe, family, becomes increasingly important. One of my granddaughters said she loves to see how much I enjoy life and her ability to see that in me is something I will always treasure. That is a gift I hope to leave with her and others whom I contact. I think I have learned to really enjoy this precious gift of life. Catherine, my friend who died at 106, taught me more about aging than any experience in my life. She still giggled like a school girl as she told me of some amusing event in her life.

CREATIVITY

Creativity is a bridge between the growing self and the transcending of self. Creativity may be the transit mechanism between self-actualization (the reaching of one's highest potential) and the step beyond, to transcend the limitations of ego. "Creativity has always been at the heart of our experience as human beings . . . this need for creativity never ends" (Perlstein, 2006, p. 5). American culture has neglected to recognize the innate creativity of older adults, who are too often viewed as debilitated, in need of medical attention, and the focus of societal problems. Promoting health in aging is more than targeting problems and developing interventions for health promotion and disease prevention. Aging encompasses potential and problems. A focus on creativity and aging and the positive impact of the arts on health, illness, and quality of life is gaining importance in our understanding of health and well-being among older adults.

The National Center for Creative Aging is dedicated to fostering the relationship between creative expression and quality of life for older adults. The *Beautiful Minds: Finding Your Lifelong Potential* campaign is an initiative from the Center that focuses on raising awareness of people who are keeping their minds beautiful and the actions people can take to maintain the brain (http://www.creativeaging.org/about-ncca-0). Research suggests that there are four dimensions to brain health: the nourished mind, the socially connected mind, the mentally active mind, and the physically active mind. These dimensions stress the importance of healthy diet, social engagement, cognitive stimulation, and physical activity to brain health.

Products of creativity are less important than creative attitudes. Curiosity, inquisitiveness, wonderment, puzzlement, and craving for understanding are creative attitudes. Much of the natural creative imagination of childhood is subdued by enculturation. As we age, some people seem able to break free of excessive enculturation and again express their free spirit when practical matters no longer demand their sole attention.

Creativity is often considered in terms of the arts, literature, and music. A truly self-actualized person may express creativity in any activity. Breaking through the habitual or traditional mode into authentic expression of self is creativity, whether it is through cooking, cleaning, planting, poetry, art, or teaching. Creative expression does not necessarily mean that the older adult has to create a work of art. Subtler ways of expressing creativity are present even in the frailest of older adults. Consider Dr. Ebersole's description of Catherine at 100 years old and living in a nursing home (Box 36.5).

Creative Arts for Older Adults

Maximizing the use of self in the later years in unique ways might be termed creative self-actualization. Many individuals will need the stimulus of an interested person to uncover latent interests and talents. Other adults will need encouragement to try new avenues of self-expression—some will be fitting for them and others not. Several ideas are presented here for nurses working with older adults who may need an introduction to creative use of leisure time.

BOX 36.5 Another View of Creativity: Catherine

Catherine was self-actualized and creative to the best possible extent. Her physical constraints were enormous: she had no material assets, her range of activity was limited to her small cubicle in a skilled nursing facility, and her body was frail. However, her spirit was strong, and she knew and used her potential. Catherine's creativity was expressed at each meal when she rearranged, mixed, and added to her food. She carefully chopped a pickle and sprinkled it on her cottage cheese and added a little honey to her applesauce. Each meal was a small adventure. Several friends would visit regularly and bring Catherine small items she enjoyed. They could always count on being entertained with creatively embroidered tales of the past. The gifts they brought were always used in extraordinary ways. A scarf might be tied around her head. Powder, perfume, books, and other things would be bartered for favors from staff members or given as gifts. Her radio brought news of the day interspersed with classical music. Catherine created a milieu in which she enjoyed life and maintained her self-esteem. That she was self-actualized was never in doubt. Her artistry overflowed in myriad small gestures.

Wikstrom suggests that art and aesthetics "help individuals know themselves, become more alive to human conditions, provide a new way of looking at themselves and the world, and offer opportunities for participation in new visual and auditory experiences" (2004, p. 30). Each person has a private, symbolic, feeling world that can be brought out by certain expressive activities.

Creative arts and expression offer great value to people with dementia and hold tremendous promise to improve quality of life. Programs of dance, storytelling (Chapter 6), music, poetry, and art should be included in activities for individuals with dementia. Killick (1997, 2000, 2008) has done beautiful work with poetry writing for persons who have dementia, and he has said that "people with dementia can often find a real solace and satisfaction and a creativity in speaking in this way and having it recognized as being of value because they're so used to being put down" (Killick, 2005).

At the Louis and Anne Green Memory and Wellness Center in the Christine E. Lynn College of Nursing at Florida Atlantic University, the "Artful Memories" program provides opportunities for individuals with mild to moderate dementia to learn techniques of artistic creation and expression in artistic media in a supportive and nonjudgmental environment (Chapter 29) (Fig. 36.1). Works created are on display at the Center and in local art museums and have also been made into calendars (Fig. 36.2). Participants have derived a great deal of pleasure, pride, stimulation, and camaraderie from the time spent creating art. More ideas for developing creative activities are presented in Box 36.6.

RECREATION

Recreation is akin to creation. The wisdom of regularly scheduled periods of recreation and recuperation following creative acts can be traced to early Jewish writings and the creation story. If God needed time to rest and recuperate, we certainly do. Inherent in creative acts is time for renewal, time for recreation. Burnout and boredom are companions of monotony and

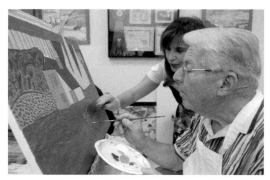

Fig. 36.1 Artful Memories Program. (Courtesy the Louis and Anne Green Memory and Wellness Center of the Christine E. Lynn College of Nursing at Florida Atlantic University.)

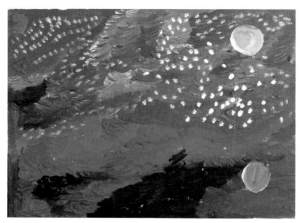

Fig. 36.2 Artwork created by Frances Hope Goldstein in the Florida Atlantic University (FAU) Louis and Anne Green Memory and Wellness Center "Artful Memories" program.

shorten the perceived life span by emptiness and vanished time. A change of scenery or companions may be exhilarating. The opportunity to be outside or look at beautiful scenery is also renewing. Many long-term care facilities are providing opportunities for gardening and enjoying nature. Retreats from routine to periods of recreation are important, as are retreats following intensive efforts. Resources that can enhance recreational activities and programs are presented in Box 36.7.

BRINGING YOUNG AND OLD TOGETHER

Larson (2006) suggests that intergenerational programs can "help older and younger people look beyond their generational stereotypes and know each other (body, mind, and spirit)" (p. 39). Intergenerational programs can be those in which older adults assist younger people (tutoring, mentoring, childcare, foster grandparent programs); those in which younger people assist older adults (social visits, meal assistance); and those in which the young and old serve together. Benefits of intergenerational programs for younger people include increased self-esteem and self-worth, improved behavior, increased involvement and success in school work, and a sense of historical and personal continuity. For older adults, contact with younger

people can promote life satisfaction, decrease isolation, help develop new skills and insights, promote fulfillment, establish new and meaningful relationships, and provide a sense of meaning and purpose. Examples of such programs include the Elders Share the Arts, Roots and Branches Theatre Company, and the Liz Lerman Dance Exchange.

Recognizing the developmental significance of contact between the generations, some long-term care facilities have included children in their milieu in various ways:

- *As residents* (children with profound developmental disabilities or severe neurological disabilities): Older adults rock, stroke, and cuddle these children, providing stimulation for both.
- *As a service to employees* (day care centers for children of employees): Older adults sometimes assist in the care and special programs for the children, such as reading stories or teaching basic skills (tying shoes, telling time).

BOX 36.7 Resources to Enhance Recreational Activities/Programs

- Local florists may present a flower show or provide a flower-arranging activity.
- Police/fire departments may give safety presentations.
- Local religious leaders may lead readings and discussions of religious/philosophical works.
- Craft suppliers may give demonstrations.
- Local pharmacists may give talks on medication use.
- Nurses or nursing students may give talks on health and well-being in aging.
- Clothing stores can sponsor fashion shows.
- Bakeries may give demonstrations of pastry decoration.
- Beauty supply houses may give makeup demonstrations.
- Travel agencies may present slide shows.
- Librarians may institute great book discussions or other activities.
- Students from community colleges may provide numerous educational events and activities.
- Garden clubs or horticultural groups may provide gardening classes.
- Collectors' clubs may talk about collecting stamps, antiques, coins, or memorabilia.
- Historical societies may give tours to historic places of interest.
- Whenever possible, events should be planned as field trips to the sites of the locals involved because trips add elements of additional interest, stimulation, and involvement in the community at large.

- *In adopt-a-grandparent programs:* One child affiliates with a resident with periodic visits, cards, and inclusion of the grandparent in some special family events.

Interesting intergenerational living programs in the Netherlands, France, and Cleveland, Ohio, offer rent-free living to college students in retirement and nursing homes. In the Netherlands, students are required to spend at least 30 hours a month acting as "good neighbors" by performing activities such as teaching new skills in use of email and social media, Skyping, walking dogs, watching sports, celebrating birthdays, and offering company. At Judson Manor in Cleveland, students from the Cleveland Institutes of Art and Music are integrated into the resident population. Students participate in the musical arts committee, assist staff therapists, volunteer at various events, and give quarterly performances to the residents (Hansman, 2015; Harris, 2016; Jansen, 2016). These innovative programs are featured in a short video (https://www.usatoday.com/videos/news/nation/2017/02/24/students-take-up-residence-retirement-homes/98342876/).

Nurses in the community may want to explore potential intergenerational experiences that might be of interest to older adults. Area Agencies on Aging can provide information on intergenerational programs available in the community. Although there are benefits to intergenerational contact when desired by the older adult, certain pitfalls must be considered. Not all older adults will enjoy contact with children. Contacts with the very young, energetic child must be brief, or the older adult is likely to become exhausted and the benefits will decrease. In intergenerational programs, young people need consistent supervision, support, and training in the developmental aspects of old age. Similarly, older adults will also benefit from education and support in understanding developmental tasks of children and effective methods of intergenerational communication.

PROMOTING HEALTHY AGING: IMPLICATIONS FOR GERONTOLOGICAL NURSING

In this chapter, we have considered what aging can be and that the last years can truly actualize the most unique capacities of older adults. Our functions as nurses who value self-actualization are (1) to continually spur our clients to ask "What is possible and suitable for me?" and (2) to assist them in finding appropriate resources and, when needed, assist in implementing activities toward self-actualization. The nature of self-actualization is self-determination and direction. Nurses are ancillary to the process but may be needed to stir the beginnings of the search. In doing so, we may move forward with our own search.

Self-actualization implies that one actualizes the potential of self through various mechanisms. We have mentioned only a few of these mechanisms in a somewhat cursory manner, knowing that these individually instituted actions have a force of their own and that once activated go far beyond the professionals' involvement. Activities such as yoga, focused meditation, the discipline of karate, and other forms of centered concentration are segued into spirituality and transcendence.

SPIRITUALITY

Spirituality is a rather indescribable need that drives individuals throughout life to seek meaning and purpose in their existence. Spirituality is difficult to define, though many people have tried. We can observe the body and we can imagine the mind in operation and measure intelligence, but there is no computed tomography scan of the spirit (Bell and Troxel, 2001). Understanding spirituality is far more elusive than learning about the pathology associated with disease and illness.

Spirituality has been defined as a "quality of a person derived from the social and cultural environment that involves faith, a search for meaning, a sense of connection with others, and a transcendence of self, resulting in a sense of inner peace and well-being" (Delgado, 2007, p. 230). The spiritual aspect of people's lives transcends the physical and psychosocial to reach the deepest individual capacity for love, hope, and meaning. "Spiritual health is an integral component of human wellbeing" (Vaineta, 2016, p. 11).

Aging as a biological process has been studied extensively. Less attention has been paid to the study of aging as a spiritual process. As people age and move closer to death, spirituality may become more important. Declining physical health, loss of loved ones, and a realization that life's end may be near often challenge older adults to reflect on the meaning of their lives. Spiritual belief and practices often play a central role in helping older adults cope with life challenges and are a source of strength in their lives. Nursing studies of spirituality and aging indicate that spirituality increases in importance and is a source of hope, aids in adaptation to illnesses, and has a positive influence on quality of life in chronically ill older adults (Edlund, 2014; Touhy, 2001a, 2001b; Touhy et al, 2005; Vaineta, 2016). Spirituality may be particularly important to healthy aging in "historically disadvantaged populations who display remarkable strength despite adversities in their lives" (Hooyman and Kiyak, 2005, p. 213).

Spirituality and Religion

Distinguishing between religion and spirituality is a concern for many health professionals. Religious beliefs and participation in religious obligations and rites are often the avenues of spiritual expression, but they are not necessarily interchangeable. "Religion can be described as a social institution that unites people in a faith in God, a higher power, and in common rituals and worshipful acts. Each religion involves a particular set of beliefs and a god, divinity, and/or soul is always included in the concept" (Strang and Strang, 2002, p. 858). For some people, particularly older adults, formalized religion helps them feel fulfilled. Spirituality is a broader concept than religion and encompasses a person's values or beliefs, search for meaning, and relationships with a higher power, with nature, and with other people. The concept of spirituality is found in all cultures and societies.

For some older adults, particularly those who are frail or cognitively impaired, meeting spiritual needs may be a greater challenge than for healthier older adults. Functional decline and dependence can threaten the sense of identity and connection with others and the world, thus causing a loss of spirit (Leetun, 1996; Touhy, 2001a). However, "although aging changes can affect the body and the mind, there is no evidence that the spirit succumbs to the aging process even in the face of debilitating physical and emotional illness" (Heriot, 1992, p. 23).

The spiritual aspect transcends the physical and psychosocial to reach the deepest individual capacity for love, hope, and meaning. The spiritual person can rise above that which is humanly expected in a situation. For example, a dying older adult in great pain who was being cared for by Dr. Ebersole (chapter author) said: "This is so hard for you." That he was able to see beyond himself at that time was difficult to believe.

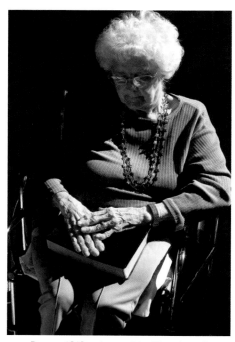

Prayer. (©iStock.com/Lisa Thornberg.)

PROMOTING HEALTHY AGING: IMPLICATIONS FOR GERONTOLOGICAL NURSING

Assessment

Assessment of spirituality is as important as assessment of physical, emotional, and social dimensions. A spiritual history opens the door to a conversation about the role of spirituality and religion in a person's life (Wittenberg et al, 2017). People often need permission to talk about these issues. Without a signal from the nurse, patients may feel that such topics are not welcome. Patients welcome a discussion of spiritual matters and want health professionals to consider their spiritual needs. The older adult may have a pressing need to talk about philosophy and spiritual development. Private time for prayer, meditation, and reflection may be needed.

Nurses may neglect to explore this issue with older adults because religion and spirituality may not seem the high priority and care focuses primarily on physical aspects (Clayton et al, 2017). The client should be assured that religious longings and rituals are important and that opportunities will be made available as desired. Nurses need to be knowledgeable and respectful about the rites and rituals of varying religions, cultural beliefs, and values (Chapter 4). Religious and spiritual resources, such as pastoral visits, should be available in all settings where older adults reside. It is important to avoid imposing one's own beliefs and to respect the person's privacy on matters of spirituality and religion (Touhy and Zerwekh, 2006).

An emphasis on spirituality in nursing is not new; nursing has encompassed the spiritual from its origin. The science of nursing was not seen as separate from the art and spirit of the discipline. Florence Nightingale's view of nursing was derived from her spiritual philosophy, and she considered nursing a spiritual experience, "intrinsic to human nature, our deepest and most potent resource for healing" (Macrae, 1995, p. 8). Many nursing theories address spirituality, including those of Neuman, Parse, and Watson (Martsolf and Mickley, 1998). Nursing and medicine are beginning to reclaim some of the essential healing values from their roots.

The essence of being spiritual is being whole or holistic, and attention to the spiritual needs of patients is a critical dimension of holistic nursing care. Yet surveys with practicing nurses suggest that most have had little, if any, education in spiritual care. Many nurses view spiritual nursing responses in religious terms and may feel that spirituality is a religious matter better left to clergy and religious leaders. Heriot (1992) suggested that nurses need to understand care of the human spirit both within and outside the context of religion. Goldberg (1998) asserted that the connection in the nurse-patient relationship is central to spiritual care but that most nurses are "carrying out spiritual interventions at an unconscious level" (p. 840). She called for education and research to help nurses become more aware of the importance of connection and use of self in relationships as ways of bringing the elements of spiritual care into conscious awareness.

An evidence-based guideline for promoting spirituality in the older adult (Gaskamp et al, 2006) provides a framework for spiritual assessment and interventions. The guideline identifies

BOX 36.8   Identifying Older Adults at Risk for Spiritual Distress

- Individuals experiencing events or conditions that affect the ability to participate in spiritual rituals
- Diagnosis and treatment of a life-threatening, chronic, or terminal illness
- Expressions of interpersonal or emotional suffering, loss of hope, lack of meaning, need to find meaning in suffering
- Evidence of depression
- Cognitive impairment
- Verbalized questioning or loss of faith
- Loss of interpersonal support

Data from Gaskamp C, Sutter R, Meraviglia M, et al: Evidence-based guideline: promoting spirituality in the older adult, *J Gerontol Nurs* 32:8–13, 2006.

BOX 36.9   Questions to Begin Dialogue About Spiritual Concerns

- Tell me more about your life.
- What has been most meaningful in your life?
- To whom do you turn when you need help?
- What brings you joy and comfort?
- What are you most proud of?
- How have you found strength throughout your life?
- What are you hopeful about?
- Is spiritual peace important to you? What would help you achieve it?
- Is your religion or God significant in your life? Can you describe how?
- Is prayer or meditation helpful?
- What spiritual or religious practices bring you comfort?
- Are there religious books or materials that you want nearby?
- What are you afraid of right now?
- What do you wish you could still do?
- What are your concerns at this time for the future?
- What matters most to you right now?

Adapted from Touhy T, Zerwekh J: Spiritual caring. In Zerwekh J, editor: *Nursing care at the end of life: palliative care for patients and families*, Philadelphia, 2006, FA Davis.

older adults who may be at risk for spiritual distress and who might be most likely to benefit from use of the guideline (Box 36.8). Spiritual distress or spiritual pain is "an individual's perception of hurt or suffering associated with that part of his or her person that seeks to transcend the realm of the material. Spiritual distress is manifested by a deep sense of hurt stemming from feelings of loss or separation from one's God or deity, a sense of personal inadequacy or sinfulness before God and man, or a pervasive condition of loneliness" (Gaskamp et al, 2006, p. 9).

The person experiencing spiritual distress is unable to experience the meaning of hope, connectedness, and transcendence. Spiritual distress may be manifested by anger, guilt, blame, hatred, expressions of alienation, turning away from family and friends, inability to derive pleasure, and inability to participate in religious activities that have previously provided comfort.

care team can respond to them. These include the Faith, Importance/Influence, Community and Address (FICA) Spiritual History (Puchalski and Romer, 2000), and the Brief Assessment of Spiritual Resources and Concerns (Koenig and Brooks, 2002; Meyer, 2003) (Box 36.10). The Joint Commission requires spiritual assessments in hospitals, nursing homes, home care organizations, and many other health care settings providing services to older adults. The process of spiritual assessment is more complex than completing a standardized form and must be done within the context of the nurse-patient relationship.

For older adults with cognitive impairment, information about the importance of spirituality and religious beliefs can be

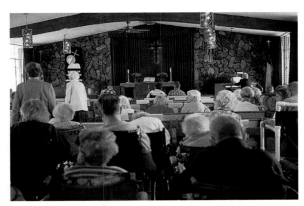

Residents attend a religious service at a nursing center. (From Sorrentino SA, Gorek B: *Mosby's textbook for long-term care assistants*, ed 5, St Louis, 2007, Mosby.)

BOX 36.10   Brief Assessment of Spiritual Resources and Concerns

Instructions: Use the following questions as an interview guide with the older adult (or caregiver if the older adult is unable to communicate).
- Does your religion/spirituality provide comfort or serve as a cause of stress? (Ask to explain in what ways spirituality is a comfort or stressor.)
- Do you have any religious or spiritual beliefs that might conflict with health care or affect health care decisions? (Ask to identify any conflicts.)
- Do you belong to a supportive church, congregation, or faith community? (Ask how the faith community is supportive.)
- Do you have any practices or rituals that help you express your spiritual or religious beliefs? (Ask to identify or describe practices.)
- Do you have any spiritual needs you would like someone to address? (Ask what those needs are and if referral to a spiritual professional is desired.)
- How can we (health care providers) help you with your spiritual needs or concerns?

From Gaskamp C, Sutter R, Meraviglia M, et al: Evidence-based guideline: promoting spirituality in the older adult, *J Gerontol Nurs* 32:10, 2006. Adapted from Meyer CL: How effectively are nurse educators preparing students to provide spiritual care? *Nurse Educ* 28(4):185–190, 2003; Koenig HG, Brooks RG: Religion, health and aging: implications for practice and public policy, *Public Policy Aging Rep* 12:13–19, 2002.

Spiritual Assessment Tools

There are formal spiritual assessments, but open-ended questions can also be used to begin dialogue about spiritual concerns (Box 36.9). Simply listening to older adults as they express their fears, hopes, and beliefs is important. Spiritual assessments are intended to elicit information about the core spiritual needs and how the nurse and other members of the health

obtained from family members. Nurses often see cognitive impairments as obstacles or excuses to providing spiritual care to people with dementia. Nurturing mind, body, and spirit is part of holistic nursing, and nurses must provide opportunities to all older adults, no matter how impaired, to live life with meaning, purpose, and hope (Touhy, 2001b).

Interventions

The caring relationship between nurses and persons nursed is the heart of nursing that touches and supports the spirit and enhances health and well-being (Research Highlights box). Knowing persons in their complexity, responding to that which matters most to them, identifying and nurturing connections, listening with one's being, using presence and silence, and fostering connections to that which is held sacred by the person are spiritual nursing responses that arise from within the caring, connected relationship (Touhy et al, 2005). Suggestions for spiritual care interventions are presented in Box 36.11.

RESEARCH HIGHLIGHTS

The study investigated the associations among hope, meaning in life, self-transcendence, and nurse-patient interaction in a sample of 202 cognitively intact Finnish nursing home residents. Residents completed the Herth Hope Index, the Purpose in Life Test, the Self-Transcendence Scale, and the Nurse-Patient Interaction Scale. Statistical analysis revealed a significant direct relationship of nurse-patient interaction on hope, meaning in life, and self-transcendence. Findings suggest that nurse-patient interaction in the nursing home setting may be a critical resource to health and well-being of residents. The researchers recommended that nursing home caregivers should be given more time for interacting with their patients and education should be provided to assist in developing and appreciating the caring interaction skills that provide hope, meaning, and self-transcendence.

From Hagan G: Nurse-patient interaction is a resource for hope, meaning in life and self-transcendence in nursing home patients, *Scand J Caring Sci* 28:74–88, 2014.

BOX 36.11 Spiritual Nursing Interventions

- Relief of physical discomfort, which permits focus on the spiritual
- Creating a peaceful environment
- Comforting touch, which fosters nurse-patient connection
- Authentic presence
- Attentive listening
- Knowing the patient as a person
- Listening to life stories
- Sharing fears and listening to self-doubts or guilt
- Fostering forgiveness and reconciliation
- Validating the person's life and ensuring persons they will be remembered
- Sharing caring words and love
- Encouraging family support and presence
- Fostering connections to that which is held sacred by the person
- Praying with and for the patient
- Respecting religious traditions and providing for access to religious objects and rituals
- Referring the person to a spiritual counselor

Data from Gaskamp C, Sutter R, Meraviglia M, et al: Evidence-based guideline: Promoting spirituality in the older adult, *J Gerontol Nurs* 32:8, 2006; Touhy T, Brown C, Smith C: Spiritual caring: end of life in a nursing home, *J Gerontol Nurs* 31:27–35, 2005.

Know that caring for an aging body is the least of the work with older adults. "Limiting care to the physical needs denies older adults the opportunity to live out their life with meaning, purpose, and hope" (Touhy, 2001a, p. 45). Recognizing the primacy of the spirit is essential. Some very spiritual individuals are unable to articulate their knowing. Therefore, do not negate that aspect of an individual's experience because it is not expressed verbally. Realizing that biopsychosocial aspects of aging are all shards of the spirit will integrate every aspect of your work in gerontological nursing.

Nurturing the Spirit of the Nurse

"Because spiritual care occurs over time and within the context of relationship, probably the most effective tool at the nurse's disposal is the use of self" (Soeken and Carson, 1987, p. 607). Nurses' ease with their own spiritualty is vital to providing spiritual care (Wittenberg et al, 2017). Nurses should attend to their own biopsychosocial and spiritual issues in the development of compassion and empathy, attributes that serve them well in caring for others' spiritual needs. Find ways to nourish your own spirit. Thinking about what gives your own life meaning and value helps in developing your spiritual self. Examples of activities include finding quiet time for meditation and reflection; keeping your own faith traditions; being with nature; appreciating the arts; spending time with those you love; and journaling. Nurses often do not take the time to do so and become dispirited. This is especially true for nurses who work with dying patients and experience grief and loss repeatedly. Having someone to talk to about feelings is important. Practicing compassion for oneself is essential to authentic practice of compassion for others (Touhy and Zerwekh, 2006) (Box 36.12).

Faith Community Nursing

Faith community nursing (FCN) is a nursing practice specialty that focuses on the intentional care of the spirit, the promotion of an integrative model of health, and the prevention and minimization of illness within the context of a faith community (American Nurses Association, 2012). Nurses can become certified in FCN through the American Nurses Credentiality Center. FCN was originally known as *parish nursing*, but the name was

BOX 36.12 Personal Spirituality Questions for Reflection for Nurses

- What do I believe in?
- How do I find purpose and meaning in my life?
- How do I take care of my physical, emotional, and spiritual needs?
- What are my hopes and dreams?
- Whom do I love, and who loves me?
- How am I with others?
- What would I change about my relationships?
- Am I willing to heal relationships that trouble me?

From Touhy T, Zerwekh J: Spiritual caring. In Zerwekh J, editor: *Nursing care at the end of life: palliative care for patients and families*, Philadelphia, 2006, FA Davis.

changed to FCN to reflect the broader scope of the practice and the full range of faiths.

In a literature review of the current state of research for FCN, Dyess et al (2010) noted that FCN began 20 years ago and is widely implemented today in many faith communities in the United States and in multiple countries around the world. These authors suggest that FCN can assist in bridging the gaps in care in the current health care system, contribute to a reduction in acute health care costs, promote health and disease prevention, and integrate faith with health care to promote positive health outcomes. Models of care such as those implemented in FCN may be particularly relevant to meeting the health maintenance needs and spiritual needs of older adults with chronic illness living in the community.

Nurses who are involved in religious organizations can also be advocates for increasing the attention given to the health needs of older adults. Nurses may even spearhead particular services to older adults, such as peer counseling, health screening activities, day care, home visitation programs, and respite for families. Many religious organizations reach out to homebound older adults in their community by offering visits from clergy or church members, involvement in prayer circles, and other activities to maintain connection with their faith community.

TRANSCENDENCE

Transcendence is the high-level emotional response to religious and spiritual life and finds expression in numerous rituals and modes of cosmic consciousness. Rituals provide a means of connecting with everyone through the ages who has observed similar rituals. These modes of thinking and feeling are sometimes unfamiliar to individuals who are immersed in the necessary materialistic concerns of young adulthood, yet moments do occur throughout life when one is deeply aware of being part of a larger scheme. Although some of the material in this chapter may be obscure, it is the springboard for learning to appreciate the full life cycle. The privilege of briefly walking alongside an older adult on the last great journey can be truly inspiring.

Transcending is roused by the desire to go beyond the self as delimited by the material and the concrete aspects of living, to expand self-boundaries and life perspectives. "Transcendence involves detachment and separation from life as it has been lived to experience a reality beyond oneself and beyond what can be seen or felt" (Touhy and Zerwekh, 2006, p. 229). Creative thought and actions are vehicles of both self-actualization and self-transcendence, the bridge to universal expression and existence. Self-transcendence is generally expressed in five modes: creative work, religious beliefs, children, identification with nature, and mystical experiences (Reed, 1991). This section of the chapter deals with various mechanisms by which one transcends the purely physical limitations of existence.

Some people may use asceticism, self-denial, and rigorous rituals to reach the peaks of human experience; many others find more prosaic approaches just as effective. The thesis of

Maslow's writings is that mystic, sacred, and transcendent experiences frequently arise from the ordinary elements of one's life (Maslow, 1970). Gardening, reading, holding an infant, dealing with loss, and numerous other normal events have elements of mystery.

With each death of a loved one, throughout life, one is reborn to a slightly altered state. When deaths of significant others abound in the later years, older adults must be given the opportunity to express how they personally have been altered by the loss. We can speculate that with each personal loss, one moves slightly closer to the universal and away from the individual until, toward the end, one feels an affiliation with all living things—animal, plant, and mineral. Some older adults have achieved a state of existence that transcends the limits of the failing body.

Gerotranscendence

The theory of gerotranscendence (Tornstam, 1994, 1996, 2005) (Chapter 3) theorizes that human aging brings about a general potential for gerotranscendence, a shift in perspective from the material world to the cosmic and, concurrent with that, an increasing life satisfaction. Gerotranscendence is thought to be a gradual and ongoing shift that is generated by the normal processes of living, sometimes hastened by serious personal disruptions (Box 36.13). An understanding of transcendence and the unique characteristics of this transformation as one ages is important to the continued growth and development of older adults.

Achieving Transcendence
Time Transcendence
Life as experienced ordinarily involves the chronological passage of time. Some types of conscious experience alter our time perception, but the unconscious destroys time. Therefore the release of the unconscious transcends the limitations of time that conscious life experience generally imposes on us. If we conquer time, we conquer annihilation and the dimensions of time that lie within the mind. Recognizing the importance of time perception, particularly in old age, is a fertile field to explore more fully. Influences on time perception include age, imminent death, level of activity, emotional state, outlook on

---

BOX 36.13 Characteristics of Individuals With a High Degree of Gerotranscendence

- Have high degrees of life satisfaction
- Engage in self-controlled social activity
- Experience satisfaction with self-selected social activities
- Social activities not essential to their well-being
- Midlife patterns and ideals no longer prime motivators
- Demonstrate complex and active coping patterns
- Have greater need for solitary philosophizing
- May appear withdrawn when engaged in inner development
- Have accelerated development of gerotranscendence fomented by life crises
- Feel shifts in perception of reality

the future, and the value attached to time. Conclusions from studies of older adults generally support the view that older adults perceive time as passing quickly and favor the past over the present or the future.

Peak Experiences

A peak experience is when one momentarily transcends the self through love, wisdom, insight, worship, commitment, or creativity. These experiences are the extraordinary events in one's life that clearly demonstrate self-actualization and personal authenticity. Peak experience is the time when restrictive boundaries seem to vanish, and one feels more aware, more complete, more ecstatic, or more concerned for others. Peak experiences include many modes of transcending one's ordinary limitations. Spiritual and paranormal experiences, creative acts, courage, and humor may all produce peak experiences. Keeping oneself open to transcendence involves finding the places in which such experiences can break through: soul-stirring concerts, sunrises, sunsets, or raging storms on mountaintops. Each individual seeks states of being in which he or she feels part of a larger whole.

Meditation

Many types and rituals of meditation have flourished in Western societies in recent years. Some methods of meditation have been used for thousands of years in Eastern cultures. Whatever the method, the goal is to quiet the mind and center oneself. When the mind slows, the body relaxes and less oxygen and nutrients are needed. Mindfulness meditation can decrease pain, improve sleep, and enhance well-being and quality of life. Meditation may also improve cognitive function.

Effective meditation requires approximately 20 minutes of focusing on a sound, a thought, or an image. Practicing two or more times daily will leave calmness, better health, and higher energy levels in its wake. Although meditation can be accomplished in any setting, a place with few distractions is helpful. People who meditate with consistency often begin to be aware of a transcendent state of being. Nurses may introduce the values of meditation to older adults and serve as guides in the beginnings of such activities. Chanting psalms, reciting poetry by rote, praying, saying the rosary, practicing yoga, and playing a musical instrument are all mechanisms of release and renewal that may bring one into higher states of awareness.

Hope as a Transcendent Mechanism

Hope is the belief in the future and the expectation of fulfillment. Hope is the anchor that sustains life in the most difficult times and in the face of doubts and ennui. Some level of hope must be maintained to survive and to die in peace. Hope embodies desires and expectations and the limitless possibilities of humans in all times and places—present, past, and future. For many older adults, hope is a major means of coping, and those who lose hope lose the capacity and desire for survival. All practicing nurses have observed how a small goal or hope for the future can sustain an older adult. The grandson's graduation from college, the daughter's return from her travels, or even a birthday may keep an older adult alive until the event is safely fulfilled.

Central to the instillation of hope is the caring relationship between nurses and patients. Caring relationships characterized by unconditional positive regard, encouragement, and competence help patients feel loved and cared about, thus inspiring hope. A patient's hope for cure may change to a hope for freedom from pain, day-to-day experiences to enjoy precious moments of life, time to accomplish life goals before life is over, sharing love with family and friends, relief of suffering, death with dignity, and eternal life. Nurses may foster hope by doing the following:

1. Presenting honestly the limits of human knowledge
2. Controlling symptoms and providing comfort
3. Encouraging patient and family to become involved in positive experiences that transcend the current situation
4. Determining significant aspects of the individual's life
5. Fostering spiritual processes and finding meaning
6. Exploring beliefs and values of the older adult
7. Promoting connection and reconciliation
8. Providing opportunities for prayer, meditation, scripture reading, clergy visits, and religious rituals, if meaningful for the older adult

Other hope-promoting experiences are presented in Box 36.14.

Transcendence in Illness

Serious illnesses influence how one perceives the meaning of life. A distinct shift in goals, relationships, and values often

---

BOX 36.14 Hope-Promoting Activities

- Feel the warmth of the sun.
- Share experiences children are having.
- See the crystal blue of the sky.
- Enjoy a garden or fresh flowers.
- Savor the richness of black coffee at breakfast.
- Feel the tartness of grapefruit to wake up the taste buds.
- Watch the activities of an animal in a tree outside the window.
- Benefit from each encounter with another person.
- Write messages to grandchildren, nieces, or nephews.
- Study a favorite painting.
- Listen to a symphony.
- Build highlights into each day such as meals, visits, Bible reading.
- Keep a journal.
- Write letters.
- Make a tape recording of your life story.
- Have hope objects or symbols nearby.
- Share hope stories.
- Focus on abilities, strengths, and past accomplishments.
- Encourage decision making about daily activities; foster a sense of control.
- Extend caring and love to others.
- Appreciate expressions of caring concern.
- Renew loving relationships.

Adapted from Jevne R: Enhancing hope in the chronically ill, *Humane Med* 9:121–130, 1993; Miller, J: *Coping with chronic illness: overcoming powerlessness,* Philadelphia, 1983, FA Davis; Touhy T, Zerwekh J: Spiritual caring. In Zerwekh J, editor: *Nursing care at the end of life: palliative care for patients and families,* Philadelphia, 2006, FA Davis.

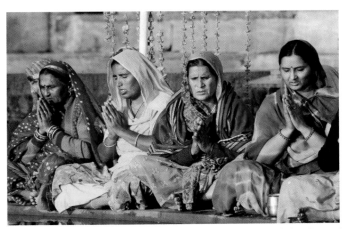

Prayer is an important spiritual practice in many cultures. (©iStock.com/ kaetana_istock.)

occurs among people who have survived life-threatening episodes. A heightened awareness of beauty and of caring relationships may occur, but a long period of emotional "splinting" may be necessary while recovering from the psychic wound of body betrayal. Newman (1994) contends that disease can be a manifestation of health as one confronts the crisis and as it reveals the special meanings.

Steeves and Kahn (1987) found from their work in hospice care that certain conditions facilitate the search for meaning in illness, noting the following:

- Suffering must be bearable and not all-consuming if one is to find meaning in the experience.
- A person must have access to and be capable of perceiving objects in the environment. Even a small window on the world may be sufficient to match the limited energy one has to attend.
- One must have time that is free of interruption and a place of solitude to experience meaning.
- Clean, comfortable surroundings and freedom from constant responsibility and decision making free the soul to search for meaning.
- An open, accepting atmosphere in which to discuss meanings with others is important.

Accompanying someone in his or her grief and quest for meaning in painful events is a privilege nurses are often given. This spiritual intimacy means being willing to suffer with another, and both the nurse and the client will reap the benefits. One of the great rewards of working with older adults is observing and participating as they turn suffering into a spiritual event.

Sister Rosemary Donley (1991) defines the nursing role in the spiritual search of suffering individuals as compassionate accompaniment, meaning entering into another's reality and quietly, attentively sharing the experience. "Nurses need to be with people who suffer, to give meaning to the reality of suffering and, in so far as possible, to remove suffering and its causes. Here lies the spiritual dimensions of health care" (Donley, 1991, p. 180). The challenge is to find meaning and some purpose in the affliction that, unchallenged, entwines and chokes identity.

LEGACIES

A legacy is one's tangible and intangible assets that are transferred to another and may be treasured as a symbol of immortality. The purpose of legacies is to supersede death. Courage, wisdom, and insights that we perceive in older adults become part of their legacy. The desire for meaning and immortality seems to be the basic motivation for leaving a legacy. Extending one's authentic self to others can be an important activity in the last years. Throughout life, shared experiences provide satisfaction, but in the last years this exchange allows one to gain a clearer perspective on how his or her movement on earth has had an impact. Older adults must be encouraged to identify that which they would like to leave and who they wish the recipients to be. This process has interpersonal significance and prepares one to leave the world with a sense of meaning. A legacy can provide a transcendent feeling of continuation and tangible or intangible ties with survivors.

Legacies are manifold and may range from memories that will live on in the minds of others to bequeathed fortunes. Box 36.15 is a partial list of legacies. The list is as diverse as individual contributions to humanity. Legacies are generative and are identified and shared best as one approaches the end of life. This activity reinforces integrity.

Certain questions allow the older person to consider a legacy if he or she is ready to do so. For example:

- What is the meaning to you of your life experience right now?
- Have you ever thought of writing an autobiography?
- If you were able to leave something to the younger generation, what would it be?
- Have you ever thought of the impact your generation has had on the world?
- What has been most meaningful in your life?
- What possessions have special meaning for you? Who else is interested in them?

BOX 36.15 Examples of Legacies

- Oral histories
- Autobiographies
- Written or video histories
- Shared memories
- Taught skills
- Works of art and music
- Publications
- Human organ donations
- Endowments
- Objects of significance
- Tangible or intangible assets
- Personal characteristics, such as courage or integrity
- Bestowed talents
- Traditions and myths perpetuated
- Philanthropic causes
- Progeny children and grandchildren
- Methods of coping
- Unique thoughts: Darwin, Einstein, Freud, Nightingale, and others

- Do you see some of your genetic traits emerging in your grandchildren?

Types of Legacies

Autobiographies and Life Histories

Oral histories are an approach to immortality. As long as one's story is told, one remains alive in the minds of others. Doers leave their products and live through them. Powerful figures are remembered in fame and infamy. The quiet, unobtrusive person survives in the memory of intimates and in family anecdotes. Everyone has a life story.

Autobiographies and recorded memoirs can serve a transcendent purpose for people who are alone—and for many who are not. Nurses can encourage older adults to write, talk, or express in other ways the meaning of their lives. The human experience and the poignant anecdotes bind people together and validate the uniqueness of each brief journey in this level of awareness and the assurance that one will not be forgotten. Dying patients can express and order their memories through audiotapes, CDs, videotapes, or DVDs, which are then bequeathed to families if the person desires.

Sharing one's personal story creates bonds of empathy, illustrates a point, conveys some of the deep wisdom that we all have, and connects us with our deepest human consciousness. "It is only when people who have loved and cared for us reach the end of life that we see the full gift we have received from them. By leaving us their reminiscences, their spirits can continue in our lives as a living memorial" (Grudzen and Soltys, 2000, p. 8). See Chapter 6 for additional discussion of storytelling, reminiscence, and life review.

Creation of Self Through Journaling

Through the personal journal, one can, in thoughtful reflection, discover meaning and patterns in daily events. The self becomes a coherent story with successive revisions as old events are reread and perceived in new contexts. The journals of older adults provide rich descriptions of the interior lives of the authors. May Sarton (1984) and Florida Scott-Maxwell (1968) are two of the best-known authors. The study of these journals and of the journals of less-known and less articulate older adults assists nurses in understanding the inner experience of older adult and, perhaps, their own.

Collective Legacies

Each person is a link in the chain of generations (Erikson, 1963) and as such may identify with generational accomplishments. An older woman may think of herself as a significant part of a generation that survived the Great Depression. A middle-aged man may identify with the generation that walked on the moon. The years of youthful idealism are impressed in one's memory by the political or ideological climate of the time. This time is the stage when one searches for a fit in the larger society.

The importance of collective legacies to nurses lies in how they use this knowledge. For instance, the nurse may ask, "Who were the great people of your time?" "Which ones were important to you?" "What events of your generation changed the world?" "What were the most important events you experienced?" Mentioning certain historical events or asking about individual reactions is sometimes helpful.

Childless individuals are becoming more prevalent with each passing generation, and they must find a way to outlive the self through a legacy. Many people choose a social legacy. Florence Nightingale would be one such person, with the grand legacy she left to nurses.

Legacies Expressed Through Other People

One's legacy can be expressed in many ways—through the development of others in a teaching or learning situation or through mentorship, patronage, shared talents, organ donations, and genetic transmission. Some creative works and research are legacies left to successive generations for continued modification and growth. In other words, one's legacy may be a product of his or her own brought to fruition through someone else who may also become an intermediary to later developments. Thus people and generations are tied in sequential progress. Some examples may illustrate this type of legacy:

- An older man cried as he talked of his grandson's talent as a violinist. Both the man and his grandson shared their love for the violin, and the grandfather believed that he had genetically and personally contributed to his grandson's development as an accomplished musician.
- A professor emeritus spoke of visiting her son in a distant state and hearing him expound ideas that had been partially developed by the professor and her father before her.
- People who amass a fortune and allocate certain funds for endowment of artists, scientific projects, and intellectual exploration are counting on others to complete their legacy.

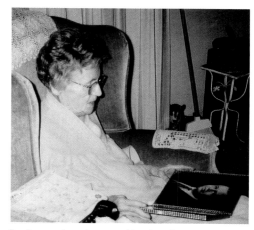

Widow reflecting on her deceased husband's legacy. (From Black JM, Hawks JH: *Medical-surgical nursing: clinical management for positive outcomes,* ed 7, St Louis, 2005, Saunders.)

Living Legacies

Many older adults wish to donate their bodies to science or donate body parts for transplant. This mechanism is a means to transcend death. Parts of the body keep another person alive, or, in the case of certain diseases, the deceased body may provide important information leading to preventive or restorative techniques in the future. Donation of body parts in old age may not be encouraged because they are often less viable than those from younger people. Nonetheless, older bodies are welcome for use as cadavers. The Dementia Brain Bank Research Program has been operated by the Alzheimer's Research Center for more than 30 years. The Brain Bank is one of the world's largest collections of brain tissue, which contributes to research on the neurochemistry, physiology, and diagnosis of dementing illnesses. People who are interested in providing such a legacy should be encouraged to call the nearest university biomedical center or Brain Bank registry and obtain more information. The nurse then has a postmortem obligation to the client to assist in carrying out his or her wishes.

Property and Assets

Wealth may be viewed as a means toward power more often than transcendence; therefore some older adults are often reluctant to disperse material goods before their death. Some use the future legacy as a means to exert power and control over offspring. One man said, "So long as I have that bankroll, they've got to treat me with respect" (Lustbader, 1996). The power to exert influence, to punish, and to reward is often bound up in an anticipated estate distribution.

Estates can be planned in certain ways that are decidedly advantageous for the planner, and the recipient, in terms of control and avoidance of lengthy probate proceedings and taxation. Because the laws are complex and ever-changing, using the services of an estate planner would be advisable. The nurse's responsibility regarding wills may be limited to advising older adults to obtain legal counsel while they are healthy and competent and plan how they would like to distribute their worldly goods.

Personal Possessions

Possessions carry more meaning as time passes; individuals change, but the possession remains much the same. A possession is a way of symbolically hanging on to individuals who are gone or times that are past. For some people, keeping personal possessions is a means of hanging on to the self that is changing with time. Cherished possessions passed on through several generations may have achieved meaning through the close family member to whom they belonged. One's personally significant items become highly charged with memories and meaning, and transferring them to friends and kin can be a tender experience. Personal possessions should never be dispersed without the individual's knowledge. Because of the uncertainty of late life lucidity, these issues should be discussed early with older individuals.

People who are approaching death must be given the opportunity to distribute their important belongings appropriately to those whom they believe will also cherish them. Nurses may encourage older adults to plan the distribution of their significant items carefully. Deciding when and how best these possessions should be given is often difficult. Some people choose to distribute possessions before dying. In these cases, nurses often need to help family members accept these gifts, appreciating the meaning and recognizing the significance.

PROMOTING HEALTHY AGING: IMPLICATIONS FOR GERONTOLOGICAL NURSING

"The responsibility of the nurse is not to make people well, or to prevent their getting sick, but to assist people to recognize the power that is within them to move to higher levels of consciousness" (Newman, 1994, p. xv). In this chapter, we have examined methods of expanding one's limited existence by developing the authentic self, transcendent self, and spiritual self and several mechanisms used to establish immortality through a legacy. These areas often become major issues in the latter part of life, and the nurse will find it a revealing, absorbing, and challenging task to be a part of this effort. An important point is that some people may avoid any such interest or concern, particularly when angry, in pain, or denying their own mortality. Nurses need not push the individual to accomplish this task but should be available to assist the person and family members.

The basic mysteries of life elude scientific researchers, yet they are the essence of existence with meaning. Remembering, feeling, dreaming, worshiping, and grasping one's connection to the universe are the realities of the human spirit. Being old is not the centrality of the self—spirit is. Spirit synthesizes the total personality and provides integration, energizing force, and immortality. It calls for a nurse who is willing to enter into meaningful spirit-sharing relationships. Such relationships have the potential to enhance inner harmony and healing. There may be no greater goal in caring for older adults than helping a person see a life well lived and meaningful to themselves and others, thus providing hope that life's journey was not in vain. Taking advantage of these opportunities will enrich our nursing, our inner selves, and the spiritual well-being of the older adults whom we nurse. As gerontological nursing scholar Sarah Gueldner (2007) so eloquently stated:

> We must help each older adult to continue to experience and express the passions that, over a lifetime, have become who they are. Older adults should continue to make their unique and precious contributions to society, and we must not fail to take note of it in even the frailest and quietest of individuals. We must give them voice and time on the center stage of life and help them connect with each other and with society in a way that fosters appreciation of the traits, talents, and memories that still define their being (p. 4).

The authors of this book hope that you find as much joy and fulfillment in your nursing with older adults as we have.

KEY CONCEPTS

- Self-actualization is a process of developing one's most authentic self. Maslow thought of self-actualization as the pinnacle of human development.
- Self-actualized individuals embody qualities of courage, humor, high moral development, and seeking to learn more about themselves and others.
- Opportunities for pursuing interests will assist individuals in developing latent talents, expressing their creativity, and rising beyond daily concerns.
- Groups working toward societal humanitarian advancement may accomplish collective actualization.
- Creativity emanates from people who are self-actualized and may be expressed in everyday activities, and the arts, music, theater, and literature.
- Transcending the material and physical limitations of existence through ritual and spiritual means is an especially important aspect of aging.
- Gerotranscendence is a theory proposed by Tornstam that implies a natural shift in concerns that occurs in the aging

process. Older adults are thought to spend more time in reflection, to spend less on materialistic concerns, and to find more satisfaction in life. This effort is an attempt to define aging not by the standards of young and middle adulthood but as having distinctive characteristics of its own.
- Illnesses that occur have the potential for altering one's fundamental beliefs and hopes. Nurses must give older adults the opportunity to discuss the meaning of an illness. Some people find that these experiences bring new insights; others are angry. Empathic nurses will provide a sounding board while the individual makes sense of an illness within a satisfactory framework.
- Nurses need not neglect discussing spirituality with older adults. Older adults will respond only if it has significance for them.
- Spiritual nursing interventions emanate from the caring relationship between the older adult and the nurse. The most important tool at the nurse's disposal is the use of self.

NURSING STUDY: SELF-ACTUALIZATION, SPIRITUALITY, AND TRANSCENDENCE

Melba had no children but had numerous nieces and nephews, though she did not feel particularly close to any of them. She had been a nursing instructor at a community college and had enjoyed her students but had not developed a sustained relationship with any of them after they had completed her courses. At her level of nursing education, the opportunity for mentorship was lacking, though she had occasionally taken students under her wing and arranged special experiences that they particularly desired. Because she had taught several courses each year, Melba never really developed a strong affiliation to a specialty but considered herself a pediatric nurse. She had not made any major contributions to the field in terms of research or publications; a few reviews, continuing education workshops, and some nursing newsletters had really been the extent of her work outside of that which was required. Melba's husband died in 1988, and she had felt very much alone since that time, especially after her retirement 3 years ago. Before her husband's death, Melba had been too busy to think about the ultimate meaning of all her years of teaching and wifely activities. With time on her hands, she began to wonder what it all meant. Had she done anything meaningful? Had she really made a difference in anything or in anyone's life? Was anyone going to remember her in any special way? So many questions were making her morose. She had never been a religious person, though her husband had been a devout Catholic. He had believed that God had a purpose for him in life, and though he was not always able to understand what it might be, he seemed to have a sense of satisfaction. She began to wonder if she should go to church—would that make her feel less depressed?

One Sunday morning, Melba had decided to attend her neighborhood Catholic church, but on her way out she slipped on the icy walkway and sustained bilateral Colles' fractures. After a brief emergency room visit for assessment,

immobilization of the wrists, and medications, Melba was sent back home with an order for home health and social service assessment on the following day. Of course, she had extreme difficulty managing the most basic self-care while keeping her wrists immobilized and was very dejected. When the home health nurse arrived the next morning, to Melba's amazement, it was a former student who had graduated 4 years previously. Melba was more chagrined than pleased and greeted her with, "Oh, I hate to have you see me so helpless. I've been feeling so useless, and, now with these wrists, I am totally useless." If you were the home health nurse, how would you begin working with Melba, knowing that you would be limited to just a few visits?

Based on the nursing study, develop a nursing care plan using the following procedure[a]:

- List Melba's comments that provide subjective data.
- List information that provides objective data.
- From these data, identify and state, using an accepted format, two nursing diagnoses you determine are most significant to Melba at this time. List two of Melba's strengths that you have identified from the data.
- Determine and state the outcome criteria for each diagnosis. These must reflect some alleviation of the problem identified in the nursing diagnosis and must be stated in concrete and measurable terms.
- Plan and state one or more interventions for each diagnosed problem. Provide specific documentation of the sources used to determine the appropriate intervention. Plan at least one intervention that incorporates Melba's existing strengths.
- Evaluate the success of the intervention. Interventions must correlate directly with the stated outcome criteria to measure the outcome success.

[a]Students are advised to refer to their nursing diagnosis text and identify possible or potential problems.

CRITICAL THINKING QUESTIONS AND ACTIVITIES

1. Discuss the meanings and the thoughts triggered by the student's and the older adult's viewpoints as expressed at the beginning of the chapter. How do they vary from your own experience?
2. How do nursing students learn about spirituality and spiritual nursing interventions?
3. What activities might be helpful in developing your own sense of spirituality?
4. How do cultural beliefs and traditions affect one's concept of spirituality?
5. How can nurses enhance spiritual care, self-actualization, and transcendence of self among older adults?

RESEARCH QUESTIONS

1. What aspects of intergenerational programs are enjoyed by younger and older individuals?
2. Who makes wills and when do they make them?
3. What are the motivating differences between gifts given during life and those given after one's death?
4. What is the perspective of the older adult related to spiritual assessment and interventions by nurses?
5. How do nurses describe the spiritual interventions they use with older adult?
6. How do nurses recognize aspects of gerotranscendence?

REFERENCES

American Nurses Association: *Faith community nursing: scope and standards of practice*, ed 2, Spring, MD, 2012, American Nurses Association.

Ardelt M: Empirical assessment of a three-dimensional wisdom scale, *Res Aging* 25(3):275–324, 2003.

Ardelt M: Wisdom as expert knowledge system: a critical review of a contemporary operationalization of an ancient concept, *Hum Dev* 47:257–285, 2004.

Bell V, Troxel D: Spirituality and the person with dementia: a view from the field, *Alzheimers Care Q* 2:31–45, 2001.

Bernstein A: *Spirituality and aging: looking at the big picture*, 2009. Aging Well. http://todaysgeriatricmedicine.com/news/septstory1.shtml. Accessed July 2014.

Clayton M, Hulettt J, Kapur K, Reblin M, Wilson A, Ellington L: Nursing support of home hospice caregivers on the day of patient death, *Oncol Nurs Forum* 44:457–464, 2017.

Cortes T: *The state of healthy aging*, 2013. http://hartfordinstitute.wordpress.com/2013/04/04/the-state-of-healthy-aging. Accessed August 2014.

Cousins N: *Anatomy of an illness*, New York, 1979, Norton.

Delgado C: Sense of coherence, spirituality, stress and quality of life in chronic illness, *J Nurs Scholarsh* 39(3):229–234, 2007.

Donley R: Spiritual dimensions of health care: nursing's mission, *Nurs Health Care* 12:178–183, 1991.

Dyess S, Chase SK, Newlin K: State of research for faith community nursing 2009, *J Relig Health* 49:188–199, 2010.

Gaskamp C, Sutter R, Meraviglia M, Adams S, Titler MG: Evidence-based guideline: promoting spirituality in the older adult, *J Gerontol Nurs* 32:8–13, 2006.

Goldberg B: Connection: an exploration of spirituality in nursing care, *J Adv Nurs* 27:836–842, 1998.

Grudzen M, Soltys FG: Reminiscence at end of life: celebrating a living legacy, *Dimensions* 7(3):4, 5, 8, 2000.

Gueldner S: Sustaining expression on identity in older adults, *J Gerontol Nurs* 33:3–4, 2007.

Hansman H: *College students are living rent-free in a Cleveland retirement home*, 2015. https://www.smithsonianmag.com/innovation/college-students-are-living-rent-free-in-cleveland-retirement-home-180956930/. Accessed December 2017.

Harris J: *Students living in nursing homes – a solution to our ageing populations?* 2016. https://www.weforum.org/agenda/2016/11/some-dutch-university-students-are-living-in-nursing-homes-this-is-why?utm_content=buffer07075&utm_medium=social&utm_source=twitter.com&utm_campaign=buffer. Accessed December 2017.

Heriot CS: Spirituality and aging, *Holist Nurs Pract* 7:22–31, 1992.

Hooyman N, Kiyak A: *Social gerontology: a multidisciplinary perspective*, Boston, 2005, Pearson.

Hudson F: *The adult years: mastering the art of self-renewal*, San Francisco, 1999, Jossey-Bass.

Jansen T: *The nursing home that's also a dorm*, 2016. https://www.citylab.com/equity/2015/10/the-nursing-home-thats-also-a-dorm/408424/. Accessed December 2017.

Killick J: *You are words*, London, 1997, Hawker.

Killick J: *Openings*, London, 2000, Hawker.

Killick J: *Dementia diary*, London, 2008, Hawker.

Koenig HG, Brooks RG: Religion, health and aging: implications for practice and public policy, *Public Policy Aging Rep* 12:13–19, 2002.

Kohlberg L, Power C: Moral development, religious thinking and the question of a seventh stage. In Kohlberg L, editor: *The philosophy of moral development* (Vol. 1), San Francisco, 1981, Harper & Row.

Kuhn M: Advocacy in this new age, *Aging* 3:297, 1979.

Larson R: Building intergenerational bonds through the arts, *Generations* 30:38, 2006.

Leetun MC: Wellness spirituality in the older adult. Assessment and intervention protocol, *Nurse Pract* 21:60, 65–70, 1996.

Lustbader W: Conflict, emotion and power surrounding legacy, *Generations* 20:54–57, 1996.

Macrae J: Nightingale's spiritual philosophy and its significance for modern nursing, *Image J Nurs Sch* 27:8–10, 1995.

Martsolf DS, Mickley JR: The concept of spirituality in nursing theories: differing world views and extent of focus, *J Adv Nurs* 27:294–303, 1998.

Maslow A: Creativity in self-actualizing people. In Anderson H, editor: *Creativity and its cultivator*, New York, 1959, Harper & Row.

Maslow A: *Religions, values and peak-experiences*, New York, 1970, Viking Press.

Metcalf CW: *Lighten up (Audiotape)*, Niles, IL, 1993, Nightingale Conant.

Meyer CL: How effectively are nurse educators preparing students to provide spiritual care? *Nurse Educ* 28(4):185–190, 2003.

Newman MA: *Health as expanding consciousness*, ed 2, New York, 1994, National League for Nursing Press.

Parisi J, Rebok G, Carlson M, et al: Can the wisdom of aging be activated and make a difference societally? *Educ Gerontol* 35:867–879, 2009.

Peck R: Psychological developments in the second half of life. In Anderson J, editor: *Psychological aspects of aging*, Washington, DC, 1955, American Psychological Association.

Perlstein S: Creative expression and quality of life: a vital relationship for elders, *Generations* 30:5–6, 2006.

Puchalski C, Romer AL: Taking a spiritual history allows clinicians to understand patients more fully, *J Palliat Med* 3:129–137, 2000.

Reed PG: Toward a nursing theory of self-transcendence: deductive reformulation using developmental theories, *Adv Nurs Sci* 13:64–77, 1991.

Reichstadt J, Sengupta G, Depp C, Palinkas LA, Jeste DV: Older adults' perspective on successful aging: qualitative interviews, *Am J Geriatr Psychiatry* 18(7):567–575, 2010.

Sarton M: *At seventy: a journal*, New York, 1984, Norton.

Scott-Maxwell F: *The measure of my days*, New York, 1968, Knopf.

Soeken KL, Carson VJ: Responding to the spiritual needs of the chronically ill, *Nurs Clin North Am* 22:603–611, 1987.

Steeves RH, Kahn DL: Experience of meaning in suffering, *Image J Nurs Sch* 19:114–116, 1987.

Strang S, Strang P: Questions posed to hospital chaplains by palliative care patients, *J Palliat Med* 5:857, 2002.

Tornstam L: Gerotranscendence: a theoretical and empirical exploration. In Thomas LE, Eisenhandler SA, editors: *Aging and the religious dimension*, Westport, CT, 1994, Greenwood Publishing Group.

Tornstam L: Gerotranscendence: a theory about maturing into old age, *J Aging Identity* 1:37–50, 1996.

Tornstam L: *Gerotranscendence: a developmental theory of positive aging*, New York, 2005, Springer.

Touhy TA: Nurturing hope and spirituality in the nursing home, *Holist Nurs Pract* 15:45–56, 2001a.

Touhy TA: Touching the spirit of elders in nursing homes: ordinary yet extraordinary care, *Int J Hum Caring* 6:12–17, 2001b.

Touhy TA, Brown C, Smith CJ: Spiritual caring: end of life in a nursing home, *J Gerontol Nurs* 31:27–35, 2005.

Touhy T, Zerwekh J: Spiritual caring. In Zerwekh J, editor: *Nursing care at the end of life: palliative care for patients and families*, Philadelphia, 2006, FA Davis.

Vaineta J: Spiritual health as an integral component of human well-being, *Appl Res Health Soc Sciences: Interface and Integration* 13(1):3–13, 2016. doi:10.1515/arhss-2016-0002.

Wikström BM: Older adults and the arts: the importance of aesthetic forms of expression in later life, *J Gerontol Nurs* 30:30–36, 2004.

Wittenberg E, Ragan SL, Ferrell B: Exploring nurse communication about spirituality, *Am J Hosp Palliat Med* 34(6):566–571, 2017.

Entry followed by *f* indicates figure, by *t* table, and by *b* box.

Quality and Safety Education for Nurses (QSEN), 241*b*
Quality Assurance Performance Improvement (QAPI), 428
Quality of life, pharmacological interventions and, 103
Questions, open-ended, 70

R
RA. *See* Rheumatoid arthritis
Race, definition of, 46
RAI. *See* Resident Assessment Instrument
Railroad Medicare, 400
Ramelteon, 225
Rapid eye movement (REM), 220
Rapid eye movement sleep behavior disorder (RBD), 227
Rapid transcranial magnetic stimulation (rTMS), for depression, 360
Readmissions, role of nursing during, 24–25, 24*b*, 25*b*
REASN project. *See* Resourcefully Enhancing Aging in Specialty Nursing project
Recreation, 495–496, 497*b*
Red blood cell count, 92–93
Red blood cells (RBCs), 91–92
Red yeast rice, 120, 120*b*
Registered nurses (RNs), in assisted living facilities, 424
Rehydration methods, 194
Reinforce teaching, medication and, 112
Relationships, 452–471
    gerontological nursing, 454, 454*b*
    in later life, 455–456
        caregiving, 461–467, 461*b*
        families, 456–460
        friendships, 455–456, 455*f*
Relaxation, 338
REM. *See* Rapid eye movement (REM)
Reminiscing, 71–72
    cognitive impairment and, 72–73
    encouraging, 71*b*
Remodeling, 284
Renal health, laboratory tests of, 99
Renal system
    age-related changes in, 202, 202*b*
    in medication excretion, 105
Renin, 202
Repositioning, for pressure injuries, 168
Rescue inhalers, 318, 318*f*
Research, on aging, 19
Resident Assessment Instrument, 86–87, 87*b*
Resident bill of rights, 427*b*, 428
Residential care/assisted living (RC/AL), 349, 423–424, 424*f*
Resilience, 345*b*
Resourcefully Enhancing Aging in Specialty Nursing (REASN) project, 18
Resourcefulness, 345*b*
Respiratory disorders, 314–317
    gerontological nursing in, 317–319, 317*b*, 318*b*, 318*f*
Respiratory health and illness, 313–320
    normal age-related changes and, 313–314
    nursing study on, 319*b*
Respiratory system, 313
Restless legs syndrome, 226–227
Restlessness, signs and symptoms of approaching death, 487*t*
Restraint-free care, 256–257, 257–258*b*, 257*b*
    suggestions from advanced practice nursing consultation on, 257*b*
Restraints, 255–257
    alternatives for, 257-258*b*
    consequences of, 256, 256*b*
    definition and history of, 255–256
Restrictive diets, in nutrition, 187–188

Retina, 133, 134*t*
Retirement, 453–454
    nursing study on, 469*b*
    planning, 453–454
    special considerations in, 453
Review of systems (ROS), 78, 79*b*
Rheumatoid arthritis (RA), 325–327, 325*t*
    complications of, 326–327
    etiology of, 326
    gerontological nursing in, 329–330, 329*b*
    nonpharmacological approaches for, 329
    pharmacological approaches for, 329–330
    risk factors for, 326*b*
    serological testing for, 326*b*
    signs and symptoms of, 326, 326*b*, 326*f*
Rivastigmine (Exelon), 299
RNA (ribonucleic acid), 33
Road Scholar program, 62
Robots, 271
Role theory, 36–37
ROS. *See* Review of systems

S
Safe conduct, 487*b*
SAFE DRIVE mnemonic, 268–269, 269*b*
Safe patient handling, falls and, 254–255, 255*b*
Safety, 261–274
    driving, 267–268, 267*b*, 267*f*, 268*b*
    emerging technologies to enhance, 270–271
    nursing study on, 273*b*
    transportation, 266–268
Salve, 118
Sarcopenia, 322
Saw palmetto, 123, 123*b*
Scabies, 156–157
Schizophrenia, 353
    consequences of, 353
    interventions for, 353–354
    prevalence of, 353
    symptoms of, 353
Scientific method, 47
Seborrheic keratosis, 157–158, 158*f*
Secondary prevention, of disease, 8–9, 9*b*
Security, 261–274
    nursing study on, 273*b*
Self, orientation to, 46–47, 46*b*
Self-actualization, 491–493
    characteristics of, 492–493, 492*b*
    collective, 493
    nursing study on, 506*b*
Self-care abilities, 25*f*
Self-care skills, diabetes mellitus and, 309–310, 309*b*
Self-determination, 407
Self-esteem, ADL care enhances, 389*f*
Self-neglect, 413
Self-renewal, 493
Senescence, 32–33
Senile miosis, 133
Senior Moment, 296
Sensorineural hearing loss, 146
Serenoa repens. See Saw palmetto
Serum albumin, 98–99
Sexual health, 437–439
    factors influencing, 437–439
        activity levels and, 438
        biological changes with age and, 438–439, 439*t*
        cohort and cultural influences and, 438
    guidelines for health care providers in talking about, 448*b*
    medications that may affect, 448*b*
Sexual response, 439–440
    female, 440
    male, 439

Sexuality, 434–447, 437*f*
    acceptance and companionship in, 437, 438*f*
    and aging women, common myths and, 438*b*
    assessment for, 447–448
    definition of, 436–437
    dementia and, 444–445
    gerontological nursing and, 447–448
    Healthy People 2020, 437*b*
    interrelationship of dimensions of, 436*f*
    interventions for, 448
    in long-term care facilities, 443–444
    nursing study on, 449*b*
    zones of, 435*f*
Shadow grief, 475, 475*b*, 475*f*
Shingles, 159
Short Michigan Alcoholism Screening Test-Geriatric Version (S-MAST-G), 364*t*
Short-term care, in nursing home, 425
Short-term memory, 58
Siblings, 460
Side rails, 256
Sildenafil, 439–440
Silence, use of, 49
Silver Alert system, 268
Silver Sneakers Program, 235
Skilled nursing care, 425
Skilled nursing facilities, 425–428
    quality of care in, 428–431, 428*b*
Skin, 155
    assessment of, guidelines for, 166, 166*b*
    care of, 154–172
    changes in
        aging and, 155, 155-156*t*
        nursing study on, 170*b*
    gerontological nursing and, 161–162
    healthy, 155
    photo damage of, 159–160
    physiological functions of, 155, 155*b*
    problems in, 156–160
    sun protection and, 162*b*
Skin cancers, 160–161
    basal cell carcinoma as, 160, 160*f*
    facts and figures of, 160
    melanoma as, 161
    squamous cell carcinoma as, 160–161, 161*f*
Skin failure, 166
Skin Tear Tool Kit, 157
Skin tears (STs), 157, 157*b*, 158*b*
Sleep, 219–229, 223*b*
    age-related changes in, 221*b*
    aging and, 220–221, 221*b*
    architecture, 220
    biorhythm and, 220
    disorders, 221–222
        abbreviations for, 225*b*
        disturbances in, risk factors for, 221*b*
    Healthy People 2020, 220-228*b*
    medications affecting, 222*b*
    nursing study on, 227-228*b*
    problems of, 219–220
    research highlights in, 223*b*
    stages of, 220*b*
Sleep apnea, 225, 225*b*
    assessment of, 226
    gerontological nursing and, 226–227
    interventions for, 226
Sleep diary, 222–223, 222*b*
Sleep disordered breathing, 225, 225*b*
    assessment of, 226
    gerontological nursing and, 226–227
    interventions for, 226
Sleep study, 226
Sleeping, increased, signs and symptoms of approaching death, 487*t*
Smallpox, centenarians and, 5
Smart homes, 270–271